D1395036

DIAGNOSTIC AND SURGICAL
IMAGING ANATOMY
MUSCULOSKELETAL

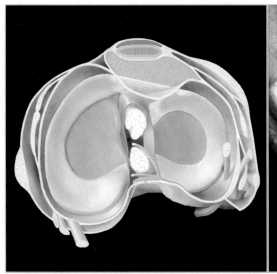

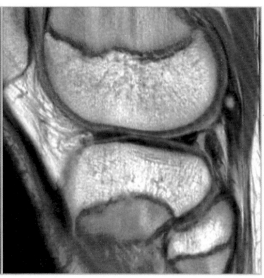

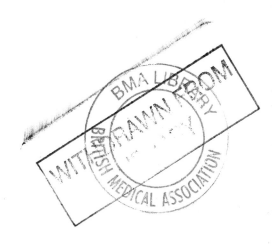

DIAGNOSTIC AND SURGICAL
IMAGING ANATOMY
MUSCULOSKELETAL

B.J. Manaster, MD, PhD, FACR

Professor and Vice Chairman
Department of Radiology
University of Colorado Denver & Health Sciences Center

Carol L. Andrews, MD

Musculoskeletal Radiology
Mink Radiologic Imaging

Julia Crim, MD

Chief of Musculoskeletal Radiology
Professor of Radiology and Orthopedics
University of Utah School of Medicine

Jeffrey W. Grossman, MD

Department of Radiology
University of Colorado Denver & Health
Sciences Center

Theodore T. Miller, MD

Attending Radiologist
Department of Radiology and Imaging
Hospital for Special Surgery
Assistant Professor
Weill Medical College of Cornell University

Cheryl A. Petersilge, MD

Chair, Department of Radiology
Marymount Hospital, Cleveland Clinic Health System
Assistant Clinical Professor of Radiology and
Orthopedic Surgery
Case Western Reserve University

Catherine C. Roberts, MD

Associate Dean, Mayo School of Health Sciences
Assistant Professor of Radiology
Consultant Radiologist
Mayo Clinic College of Medicine

Zehava Sadka Rosenberg, MD

Professor of Radiology
New York University School of Medicine
NYU - Hospital for Joint Diseases

Managing Editor
R. Kent Sanders, MD

Assistant Professor of Radiology
University of Utah School of Medicine

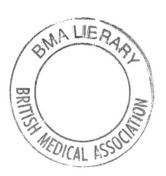

AMIRSYS®
Names you know, content you trust

AMIRSYS®

Names you know, content you trust®

First Edition

Text - Copyright B.J. Manaster MD, PhD, FACR 2006

Drawings - Copyright Amirsys Inc 2006

Compilation - Copyright Amirsys Inc 2006

Composition by Amirsys Inc, Salt Lake City, Utah

Printed in Canada by Friesens, Altona, Manitoba, Canada

ISBN-13: 978-1-931884-31-0
ISBN-10: 1-931884-31-5
ISBN-13: 978-1-931884-32-7 (International English Edition)
ISBN-10: 1-931884-32-3 (International English Edition)

Notice and Disclaimer

Library of Congress Cataloging-in-Publication Data

Diagnostic and surgical imaging anatomy. Musculoskeletal / B.J.
    Manaster ... [et al.] ; managing editor, R. Kent Sanders. — 1st ed.
      p. ; cm.
    Includes index.
    ISBN-13: 978-1-931884-31-0
    ISBN-10: 1-931884-31-5
    ISBN-13: 978-1-931884-32-7 (international English ed.)
    ISBN-10: 1-931884-32-3 (international English ed.)
    1. Musculoskeletal system—Anatomy—Atlases. 2. Musculoskeletal
system—Imaging—Atlases.   I. Manaster, B. J. II. Title: Musculoskeletal.
    [DNLM: 1. Musculoskeletal System—anatomy & histology—Atlases.
2. Magnetic Resonance Spectroscopy—Atlases. 3. Tomography,
X-Ray Computed—Atlases.   WE 17 D5365 2006]
QM100.D53 2006
611'.700222—dc22

                                    2006030832

Dedicated with love to our families:

Steve, Tracy Joy, and Katy Rose
John, Sara, and Jenna
Lester, Philip, and Eleanor
Mandy, Aidan, and Kara-Elise
Terry, Jack, Elissa, Benjamin, and Landon
Will, Melissa, and Stephen
John, Emma Patricia, and Austin Justice
Ron and Leora
Micki

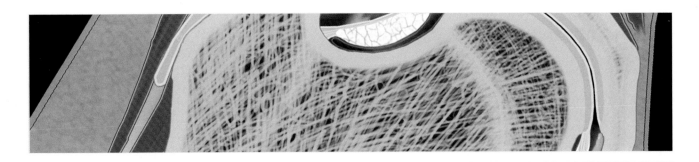

DIAGNOSTIC AND SURGICAL IMAGING ANATOMY: MUSCULOSKELETAL

We at Amirsys, together with our distribution colleagues at LWW, are proud to present _Diagnostic and Surgical Imaging Anatomy: Musculoskeletal_, the second in our brand-new series of anatomy reference titles. All books in the series are designed specifically to serve clinicians in medical imaging and each area's related surgical subspecialties. We focus on anatomy that is generally visible on imaging studies, crossing modalities and presenting bulleted brief introductory text descriptions along with a glorious, rich offering of color normal anatomy graphics together with in-depth multimodality, multiplanar high-resolution imaging.

Each imaging anatomy textbook contains over 2,500 labeled color graphics and high resolution radiologic images, with heavy emphasis on 3 Tesla MR and state-of-the-art multi-detector CT. It is designed to give the busy medical professional rapid answers to imaging anatomy questions. Each normal anatomy sequence provides detailed views of anatomic structures never before seen and discussed in an anatomy reference textbook. For easy reference, _Musculoskeletal_ is subdivided into separate sections that cover detailed normal anatomy of each major joint with adjacent long bones (such as shoulder, hip and pelvis, knee, etc.).

In summary, _Diagnostic and Surgical Imaging Anatomy: Musculoskeletal_ is a product designed with you, the reader, in mind. Today's typical radiologic, surgical, and sports medicine practice settings demand both accuracy and efficiency in image interpretation for clinical decision-making. We think you'll find this new approach to anatomy a highly efficient and wonderfully rich resource that will be the core of your reference collection in musculoskeletal anatomy. The new _Diagnostic and Surgical Imaging Anatomy: Chest, Abdomen, and Pelvis_ is also now available. Coming in 2007 are volumes on Ultrasound as well as a subspecialty- and podiatry-oriented text on Knee, Ankle, and Foot.

We hope that you will sit back, dig in, and enjoy seeing anatomy and imaging with a whole different eye.

Anne G. Osborn, MD
Executive Vice President and Editor-in-Chief, Amirsys Inc.

H. Ric Harnsberger, MD
CEO & Chairman, Amirsys Inc.

Paula J. Woodward, MD
Senior Vice President & Medical Director, Amirsys Inc.

B.J. Manaster, MD
Vice President & Associate Medical Director, Amirsys Inc.

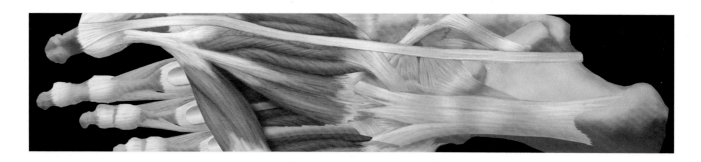

FOREWORD

Depiction of the musculoskeletal system is a dynamic process which utilizes the latest innovations of imaging technology to elucidate anatomy, both structural and functional. Although there has been no change in the bones, ligaments, muscles, and tendons, there has been a revolution in the way they are evaluated. Even the most accomplished clinician will benefit from an all-inclusive resource providing the details of the musculoskeletal system. Compilation of a comprehensive musculoskeletal imaging atlas, covering the different imaging modalities-from radiographs to MR arthrography, as well as having three dimensional musculoskeletal anatomy of the whole body-was, until now, lacking.

This new atlas is a timely addition which solves all of the problems of previous atlases with its novel, multifunctional layout. The highly regarded editor, B.J. Manaster, her managing editor, Kent Sanders, as well as the authors, Zehava Rosenberg, Julia Crim, Cheryl Petersilge, Carol Andrews, Catherine Roberts, Jeff Grossman and Ted Miller are all well known authorities in the field of musculoskeletal imaging.

Beautiful black and white as well as color images and illustrations are present throughout this work along with an outlined text that covers those details which both radiologists and clinicians want to know in an easy-to-read format. The multimodality approach is a breath of fresh air that puts immensely valuable information into a single text.

Anatomy is shown with the use of radiographs, arthrography, CT, CT arthrography, MRI and MR arthrography. The radiographs utilize the standard imaging positions, allowing the reader to understand the osseous anatomy that is best depicted in each position. A very valuable feature is the inclusion of left and right mirror images for MRI, which makes it easier to identify structures within the extremities without having to transpose. Most atlases provide images for only one side, forcing the reader to mentally create the contralateral side. Such exercises can lead to errors in structure identification. Three dimensional graphics that depict muscles, nerves and vessels are rendered in detail that is invaluable to the practicing clinician. Intricate anatomy defined by multiple small structures, such as the ligaments seen in the posterolateral corner of the knee, is nicely demonstrated in diagramatic form as well as on MRI.

This book shall prove to be extremely useful for radiologists, orthopedic surgeons, rheumatologists, physiatrists, physical therapists and clinicians, whether in training or in practice. It is the atlas to purchase for those who seek answers related to musculoskeletal anatomy and its imaging. These authors are to be congratulated for compiling such a comprehensive work.

Lynne Steinbach, MD
Professor of Clinical Radiology and Orthopaedic Surgery
Chief, Musculoskeletal Imaging
University of California San Francisco

x

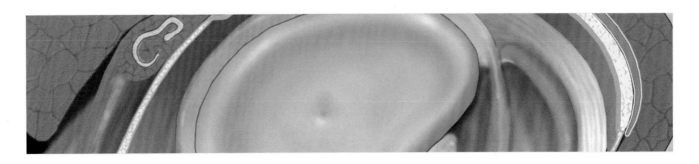

PREFACE

We are pleased to present to our colleagues a comprehensive atlas of musculoskeletal imaging. The user will find the information in this book to be easily accessible on many levels. First, for the traditional quick "identify or locate the structure" question, all musculoskeletal body parts are presented in the traditional three planes with extensive labeling. A unique feature is that, for the coronal and axial planes, the right and left side of the body are shown on facing pages. Additionally, not only the joints but also the long bones and associated structures are shown in detail in all planes. For those joints where special positioning or planes are utilized, these are demonstrated and labeled as well.

The second unique feature of the atlas is the addition of text and over 300 full color graphics which will assist the reader in furthering their understanding of anatomical structures and pathways in the musculoskeletal system. These graphics are matched with images to more fully illustrate anatomical relationships.

Finally, the authors have chosen several uniquely difficult anatomic or functional regions of the musculoskeletal system for amplification. Some examples of these include the posterolateral corner of the knee, rotator interval of the shoulder, pulley and ligament/tendon system of the finger, and ligaments of the wrist. Each of these is presented as a sub module, with its own set of text, graphics, images, and is often supplemented with MR arthrographic or CT images. We trust that this additional material can be used to gain an in-depth understanding of the musculoskeletal system.

We hope and expect our readers will find our "labor of love" useful in their work.

B.J. Manaster, MD, PhD, FACR
Professor and Vice Chairman
Department of Radiology
University of Colorado Denver & Health Sciences Center

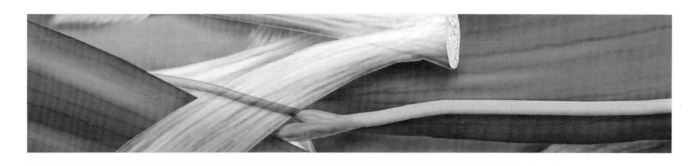

ACKNOWLEDGMENTS

Illustrations
Richard Coombs, MS

Image/Text Editing
Kaerli Main
Douglas Grant Jackson
Amanda Hurtado
Melanie Hall

Medical Text Editing
R. Kent Sanders, MD

Case Management
Roth LaFleur
Christopher Odekirk

Production Lead
Melissa A. Hoopes

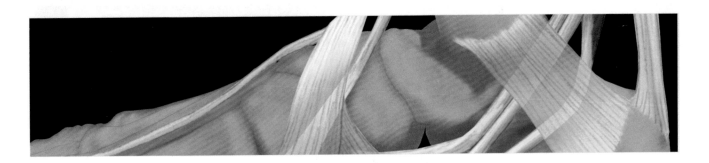

SECTIONS

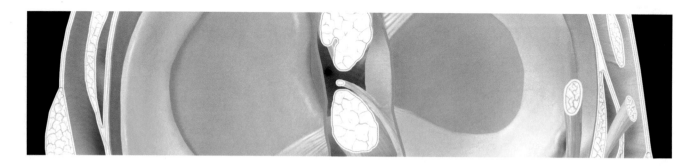

TABLE OF CONTENTS

DIAGNOSTIC AND SURGICAL
IMAGING ANATOMY
MUSCULOSKELETAL

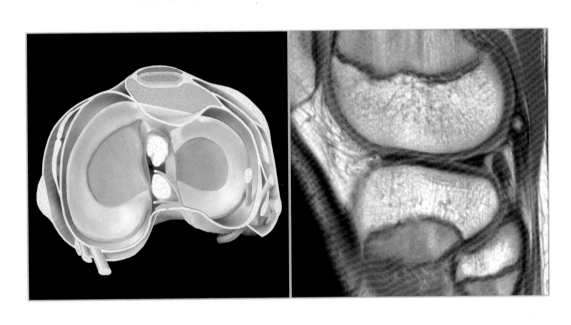

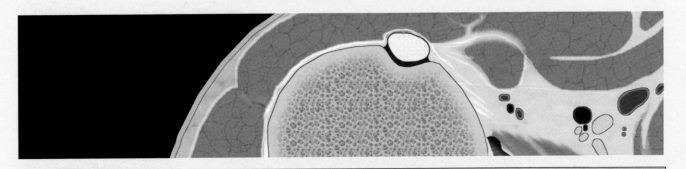

SECTION I: Shoulder

SHOULDER OVERVIEW

Gross Anatomy

Overview

- Multiaxial ball-and-socket joint
- Hemispheric humeral head articulates with shallow pear-shaped glenoid fossa
  - Joint surrounded by a synovial-lined fibrous capsule
  - Glenoid deepened by labrum, a fibrocartilage rim of tissue
  - Cartilage thins in central glenoid and in periphery of humeral head
- **Range of motion**: Flexion, extension, abduction, adduction, circumduction, medial rotation & lateral rotation
  - **Flexion**: Pectoralis major, deltoid, coracobrachialis & biceps muscles
  - **Extension**: Deltoid & teres major muscles
    - If against resistance, also latissimus dorsi & pectoralis major
  - **Abduction**: Deltoid & supraspinatus muscles
    - Subscapularis, infraspinatus & teres minor exert downward traction
    - Supraspinatus contribution controversial
  - **Medial rotation**: Pectoralis major, deltoid, latissimus dorsi & teres major muscles
    - Subscapularis when arm at side
  - **Lateral rotation**: Infraspinatus, deltoid & teres minor muscles
- **Joint stabilizers**
  - Skeletally unstable joint
  - Superior support by coracoacromial arch
  - Anterior support by subscapularis tendon, anterior capsule, synovial membrane, anterior labrum and superior, middle & inferior glenohumeral ligaments
  - Posterior support by infraspinatus and teres minor tendons, posterior capsule, synovial membrane, posterior labrum & inferior glenohumeral ligament
- **Vascular supply**
  - Articular branches of anterior and posterior humeral circumflex arteries and transverse scapular artery
- **Innervation**
  - Axillary and suprascapular nerves

Imaging Anatomy

Overview

- **Humerus**
  - Eight ossification centers: Shaft, head, greater tuberosity, lesser tuberosity, capitulum, trochlea, medial & lateral epicondyles
  - Anatomic neck located along base of the articular surface, region of fused epiphyseal plate and attachment of joint capsule
  - Surgical neck located 2 cm distal to anatomic neck, below greater and lesser tuberosities, extracapsular, most common site of fracture
  - **Greater tuberosity** anterolateral on humeral head
    - Attachment of supraspinatus, infraspinatus & teres minor tendons
  - **Lesser tuberosity** located along proximal anterior humeral head, medial to greater tuberosity
    - Attachment of subscapularis tendon
  - Intertubercular or bicipital groove
    - Between greater and lesser tuberosities
    - Transverse ligament, an extension of subscapularis tendon, forms roof of groove
    - Contains long head of biceps tendon & anterolateral branch of anterior circumflex humeral artery and vein
- **Scapula**
  - **Acromion**
    - Acromion orientation ranges from flat to sloping, mediolaterally
    - Roughly classified into 4 types based on posterior to anterior shape
    - Type I: Flat
    - Type II: Curved, paralleling humeral head
    - Type III: Anterior hooked
    - Type IV: Convex undersurface
    - Low-lying, anterior downsloping or inferolateral tilt decreases volume of coracoacromial outlet
  - **Os acromiale**
    - Un-united acromial ossification center
    - Should fuse by 25 years of age
    - Incidence: 2-10%
    - 60% bilateral
    - Four types: Mesoacromion, metaacromion, preacromion, basiacromion
  - **Glenoid**
    - Shallow, oval recess
    - Fibrocartilage labrum increases depth
  - **Coracoid process**
    - May extend lateral to plane of glenoid
    - Normal distance between coracoid and lesser tuberosity > 11 mm with arm in internal rotation
- **Clavicle**
  - Acromioclavicular joint between distal clavicle & acromion
    - 20 degree range of motion
  - Synovial-lined joint capsule
  - Fibrocartilage-covered ends of bone & central fibrocartilage disk
- **Bone marrow**
  - Predominantly yellow marrow in adults with residual hematopoietic red marrow in glenoid and proximal humeral metaphysis
- **Glenohumeral joint space**
  - 1-2 ml synovial fluid
  - Normal communication with biceps tendon sheath
  - Normal communication with subscapular recess
  - Posterior joint capsule typically inserts on base of labrum
  - Anterior joint capsule has variable insertion
- **Anterior joint capsule insertion**
  - Type 1: Inserts at tip or base of labrum
  - Type 2: Inserts scapular neck < 1 cm from labrum
  - Type 3: Inserts scapular neck > 1 cm from labrum
- **Subscapular recess**
  - Between scapula & subscapularis muscle and tendon
  - Joint communication via foramen of Weitbrecht: Between superior and middle glenohumeral ligaments
  - Joint communication via foramen of Rouviere: Between middle and inferior glenohumeral ligaments

SHOULDER OVERVIEW

- o Normally opacified during arthrography
- **Rotator cuff**
  - o Supraspinatus, infraspinatus, subscapularis & teres minor
  - o Tendons interdigitate forming a continuous band at attachment to humerus
  - o **Origins**
    - Supraspinatus: Supraspinatus fossa of scapula
    - Infraspinatus: Infraspinatus fossa of scapula
    - Teres minor: Lateral scapular border, middle
    - Subscapularis: Anterior scapular surface
  - o **Insertions**
    - Supraspinatus, infraspinatus & teres minor insert on the greater tuberosity
    - Supraspinatus has a direct component which inserts on anterior portion of tuberosity & posterior oblique component which undercuts the infraspinatus at the posterior portion of tuberosity
    - Subscapularis inserts on the lesser tuberosity
- **Ligaments**
  - o Coracoacromial ligament
    - Anterior 2/3 of coracoid to tip of acromion
  - o Coracoclavicular ligament
    - Base of coracoid process to clavicle
    - Stabilizes acromioclavicular joint
    - Conoid & trapezoid portions merge to form a V
  - o Coracohumeral ligament
    - Lateral base of coracoid to lesser & greater tuberosities
    - Blends with subscapularis tendon, supraspinatus tendon, joint capsule & superior glenohumeral ligament
  - o Superior & inferior acromioclavicular ligaments
  - o Superior, middle & inferior glenohumeral ligaments
    - Superior and middle glenohumeral ligaments extend from superior glenoid region to lesser tuberosity
    - Congenitally absent or diminutive middle glenohumeral ligament in 30% of population
    - Inferior glenohumeral ligament (anterior band, posterior band & axillary pouch) extends from inferior labrum to humeral anatomic neck
- **Capsulolabral complex**
  - o Labrum
    - Oval fibrocartilage tissue along glenoid rim
    - Hyaline cartilage may lie between labrum & bone
    - Varies in shape, size and appearance
    - Anatomic variants, most common in anterosuperior region, include sublabral foramen & Buford complex
  - o Biceps tendon
    - Long head arises from supraglenoid tubercle or superior labrum
    - Long head may be congenitally absent
    - Long head may arise from intertubercular groove or joint capsule
    - Short head originates at coracoid process as conjoined tendon with coracobrachialis
    - Additional heads are rarely present and arise from brachialis muscle, intertubercular groove or greater tubercle
- **Bursae**
  - o Subacromial-subdeltoid bursa

- Normally contains a minimal amount of fluid
- Adherent to undersurface of acromion
- Lies superficial to the rotator cuff
  - o Subcoracoid bursa
    - Separate from the normal subscapular recess of joint
    - Between subscapularis tendon and coracobrachialis/short head of biceps tendon
    - Can communicate with subacromial-subdeltoid bursa
    - Does not normally communicate with joint
  - o Infraspinatus bursa
    - Between infraspinatus tendon and joint capsule
    - Can rarely communicate with joint
  - o Other less common bursae
    - Deep to coracobrachialis muscle
    - Between teres major & long head of triceps
    - Anterior & posterior to latissimus dorsi tendon
    - Superior to acromion
- **Additional muscles of upper arm**
  - o Deltoid, biceps, coracobrachialis, triceps
- **Extrinsic shoulder muscles**
  - o Trapezius, latissimus dorsi, levator scapulae, major & minor rhomboids, serratus anterior, subclavius, omohyoid, pectoralis major, pectoralis minor

Internal Structures-Critical Contents

- **Quadrilateral or quadrangular space**
  - o Teres minor, superior border
  - o Teres major, inferior border
  - o Humerus, lateral border
  - o Long head triceps, medial border
  - o Contains axillary nerve and posterior circumflex humeral artery
- **Coracoacromial arch**
  - o Acromion, superior border
  - o Humeral head, posterior border
  - o Coracoid process and coracoacromial ligament, anterior border
  - o Contains subacromial-subdeltoid bursa, supraspinatus muscle/tendon, long head of biceps
- **Rotator interval**
  - o Triangular space between the inferior border of supraspinatus muscle/tendon and superior border of subscapularis muscle/tendon
  - o Medially bordered by coracoid process
  - o Laterally bordered by transverse humeral ligament
  - o Anterior border formed by coracohumeral ligament, superior glenohumeral ligament & joint capsule

Anatomy-Based Imaging Issues

Imaging Approaches

- **Radiographs**
  - o Standard views include AP internal rotation, AP external rotation and axillary views
  - o Scapular Y-view to evaluate supraspinatus outlet and assess for dislocation
  - o Rockwood view, 30 degrees caudal tilt AP, to evaluate acromion
  - o Zanca view, 10-20 degrees cephalic tilt AP, to evaluate acromioclavicular joint

- Garth apical oblique or West Point axillary view to assess anteroinferior glenoid rim
  - Garth: Patient seated, arm at side, cassette posterior lying parallel to the spine of the scapula, beam centered at glenohumeral joint angled 45 degrees to the plane of the thorax and 45 degrees caudal
  - West Point axillary: Patient prone, head turned away from involved side, cassette held against superior aspect of shoulder, beam centered at axilla angled 25 degrees downward from horizontal and 25 degrees medial
  - Stryker notch view to assess humeral head and base of coracoid process
    - Patient supine, cassette under involved shoulder, palm of hand on top of head with fingers toward back of head
- **Computed tomography (CT)**
  - Best evaluates bone contour
- **Magnetic resonance (MR) imaging**
  - High field MR scanner
  - Low-field dedicated extremity MR scanners improving in quality
  - Dedicated shoulder coil centered on region of interest
  - Patient positioning
    - Supine, arm neutral to slight external rotation, avoid internal rotation
    - Arm at side and slightly away from side of body
  - Scout images in coronal plane
  - Axial gradient echo or T2 FS from acromion through inferior glenoid fossa
  - Coronal oblique T2 FS or proton density & T1 sequences oriented parallel to supraspinatus tendon
    - From subscapularis muscle anteriorly through infraspinatus muscle posteriorly
  - Sagittal oblique T2 FS oriented perpendicular to supraspinatus tendon
    - Scapular neck through lateral border of greater tuberosity
    - T1 sagittal oblique sequence helpful for assessing muscle atrophy
- **Arthrography**
  - Conventional arthrography
    - Needle placed into glenohumeral joint under fluoroscopic guidance
    - Administer 10 to 12 ml contrast
    - Contrast should remain within joint, without extension into rotator cuff or subacromial-subdeltoid bursa
    - Opacification of subscapular recess & biceps tendon sheath is normal
  - CT arthrography helpful in patients with contraindication to MR
  - MR arthrography
    - Best evaluates capsulolabral complex
    - Intraarticular 12 ml dilute gadopentetate dimeglumine (2 mmol/L) mixed with iodinated contrast, Marcaine & epinephrine according to institutional preference
    - Avoid shoulder exercise prior to imaging to minimize contrast leakage
    - Indirect method utilizes IV gadopentetate dimeglumine
    - T1 FS sequences in axial, coronal oblique & sagittal oblique planes
    - Optional abduction-external rotation (ABER)
    - Injection of air can simulate loose bodies

Imaging Pitfalls

- **Magic angle phenomenon on MR**
  - 55° to main magnetic field when image TE < 30 ms
  - Increases signal intensity in otherwise normal structures
  - Most often seen in supraspinatus tendon, commonly in "critical zone," 1 cm from greater tuberosity
  - Can be seen in glenoid labrum and biceps tendon proximal to bicipital groove
  - Avoid pitfall by comparing with images acquired with longer TE
- **Interdigitation of muscle or fibrous tissue between supraspinatus and infraspinatus tendons**
  - Simulates increased T2 MR signal within supraspinatus tendon
  - Exaggerated if imaged in internal rotation
- **Volume averaging of rotator interval contents on coronal oblique images**
  - Simulates increased T2 MR signal within supraspinatus tendon
- **Normal flattening or slight concavity of posterolateral humeral head**
  - Proximal to teres minor tendon insertion
  - Can be confused with Hill-Sachs lesion, which is located more proximally, above the level of the coracoid process
- **Acromial pseudospurs mimicking osteophytes**
  - Fibrocartilaginous hypertrophy at insertion of coracoacromial ligament on inferior acromion
  - Superior and inferior tendon slips of deltoid muscle
- **Normal residual red bone marrow in glenoid and proximal humeral metaphysis can mimic neoplastic process**
  - Red marrow has higher T1 signal than adjacent muscle
  - Red marrow typically decreases in signal on out of phase images, compared with in phase images
- **Anterolateral branch of anterior circumflex humeral artery & vein in lateral bicipital groove**
  - Can be mistaken for biceps tendon longitudinal tear
- **Hyaline cartilage undercutting of superior labrum simulating labral tear**
- **Vacuum effect simulating loose bodies or chondrocalcinosis**
  - Exaggerated on gradient echo MR sequences & with external rotation positioning
- **General imaging artifacts**
  - Motion artifact can be decreased by positioning the arm away from patient's body
  - Avoid superior to inferior phase encoding to decrease artifact from axillary vessels
  - Metal susceptibility artifact
    - Increase bandwidth on all sequences
    - Use fast spin echo rather than conventional spin echo sequences

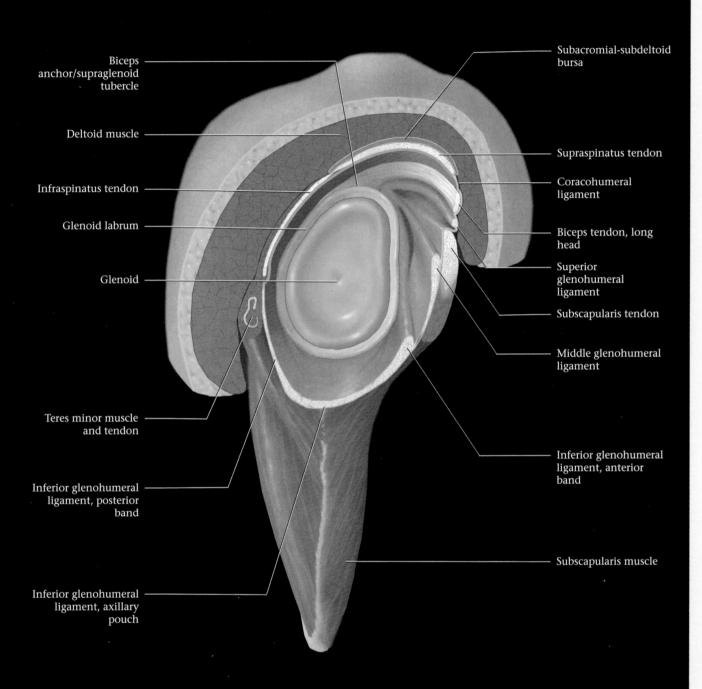

Biceps anchor/supraglenoid tubercle

Deltoid muscle

Infraspinatus tendon

Glenoid labrum

Glenoid

Teres minor muscle and tendon

Inferior glenohumeral ligament, posterior band

Inferior glenohumeral ligament, axillary pouch

Subacromial-subdeltoid bursa

Supraspinatus tendon

Coracohumeral ligament

Biceps tendon, long head

Superior glenohumeral ligament

Subscapularis tendon

Middle glenohumeral ligament

Inferior glenohumeral ligament, anterior band

Subscapularis muscle

Sagittal graphic of the shoulder with the humerus removed.

ANTERIOR GRAPHIC

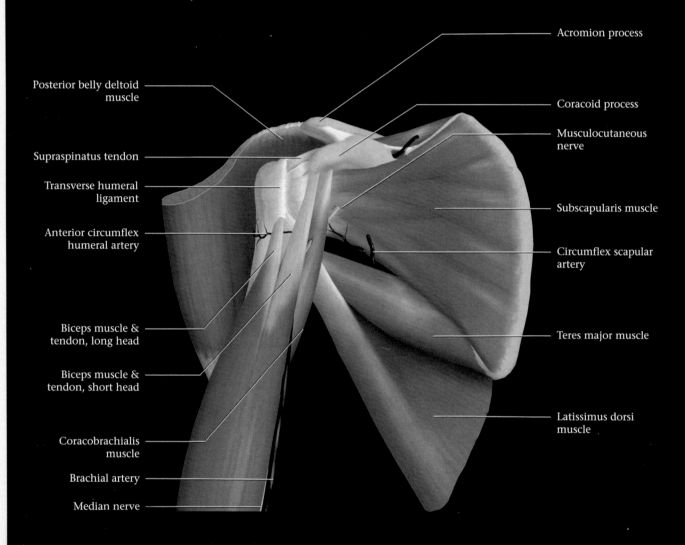

Posterior belly deltoid muscle

Supraspinatus tendon

Transverse humeral ligament

Anterior circumflex humeral artery

Biceps muscle & tendon, long head

Biceps muscle & tendon, short head

Coracobrachialis muscle

Brachial artery

Median nerve

Acromion process

Coracoid process

Musculocutaneous nerve

Subscapularis muscle

Circumflex scapular artery

Teres major muscle

Latissimus dorsi muscle

Anterior graphic of the shoulder shows a superficial scapulohumeral dissection.

SHOULDER OVERVIEW

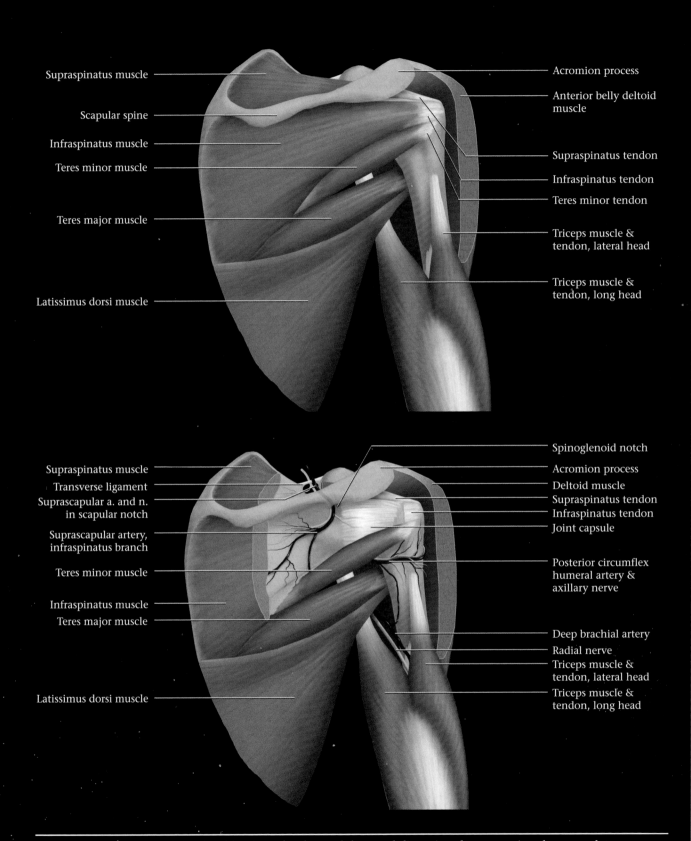

Supraspinatus muscle

Scapular spine

Infraspinatus muscle

Teres minor muscle

Teres major muscle

Latissimus dorsi muscle

Acromion process

Anterior belly deltoid muscle

Supraspinatus tendon

Infraspinatus tendon

Teres minor tendon

Triceps muscle & tendon, lateral head

Triceps muscle & tendon, long head

Supraspinatus muscle

Transverse ligament

Suprascapular a. and n. in scapular notch

Suprascapular artery, infraspinatus branch

Teres minor muscle

Infraspinatus muscle

Teres major muscle

Latissimus dorsi muscle

Spinoglenoid notch

Acromion process

Deltoid muscle

Supraspinatus tendon

Infraspinatus tendon

Joint capsule

Posterior circumflex humeral artery & axillary nerve

Deep brachial artery

Radial nerve

Triceps muscle & tendon, lateral head

Triceps muscle & tendon, long head

(Top) Posterior graphic of the shoulder. Superficial scapulohumeral dissection demonstrating the musculature. **(Bottom)** Deep scapulohumeral dissection demonstrates the major neurovascular structures.

VASCULAR GRAPHICS

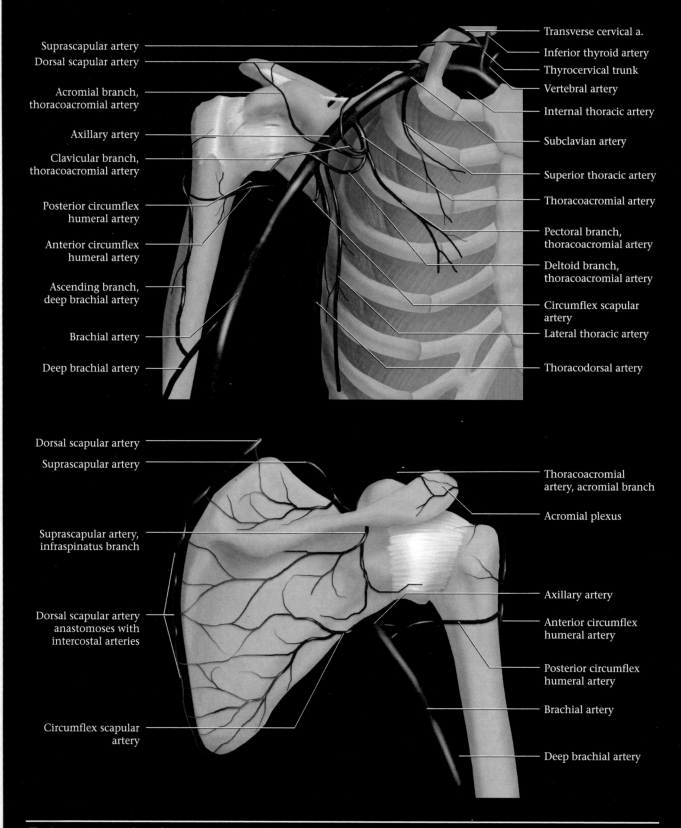

Suprascapular artery
Dorsal scapular artery

Acromial branch, thoracoacromial artery

Axillary artery

Clavicular branch, thoracoacromial artery

Posterior circumflex humeral artery

Anterior circumflex humeral artery

Ascending branch, deep brachial artery

Brachial artery

Deep brachial artery

Transverse cervical a.
Inferior thyroid artery
Thyrocervical trunk
Vertebral artery
Internal thoracic artery
Subclavian artery
Superior thoracic artery
Thoracoacromial artery
Pectoral branch, thoracoacromial artery
Deltoid branch, thoracoacromial artery
Circumflex scapular artery
Lateral thoracic artery
Thoracodorsal artery

Dorsal scapular artery
Suprascapular artery

Suprascapular artery, infraspinatus branch

Dorsal scapular artery anastomoses with intercostal arteries

Circumflex scapular artery

Thoracoacromial artery, acromial branch
Acromial plexus

Axillary artery
Anterior circumflex humeral artery
Posterior circumflex humeral artery
Brachial artery
Deep brachial artery

(Top) Anterior graphic of arterial supply to shoulder. The shoulder is predominantly supplied by anterior and posterior circumflex humeral, suprascapular and circumflex scapular arteries. **(Bottom)** Posterior graphic of arterial supply to shoulder. Extensive collateral blood vessels include anastomoses with intercostal arteries.

SHOULDER OVERVIEW

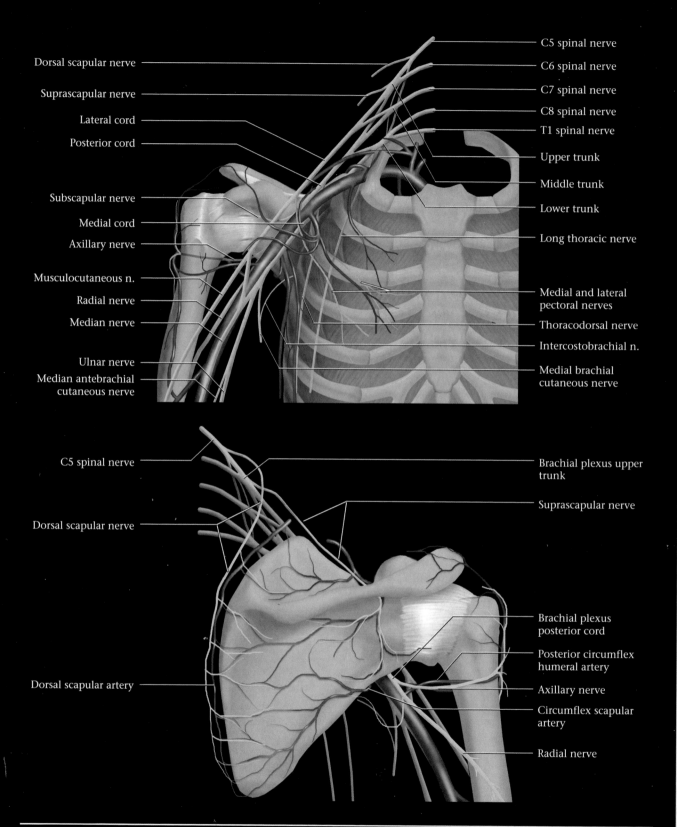

Dorsal scapular nerve

Suprascapular nerve

Lateral cord

Posterior cord

Subscapular nerve

Medial cord

Axillary nerve

Musculocutaneous n.

Radial nerve

Median nerve

Ulnar nerve

Median antebrachial cutaneous nerve

C5 spinal nerve

C6 spinal nerve

C7 spinal nerve

C8 spinal nerve

T1 spinal nerve

Upper trunk

Middle trunk

Lower trunk

Long thoracic nerve

Medial and lateral pectoral nerves

Thoracodorsal nerve

Intercostobrachial n.

Medial brachial cutaneous nerve

C5 spinal nerve

Dorsal scapular nerve

Dorsal scapular artery

Brachial plexus upper trunk

Suprascapular nerve

Brachial plexus posterior cord

Posterior circumflex humeral artery

Axillary nerve

Circumflex scapular artery

Radial nerve

(Top) Anterior graphic of the brachial plexus. **(Bottom)** Posterior graphic of the brachial plexus branches innervating the shoulder.

SHOULDER OVERVIEW

EXTERNAL & INTERNAL ROTATION RADIOGRAPHS

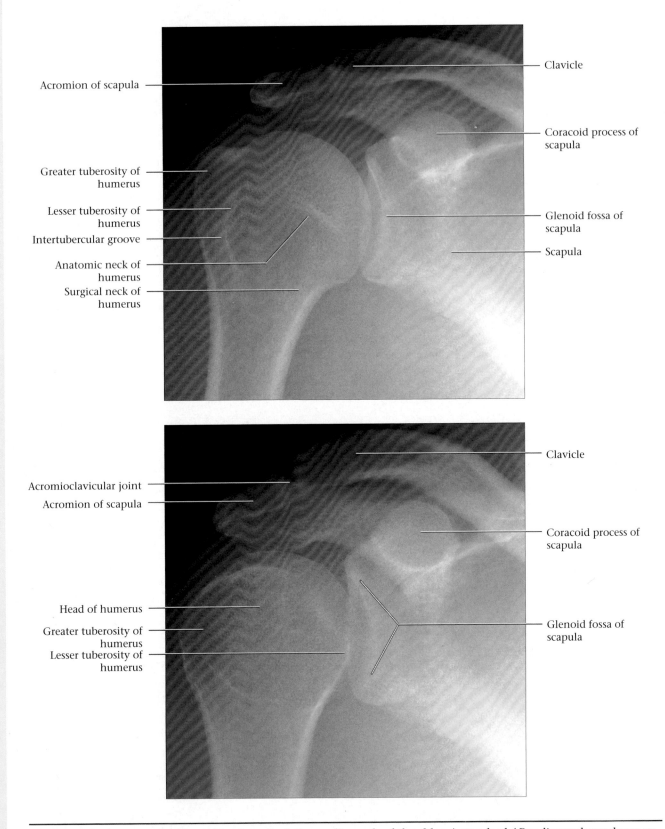

Acromion of scapula

Greater tuberosity of humerus

Lesser tuberosity of humerus

Intertubercular groove

Anatomic neck of humerus

Surgical neck of humerus

Clavicle

Coracoid process of scapula

Glenoid fossa of scapula

Scapula

Acromioclavicular joint

Acromion of scapula

Head of humerus

Greater tuberosity of humerus

Lesser tuberosity of humerus

Clavicle

Coracoid process of scapula

Glenoid fossa of scapula

(Top) Standard anteroposterior (AP) external rotation radiograph of shoulder. A standard AP radiograph produces an oblique view of the glenohumeral joint, which has a normal anterior angle of approximately 40 degrees. The standard AP view can be obtained in neutral position, internal rotation or external rotation. With the arm in external rotation, the greater tuberosity projects at the lateral aspect of the humeral head. **(Bottom)** Standard AP internal rotation radiograph of shoulder. The lesser tuberosity projects at the medial aspect of the humeral head. The greater tuberosity has rotated anterior and is partially obscured. The posterolateral aspect of the humeral head projects laterally.

SHOULDER OVERVIEW

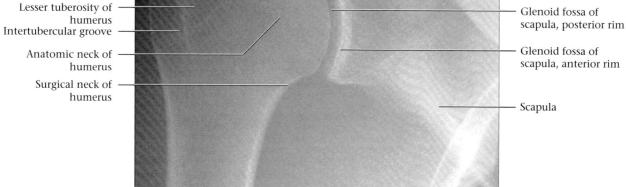

Acromion of scapula

Clavicle

Greater tuberosity of humerus

Coracoid process of scapula

Lesser tuberosity of humerus
Intertubercular groove

Glenoid fossa of scapula, posterior rim

Anatomic neck of humerus

Glenoid fossa of scapula, anterior rim

Surgical neck of humerus

Scapula

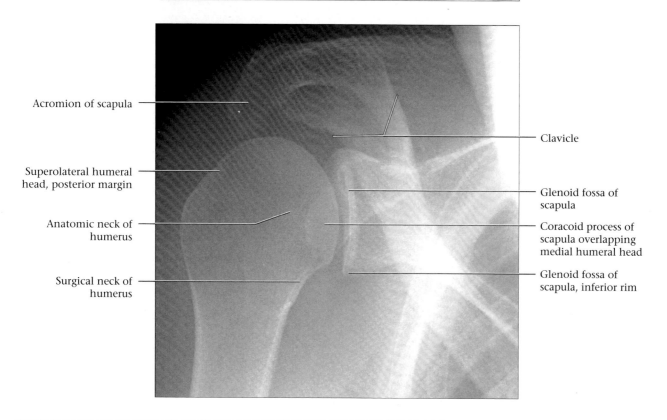

Acromion of scapula

Clavicle

Superolateral humeral head, posterior margin

Glenoid fossa of scapula

Anatomic neck of humerus

Coracoid process of scapula overlapping medial humeral head

Surgical neck of humerus

Glenoid fossa of scapula, inferior rim

(Top) Grashey or true AP view of shoulder. A true AP view of the shoulder is obtained by tilting the X-ray beam approximately 45 degrees laterally from the standard AP view. This produces a true AP view of the anteriorly angled glenohumeral joint. The anterior and posterior rims of the glenoid should nearly overlap on this view. The Grashey view is helpful for evaluating joint congruity, joint space narrowing and humeral head subluxation. (Bottom) Garth view of shoulder. The Garth view is obtained by angling the X-ray beam 45 degrees caudally from a standard AP view. The inferior glenohumeral rim and posterior margin of the superolateral humeral head are well demonstrated. In patients with acute or chronic anterior humeral head dislocations, this view may assist in detection of Bankart fractures of the inferior glenoid and Hill-Sachs deformities of the humeral head.

SHOULDER OVERVIEW

AXILLARY & WEST POINT RADIOGRAPHS

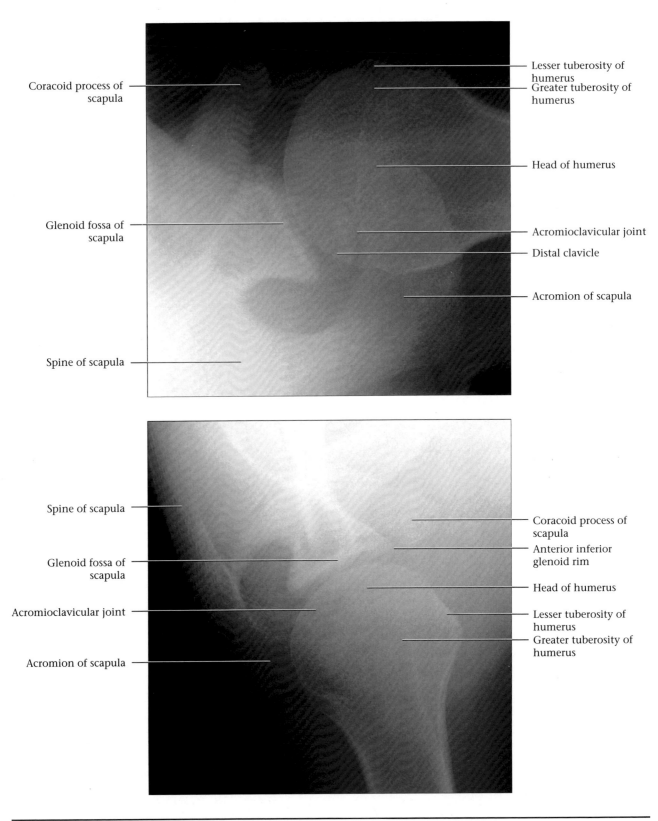

Coracoid process of scapula

Lesser tuberosity of humerus

Greater tuberosity of humerus

Head of humerus

Glenoid fossa of scapula

Acromioclavicular joint

Distal clavicle

Acromion of scapula

Spine of scapula

Spine of scapula

Coracoid process of scapula

Anterior inferior glenoid rim

Glenoid fossa of scapula

Head of humerus

Acromioclavicular joint

Lesser tuberosity of humerus

Acromion of scapula

Greater tuberosity of humerus

(Top) Standard axillary view of shoulder. This view is obtained with the patient supine, the arm abducted to 90 degrees and the X-ray beam angled 15 to 30 degrees medially to compensate for rotation of the scapula. The resultant image is tangential to the glenohumeral joint. This view is helpful for identification of humeral head dislocation and anterior or posterior glenoid rim fractures. **(Bottom)** West Point axillary view of shoulder. This variation on the standard axillary view is acquired with the patient prone and the abducted forearm hanging off the edge of the table. The X-ray beam is angled 25 degrees medially and anteriorly. The West Point view better demonstrates the anterior inferior glenoid, making it useful for detection of Bankart fractures.

SHOULDER OVERVIEW

STRYKER NOTCH & SUPRASPINATUS OUTLET RADIOGRAPHS

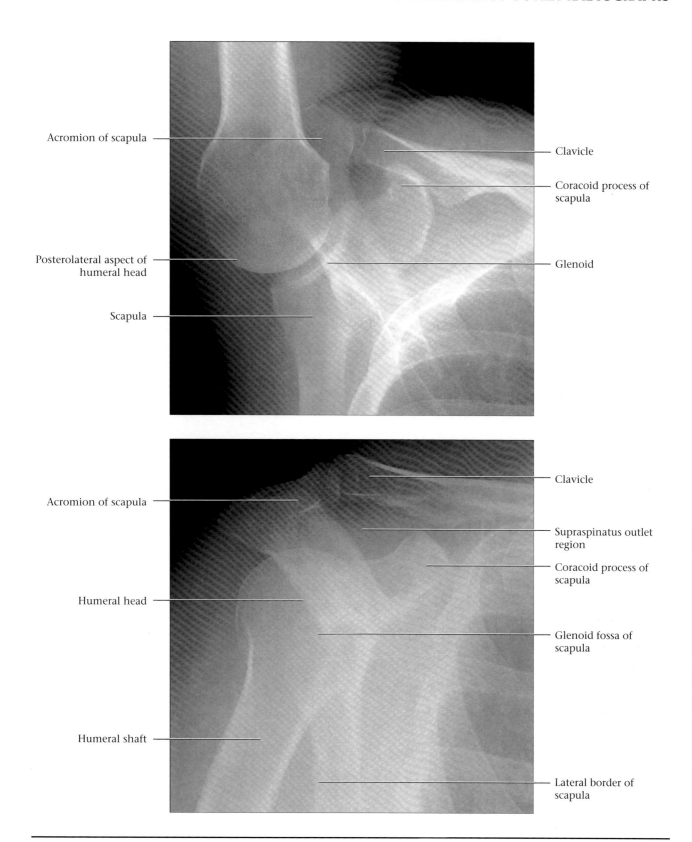

(Top) Stryker notch view of shoulder. This view is obtained with the patient supine and the arm in an abducted and externally rotated (ABER) position. The X-ray beam is angled 10 degrees cephalic. The posterolateral aspect of the humeral head, where a Hill-Sachs deformity could be located, is well demonstrated. **(Bottom)** Supraspinatus outlet view of the shoulder. This view is obtained by placing the anterior aspect of the affected shoulder against the X-ray plate, rotating the opposite shoulder approximately 40 degrees away from the plate then tilting the X-ray beam 5 to 10 degrees caudally. The acromion and subacromial space are imaged in profile. The supraspinatus outlet view is helpful for assessing acromial morphology and humeral head subluxation.

SHOULDER OVERVIEW

SCAPULAR Y VIEW & AP SCAPULA RADIOGRAPHS

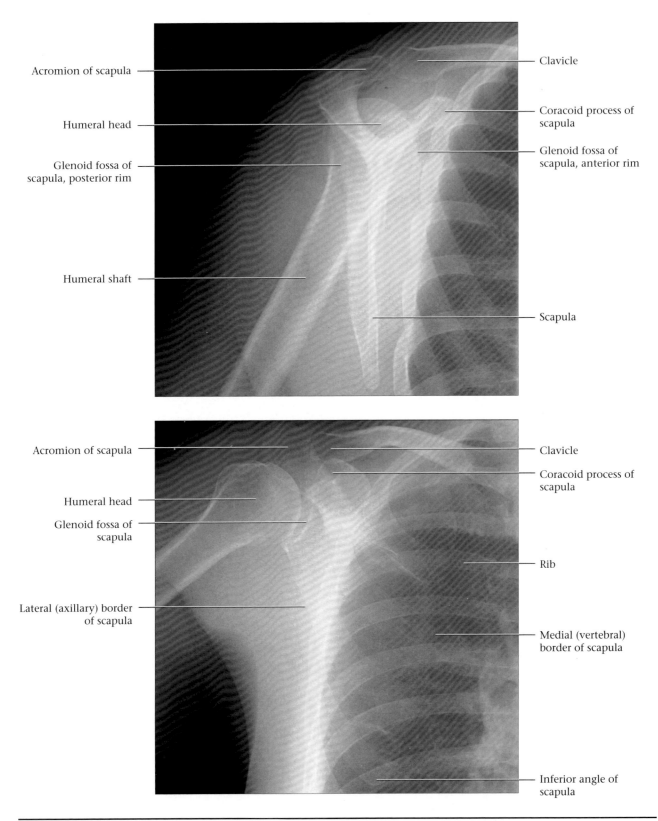

Acromion of scapula — ... — Clavicle

Humeral head —

Coracoid process of scapula

Glenoid fossa of scapula, posterior rim —

Glenoid fossa of scapula, anterior rim

Humeral shaft —

Scapula

Acromion of scapula — ... — Clavicle

Coracoid process of scapula

Humeral head —

Glenoid fossa of scapula —

Rib

Lateral (axillary) border of scapula —

Medial (vertebral) border of scapula

Inferior angle of scapula

(Top) Scapular Y view of shoulder. The anterior aspect of the affected shoulder is placed against the X-ray plate and the opposite shoulder rotated approximately 45 to 60 degrees away from the plate. The x-ray beam is directed along the scapular spine producing a true lateral view of the shoulder. The scapula is shaped like the letter Y in this projection. The humeral head should be located at the center of the Y. Anteriorly dislocated shoulders will show the humeral head lying below the coracoid process. Posteriorly dislocated shoulders will show the humeral head lying posterior to the glenoid. **(Bottom)** AP view of scapula. This is obtained standing or supine with the arm abducted and hand supinated. The medial (vertebral) border of the scapula is shown through the upper lung.

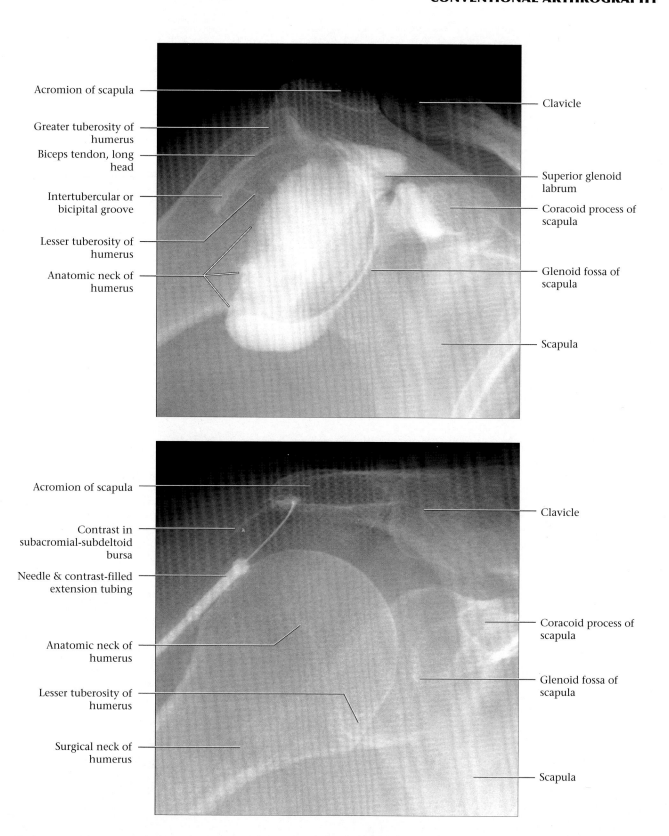

Acromion of scapula

Greater tuberosity of humerus

Biceps tendon, long head

Intertubercular or bicipital groove

Lesser tuberosity of humerus

Anatomic neck of humerus

Clavicle

Superior glenoid labrum

Coracoid process of scapula

Glenoid fossa of scapula

Scapula

Acromion of scapula

Contrast in subacromial-subdeltoid bursa

Needle & contrast-filled extension tubing

Anatomic neck of humerus

Lesser tuberosity of humerus

Surgical neck of humerus

Clavicle

Coracoid process of scapula

Glenoid fossa of scapula

Scapula

(Top) Conventional shoulder arthrogram. Intraarticular contrast outlines the confines of the joint. Contrast extends to the anatomic neck of the humerus, where the joint capsule inserts. Contrast can normally extend into the biceps tendon sheath and subscapular recess. **(Bottom)** Subacromial-subdeltoid bursa injection. A 25g needle is placed just below the acromion process. Administered contrast will have a curvilinear configuration as it tracks within the subacromial-subdeltoid bursa. The shoulder is internally rotated on this image.

Shoulder

3D CT RECONSTRUCTION

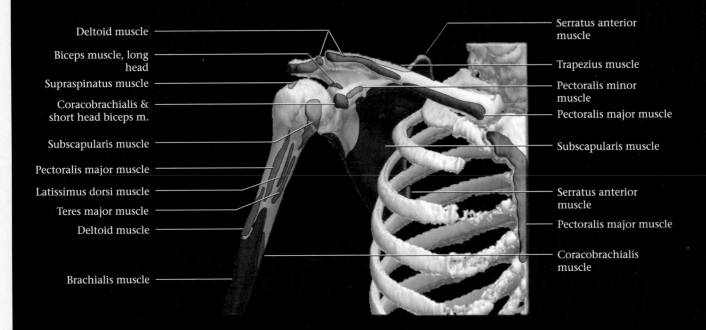

Deltoid muscle

Biceps muscle, long head

Supraspinatus muscle

Coracobrachialis & short head biceps m.

Subscapularis muscle

Pectoralis major muscle

Latissimus dorsi muscle

Teres major muscle

Deltoid muscle

Brachialis muscle

Serratus anterior muscle

Trapezius muscle

Pectoralis minor muscle

Pectoralis major muscle

Subscapularis muscle

Serratus anterior muscle

Pectoralis major muscle

Coracobrachialis muscle

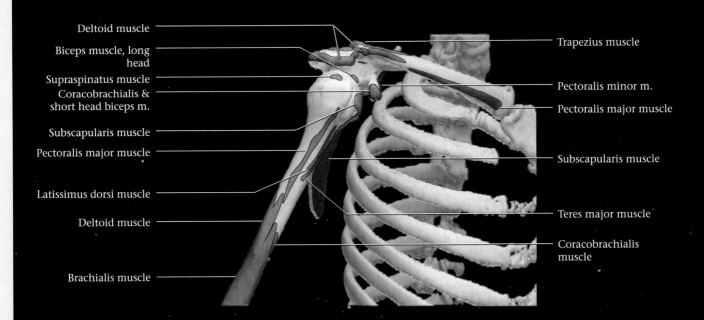

Deltoid muscle

Biceps muscle, long head

Supraspinatus muscle

Coracobrachialis & short head biceps m.

Subscapularis muscle

Pectoralis major muscle

Latissimus dorsi muscle

Deltoid muscle

Brachialis muscle

Trapezius muscle

Pectoralis minor m.

Pectoralis major muscle

Subscapularis muscle

Teres major muscle

Coracobrachialis muscle

(Top) Anterior view of the right shoulder from a 3D CT reconstruction. Muscle origins are shown in red. Muscle insertions are shown in blue. **(Bottom)** Anterior oblique view of the shoulder.

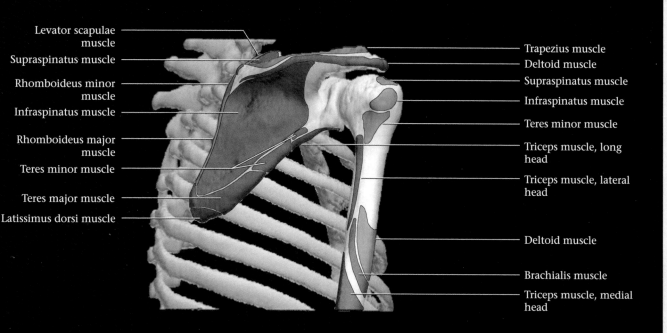

Levator scapulae muscle
Supraspinatus muscle
Rhomboideus minor muscle
Infraspinatus muscle
Rhomboideus major muscle
Teres minor muscle
Teres major muscle
Latissimus dorsi muscle

Trapezius muscle
Deltoid muscle
Supraspinatus muscle
Infraspinatus muscle
Teres minor muscle
Triceps muscle, long head
Triceps muscle, lateral head
Deltoid muscle
Brachialis muscle
Triceps muscle, medial head

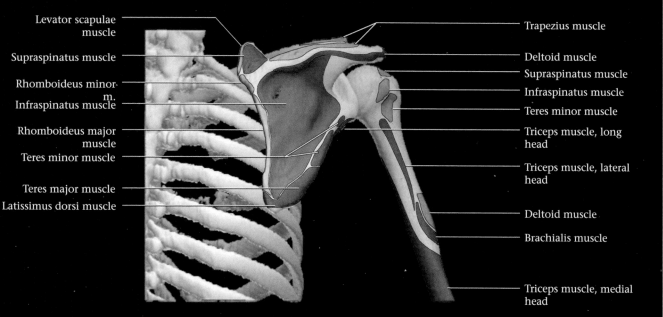

Levator scapulae muscle
Supraspinatus muscle
Rhomboideus minor m.
Infraspinatus muscle
Rhomboideus major muscle
Teres minor muscle
Teres major muscle
Latissimus dorsi muscle

Trapezius muscle
Deltoid muscle
Supraspinatus muscle
Infraspinatus muscle
Teres minor muscle
Triceps muscle, long head
Triceps muscle, lateral head
Deltoid muscle
Brachialis muscle
Triceps muscle, medial head

(Top) Posterior oblique view of the shoulder from a 3D CT reconstruction. Muscle origins are shown in red. Muscle insertions are shown in blue. **(Bottom)** Posterior view of the shoulder.

Shoulder

I

AXIAL T1 MR, RIGHT SHOULDER

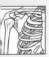

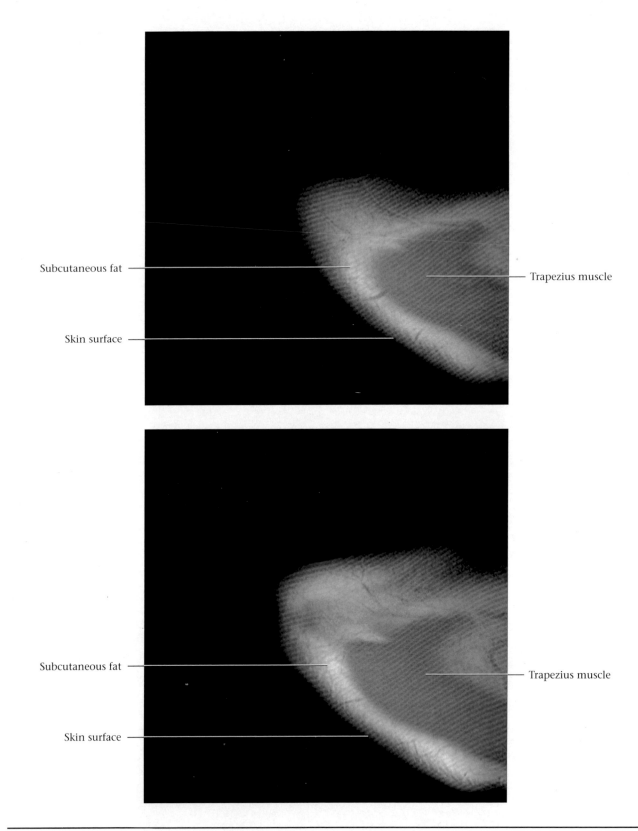

Subcutaneous fat ————— ————— Trapezius muscle

Skin surface —————

Subcutaneous fat ————— ————— Trapezius muscle

Skin surface —————

(Top) First in series of T1 MR images of the right shoulder displayed superior to inferior. Images were acquired using a shoulder coil on a 3T MR scanner. **(Bottom)** The trapezius muscle covers the superior and posterior aspect of the upper shoulder. It originates from occipital bone, ligamentum nuchae and the spinous processes of C7 to T12. It inserts on the posterior border of the lateral clavicle, the medial border of the acromion and the spine of the scapula.

SHOULDER OVERVIEW

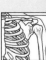

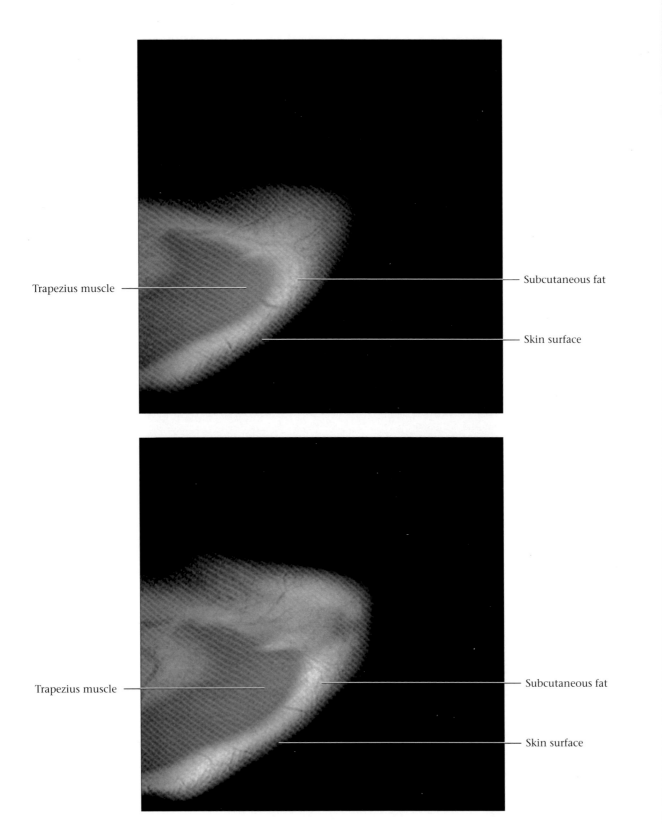

Trapezius muscle ——————————————— Subcutaneous fat

————————————— Skin surface

Trapezius muscle ——————————————— Subcutaneous fat

————————————— Skin surface

(Top) First in series of T1 MR images of the left shoulder displayed superior to inferior. Images were acquired using a shoulder coil on a 3T MR scanner. **(Bottom)** The trapezius muscle covers the superior and posterior aspect of the upper shoulder. It originates from occipital bone, ligamentum nuchae and the spinous processes of C7 to T12. It inserts on the posterior border of the lateral clavicle, the medial border of the acromion and the spine of the scapula.

AXIAL T1 MR, RIGHT SHOULDER

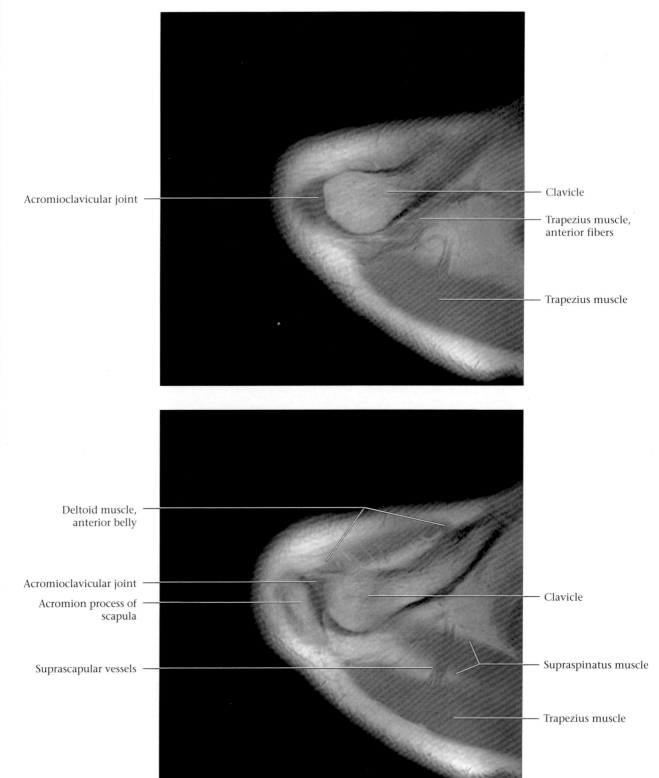

Acromioclavicular joint ——————————————————— Clavicle

——————————————————— Trapezius muscle, anterior fibers

——————————————————— Trapezius muscle

Deltoid muscle, anterior belly ——————

Acromioclavicular joint ——————

Acromion process of scapula ——————

——————————————————— Clavicle

Suprascapular vessels ——————

——————————————————— Supraspinatus muscle

——————————————————— Trapezius muscle

(Top) The distal clavicle is visible at this level. The trapezius muscle is present posteriorly and a few of the anterior trapezius fibers are inserting along the posterior border of the distal clavicle. **(Bottom)** The acromion and distal clavicle form the bony roof of the superior shoulder. The supraspinatus muscle becomes visible beneath branches of the suprascapular vessels.

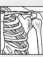

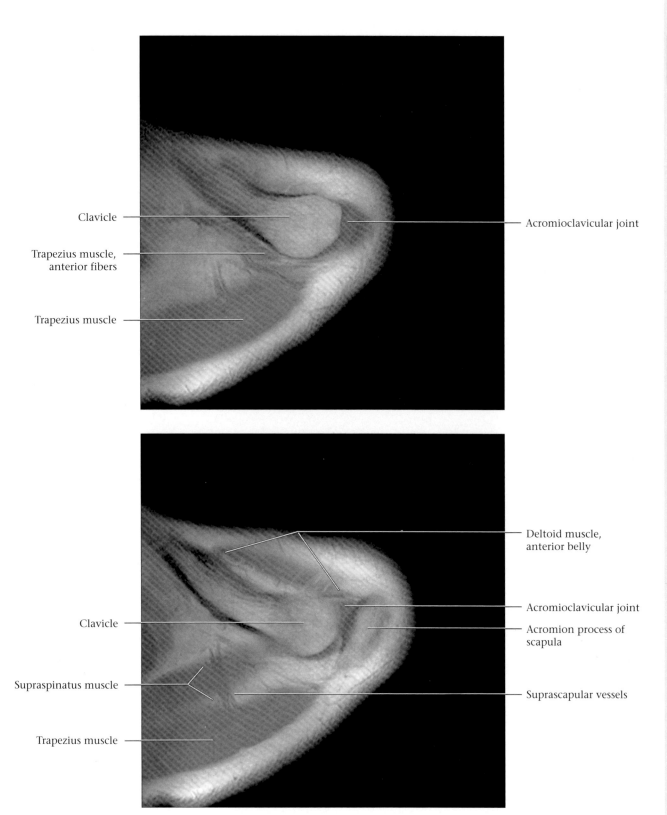

Clavicle — — Acromioclavicular joint

Trapezius muscle, anterior fibers

Trapezius muscle

Deltoid muscle, anterior belly

Clavicle — — Acromioclavicular joint

— Acromion process of scapula

Supraspinatus muscle

Trapezius muscle — — Suprascapular vessels

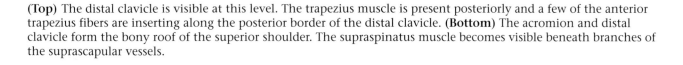

(Top) The distal clavicle is visible at this level. The trapezius muscle is present posteriorly and a few of the anterior trapezius fibers are inserting along the posterior border of the distal clavicle. **(Bottom)** The acromion and distal clavicle form the bony roof of the superior shoulder. The supraspinatus muscle becomes visible beneath branches of the suprascapular vessels.

AXIAL T1 MR, RIGHT SHOULDER

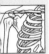

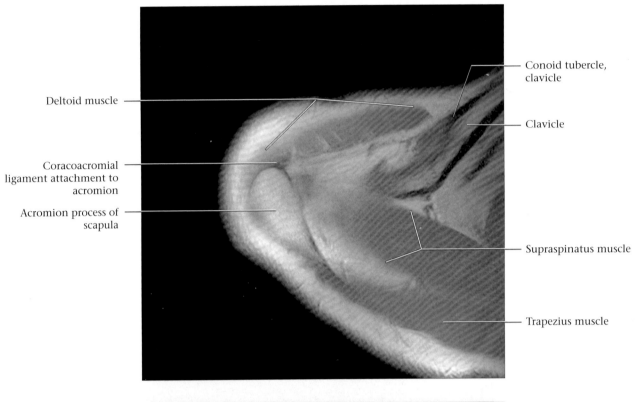

Deltoid muscle

Coracoacromial ligament attachment to acromion

Acromion process of scapula

Conoid tubercle, clavicle

Clavicle

Supraspinatus muscle

Trapezius muscle

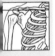

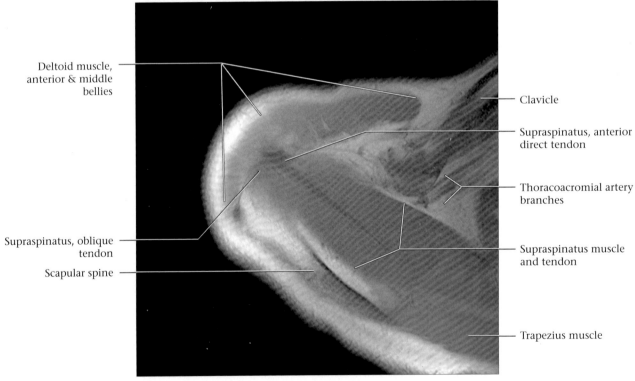

Deltoid muscle, anterior & middle bellies

Supraspinatus, oblique tendon

Scapular spine

Clavicle

Supraspinatus, anterior direct tendon

Thoracoacromial artery branches

Supraspinatus muscle and tendon

Trapezius muscle

(Top) The majority of the acromion process of the scapula is visible on this axial image. This is the level to assess for the presence of an os acromiale, an unfused acromial apophysis that can be symptomatic. **(Bottom)** Image is just below the acromion process. The supraspinatus tendon arcs over the humeral head toward the attachment on the greater tuberosity. The deltoid muscle covers the anterior, lateral and posterior aspect of the shoulder. It originates from the lateral third of the clavicle, lateral margin of the acromion and posterior border of the scapular spine.

SHOULDER OVERVIEW

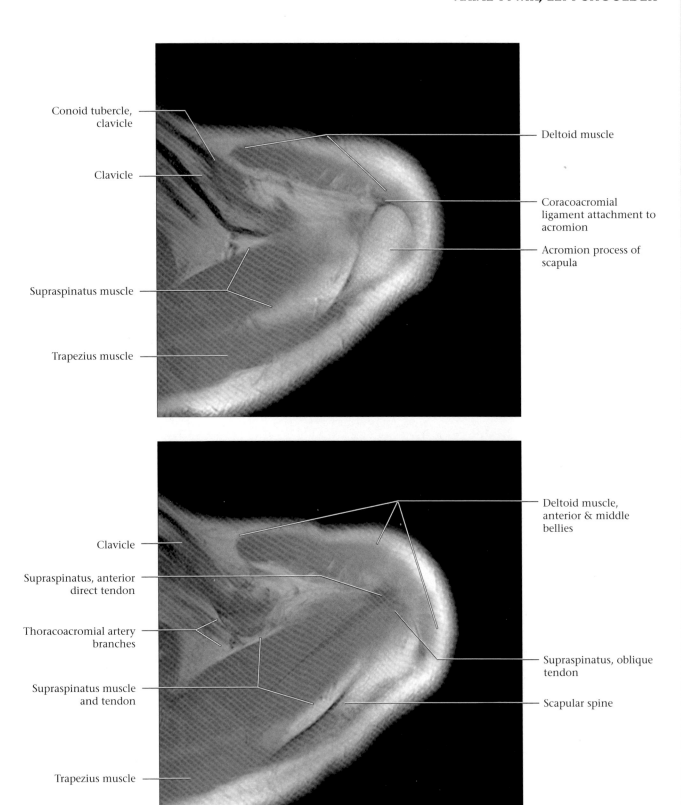
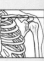

Conoid tubercle, clavicle

Clavicle

Supraspinatus muscle

Trapezius muscle

Deltoid muscle

Coracoacromial ligament attachment to acromion

Acromion process of scapula

Clavicle

Supraspinatus, anterior direct tendon

Thoracoacromial artery branches

Supraspinatus muscle and tendon

Trapezius muscle

Deltoid muscle, anterior & middle bellies

Supraspinatus, oblique tendon

Scapular spine

(Top) The majority of the acromion process of the scapula is visible on this axial image. This is the level to assess for the presence of an os acromiale, an unfused acromial apophysis that can be symptomatic. **(Bottom)** Image is just below the acromion process. The supraspinatus tendon arcs over the humeral head toward the attachment on the greater tuberosity. The deltoid muscle covers the anterior, lateral and posterior aspect of the shoulder. It originates from the lateral third of the clavicle, lateral margin of the acromion and posterior border of the scapular spine.

AXIAL T1 MR, RIGHT SHOULDER

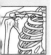

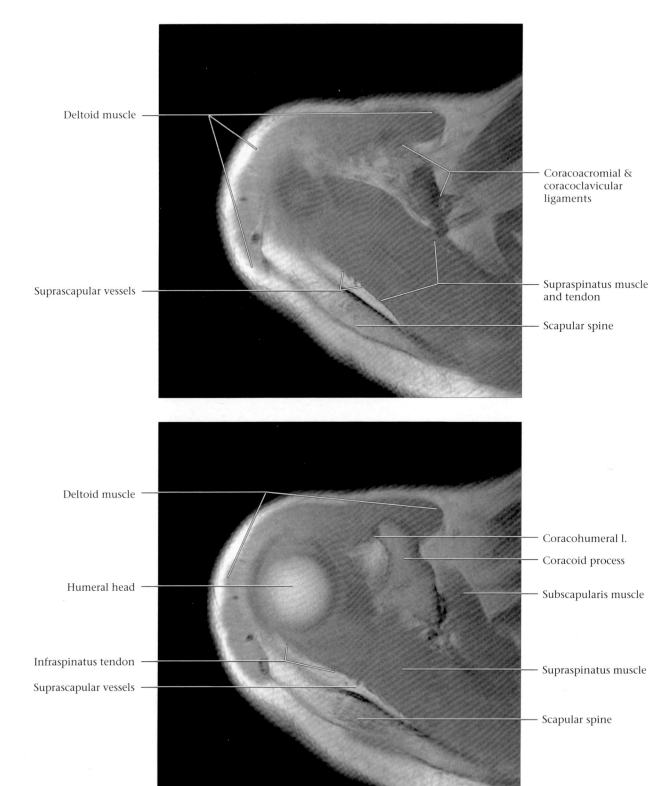

Deltoid muscle

Coracoacromial & coracoclavicular ligaments

Suprascapular vessels

Supraspinatus muscle and tendon

Scapular spine

Deltoid muscle

Coracohumeral l.

Coracoid process

Humeral head

Subscapularis muscle

Infraspinatus tendon

Suprascapular vessels

Supraspinatus muscle

Scapular spine

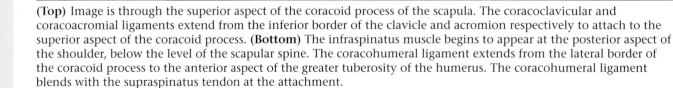

(Top) Image is through the superior aspect of the coracoid process of the scapula. The coracoclavicular and coracoacromial ligaments extend from the inferior border of the clavicle and acromion respectively to attach to the superior aspect of the coracoid process. **(Bottom)** The infraspinatus muscle begins to appear at the posterior aspect of the shoulder, below the level of the scapular spine. The coracohumeral ligament extends from the lateral border of the coracoid process to the anterior aspect of the greater tuberosity of the humerus. The coracohumeral ligament blends with the supraspinatus tendon at the attachment.

SHOULDER OVERVIEW

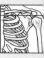

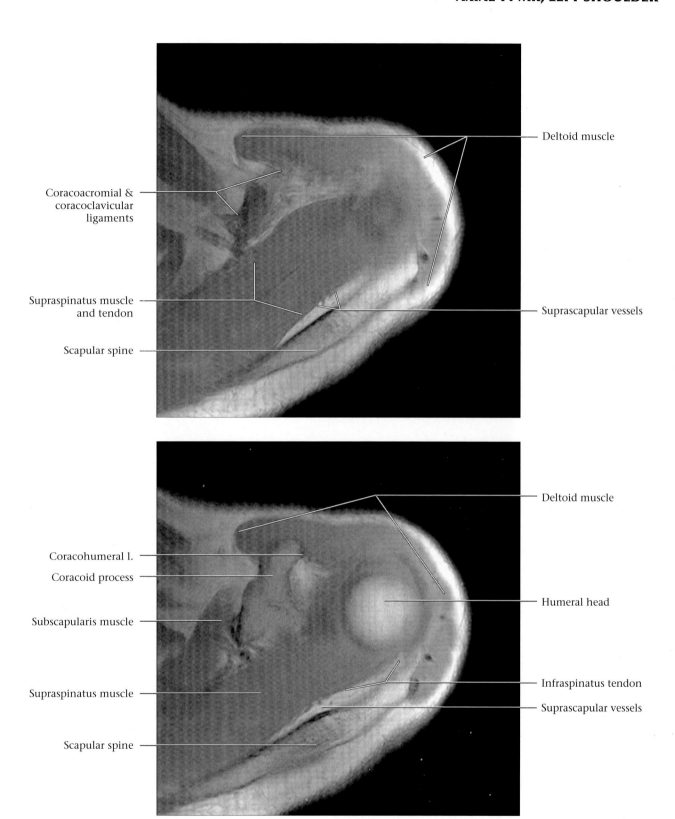

Coracoacromial & coracoclavicular ligaments

Supraspinatus muscle and tendon

Scapular spine

Deltoid muscle

Suprascapular vessels

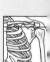

Coracohumeral l.

Coracoid process

Subscapularis muscle

Supraspinatus muscle

Scapular spine

Deltoid muscle

Humeral head

Infraspinatus tendon

Suprascapular vessels

(Top) Image is through the superior aspect of the coracoid process of the scapula. The coracoclavicular and coracoacromial ligaments extend from the inferior border of the clavicle and acromion respectively to attach to the superior aspect of the coracoid process. (Bottom) The infraspinatus muscle begins to appear at the posterior aspect of the shoulder, below the level of the scapular spine. The coracohumeral ligament extends from the lateral border of the coracoid process to the anterior aspect of the greater tuberosity of the humerus. The coracohumeral ligament blends with the supraspinatus tendon at the attachment.

Shoulder

I

25

AXIAL T1 MR, RIGHT SHOULDER

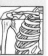

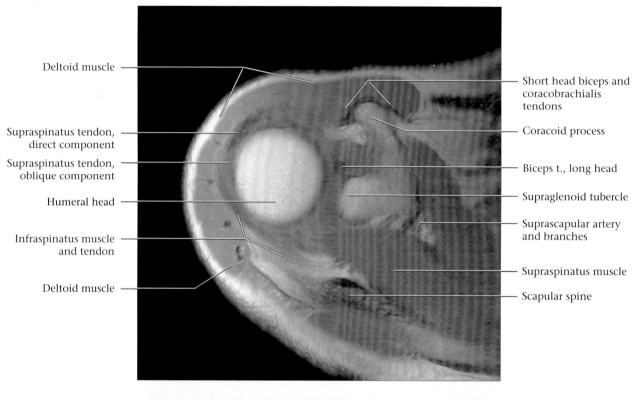

Deltoid muscle

Supraspinatus tendon, direct component

Supraspinatus tendon, oblique component

Humeral head

Infraspinatus muscle and tendon

Deltoid muscle

Short head biceps and coracobrachialis tendons

Coracoid process

Biceps t., long head

Supraglenoid tubercle

Suprascapular artery and branches

Supraspinatus muscle

Scapular spine

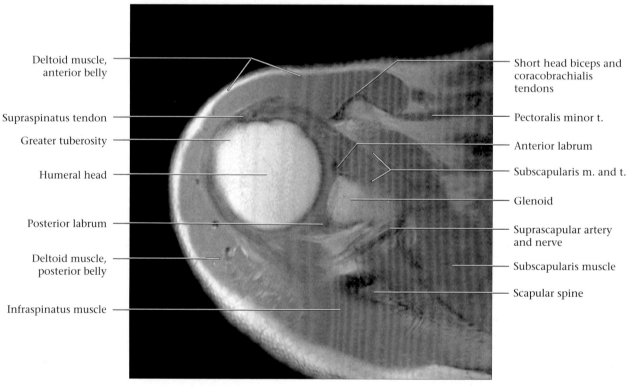

Deltoid muscle, anterior belly

Supraspinatus tendon

Greater tuberosity

Humeral head

Posterior labrum

Deltoid muscle, posterior belly

Infraspinatus muscle

Short head biceps and coracobrachialis tendons

Pectoralis minor t.

Anterior labrum

Subscapularis m. and t.

Glenoid

Suprascapular artery and nerve

Subscapularis muscle

Scapular spine

(Top) The long head of the biceps tendon originates from the superior glenoid labrum and supraglenoid tuberosity of the scapula. The short head of the biceps and coracobrachialis muscles originate from the tip of the coracoid process. **(Bottom)** The suprascapular artery and nerve branches course along the posterior glenoid fossa. The point labeled "supraspinatus tendon" represents the most lateral extent of rotator cuff interval, where the transverse ligament component of subscapularis meets the anterior edge of supraspinatus (direct tendon).

SHOULDER OVERVIEW

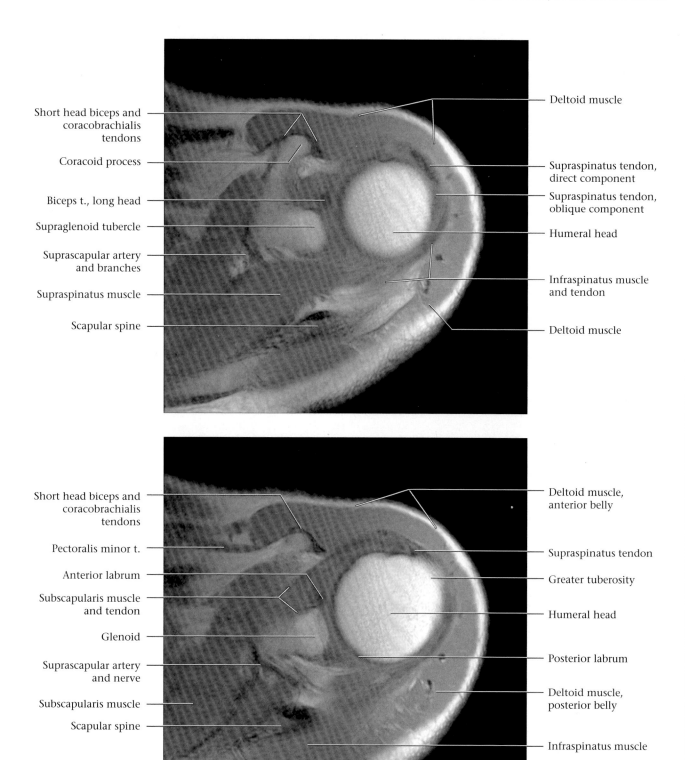
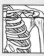
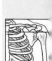

Short head biceps and coracobrachialis tendons

Coracoid process

Biceps t., long head

Supraglenoid tubercle

Suprascapular artery and branches

Supraspinatus muscle

Scapular spine

Deltoid muscle

Supraspinatus tendon, direct component

Supraspinatus tendon, oblique component

Humeral head

Infraspinatus muscle and tendon

Deltoid muscle

Short head biceps and coracobrachialis tendons

Pectoralis minor t.

Anterior labrum

Subscapularis muscle and tendon

Glenoid

Suprascapular artery and nerve

Subscapularis muscle

Scapular spine

Deltoid muscle, anterior belly

Supraspinatus tendon

Greater tuberosity

Humeral head

Posterior labrum

Deltoid muscle, posterior belly

Infraspinatus muscle

(Top) The long head of the biceps tendon originates from the superior glenoid labrum and supraglenoid tuberosity of the scapula. The short head of the biceps and coracobrachialis muscles originate from the tip of the coracoid process. **(Bottom)** The suprascapular artery and nerve branches course along the posterior glenoid fossa. The point labeled "supraspinatus tendon" represents the most lateral extent of rotator cuff interval, where the transverse ligament component of subscapularis meets the anterior edge of supraspinatus (direct tendon).

AXIAL T1 MR, RIGHT SHOULDER

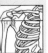

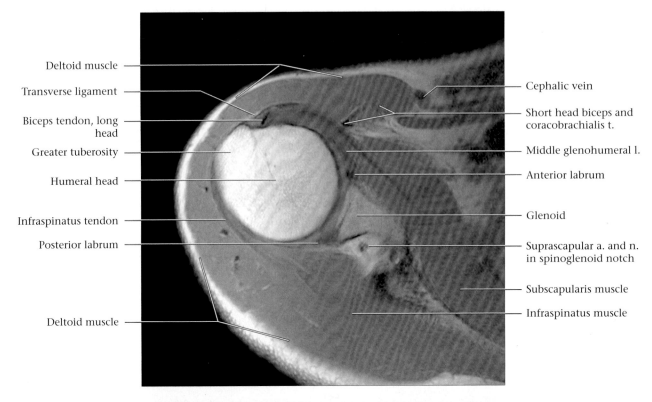

Deltoid muscle

Transverse ligament

Biceps tendon, long head

Greater tuberosity

Humeral head

Infraspinatus tendon

Posterior labrum

Deltoid muscle

Cephalic vein

Short head biceps and coracobrachialis t.

Middle glenohumeral l.

Anterior labrum

Glenoid

Suprascapular a. and n. in spinoglenoid notch

Subscapularis muscle

Infraspinatus muscle

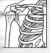

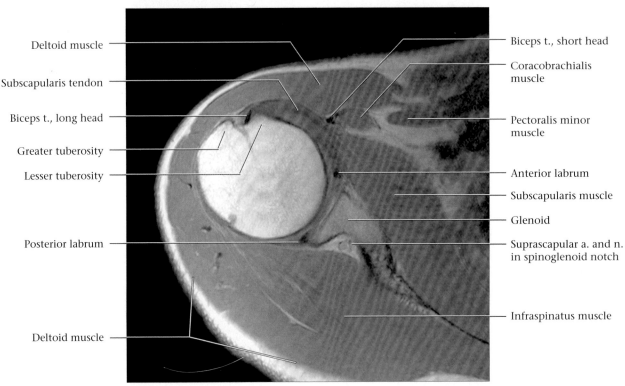

Deltoid muscle

Subscapularis tendon

Biceps t., long head

Greater tuberosity

Lesser tuberosity

Posterior labrum

Deltoid muscle

Biceps t., short head

Coracobrachialis muscle

Pectoralis minor muscle

Anterior labrum

Subscapularis muscle

Glenoid

Suprascapular a. and n. in spinoglenoid notch

Infraspinatus muscle

(Top) The middle glenohumeral joint is seen as a dark band near the anterior labrum. This extends from the anterior glenoid to the lower part of the lesser tuberosity. **(Bottom)** The glenoid labrum is seen as low signal triangles at the anterior and posterior rim of the glenoid.

SHOULDER OVERVIEW

AXIAL T1 MR, LEFT SHOULDER

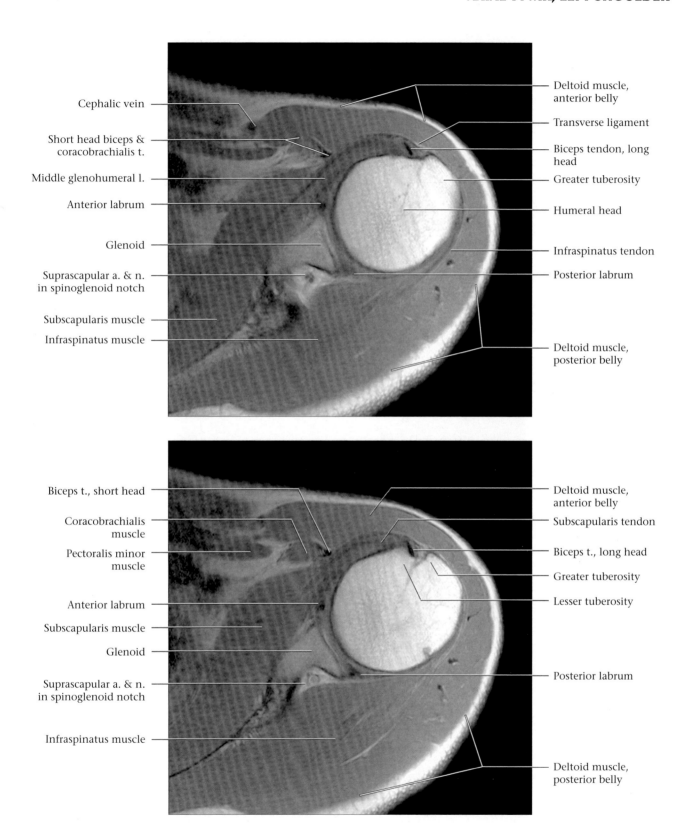

Cephalic vein

Short head biceps &
coracobrachialis t.

Middle glenohumeral l.

Anterior labrum

Glenoid

Suprascapular a. & n.
in spinoglenoid notch

Subscapularis muscle

Infraspinatus muscle

Deltoid muscle,
anterior belly

Transverse ligament

Biceps tendon, long
head

Greater tuberosity

Humeral head

Infraspinatus tendon

Posterior labrum

Deltoid muscle,
posterior belly

Biceps t., short head

Coracobrachialis
muscle

Pectoralis minor
muscle

Anterior labrum

Subscapularis muscle

Glenoid

Suprascapular a. & n.
in spinoglenoid notch

Infraspinatus muscle

Deltoid muscle,
anterior belly

Subscapularis tendon

Biceps t., long head

Greater tuberosity

Lesser tuberosity

Posterior labrum

Deltoid muscle,
posterior belly

(Top) The middle glenohumeral joint is seen as a dark band near the anterior labrum. This extends from the anterior glenoid to the lower part of the lesser tuberosity. **(Bottom)** The glenoid labrum is seen as low signal triangles at the anterior and posterior rim of the glenoid.

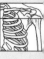

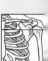

Shoulder

I

29

AXIAL T1 MR, RIGHT SHOULDER

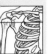

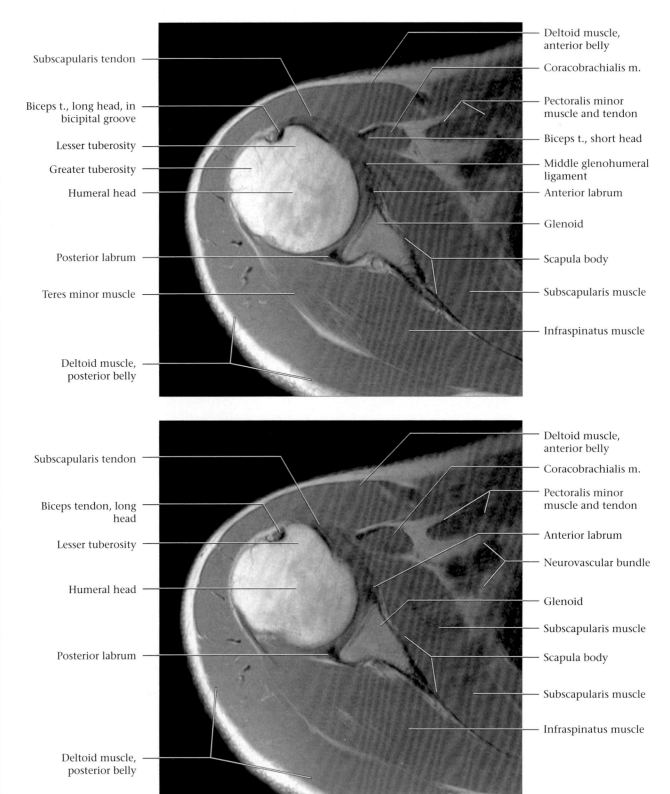

Subscapularis tendon

Biceps t., long head, in bicipital groove

Lesser tuberosity

Greater tuberosity

Humeral head

Posterior labrum

Teres minor muscle

Deltoid muscle, posterior belly

Deltoid muscle, anterior belly

Coracobrachialis m.

Pectoralis minor muscle and tendon

Biceps t., short head

Middle glenohumeral ligament

Anterior labrum

Glenoid

Scapula body

Subscapularis muscle

Infraspinatus muscle

Subscapularis tendon

Biceps tendon, long head

Lesser tuberosity

Humeral head

Posterior labrum

Deltoid muscle, posterior belly

Deltoid muscle, anterior belly

Coracobrachialis m.

Pectoralis minor muscle and tendon

Anterior labrum

Neurovascular bundle

Glenoid

Subscapularis muscle

Scapula body

Subscapularis muscle

Infraspinatus muscle

(Top) The lesser tuberosity is located at the anterior aspect of the humeral head in this position. The subscapularis tendon is seen inserting on the lesser tuberosity. The long head of the biceps tendon is within the bicipital groove. **(Bottom)** The neurovascular bundle lies deep to the pectoralis minor muscle. The subclavian artery becomes the axillary artery when it extends beyond the first rib below the clavicle.

SHOULDER OVERVIEW

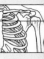
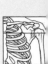
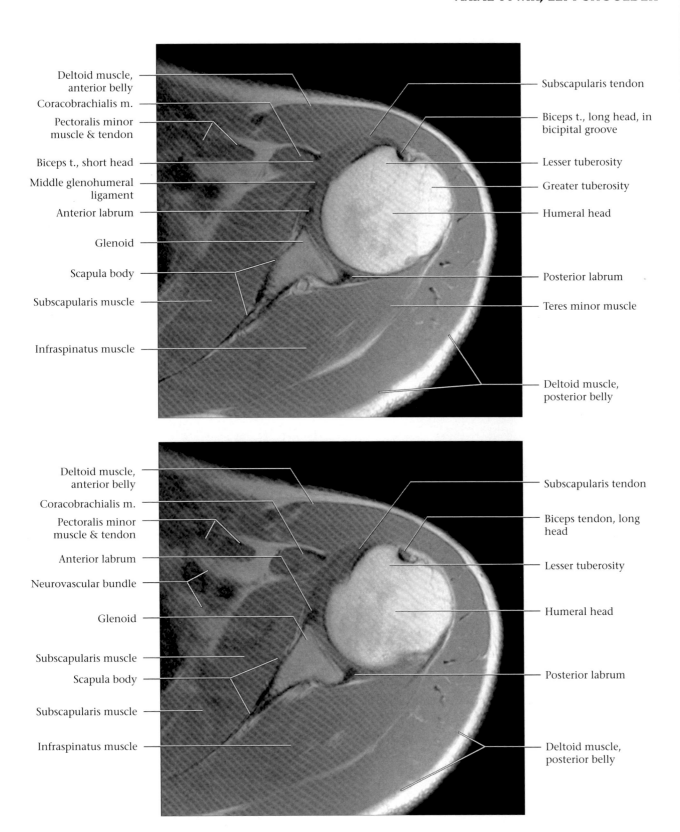

Deltoid muscle, anterior belly

Coracobrachialis m.

Pectoralis minor muscle & tendon

Biceps t., short head

Middle glenohumeral ligament

Anterior labrum

Glenoid

Scapula body

Subscapularis muscle

Infraspinatus muscle

Subscapularis tendon

Biceps t., long head, in bicipital groove

Lesser tuberosity

Greater tuberosity

Humeral head

Posterior labrum

Teres minor muscle

Deltoid muscle, posterior belly

Deltoid muscle, anterior belly

Coracobrachialis m.

Pectoralis minor muscle & tendon

Anterior labrum

Neurovascular bundle

Glenoid

Subscapularis muscle

Scapula body

Subscapularis muscle

Infraspinatus muscle

Subscapularis tendon

Biceps tendon, long head

Lesser tuberosity

Humeral head

Posterior labrum

Deltoid muscle, posterior belly

(Top) The lesser tuberosity is located at the anterior aspect of the humeral head in this position. The subscapularis tendon is seen inserting on the lesser tuberosity. The long head of the biceps tendon is within the bicipital groove. **(Bottom)** The neurovascular bundle lies deep to the pectoralis minor muscle. The subclavian artery becomes the axillary artery when it extends beyond the first rib below the clavicle.

AXIAL T1 MR, RIGHT SHOULDER

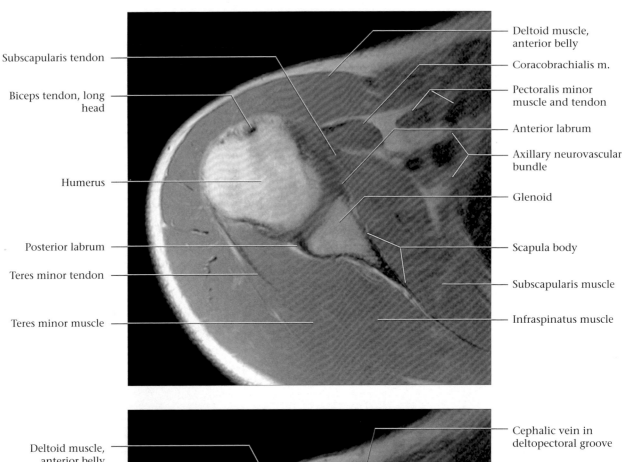

Subscapularis tendon

Biceps tendon, long head

Humerus

Posterior labrum

Teres minor tendon

Teres minor muscle

Deltoid muscle, anterior belly

Coracobrachialis m.

Pectoralis minor muscle and tendon

Anterior labrum

Axillary neurovascular bundle

Glenoid

Scapula body

Subscapularis muscle

Infraspinatus muscle

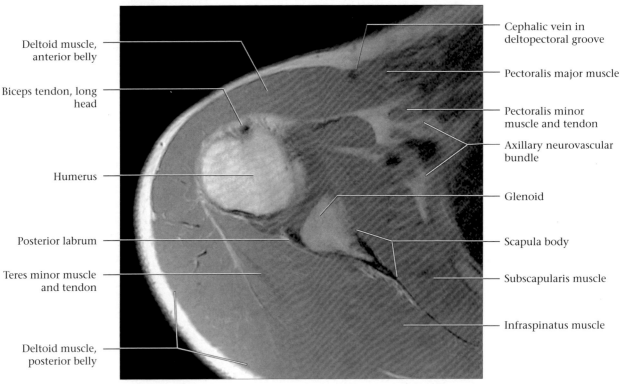

Deltoid muscle, anterior belly

Biceps tendon, long head

Humerus

Posterior labrum

Teres minor muscle and tendon

Deltoid muscle, posterior belly

Cephalic vein in deltopectoral groove

Pectoralis major muscle

Pectoralis minor muscle and tendon

Axillary neurovascular bundle

Glenoid

Scapula body

Subscapularis muscle

Infraspinatus muscle

(Top) The teres minor and infraspinatus muscles are difficult to separate at this level. The teres minor muscle is lying more lateral than what remains of the infraspinatus muscle, lying more medial. **(Bottom)** The cephalic vein anteriorly, lies within the deltopectoral groove.

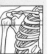
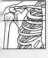

SHOULDER OVERVIEW

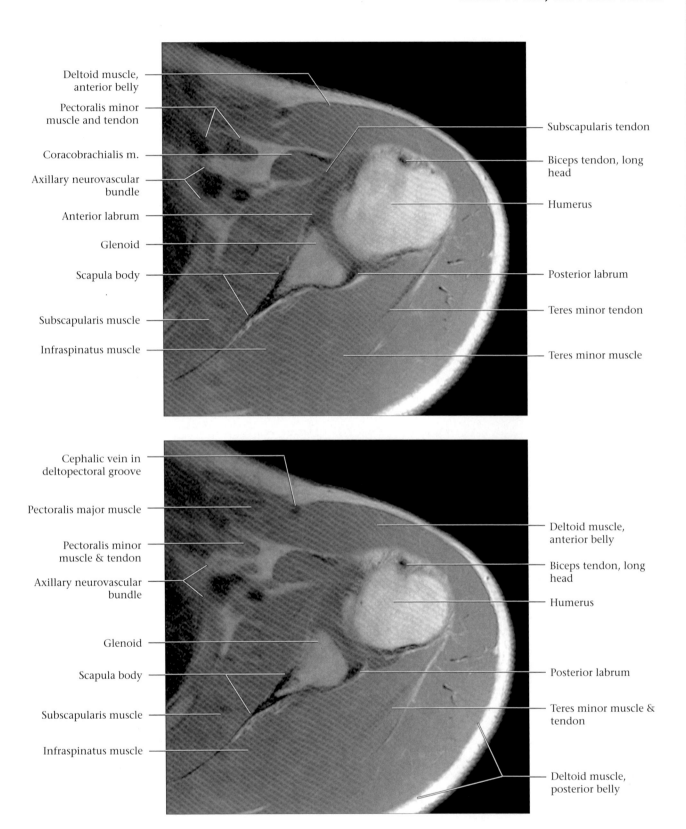

Deltoid muscle, anterior belly

Pectoralis minor muscle and tendon

Coracobrachialis m.

Axillary neurovascular bundle

Anterior labrum

Glenoid

Scapula body

Subscapularis muscle

Infraspinatus muscle

Subscapularis tendon

Biceps tendon, long head

Humerus

Posterior labrum

Teres minor tendon

Teres minor muscle

Cephalic vein in deltopectoral groove

Pectoralis major muscle

Pectoralis minor muscle & tendon

Axillary neurovascular bundle

Glenoid

Scapula body

Subscapularis muscle

Infraspinatus muscle

Deltoid muscle, anterior belly

Biceps tendon, long head

Humerus

Posterior labrum

Teres minor muscle & tendon

Deltoid muscle, posterior belly

(Top) The teres minor and infraspinatus muscles are difficult to separate at this level. The teres minor muscle is lying more lateral than what remains of the infraspinatus muscle, lying more medial. **(Bottom)** The cephalic vein anteriorly, lies within the deltopectoral groove.

AXIAL T1 MR, RIGHT SHOULDER

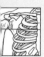

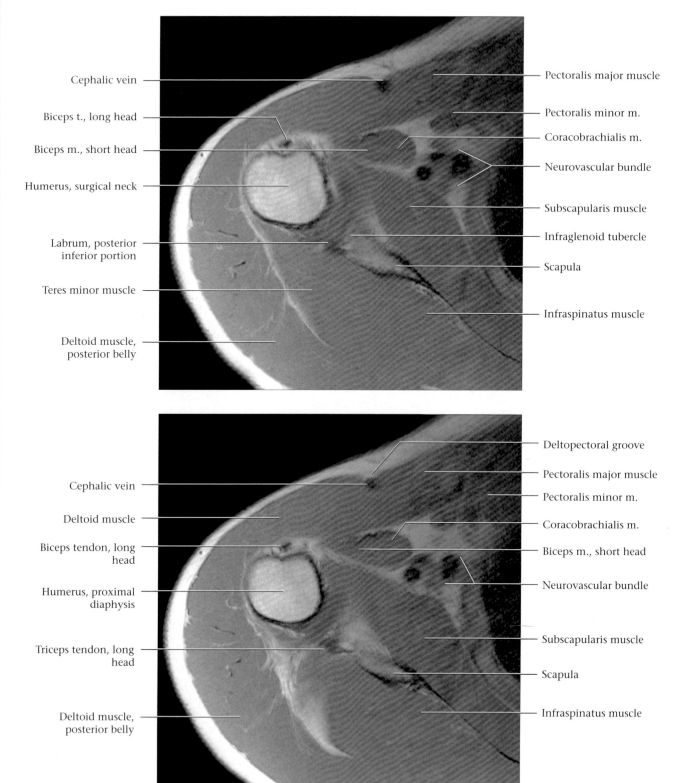

Cephalic vein — Pectoralis major muscle

Biceps t., long head — Pectoralis minor m.

Biceps m., short head — Coracobrachialis m.

Humerus, surgical neck — Neurovascular bundle

Subscapularis muscle

Labrum, posterior inferior portion — Infraglenoid tubercle

Scapula

Teres minor muscle — Infraspinatus muscle

Deltoid muscle, posterior belly

Deltopectoral groove

Cephalic vein — Pectoralis major muscle

Pectoralis minor m.

Deltoid muscle — Coracobrachialis m.

Biceps tendon, long head — Biceps m., short head

Humerus, proximal diaphysis — Neurovascular bundle

Triceps tendon, long head — Subscapularis muscle

Scapula

Deltoid muscle, posterior belly — Infraspinatus muscle

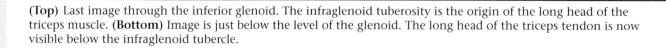

(Top) Last image through the inferior glenoid. The infraglenoid tuberosity is the origin of the long head of the triceps muscle. **(Bottom)** Image is just below the level of the glenoid. The long head of the triceps tendon is now visible below the infraglenoid tubercle.

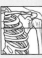

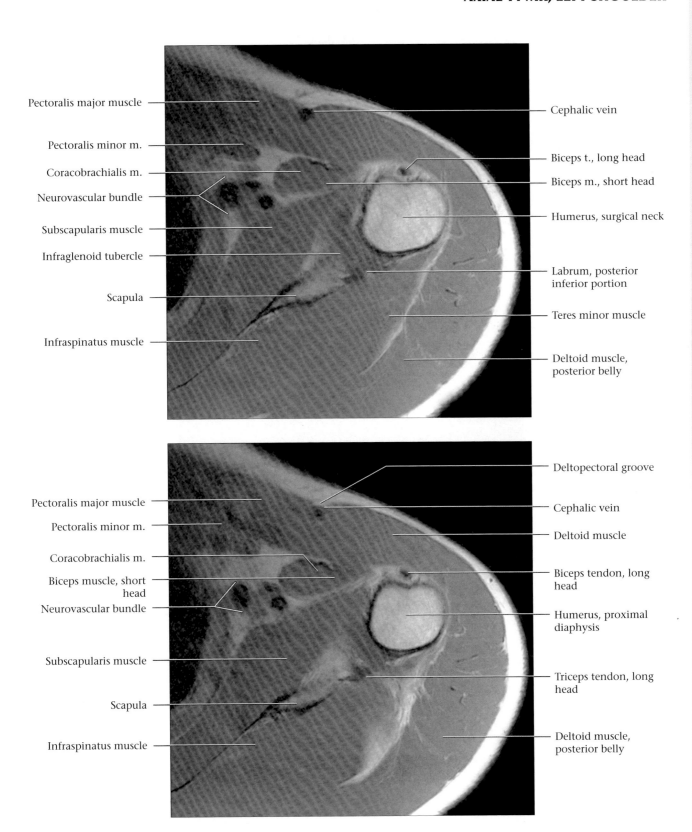

Pectoralis major muscle — Cephalic vein

Pectoralis minor m. — Biceps t., long head

Coracobrachialis m. — Biceps m., short head

Neurovascular bundle — Humerus, surgical neck

Subscapularis muscle

Infraglenoid tubercle — Labrum, posterior inferior portion

— Teres minor muscle

Scapula

— Deltoid muscle, posterior belly

Infraspinatus muscle

— Deltopectoral groove

Pectoralis major muscle — Cephalic vein

Pectoralis minor m. — Deltoid muscle

Coracobrachialis m.

Biceps muscle, short head — Biceps tendon, long head

Neurovascular bundle — Humerus, proximal diaphysis

Subscapularis muscle

Scapula — Triceps tendon, long head

Infraspinatus muscle — Deltoid muscle, posterior belly

(Top) Last image through the inferior glenoid. The infraglenoid tuberosity is the origin of the long head of the triceps muscle. **(Bottom)** Image is just below the level of the glenoid. The long head of the triceps tendon is now visible below the infraglenoid tubercle.

AXIAL T1 MR, RIGHT SHOULDER

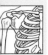

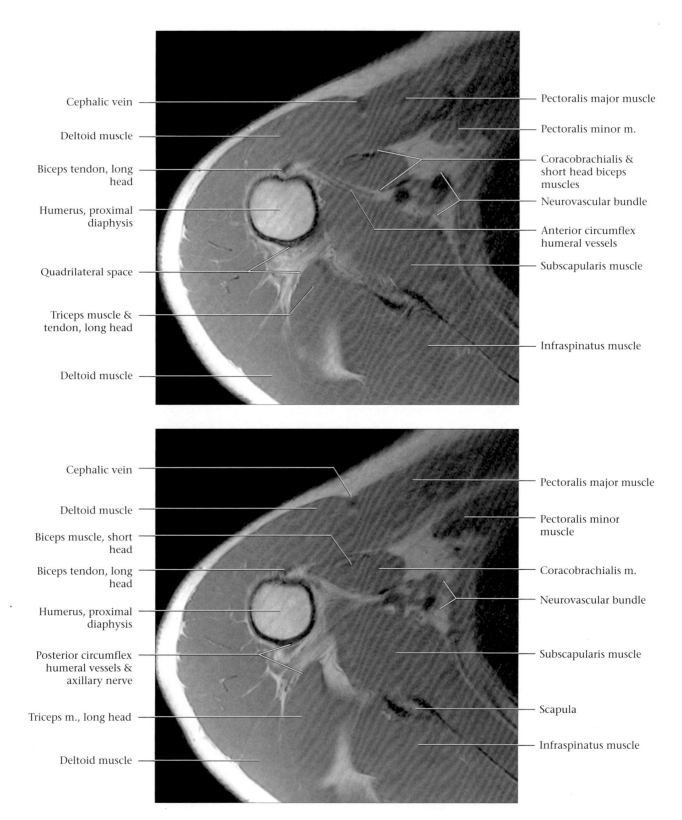

Cephalic vein

Deltoid muscle

Biceps tendon, long head

Humerus, proximal diaphysis

Quadrilateral space

Triceps muscle & tendon, long head

Deltoid muscle

Pectoralis major muscle

Pectoralis minor m.

Coracobrachialis & short head biceps muscles

Neurovascular bundle

Anterior circumflex humeral vessels

Subscapularis muscle

Infraspinatus muscle

Cephalic vein

Deltoid muscle

Biceps muscle, short head

Biceps tendon, long head

Humerus, proximal diaphysis

Posterior circumflex humeral vessels & axillary nerve

Triceps m., long head

Deltoid muscle

Pectoralis major muscle

Pectoralis minor muscle

Coracobrachialis m.

Neurovascular bundle

Subscapularis muscle

Scapula

Infraspinatus muscle

(Top) The posterior circumflex humeral vessels and axillary nerve traverse the quadrilateral space. This space is formed by the subscapularis and teres minor muscles superiorly, the teres major inferiorly, the long head of the triceps medially and the surgical neck of the humerus laterally. **(Bottom)** The short head of the biceps muscle and the coracobrachialis muscle can be difficult to distinguish as separate structures in the anterior shoulder. The coracobrachialis muscle originates from the coracoid process more laterally than the short head of the biceps muscle. The coracobrachialis muscle then swings posterior to the short head of the biceps muscle as it enters the upper arm.

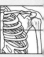

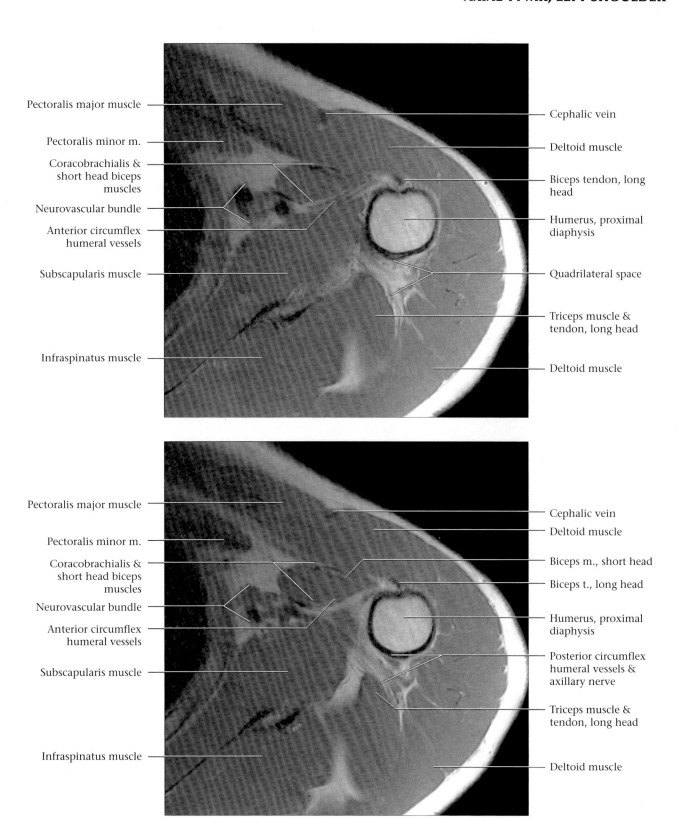

Pectoralis major muscle

Pectoralis minor m.

Coracobrachialis & short head biceps muscles

Neurovascular bundle

Anterior circumflex humeral vessels

Subscapularis muscle

Infraspinatus muscle

Cephalic vein

Deltoid muscle

Biceps tendon, long head

Humerus, proximal diaphysis

Quadrilateral space

Triceps muscle & tendon, long head

Deltoid muscle

Pectoralis major muscle

Pectoralis minor m.

Coracobrachialis & short head biceps muscles

Neurovascular bundle

Anterior circumflex humeral vessels

Subscapularis muscle

Infraspinatus muscle

Cephalic vein

Deltoid muscle

Biceps m., short head

Biceps t., long head

Humerus, proximal diaphysis

Posterior circumflex humeral vessels & axillary nerve

Triceps muscle & tendon, long head

Deltoid muscle

(Top) The posterior circumflex humeral vessels and axillary nerve traverse the quadrilateral space. This space is formed by the subscapularis and teres minor muscles superiorly, the teres major inferiorly, the long head of the triceps medially and the surgical neck of the humerus laterally. **(Bottom)** The short head of the biceps muscle and the coracobrachialis muscle can be difficult to distinguish as separate structures in the anterior shoulder. The coracobrachialis muscle originates from the coracoid process more laterally than the short head of the biceps muscle. The coracobrachialis muscle then swings posterior to the short head of the biceps muscle as it enters the upper arm.

AXIAL T1 MR, RIGHT SHOULDER

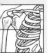

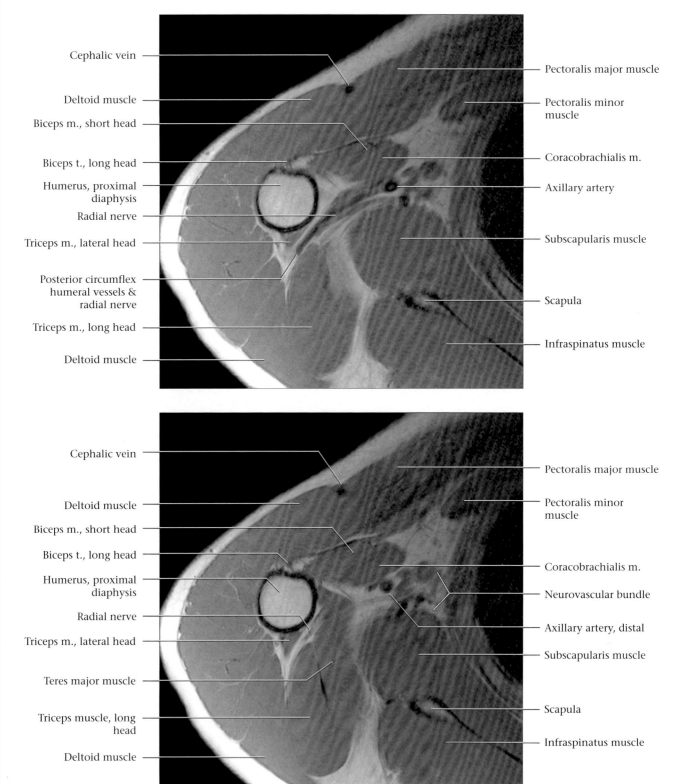

Cephalic vein — Pectoralis major muscle

Deltoid muscle — Pectoralis minor muscle

Biceps m., short head — Coracobrachialis m.

Biceps t., long head — Axillary artery

Humerus, proximal diaphysis — Subscapularis muscle

Radial nerve

Triceps m., lateral head

Posterior circumflex humeral vessels & radial nerve — Scapula

Triceps m., long head — Infraspinatus muscle

Deltoid muscle

Cephalic vein — Pectoralis major muscle

Deltoid muscle — Pectoralis minor muscle

Biceps m., short head

Biceps t., long head — Coracobrachialis m.

Humerus, proximal diaphysis — Neurovascular bundle

Radial nerve — Axillary artery, distal

Triceps m., lateral head — Subscapularis muscle

Teres major muscle

Triceps muscle, long head — Scapula

Deltoid muscle — Infraspinatus muscle

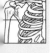

(Top) The lateral head of the triceps muscle arises directly from the posterior surface of the humeral shaft. **(Bottom)** The teres major muscle arises from the inferior angle of the scapula and inserts below the lesser tuberosity on the anteromedial humeral shaft.

AXIAL T1 MR, LEFT SHOULDER

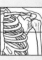

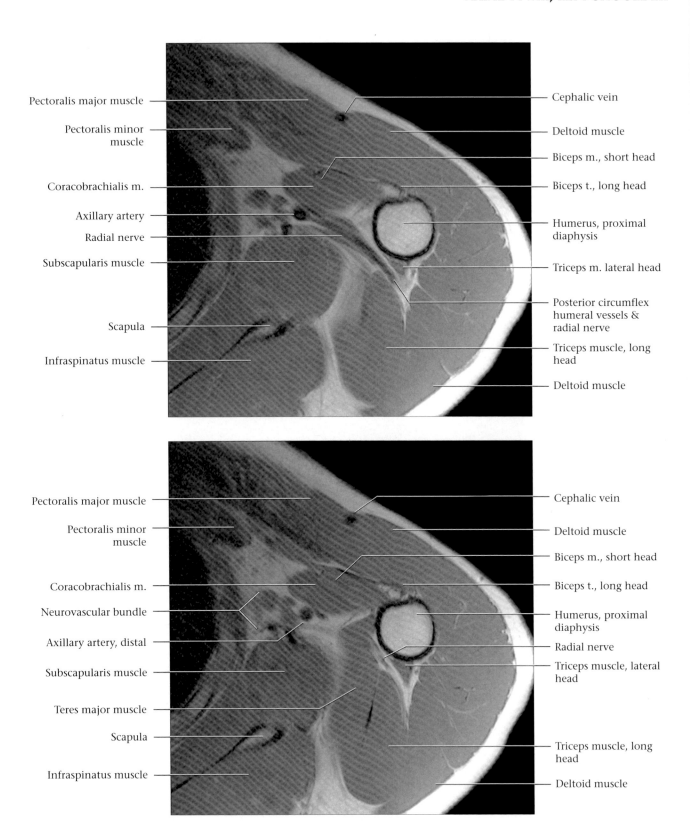

Pectoralis major muscle — Cephalic vein

Pectoralis minor muscle — Deltoid muscle

— Biceps m., short head

Coracobrachialis m. — Biceps t., long head

Axillary artery — Humerus, proximal diaphysis

Radial nerve

Subscapularis muscle — Triceps m. lateral head

— Posterior circumflex humeral vessels & radial nerve

Scapula — Triceps muscle, long head

Infraspinatus muscle — Deltoid muscle

Pectoralis major muscle — Cephalic vein

Pectoralis minor muscle — Deltoid muscle

— Biceps m., short head

Coracobrachialis m. — Biceps t., long head

Neurovascular bundle — Humerus, proximal diaphysis

Axillary artery, distal — Radial nerve

Subscapularis muscle — Triceps muscle, lateral head

Teres major muscle

Scapula — Triceps muscle, long head

Infraspinatus muscle — Deltoid muscle

(Top) The lateral head of the triceps muscle arises directly from the posterior surface of the humeral shaft. **(Bottom)** The teres major muscle arises from the inferior angle of the scapula and inserts below the lesser tuberosity on the anteromedial humeral shaft.

Shoulder

I

39

AXIAL T1 MR, RIGHT SHOULDER

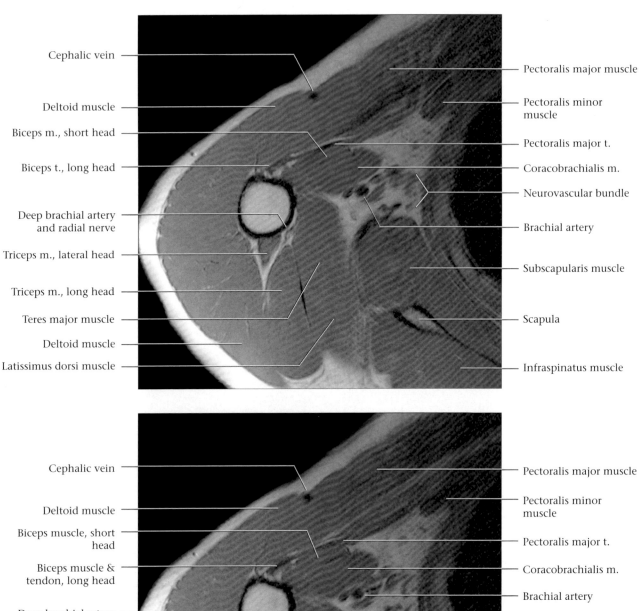

Cephalic vein — Pectoralis major muscle

Deltoid muscle — Pectoralis minor muscle

Biceps m., short head — Pectoralis major t.

Biceps t., long head — Coracobrachialis m.

— Neurovascular bundle

Deep brachial artery and radial nerve — Brachial artery

Triceps m., lateral head — Subscapularis muscle

Triceps m., long head

Teres major muscle — Scapula

Deltoid muscle

Latissimus dorsi muscle — Infraspinatus muscle

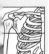

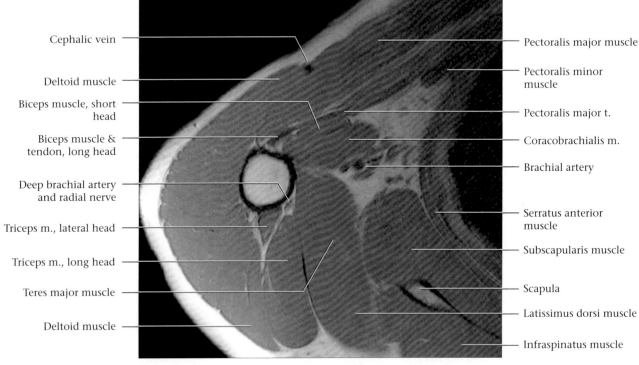

Cephalic vein — Pectoralis major muscle

Deltoid muscle — Pectoralis minor muscle

Biceps muscle, short head — Pectoralis major t.

Biceps muscle & tendon, long head — Coracobrachialis m.

— Brachial artery

Deep brachial artery and radial nerve

Triceps m., lateral head — Serratus anterior muscle

— Subscapularis muscle

Triceps m., long head

Teres major muscle — Scapula

— Latissimus dorsi muscle

Deltoid muscle — Infraspinatus muscle

(Top) The axillary artery becomes the brachial artery at the lower margin of the teres major muscle. The brachial artery has paired brachial veins, lying on each side of the artery. The pectoralis major muscle has a long insertion along the lateral aspect of the bicipital groove. In some places it fuses with the joint capsule, deltoid tendon and fascia of the upper arm. **(Bottom)** The deep brachial artery is the first branch of the brachial artery. The deep brachial artery travels with the radial nerve between the lateral and long heads of the triceps in the upper arm.

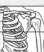

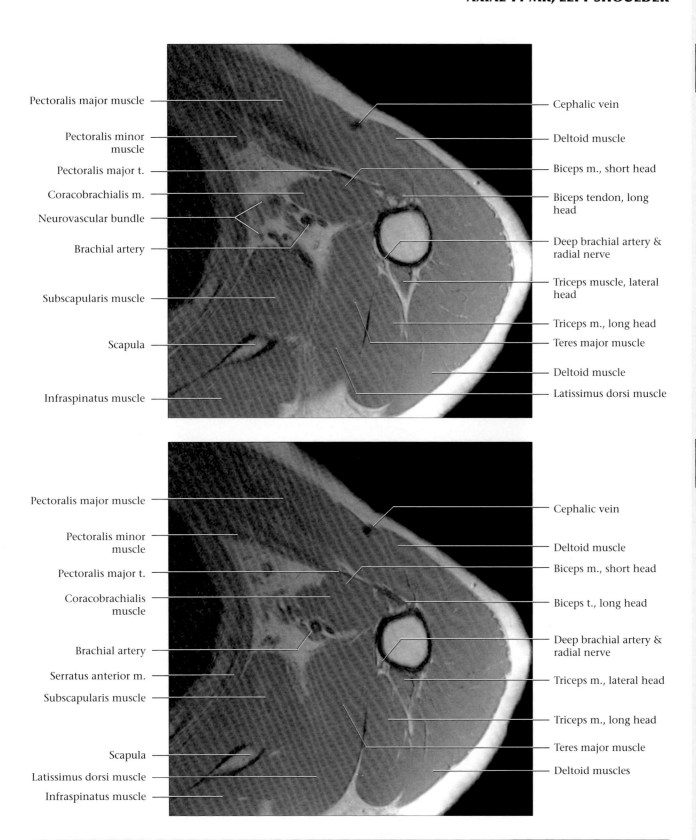

Pectoralis major muscle

Pectoralis minor muscle

Pectoralis major t.

Coracobrachialis m.

Neurovascular bundle

Brachial artery

Subscapularis muscle

Scapula

Infraspinatus muscle

Cephalic vein

Deltoid muscle

Biceps m., short head

Biceps tendon, long head

Deep brachial artery & radial nerve

Triceps muscle, lateral head

Triceps m., long head

Teres major muscle

Deltoid muscle

Latissimus dorsi muscle

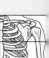

Pectoralis major muscle

Pectoralis minor muscle

Pectoralis major t.

Coracobrachialis muscle

Brachial artery

Serratus anterior m.

Subscapularis muscle

Scapula

Latissimus dorsi muscle

Infraspinatus muscle

Cephalic vein

Deltoid muscle

Biceps m., short head

Biceps t., long head

Deep brachial artery & radial nerve

Triceps m., lateral head

Triceps m., long head

Teres major muscle

Deltoid muscles

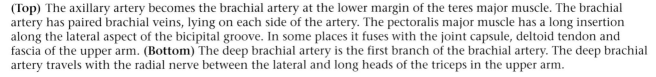

(Top) The axillary artery becomes the brachial artery at the lower margin of the teres major muscle. The brachial artery has paired brachial veins, lying on each side of the artery. The pectoralis major muscle has a long insertion along the lateral aspect of the bicipital groove. In some places it fuses with the joint capsule, deltoid tendon and fascia of the upper arm. **(Bottom)** The deep brachial artery is the first branch of the brachial artery. The deep brachial artery travels with the radial nerve between the lateral and long heads of the triceps in the upper arm.

Shoulder

I

41

AXIAL T1 MR, RIGHT SHOULDER

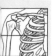

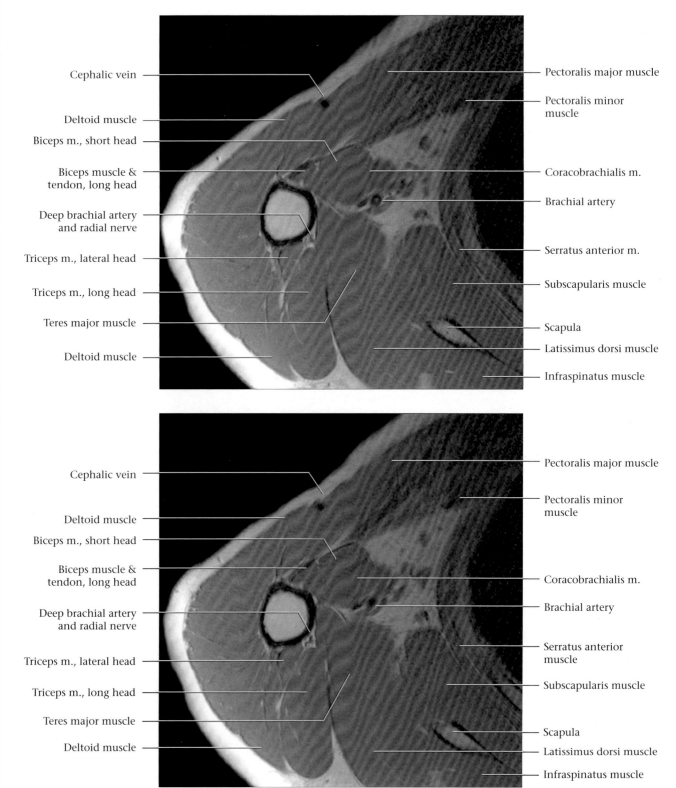

Cephalic vein

Deltoid muscle

Biceps m., short head

Biceps muscle & tendon, long head

Deep brachial artery and radial nerve

Triceps m., lateral head

Triceps m., long head

Teres major muscle

Deltoid muscle

Pectoralis major muscle

Pectoralis minor muscle

Coracobrachialis m.

Brachial artery

Serratus anterior m.

Subscapularis muscle

Scapula

Latissimus dorsi muscle

Infraspinatus muscle

Cephalic vein

Deltoid muscle

Biceps m., short head

Biceps muscle & tendon, long head

Deep brachial artery and radial nerve

Triceps m., lateral head

Triceps m., long head

Teres major muscle

Deltoid muscle

Pectoralis major muscle

Pectoralis minor muscle

Coracobrachialis m.

Brachial artery

Serratus anterior muscle

Subscapularis muscle

Scapula

Latissimus dorsi muscle

Infraspinatus muscle

(Top) The latissimus dorsi muscle courses superiorly from the lower back, around the inferior border of the teres major muscle, to insert along the inferior aspect of the bicipital groove. **(Bottom)** The subscapularis muscle covers the entire ventral surface of the scapula.

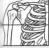

Shoulder

SHOULDER OVERVIEW

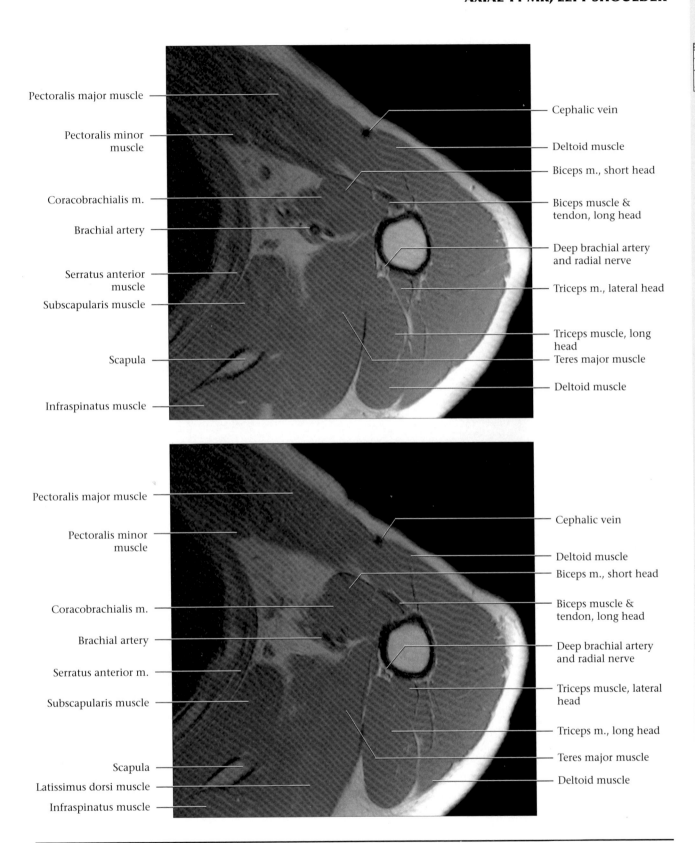

Pectoralis major muscle

Pectoralis minor muscle

Coracobrachialis m.

Brachial artery

Serratus anterior muscle

Subscapularis muscle

Scapula

Infraspinatus muscle

Cephalic vein

Deltoid muscle

Biceps m., short head

Biceps muscle & tendon, long head

Deep brachial artery and radial nerve

Triceps m., lateral head

Triceps muscle, long head

Teres major muscle

Deltoid muscle

Pectoralis major muscle

Pectoralis minor muscle

Coracobrachialis m.

Brachial artery

Serratus anterior m.

Subscapularis muscle

Scapula

Latissimus dorsi muscle

Infraspinatus muscle

Cephalic vein

Deltoid muscle

Biceps m., short head

Biceps muscle & tendon, long head

Deep brachial artery and radial nerve

Triceps muscle, lateral head

Triceps m., long head

Teres major muscle

Deltoid muscle

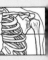

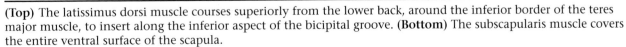

(Top) The latissimus dorsi muscle courses superiorly from the lower back, around the inferior border of the teres major muscle, to insert along the inferior aspect of the bicipital groove. (Bottom) The subscapularis muscle covers the entire ventral surface of the scapula.

AXIAL T1 MR, RIGHT SHOULDER

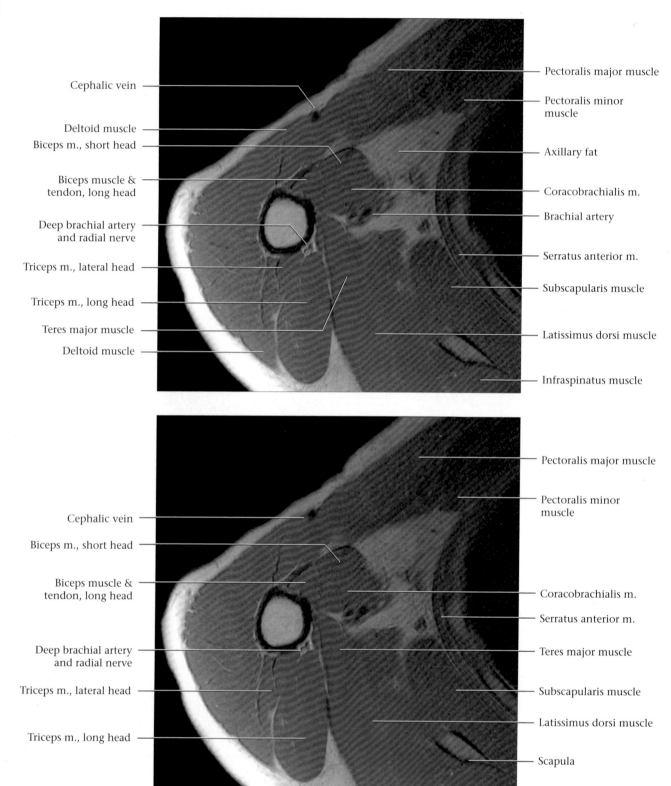

Cephalic vein

Deltoid muscle

Biceps m., short head

Biceps muscle & tendon, long head

Deep brachial artery and radial nerve

Triceps m., lateral head

Triceps m., long head

Teres major muscle

Deltoid muscle

Pectoralis major muscle

Pectoralis minor muscle

Axillary fat

Coracobrachialis m.

Brachial artery

Serratus anterior m.

Subscapularis muscle

Latissimus dorsi muscle

Infraspinatus muscle

Cephalic vein

Biceps m., short head

Biceps muscle & tendon, long head

Deep brachial artery and radial nerve

Triceps m., lateral head

Triceps m., long head

Pectoralis major muscle

Pectoralis minor muscle

Coracobrachialis m.

Serratus anterior m.

Teres major muscle

Subscapularis muscle

Latissimus dorsi muscle

Scapula

(Top) The pectoralis major and minor form the anterior wall of the axilla. **(Bottom)** The serratus anterior muscle is a thin band of muscle that lies between the ribs and scapula at the posterolateral aspect of the upper chest.

SHOULDER OVERVIEW

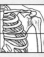

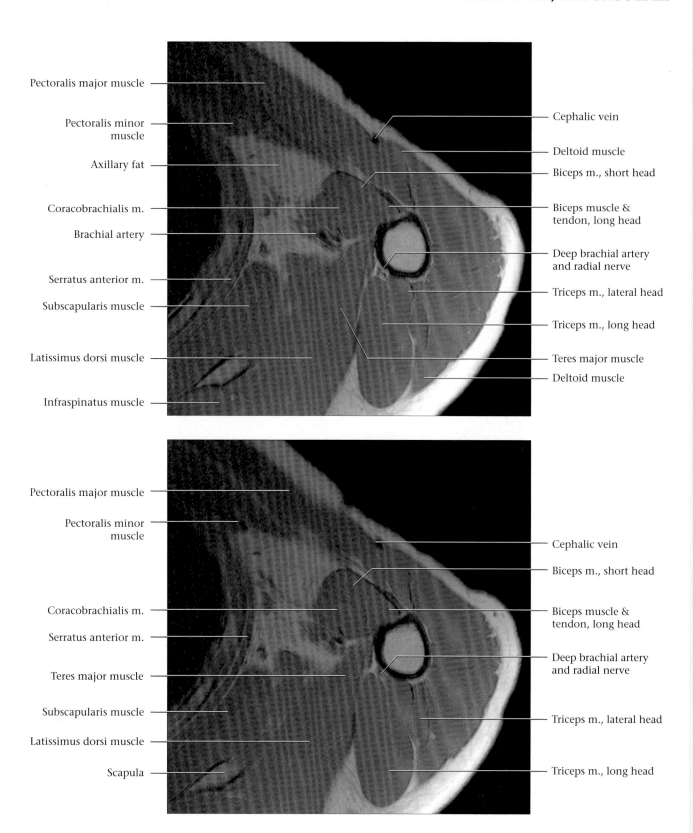

Pectoralis major muscle

Pectoralis minor muscle

Axillary fat

Coracobrachialis m.

Brachial artery

Serratus anterior m.

Subscapularis muscle

Latissimus dorsi muscle

Infraspinatus muscle

Cephalic vein

Deltoid muscle

Biceps m., short head

Biceps muscle & tendon, long head

Deep brachial artery and radial nerve

Triceps m., lateral head

Triceps m., long head

Teres major muscle

Deltoid muscle

Pectoralis major muscle

Pectoralis minor muscle

Coracobrachialis m.

Serratus anterior m.

Teres major muscle

Subscapularis muscle

Latissimus dorsi muscle

Scapula

Cephalic vein

Biceps m., short head

Biceps muscle & tendon, long head

Deep brachial artery and radial nerve

Triceps m., lateral head

Triceps m., long head

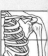

(Top) The pectoralis major and minor form the anterior wall of the axilla. **(Bottom)** The serratus anterior muscle is a thin band of muscle that lies between the ribs and scapula at the posterolateral aspect of the upper chest.

CORONAL OBLIQUE T1 MR, RIGHT SHOULDER

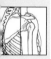

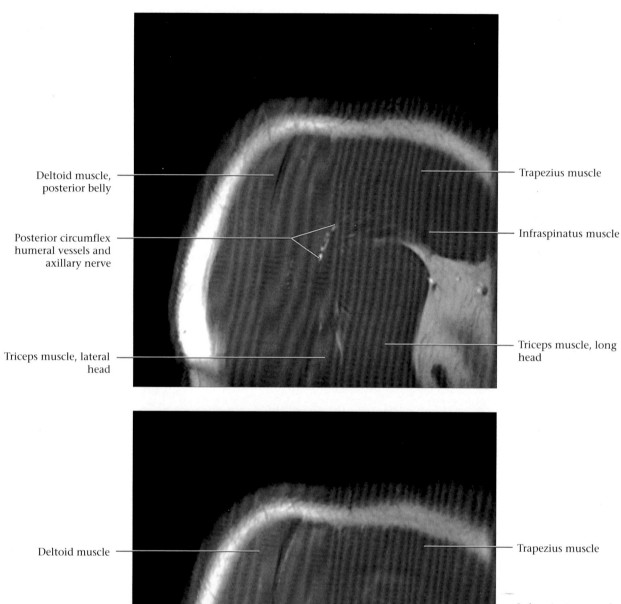

Deltoid muscle, posterior belly

Posterior circumflex humeral vessels and axillary nerve

Triceps muscle, lateral head

Trapezius muscle

Infraspinatus muscle

Triceps muscle, long head

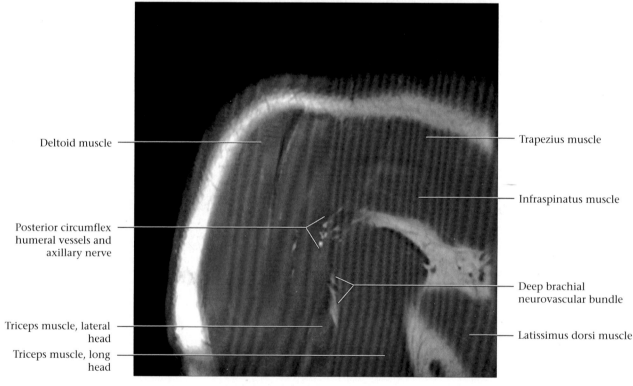

Deltoid muscle

Posterior circumflex humeral vessels and axillary nerve

Triceps muscle, lateral head

Triceps muscle, long head

Trapezius muscle

Infraspinatus muscle

Deep brachial neurovascular bundle

Latissimus dorsi muscle

(Top) First in series of coronal oblique T1 MR images of right shoulder displayed posterior to anterior. Images were obtained with a shoulder coil on a 3T MR scanner. At the most posterior aspect of the shoulder, the deltoid muscle covers the majority of the shoulder joint. The trapezius muscle covers the superomedial aspect of the shoulder girdle. (Bottom) The radial nerve supplies the triceps muscle. It is part of the deep brachial neurovascular bundle.

SHOULDER OVERVIEW

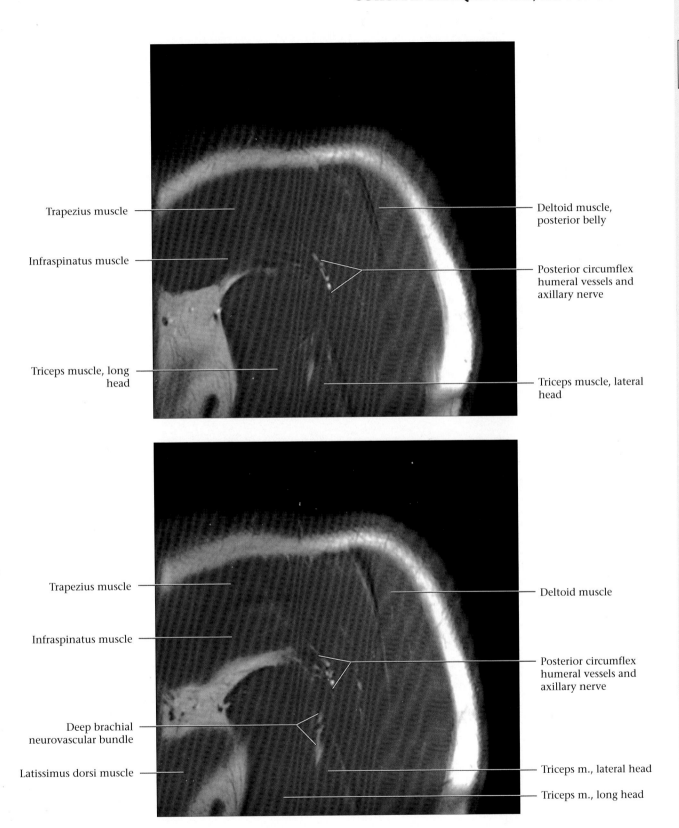

Trapezius muscle

Infraspinatus muscle

Triceps muscle, long head

Deltoid muscle, posterior belly

Posterior circumflex humeral vessels and axillary nerve

Triceps muscle, lateral head

Trapezius muscle

Infraspinatus muscle

Deep brachial neurovascular bundle

Latissimus dorsi muscle

Deltoid muscle

Posterior circumflex humeral vessels and axillary nerve

Triceps m., lateral head

Triceps m., long head

(Top) First in series of coronal oblique T1 MR images of left shoulder displayed posterior to anterior. Images were obtained with a shoulder coil on a 3T MR scanner. At the most posterior aspect of the shoulder, the deltoid muscle covers the majority of the shoulder joint. The trapezius muscle covers the superomedial aspect of the shoulder girdle. **(Bottom)** The radial nerve supplies the triceps muscle. It is part of the deep brachial neurovascular bundle.

SHOULDER OVERVIEW

CORONAL OBLIQUE T1 MR, RIGHT SHOULDER

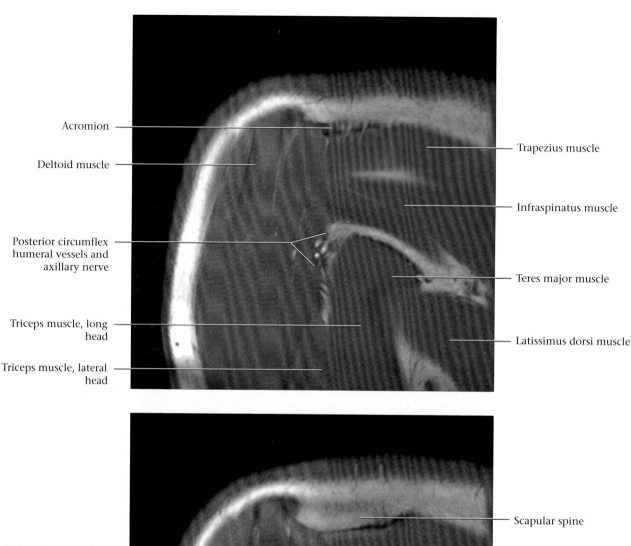

Acromion

Deltoid muscle

Posterior circumflex
humeral vessels and
axillary nerve

Triceps muscle, long
head

Triceps muscle, lateral
head

Trapezius muscle

Infraspinatus muscle

Teres major muscle

Latissimus dorsi muscle

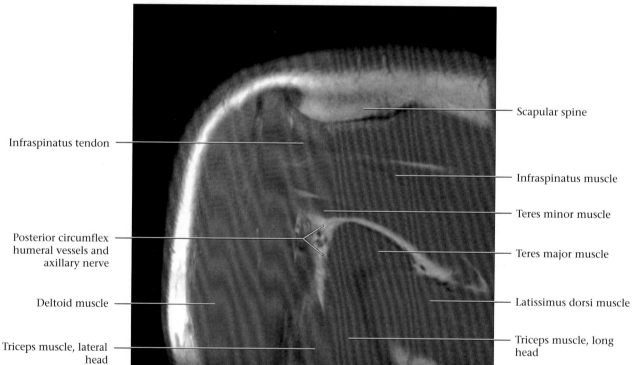

Infraspinatus tendon

Posterior circumflex
humeral vessels and
axillary nerve

Deltoid muscle

Triceps muscle, lateral
head

Scapular spine

Infraspinatus muscle

Teres minor muscle

Teres major muscle

Latissimus dorsi muscle

Triceps muscle, long
head

(Top) The long head of the triceps muscle is the most medial muscle of the posterior upper arm. Axillary nerve branches supply the skin and shoulder joint. **(Bottom)** The infraspinatus tendon arches over the posterosuperior aspect of the humeral head to insert on the greater tuberosity.

CORONAL OBLIQUE T1 MR, LEFT SHOULDER

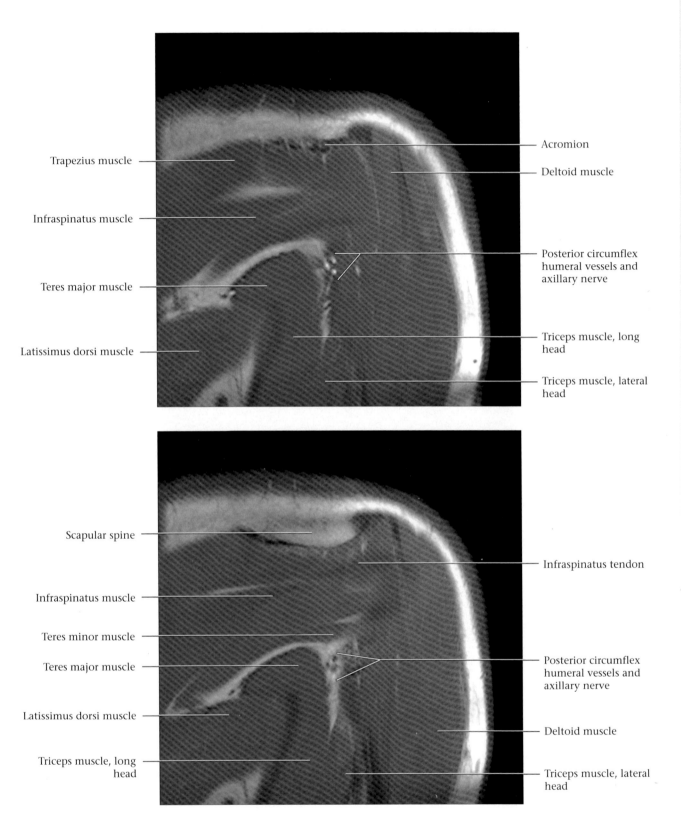

(Top) The long head of the triceps muscle is the most medial muscle of the posterior upper arm. Axillary nerve branches supply the skin and shoulder joint. **(Bottom)** The infraspinatus tendon arches over the posterosuperior aspect of the humeral head to insert on the greater tuberosity.

CORONAL OBLIQUE T1 MR, RIGHT SHOULDER

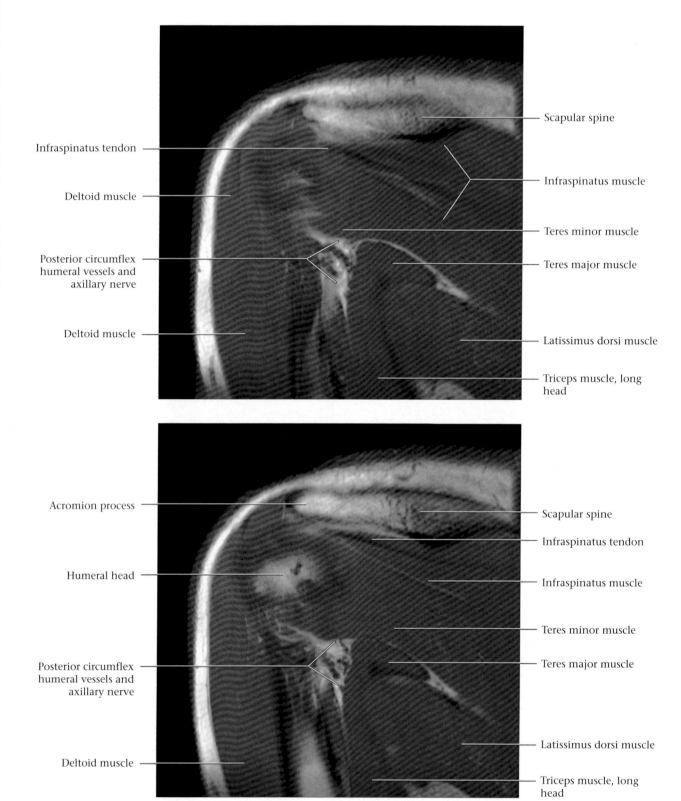

Infraspinatus tendon

Deltoid muscle

Posterior circumflex
humeral vessels and
axillary nerve

Deltoid muscle

Scapular spine

Infraspinatus muscle

Teres minor muscle

Teres major muscle

Latissimus dorsi muscle

Triceps muscle, long
head

Acromion process

Humeral head

Posterior circumflex
humeral vessels and
axillary nerve

Deltoid muscle

Scapular spine

Infraspinatus tendon

Infraspinatus muscle

Teres minor muscle

Teres major muscle

Latissimus dorsi muscle

Triceps muscle, long
head

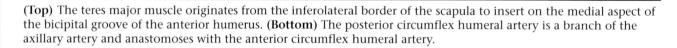

(Top) The teres major muscle originates from the inferolateral border of the scapula to insert on the medial aspect of the bicipital groove of the anterior humerus. **(Bottom)** The posterior circumflex humeral artery is a branch of the axillary artery and anastomoses with the anterior circumflex humeral artery.

CORONAL OBLIQUE T1 MR, LEFT SHOULDER

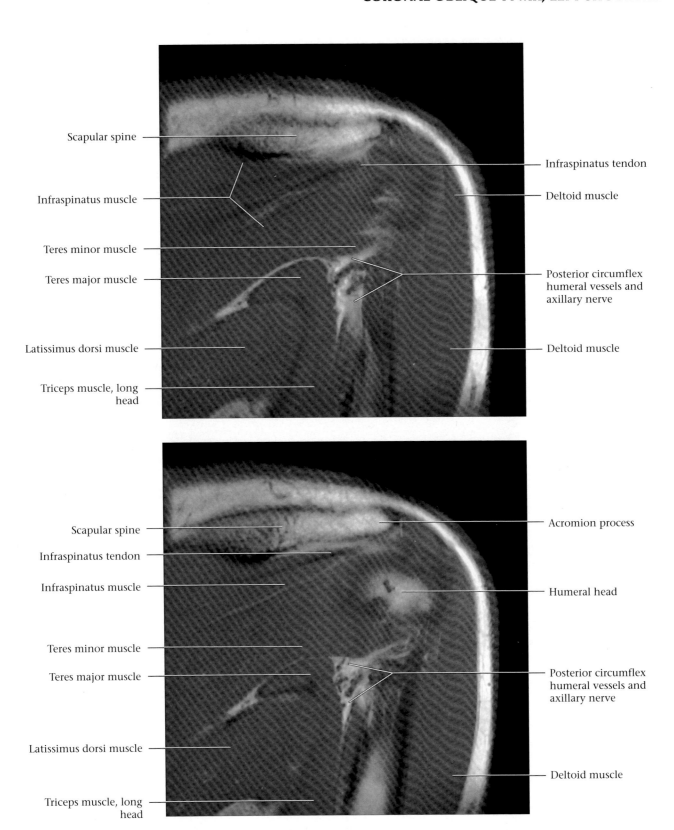

Scapular spine

Infraspinatus muscle

Teres minor muscle

Teres major muscle

Latissimus dorsi muscle

Triceps muscle, long head

Infraspinatus tendon

Deltoid muscle

Posterior circumflex humeral vessels and axillary nerve

Deltoid muscle

Scapular spine

Infraspinatus tendon

Infraspinatus muscle

Teres minor muscle

Teres major muscle

Latissimus dorsi muscle

Triceps muscle, long head

Acromion process

Humeral head

Posterior circumflex humeral vessels and axillary nerve

Deltoid muscle

(Top) The teres major muscle originates from the inferolateral border of the scapula to insert on the medial aspect of the bicipital groove of the anterior humerus. **(Bottom)** The posterior circumflex humeral artery is a branch of the axillary artery and anastomoses with the anterior circumflex humeral artery.

Shoulder

I

CORONAL OBLIQUE T1 MR, RIGHT SHOULDER

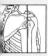

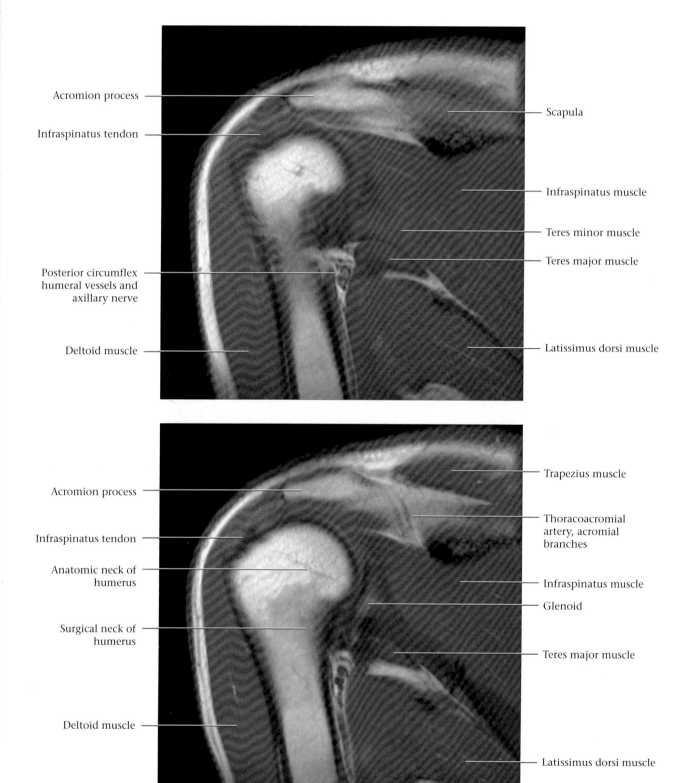

Acromion process

Infraspinatus tendon

Posterior circumflex humeral vessels and axillary nerve

Deltoid muscle

Scapula

Infraspinatus muscle

Teres minor muscle

Teres major muscle

Latissimus dorsi muscle

Acromion process

Infraspinatus tendon

Anatomic neck of humerus

Surgical neck of humerus

Deltoid muscle

Trapezius muscle

Thoracoacromial artery, acromial branches

Infraspinatus muscle

Glenoid

Teres major muscle

Latissimus dorsi muscle

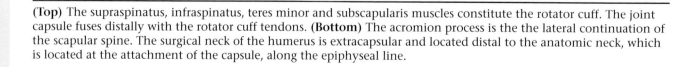

(Top) The supraspinatus, infraspinatus, teres minor and subscapularis muscles constitute the rotator cuff. The joint capsule fuses distally with the rotator cuff tendons. (Bottom) The acromion process is the the lateral continuation of the scapular spine. The surgical neck of the humerus is extracapsular and located distal to the anatomic neck, which is located at the attachment of the capsule, along the epiphyseal line.

CORONAL OBLIQUE T1 MR, LEFT SHOULDER

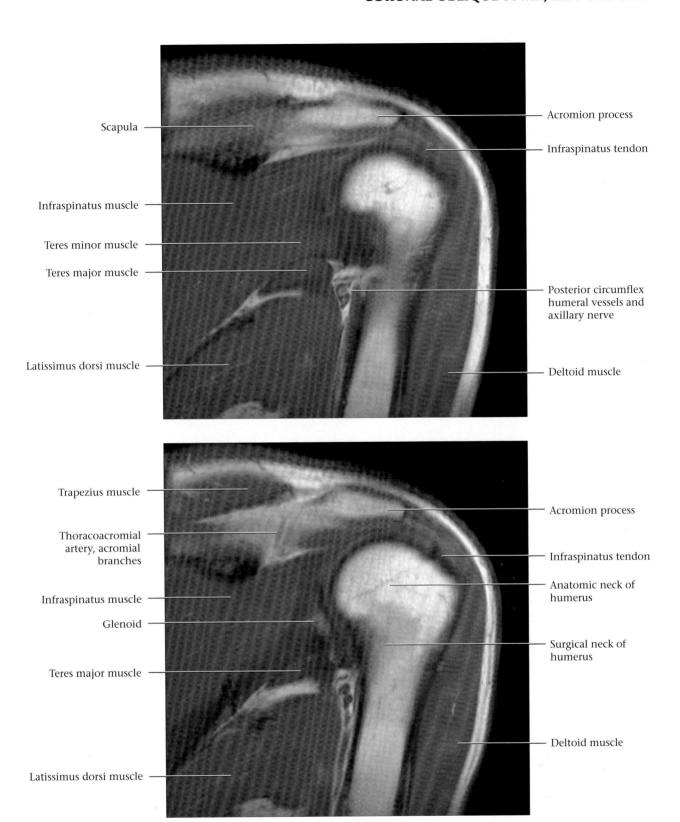

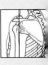

Scapula

Infraspinatus muscle

Teres minor muscle

Teres major muscle

Latissimus dorsi muscle

Acromion process

Infraspinatus tendon

Posterior circumflex humeral vessels and axillary nerve

Deltoid muscle

Trapezius muscle

Thoracoacromial artery, acromial branches

Infraspinatus muscle

Glenoid

Teres major muscle

Latissimus dorsi muscle

Acromion process

Infraspinatus tendon

Anatomic neck of humerus

Surgical neck of humerus

Deltoid muscle

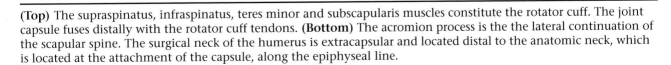

(Top) The supraspinatus, infraspinatus, teres minor and subscapularis muscles constitute the rotator cuff. The joint capsule fuses distally with the rotator cuff tendons. **(Bottom)** The acromion process is the the lateral continuation of the scapular spine. The surgical neck of the humerus is extracapsular and located distal to the anatomic neck, which is located at the attachment of the capsule, along the epiphyseal line.

CORONAL OBLIQUE T1 MR, RIGHT SHOULDER

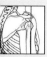

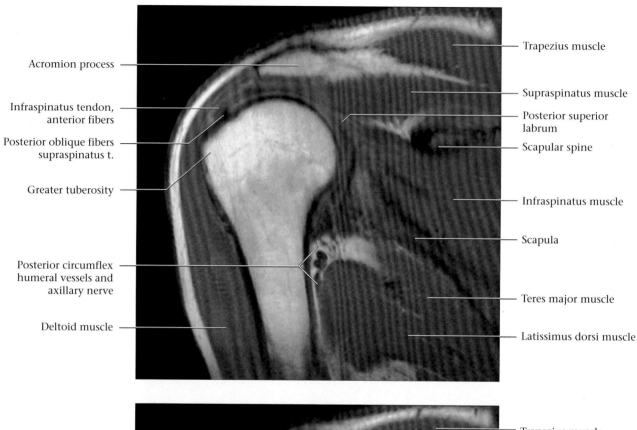

Acromion process

Infraspinatus tendon, anterior fibers

Posterior oblique fibers supraspinatus t.

Greater tuberosity

Posterior circumflex humeral vessels and axillary nerve

Deltoid muscle

Trapezius muscle

Supraspinatus muscle

Posterior superior labrum

Scapular spine

Infraspinatus muscle

Scapula

Teres major muscle

Latissimus dorsi muscle

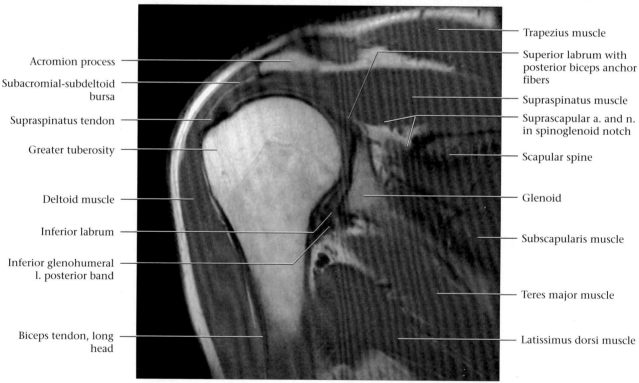

Acromion process

Subacromial-subdeltoid bursa

Supraspinatus tendon

Greater tuberosity

Deltoid muscle

Inferior labrum

Inferior glenohumeral l. posterior band

Biceps tendon, long head

Trapezius muscle

Superior labrum with posterior biceps anchor fibers

Supraspinatus muscle

Suprascapular a. and n. in spinoglenoid notch

Scapular spine

Glenoid

Subscapularis muscle

Teres major muscle

Latissimus dorsi muscle

(Top) The scapular spine divides the posterior border of the scapula into the supraspinatus fossa and infraspinatus fossa. The supraspinatus outlet refers to the area of the lateral third of the supraspinatus muscle and tendon.
(Bottom) The superior and inferior glenoid labrum are shown here. The labrum varies in shape and size but typically has a triangular shape of uniformly low signal.

CORONAL OBLIQUE T1 MR, LEFT SHOULDER

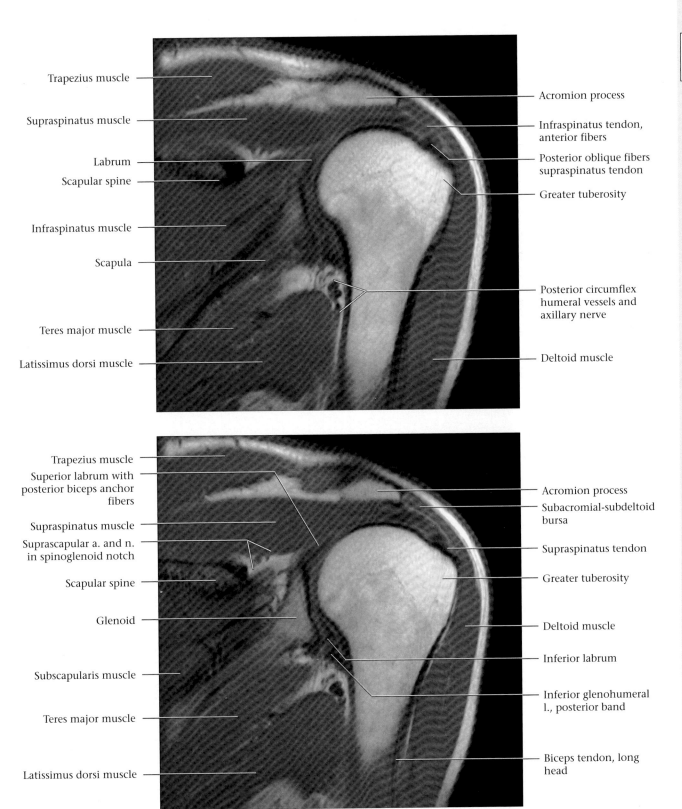

Trapezius muscle

Supraspinatus muscle

Labrum

Scapular spine

Infraspinatus muscle

Scapula

Teres major muscle

Latissimus dorsi muscle

Acromion process

Infraspinatus tendon, anterior fibers

Posterior oblique fibers supraspinatus tendon

Greater tuberosity

Posterior circumflex humeral vessels and axillary nerve

Deltoid muscle

Trapezius muscle

Superior labrum with posterior biceps anchor fibers

Supraspinatus muscle

Suprascapular a. and n. in spinoglenoid notch

Scapular spine

Glenoid

Subscapularis muscle

Teres major muscle

Latissimus dorsi muscle

Acromion process

Subacromial-subdeltoid bursa

Supraspinatus tendon

Greater tuberosity

Deltoid muscle

Inferior labrum

Inferior glenohumeral l., posterior band

Biceps tendon, long head

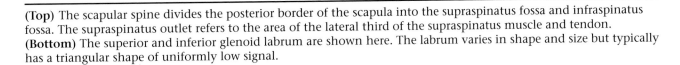

(Top) The scapular spine divides the posterior border of the scapula into the supraspinatus fossa and infraspinatus fossa. The supraspinatus outlet refers to the area of the lateral third of the supraspinatus muscle and tendon.
(Bottom) The superior and inferior glenoid labrum are shown here. The labrum varies in shape and size but typically has a triangular shape of uniformly low signal.

CORONAL OBLIQUE T1 MR, RIGHT SHOULDER

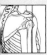

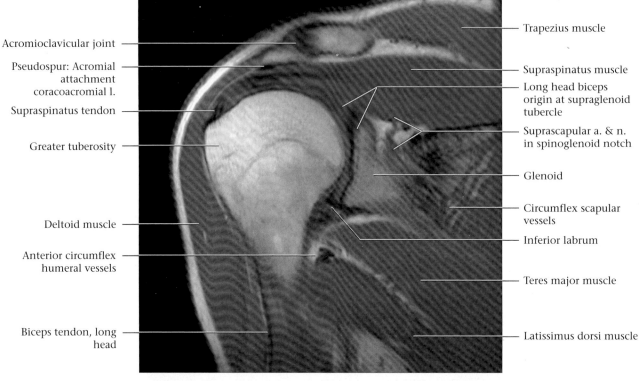

Acromioclavicular joint

Pseudospur: Acromial attachment coracoacromial l.

Supraspinatus tendon

Greater tuberosity

Deltoid muscle

Anterior circumflex humeral vessels

Biceps tendon, long head

Trapezius muscle

Supraspinatus muscle

Long head biceps origin at supraglenoid tubercle

Suprascapular a. & n. in spinoglenoid notch

Glenoid

Circumflex scapular vessels

Inferior labrum

Teres major muscle

Latissimus dorsi muscle

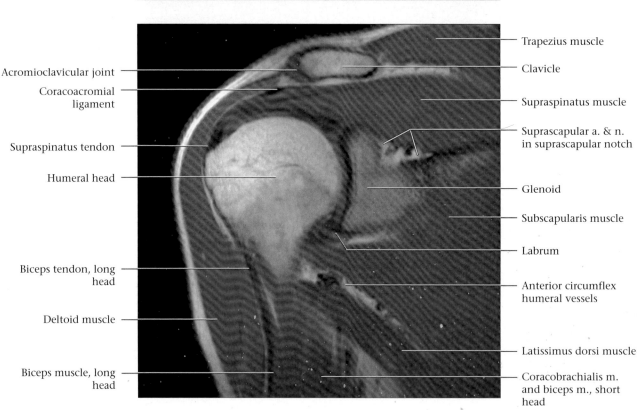

Acromioclavicular joint

Coracoacromial ligament

Supraspinatus tendon

Humeral head

Biceps tendon, long head

Deltoid muscle

Biceps muscle, long head

Trapezius muscle

Clavicle

Supraspinatus muscle

Suprascapular a. & n. in suprascapular notch

Glenoid

Subscapularis muscle

Labrum

Anterior circumflex humeral vessels

Latissimus dorsi muscle

Coracobrachialis m. and biceps m., short head

(Top) Anterior circumflex artery is a branch of the axillary artery. **(Bottom)** The spinoglenoid notch contains fat and the suprascapular artery and nerve. A mass in this region can impinge the nerve and produce focal atrophy of the infraspinatus muscle.

SHOULDER OVERVIEW

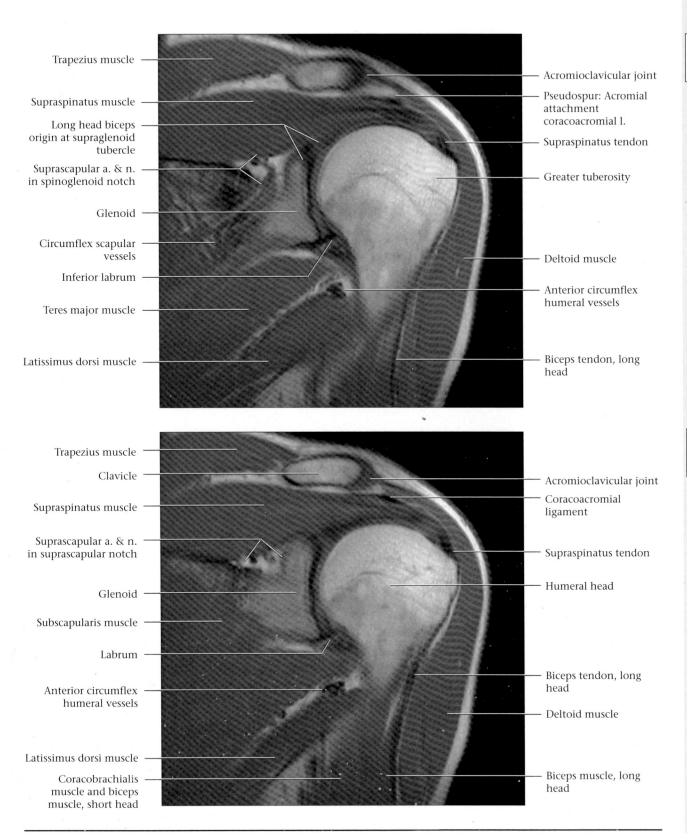

Trapezius muscle

Supraspinatus muscle

Long head biceps origin at supraglenoid tubercle

Suprascapular a. & n. in spinoglenoid notch

Glenoid

Circumflex scapular vessels

Inferior labrum

Teres major muscle

Latissimus dorsi muscle

Acromioclavicular joint

Pseudospur: Acromial attachment coracoacromial l.

Supraspinatus tendon

Greater tuberosity

Deltoid muscle

Anterior circumflex humeral vessels

Biceps tendon, long head

Trapezius muscle

Clavicle

Supraspinatus muscle

Suprascapular a. & n. in suprascapular notch

Glenoid

Subscapularis muscle

Labrum

Anterior circumflex humeral vessels

Latissimus dorsi muscle

Coracobrachialis muscle and biceps muscle, short head

Acromioclavicular joint

Coracoacromial ligament

Supraspinatus tendon

Humeral head

Biceps tendon, long head

Deltoid muscle

Biceps muscle, long head

(Top) Anterior circumflex artery is a branch of the axillary artery. **(Bottom)** The spinoglenoid notch contains fat and the suprascapular artery and nerve. A mass in this region can impinge the nerve and produce focal atrophy of the infraspinatus muscle.

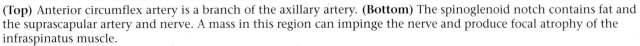

CORONAL OBLIQUE T1 MR, RIGHT SHOULDER

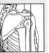

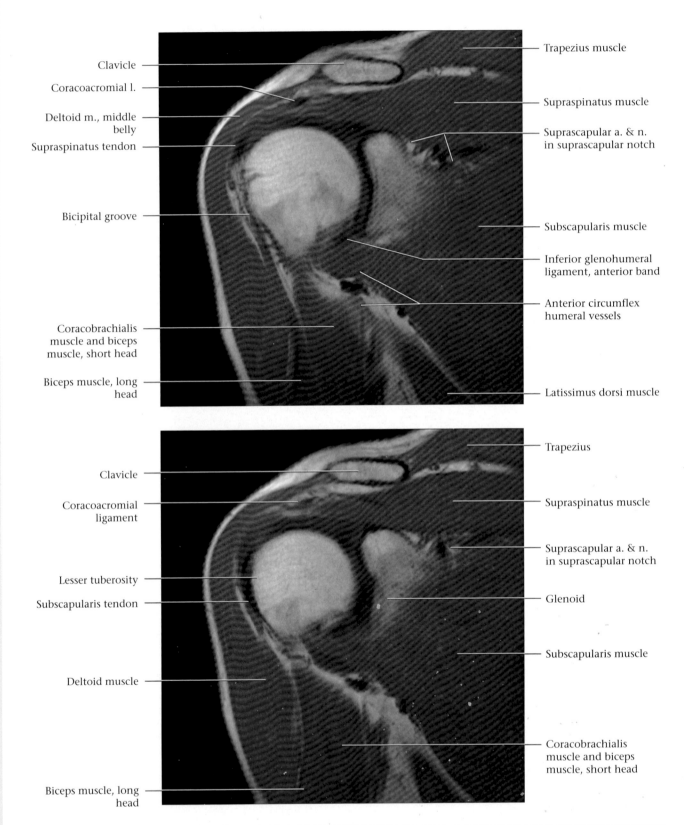

Clavicle

Coracoacromial l.

Deltoid m., middle belly

Supraspinatus tendon

Bicipital groove

Coracobrachialis muscle and biceps muscle, short head

Biceps muscle, long head

Trapezius muscle

Supraspinatus muscle

Suprascapular a. & n. in suprascapular notch

Subscapularis muscle

Inferior glenohumeral ligament, anterior band

Anterior circumflex humeral vessels

Latissimus dorsi muscle

Clavicle

Coracoacromial ligament

Lesser tuberosity

Subscapularis tendon

Deltoid muscle

Biceps muscle, long head

Trapezius

Supraspinatus muscle

Suprascapular a. & n. in suprascapular notch

Glenoid

Subscapularis muscle

Coracobrachialis muscle and biceps muscle, short head

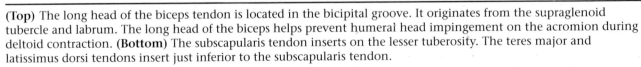

(Top) The long head of the biceps tendon is located in the bicipital groove. It originates from the supraglenoid tubercle and labrum. The long head of the biceps helps prevent humeral head impingement on the acromion during deltoid contraction. (Bottom) The subscapularis tendon inserts on the lesser tuberosity. The teres major and latissimus dorsi tendons insert just inferior to the subscapularis tendon.

SHOULDER OVERVIEW

CORONAL OBLIQUE T1 MR, LEFT SHOULDER

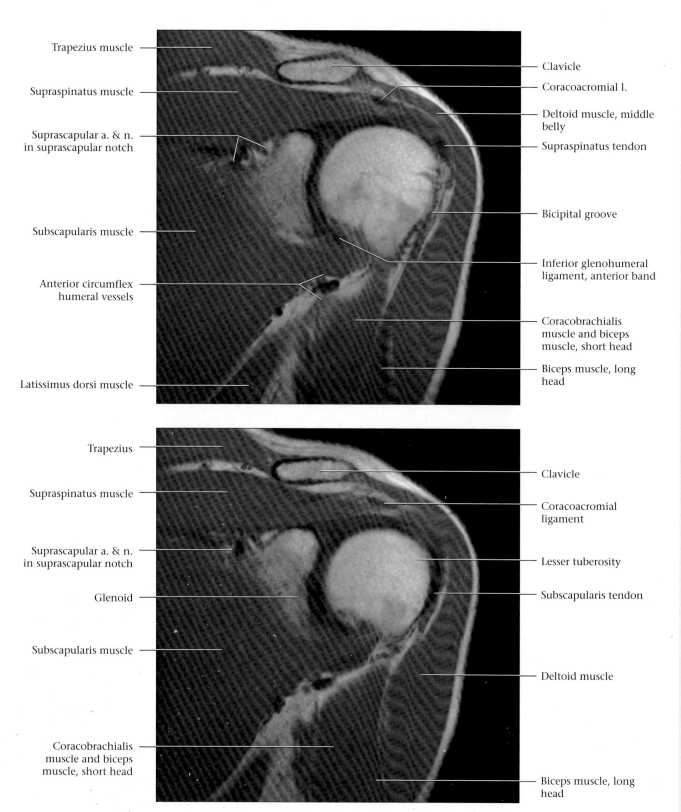

Trapezius muscle

Supraspinatus muscle

Suprascapular a. & n. in suprascapular notch

Subscapularis muscle

Anterior circumflex humeral vessels

Latissimus dorsi muscle

Clavicle

Coracoacromial l.

Deltoid muscle, middle belly

Supraspinatus tendon

Bicipital groove

Inferior glenohumeral ligament, anterior band

Coracobrachialis muscle and biceps muscle, short head

Biceps muscle, long head

Trapezius

Supraspinatus muscle

Suprascapular a. & n. in suprascapular notch

Glenoid

Subscapularis muscle

Coracobrachialis muscle and biceps muscle, short head

Clavicle

Coracoacromial ligament

Lesser tuberosity

Subscapularis tendon

Deltoid muscle

Biceps muscle, long head

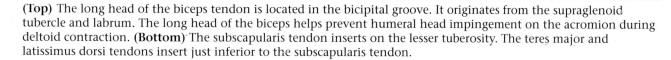

(Top) The long head of the biceps tendon is located in the bicipital groove. It originates from the supraglenoid tubercle and labrum. The long head of the biceps helps prevent humeral head impingement on the acromion during deltoid contraction. **(Bottom)** The subscapularis tendon inserts on the lesser tuberosity. The teres major and latissimus dorsi tendons insert just inferior to the subscapularis tendon.

Shoulder

I

CORONAL OBLIQUE T1 MR, RIGHT SHOULDER

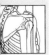

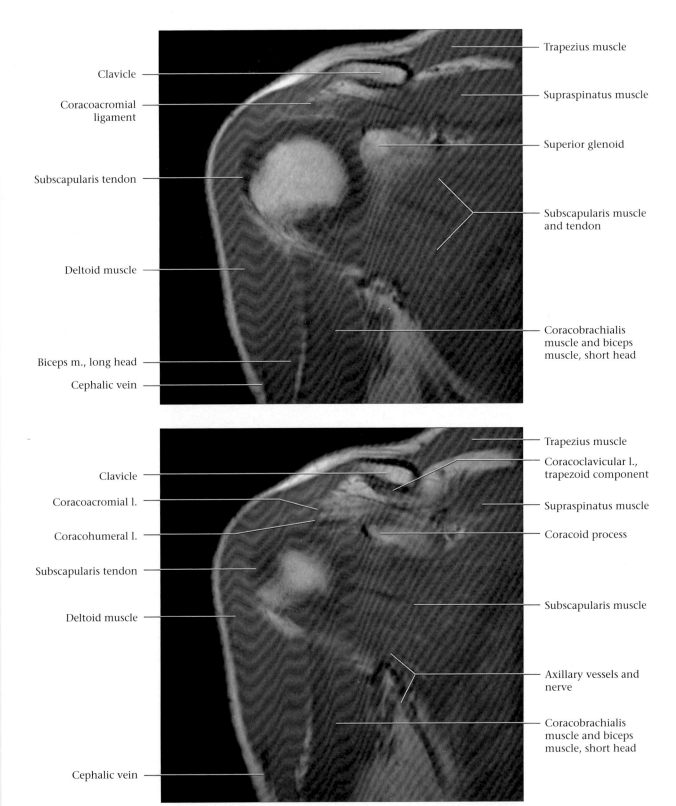

Clavicle

Coracoacromial ligament

Subscapularis tendon

Deltoid muscle

Biceps m., long head

Cephalic vein

Trapezius muscle

Supraspinatus muscle

Superior glenoid

Subscapularis muscle and tendon

Coracobrachialis muscle and biceps muscle, short head

Clavicle

Coracoacromial l.

Coracohumeral l.

Subscapularis tendon

Deltoid muscle

Cephalic vein

Trapezius muscle

Coracoclavicular l., trapezoid component

Supraspinatus muscle

Coracoid process

Subscapularis muscle

Axillary vessels and nerve

Coracobrachialis muscle and biceps muscle, short head

(Top) The deltoid and trapezius muscles attach to the scapular spine, lateral third of clavicle and acromion. Anterior compartment muscles are innervated by the musculocutaneous nerve. **(Bottom)** The axillary artery becomes the brachial artery below the level of the teres major muscle. On this image the bundle still consists of the axillary neurovascular structures. The brachial artery (not shown on this image) will course along the medial border of the coracobrachialis muscle.

SHOULDER OVERVIEW

CORONAL OBLIQUE T1 MR, LEFT SHOULDER

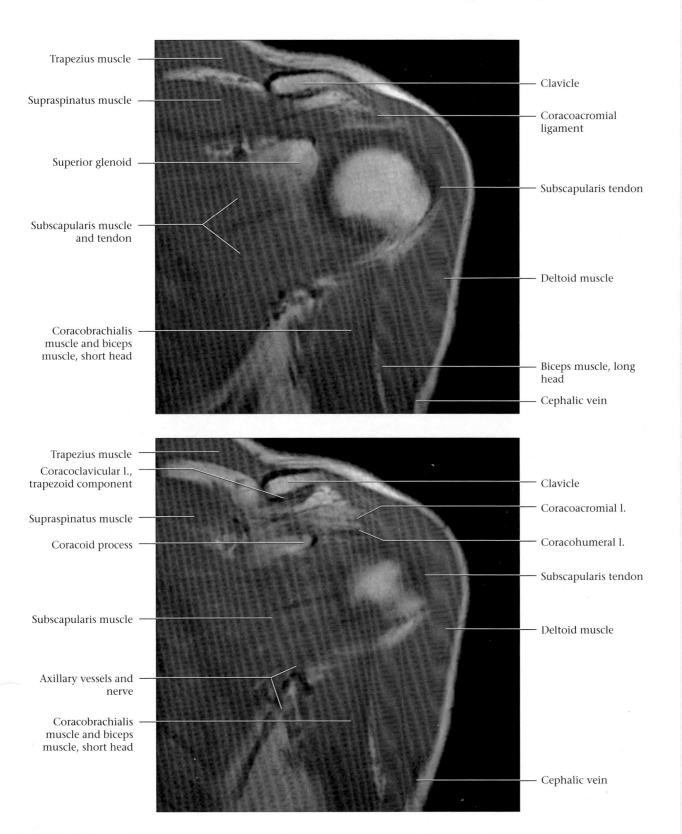

Trapezius muscle

Supraspinatus muscle

Superior glenoid

Subscapularis muscle and tendon

Coracobrachialis muscle and biceps muscle, short head

Clavicle

Coracoacromial ligament

Subscapularis tendon

Deltoid muscle

Biceps muscle, long head

Cephalic vein

Trapezius muscle

Coracoclavicular l., trapezoid component

Supraspinatus muscle

Coracoid process

Subscapularis muscle

Axillary vessels and nerve

Coracobrachialis muscle and biceps muscle, short head

Clavicle

Coracoacromial l.

Coracohumeral l.

Subscapularis tendon

Deltoid muscle

Cephalic vein

(Top) The deltoid and trapezius muscles attach to the scapular spine, lateral third of clavicle and acromion. Anterior compartment muscles are innervated by the musculocutaneous nerve. **(Bottom)** The axillary artery becomes the brachial artery below the level of the teres major muscle. On this image the bundle still consists of the axillary neurovascular structures. The brachial artery (not shown on this image) will course along the medial border of the coracobrachialis muscle.

CORONAL OBLIQUE T1 MR, RIGHT SHOULDER

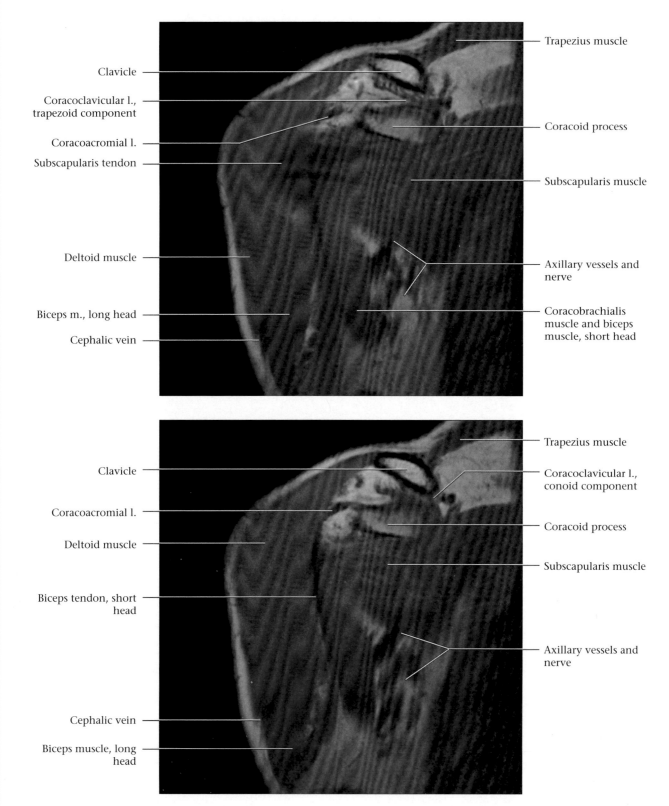

Top image labels:
- Clavicle
- Coracoclavicular l., trapezoid component
- Coracoacromial l.
- Subscapularis tendon
- Deltoid muscle
- Biceps m., long head
- Cephalic vein
- Trapezius muscle
- Coracoid process
- Subscapularis muscle
- Axillary vessels and nerve
- Coracobrachialis muscle and biceps muscle, short head

Bottom image labels:
- Clavicle
- Coracoacromial l.
- Deltoid muscle
- Biceps tendon, short head
- Cephalic vein
- Biceps muscle, long head
- Trapezius muscle
- Coracoclavicular l., conoid component
- Coracoid process
- Subscapularis muscle
- Axillary vessels and nerve

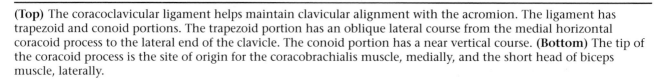

(Top) The coracoclavicular ligament helps maintain clavicular alignment with the acromion. The ligament has trapezoid and conoid portions. The trapezoid portion has an oblique lateral course from the medial horizontal coracoid process to the lateral end of the clavicle. The conoid portion has a near vertical course. (Bottom) The tip of the coracoid process is the site of origin for the coracobrachialis muscle, medially, and the short head of biceps muscle, laterally.

CORONAL OBLIQUE T1 MR, LEFT SHOULDER

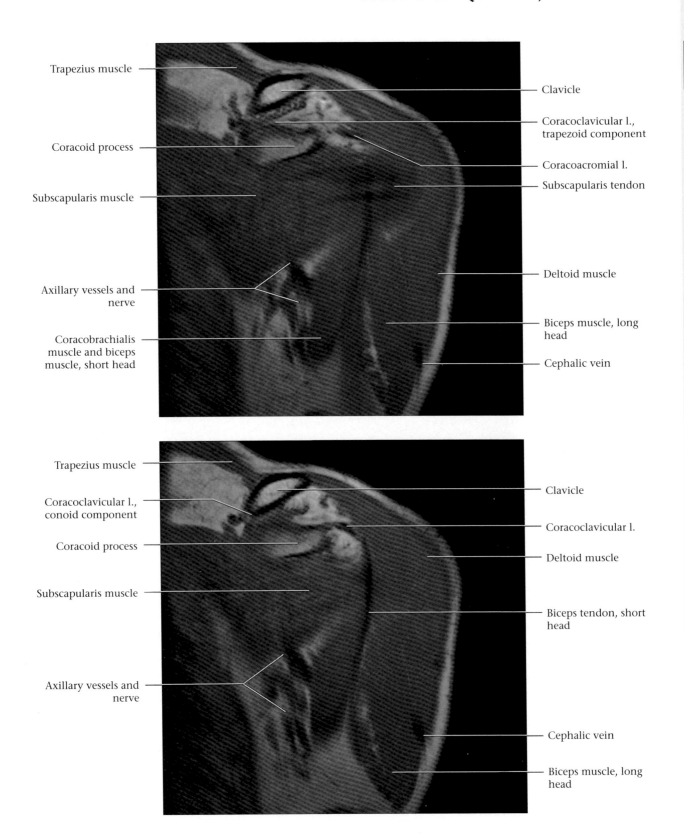

Trapezius muscle

Coracoid process

Subscapularis muscle

Axillary vessels and nerve

Coracobrachialis muscle and biceps muscle, short head

Clavicle

Coracoclavicular l., trapezoid component

Coracoacromial l.

Subscapularis tendon

Deltoid muscle

Biceps muscle, long head

Cephalic vein

Trapezius muscle

Coracoclavicular l., conoid component

Coracoid process

Subscapularis muscle

Axillary vessels and nerve

Clavicle

Coracoclavicular l.

Deltoid muscle

Biceps tendon, short head

Cephalic vein

Biceps muscle, long head

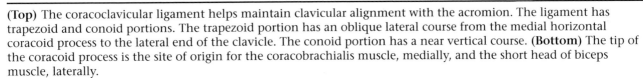

(Top) The coracoclavicular ligament helps maintain clavicular alignment with the acromion. The ligament has trapezoid and conoid portions. The trapezoid portion has an oblique lateral course from the medial horizontal coracoid process to the lateral end of the clavicle. The conoid portion has a near vertical course. **(Bottom)** The tip of the coracoid process is the site of origin for the coracobrachialis muscle, medially, and the short head of biceps muscle, laterally.

Shoulder

I

SAGITTAL OBLIQUE T1 MR, RIGHT SHOULDER

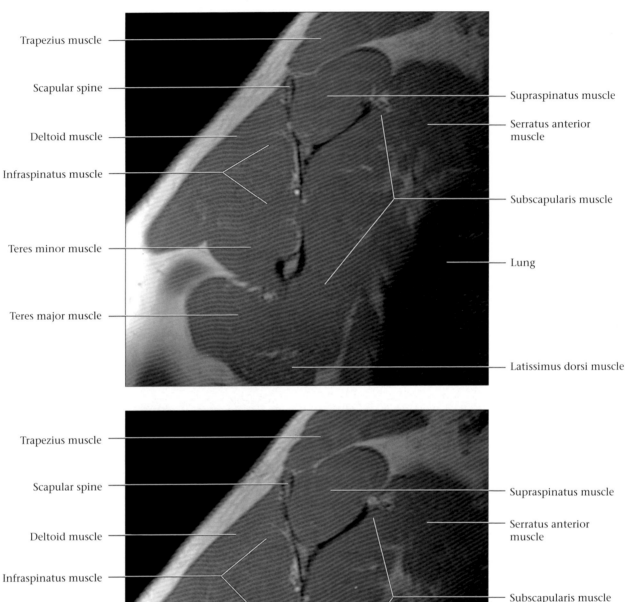

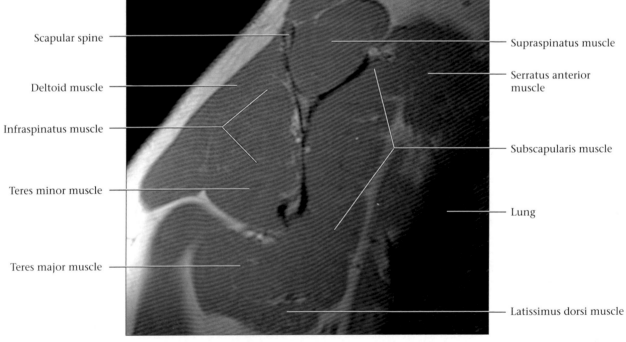

(**Top**) First of 24 sequential sagittal oblique T1 MR images of the right shoulder displayed medial to lateral. Images were obtained with a shoulder coil on a 3T MR scanner. Image is far medial, including a portion of the lateral lung and chest wall. (**Bottom**) The latissimus dorsi muscle wraps around the inferior aspect of the teres major muscle. These two muscles can be difficult to differentiate as separate structures. Each courses superiorly and laterally to insert on the crest of the lesser tuberosity.

SHOULDER OVERVIEW

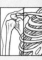

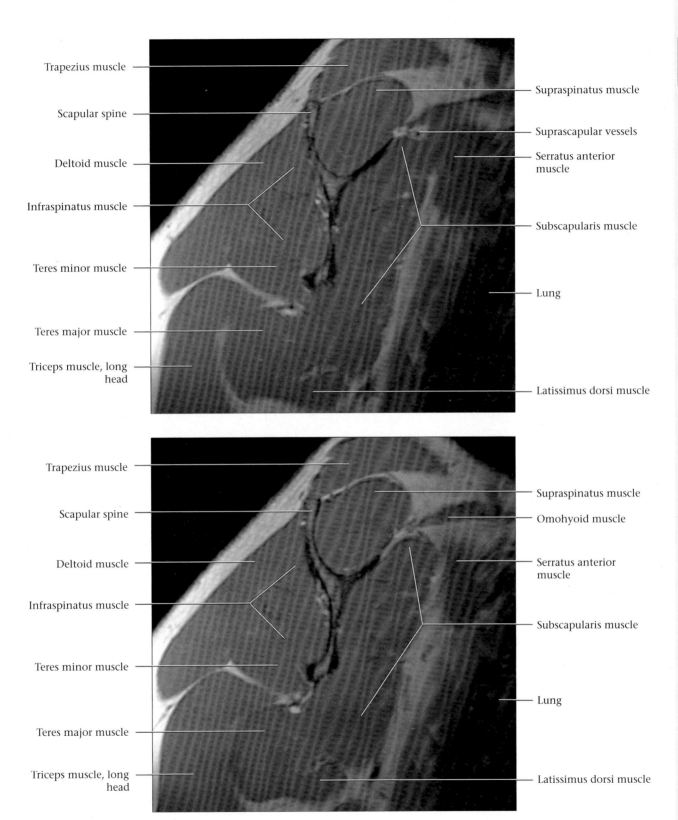

Trapezius muscle

Scapular spine

Deltoid muscle

Infraspinatus muscle

Teres minor muscle

Teres major muscle

Triceps muscle, long head

Supraspinatus muscle

Suprascapular vessels

Serratus anterior muscle

Subscapularis muscle

Lung

Latissimus dorsi muscle

Trapezius muscle

Scapular spine

Deltoid muscle

Infraspinatus muscle

Teres minor muscle

Teres major muscle

Triceps muscle, long head

Supraspinatus muscle

Omohyoid muscle

Serratus anterior muscle

Subscapularis muscle

Lung

Latissimus dorsi muscle

(Top) The rotator cuff muscles consist of the supraspinatus, infraspinatus, teres minor and subscapularis. All of the rotator cuff muscles originate from the scapula. **(Bottom)** The omohyoid muscle originates from the superior border of the scapula. It has an inferior belly and a superior belly. The superior portion inserts on the lower border of the hyoid bone.

SAGITTAL OBLIQUE T1 MR, RIGHT SHOULDER

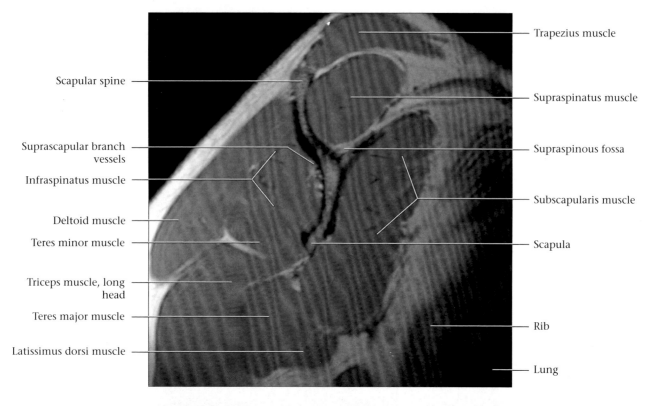

Scapular spine

Suprascapular branch vessels

Infraspinatus muscle

Deltoid muscle

Teres minor muscle

Triceps muscle, long head

Teres major muscle

Latissimus dorsi muscle

Trapezius muscle

Supraspinatus muscle

Supraspinous fossa

Subscapularis muscle

Scapula

Rib

Lung

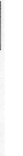

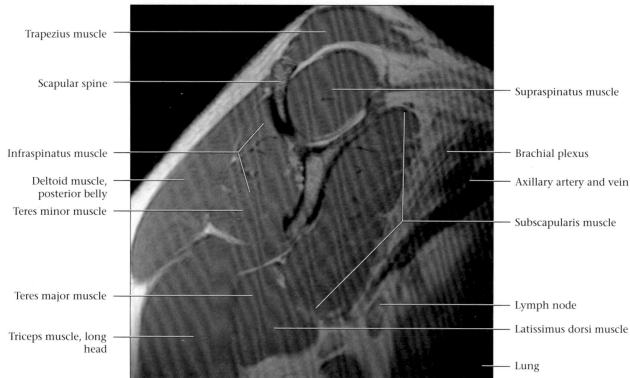

Trapezius muscle

Scapular spine

Infraspinatus muscle

Deltoid muscle, posterior belly

Teres minor muscle

Teres major muscle

Triceps muscle, long head

Supraspinatus muscle

Brachial plexus

Axillary artery and vein

Subscapularis muscle

Lymph node

Latissimus dorsi muscle

Lung

(Top) The scapula has a Y-shaped configuration due to the posterior extent of the scapular spine. The supraspinatus muscle is contained entirely within the crux of the "Y" and should roughly fill this area unless the muscle is atrophied. **(Bottom)** A portion of the trapezius muscle is seen at the superior aspect of the shoulder. The trapezius inserts on the superior border of the lateral clavicle, the medial border of the acromion and the superior border of the scapular spine. The deltoid originates at the same osseous sites, adjacent to the trapezius, but on the opposite border of each of the bones (inferior border of lateral clavicle, lateral border of acromion, inferior border of scapular spine).

SAGITTAL OBLIQUE T1 MR, RIGHT SHOULDER

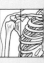

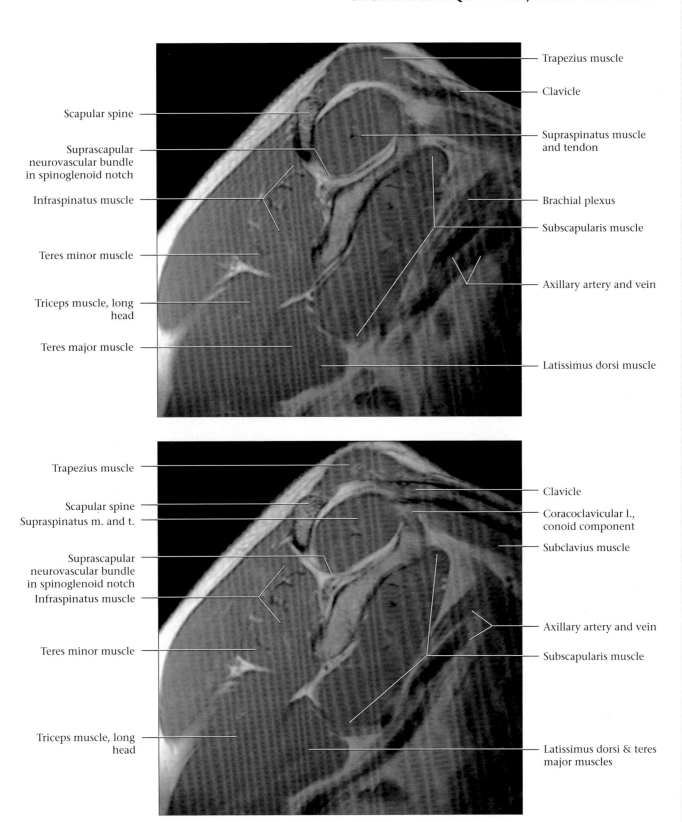

Scapular spine

Suprascapular neurovascular bundle in spinoglenoid notch

Infraspinatus muscle

Teres minor muscle

Triceps muscle, long head

Teres major muscle

Trapezius muscle

Clavicle

Supraspinatus muscle and tendon

Brachial plexus

Subscapularis muscle

Axillary artery and vein

Latissimus dorsi muscle

Trapezius muscle

Scapular spine
Supraspinatus m. and t.

Suprascapular neurovascular bundle in spinoglenoid notch
Infraspinatus muscle

Teres minor muscle

Triceps muscle, long head

Clavicle

Coracoclavicular l., conoid component

Subclavius muscle

Axillary artery and vein

Subscapularis muscle

Latissimus dorsi & teres major muscles

(Top) The subscapularis muscle fills the subscapular fossa of the scapula. **(Bottom)** The infraspinatus and teres minor muscles are located below the scapular spine. The infraspinatus muscle is the larger and is located more superiorly than teres minor.

SHOULDER OVERVIEW

SAGITTAL OBLIQUE T1 MR, RIGHT SHOULDER

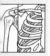

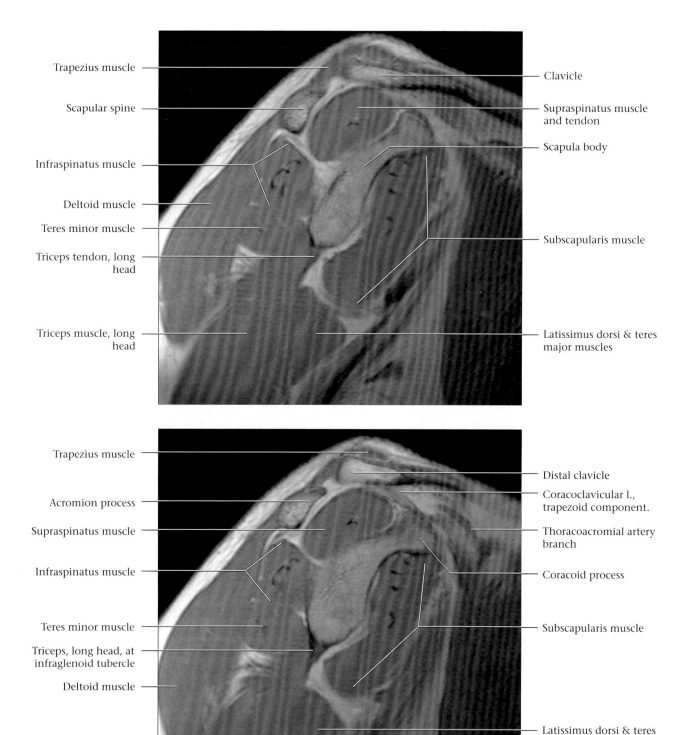

Trapezius muscle — Clavicle

Scapular spine — Supraspinatus muscle and tendon

— Scapula body

Infraspinatus muscle —

Deltoid muscle —

Teres minor muscle —

Triceps tendon, long head — Subscapularis muscle

Triceps muscle, long head — Latissimus dorsi & teres major muscles

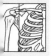

Trapezius muscle — Distal clavicle

Acromion process — Coracoclavicular l., trapezoid component.

Supraspinatus muscle — Thoracoacromial artery branch

Infraspinatus muscle — Coracoid process

Teres minor muscle —

Triceps, long head, at infraglenoid tubercle — Subscapularis muscle

Deltoid muscle —

Triceps muscle, long head — Latissimus dorsi & teres major muscles

(Top) The supraspinatus, subscapularis, teres minor and infraspinatus (clockwise) continue to course laterally. The tendons of these muscles will conjoin as they reach the lateral aspect of the humeral head. **(Bottom)** The scapular spine ends as the acromion process. The acromioclavicular joint is becoming visible. The neurovascular bundle lies along the anterior surface of the subscapularis muscle.

SAGITTAL OBLIQUE T1 MR, RIGHT SHOULDER

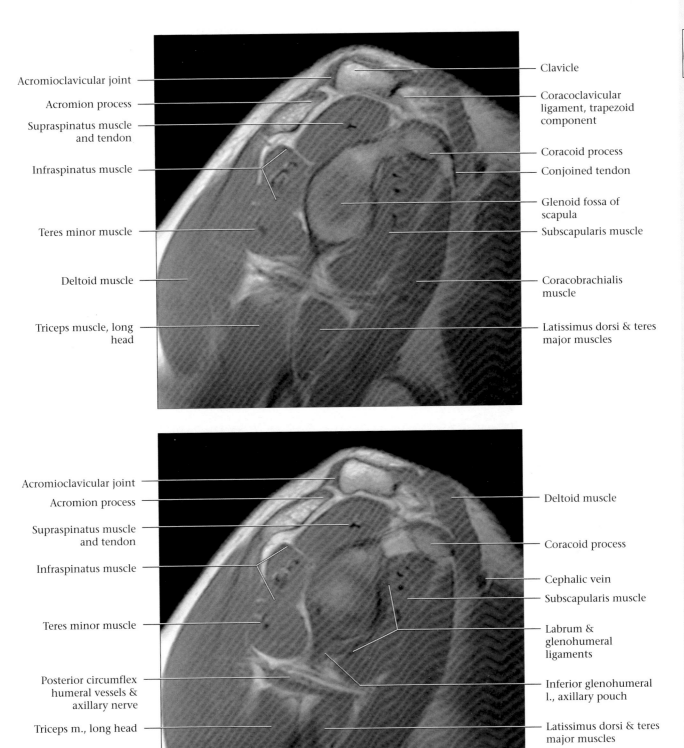

Acromioclavicular joint

Acromion process

Supraspinatus muscle and tendon

Infraspinatus muscle

Teres minor muscle

Deltoid muscle

Triceps muscle, long head

Clavicle

Coracoclavicular ligament, trapezoid component

Coracoid process

Conjoined tendon

Glenoid fossa of scapula

Subscapularis muscle

Coracobrachialis muscle

Latissimus dorsi & teres major muscles

Acromioclavicular joint

Acromion process

Supraspinatus muscle and tendon

Infraspinatus muscle

Teres minor muscle

Posterior circumflex humeral vessels & axillary nerve

Triceps m., long head

Deltoid muscle

Deltoid muscle

Coracoid process

Cephalic vein

Subscapularis muscle

Labrum & glenohumeral ligaments

Inferior glenohumeral l., axillary pouch

Latissimus dorsi & teres major muscles

(Top) Image is at the level of the glenoid fossa of the scapula. The dark surrounding rim of the glenoid labrum is becoming visible. The coracoid process is the origin of the coracobrachialis and short head of the biceps tendon. **(Bottom)** The glenohumeral ligaments are seen as low signal bands of tissue surrounding the anterior, inferior and posteroinferior aspects of the shoulder joint. The glenohumeral ligaments strengthen the joint capsule.

SAGITTAL OBLIQUE T1 MR, RIGHT SHOULDER

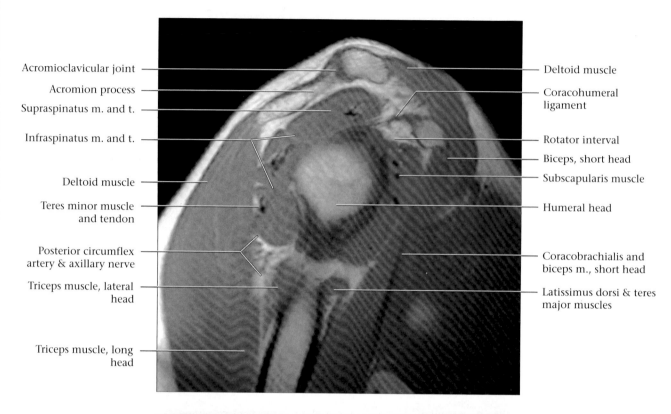

Acromioclavicular joint

Acromion process

Supraspinatus m. and t.

Infraspinatus m. and t.

Deltoid muscle

Teres minor muscle and tendon

Posterior circumflex artery & axillary nerve

Triceps muscle, lateral head

Triceps muscle, long head

Deltoid muscle

Coracohumeral ligament

Rotator interval

Biceps, short head

Subscapularis muscle

Humeral head

Coracobrachialis and biceps m., short head

Latissimus dorsi & teres major muscles

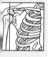

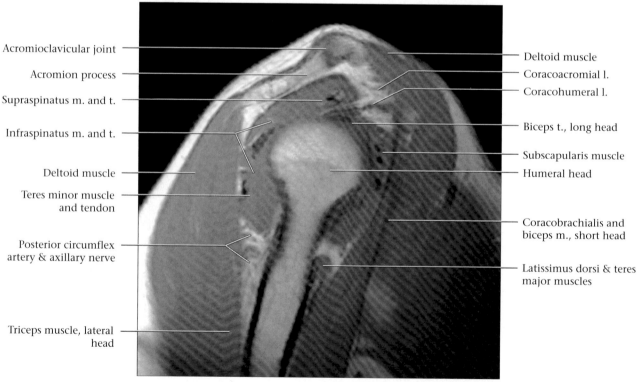

Acromioclavicular joint

Acromion process

Supraspinatus m. and t.

Infraspinatus m. and t.

Deltoid muscle

Teres minor muscle and tendon

Posterior circumflex artery & axillary nerve

Triceps muscle, lateral head

Deltoid muscle

Coracoacromial l.

Coracohumeral l.

Biceps t., long head

Subscapularis muscle

Humeral head

Coracobrachialis and biceps m., short head

Latissimus dorsi & teres major muscles

(Top) Image is at the medial border of the humeral head. The posterior circumflex humeral artery winds around the neck of the humerus to anastomose with the anterior circumflex humeral artery. **(Bottom)** The rotator interval is a triangular space bordered superiorly by the supraspinatus tendon anterior margin, inferiorly by the subscapularis tendon superior border, medially by the coracoid base and laterally by the long head of the biceps tendon bicipital groove.

SHOULDER OVERVIEW

SAGITTAL OBLIQUE T1 MR, RIGHT SHOULDER

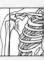

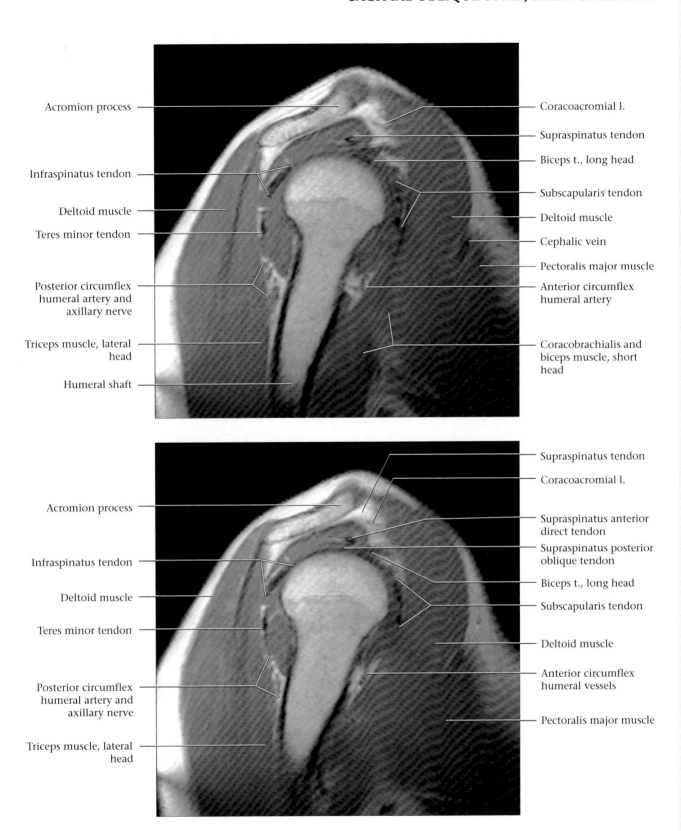

Acromion process — Coracoacromial l.

Supraspinatus tendon

Biceps t., long head

Infraspinatus tendon — Subscapularis tendon

Deltoid muscle — Deltoid muscle

Teres minor tendon — Cephalic vein

Pectoralis major muscle

Posterior circumflex humeral artery and axillary nerve — Anterior circumflex humeral artery

Triceps muscle, lateral head — Coracobrachialis and biceps muscle, short head

Humeral shaft

Supraspinatus tendon

Coracoacromial l.

Acromion process — Supraspinatus anterior direct tendon

Supraspinatus posterior oblique tendon

Infraspinatus tendon — Biceps t., long head

Deltoid muscle — Subscapularis tendon

Teres minor tendon — Deltoid muscle

Anterior circumflex humeral vessels

Posterior circumflex humeral artery and axillary nerve — Pectoralis major muscle

Triceps muscle, lateral head

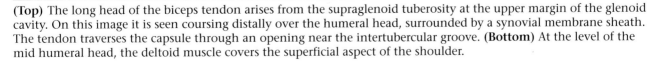

(Top) The long head of the biceps tendon arises from the supraglenoid tuberosity at the upper margin of the glenoid cavity. On this image it is seen coursing distally over the humeral head, surrounded by a synovial membrane sheath. The tendon traverses the capsule through an opening near the intertubercular groove. **(Bottom)** At the level of the mid humeral head, the deltoid muscle covers the superficial aspect of the shoulder.

SAGITTAL OBLIQUE T1 MR, RIGHT SHOULDER

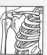

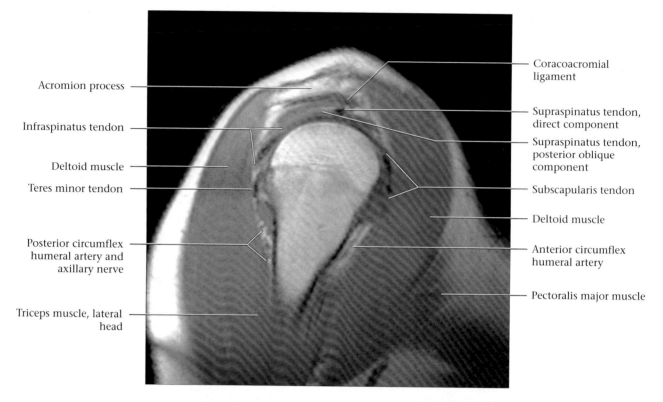

Acromion process

Infraspinatus tendon

Deltoid muscle

Teres minor tendon

Posterior circumflex humeral artery and axillary nerve

Triceps muscle, lateral head

Coracoacromial ligament

Supraspinatus tendon, direct component

Supraspinatus tendon, posterior oblique component

Subscapularis tendon

Deltoid muscle

Anterior circumflex humeral artery

Pectoralis major muscle

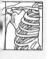

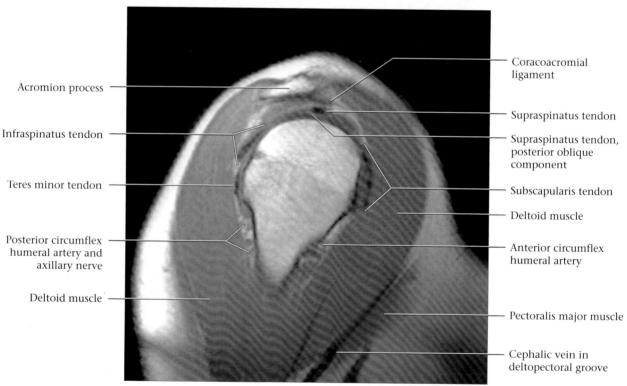

Acromion process

Infraspinatus tendon

Teres minor tendon

Posterior circumflex humeral artery and axillary nerve

Deltoid muscle

Coracoacromial ligament

Supraspinatus tendon

Supraspinatus tendon, posterior oblique component

Subscapularis tendon

Deltoid muscle

Anterior circumflex humeral artery

Pectoralis major muscle

Cephalic vein in deltopectoral groove

(**Top**) Evaluating the morphologic type of acromion is best assessed on the first image lateral to the acromioclavicular joint. (**Bottom**) The rotator cuff is predominantly tendinous as it passes toward the lateral aspect of the humeral head. The tendons are beginning to fuse with each other and the joint capsule.

SAGITTAL OBLIQUE T1 MR, RIGHT SHOULDER

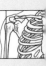

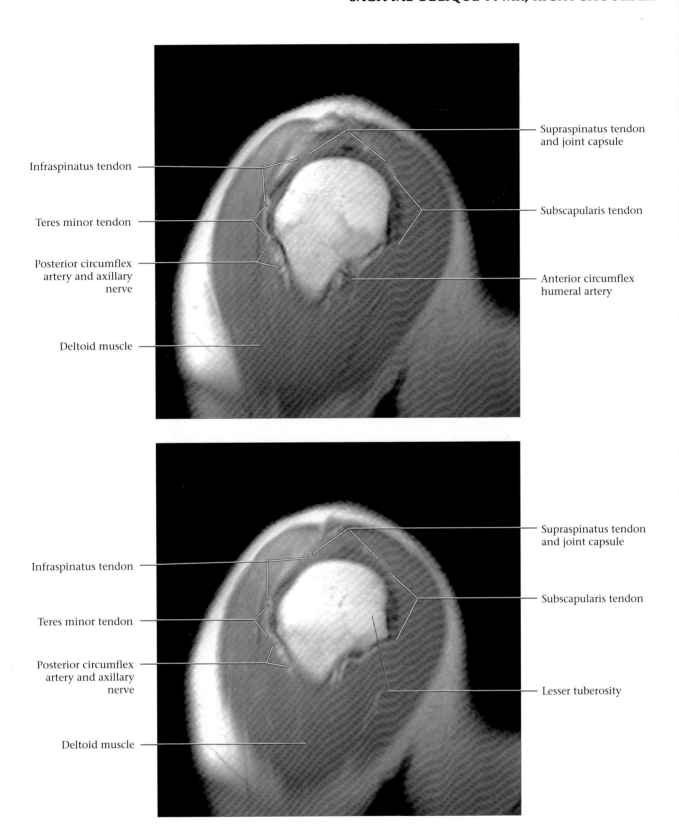

Infraspinatus tendon

Teres minor tendon

Posterior circumflex artery and axillary nerve

Deltoid muscle

Supraspinatus tendon and joint capsule

Subscapularis tendon

Anterior circumflex humeral artery

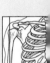

Infraspinatus tendon

Teres minor tendon

Posterior circumflex artery and axillary nerve

Deltoid muscle

Supraspinatus tendon and joint capsule

Subscapularis tendon

Lesser tuberosity

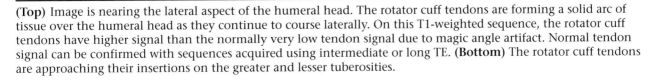

(Top) Image is nearing the lateral aspect of the humeral head. The rotator cuff tendons are forming a solid arc of tissue over the humeral head as they continue to course laterally. On this T1-weighted sequence, the rotator cuff tendons have higher signal than the normally very low tendon signal due to magic angle artifact. Normal tendon signal can be confirmed with sequences acquired using intermediate or long TE. **(Bottom)** The rotator cuff tendons are approaching their insertions on the greater and lesser tuberosities.

Shoulder

I

SHOULDER OVERVIEW

SAGITTAL OBLIQUE T1 MR, RIGHT SHOULDER

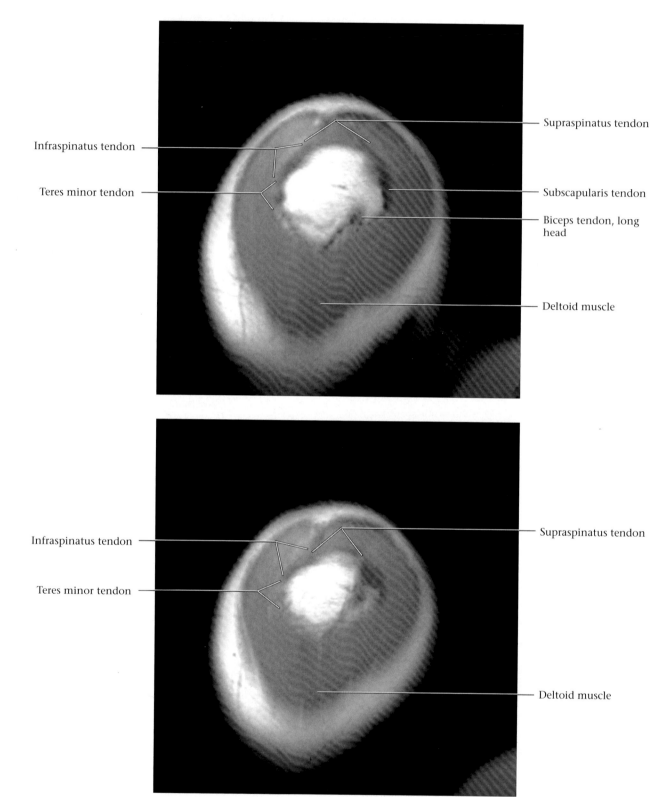

Infraspinatus tendon

Teres minor tendon

Supraspinatus tendon

Subscapularis tendon

Biceps tendon, long head

Deltoid muscle

Infraspinatus tendon

Teres minor tendon

Supraspinatus tendon

Deltoid muscle

(Top) The subscapularis tendon inserts on the lesser tuberosity and forms the roof of the bicipital groove. **(Bottom)** The supraspinatus, infraspinatus and teres minor tendons insert on the greater tuberosity superior facet, middle facet and inferior facet respectively.

SHOULDER OVERVIEW

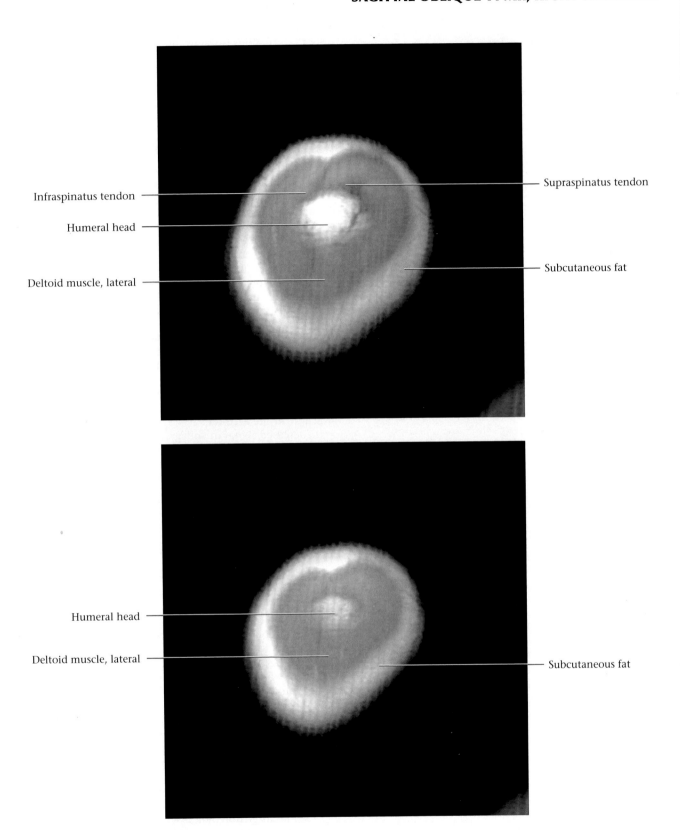

Infraspinatus tendon — Supraspinatus tendon

Humeral head

Deltoid muscle, lateral — Subcutaneous fat

Humeral head

Deltoid muscle, lateral — Subcutaneous fat

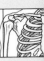

(Top) Small portions of the supraspinatus and infraspinatus tendons are still visible inserting on the greater tuberosity. (Bottom) The far lateral, superficial aspect of the shoulder is entirely covered by the middle belly of deltoid muscle.

ROTATOR CUFF AND BICEPS TENDON

Imaging Anatomy

Overview
- **Rotator cuff**
  - Consists of supraspinatus, infraspinatus, teres minor and subscapularis muscles and tendons
  - Uniform, hypointense tendons on all sequences
  - Cuff tendons blend with shoulder joint capsule
- **Supraspinatus muscle**
  - Origin: Supraspinatus fossa of scapula
  - Insertion: Superior facet (horizontal orientation) and portion of middle facet of greater tuberosity
  - Nerve supply: Suprascapular nerve
  - Blood supply: Suprascapular artery and circumflex scapular branches of subscapular artery
  - Action: Abduction of humerus
  - Anterior and posterior muscle bellies
    - Anterior belly is larger, has central tendon and is more likely to tear
    - Posterior belly is strap-like & has terminal tendon
  - Most commonly injured rotator cuff muscle
- **Infraspinatus muscle**
  - Origin: Infraspinatus fossa of scapula
  - Insertion: Middle facet greater tuberosity
  - Nerve supply: Suprascapular nerve, distal fibers
  - Blood supply: Suprascapular artery and circumflex scapular branches of subscapular artery
  - Action: External rotation of humerus and resists posterior subluxation
- **Teres minor muscle**
  - Origin: Lateral scapular border, middle half
  - Insertion: Inferior facet (vertical orientation) of humerus greater tuberosity
  - Nerve supply: Axillary nerve
  - Blood supply: Posterior circumflex humeral artery & circumflex scapular branches of subscapular artery
  - Action: External rotation of humerus
  - Least commonly injured rotator cuff muscle
- **Subscapularis muscle**
  - Origin: Subscapular fossa of scapula
  - Insertion: Lesser tuberosity and up to 40% may insert at surgical neck
  - Nerve supply: Subscapular nerve, upper and lower
  - Blood supply: Subscapularis artery
  - Action: Internal rotation of humerus, also adduction, extension, depression and flexion
  - 4-6 tendon slips converge into main tendon; multipennate morphology increases strength
- **Rotator cuff tendon blood supply**
  - Derived from adjacent muscle, bone and bursae
  - Normal hypovascular regions in tendons
    - Termed "critical zone"
    - Vulnerable to degeneration
    - However, not the most common region of tearing
- **Biceps tendon, long head**
  - Low signal intensity on all sequences
  - Origin: Superior glenoid labrum
    - Portions may attach to supraglenoid tubercle, anterosuperior labrum, posterosuperior labrum and coracoid base
  - Courses through superior shoulder joint to intertubercular or bicipital groove
  - Action: Stabilizes and depresses humeral head
  - Anatomic variants
    - Anomalous intra-articular and extra-articular origins from rotator cuff and joint capsule
    - May be bifid or absent
  - **Tendon sheath** communicates with joint and normally contains a small amount of fluid

Anatomy-Based Imaging Issues

Imaging Recommendations
- **Radiographs**: AP and supraspinatus outlet views to assess humeral head position and thus indirectly assess supraspinatus tendon
- **MR**: Best study for evaluation of rotator cuff
  - T1 sequences without fat suppression helpful for evaluating muscle mass
- **MR arthrography**: Improves evaluation of rotator cuff and capsulolabral complex
  - Improved visualization of cuff articular surface

Imaging Pitfalls
- **Increased signal in supraspinatus tendon approximately 1 cm from insertion**
  - Present in asymptomatic patients
  - Attributed to magic angle artifact, tendon degeneration, partial volume effect and positioning artifacts
- **Magic angle artifact**
  - Increased signal in collagen fibers oriented 55° to main magnetic field on short TE images
  - Can occur in rotator cuff and biceps tendon
  - Recognize by comparing with long TE images
- **Partial volume averaging**
  - Anterior supraspinatus may volume average with fluid in subscapularis bursa or biceps tendon sheath simulating tear
    - Avoid excessive external arm rotation
  - Posterior oblique fibers of supraspinatus attach deep to overlapping anterior fibers of infraspinatus; cuff may appear thin in this zone, sometimes with increased linear signal
    - Most pronounced with internal arm rotation
  - Mid supraspinatus may average with thickened region of humeral head cartilage
  - Tendons may average with normal variant muscle slips extending above or below tendon
    - Follow muscle slips back to the muscle belly
- **Motion artifact**
  - Recognize by propagation across image in phase encoding direction
- **Dilated veins in supraspinatus muscle**
  - Usually in the periphery of muscle
  - May simulate intramuscular ganglion cysts
- **Interruption of subacromial-subdeltoid fat plane**
  - Fat plane is superficial to bursa
  - Can be interrupted or absent in normal patients
  - Not a reliable sign of rotator cuff abnormality
- **Increased signal in lateral bicipital groove**
  - Due to anterolateral branch of anterior circumflex humeral artery and vein
  - Do not confuse with fluid from tenosynovitis or tendon tear

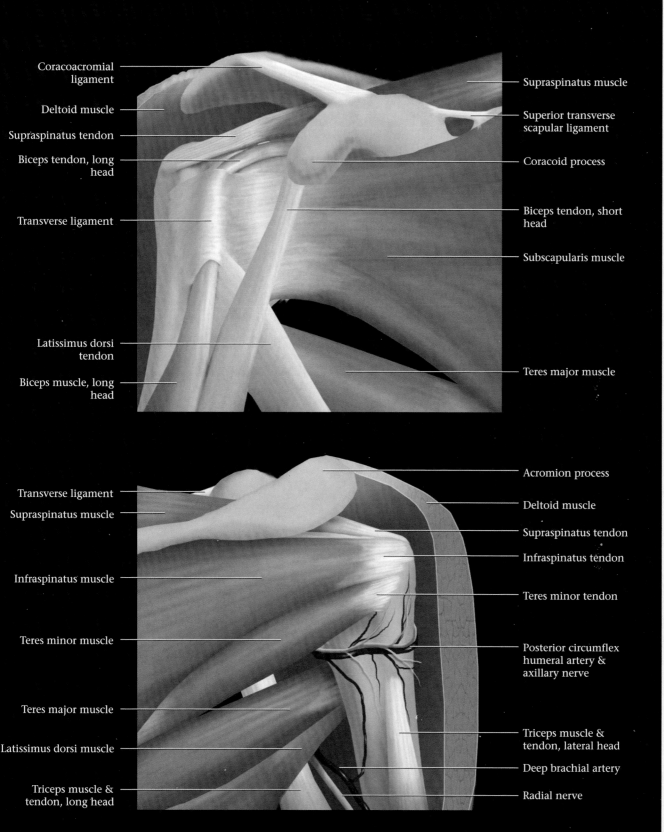

Coracoacromial ligament

Deltoid muscle

Supraspinatus tendon

Biceps tendon, long head

Transverse ligament

Latissimus dorsi tendon

Biceps muscle, long head

Supraspinatus muscle

Superior transverse scapular ligament

Coracoid process

Biceps tendon, short head

Subscapularis muscle

Teres major muscle

Transverse ligament

Supraspinatus muscle

Infraspinatus muscle

Teres minor muscle

Teres major muscle

Latissimus dorsi muscle

Triceps muscle & tendon, long head

Acromion process

Deltoid muscle

Supraspinatus tendon

Infraspinatus tendon

Teres minor tendon

Posterior circumflex humeral artery & axillary nerve

Triceps muscle & tendon, lateral head

Deep brachial artery

Radial nerve

(Top) Anterior graphic of right shoulder demonstrating the rotator cuff and adjacent structures. **(Bottom)** Posterior graphic of right shoulder demonstrating the rotator cuff and adjacent structures.

SAGITTAL T2 FS MR, RIGHT SHOULDER

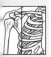

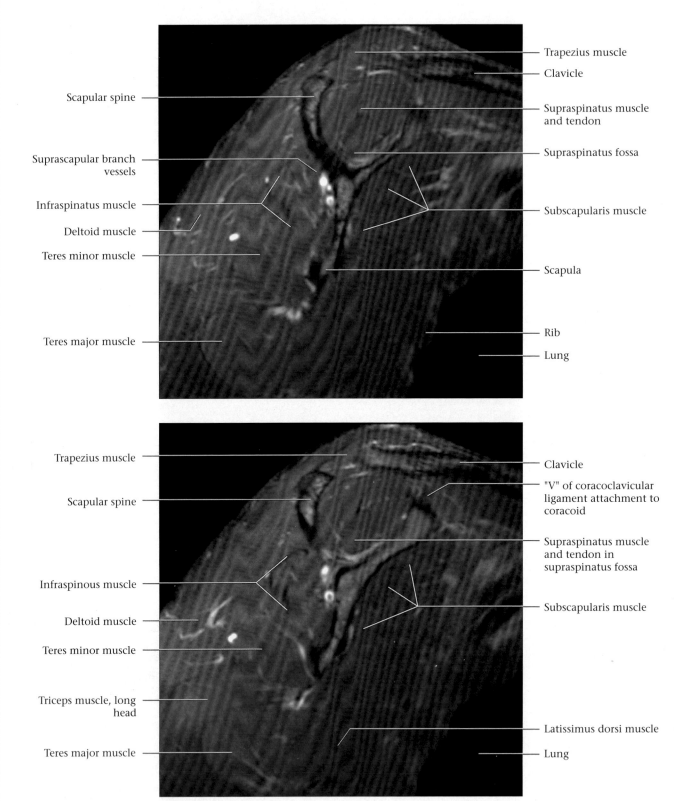

(Top) First of eighteen sequential sagittal oblique T2 FS MR images of the right shoulder displayed medial to lateral. Images were acquired at 1.5 T with a shoulder coil. **(Bottom)** The supraspinatus muscle fills the supraspinatus fossa of the scapula. The normal muscle should fill or extend slightly above a line drawn along the top border of the Y of the scapula. When the muscle atrophies, the muscle will be replaced by fat. With atrophy, the supraspinatus tendon may become eccentric in location, approaching the superior border of the muscle.

ROTATOR CUFF AND BICEPS TENDON

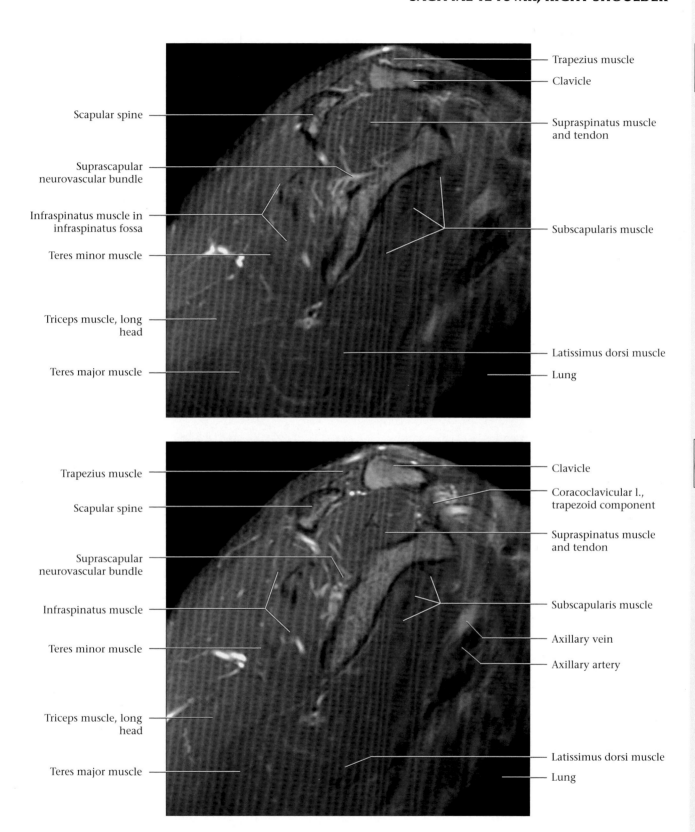
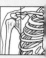
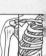

(Top) The infraspinatus muscle fills the infraspinatus fossa of the scapula. A normal infraspinatus muscle should fill the fossa and extend posterior to a line drawn from from the posterior aspect of the scapular spine to the inferior border of the scapula. Infraspinatus muscle atrophy may occur in the absence of tendon abnormality. **(Bottom)** The normal subscapularis muscle should fill the subscapular fossa. The muscle should have a convex anterior border.

SAGITTAL T2 FS MR, RIGHT SHOULDER

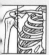

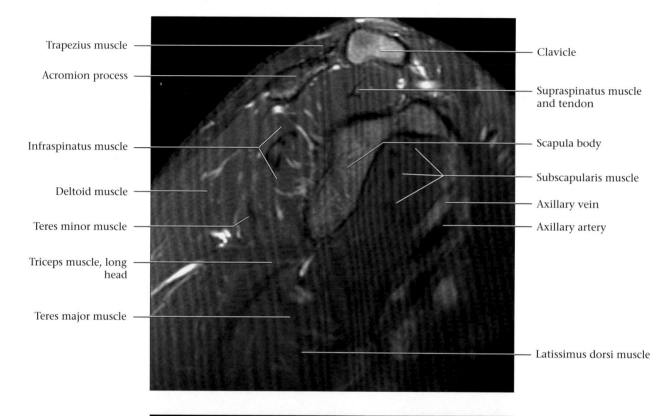

Trapezius muscle

Acromion process

Infraspinatus muscle

Deltoid muscle

Teres minor muscle

Triceps muscle, long head

Teres major muscle

Clavicle

Supraspinatus muscle and tendon

Scapula body

Subscapularis muscle

Axillary vein

Axillary artery

Latissimus dorsi muscle

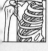

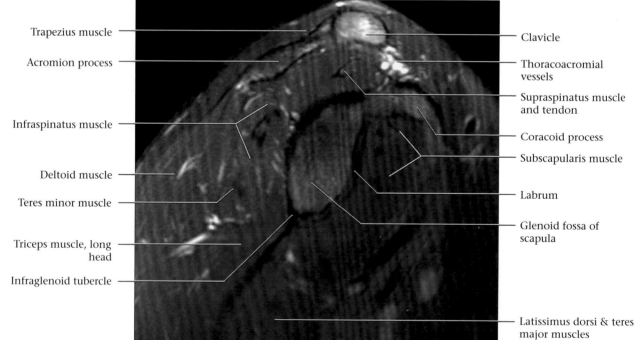

Trapezius muscle

Acromion process

Infraspinatus muscle

Deltoid muscle

Teres minor muscle

Triceps muscle, long head

Infraglenoid tubercle

Clavicle

Thoracoacromial vessels

Supraspinatus muscle and tendon

Coracoid process

Subscapularis muscle

Labrum

Glenoid fossa of scapula

Latissimus dorsi & teres major muscles

(Top) The teres muscle lies inferior to the infraspinatus muscle. It assists in external rotation of humerus. The teres minor also resists posterior subluxation of the humeral head. **(Bottom)** All of the rotator cuff muscles originate from the scapula and insert on the humeral head.

ROTATOR CUFF AND BICEPS TENDON

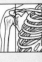

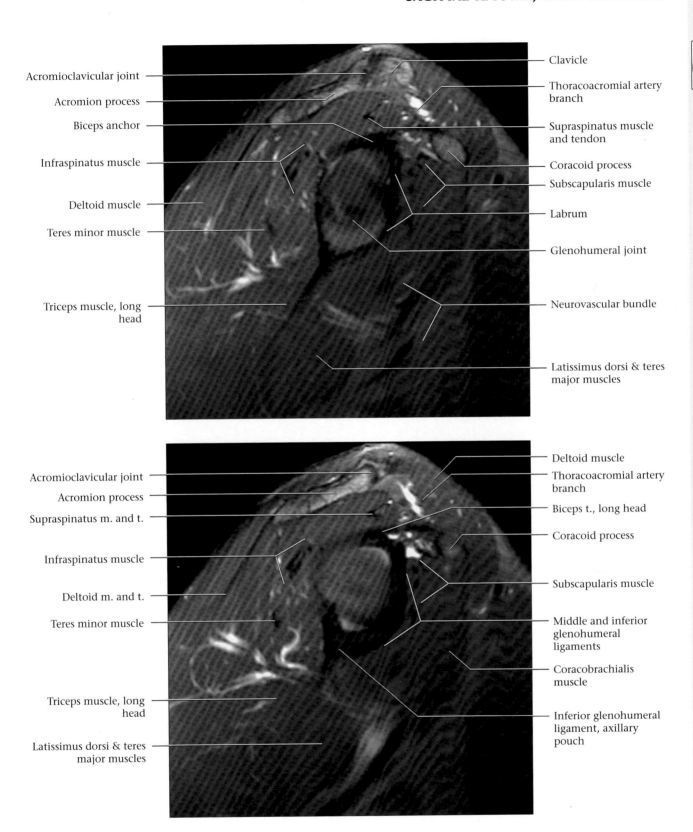

Top image labels:

Left side:
- Acromioclavicular joint
- Acromion process
- Biceps anchor
- Infraspinatus muscle
- Deltoid muscle
- Teres minor muscle
- Triceps muscle, long head

Right side:
- Clavicle
- Thoracoacromial artery branch
- Supraspinatus muscle and tendon
- Coracoid process
- Subscapularis muscle
- Labrum
- Glenohumeral joint
- Neurovascular bundle
- Latissimus dorsi & teres major muscles

Bottom image labels:

Left side:
- Acromioclavicular joint
- Acromion process
- Supraspinatus m. and t.
- Infraspinatus muscle
- Deltoid m. and t.
- Teres minor muscle
- Triceps muscle, long head
- Latissimus dorsi & teres major muscles

Right side:
- Deltoid muscle
- Thoracoacromial artery branch
- Biceps t., long head
- Coracoid process
- Subscapularis muscle
- Middle and inferior glenohumeral ligaments
- Coracobrachialis muscle
- Inferior glenohumeral ligament, axillary pouch

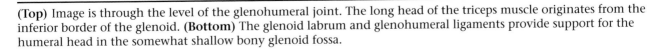

(Top) Image is through the level of the glenohumeral joint. The long head of the triceps muscle originates from the inferior border of the glenoid. **(Bottom)** The glenoid labrum and glenohumeral ligaments provide support for the humeral head in the somewhat shallow bony glenoid fossa.

SAGITTAL T2 FS MR, RIGHT SHOULDER

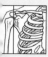

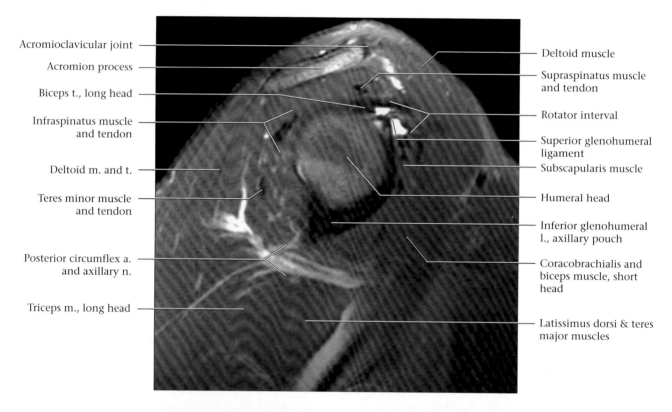

Acromioclavicular joint

Acromion process

Biceps t., long head

Infraspinatus muscle and tendon

Deltoid m. and t.

Teres minor muscle and tendon

Posterior circumflex a. and axillary n.

Triceps m., long head

Deltoid muscle

Supraspinatus muscle and tendon

Rotator interval

Superior glenohumeral ligament

Subscapularis muscle

Humeral head

Inferior glenohumeral l., axillary pouch

Coracobrachialis and biceps muscle, short head

Latissimus dorsi & teres major muscles

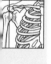

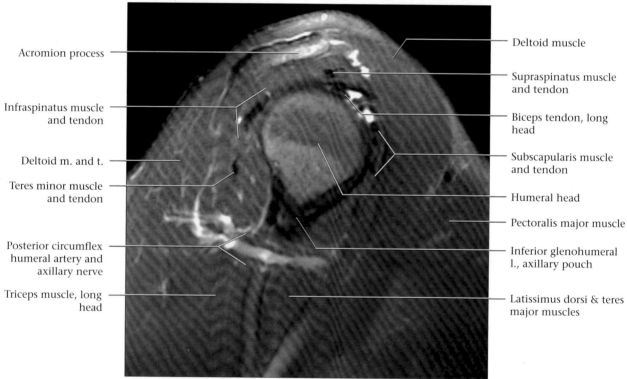

Acromion process

Infraspinatus muscle and tendon

Deltoid m. and t.

Teres minor muscle and tendon

Posterior circumflex humeral artery and axillary nerve

Triceps muscle, long head

Deltoid muscle

Supraspinatus muscle and tendon

Biceps tendon, long head

Subscapularis muscle and tendon

Humeral head

Pectoralis major muscle

Inferior glenohumeral l., axillary pouch

Latissimus dorsi & teres major muscles

(Top) The rotator interval is a triangular space between the supraspinatus and subscapularis tendons. The long head of the biceps traverses the rotator interval. The coracohumeral ligament and superior glenohumeral ligament provide support for the long head of the biceps tendon in the rotator interval. **(Bottom)** The long head of the biceps in this region is intra-articular but extrasynovial.

SAGITTAL T2 FS MR, RIGHT SHOULDER

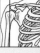

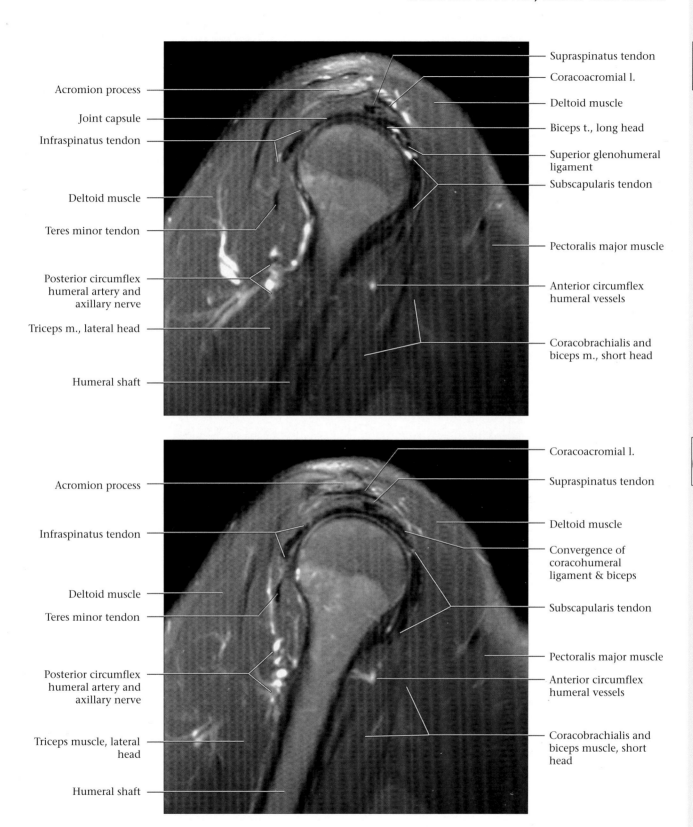

Acromion process

Joint capsule

Infraspinatus tendon

Deltoid muscle

Teres minor tendon

Posterior circumflex humeral artery and axillary nerve

Triceps m., lateral head

Humeral shaft

Supraspinatus tendon

Coracoacromial l.

Deltoid muscle

Biceps t., long head

Superior glenohumeral ligament

Subscapularis tendon

Pectoralis major muscle

Anterior circumflex humeral vessels

Coracobrachialis and biceps m., short head

Acromion process

Infraspinatus tendon

Deltoid muscle

Teres minor tendon

Posterior circumflex humeral artery and axillary nerve

Triceps muscle, lateral head

Humeral shaft

Coracoacromial l.

Supraspinatus tendon

Deltoid muscle

Convergence of coracohumeral ligament & biceps

Subscapularis tendon

Pectoralis major muscle

Anterior circumflex humeral vessels

Coracobrachialis and biceps muscle, short head

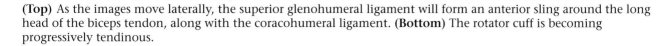

(Top) As the images move laterally, the superior glenohumeral ligament will form an anterior sling around the long head of the biceps tendon, along with the coracohumeral ligament. **(Bottom)** The rotator cuff is becoming progressively tendinous.

Shoulder

83

SAGITTAL T2 FS MR, RIGHT SHOULDER

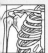

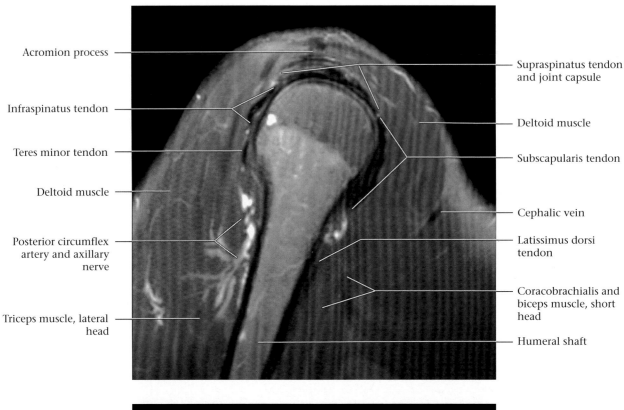

Acromion process — Supraspinatus tendon and joint capsule

Infraspinatus tendon — Deltoid muscle

Teres minor tendon — Subscapularis tendon

Deltoid muscle — Cephalic vein

Posterior circumflex artery and axillary nerve — Latissimus dorsi tendon

— Coracobrachialis and biceps muscle, short head

Triceps muscle, lateral head — Humeral shaft

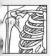

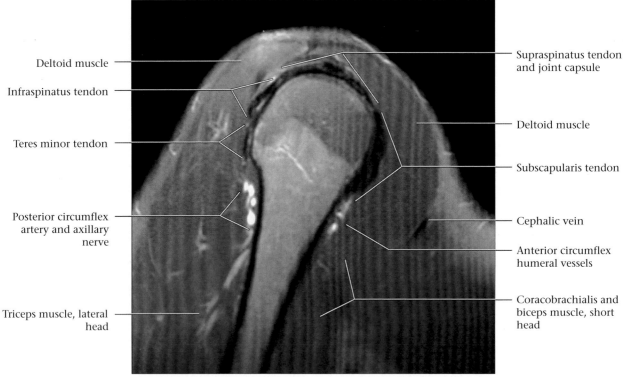

Deltoid muscle — Supraspinatus tendon and joint capsule

Infraspinatus tendon — Deltoid muscle

Teres minor tendon — Subscapularis tendon

Posterior circumflex artery and axillary nerve — Cephalic vein

— Anterior circumflex humeral vessels

Triceps muscle, lateral head — Coracobrachialis and biceps muscle, short head

(Top) The rotator cuff tendons fuse with the joint capsule. The coracohumeral ligament fuses with the supraspinatus and subscapularis tendons, spanning the gap between the two tendons. **(Bottom)** Anterior and posterior circumflex humeral vessels anastomose at the lateral aspect of the humeral neck.

ROTATOR CUFF AND BICEPS TENDON

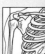
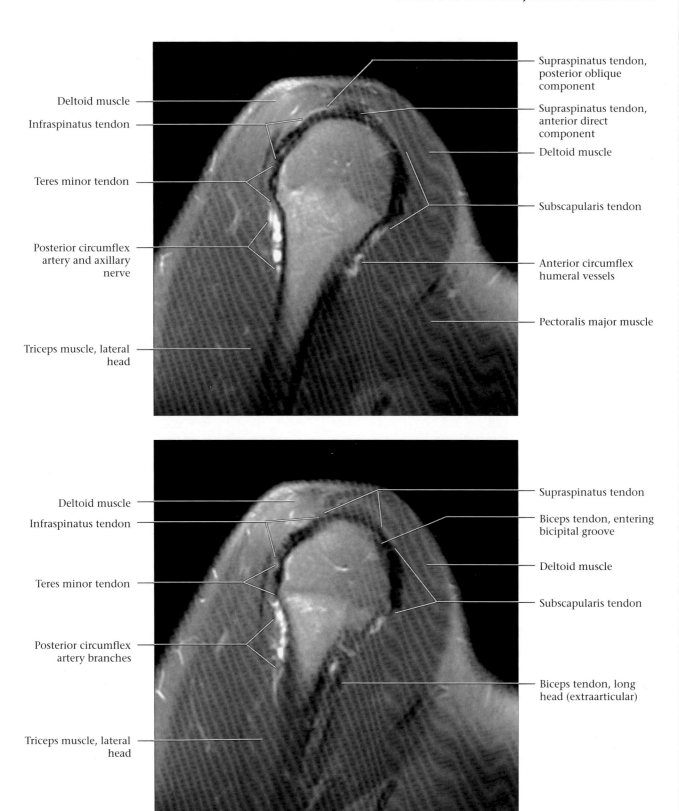

Top image labels:
- Deltoid muscle
- Infraspinatus tendon
- Teres minor tendon
- Posterior circumflex artery and axillary nerve
- Triceps muscle, lateral head
- Supraspinatus tendon, posterior oblique component
- Supraspinatus tendon, anterior direct component
- Deltoid muscle
- Subscapularis tendon
- Anterior circumflex humeral vessels
- Pectoralis major muscle

Bottom image labels:
- Deltoid muscle
- Infraspinatus tendon
- Teres minor tendon
- Posterior circumflex artery branches
- Triceps muscle, lateral head
- Supraspinatus tendon
- Biceps tendon, entering bicipital groove
- Deltoid muscle
- Subscapularis tendon
- Biceps tendon, long head (extraarticular)

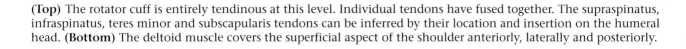

(Top) The rotator cuff is entirely tendinous at this level. Individual tendons have fused together. The supraspinatus, infraspinatus, teres minor and subscapularis tendons can be inferred by their location and insertion on the humeral head. **(Bottom)** The deltoid muscle covers the superficial aspect of the shoulder anteriorly, laterally and posteriorly.

ROTATOR CUFF AND BICEPS TENDON

SAGITTAL T2 FS MR, RIGHT SHOULDER

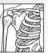
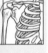
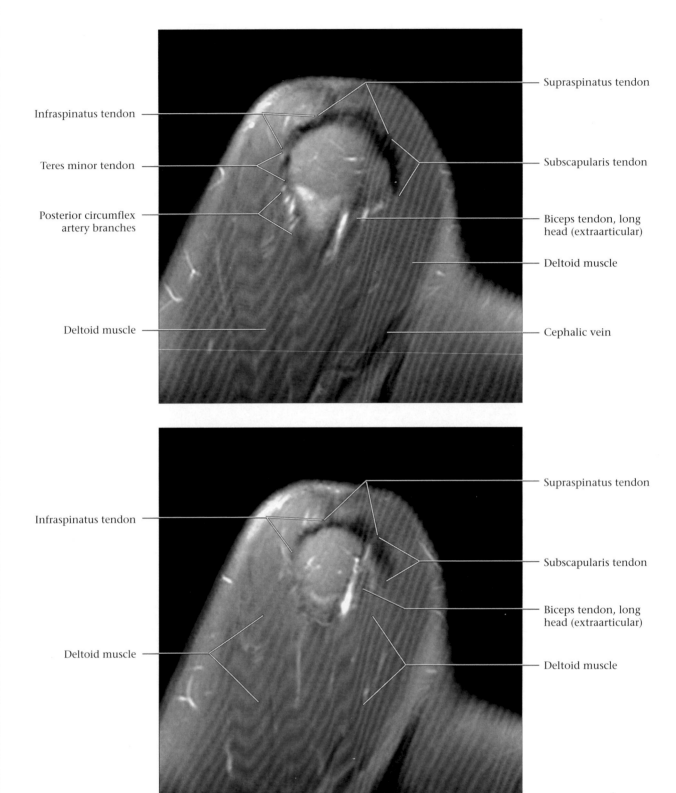

Infraspinatus tendon

Teres minor tendon

Posterior circumflex artery branches

Deltoid muscle

Supraspinatus tendon

Subscapularis tendon

Biceps tendon, long head (extraarticular)

Deltoid muscle

Cephalic vein

Infraspinatus tendon

Deltoid muscle

Supraspinatus tendon

Subscapularis tendon

Biceps tendon, long head (extraarticular)

Deltoid muscle

(Top) There are three facets of the greater tuberosity. The superior facet is horizontally oriented. The middle facet is obliquely oriented. The inferior facet is vertically oriented. The supraspinatus, infraspinatus and teres minor tendons insert on the superior, middle and inferior facets of the greater tuberosity respectively. The supraspinatus partially inserts on the middle facet, as as well as on the superior facet. **(Bottom)** The subscapularis tendon inserts on the lesser tuberosity.

ROTATOR CUFF AND BICEPS TENDON

MR IMAGING PITFALL, INCREASED SIGNAL IN SUPRASPINATUS TENDON

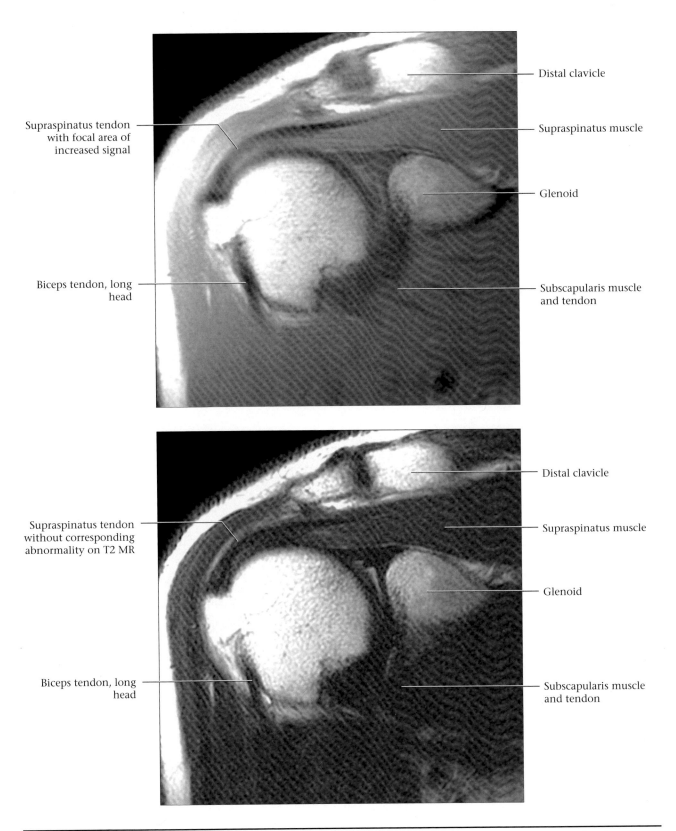

Supraspinatus tendon with focal area of increased signal

Biceps tendon, long head

Distal clavicle

Supraspinatus muscle

Glenoid

Subscapularis muscle and tendon

Supraspinatus tendon without corresponding abnormality on T2 MR

Biceps tendon, long head

Distal clavicle

Supraspinatus muscle

Glenoid

Subscapularis muscle and tendon

(Top) First of two coronal oblique images through the same level in the same patient. Image is proton density weighted with a TE of 11. A focal area of increased signal in the supraspinatus tendon is located approximately 1 cm from the insertion on the greater tuberosity. **(Bottom)** Image is T2 weighted with a TE of 93. There is no corresponding abnormal signal on this sequence. Abnormal signal in this area of the supraspinatus tendon has been attributed to many different entities including magic angle artifact, tendon degeneration and partial volume effect. The resolution of the abnormal signal when the TE of the sequence was increased favors magic angle artifact.

MR IMAGING PITFALL, OBSCURED SUBACROMIAL-SUBDELTOID FAT PLANE

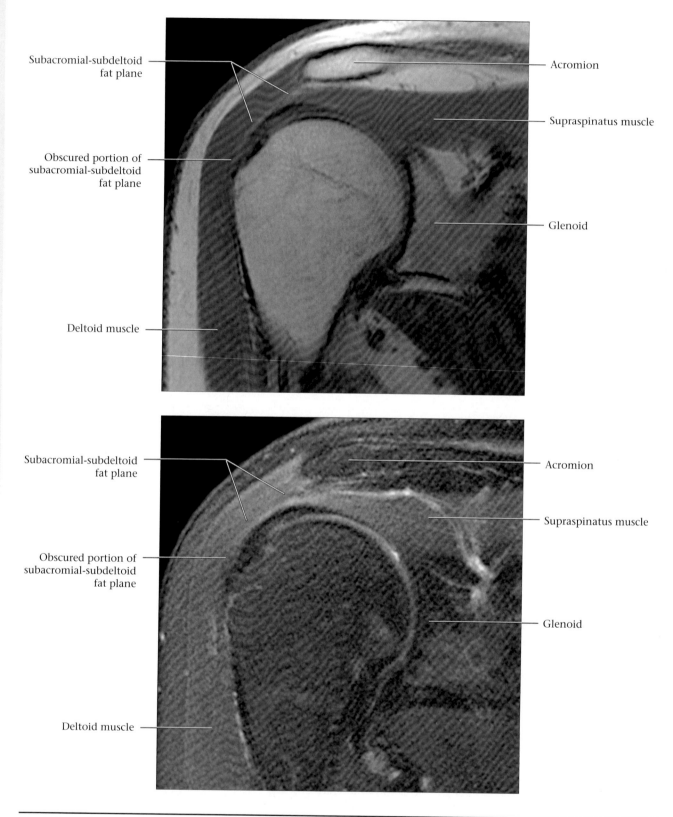

Subacromial-subdeltoid fat plane

Obscured portion of subacromial-subdeltoid fat plane

Deltoid muscle

Acromion

Supraspinatus muscle

Glenoid

Subacromial-subdeltoid fat plane

Obscured portion of subacromial-subdeltoid fat plane

Deltoid muscle

Acromion

Supraspinatus muscle

Glenoid

(Top) First of two coronal oblique images in the same patient demonstrating a partially obscured subacromial-subdeltoid fat plane. T1 MR image shows the high signal fat plane to be partially absent adjacent to the supraspinatus tendon insertion on the greater tuberosity. This fat plane is normally located superficially along the course of the bursa. Absence of this fat plane has been described as an indicator of injury or inflammation in the surrounding soft tissues. This sign is inconsistently seen. The fat plane may be completely or partially absent in normal patients. (Bottom) Coronal oblique T2 FS MR image is obtained at the same location as the previous T1 MR image. The area where the fat plane is absent shows no increased signal to indicate injury or inflammation.

ROTATOR CUFF AND BICEPS TENDON

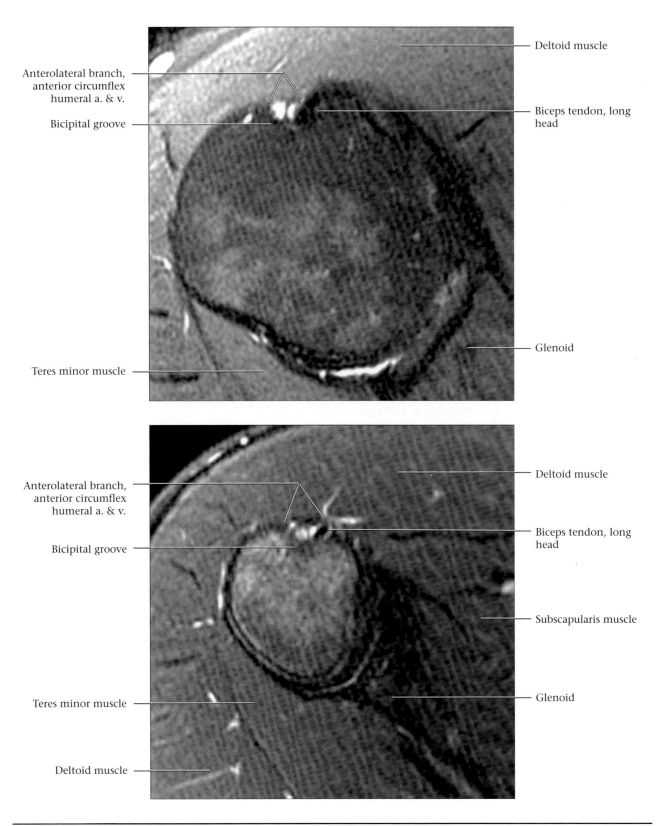

Deltoid muscle

Anterolateral branch, anterior circumflex humeral a. & v.

Bicipital groove

Biceps tendon, long head

Glenoid

Teres minor muscle

Deltoid muscle

Anterolateral branch, anterior circumflex humeral a. & v.

Bicipital groove

Biceps tendon, long head

Subscapularis muscle

Teres minor muscle

Glenoid

Deltoid muscle

(Top) Increased signal within lateral aspect of bicipital groove on axial T2 FS MR image. The anterolateral branch of the anterior circumflex humeral artery and vein lie within the groove. These vessels should not be confused with fluid from tenosynovitis or a tear of the biceps tendon. **(Bottom)** Companion case showing the anterolateral branch of the anterior circumflex humeral artery and vein within lateral aspect of bicipital groove on axial T2 FS MR image.

ROTATOR INTERVAL

Terminology

Abbreviations
- Coracohumeral ligament (CHL)
- Superior glenohumeral ligament (SGHL)
- Long head, biceps tendon (LBT)

Imaging Anatomy

Overview
- **Triangular space between supraspinatus and subscapularis tendons**
  - Base of triangle at coracoid process
  - Tip of triangle at transverse ligament
- **Borders of rotator interval**
  - Medial extent: Coracoid base
  - Lateral extent: Entrance to bicipital groove, transverse ligament
  - Floor: Humeral head cartilage
  - Roof: Joint capsule
    - Coracohumeral ligament on bursal surface
    - Fasciculus obliquus on articular surface
    - Synovial lining
- **Contents of rotator interval**
  - Coracohumeral ligament
  - Superior glenohumeral ligament
  - Biceps tendon, long head
- Coracohumeral ligament and superior glenohumeral ligament stabilize long head of biceps tendon as it enters bicipital groove

Internal Structures-Critical Contents
- **Coracohumeral ligament**
  - Origin: Base of coracoid process
  - Insertion: Lesser and greater tuberosities, humerus
    - Forms two bands laterally
    - Larger inserts on greater tuberosity and supraspinatus anterior border
    - Smaller band inserts on lesser tuberosity, transverse ligament and superior subscapularis tendon
  - **Histologically more similar to a capsule than a true ligament**
  - **Blends with superficial and deep layers of rotator cuff tendons and joint capsule**
  - Forms a solid layer of tissue between supraspinatus and subscapularis tendons
  - Covers the intra-articular portion of LBT
  - Optimal imaging plane: Sagittal oblique but should be visible in all planes
  - Homogeneous low signal on all sequences
  - Cannot be differentiated from supraspinatus and subscapularis tendons where it is fused
- **Superior glenohumeral ligament**
  - Origin: Superior tubercle of glenoid, anterior to biceps
  - Insertion: Superolateral lesser tuberosity, deep to superior border of subscapularis tendon
  - **May not be possible to differentiate from coracohumeral ligament in absence intra-articular contrast or joint effusion**
  - Changes configuration through course of interval
    - Medial: Tubular, anterior to LBT
    - Mid portion: Flattened anterior band with T-shaped connection to CHL
    - Lateral: Fuses with CHL to form sling around LBT
  - **On axial images, may be seen as band anterior to biceps tendon**
  - Optimal imaging plane: Sagittal oblique MR arthrogram or MR with joint effusion
- **Biceps tendon, long head**
  - Origin: Superior glenoid labrum
    - May also have origin from supraglenoid tubercle, rotator cuff, joint capsule and coracoid base
  - Courses through superior shoulder joint to intertubercular or bicipital groove
    - Traction zone: Intra-articular, extra-synovial, tendon histology
    - Sliding zone: Contacts humerus, fibrocartilage histology
  - Action: Stabilizes and depresses humeral head
  - Uniform low signal intensity on all sequences

Other
- **Lower rotator interval**
  - Separate entity from the classic rotator interval described above
  - Located between teres minor and subscapularis tendons
  - Instability may disrupt this region
  - Encompasses the axillary sling

Anatomy-Based Imaging Issues

Imaging Recommendations
- MR: Sagittal oblique T2 FS images to accentuate fluid in rotator interval
- **MR arthrography (direct)**
  - **Best imaging study for rotator interval**
  - Sagittal oblique T1 arthrogram
- CT arthrography: May be useful for patients with contraindication to MR

Imaging Pitfalls
- **Synovium and capsule may herniate into interval**
  - Present in asymptomatic shoulders
  - Causes focal fluid signal intensity
  - May simulate tear
- **Iatrogenic disruption of rotator interval**
  - Arthroscopic surgery with probe placed through rotator interval
  - Arthrography using a rotator interval approach

Clinical Implications

Clinical Importance
- Provides passive shoulder stability
- Injury to one structure associated with injuries to other structures within rotator interval
- Rotator interval injury predisposes to additional injuries due to humeral head instability

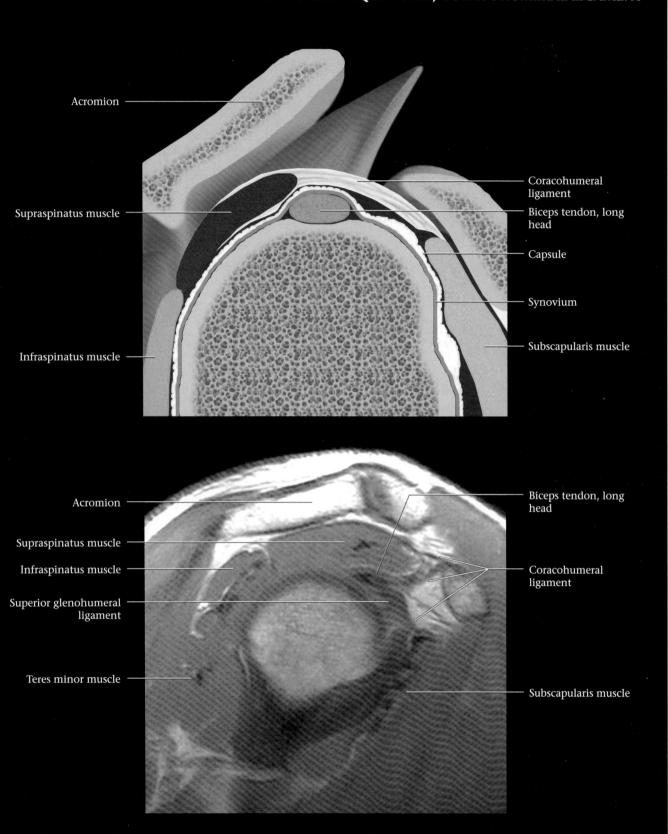

Acromion

Coracohumeral ligament

Supraspinatus muscle

Biceps tendon, long head

Capsule

Synovium

Infraspinatus muscle

Subscapularis muscle

Acromion

Biceps tendon, long head

Supraspinatus muscle

Infraspinatus muscle

Coracohumeral ligament

Superior glenohumeral ligament

Teres minor muscle

Subscapularis muscle

(Top) Relationship of coracohumeral ligament with the rotator cuff muscles. Portions of the CHL pass superficial and deep to the supraspinatus muscle. The CHL attaches to the superior border of the subscapularis muscle. **(Bottom)** Sagittal oblique T1 MR image through the rotator interval of the right shoulder. Portions of the coracohumeral ligament blend with the superficial and deep aspects of the supraspinatus. A portion also blends with the superficial subscapularis. The superior glenohumeral ligament is seen as globular low signal anterior to the long head of the biceps tendon. Without fluid in the joint, the superior glenohumeral ligament can be difficult to differentiate as a separate structure from the coracohumeral ligament.

ROTATOR INTERVAL ANATOMY GRAPHIC

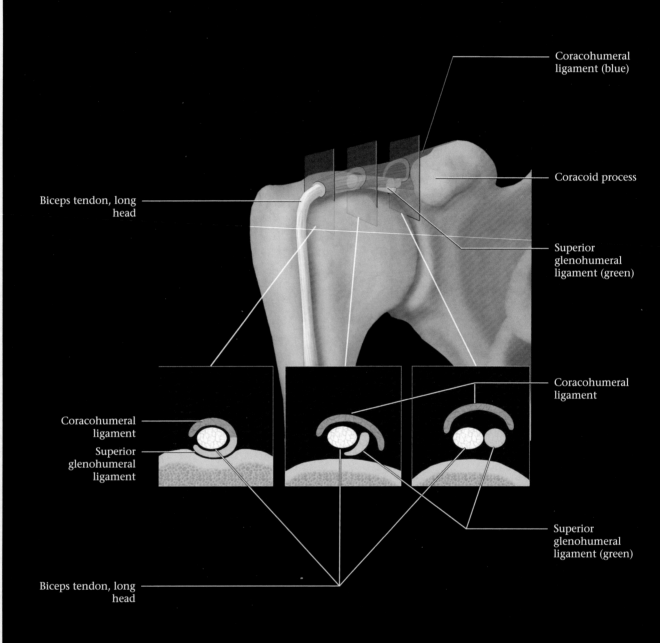

Coracohumeral ligament (blue)

Coracoid process

Biceps tendon, long head

Superior glenohumeral ligament (green)

Coracohumeral ligament

Coracohumeral ligament

Superior glenohumeral ligament

Superior glenohumeral ligament (green)

Biceps tendon, long head

Normal rotator interval anatomy graphic. Cross section images at the lateral, mid and medial portions of the rotator interval are located along the bottom of the image. At the lateral aspect of the rotator interval, just proximal to the entrance to the bicipital groove, the coracohumeral ligament (blue) and superior glenohumeral ligament (green) form a sling around the long head of the biceps tendon. At the mid portion of the rotator interval, the CHL covers the superior aspect of the LBT, with the SGHL forming a T-shaped junction with the CHL. Near the medial border of the rotator interval, the SGHL is a round structure lying anterior to the LBT. The CHL forms a U-shaped roof over the LBT and SGHL. (Graphic modified from OP Krief: MRI of the Rotator Interval Capsule, AJR(2005) 184: 1490).

ROTATOR INTERVAL

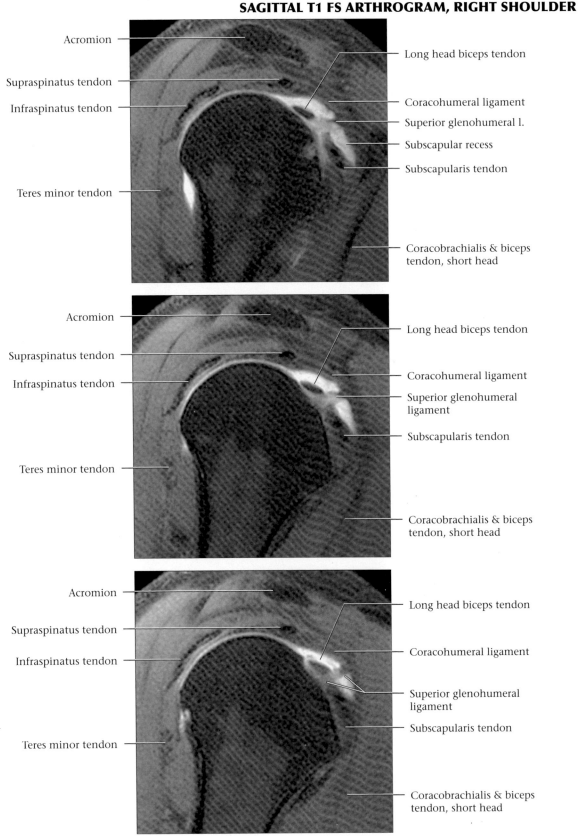

Acromion

Supraspinatus tendon

Infraspinatus tendon

Teres minor tendon

Long head biceps tendon

Coracohumeral ligament

Superior glenohumeral l.

Subscapular recess

Subscapularis tendon

Coracobrachialis & biceps tendon, short head

Acromion

Supraspinatus tendon

Infraspinatus tendon

Teres minor tendon

Long head biceps tendon

Coracohumeral ligament

Superior glenohumeral ligament

Subscapularis tendon

Coracobrachialis & biceps tendon, short head

Acromion

Supraspinatus tendon

Infraspinatus tendon

Teres minor tendon

Long head biceps tendon

Coracohumeral ligament

Superior glenohumeral ligament

Subscapularis tendon

Coracobrachialis & biceps tendon, short head

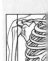

(Top) First of three sagittal oblique T1 FS MR arthrogram images of the right shoulder. Images are displayed medial to lateral. The sagittal oblique plane is the optimal plane for evaluating the rotator interval. These images were chosen to match the cross section graphics on the prior page. The coracohumeral ligament forms the roof of the rotator interval on all three images. **(Middle)** The superior glenohumeral ligament has a T-shaped junction with the coracohumeral ligament at the mid portion of the rotator interval. **(Bottom)** At the lateral aspect of the rotator interval, the superior glenohumeral ligament forms the inferior portion of the sling around the long head of the biceps tendon.

ROTATOR INTERVAL

AXIAL T2 MR ARTHROGRAM, ROTATOR INTERVAL

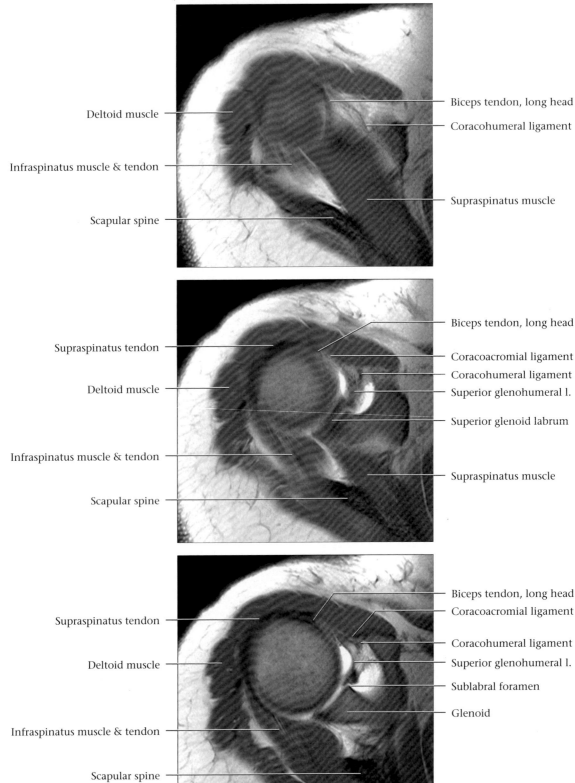

Deltoid muscle

Infraspinatus muscle & tendon

Scapular spine

Biceps tendon, long head

Coracohumeral ligament

Supraspinatus muscle

Supraspinatus tendon

Deltoid muscle

Infraspinatus muscle & tendon

Scapular spine

Biceps tendon, long head

Coracoacromial ligament

Coracohumeral ligament

Superior glenohumeral l.

Superior glenoid labrum

Supraspinatus muscle

Supraspinatus tendon

Deltoid muscle

Infraspinatus muscle & tendon

Scapular spine

Biceps tendon, long head

Coracoacromial ligament

Coracohumeral ligament

Superior glenohumeral l.

Sublabral foramen

Glenoid

(Top) First of three consecutive axial T2 MR arthrogram images through the rotator interval. Axial imaging is not the optimal plane for evaluating the rotator interval, but can be useful. The long head of the biceps tendon is seen traversing the superomedial humeral head. **(Middle)** The superior glenohumeral ligament has a roughly parallel course to the long head of the biceps tendon on axial images. **(Bottom)** The superior glenohumeral ligament fuses with the coracohumeral ligament. These in turn will fuse with the joint capsule and rotator cuff tendons. These images are T2WI and have intra-articular contrast. The fat and bone marrow are near the intensity of a T1WI study due to a relatively short TE.

ROTATOR INTERVAL

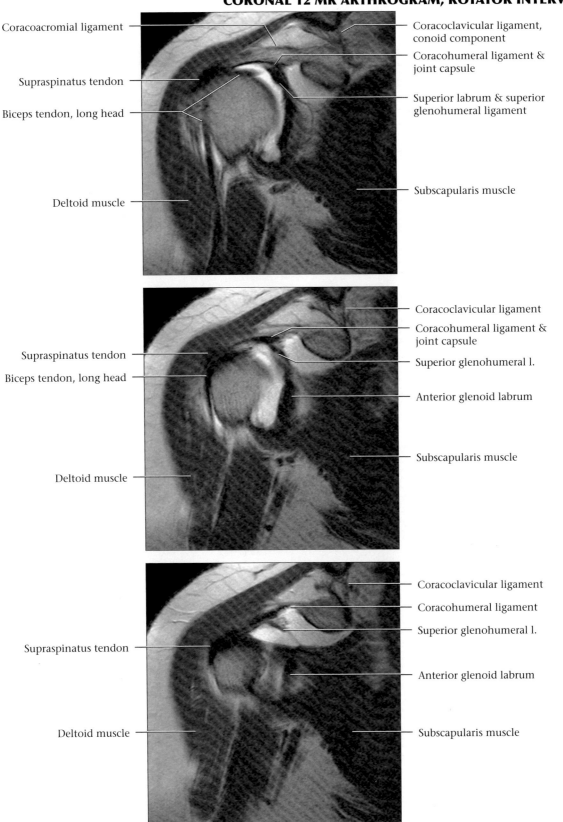

Coracoacromial ligament

Supraspinatus tendon

Biceps tendon, long head

Deltoid muscle

Coracoclavicular ligament, conoid component

Coracohumeral ligament & joint capsule

Superior labrum & superior glenohumeral ligament

Subscapularis muscle

Supraspinatus tendon

Biceps tendon, long head

Deltoid muscle

Coracoclavicular ligament

Coracohumeral ligament & joint capsule

Superior glenohumeral l.

Anterior glenoid labrum

Subscapularis muscle

Supraspinatus tendon

Deltoid muscle

Coracoclavicular ligament

Coracohumeral ligament

Superior glenohumeral l.

Anterior glenoid labrum

Subscapularis muscle

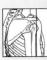
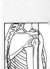

(Top) First of three consecutive coronal oblique T2 MR images through the rotator interval. Images are displayed posterior to anterior. The rotator interval is best evaluated in the sagittal oblique plane. **(Middle)** The long head of the biceps tendon is exiting the rotator interval as it enters the bicipital groove. **(Bottom)** In any plane, it may be difficult to separate the superior glenohumeral ligament, coracohumeral ligament, joint capsule and rotator cuff tendons, especially at the anterolateral aspect of the rotator interval.

Shoulder

I

SAGITTAL T1 FS MR ARTHROGRAM, RIGHT SHOULDER

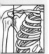

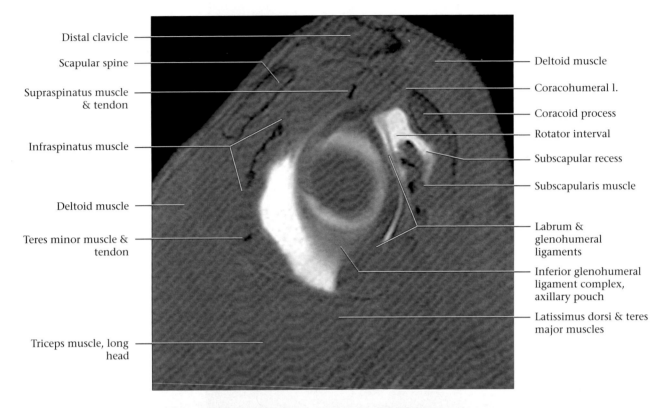

Distal clavicle

Scapular spine

Supraspinatus muscle & tendon

Infraspinatus muscle

Deltoid muscle

Teres minor muscle & tendon

Triceps muscle, long head

Deltoid muscle

Coracohumeral l.

Coracoid process

Rotator interval

Subscapular recess

Subscapularis muscle

Labrum & glenohumeral ligaments

Inferior glenohumeral ligament complex, axillary pouch

Latissimus dorsi & teres major muscles

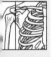

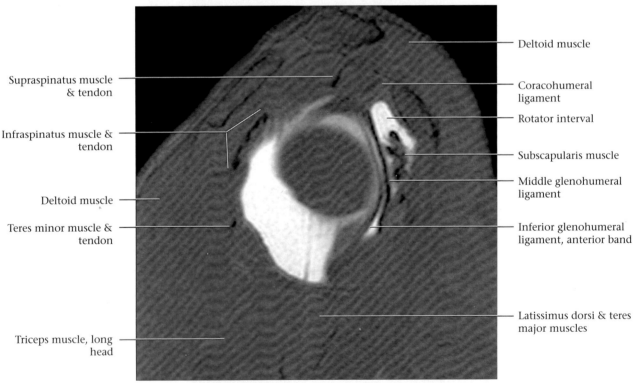

Supraspinatus muscle & tendon

Infraspinatus muscle & tendon

Deltoid muscle

Teres minor muscle & tendon

Triceps muscle, long head

Deltoid muscle

Coracohumeral ligament

Rotator interval

Subscapularis muscle

Middle glenohumeral ligament

Inferior glenohumeral ligament, anterior band

Latissimus dorsi & teres major muscles

(Top) First of twelve sagittal oblique T1 FS MR arthrogram images of the right shoulder displayed medial to lateral. Images were acquired at 1.5 T with a shoulder coil. This image is through the level of the glenohumeral joint. The glenoid labrum forms an oval low signal band around the medial aspect of the humeral head. (Bottom) The rotator interval is the space between the supraspinatus and subscapularis tendons. The medial extent is the coracoid process.

ROTATOR INTERVAL

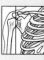

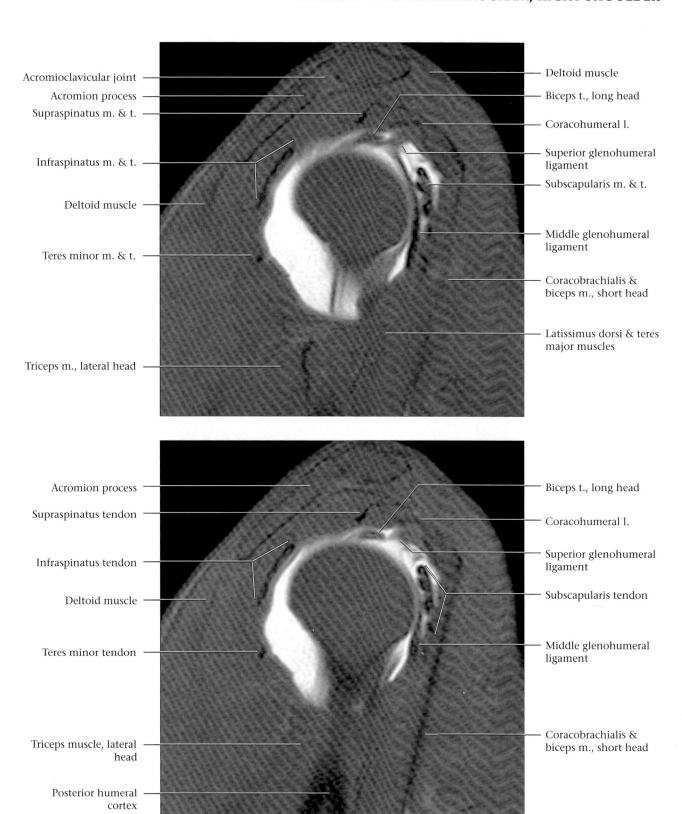

Acromioclavicular joint

Acromion process

Supraspinatus m. & t.

Infraspinatus m. & t.

Deltoid muscle

Teres minor m. & t.

Triceps m., lateral head

Deltoid muscle

Biceps t., long head

Coracohumeral l.

Superior glenohumeral ligament

Subscapularis m. & t.

Middle glenohumeral ligament

Coracobrachialis & biceps m., short head

Latissimus dorsi & teres major muscles

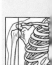

Acromion process

Supraspinatus tendon

Infraspinatus tendon

Deltoid muscle

Teres minor tendon

Triceps muscle, lateral head

Posterior humeral cortex

Biceps t., long head

Coracohumeral l.

Superior glenohumeral ligament

Subscapularis tendon

Middle glenohumeral ligament

Coracobrachialis & biceps m., short head

(Top) The superior glenohumeral ligament has a T-shaped connection with the coracohumeral ligament at this level. **(Bottom)** The coracohumeral ligament forms the roof of the rotator interval. Portions of the coracohumeral ligament fuse with the joint capsule, supraspinatus tendon and subscapularis tendons. Note that at this level the coracohumeral ligament extends to the articular surface of supraspinatus and is medial to the origin of the more superficial coracoacromial ligament (shown on the next lateral image).

Shoulder

I

97

SAGITTAL T1 FS MR ARTHROGRAM, RIGHT SHOULDER

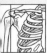

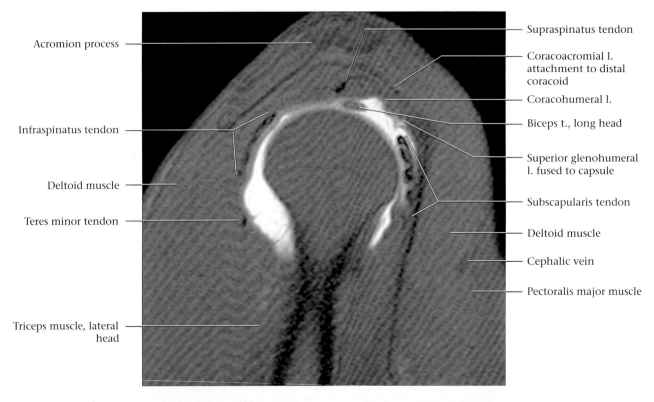

Acromion process

Infraspinatus tendon

Deltoid muscle

Teres minor tendon

Triceps muscle, lateral head

Supraspinatus tendon

Coracoacromial l. attachment to distal coracoid

Coracohumeral l.

Biceps t., long head

Superior glenohumeral l. fused to capsule

Subscapularis tendon

Deltoid muscle

Cephalic vein

Pectoralis major muscle

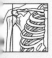

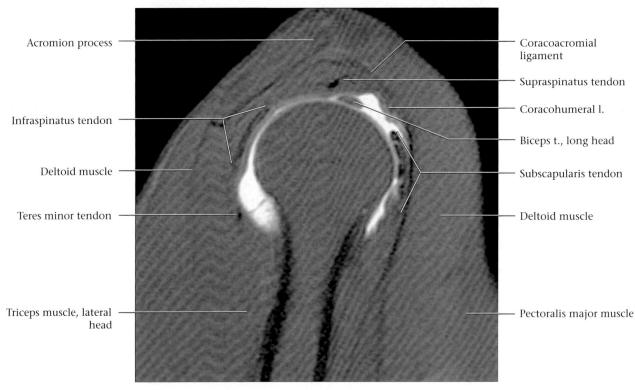

Acromion process

Infraspinatus tendon

Deltoid muscle

Teres minor tendon

Triceps muscle, lateral head

Coracoacromial ligament

Supraspinatus tendon

Coracohumeral l.

Biceps t., long head

Subscapularis tendon

Deltoid muscle

Pectoralis major muscle

(Top) The long head of the biceps tendon courses over the top of the humeral head. **(Bottom)** The floor of the rotator interval is the humeral head cartilage.

SAGITTAL T1 FS MR ARTHROGRAM, RIGHT SHOULDER

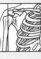

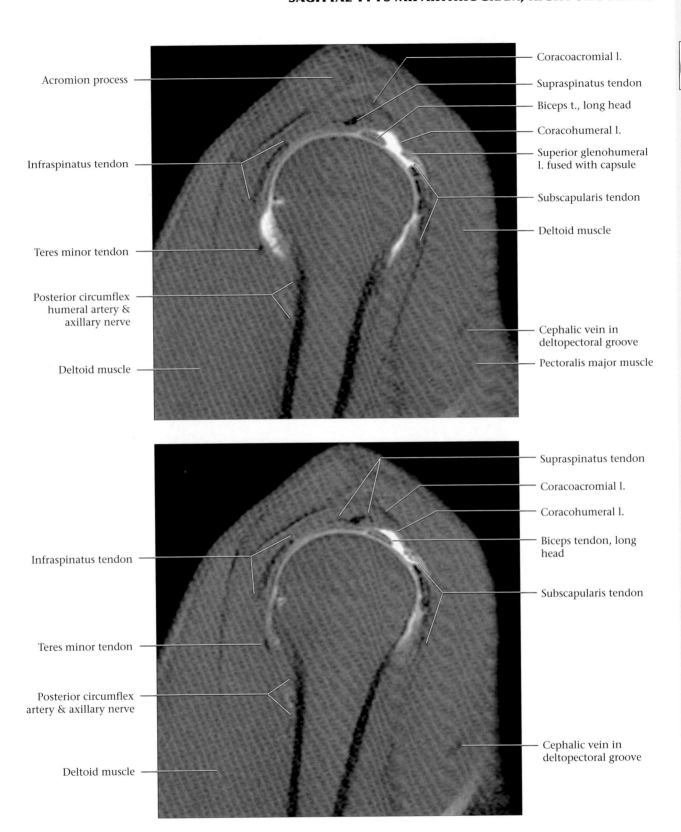

Acromion process

Coracoacromial l.

Supraspinatus tendon

Biceps t., long head

Coracohumeral l.

Superior glenohumeral l. fused with capsule

Infraspinatus tendon

Subscapularis tendon

Deltoid muscle

Teres minor tendon

Posterior circumflex humeral artery & axillary nerve

Cephalic vein in deltopectoral groove

Pectoralis major muscle

Deltoid muscle

Supraspinatus tendon

Coracoacromial l.

Coracohumeral l.

Infraspinatus tendon

Biceps tendon, long head

Subscapularis tendon

Teres minor tendon

Posterior circumflex artery & axillary nerve

Cephalic vein in deltopectoral groove

Deltoid muscle

(Top) The rotator cuff becomes progressively tendinous as it extends laterally. **(Bottom)** The cuff tendons will fuse with the joint capsule, as will the coracohumeral ligament. The coracohumeral ligament will span the rotator interval roof to fill the space between the supraspinatus and subscapularis tendons. The coracohumeral ligament will not be distinguishable from the rotator cuff tendons or joint capsule when it fuses.

ROTATOR INTERVAL

SAGITTAL T1 FS MR ARTHROGRAM, RIGHT SHOULDER

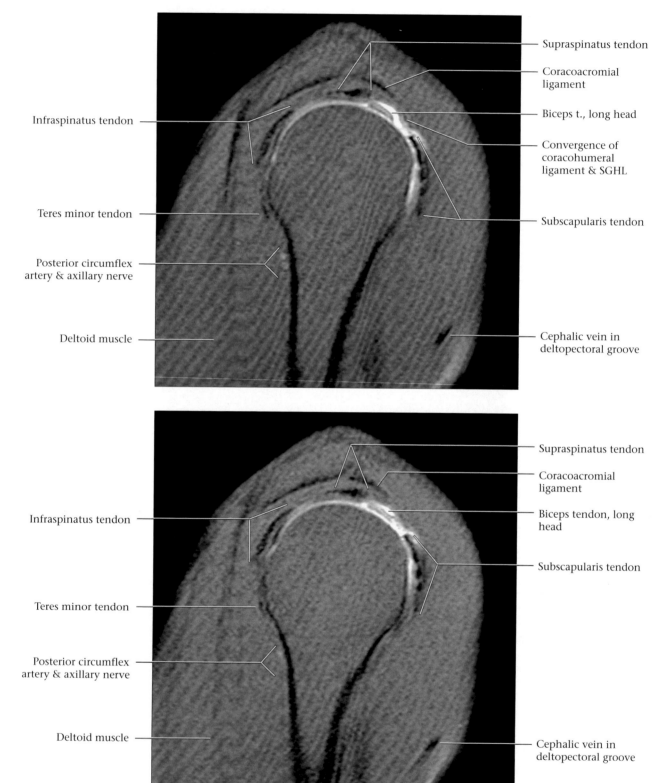

Top image labels:
- Supraspinatus tendon
- Coracoacromial ligament
- Biceps t., long head
- Convergence of coracohumeral ligament & SGHL
- Subscapularis tendon
- Cephalic vein in deltopectoral groove
- Infraspinatus tendon
- Teres minor tendon
- Posterior circumflex artery & axillary nerve
- Deltoid muscle

Bottom image labels:
- Supraspinatus tendon
- Coracoacromial ligament
- Biceps tendon, long head
- Subscapularis tendon
- Cephalic vein in deltopectoral groove
- Infraspinatus tendon
- Teres minor tendon
- Posterior circumflex artery & axillary nerve
- Deltoid muscle

(Top) The long head of the biceps tendon is nearing the entrance into the bicipital groove. The coracohumeral ligament and superior glenohumeral ligament can be difficult to appreciate but are within the globular soft tissue anterior to the biceps tendon. **(Bottom)** The cotacohumeral ligament and superior glenohumeral ligament provide support to the long head of the biceps tendon.

ROTATOR INTERVAL

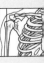

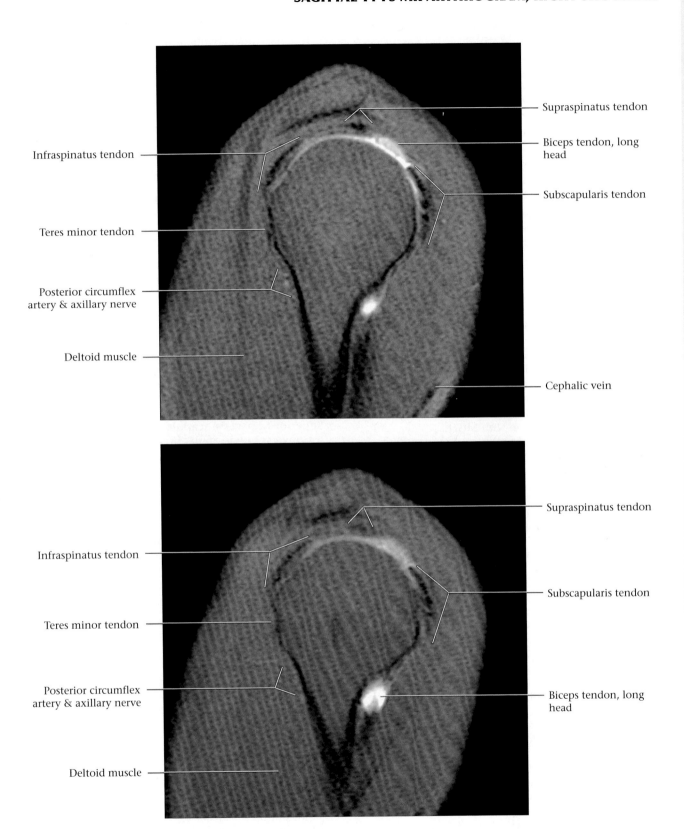

Supraspinatus tendon

Biceps tendon, long head

Infraspinatus tendon

Subscapularis tendon

Teres minor tendon

Posterior circumflex artery & axillary nerve

Deltoid muscle

Cephalic vein

Supraspinatus tendon

Infraspinatus tendon

Subscapularis tendon

Teres minor tendon

Posterior circumflex artery & axillary nerve

Biceps tendon, long head

Deltoid muscle

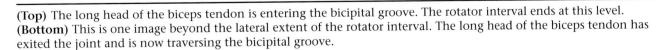

(Top) The long head of the biceps tendon is entering the bicipital groove. The rotator interval ends at this level. **(Bottom)** This is one image beyond the lateral extent of the rotator interval. The long head of the biceps tendon has exited the joint and is now traversing the bicipital groove.

LIGAMENTS

Terminology

Abbreviations
- Acromioclavicular (AC)
- Coracohumeral (CH)
- Superior glenohumeral ligament (SGHL)
- Middle glenohumeral ligament (MGHL)
- Inferior glenohumeral ligament (IGHL)

Imaging Anatomy

Anatomy Relationships
- **Glenohumeral ligaments**
  - Strengthen and fuse with joint capsule
  - **Presence of true ligaments debated**
    - May represent folds in joint capsule
    - Termed glenolabral periarticular fiber complex
  - **Vary in number and size**
    - Type I: Classic three ligaments (SGHL, MGHL, IGHL)
    - Type II: MGHL cord, pseudo-Buford
    - Type III: Combined MGHL/IGHL cord, pseudo-Buford
    - Type IV: No ligaments
  - **Superior glenohumeral ligament**
    - Stabilizes shoulder in adduction
    - May originate from biceps tendon, anterior labrum, or in common with MGHL
    - Extends to lesser tuberosity
    - Fuses with coracohumeral ligament
    - Transverse orientation
    - Gentle curving shape on axial images at level of superior coracoid process
    - Almost always anatomically present
    - Visible on 30% conventional MR, 85% MR arthrograms
  - **Middle glenohumeral ligament**
    - Stabilizes shoulder in abduction
    - Originates from anterior labrum or scapular neck
    - Extends along deep surface of subscapularis to lesser tuberosity
    - Oblique orientation
    - Blends with joint capsule and labrum anteriorly
    - Absent or small MGHL in 30%
    - May be enlarged and cord-like
    - Buford complex: Thick or cord-like MGHL and absent anterosuperior labrum
    - Can fuse with the anterior band of IGHL
  - **Inferior glenohumeral ligament**
    - Resists anterior dislocation and stabilizes in abduction
    - More accurately termed IGHL complex
    - Anterior band, fascicles of axillary pouch and posterior band
    - Extends from inferior glenoid labrum to inferior humeral anatomic neck
    - Vertical orientation of anterior & posterior bands
    - Anterior band is usually larger than posterior band
- **Coracohumeral ligament**
  - Coracoid process base to greater & lesser tuberosities
  - Horizontal orientation
  - **Forms roof of rotator interval**
    - Stabilizes long head of biceps tendon from subluxing medially into subscapularis
  - Strengthens transverse ligament covering bicipital groove
  - Fuses with supraspinatus tendon, subscapularis tendon, joint capsule and SGHL
- **Coracoacromial ligament**
  - Forms the coracoacromial arch along with acromion and coracoid process
  - Reinforces inferior aspect of acromioclavicular joint
  - Extends from distal two-thirds of coracoid to acromion tip
  - Two conjoined or closely associated bands
  - May have a broad acromial insertion
- **Coracoclavicular ligament**
  - Major stabilizer of acromioclavicular joint
  - Extends from base of coracoid process to undersurface of clavicle
  - Fan-shaped complex with two fasciculi
    - Conoid ligament: Posteromedial, vertical
    - Trapezoid ligament: Anterolateral, oblique
- **Acromioclavicular ligaments**
  - Superior and inferior AC ligaments
  - Reinforce acromioclavicular joint capsule
- **Transverse humeral ligament**
  - Extends between greater and lesser tuberosities
  - Contains fibers from the subscapularis tendon
  - Covers bicipital groove
- **Superior transverse scapular ligament**
  - Converts suprascapular notch into a foramen
  - Suprascapular nerve passes below the ligament
    - Potential for suprascapular nerve entrapment
  - Suprascapular vessels pass above the ligament
- **Inferior transverse scapular ligament**
  - Extends from scapular spine to glenoid rim
  - Lateral to spinoglenoid notch
  - Subscapular nerve passes beneath the ligament
  - Inconsistently present

Anatomy-Based Imaging Issues

Imaging Recommendations
- MR: Ligaments have low signal intensity on all imaging sequences
- **MR arthrography**
  - **Best imaging study for glenohumeral ligaments**
    - Sagittal oblique for MGHL and IGHL
    - Axial for SGHL and MGHL

Imaging Pitfalls
- **Subacromial pseudospur**
  - **Coracoacromial ligament hypertrophy**
    - Located at insertion on acromion
  - **Hypertrophied deltoid muscle inferior tendon slip**
  - Can simulate a subacromial enthesophyte
  - On T1 MR, mature osteophytes should demonstrate fatty bone marrow
  - Sclerotic or immature osteophytes may not have marrow fat, so compare with radiographs
- **MGHL origin from scapular neck** (uncommon)
  - May simulate stripping of anterior capsule

LIGAMENTS

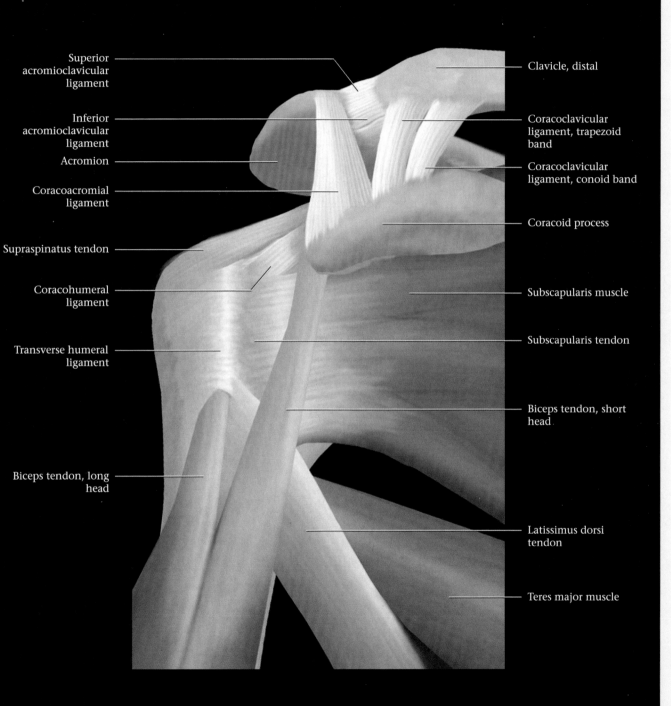

Superior acromioclavicular ligament

Inferior acromioclavicular ligament

Acromion

Coracoacromial ligament

Supraspinatus tendon

Coracohumeral ligament

Transverse humeral ligament

Biceps tendon, long head

Clavicle, distal

Coracoclavicular ligament, trapezoid band

Coracoclavicular ligament, conoid band

Coracoid process

Subscapularis muscle

Subscapularis tendon

Biceps tendon, short head

Latissimus dorsi tendon

Teres major muscle

Anterior lordotic graphic of the shoulder, superficial dissection.

ANTERIOR & SAGITTAL GRAPHICS, GLENOHUMERAL LIGAMENTS

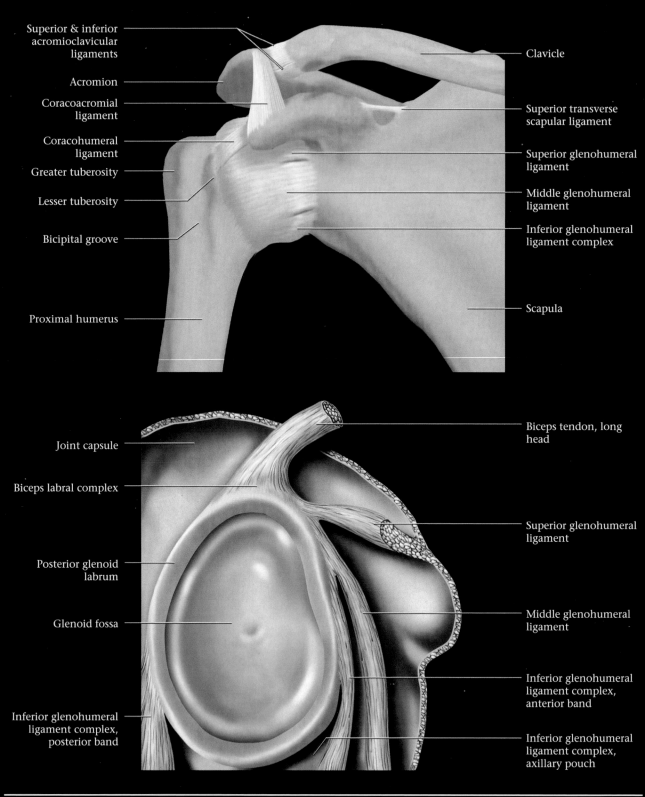

Superior & inferior acromioclavicular ligaments

Acromion

Coracoacromial ligament

Coracohumeral ligament

Greater tuberosity

Lesser tuberosity

Bicipital groove

Proximal humerus

Clavicle

Superior transverse scapular ligament

Superior glenohumeral ligament

Middle glenohumeral ligament

Inferior glenohumeral ligament complex

Scapula

Joint capsule

Biceps labral complex

Posterior glenoid labrum

Glenoid fossa

Inferior glenohumeral ligament complex, posterior band

Biceps tendon, long head

Superior glenohumeral ligament

Middle glenohumeral ligament

Inferior glenohumeral ligament complex, anterior band

Inferior glenohumeral ligament complex, axillary pouch

(Top) Anterior graphic of the right shoulder, deep dissection. The muscles have been removed. **(Bottom)** Sagittal graphic of the intra-articular portion of the shoulder. The humeral head has been removed.

LIGAMENTS

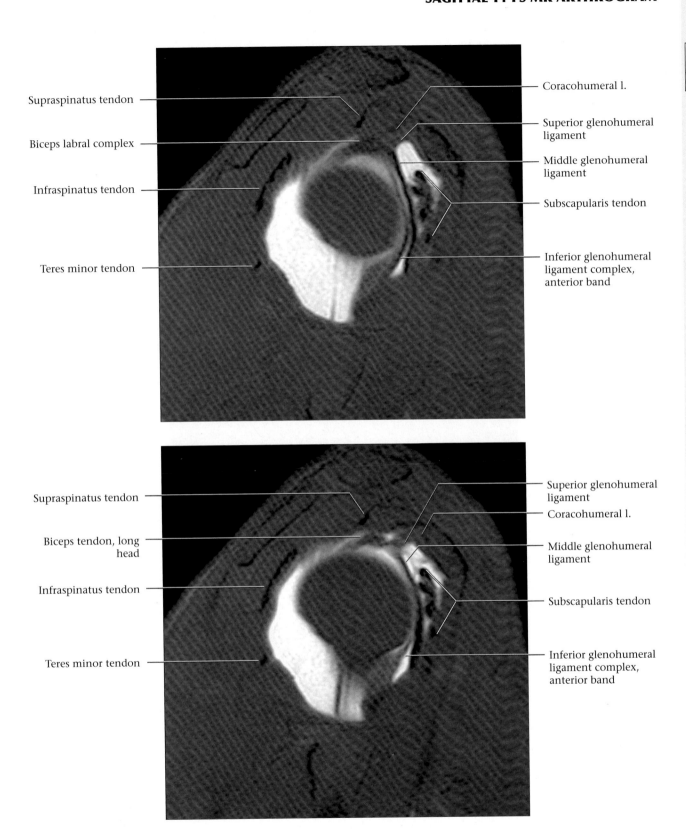
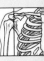
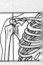

Supraspinatus tendon

Biceps labral complex

Infraspinatus tendon

Teres minor tendon

Coracohumeral l.

Superior glenohumeral ligament

Middle glenohumeral ligament

Subscapularis tendon

Inferior glenohumeral ligament complex, anterior band

Supraspinatus tendon

Biceps tendon, long head

Infraspinatus tendon

Teres minor tendon

Superior glenohumeral ligament

Coracohumeral l.

Middle glenohumeral ligament

Subscapularis tendon

Inferior glenohumeral ligament complex, anterior band

(Top) First of two sequential sagittal oblique T1 FS MR arthrogram images of the right shoulder. Image is through the medial aspect of the humeral head. The middle and inferior glenohumeral ligaments have an oblique to vertical course. (Bottom) This image is located just lateral to the previous image. The superior glenohumeral ligament is the rounded soft tissue density located anterior to the long head of the biceps tendon.

Shoulder

I

AXIAL T1 FS MR ARTHROGRAM, SUPERIOR GLENOHUMERAL LIGAMENT

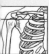

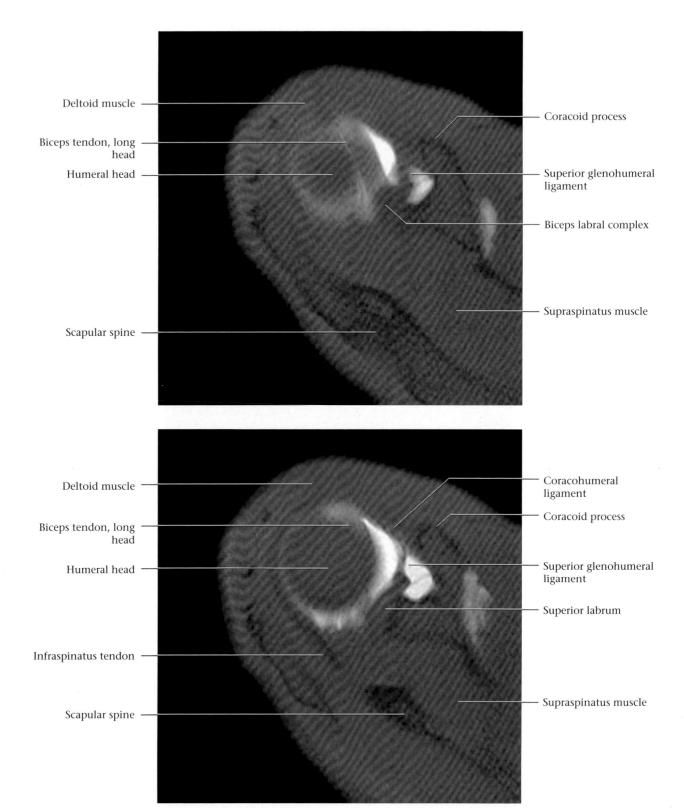

Deltoid muscle

Biceps tendon, long head

Humeral head

Scapular spine

Coracoid process

Superior glenohumeral ligament

Biceps labral complex

Supraspinatus muscle

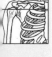

Deltoid muscle

Biceps tendon, long head

Humeral head

Infraspinatus tendon

Scapular spine

Coracohumeral ligament

Coracoid process

Superior glenohumeral ligament

Superior labrum

Supraspinatus muscle

(Top) First of two axial T1 FS MR arthrogram images of the right shoulder. The long head of the biceps tendon has an oblique course across the top of the humeral head. The superior glenohumeral ligament is located medial to the long head of the biceps and has a roughly parallel course on axial images. **(Bottom)** This image is located below the previous image. The biceps tendon is curving along the anterior humeral head toward the bicipital groove. The superior glenohumeral ligament fuses with the coracohumeral ligament anteriorly. These structures in turn fuse with the joint capsule, supraspinatus tendon and subscapularis tendon to form the rotator interval.

LIGAMENTS

AXIAL T1 FS MR & CT ARTHROGRAM, MIDDLE GLENOHUMERAL LIGAMENT

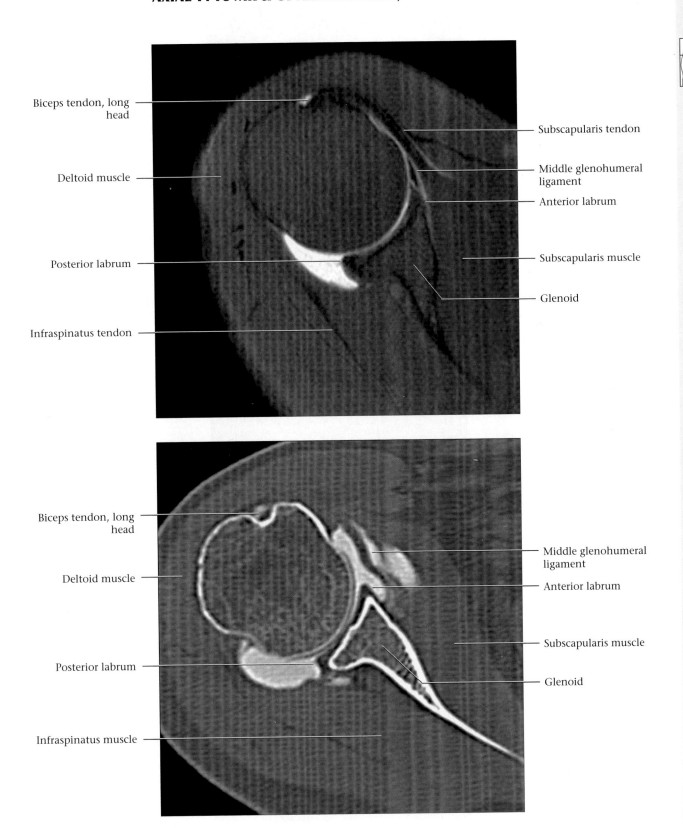

Biceps tendon, long head

Deltoid muscle

Posterior labrum

Infraspinatus tendon

Subscapularis tendon

Middle glenohumeral ligament

Anterior labrum

Subscapularis muscle

Glenoid

Biceps tendon, long head

Deltoid muscle

Posterior labrum

Infraspinatus muscle

Middle glenohumeral ligament

Anterior labrum

Subscapularis muscle

Glenoid

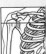

(Top) Axial T1 FS MR arthrogram image. The middle glenohumeral ligament lies anterior to the anterior labrum. (Bottom) Axial CT arthrogram image. The middle glenohumeral ligament is displaced further from the anterior labrum due to better distension of the joint.

LIGAMENTS

AXIAL T1 FS MR ARTHROGRAM, BUFORD COMPLEX

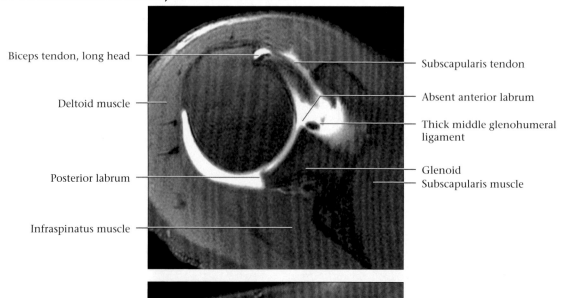

Biceps tendon, long head

Deltoid muscle

Posterior labrum

Infraspinatus muscle

Subscapularis tendon

Absent anterior labrum

Thick middle glenohumeral ligament

Glenoid
Subscapularis muscle

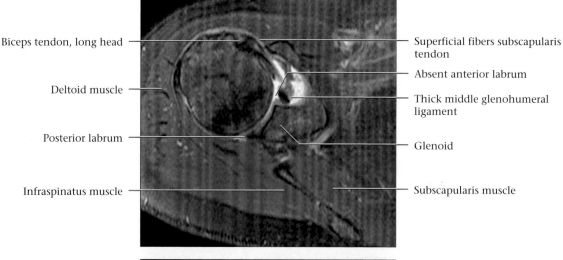

Biceps tendon, long head

Deltoid muscle

Posterior labrum

Infraspinatus muscle

Superficial fibers subscapularis tendon

Absent anterior labrum

Thick middle glenohumeral ligament

Glenoid

Subscapularis muscle

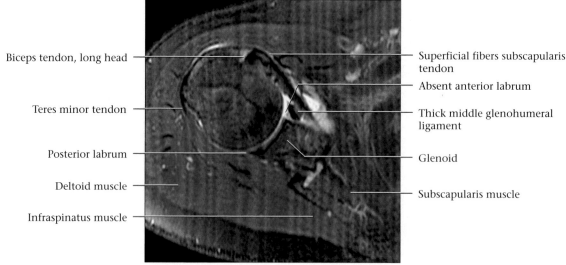

Biceps tendon, long head

Teres minor tendon

Posterior labrum

Deltoid muscle

Infraspinatus muscle

Superficial fibers subscapularis tendon

Absent anterior labrum

Thick middle glenohumeral ligament

Glenoid

Subscapularis muscle

(Top) Axial T1 FS MR arthrogram image of a Buford complex. The middle glenohumeral ligament is thick and cord-like. The anterior glenoid labrum is absent. **(Middle)** First of two sequential axial T1 FS MR arthrogram images of a Buford complex. **(Bottom)** Image is located distal to the previous image. A thick middle glenohumeral ligament is a relatively common normal variant.

LIGAMENTS

SAGITTAL T1 FS MR ARTHROGRAM, VARIANT GHL CONFIGURATION

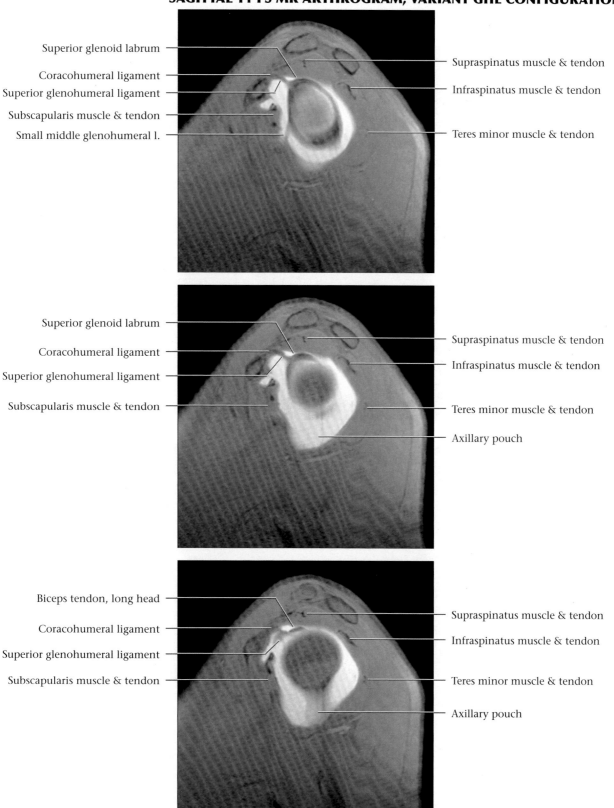

Superior glenoid labrum — Supraspinatus muscle & tendon

Coracohumeral ligament — Infraspinatus muscle & tendon

Superior glenohumeral ligament

Subscapularis muscle & tendon — Teres minor muscle & tendon

Small middle glenohumeral l.

Superior glenoid labrum — Supraspinatus muscle & tendon

Coracohumeral ligament — Infraspinatus muscle & tendon

Superior glenohumeral ligament

Subscapularis muscle & tendon — Teres minor muscle & tendon

— Axillary pouch

Biceps tendon, long head — Supraspinatus muscle & tendon

Coracohumeral ligament — Infraspinatus muscle & tendon

Superior glenohumeral ligament

Subscapularis muscle & tendon — Teres minor muscle & tendon

— Axillary pouch

(**Top**) First of three T1 FS MR arthrogram images of the left shoulder displayed medial to lateral. Glenohumeral ligaments can normally vary in size and presence. The superior and middle glenohumeral ligaments are outlined by contrast in this image. The middle glenohumeral ligament is smaller than is typically seen. (**Middle**) The superior glenohumeral ligament is larger than usual and blends with the coracohumeral ligament and joint capsule in this image. These structures will also fuse with the supraspinatus and subscapularis tendons as they extend laterally. (**Bottom**) Anterior and posterior bands of the inferior glenohumeral ligament complex are absent. Fascicles of the axillary pouch are present.

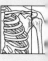

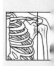

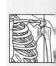

Shoulder

LIGAMENTS

SAGITTAL T1 FS MR & CT ARTHROGRAM, INFERIOR GLENOHUMERAL LIGAMENT COMPLEX

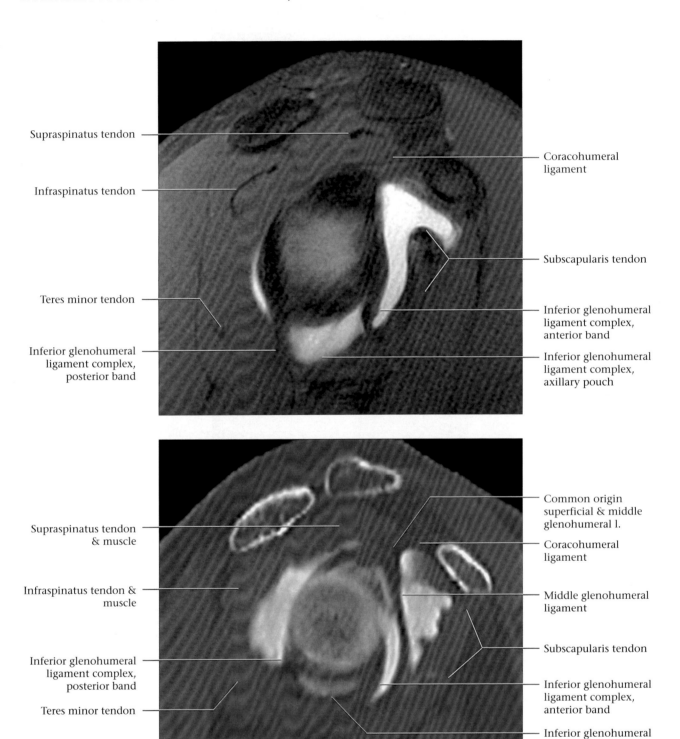

Supraspinatus tendon

Infraspinatus tendon

Teres minor tendon

Inferior glenohumeral ligament complex, posterior band

Coracohumeral ligament

Subscapularis tendon

Inferior glenohumeral ligament complex, anterior band

Inferior glenohumeral ligament complex, axillary pouch

Supraspinatus tendon & muscle

Infraspinatus tendon & muscle

Inferior glenohumeral ligament complex, posterior band

Teres minor tendon

Common origin superficial & middle glenohumeral l.

Coracohumeral ligament

Middle glenohumeral ligament

Subscapularis tendon

Inferior glenohumeral ligament complex, anterior band

Inferior glenohumeral ligament complex, axillary pouch

(Top) Sagittal oblique T1 FS MR arthrogram image of the right shoulder shows the inferior glenohumeral ligament complex. **(Bottom)** Sagittal oblique CT arthrogram image of the right shoulder shows the inferior glenohumeral ligament complex and middle glenohumeral ligament.

LIGAMENTS

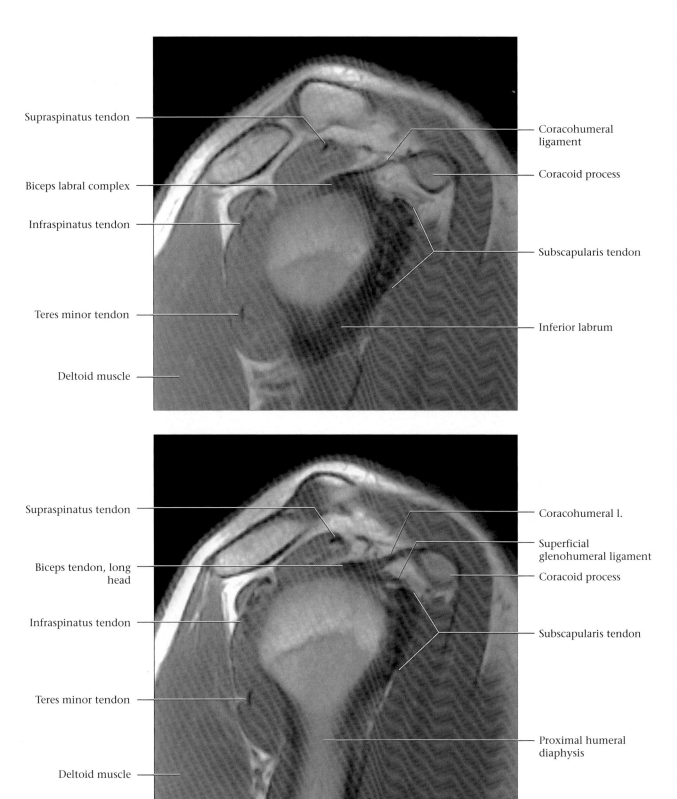

Supraspinatus tendon

Biceps labral complex

Infraspinatus tendon

Teres minor tendon

Deltoid muscle

Coracohumeral ligament

Coracoid process

Subscapularis tendon

Inferior labrum

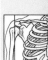

Supraspinatus tendon

Biceps tendon, long head

Infraspinatus tendon

Teres minor tendon

Deltoid muscle

Coracohumeral l.

Superficial glenohumeral ligament

Coracoid process

Subscapularis tendon

Proximal humeral diaphysis

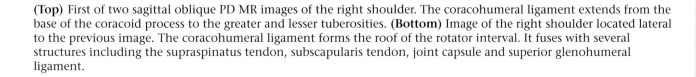

(Top) First of two sagittal oblique PD MR images of the right shoulder. The coracohumeral ligament extends from the base of the coracoid process to the greater and lesser tuberosities. **(Bottom)** Image of the right shoulder located lateral to the previous image. The coracohumeral ligament forms the roof of the rotator interval. It fuses with several structures including the supraspinatus tendon, subscapularis tendon, joint capsule and superior glenohumeral ligament.

AXIAL PD MR, CORACOHUMERAL LIGAMENT

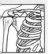

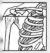

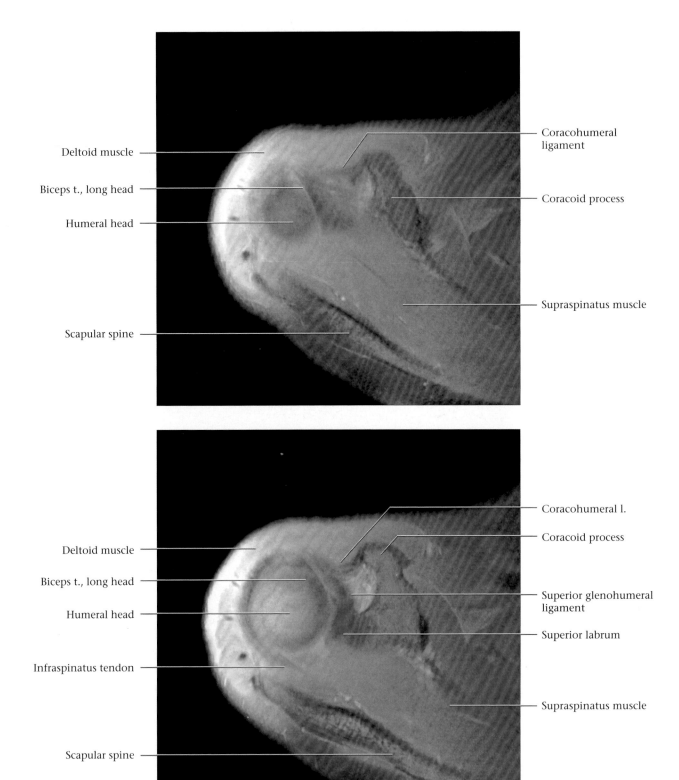

(Top) First of two sequential axial PD MR images of the right shoulder. The coracohumeral ligament arcs between the coracoid process and anterior humeral head. **(Bottom)** This image is located below the previous image. The coracohumeral ligament is fusing with the superior glenohumeral ligament and joint capsule.

LIGAMENTS

CORONAL OBLIQUE PD & T2 MR, CORACOHUMERAL LIGAMENT

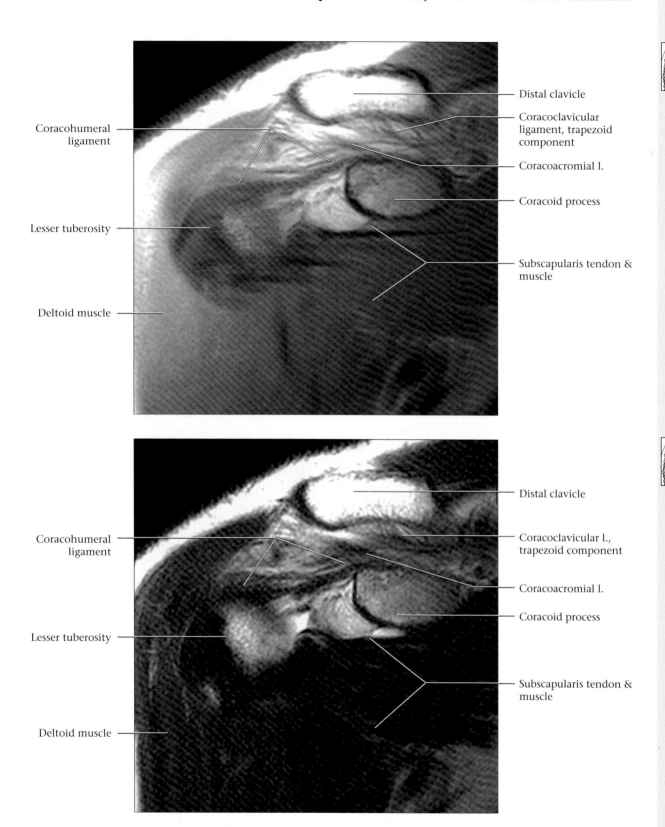

Coracohumeral ligament

Lesser tuberosity

Deltoid muscle

Distal clavicle

Coracoclavicular ligament, trapezoid component

Coracoacromial l.

Coracoid process

Subscapularis tendon & muscle

Coracohumeral ligament

Lesser tuberosity

Deltoid muscle

Distal clavicle

Coracoclavicular l., trapezoid component

Coracoacromial l.

Coracoid process

Subscapularis tendon & muscle

(Top) First of two coronal oblique images through the same level. The coracohumeral ligament has a roughly transverse course on coronal oblique images. **(Bottom)** Coronal T2 MR is through the same level as the previous image. Surrounding fat outlines the coracohumeral ligament. When this ligament fuses with the supraspinatus tendon, subscapularis tendon and joint capsule, the structures cannot be differentiated from each other.

LIGAMENTS

CORONAL OBLIQUE T1 MR, CORACOCLAVICULAR LIGAMENT

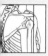

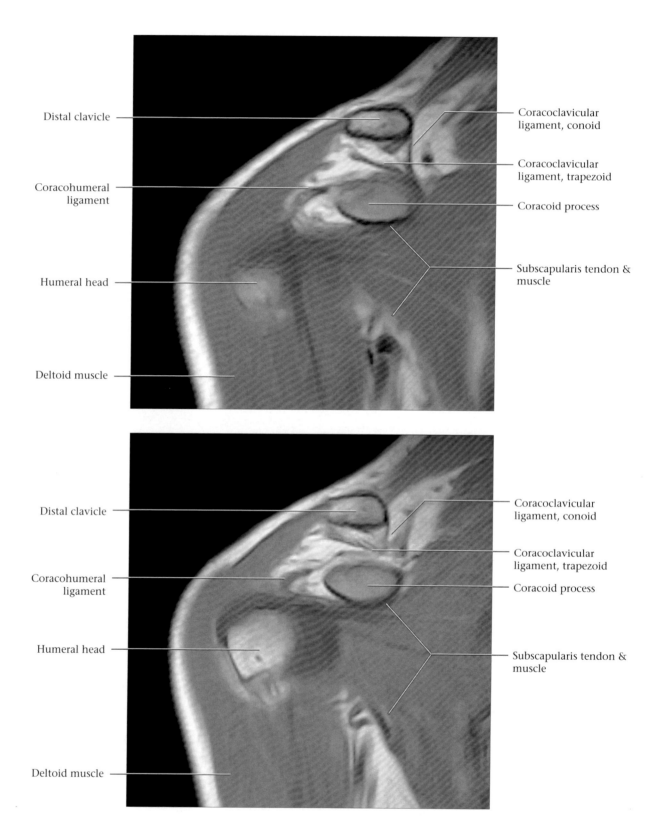

(Top) First of two coronal oblique T1 MR images. The coracoclavicular ligament has two fasciculi, the conoid ligament and the trapezoid ligament. The conoid ligament is located medially and is more vertical in orientation. The trapezoid ligament is more laterally located and has an oblique course. (Bottom) The coracoclavicular ligament extends from the base of the coracoid process to the undersurface of the clavicle. It acts to stabilize the acromioclavicular joint.

LIGAMENTS

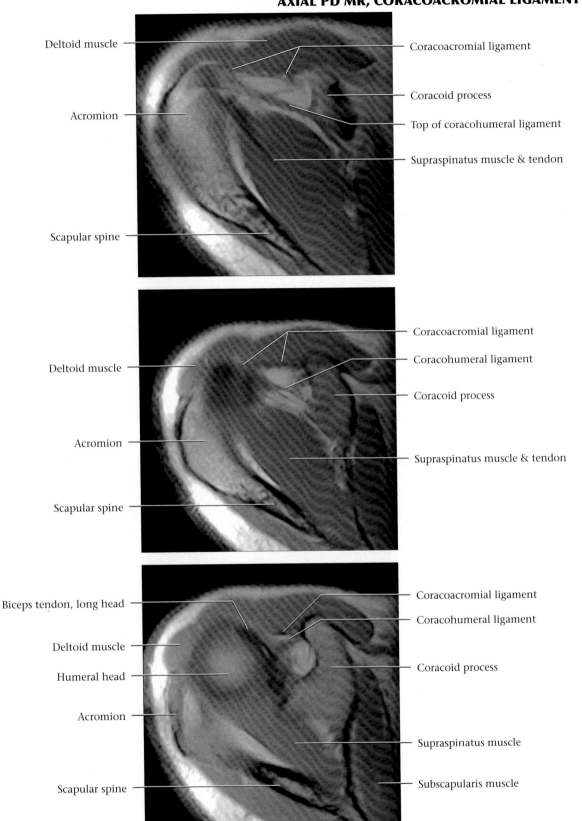

Deltoid muscle — Coracoacromial ligament

Coracoid process

Acromion — Top of coracohumeral ligament

Supraspinatus muscle & tendon

Scapular spine —

Deltoid muscle — Coracoacromial ligament

Coracohumeral ligament

Acromion — Coracoid process

Supraspinatus muscle & tendon

Scapular spine —

Biceps tendon, long head — Coracoacromial ligament

Coracohumeral ligament

Deltoid muscle —

Humeral head — Coracoid process

Acromion —

Supraspinatus muscle

Subscapularis muscle

Scapular spine —

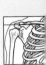

(Top) First of three axial PD MR images of the right shoulder. Image is through the level of the acromion. The coracoacromial ligament extends from the coracoid process to the anterior aspect of the acromion. **(Middle)** Strands of the coracoacromial ligament are visible in this obliquely oriented structure. **(Bottom)** Image is below the level of the coracoacromial ligament. The coracohumeral ligament is becoming visible.

Shoulder

I

115

LIGAMENTS

CORONAL OBLIQUE T1 MR, ACROMIOCLAVICULAR LIGAMENTS

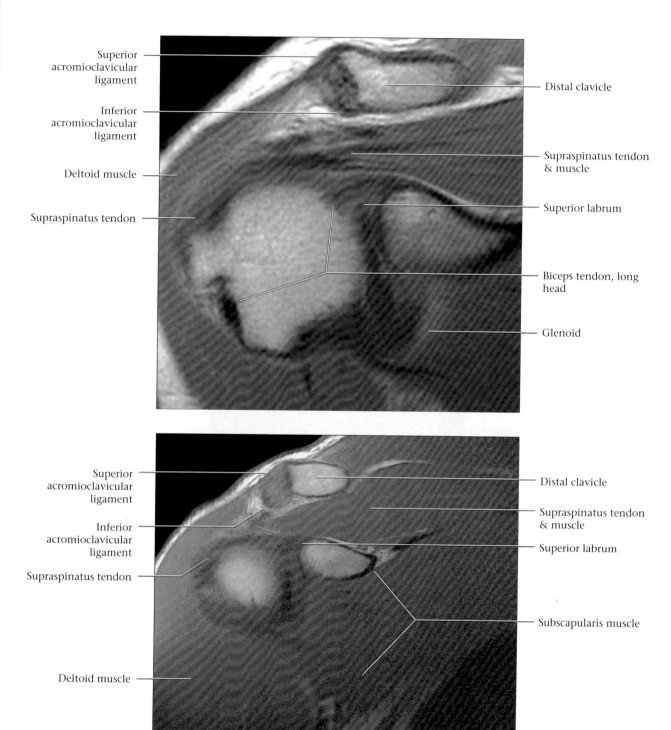

Superior acromioclavicular ligament — Distal clavicle

Inferior acromioclavicular ligament

Deltoid muscle — Supraspinatus tendon & muscle

Supraspinatus tendon — Superior labrum

Biceps tendon, long head

Glenoid

Superior acromioclavicular ligament — Distal clavicle

Inferior acromioclavicular ligament — Supraspinatus tendon & muscle

Supraspinatus tendon — Superior labrum

Deltoid muscle — Subscapularis muscle

(Top) Coronal oblique T1 MR image through the anterior right shoulder. Superior and inferior ligaments reinforce the acromioclavicular joint. **(Bottom)** Coronal oblique T1 MR image in a different patient from previous image shows the superior and inferior acromioclavicular ligaments.

Shoulder

LIGAMENTS

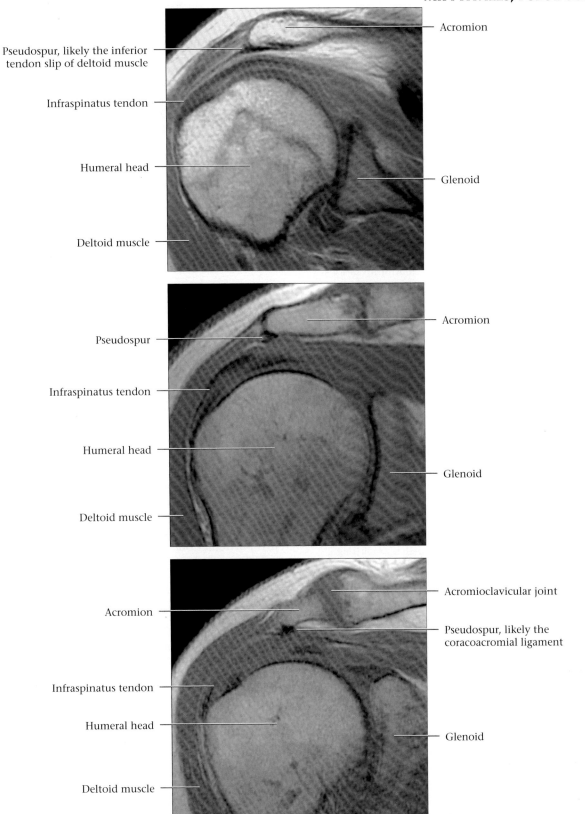

Pseudospur, likely the inferior tendon slip of deltoid muscle

Infraspinatus tendon

Humeral head

Deltoid muscle

Acromion

Glenoid

Pseudospur

Infraspinatus tendon

Humeral head

Deltoid muscle

Acromion

Glenoid

Acromion

Infraspinatus tendon

Humeral head

Deltoid muscle

Acromioclavicular joint

Pseudospur, likely the coracoacromial ligament

Glenoid

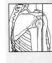
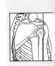

(Top) First of three coronal oblique T1 MR images of the right shoulder in three different patients with subacromial pseudospurs. None of the patients had a bony spur on radiographs. The low signal subacromial pseudospur in this patient is oriented laterally and likely represents a the inferior tendon slip of the deltoid muscle. (Middle) In this patient, the low signal subacromial pseudospur is globular. It could be due to hypertrophy of the inferior tendon slip of the deltoid muscle or the coracoacromial ligament. (Bottom) In this patient, the low signal subacromial pseudospur is oriented medially. It is likely due to coracoacromial ligament hypertrophy.

Shoulder

I

117

LABRUM

Terminology

Abbreviations
- Biceps labral complex (BLC)

Imaging Anatomy

Overview
- **Glenoid labrum consists of hyaline cartilage, fibrocartilage and fibrous tissue**
  - Increases joint circumference and depth
  - Increases surface area and surface contact
  - Approximately 4 mm wide
  - Provides increased rotational stability
- **Variable size, shape and signal intensity**
  - Classic triangle or wedge shape on axial imaging is present in less than 50% of normal anterior labra and less than 80% of posterior labra
  - Normal shapes include round, blunted, crescentic, flat, notched and cleaved
  - May be small or absent anteriorly
  - Not always symmetric anterior to posterior
  - Can vary in signal intensity due to mucinous and myxoid contents
- **Portions of labrum described as positions on face of clock** (either shoulder)
  - 12:00: Superior
  - 3:00: Anterior
  - 6:00: Inferior
  - 9:00: Posterior
- Blood supply via periosteal and capsular vessels

Anatomy Relationships
- **Labral attachment types**
  - Type A: Detached free edge overlying glenoid articular cartilage (meniscoid)
  - Type B: Adherent to the glenoid articular cartilage
- **Biceps labral complex**
  - Biceps tendon attachment to labrum
  - Type 1 BLC: Firmly adherent to glenoid and superior labrum, slab type
  - Type 2 BLC: Small sulcus between biceps/labrum and glenoid, may be continuous with sublabral foramen, intermediate type
  - Type 3 BLC: Large sulcus between biceps/labrum and glenoid, labrum often continues as sublabral foramen, meniscoid type
- **Buford complex**
  - Diminutive or absent anterosuperior labrum
  - Thick or cord-like middle glenohumeral ligament
  - Present in 1-6.5% population
  - Pseudo-Buford appearance can occur when middle and inferior glenohumeral ligaments are combined
- **Superior sublabral recess (sulcus)**
  - Located along superior labrum
    - 1-2 mm in thickness along the full anterior to posterior extent
    - Does not extend posterior to biceps tendon
  - Fluid may extend into recess simulating tear
    - Medial or vertical orientation of fluid between base of labrum & cartilaginous margin of glenoid rim suggests recess

- Laterally angulated, irregular fluid cleft distal to glenolabral attachment suggests tear
  - May be continuous with sublabral foramen
- **Sublabral foramen (hole)**
  - Present in 8-18% population
  - Anterosuperior quadrant of labrum only
  - Can mimic tear if filled with fluid or contrast
  - Foramen is smooth and tapered
  - Tears are irregular and displace labrum away from glenoid when filled with fluid
- **Sublabral foramen with sulcus between biceps tendon and superior labrum**
  - "Double oreo cookie" sign on coronal oblique MR
  - Glenoid cortex (black) + sublabral recess (white) + labrum (black) + biceps/superior labrum sulcus (white) + biceps tendon (black)
  - Similar appearance can be seen with superior labral tear instead of biceps/superior labrum sulcus

Anatomy-Based Imaging Issues

Imaging Recommendations
- **MR arthrography (direct)**
  - Coronal oblique plane best demonstrates biceps labral complex
  - Fibrocartilaginous labrum outlined by contrast
- CT arthrography can be useful in patients with contraindication to MR

Imaging Pitfalls
- **Variant anatomy**
  - Many normal variants of labral anatomy can be confused with pathology
  - Most normal variants occur at 11:00-3:00 position
- **Magic angle artifact**
  - Anteroinferior and posterosuperior labrum
- **Intra-articular biceps tendon dislocation**
  - Dislocated tendon lies adjacent to labrum
  - May simulate tear
- **Hyaline cartilage undercutting**
  - Cartilage lying beneath labrum may simulate tear
  - Cartilage signal intensity is higher than fibrous labrum
  - Differentiate by smooth, even character of cartilage
    - Tears tend to be irregular
  - Cartilage does not extend through to opposite labral surface
- **Confusion with middle glenohumeral ligament**
  - On axial images, middle glenohumeral ligament lies adjacent to anterior labrum
    - May appear to be fragment of anterior labrum
  - Crescent of fluid between labrum and middle glenohumeral ligament can simulate tear
  - A "pseudo-sublabral foramen" appearance may occur when oblique sagittal images are improperly oriented
  - Follow oblique course of middle glenohumeral ligament on consecutive images to confirm that it is a separate structure from labrum
  - Confirm normal signal in the underlying labrum
- **Volume averaging with contrast in sublabral foramen on MR arthrogram may simulate tear**

SAGITTAL GRAPHIC, NORMAL LABRUM

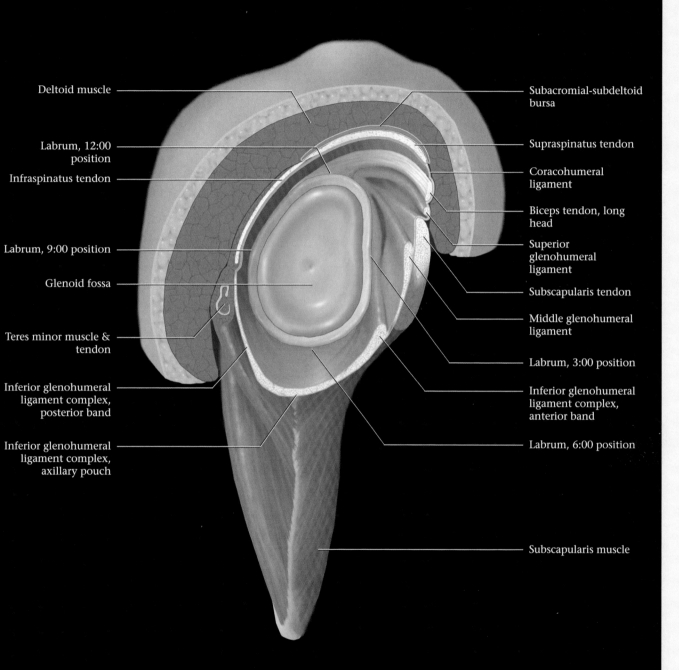

Deltoid muscle

Labrum, 12:00 position

Infraspinatus tendon

Labrum, 9:00 position

Glenoid fossa

Teres minor muscle & tendon

Inferior glenohumeral ligament complex, posterior band

Inferior glenohumeral ligament complex, axillary pouch

Subacromial-subdeltoid bursa

Supraspinatus tendon

Coracohumeral ligament

Biceps tendon, long head

Superior glenohumeral ligament

Subscapularis tendon

Middle glenohumeral ligament

Labrum, 3:00 position

Inferior glenohumeral ligament complex, anterior band

Labrum, 6:00 position

Subscapularis muscle

Sagittal graphic of the glenoid fossa. The labrum lines the edge of the glenoid, increasing the circumference and depth of the shoulder joint.

SAGITTAL GRAPHICS, LABRAL VARIANTS

Deltoid muscle

Infraspinatus tendon

Glenoid labrum

Glenoid

Sublabral foramen

Teres minor muscle & tendon

Inferior glenohumeral ligament complex, posterior band

Inferior glenohumeral ligament complex, axillary pouch

Subacromial-subdeltoid bursa

Supraspinatus tendon

Biceps t., long head

Superior glenohumeral ligament

Subscapularis tendon

Middle glenohumeral ligament

Inferior glenohumeral ligament complex, anterior band

Subscapularis muscle

Deltoid muscle

Absent superior labrum

Infraspinatus tendon

Glenoid labrum

Glenoid

Teres minor muscle & tendon

Inferior glenohumeral ligament complex, posterior band

Inferior glenohumeral ligament complex, axillary pouch

Subacromial-subdeltoid bursa

Supraspinatus tendon

Biceps tendon, long head

Superior glenohumeral ligament

Subscapularis tendon

Middle glenohumeral ligament, thick

Inferior glenohumeral ligament complex, anterior band

Subscapularis muscle

(Top) Sagittal graphic shows a sublabral foramen. The anterior superior labrum is not firmly adherent to the glenoid. (Bottom) Sagittal graphic shows a Buford complex. The anterior superior glenoid labrum is absent. The middle glenohumeral ligament is enlarged and cord-like.

LABRUM

AXIAL & SAGITTAL T1 MR ARTHROGRAM, BUFORD COMPLEX

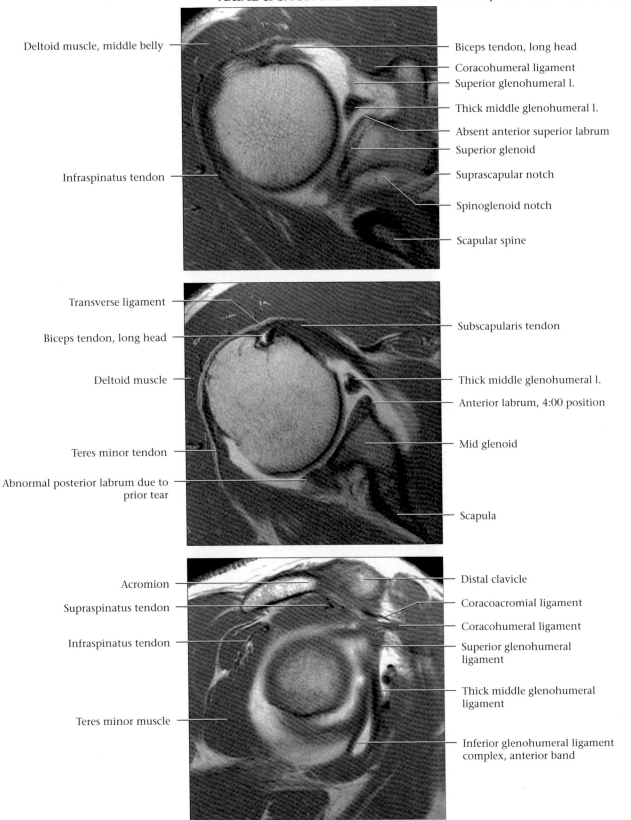

(Top) First of two non-sequential axial T1 MR arthrogram images of the right shoulder with Buford complex normal variant. The anterior superior glenoid labrum is absent. The middle glenohumeral ligament is thickened. The posterior labrum has abnormal size and shape due to a tear. This is unrelated to the Buford complex. **(Middle)** Image at the mid-glenoid level. The middle glenohumeral ligament is still thick and cord-like. Labral tissue has reappeared anteriorly. **(Bottom)** Sagittal oblique T1 MR arthrogram image of the same patient in previous images. The middle glenohumeral ligament is enlarged.

LABRUM

SAGITTAL OBLIQUE T1 FS MR ARTHROGRAM, NORMAL LABRUM

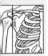

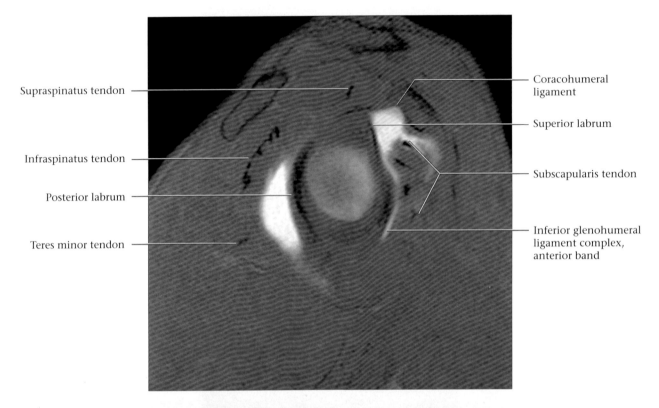

Supraspinatus tendon

Infraspinatus tendon

Posterior labrum

Teres minor tendon

Coracohumeral ligament

Superior labrum

Subscapularis tendon

Inferior glenohumeral ligament complex, anterior band

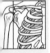

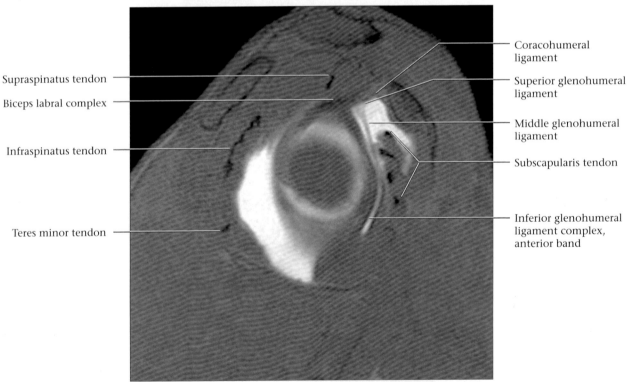

Supraspinatus tendon

Biceps labral complex

Infraspinatus tendon

Teres minor tendon

Coracohumeral ligament

Superior glenohumeral ligament

Middle glenohumeral ligament

Subscapularis tendon

Inferior glenohumeral ligament complex, anterior band

(Top) First of two sagittal oblique T1 FS MR arthrogram images of the right shoulder. This image through the glenohumeral joint. The labrum is a low signal, pear-shaped structure lining the edge of the glenoid fossa. **(Bottom)** Image located just lateral to the previous image. The medial aspect of the humeral head is coming in to view. The long head of the biceps tendon fuses with the superior labrum to form the biceps labral complex.

LABRUM

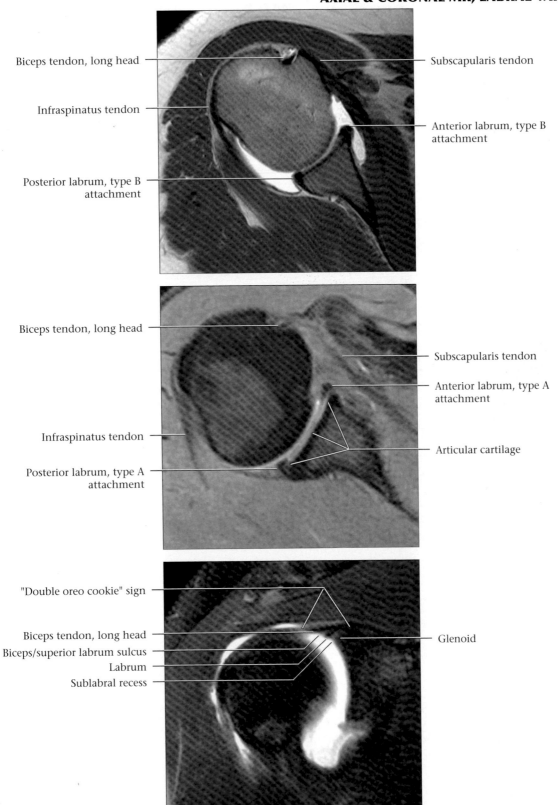

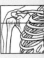

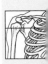

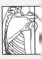

Biceps tendon, long head

Infraspinatus tendon

Posterior labrum, type B attachment

Subscapularis tendon

Anterior labrum, type B attachment

Biceps tendon, long head

Infraspinatus tendon

Posterior labrum, type A attachment

Subscapularis tendon

Anterior labrum, type A attachment

Articular cartilage

"Double oreo cookie" sign

Biceps tendon, long head

Biceps/superior labrum sulcus

Labrum

Sublabral recess

Glenoid

(Top) First of three MR images of glenoid labral variants in three different patients. Axial T1 MR arthrogram without fat suppression. The anterior and posterior labrum are firmly adherent to the articular cartilage. This is referred to as a type B attachment. **(Middle)** Axial PD MR in a different patient from previous image. The anterior and posterior labrum overlie the articular cartilage. This is referred to as a type A attachment. **(Bottom)** The "double oreo cookie" sign in a different patient from previous image on coronal T2 FS arthrogram. From medial to lateral, the layers of the cookie correspond to the glenoid cortex (black) + sublabral recess (white) + labrum (black) + biceps/superior labrum sulcus (white) + biceps tendon (black). This sign can also be seen when a superior labral tear is present in place of the biceps/superior labrum sulcus.

Shoulder

I

123

CORONAL GRAPHICS: BICEPS LABRAL COMPLEX, NORMAL VARIANTS

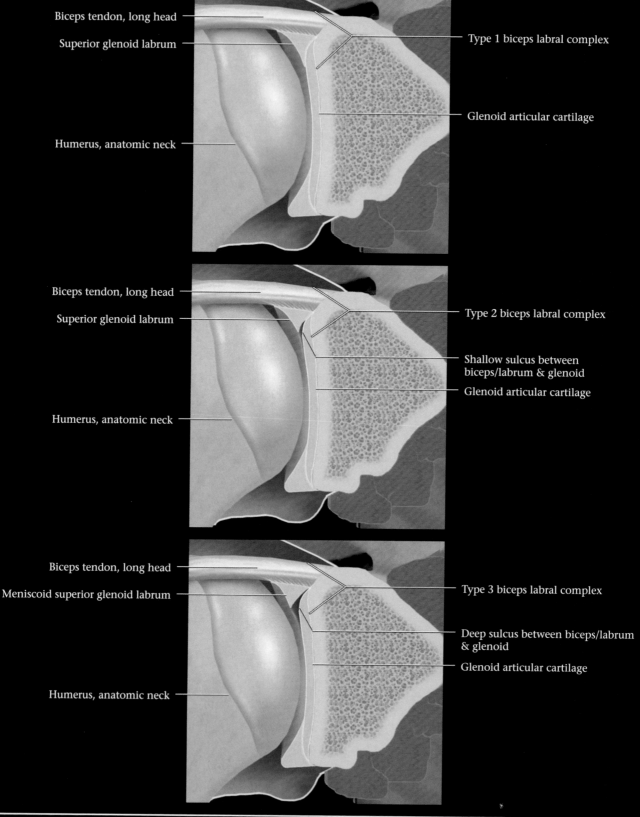

Biceps tendon, long head

Superior glenoid labrum

Humerus, anatomic neck

Type 1 biceps labral complex

Glenoid articular cartilage

Biceps tendon, long head

Superior glenoid labrum

Humerus, anatomic neck

Type 2 biceps labral complex

Shallow sulcus between biceps/labrum & glenoid

Glenoid articular cartilage

Biceps tendon, long head

Meniscoid superior glenoid labrum

Humerus, anatomic neck

Type 3 biceps labral complex

Deep sulcus between biceps/labrum & glenoid

Glenoid articular cartilage

(Top) First of three coronal graphics shows biceps labral complex normal variants. The type 1 biceps labral complex is firmly adherent to the glenoid. This is also referred to as the slab type BLC. **(Middle)** The type 2 BLC has a shallow sulcus between the glenoid and biceps/labrum. This morphology is also referred to as intermediate type BLC. **(Bottom)** The type 3 BLC has a deep sulcus between the glenoid and biceps/labrum. The superior glenoid labrum is meniscoid, thus this normal variant is also called the meniscoid type BLC. This deep sulcus often continues anteriorly as a sublabral foramen.

LABRUM

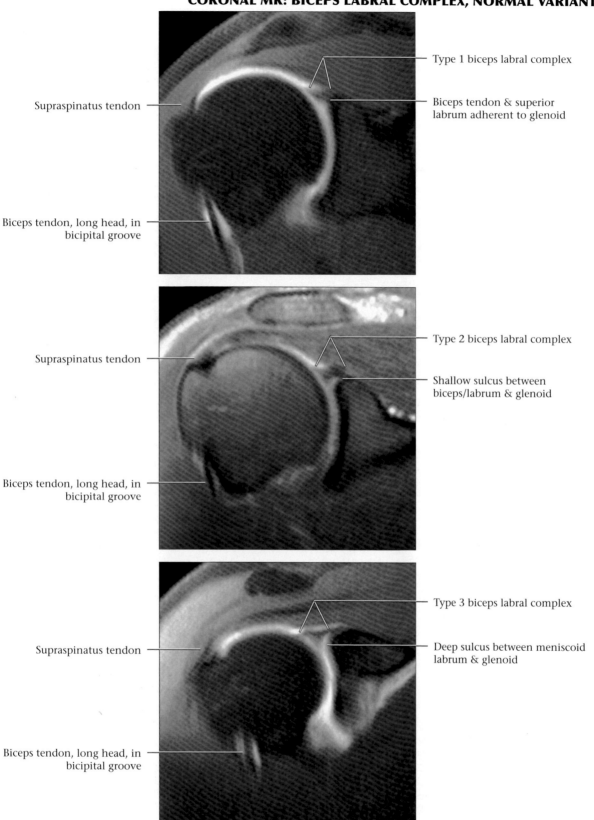

Supraspinatus tendon

Biceps tendon, long head, in bicipital groove

Type 1 biceps labral complex

Biceps tendon & superior labrum adherent to glenoid

Supraspinatus tendon

Biceps tendon, long head, in bicipital groove

Type 2 biceps labral complex

Shallow sulcus between biceps/labrum & glenoid

Supraspinatus tendon

Biceps tendon, long head, in bicipital groove

Type 3 biceps labral complex

Deep sulcus between meniscoid labrum & glenoid

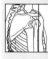

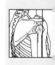

(Top) First of three coronal MR images of the right shoulder in three different patients shows biceps labral complex normal variants. Coronal oblique T1 FS MR arthrogram. The biceps tendon is firmly adherent to the labrum and superior glenoid. This is a type 1 or slab type BLC. **(Middle)** Coronal oblique T1 MR. A relatively shallow sulcus lies between the biceps/labrum and glenoid. This is a type 2 or intermediate type BLC. **(Bottom)** Coronal oblique T1 FS MR arthrogram. A deep sulcus lies between the biceps/labrum and glenoid. This is a type 3 or meniscoid type BLC.

LABRUM

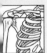

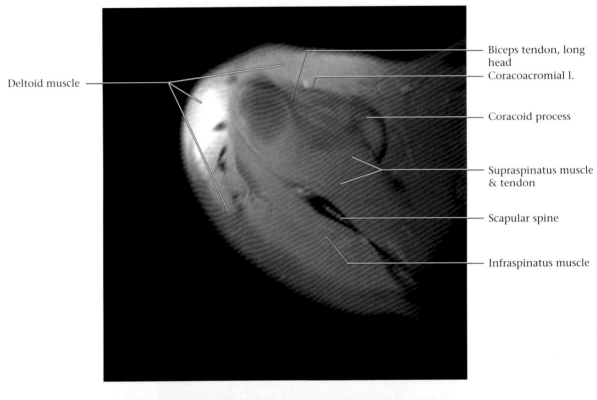

Deltoid muscle

Biceps tendon, long head

Coracoacromial l.

Coracoid process

Supraspinatus muscle & tendon

Scapular spine

Infraspinatus muscle

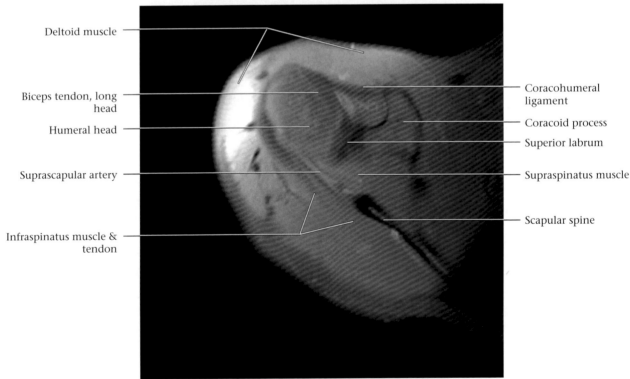

Deltoid muscle

Biceps tendon, long head

Humeral head

Suprascapular artery

Infraspinatus muscle & tendon

Coracohumeral ligament

Coracoid process

Superior labrum

Supraspinatus muscle

Scapular spine

(**Top**) First of twelve axial PD FS MR images of the right shoulder presented from proximal to distal. Image is above the level of the glenoid labrum. The fibrous labrum increases the stability of the glenohumeral joint and is an important attachment site for the glenohumeral ligaments and long head of the biceps tendon. (**Bottom**) The superior glenoid labrum comes into view on this image. It has normal low signal. The long head of the biceps tendon attaches to the superior labrum, forming the biceps labral complex. Note that the coracohumeral ligament is unusually taut and well demonstrated in this hyper-externally rotated shoulder.

LABRUM

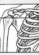

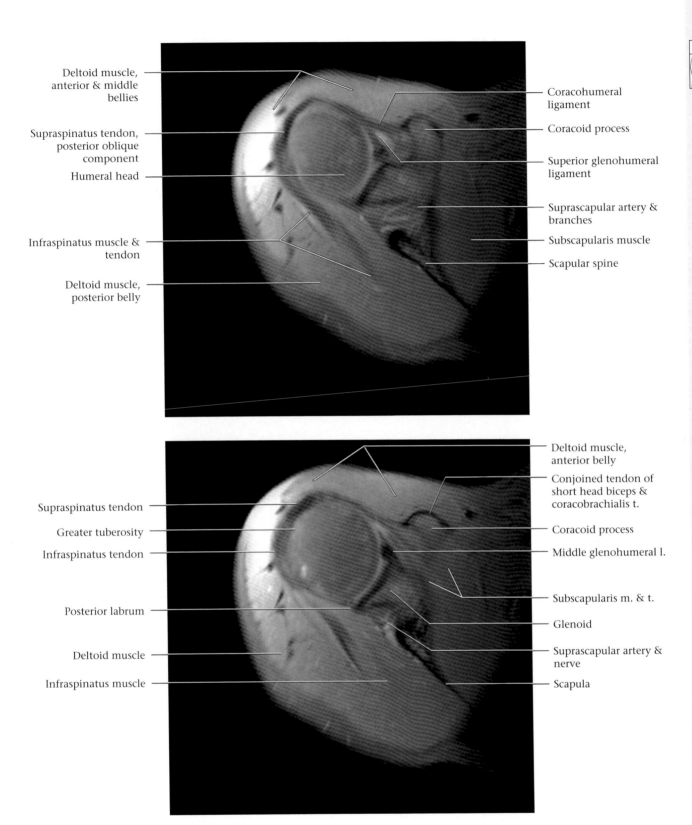

Deltoid muscle, anterior & middle bellies

Supraspinatus tendon, posterior oblique component

Humeral head

Infraspinatus muscle & tendon

Deltoid muscle, posterior belly

Coracohumeral ligament

Coracoid process

Superior glenohumeral ligament

Suprascapular artery & branches

Subscapularis muscle

Scapular spine

Supraspinatus tendon

Greater tuberosity

Infraspinatus tendon

Posterior labrum

Deltoid muscle

Infraspinatus muscle

Deltoid muscle, anterior belly

Conjoined tendon of short head biceps & coracobrachialis t.

Coracoid process

Middle glenohumeral l.

Subscapularis m. & t.

Glenoid

Suprascapular artery & nerve

Scapula

(Top) The superior glenohumeral ligament attachment to the anterior superior labrum is shown on this image. The glenohumeral ligaments may actually represent folds of the joint capsule, as opposed to true ligaments. The superior glenohumeral ligament will fuse with the coracohumeral ligament form a supportive sling around the long head of the biceps tendon. **(Bottom)** The middle glenohumeral ligament also arises anteriorly. It is larger than the superior glenohumeral ligament and can be confused for a torn fragment of labrum if it is not followed along its oblique course.

LABRUM

AXIAL PD FS MR

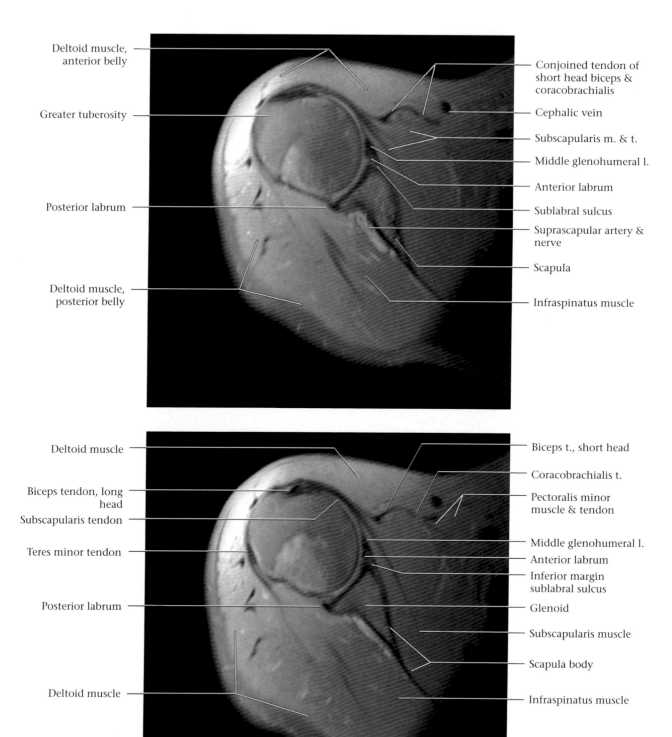

Deltoid muscle, anterior belly

Greater tuberosity

Posterior labrum

Deltoid muscle, posterior belly

Conjoined tendon of short head biceps & coracobrachialis

Cephalic vein

Subscapularis m. & t.

Middle glenohumeral l.

Anterior labrum

Sublabral sulcus

Suprascapular artery & nerve

Scapula

Infraspinatus muscle

Deltoid muscle

Biceps tendon, long head

Subscapularis tendon

Teres minor tendon

Posterior labrum

Deltoid muscle

Biceps t., short head

Coracobrachialis t.

Pectoralis minor muscle & tendon

Middle glenohumeral l.

Anterior labrum

Inferior margin sublabral sulcus

Glenoid

Subscapularis muscle

Scapula body

Infraspinatus muscle

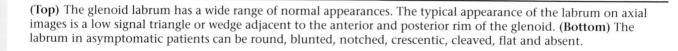

(Top) The glenoid labrum has a wide range of normal appearances. The typical appearance of the labrum on axial images is a low signal triangle or wedge adjacent to the anterior and posterior rim of the glenoid. **(Bottom)** The labrum in asymptomatic patients can be round, blunted, notched, crescentic, cleaved, flat and absent.

LABRUM

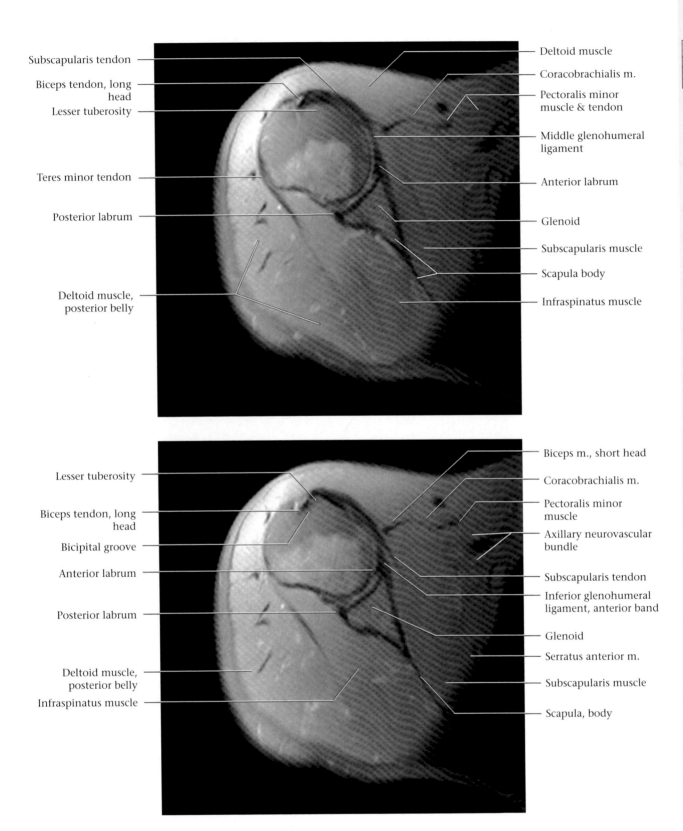
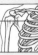

Top image labels (left):
- Subscapularis tendon
- Biceps tendon, long head
- Lesser tuberosity
- Teres minor tendon
- Posterior labrum
- Deltoid muscle, posterior belly

Top image labels (right):
- Deltoid muscle
- Coracobrachialis m.
- Pectoralis minor muscle & tendon
- Middle glenohumeral ligament
- Anterior labrum
- Glenoid
- Subscapularis muscle
- Scapula body
- Infraspinatus muscle

Bottom image labels (left):
- Lesser tuberosity
- Biceps tendon, long head
- Bicipital groove
- Anterior labrum
- Posterior labrum
- Deltoid muscle, posterior belly
- Infraspinatus muscle

Bottom image labels (right):
- Biceps m., short head
- Coracobrachialis m.
- Pectoralis minor muscle
- Axillary neurovascular bundle
- Subscapularis tendon
- Inferior glenohumeral ligament, anterior band
- Glenoid
- Serratus anterior m.
- Subscapularis muscle
- Scapula, body

(Top) The inferior glenohumeral ligament complex consists of an anterior band, axillary pouch and posterior band. This complex represents the thickest portion of the joint capsule. A distinct site of origin of this triangular shaped complex is more difficult to identify than the superior and middle glenohumeral ligament origins. **(Bottom)** The anterior and posterior labrum can normally have asymmetric shapes. Hyaline cartilage undercutting of the labrum, seen anteriorly in this case, can simulate a tear due the relatively increased signal of cartilage compared with the fibrous labrum.

Shoulder

I

AXIAL PD FS MR

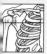

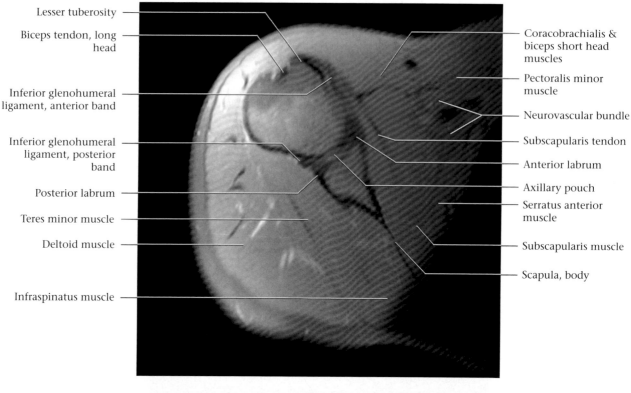

Lesser tuberosity

Biceps tendon, long head

Inferior glenohumeral ligament, anterior band

Inferior glenohumeral ligament, posterior band

Posterior labrum

Teres minor muscle

Deltoid muscle

Infraspinatus muscle

Coracobrachialis & biceps short head muscles

Pectoralis minor muscle

Neurovascular bundle

Subscapularis tendon

Anterior labrum

Axillary pouch

Serratus anterior muscle

Subscapularis muscle

Scapula, body

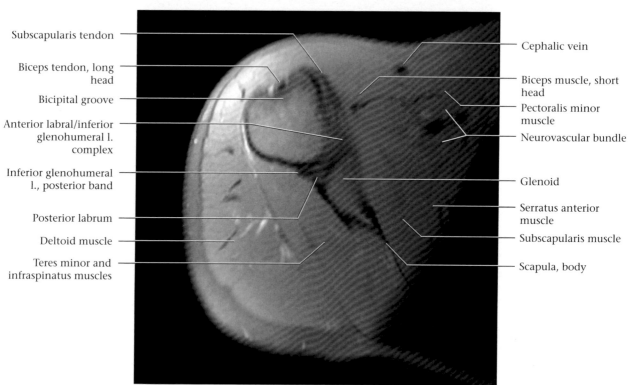

Subscapularis tendon

Biceps tendon, long head

Bicipital groove

Anterior labral/inferior glenohumeral l. complex

Inferior glenohumeral l., posterior band

Posterior labrum

Deltoid muscle

Teres minor and infraspinatus muscles

Cephalic vein

Biceps muscle, short head

Pectoralis minor muscle

Neurovascular bundle

Glenoid

Serratus anterior muscle

Subscapularis muscle

Scapula, body

(Top) Near the inferior aspect of the glenohumeral joint, the axillary pouch normally contains a small amount of joint fluid. The joint capsule may become redundant in this area, simulating loose bodies. **(Bottom)** Magic angle artifact can cause increased signal in the labrum. This is most commonly seen in the superior and inferior aspects of both the anterior and posterior labrum on short TE images. Any abnormal labral signal should be confirmed on T2 sequences.

Shoulder

I

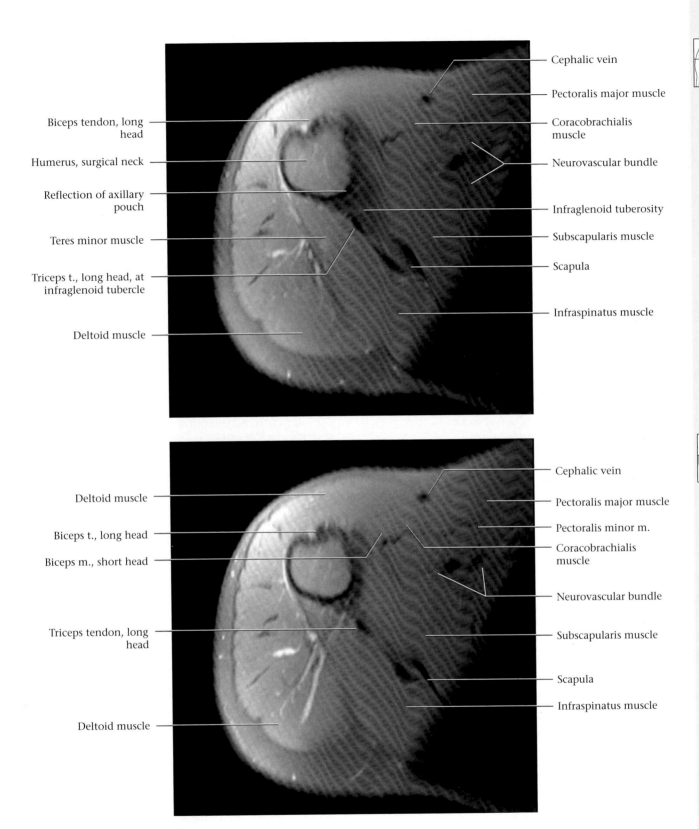

Top image labels (left): Biceps tendon, long head; Humerus, surgical neck; Reflection of axillary pouch; Teres minor muscle; Triceps t., long head, at infraglenoid tubercle; Deltoid muscle

Top image labels (right): Cephalic vein; Pectoralis major muscle; Coracobrachialis muscle; Neurovascular bundle; Infraglenoid tuberosity; Subscapularis muscle; Scapula; Infraspinatus muscle

Bottom image labels (left): Deltoid muscle; Biceps t., long head; Biceps m., short head; Triceps tendon, long head; Deltoid muscle

Bottom image labels (right): Cephalic vein; Pectoralis major muscle; Pectoralis minor m.; Coracobrachialis muscle; Neurovascular bundle; Subscapularis muscle; Scapula; Infraspinatus muscle

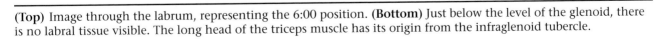

(Top) Image through the labrum, representing the 6:00 position. **(Bottom)** Just below the level of the glenoid, there is no labral tissue visible. The long head of the triceps muscle has its origin from the infraglenoid tubercle.

CLINICALLY RELEVANT REGIONS

Terminology

Abbreviations
- Coracoacromial arch (CCA)
- Superior transverse scapular ligament (STSL)
- Inferior transverse scapular ligament (ITSL)

Imaging Anatomy

Overview
- Several regions of the shoulder are of particular clinical importance

Anatomy Relationships
- **Quadrilateral space**
  - Superior border: Teres minor muscle
  - Inferior border: Teres major muscle
  - Lateral border: Surgical neck of humerus
  - Medial border: Long head of triceps muscle
  - Contents: Axillary nerve and posterior circumflex humeral artery
    - Axillary nerve supplies teres minor muscle, deltoid muscle, posterolateral cutaneous region of shoulder and upper arm
  - Can have complications that are purely neurologic, purely vascular or both
- **Triangular space**
  - Located medial to quadrilateral space
  - Superior border: Teres minor muscle
  - Inferior border: Teres major muscle
  - Lateral border: Long head of triceps muscle
  - Contents: Circumflex scapular artery
    - Branch of subscapular artery supplying infraspinatus fossa
- **Suprascapular notch**
  - Roof of notch covered by superior transverse scapular ligament
  - Contents: Suprascapular nerve
    - Arises from brachial plexus superior trunk, 4th-6th cervical nerve roots
    - Motor and sensory fibers
    - Supplies supraspinatus and infraspinatus muscles
  - Anterior compression causes supraspinatus and infraspinatus atrophy
  - Posterior compression causes infraspinatus atrophy
  - Suprascapular artery and vein pass above superior transverse scapular ligament
- **Spinoglenoid notch**
  - Located inferior to suprascapular notch, between scapular spine and posterior surface of glenoid body
  - Contains infraspinatus branch of suprascapular nerve
    - Supplies infraspinatus muscle
  - Also contains suprascapular vessels
  - Neurovascular bundle passes beneath inferior transverse scapular ligament
    - Ligament present in 50% population
- **Coracoacromial arch**
  - **Borders**
    - Superior border: Acromion
    - Anterior border: Coracoacromial ligament
    - Anterior border: Coracoid process
    - Posterior border: Humeral head
  - **Contents**
    - Subacromial-subdeltoid bursa
    - Supraspinatus muscle and tendon
    - Biceps tendon, long head
  - **Os acromiale**
    - Normal variant anatomy 5%
    - Unfused acromial apophysis
    - Normally fused by age 25
    - Mobile and decreases coracoacromial space during motion
    - Differentiate from acromioclavicular joint by location within the acromion process
    - Predisposes to impingement & rotator cuff tear
    - Best imaged by radiographs, CT or axial plane MR

Anatomy-Based Imaging Issues

Key Concepts or Questions
- **Suprascapular neuropathies**
  - Due to lesions in or near suprascapular or spinoglenoid notch
  - **Causes atrophy of supraspinatus, infraspinatus or both muscles**
  - Paralabral cysts
    - Most common cause of mass in this region
    - High association with labral tears
    - May cause bone erosion
  - Distal clavicle osteolysis
    - Course of nerve closely associated with posterior aspect of distal clavicle & acromioclavicular joint
  - Anomalous or calcified ligaments
  - Scapular fracture
  - Blunt or penetrating trauma
  - Glenohumeral joint dislocation
  - Radical neck dissection
  - Supraclavicular lymph node biopsy
  - Stretching or mechanical irritation
  - Tumor
  - Varices
- **Axillary neuropathies**
  - Due to abnormalities in quadrilateral space
    - Paralabral cysts
    - Fibrous bands
    - Glenohumeral joint dislocation
    - Humeral fracture
    - Extreme or prolonged abduction of arm during sleep
  - **Atrophy of teres minor muscle**
  - May affect deltoid muscle
- **Shoulder impingement**
  - Any lesion or anatomic variant that narrows the coracoacromial arch predisposes to impingement

Imaging Recommendations
- **MR**: Best demonstrates the anatomic spaces and assesses for the presence of lesions
- **Arteriography**: To assess for occlusion of posterior circumflex humeral artery when in abducted, externally rotated position
- **Radiographs and CT**: To assess for fracture or bone tumor

CLINICALLY RELEVANT REGIONS

GRAPHICS, SUPRASCAPULAR & SPINOGLENOID NOTCH

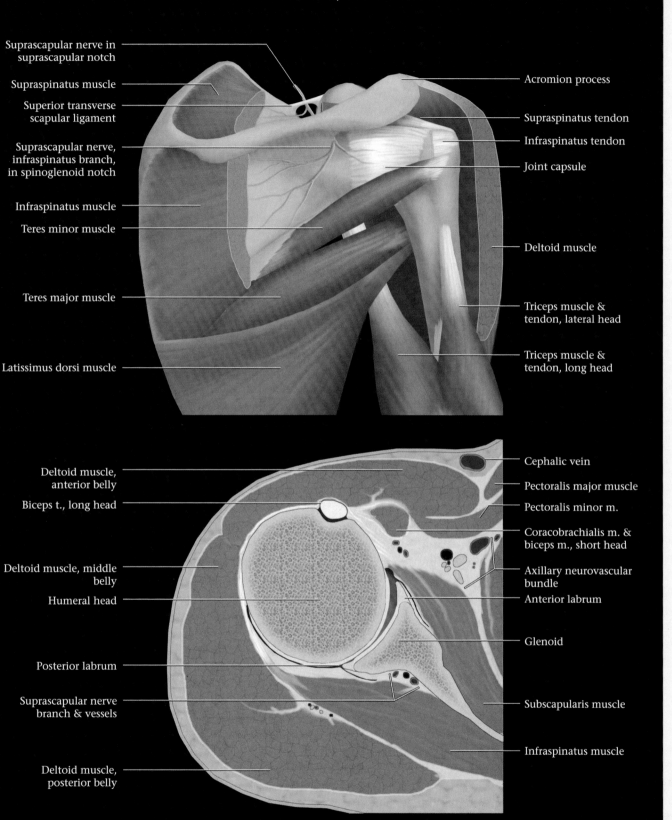

Suprascapular nerve in suprascapular notch

Supraspinatus muscle

Superior transverse scapular ligament

Suprascapular nerve, infraspinatus branch, in spinoglenoid notch

Infraspinatus muscle

Teres minor muscle

Teres major muscle

Latissimus dorsi muscle

Acromion process

Supraspinatus tendon

Infraspinatus tendon

Joint capsule

Deltoid muscle

Triceps muscle & tendon, lateral head

Triceps muscle & tendon, long head

Deltoid muscle, anterior belly

Biceps t., long head

Deltoid muscle, middle belly

Humeral head

Posterior labrum

Suprascapular nerve branch & vessels

Deltoid muscle, posterior belly

Cephalic vein

Pectoralis major muscle

Pectoralis minor m.

Coracobrachialis m. & biceps m., short head

Axillary neurovascular bundle

Anterior labrum

Glenoid

Subscapularis muscle

Infraspinatus muscle

(Top) Deep scapulohumeral dissection shows the course of the suprascapular nerve. (Bottom) Axial graphic shows the location of the suprascapular artery, nerve and vein branches, just below the level of the spinoglenoid notch.

CLINICALLY RELEVANT REGIONS

GRAPHICS, QUADRILATERAL SPACE

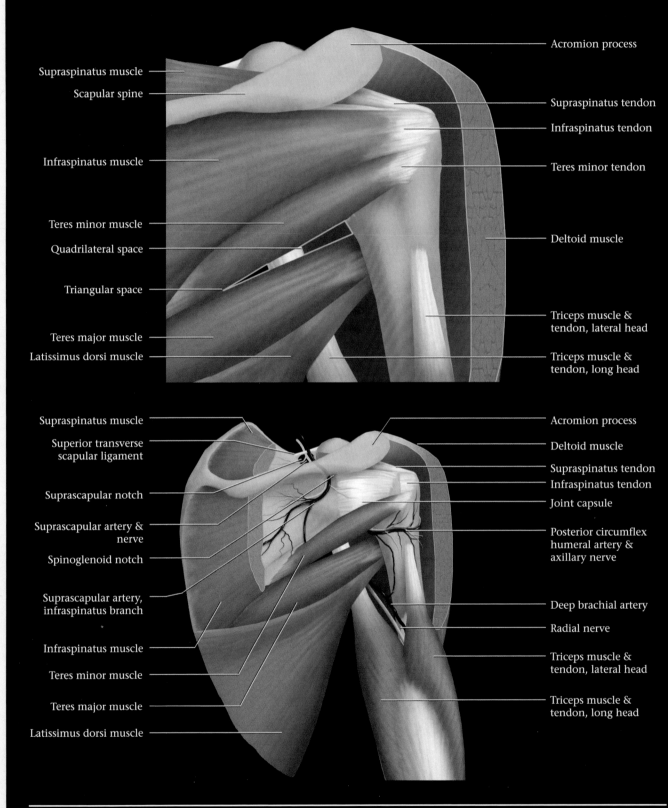

Supraspinatus muscle
Scapular spine
Infraspinatus muscle
Teres minor muscle
Quadrilateral space
Triangular space
Teres major muscle
Latissimus dorsi muscle

Acromion process
Supraspinatus tendon
Infraspinatus tendon
Teres minor tendon
Deltoid muscle
Triceps muscle & tendon, lateral head
Triceps muscle & tendon, long head

Supraspinatus muscle
Superior transverse scapular ligament
Suprascapular notch
Suprascapular artery & nerve
Spinoglenoid notch
Suprascapular artery, infraspinatus branch
Infraspinatus muscle
Teres minor muscle
Teres major muscle
Latissimus dorsi muscle

Acromion process
Deltoid muscle
Supraspinatus tendon
Infraspinatus tendon
Joint capsule
Posterior circumflex humeral artery & axillary nerve
Deep brachial artery
Radial nerve
Triceps muscle & tendon, lateral head
Triceps muscle & tendon, long head

(Top) Posterior graphic of the shoulder. Superficial scapulohumeral dissection shows the location of the quadrilateral space and triangular space (each outlined in green). **(Bottom)** Deep scapulohumeral dissection shows the major neurovascular structures, including those in the quadrilateral space.

AXIAL PD FS MR, QUADRILATERAL SPACE

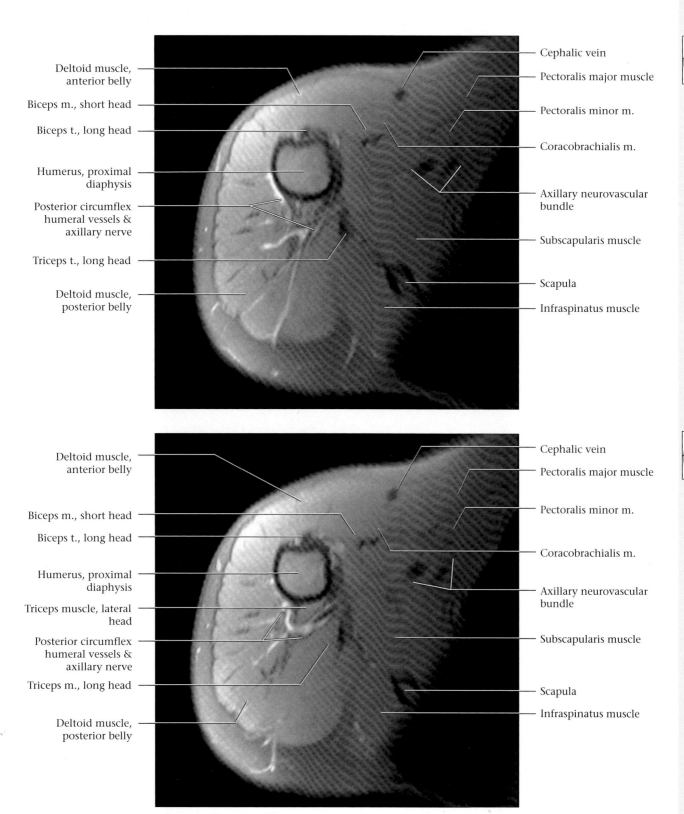

Deltoid muscle, anterior belly

Biceps m., short head

Biceps t., long head

Humerus, proximal diaphysis

Posterior circumflex humeral vessels & axillary nerve

Triceps t., long head

Deltoid muscle, posterior belly

Cephalic vein

Pectoralis major muscle

Pectoralis minor m.

Coracobrachialis m.

Axillary neurovascular bundle

Subscapularis muscle

Scapula

Infraspinatus muscle

Deltoid muscle, anterior belly

Biceps m., short head

Biceps t., long head

Humerus, proximal diaphysis

Triceps muscle, lateral head

Posterior circumflex humeral vessels & axillary nerve

Triceps m., long head

Deltoid muscle, posterior belly

Cephalic vein

Pectoralis major muscle

Pectoralis minor m.

Coracobrachialis m.

Axillary neurovascular bundle

Subscapularis muscle

Scapula

Infraspinatus muscle

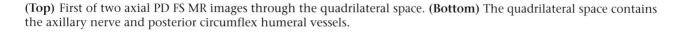

(Top) First of two axial PD FS MR images through the quadrilateral space. **(Bottom)** The quadrilateral space contains the axillary nerve and posterior circumflex humeral vessels.

Shoulder

I

CORONAL T1 MR, SCAPULA

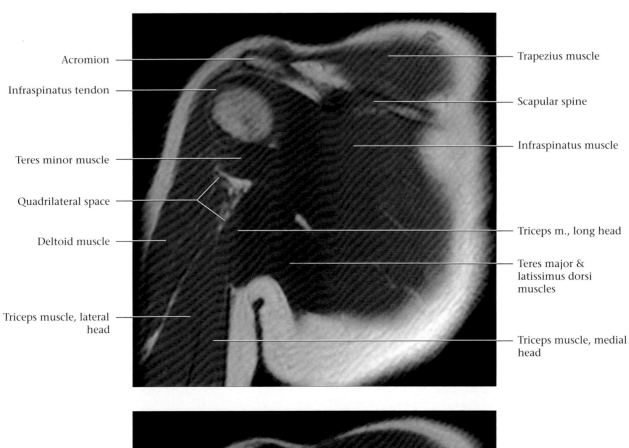

Acromion — Trapezius muscle

Infraspinatus tendon — Scapular spine

Infraspinatus muscle

Teres minor muscle —

Quadrilateral space —

Deltoid muscle — Triceps m., long head

Teres major & latissimus dorsi muscles

Triceps muscle, lateral head —

Triceps muscle, medial head

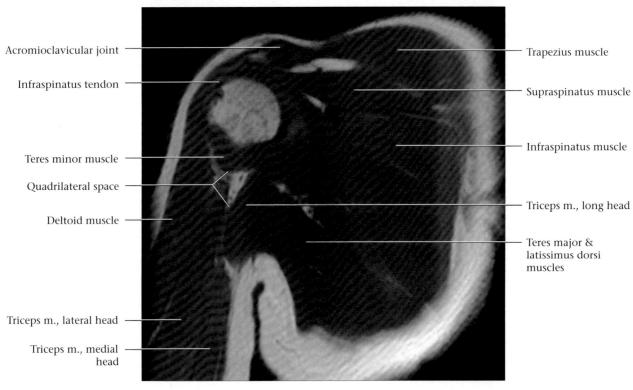

Acromioclavicular joint — Trapezius muscle

Infraspinatus tendon — Supraspinatus muscle

Infraspinatus muscle

Teres minor muscle —

Quadrilateral space —

Deltoid muscle — Triceps m., long head

Teres major & latissimus dorsi muscles

Triceps m., lateral head —

Triceps m., medial head —

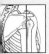

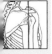

(Top) First of four coronal T1 MR images of the right scapula, presented from posterior to anterior. The quadrilateral space contains the axillary nerve and posterior circumflex humeral artery. (Bottom) The quadrilateral space lies between the teres minor and teres major muscles, superiorly and inferiorly, and between the long head of the triceps muscle and humerus surgical neck, medially and laterally.

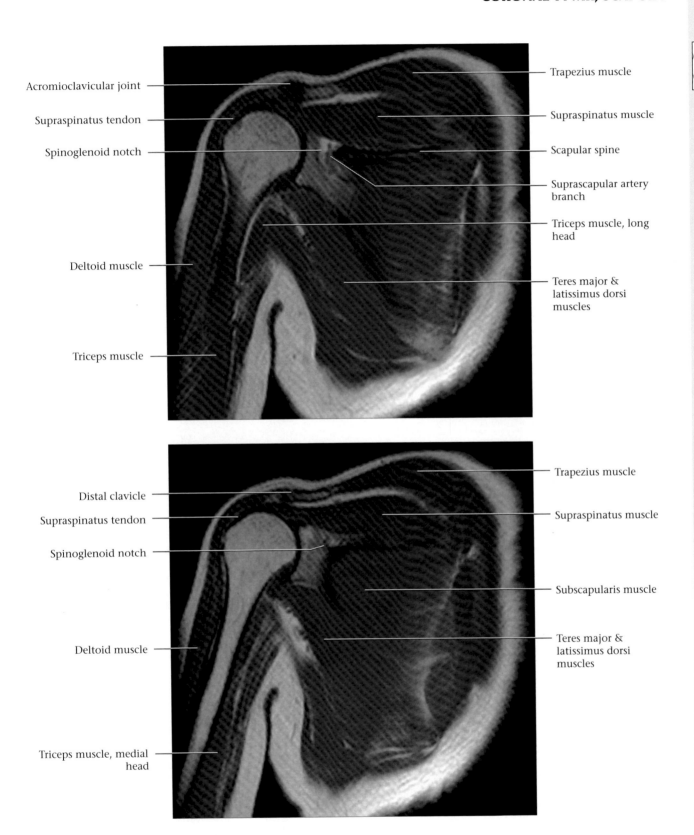

(Top) The spinoglenoid notch lies between the scapular spine and glenoid. **(Bottom)** The infraspinatus branch of the suprascapular nerve and branches of the suprascapular vessels traverse the spinoglenoid notch.

Labels (top image):
- Acromioclavicular joint
- Supraspinatus tendon
- Spinoglenoid notch
- Deltoid muscle
- Triceps muscle
- Trapezius muscle
- Supraspinatus muscle
- Scapular spine
- Suprascapular artery branch
- Triceps muscle, long head
- Teres major & latissimus dorsi muscles

Labels (bottom image):
- Distal clavicle
- Supraspinatus tendon
- Spinoglenoid notch
- Deltoid muscle
- Triceps muscle, medial head
- Trapezius muscle
- Supraspinatus muscle
- Subscapularis muscle
- Teres major & latissimus dorsi muscles

AXILLARY RADIOGRAPH & AXIAL CT, OS ACROMIALE

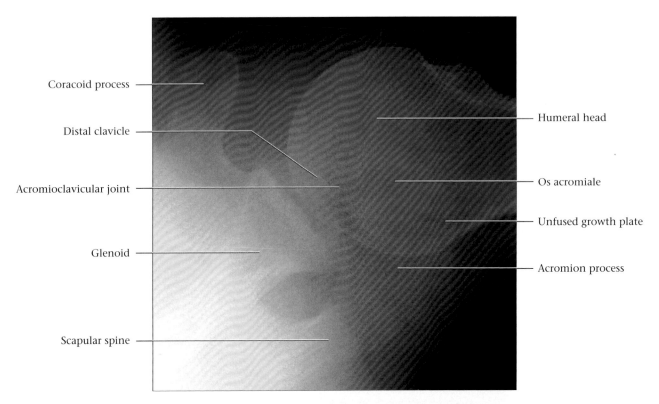

Coracoid process

Distal clavicle

Acromioclavicular joint

Glenoid

Scapular spine

Humeral head

Os acromiale

Unfused growth plate

Acromion process

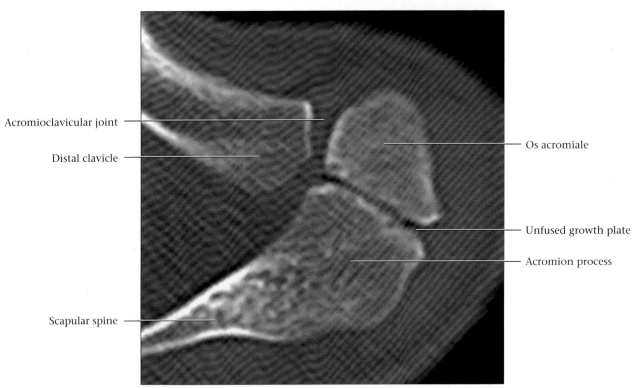

Acromioclavicular joint

Distal clavicle

Scapular spine

Os acromiale

Unfused growth plate

Acromion process

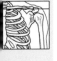

(Top) Os acromiale, the most common normal anatomic variant of the shoulder. An axillary radiograph demonstrates an accessory articulation within the acromion process, representing an unfused ossification center. **(Bottom)** An axial unenhanced CT in the same patient better demonstrates the os acromiale.

CLINICALLY RELEVANT REGIONS

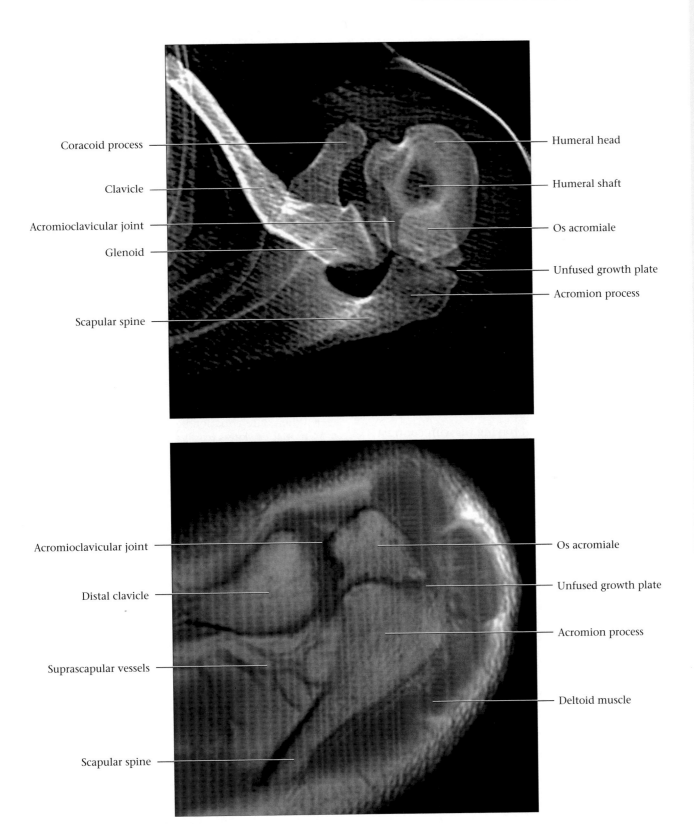

Coracoid process — Humeral head

Clavicle — Humeral shaft

Acromioclavicular joint — Os acromiale

Glenoid — Unfused growth plate

— Acromion process

Scapular spine

Acromioclavicular joint — Os acromiale

Distal clavicle — Unfused growth plate

— Acromion process

Suprascapular vessels

— Deltoid muscle

Scapular spine

(Top) 3D CT volume rendered image of an os acromiale in the same patient as on the previous image. The image is oriented as if it were being viewed from below. **(Bottom)** Axial T1 MR of an arthritic os acromiale in a different patient.

ABER POSITIONING

Terminology

Abbreviations
- Abduction external rotation (ABER)

Imaging Anatomy

Overview
- **An optional patient position for MR arthrography**

Anatomy Relationships
- **Bicipital groove rotated to lie at superior aspect of humeral head**
  - Externally rotated and elevated
  - Above spinoglenoid notch
- **Inferior glenohumeral ligament is pulled taut**
  - Exerts traction on anterior labral ligamentous complex
  - Allows intra-articular contrast to flow into tears
- **Coracoid process tip indicates approximately 2:00-3:00 position of anterior labrum**
- Inferior images show the 5:00-7:00 position of labrum, depending on alignment

Internal Structures-Critical Contents
- **Articular surface of rotator cuff and rotator cuff "footprint"**
  - Relieved of tension, kinks
  - **Undersurface tears and fraying fill with contrast**
- **Labrum**
  - **Anterior labrum under tension**
  - Posterior labrum in contact with articular surface of rotator cuff

Anatomy-Based Imaging Issues

Imaging Recommendations
- High field strength MR scanner
- Flexible shoulder coil or phased array coil

Imaging Approaches
- Standard MR arthrogram injection performed
  - 12 ml dilute gadopentetate dimeglumine (2 mmol/L) mixed with iodinated contrast, Marcaine & epinephrine according to institutional preference
- Indirect MR arthrogram IV injection also useful when direct injection not performed
- **Arm abducted greater than 90°**, unless imaging with an open MR system
- **Hand placed on top of head, over head or behind neck**
  - Elbow flexed
- Scout view obtained in coronal plane
- **Images aligned with shaft of humerus**
  - Humerus long axis images
  - Oblique axial images through joint
  - Oblique sagittal images with respect to body

Imaging Pitfalls
- **Improper positioning**
  - Patients unwilling or unable to hold this position due to pain or apprehension
  - Unfamiliar position for technologists
    - Requires extra time positioning patient and coil
- **Improper alignment of axial images**
  - **Images need to be prescribed along shaft of humerus from orthogonal coronal plane scout**
  - This nonstandard alignment may be difficult to achieve when not part of routine study
- **Wrap artifact**
  - Saturation band can be placed over medial chest wall
- **Inadequate signal**
  - Clamshell coil vs. multi element array
  - Malposition of array elements
- **Meniscoid (type 3) labrum**
  - Contrast extends into a normal gap between meniscoid labrum and cartilage

Clinical Implications

Clinical Importance
- **ABER position for MR imaging improves visualization of several regions**
  - **Anterior and posterior labrum**
    - Especially non-detached tears of anterior labrum
  - **Anterior capsular attachment**
  - **Inferior glenohumeral ligament**
  - **Undersurface of rotator cuff**
    - When differentiation between tendinosis and partial thickness tear is clinically important
    - Throwing athletes
  - **Intrasubstance or horizontal component tears of rotator cuff**
  - **Coracohumeral ligament**

Selected References

1. Herold T et al: Indirect MR Arthrography of the Shoulder: Use of Abduction and External Rotation to Detect Full- and Partial-Thickness Tears of the Supraspinatus Tendon. Radiology. 2006
2. Lee SY et al: Horizontal component of partial-thickness tears of rotator cuff: imaging characteristics and comparison of ABER view with oblique coronal view at MR arthrography initial results. Radiology. 224(2):470-6, 2002
3. Choi JA et al: Comparison between conventional MR arthrography and abduction and external rotation MR arthrography in revealing tears of the antero-inferior glenoid labrum. Korean J Radiol. 2(4):216-21, 2001
4. Kwak SM et al: Glenohumeral joint: comparison of shoulder positions at MR arthrography. Radiology. 208(2):375-80, 1998
5. Wintzell G et al: Indirect MR arthrography of anterior shoulder instability in the ABER and the apprehension test positions: a prospective comparative study of two different shoulder positions during MRI using intravenous gadodiamide contrast for enhancement of the joint fluid. Skeletal Radiol. 27(9):488-94, 1998
6. Cvitanic O et al: Using abduction and external rotation of the shoulder to increase the sensitivity of MR arthrography in revealing tears of the anterior glenoid labrum. AJR Am J Roentgenol. 169(3):837-44, 1997
7. Tirman PF et al: MR arthrographic depiction of tears of the rotator cuff: benefit of abduction and external rotation of the arm. Radiology. 192(3):851-6, 1994

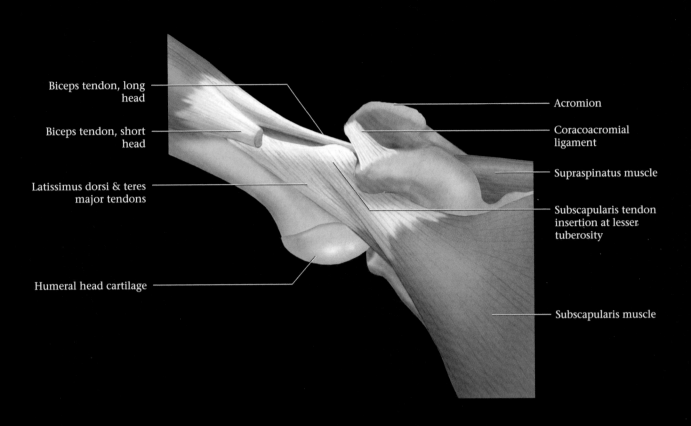

Biceps tendon, long head

Biceps tendon, short head

Latissimus dorsi & teres major tendons

Humeral head cartilage

Acromion

Coracoacromial ligament

Supraspinatus muscle

Subscapularis tendon insertion at lesser tuberosity

Subscapularis muscle

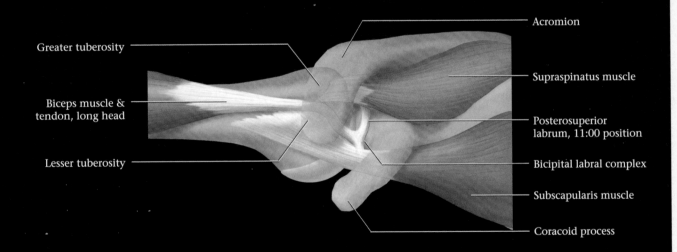

Greater tuberosity

Biceps muscle & tendon, long head

Lesser tuberosity

Acromion

Supraspinatus muscle

Posterosuperior labrum, 11:00 position

Bicipital labral complex

Subscapularis muscle

Coracoid process

(Top) Anterior graphic of the shoulder in the ABER position. **(Bottom)** Graphic of the shoulder in the ABER position, as seen from the superior aspect of the shoulder.

ABER POSITIONING

ABER T1 FS MR ARTHROGRAM

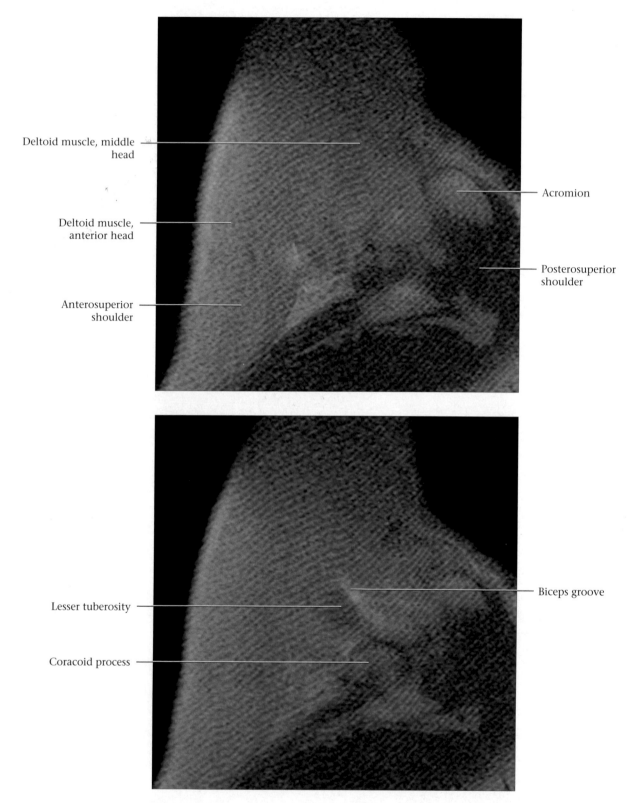

Deltoid muscle, middle head

Deltoid muscle, anterior head

Anterosuperior shoulder

Acromion

Posterosuperior shoulder

Lesser tuberosity

Coracoid process

Biceps groove

(Top) First of twenty T1 FS MR arthrogram images of the shoulder in the ABER position presented superior to inferior. **(Bottom)** The patient is positioned with the arm held behind the neck or head. An orthogonal coronal scout image is obtained and axial oblique images are prescribed along the long axis of the humeral shaft.

ABER POSITIONING

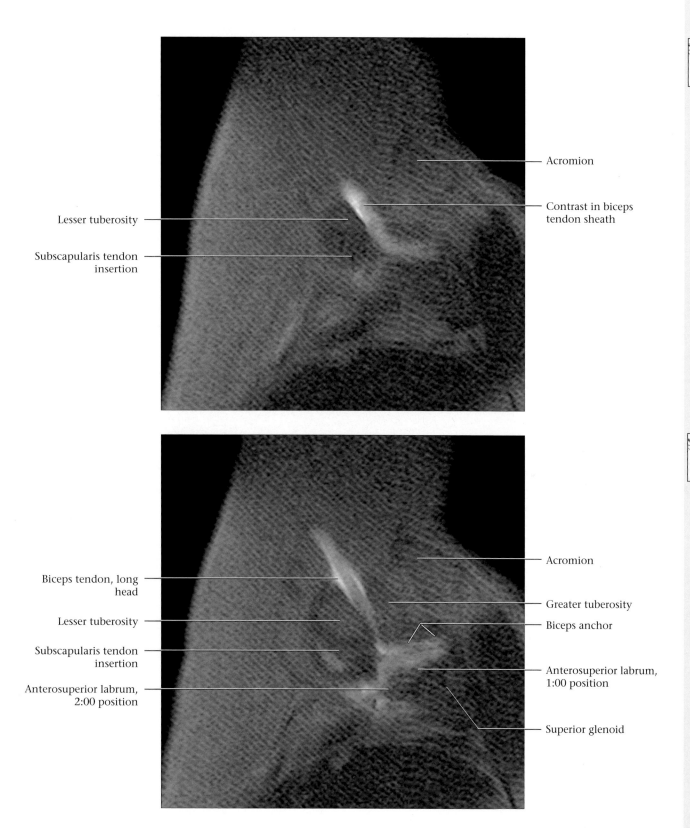

Top image labels:
- Lesser tuberosity
- Subscapularis tendon insertion
- Acromion
- Contrast in biceps tendon sheath

Bottom image labels:
- Biceps tendon, long head
- Lesser tuberosity
- Subscapularis tendon insertion
- Anterosuperior labrum, 2:00 position
- Acromion
- Greater tuberosity
- Biceps anchor
- Anterosuperior labrum, 1:00 position
- Superior glenoid

(Top) The subscapularis tendon insertion on the lesser tuberosity is shown on this image. Intra-articular contrast can normally extend into the biceps tendon sheath. **(Bottom)** The long head of the biceps tendon is shown along the length of the proximal bicipital groove.

ABER T1 FS MR ARTHROGRAM

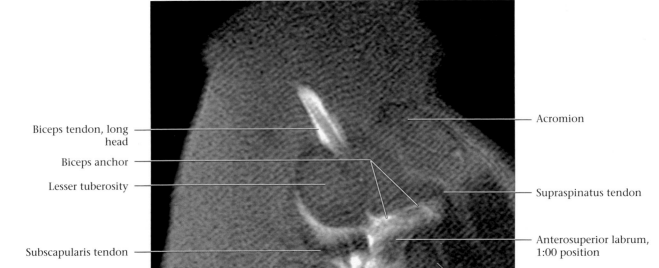

Biceps tendon, long head — Acromion

Biceps anchor —

Lesser tuberosity — Supraspinatus tendon

Subscapularis tendon — Anterosuperior labrum, 1:00 position

— Superior glenoid

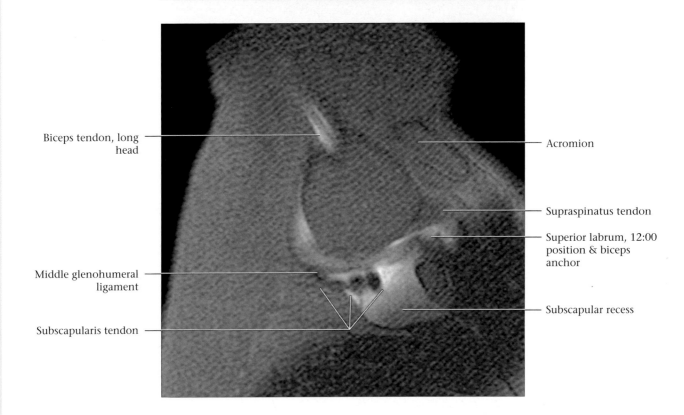

Biceps tendon, long head — Acromion

— Supraspinatus tendon

Middle glenohumeral ligament — Superior labrum, 12:00 position & biceps anchor

Subscapularis tendon — Subscapular recess

(Top) The most superior images through the shoulder joint show the long head of the biceps tendon. The biceps anchor to the labrum is also demonstrated. This position is relatively insensitive for the detection of superior labral anterior to posterior (SLAP) tears. **(Bottom)** The biceps tendon, just proximal to the labral attachment, can be kinked due to positioning. Kinking of the biceps tendon can sometimes indicate a SLAP tear.

ABER T1 FS MR ARTHROGRAM

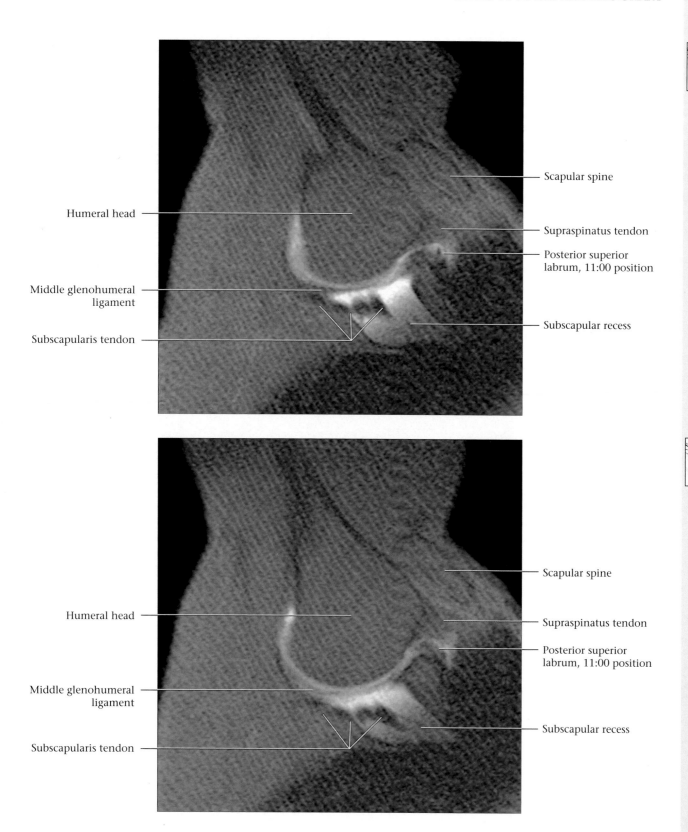

Humeral head

Middle glenohumeral ligament

Subscapularis tendon

Scapular spine

Supraspinatus tendon

Posterior superior labrum, 11:00 position

Subscapular recess

Humeral head

Middle glenohumeral ligament

Subscapularis tendon

Scapular spine

Supraspinatus tendon

Posterior superior labrum, 11:00 position

Subscapular recess

(Top) The posterosuperior labrum is partially visualized. The ABER position best shows the 2:00-10:00 position of the labrum. **(Bottom)** The middle glenohumeral ligament is demonstrated at the attachment to the subscapularis tendon. The presence of true glenohumeral ligaments is debated. The glenohumeral ligaments may represent folds of the joint capsule.

ABER T1 FS MR ARTHROGRAM

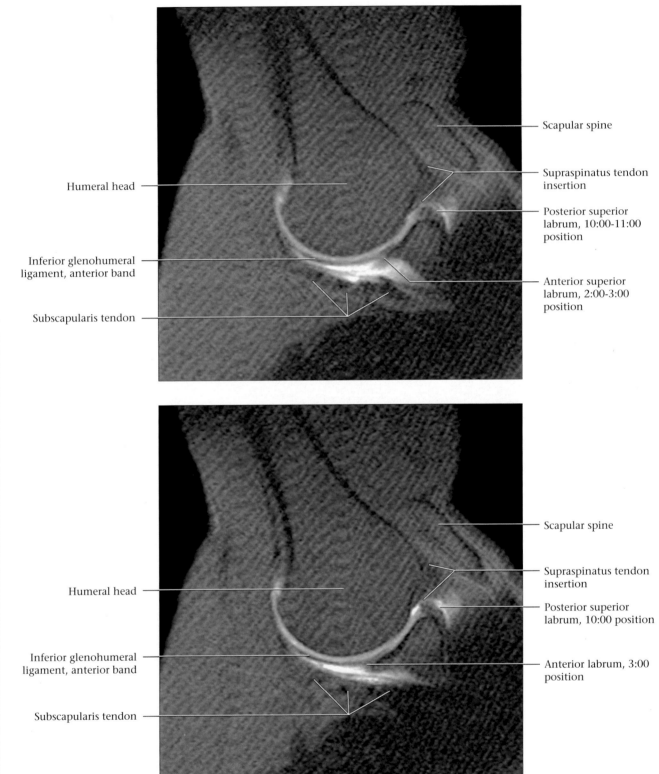

(Top image labels)
- Humeral head
- Inferior glenohumeral ligament, anterior band
- Subscapularis tendon
- Scapular spine
- Supraspinatus tendon insertion
- Posterior superior labrum, 10:00-11:00 position
- Anterior superior labrum, 2:00-3:00 position

(Bottom image labels)
- Humeral head
- Inferior glenohumeral ligament, anterior band
- Subscapularis tendon
- Scapular spine
- Supraspinatus tendon insertion
- Posterior superior labrum, 10:00 position
- Anterior labrum, 3:00 position

(Top) The anterior band of the inferior glenohumeral ligament is under traction and is seen curving around the anterior border of the humeral head. The traction force is transmitted to the anterior labrum, increasing the likelihood of contrast to enter a small tear. **(Bottom)** If posterosuperior subglenoid impingement of the humeral head were present, it may be seen at this level. Contact between the rotator cuff undersurface and labrum can be seen in asymptomatic patients.

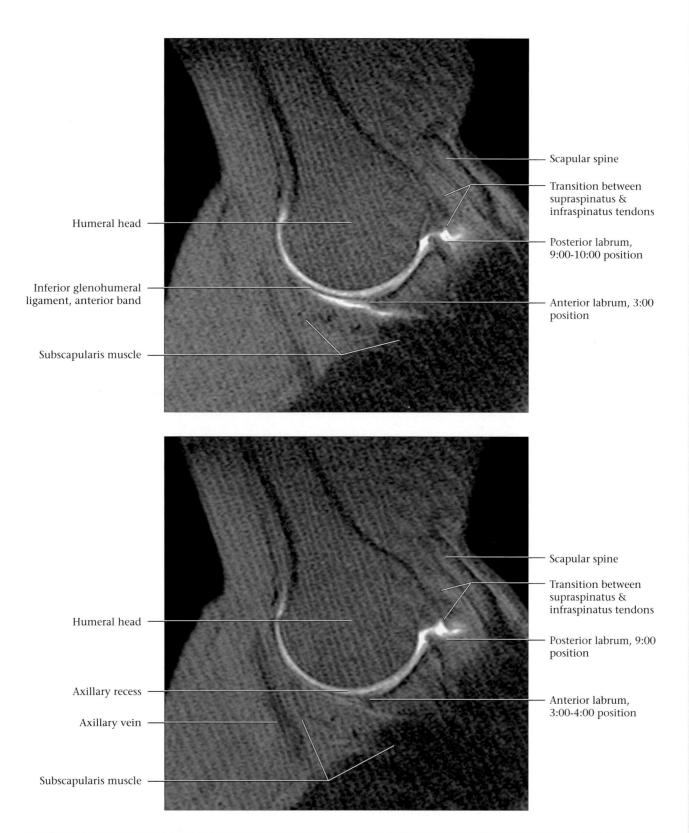

Scapular spine

Transition between supraspinatus & infraspinatus tendons

Posterior labrum, 9:00-10:00 position

Anterior labrum, 3:00 position

Humeral head

Inferior glenohumeral ligament, anterior band

Subscapularis muscle

Scapular spine

Transition between supraspinatus & infraspinatus tendons

Posterior labrum, 9:00 position

Anterior labrum, 3:00-4:00 position

Humeral head

Axillary recess

Axillary vein

Subscapularis muscle

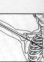

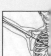

(Top) The traction of the anterior band of the inferior glenohumeral ligament also increases visualization of labral tears that have partially healed or have been resynovialized. **(Bottom)** The ABER position allows the anteroinferior labrum to be imaged without magic angle artifact that can be present with standard, adducted postioning.

ABER POSITIONING

ABER T1 FS MR ARTHROGRAM

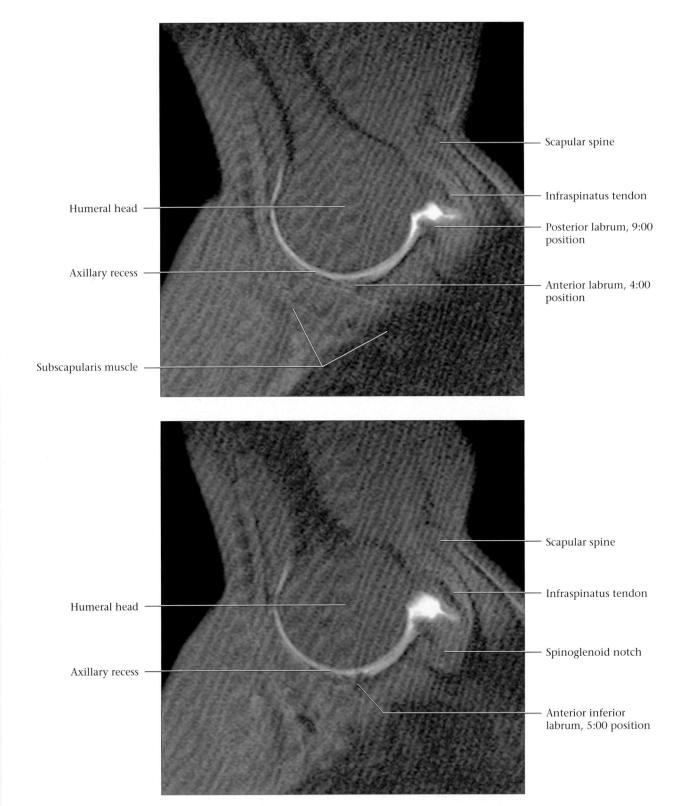

Scapular spine

Infraspinatus tendon

Posterior labrum, 9:00 position

Anterior labrum, 4:00 position

Humeral head

Axillary recess

Subscapularis muscle

Scapular spine

Infraspinatus tendon

Spinoglenoid notch

Anterior inferior labrum, 5:00 position

Humeral head

Axillary recess

(Top) Osteochondral injuries of the posterosuperior humeral head, not present in this case, are accentuated in the ABER position. **(Bottom)** Detection of anteroinferior labral tears is improved in the ABER position.

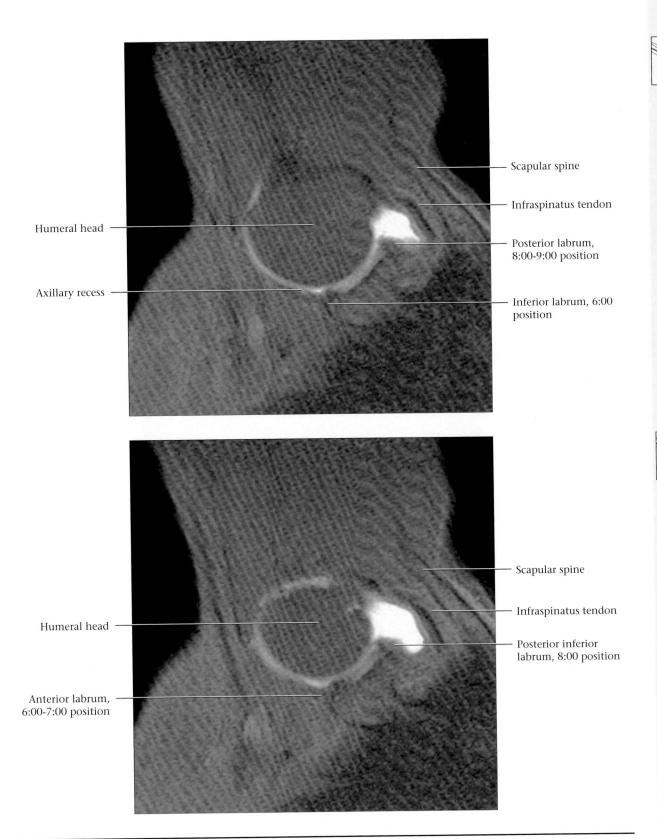

(Top) The smooth undersurface of the infraspinatus tendon is shown. (Bottom) The ABER position allows the supraspinatus, infraspinatus and teres minor tendons to kink. This would potentially allow contrast to fill small undersurface tears. The ABER position is very helpful for detection of delaminated rotator cuff tears.

ABER T1 FS MR ARTHROGRAM

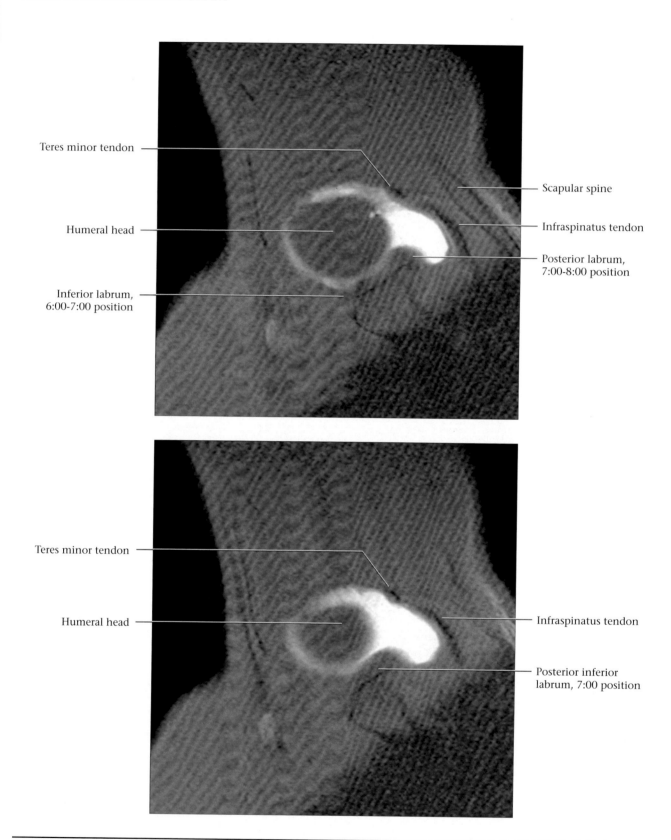

Teres minor tendon

Humeral head

Inferior labrum,
6:00-7:00 position

Scapular spine

Infraspinatus tendon

Posterior labrum,
7:00-8:00 position

Teres minor tendon

Humeral head

Infraspinatus tendon

Posterior inferior
labrum, 7:00 position

(Top) Undersurface tears of the teres minor can be accentuated in this position, when compared with standard adducted MR images. (Bottom) The most inferior image through the glenoid labrum ranges from the 5:00-7:00 position. The exact location depends on patient positioning and image alignment.

Shoulder

ABER POSITIONING

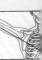

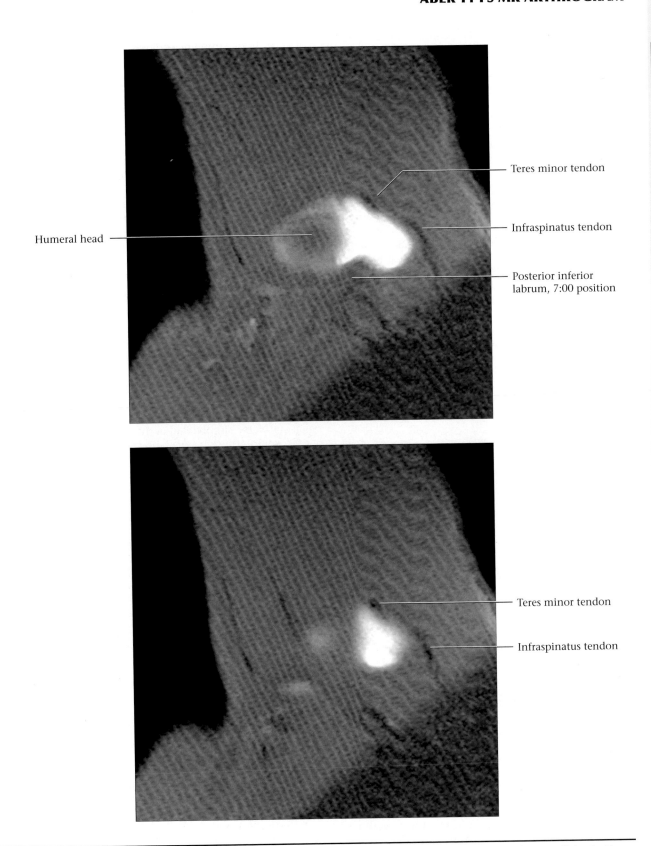

Teres minor tendon

Infraspinatus tendon

Posterior inferior labrum, 7:00 position

Humeral head

Teres minor tendon

Infraspinatus tendon

(Top) Although ABER positioning may improve visualization of some anatomic structures and abnormalities in the shoulder, there are limitations. The most significant limitation is that many patients with shoulder pain will not be able to tolerate this position. Additionally, proper placement of the shoulder coil and alignment of the images can be challenging for technologist unfamiliar with this technique. **(Bottom)** The ABER position should be an optional addition to routine shoulder imaging, balancing the increased imaging time and patient discomfort with the potential for improved visualization of otherwise subtle abnormalities.

ARM OVERVIEW

Imaging Anatomy

Overview
- Muscles of the upper arm are divided into anterior and posterior compartments

Anatomy Relationships
- **Anterior compartment of arm**
  - **Coracobrachialis muscle**
    - Origin: Coracoid process tip, in common with and medial to short head biceps tendon
    - Insertion: Medial surface of humeral mid shaft, between brachialis and triceps muscle origins
    - Nerve supply: Musculocutaneous nerve, perforates muscle
    - Blood supply: Brachial artery, muscular branches
    - Action: Flexes and adducts shoulder, supports humeral head in glenoid
    - Variants: Bony head extending to medial epicondyle, short head extending to lesser tuberosity
  - **Biceps muscle, short head**
    - Origin: Coracoid process tip, in common with and lateral to coracobrachialis tendon
    - Insertion: Radial tuberosity after joining long head
    - Nerve supply: Musculocutaneous nerve
    - Blood supply: Brachial artery, muscular branches
    - Action: Flexes elbow & shoulder, supinates forearm
  - **Biceps muscle, long head**
    - Origin: Predominantly supraglenoid tubercle; also superior glenoid labrum and coracoid base
    - Insertion: Radial tuberosity after joining with short head
    - Nerve supply: Musculocutaneous nerve
    - Blood supply: Brachial artery, muscular branches
    - Action: Flexes elbow & shoulder, supinates forearm
    - Lacertus fibrosus (distal bicipital fascia/aponeurosis) provides traction on deep fascia of forearm
    - Variants, biceps muscle: Third head in 10% arising at upper medial aspect of brachialis muscle, fourth head can arise from lateral humerus, bicipital groove or greater tuberosity
  - **Brachialis muscle**
    - Origin: Distal half of anterior humeral shaft and two intermuscular septae
    - Insertion: Tuberosity of ulna and anterior surface of coronoid process
    - Nerve supply: Musculocutaneous nerve plus branch of radial nerve
    - Blood supply: Brachial artery, muscular branches and recurrent radial artery
    - Action: Flexes forearm
    - Covers anterior aspect of elbow joint
    - Variants: Doubled; slips to supinator, pronator teres, biceps, lacertus fibrosus or radius
- **Posterior compartment of arm**
  - **Triceps muscle, long head**
    - Origin: Infraglenoid tubercle of scapula
    - Insertion: Proximal olecranon and deep fascia of arm after joining with lateral and medial heads

- Nerve supply: Radial nerve
- Blood supply: Deep brachial artery branches
- Action: Elbow extension, adducts humerus when arm is extended
  - **Triceps muscle, lateral head**
    - Origin: Posterior and lateral humeral shaft, lateral intermuscular septum
    - Insertion: Proximal olecranon and deep fascia of arm after joining with long and medial heads
    - Nerve supply: Radial nerve
    - Blood supply: Deep brachial artery branches
    - Action: Elbow extension
  - **Triceps muscle, medial head**
    - Origin: Posterior humeral shaft from teres major insertion to near trochlea, medial intermuscular septum
    - Insertion: Proximal olecranon and deep fascia of arm after joining with lateral and long heads
    - Nerve supply: Radial & branches of ulnar nerve
    - Blood supply: Deep brachial artery branches
    - Action: Elbow extension
    - Variants, triceps muscle: Fourth head from medial humerus, slip termed the dorso-epitrochlearis extending between triceps and latissimus dorsi
  - **Anconeus muscle**
    - Origin: Lateral epicondyle of humerus
    - Insertion: Lateral olecranon and posterior one-fourth of ulna
    - Nerve supply: Radial nerve
    - Blood supply: Deep brachial artery, middle collateral branch
    - Action: Assists elbow extension, abducts ulna
- **Fascia**
  - **Brachial fascia**
    - Continuous with fascia covering deltoid and pectoralis major
    - Varies in thickness being thin over biceps and thick over triceps muscles
    - Lateral intermuscular septum from lower aspect of greater tuberosity to lateral epicondyle
    - Medial intermuscular septum from lower aspect of lesser tuberosity to medial epicondyle
    - Perforated by ulnar nerve, superior ulnar collateral artery and posterior branch of inferior ulnar collateral artery
  - **Bicipital fascia**
    - Also known as lacertus fibrosus
    - Arises from medial side of distal biceps tendon at level of elbow joint
    - Passes superficial to brachial artery
    - Continuous with deep fascia of forearm

Anatomy-Based Imaging Issues

Imaging Recommendations
- **Radiographs and CT**: Evaluation of bone cortex and matrix of any identified bone lesion
- **MR**: Axial plane most helpful to delineate borders of anterior and posterior compartments and relationship to neurovascular structures

ARM OVERVIEW

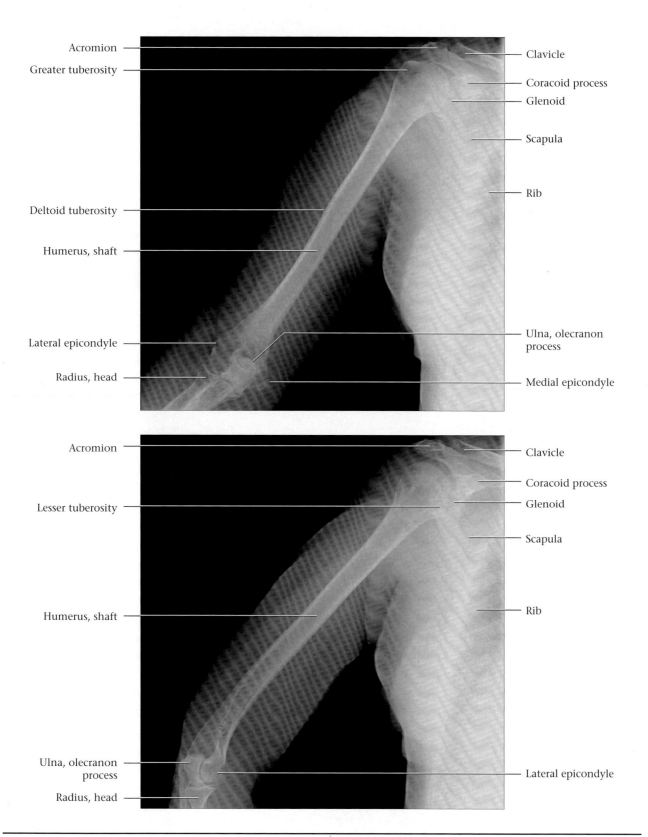

Acromion

Greater tuberosity

Deltoid tuberosity

Humerus, shaft

Lateral epicondyle

Radius, head

Clavicle

Coracoid process

Glenoid

Scapula

Rib

Ulna, olecranon process

Medial epicondyle

Acromion

Lesser tuberosity

Humerus, shaft

Ulna, olecranon process

Radius, head

Clavicle

Coracoid process

Glenoid

Scapula

Rib

Lateral epicondyle

(Top) Normal AP radiograph of right humerus, externally rotated. The patient is positioned with the shoulder mildly abducted, the elbow extended and the hand supinated. Both the shoulder and elbow joints should be visible on the radiograph. (Bottom) Normal internally rotated lateral radiograph of right humerus. The patient is positioned with the shoulder internally rotated and mildly abducted. If obtained lateromedial, as in this case, the elbow is partially flexed. If obtained mediolateral, then the elbow would be flexed 90°.

ANTERIOR GRAPHICS

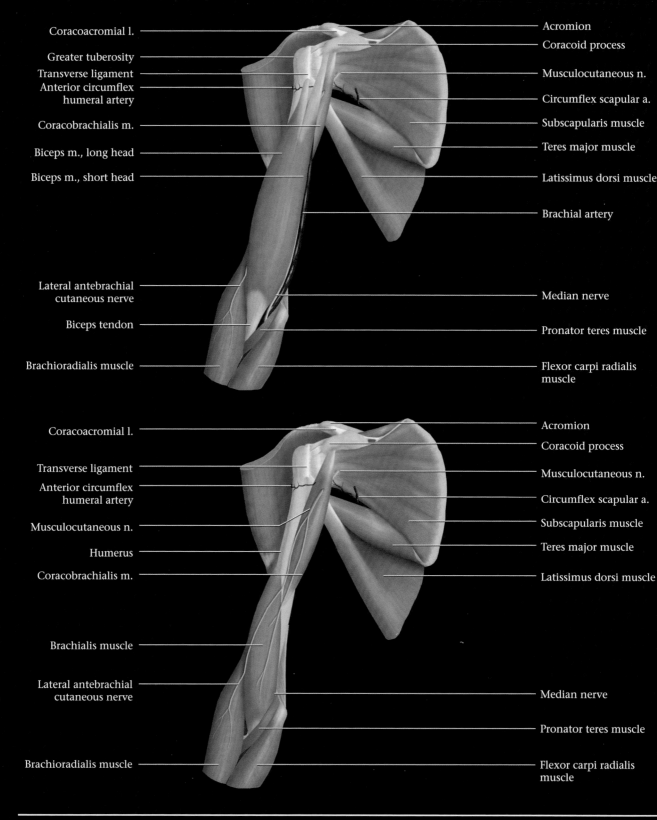

Coracoacromial l.

Greater tuberosity

Transverse ligament

Anterior circumflex humeral artery

Coracobrachialis m.

Biceps m., long head

Biceps m., short head

Lateral antebrachial cutaneous nerve

Biceps tendon

Brachioradialis muscle

Acromion

Coracoid process

Musculocutaneous n.

Circumflex scapular a.

Subscapularis muscle

Teres major muscle

Latissimus dorsi muscle

Brachial artery

Median nerve

Pronator teres muscle

Flexor carpi radialis muscle

Coracoacromial l.

Transverse ligament

Anterior circumflex humeral artery

Musculocutaneous n.

Humerus

Coracobrachialis m.

Brachialis muscle

Lateral antebrachial cutaneous nerve

Brachioradialis muscle

Acromion

Coracoid process

Musculocutaneous n.

Circumflex scapular a.

Subscapularis muscle

Teres major muscle

Latissimus dorsi muscle

Median nerve

Pronator teres muscle

Flexor carpi radialis muscle

(Top) First of two anterior graphics of the right arm. Superficial dissection. **(Bottom)** Deep dissection.

ARM OVERVIEW

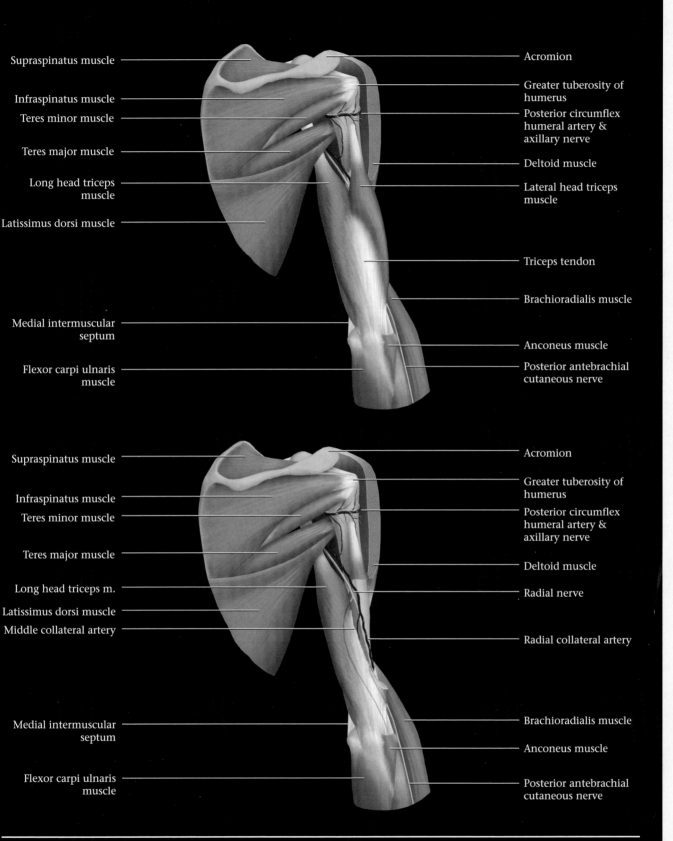

Supraspinatus muscle

Infraspinatus muscle

Teres minor muscle

Teres major muscle

Long head triceps muscle

Latissimus dorsi muscle

Medial intermuscular septum

Flexor carpi ulnaris muscle

Acromion

Greater tuberosity of humerus

Posterior circumflex humeral artery & axillary nerve

Deltoid muscle

Lateral head triceps muscle

Triceps tendon

Brachioradialis muscle

Anconeus muscle

Posterior antebrachial cutaneous nerve

Supraspinatus muscle

Infraspinatus muscle

Teres minor muscle

Teres major muscle

Long head triceps m.

Latissimus dorsi muscle

Middle collateral artery

Medial intermuscular septum

Flexor carpi ulnaris muscle

Acromion

Greater tuberosity of humerus

Posterior circumflex humeral artery & axillary nerve

Deltoid muscle

Radial nerve

Radial collateral artery

Brachioradialis muscle

Anconeus muscle

Posterior antebrachial cutaneous nerve

(Top) First of two posterior graphics of the right arm. Superficial dissection. **(Bottom)** Deep dissection.

AXIAL GRAPHICS

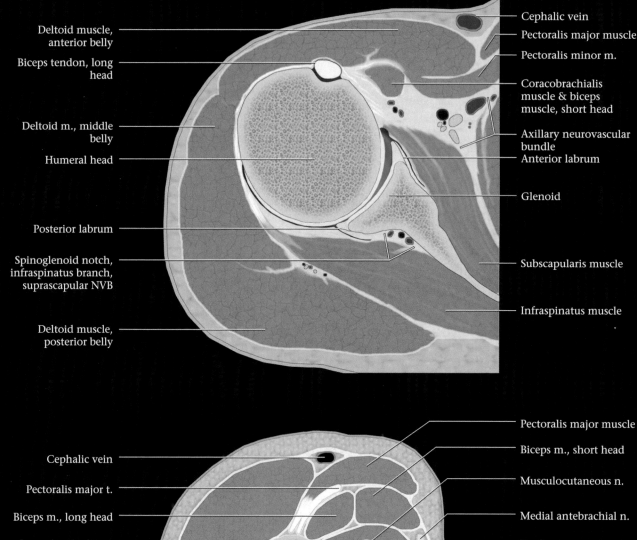

Deltoid muscle, anterior belly

Biceps tendon, long head

Deltoid m., middle belly

Humeral head

Posterior labrum

Spinoglenoid notch, infraspinatus branch, suprascapular NVB

Deltoid muscle, posterior belly

Cephalic vein

Pectoralis major muscle

Pectoralis minor m.

Coracobrachialis muscle & biceps muscle, short head

Axillary neurovascular bundle

Anterior labrum

Glenoid

Subscapularis muscle

Infraspinatus muscle

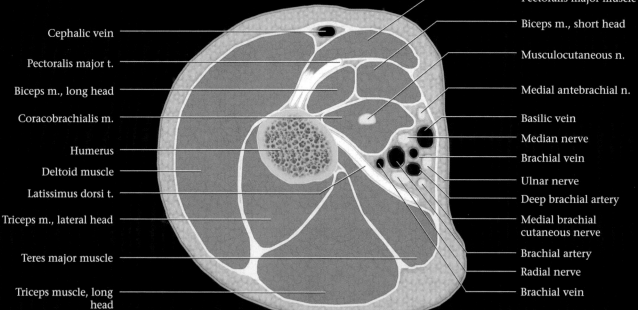

Cephalic vein

Pectoralis major t.

Biceps m., long head

Coracobrachialis m.

Humerus

Deltoid muscle

Latissimus dorsi t.

Triceps m., lateral head

Teres major muscle

Triceps muscle, long head

Pectoralis major muscle

Biceps m., short head

Musculocutaneous n.

Medial antebrachial n.

Basilic vein

Median nerve

Brachial vein

Ulnar nerve

Deep brachial artery

Medial brachial cutaneous nerve

Brachial artery

Radial nerve

Brachial vein

(Top) First of four axial graphics of the right arm. Shoulder level. **(Bottom)** Upper humeral level.

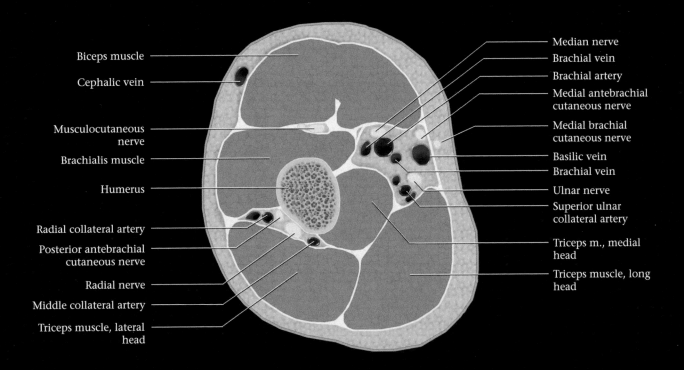

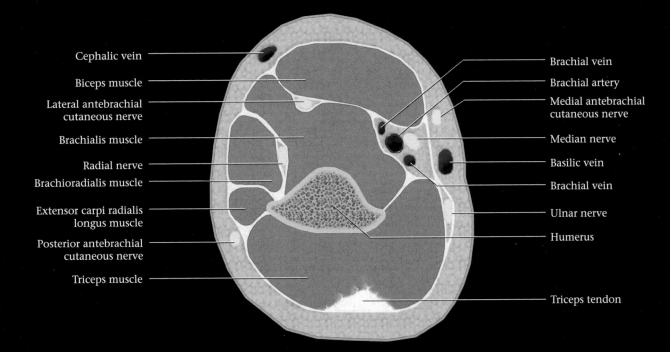

(Top) Axial graphic of the right arm. Mid humeral level. **(Bottom)** Distal humeral level.

AXIAL T1 MR, RIGHT ARM

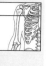

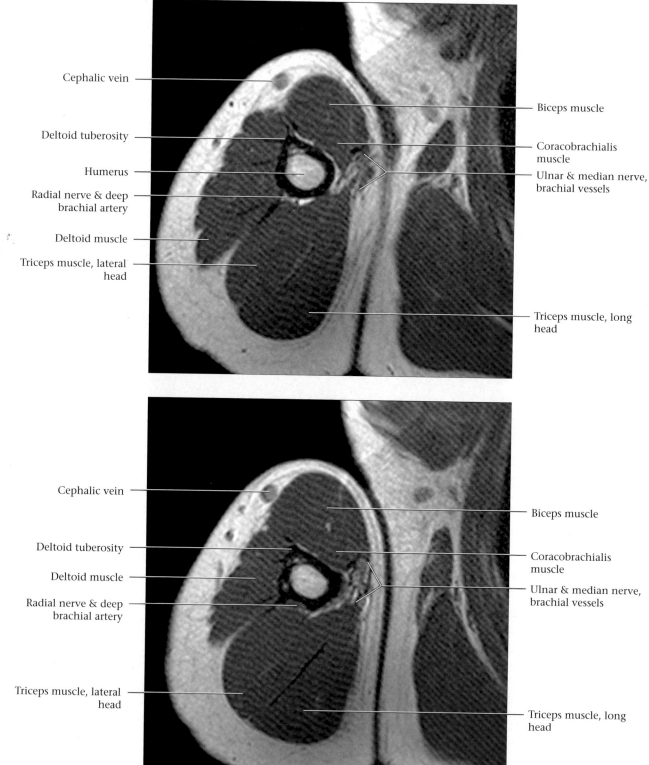

Cephalic vein

Biceps muscle

Deltoid tuberosity

Coracobrachialis muscle

Humerus

Ulnar & median nerve, brachial vessels

Radial nerve & deep brachial artery

Deltoid muscle

Triceps muscle, lateral head

Triceps muscle, long head

Cephalic vein

Biceps muscle

Deltoid tuberosity

Coracobrachialis muscle

Deltoid muscle

Ulnar & median nerve, brachial vessels

Radial nerve & deep brachial artery

Triceps muscle, lateral head

Triceps muscle, long head

(Top) First in series of axial T1 MR images of the right arm displayed proximal to distal. Images were acquired at 3T. This image is located just distal to the axilla. (Bottom) The deltoid muscle inserts on the deltoid tuberosity.

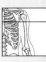

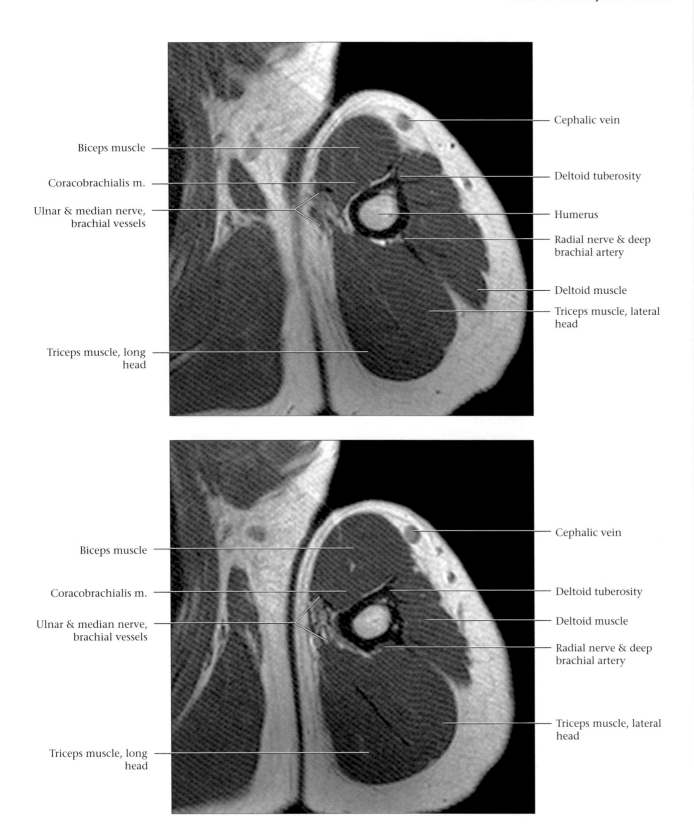

Biceps muscle

Coracobrachialis m.

Ulnar & median nerve, brachial vessels

Triceps muscle, long head

Cephalic vein

Deltoid tuberosity

Humerus

Radial nerve & deep brachial artery

Deltoid muscle

Triceps muscle, lateral head

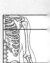

Biceps muscle

Coracobrachialis m.

Ulnar & median nerve, brachial vessels

Triceps muscle, long head

Cephalic vein

Deltoid tuberosity

Deltoid muscle

Radial nerve & deep brachial artery

Triceps muscle, lateral head

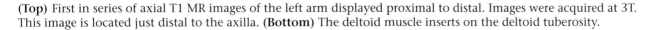

(Top) First in series of axial T1 MR images of the left arm displayed proximal to distal. Images were acquired at 3T. This image is located just distal to the axilla. **(Bottom)** The deltoid muscle inserts on the deltoid tuberosity.

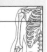

ARM OVERVIEW

AXIAL T1 MR, RIGHT ARM

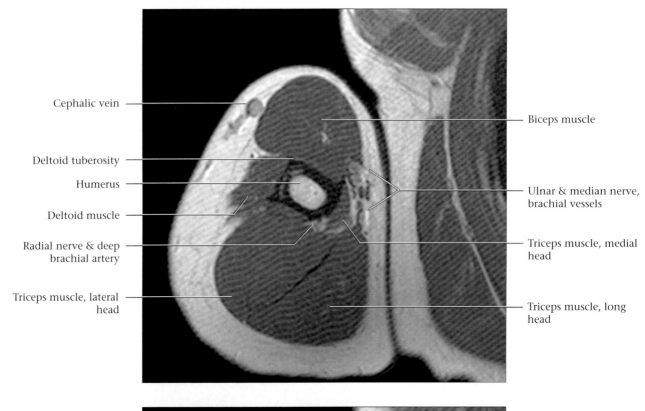

Cephalic vein — Biceps muscle

Deltoid tuberosity

Humerus — Ulnar & median nerve, brachial vessels

Deltoid muscle

Radial nerve & deep brachial artery — Triceps muscle, medial head

Triceps muscle, lateral head — Triceps muscle, long head

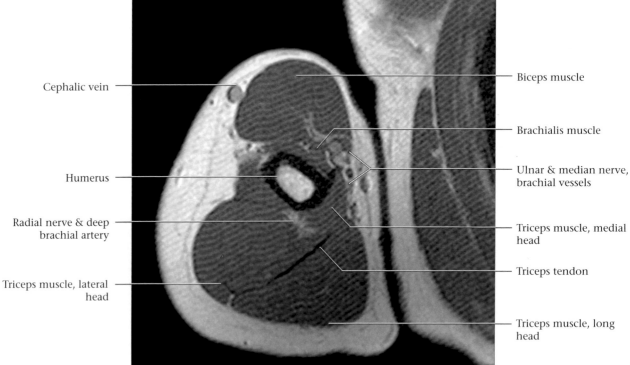

Cephalic vein — Biceps muscle

— Brachialis muscle

Humerus — Ulnar & median nerve, brachial vessels

Radial nerve & deep brachial artery — Triceps muscle, medial head

— Triceps tendon

Triceps muscle, lateral head

— Triceps muscle, long head

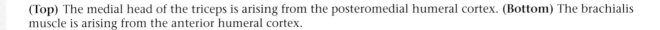

(Top) The medial head of the triceps is arising from the posteromedial humeral cortex. **(Bottom)** The brachialis muscle is arising from the anterior humeral cortex.

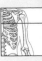

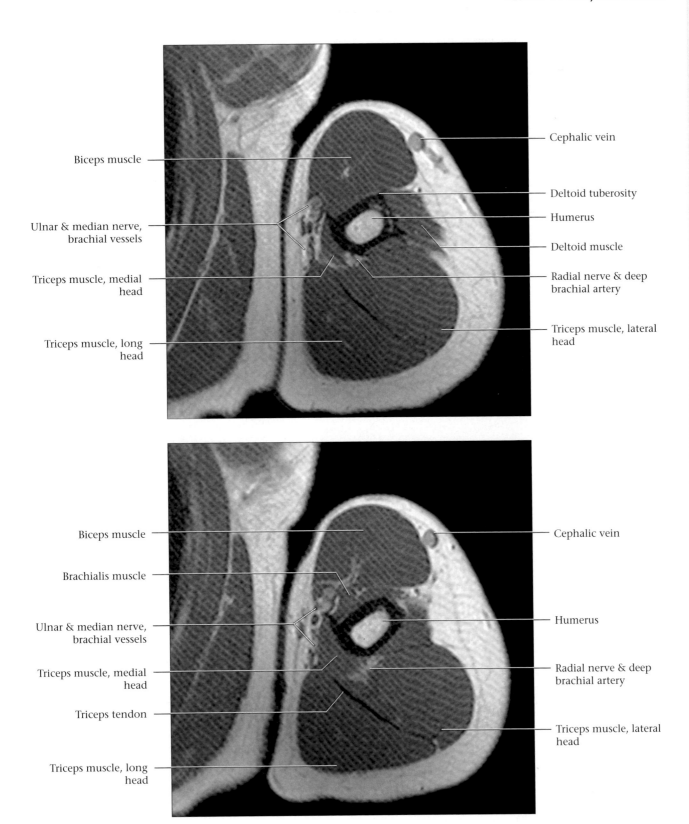

Biceps muscle

Ulnar & median nerve, brachial vessels

Triceps muscle, medial head

Triceps muscle, long head

Cephalic vein

Deltoid tuberosity

Humerus

Deltoid muscle

Radial nerve & deep brachial artery

Triceps muscle, lateral head

Biceps muscle

Brachialis muscle

Ulnar & median nerve, brachial vessels

Triceps muscle, medial head

Triceps tendon

Triceps muscle, long head

Cephalic vein

Humerus

Radial nerve & deep brachial artery

Triceps muscle, lateral head

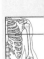

(Top) The medial head of the triceps is arising from the posteromedial humeral cortex. **(Bottom)** The brachialis muscle is arising from the anterior humeral cortex.

Shoulder

I

AXIAL T1 MR, RIGHT ARM

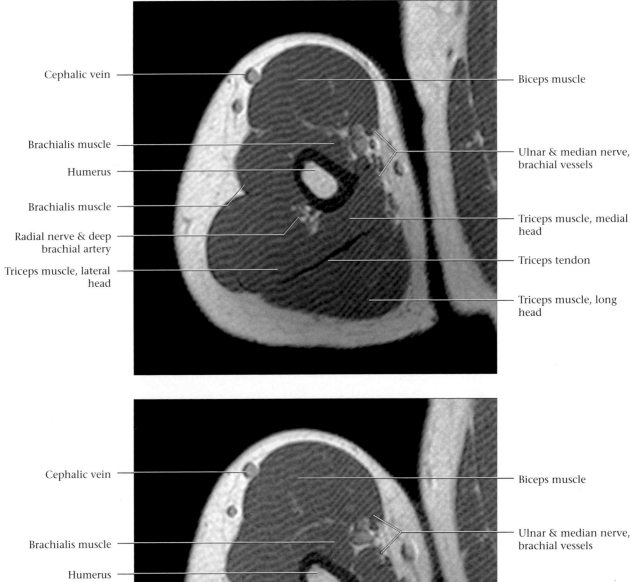

Cephalic vein — Biceps muscle

Brachialis muscle — Ulnar & median nerve, brachial vessels

Humerus —

Brachialis muscle —

Radial nerve & deep brachial artery — Triceps muscle, medial head

Triceps muscle, lateral head — Triceps tendon

Triceps muscle, long head

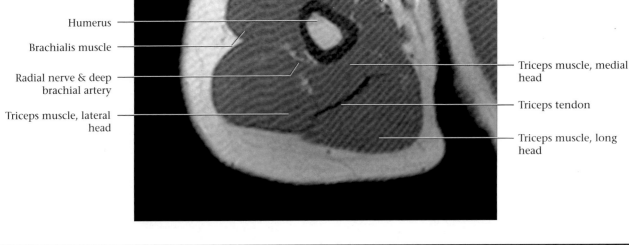

Cephalic vein — Biceps muscle

Brachialis muscle — Ulnar & median nerve, brachial vessels

Humerus —

Brachialis muscle —

Radial nerve & deep brachial artery — Triceps muscle, medial head

Triceps muscle, lateral head — Triceps tendon

Triceps muscle, long head

(Top) The posterior compartment of the arm consists of the three heads of the triceps muscle. **(Bottom)** The deep brachial artery and radial nerve course along the posterolateral humerus.

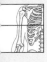
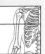

Shoulder

I

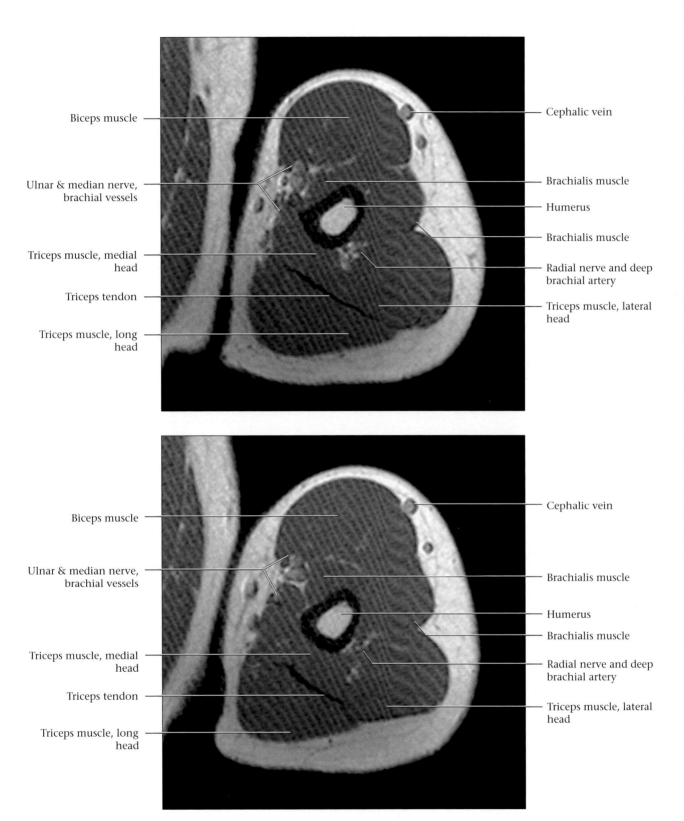

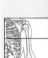

(Top) The posterior compartment of the arm consists of the three heads of the triceps muscle. **(Bottom)** The deep brachial artery and radial nerve course along the posterolateral humerus.

ARM OVERVIEW

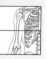

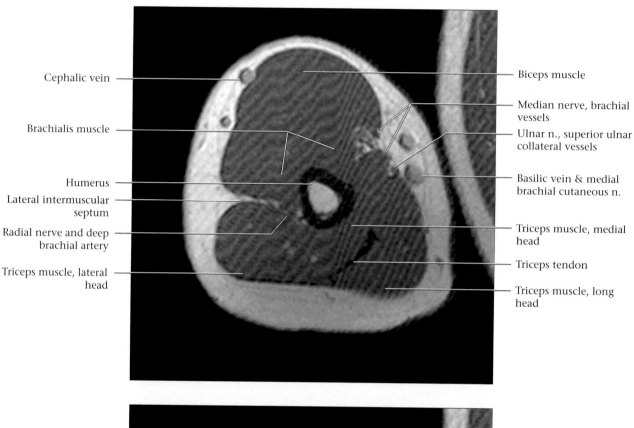

Cephalic vein —

Brachialis muscle —

Humerus —

Lateral intermuscular septum —

Radial nerve and deep brachial artery —

Triceps muscle, lateral head —

— Biceps muscle

— Median nerve, brachial vessels

— Ulnar n., superior ulnar collateral vessels

— Basilic vein & medial brachial cutaneous n.

— Triceps muscle, medial head

— Triceps tendon

— Triceps muscle, long head

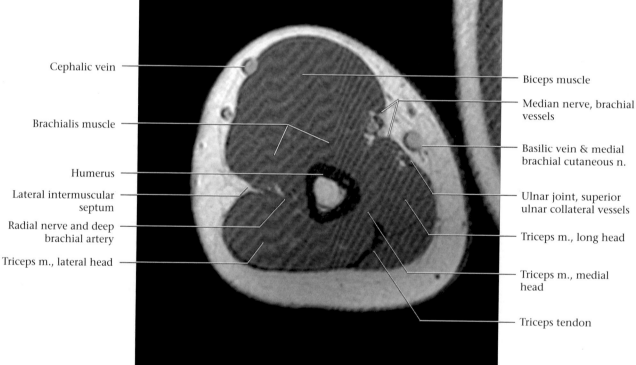

Cephalic vein —

Brachialis muscle —

Humerus —

Lateral intermuscular septum —

Radial nerve and deep brachial artery —

Triceps m., lateral head —

— Biceps muscle

— Median nerve, brachial vessels

— Basilic vein & medial brachial cutaneous n.

— Ulnar joint, superior ulnar collateral vessels

— Triceps m., long head

— Triceps m., medial head

— Triceps tendon

(Top) Branches of the radial nerve innervate the lateral, long and medial heads of the triceps muscle. **(Bottom)** The neurovascular bundle containing the median nerve and brachial vessels denotes the location of the medial intermuscular septum.

ARM OVERVIEW

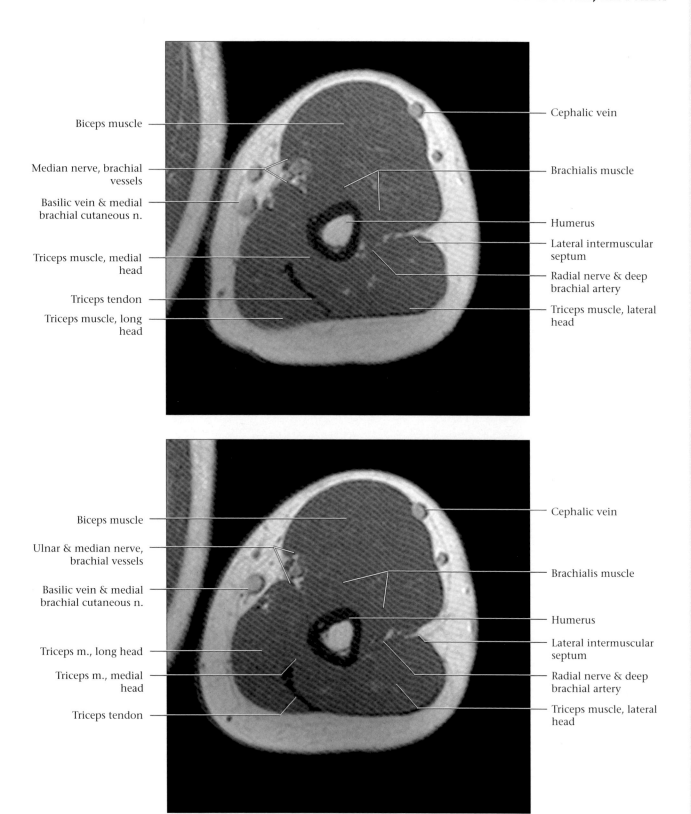

Biceps muscle

Median nerve, brachial vessels

Basilic vein & medial brachial cutaneous n.

Triceps muscle, medial head

Triceps tendon

Triceps muscle, long head

Cephalic vein

Brachialis muscle

Humerus

Lateral intermuscular septum

Radial nerve & deep brachial artery

Triceps muscle, lateral head

Biceps muscle

Ulnar & median nerve, brachial vessels

Basilic vein & medial brachial cutaneous n.

Triceps m., long head

Triceps m., medial head

Triceps tendon

Cephalic vein

Brachialis muscle

Humerus

Lateral intermuscular septum

Radial nerve & deep brachial artery

Triceps muscle, lateral head

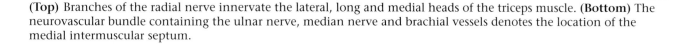

(Top) Branches of the radial nerve innervate the lateral, long and medial heads of the triceps muscle. (Bottom) The neurovascular bundle containing the ulnar nerve, median nerve and brachial vessels denotes the location of the medial intermuscular septum.

AXIAL T1 MR, RIGHT ARM

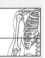

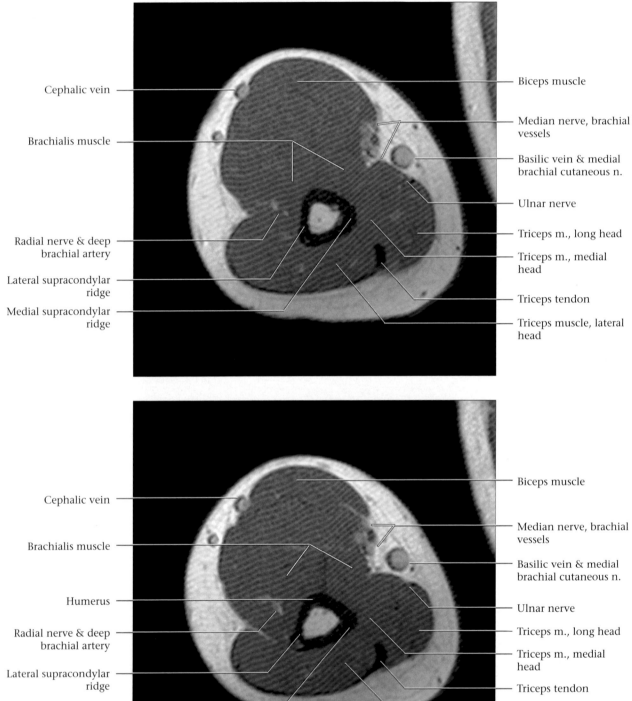

Cephalic vein

Brachialis muscle

Radial nerve & deep brachial artery

Lateral supracondylar ridge

Medial supracondylar ridge

Biceps muscle

Median nerve, brachial vessels

Basilic vein & medial brachial cutaneous n.

Ulnar nerve

Triceps m., long head

Triceps m., medial head

Triceps tendon

Triceps muscle, lateral head

Cephalic vein

Brachialis muscle

Humerus

Radial nerve & deep brachial artery

Lateral supracondylar ridge

Medial supracondylar ridge

Biceps muscle

Median nerve, brachial vessels

Basilic vein & medial brachial cutaneous n.

Ulnar nerve

Triceps m., long head

Triceps m., medial head

Triceps tendon

Triceps muscle, lateral head

(Top) The thick triceps tendon lies between the triceps lateral and long heads. **(Bottom)** The biceps muscle is thinning anteriorly.

ARM OVERVIEW

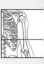

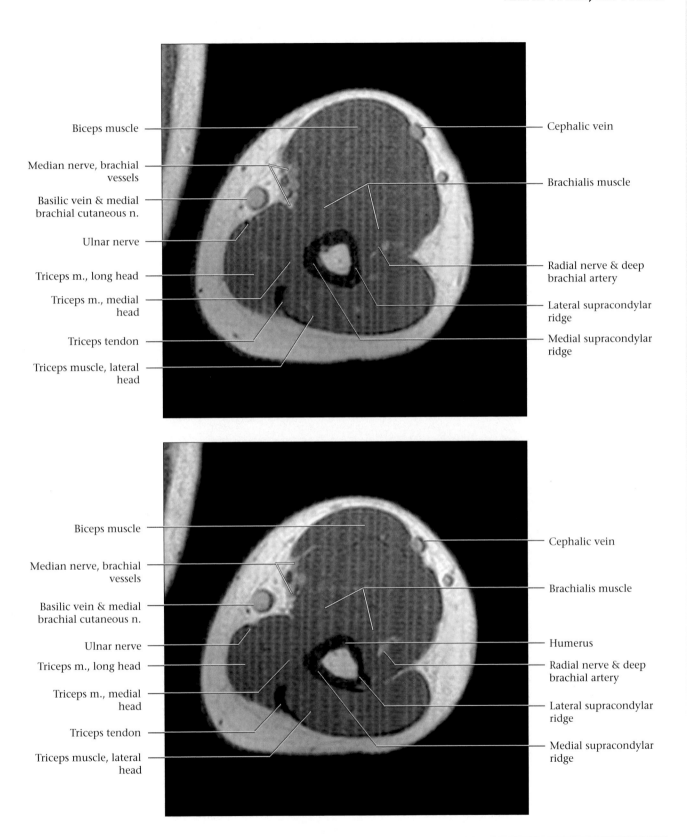

Biceps muscle — Cephalic vein

Median nerve, brachial vessels — Brachialis muscle

Basilic vein & medial brachial cutaneous n.

Ulnar nerve — Radial nerve & deep brachial artery

Triceps m., long head — Lateral supracondylar ridge

Triceps m., medial head — Medial supracondylar ridge

Triceps tendon

Triceps muscle, lateral head

Biceps muscle — Cephalic vein

Median nerve, brachial vessels — Brachialis muscle

Basilic vein & medial brachial cutaneous n.

Ulnar nerve — Humerus

Triceps m., long head — Radial nerve & deep brachial artery

Triceps m., medial head — Lateral supracondylar ridge

Triceps tendon — Medial supracondylar ridge

Triceps muscle, lateral head

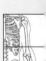

(Top) The thick triceps tendon lies between the triceps lateral and long heads. **(Bottom)** The biceps muscle is thinning anteriorly.

Shoulder I

167

AXIAL T1 MR, RIGHT ARM

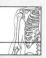

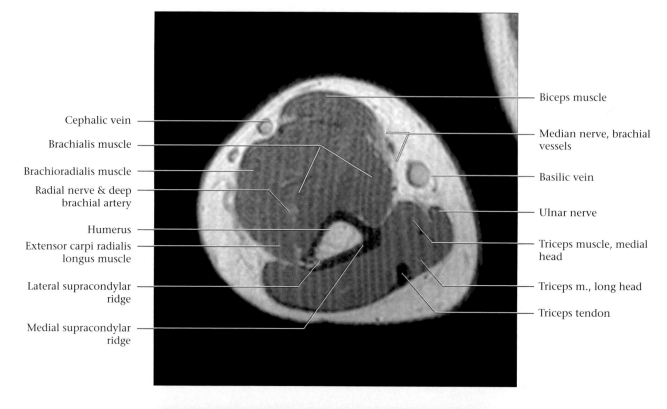

Cephalic vein

Brachialis muscle

Brachioradialis muscle

Radial nerve & deep brachial artery

Humerus

Extensor carpi radialis longus muscle

Lateral supracondylar ridge

Medial supracondylar ridge

Biceps muscle

Median nerve, brachial vessels

Basilic vein

Ulnar nerve

Triceps muscle, medial head

Triceps m., long head

Triceps tendon

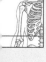

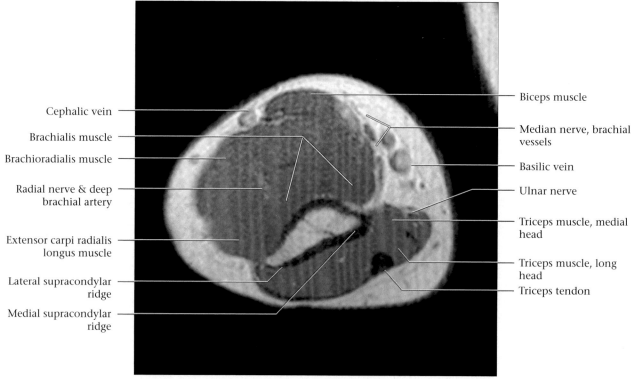

Cephalic vein

Brachialis muscle

Brachioradialis muscle

Radial nerve & deep brachial artery

Extensor carpi radialis longus muscle

Lateral supracondylar ridge

Medial supracondylar ridge

Biceps muscle

Median nerve, brachial vessels

Basilic vein

Ulnar nerve

Triceps muscle, medial head

Triceps muscle, long head

Triceps tendon

(Top) The extensor carpi radialis longus muscle originates from the distal lateral supracondylar ridge. **(Bottom)** The brachioradialis has become the largest muscle in the anterior compartment.

ARM OVERVIEW

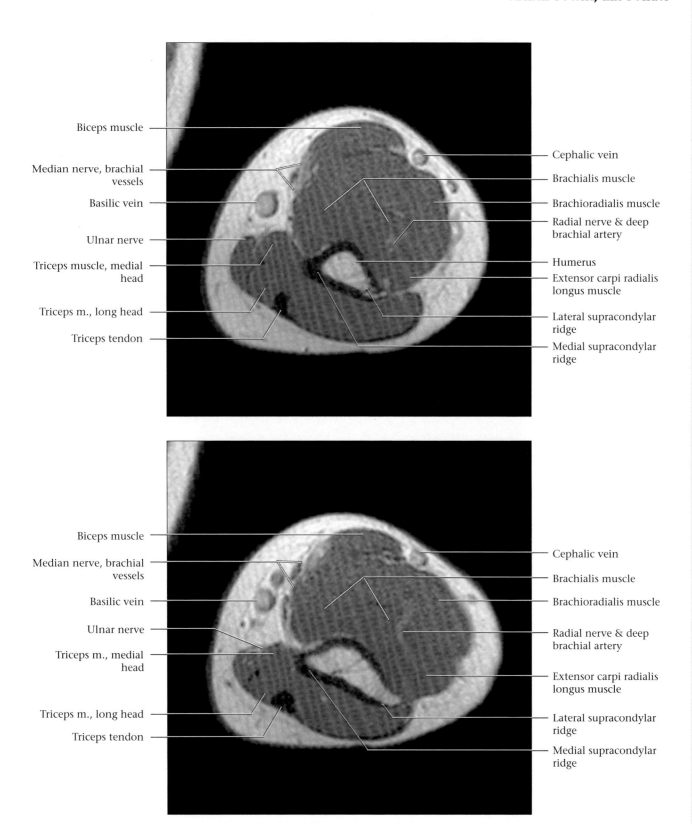

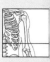
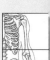

Top image labels (left): Biceps muscle; Median nerve, brachial vessels; Basilic vein; Ulnar nerve; Triceps muscle, medial head; Triceps m., long head; Triceps tendon

Top image labels (right): Cephalic vein; Brachialis muscle; Brachioradialis muscle; Radial nerve & deep brachial artery; Humerus; Extensor carpi radialis longus muscle; Lateral supracondylar ridge; Medial supracondylar ridge

Bottom image labels (left): Biceps muscle; Median nerve, brachial vessels; Basilic vein; Ulnar nerve; Triceps m., medial head; Triceps m., long head; Triceps tendon

Bottom image labels (right): Cephalic vein; Brachialis muscle; Brachioradialis muscle; Radial nerve & deep brachial artery; Extensor carpi radialis longus muscle; Lateral supracondylar ridge; Medial supracondylar ridge

(Top) The extensor carpi radialis longus muscle originates from the distal lateral supracondylar ridge. **(Bottom)** The brachioradialis has become the largest muscle in the anterior compartment.

Shoulder

I

169

AXIAL T1 MR, RIGHT ARM

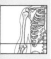

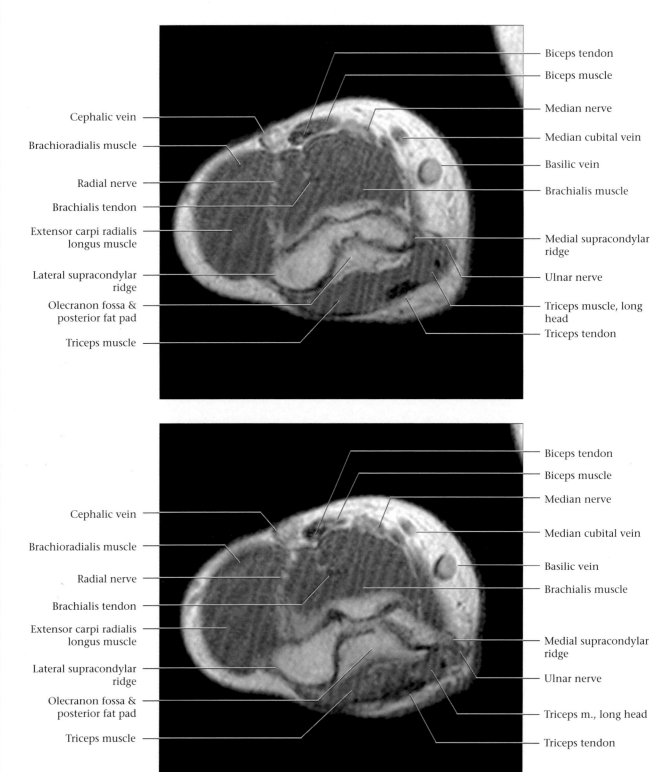

Cephalic vein

Brachioradialis muscle

Radial nerve

Brachialis tendon

Extensor carpi radialis longus muscle

Lateral supracondylar ridge

Olecranon fossa & posterior fat pad

Triceps muscle

Biceps tendon

Biceps muscle

Median nerve

Median cubital vein

Basilic vein

Brachialis muscle

Medial supracondylar ridge

Ulnar nerve

Triceps muscle, long head

Triceps tendon

Cephalic vein

Brachioradialis muscle

Radial nerve

Brachialis tendon

Extensor carpi radialis longus muscle

Lateral supracondylar ridge

Olecranon fossa & posterior fat pad

Triceps muscle

Biceps tendon

Biceps muscle

Median nerve

Median cubital vein

Basilic vein

Brachialis muscle

Medial supracondylar ridge

Ulnar nerve

Triceps m., long head

Triceps tendon

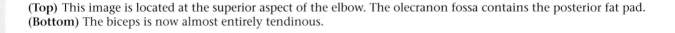

(Top) This image is located at the superior aspect of the elbow. The olecranon fossa contains the posterior fat pad. **(Bottom)** The biceps is now almost entirely tendinous.

AXIAL T1 MR, LEFT ARM

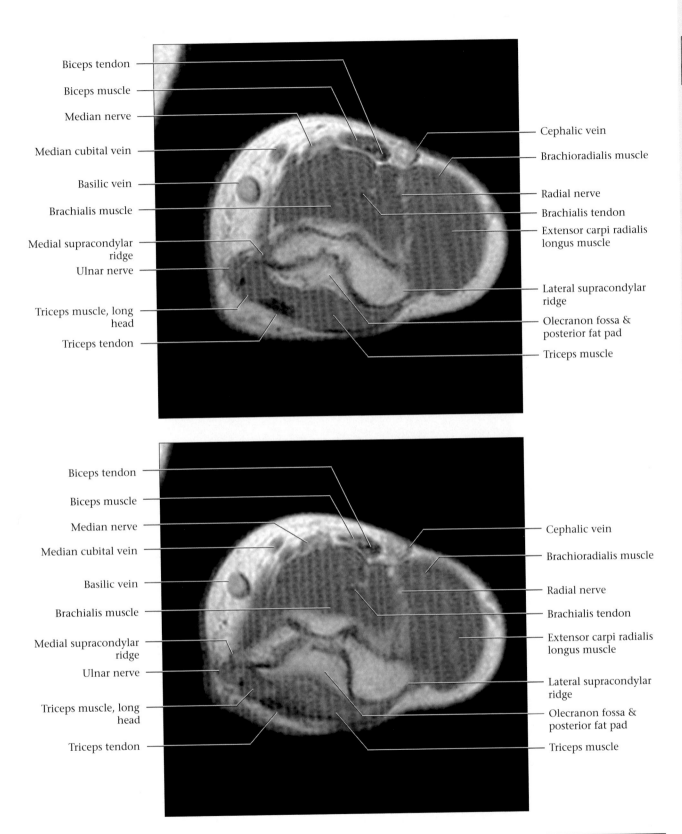

Biceps tendon

Biceps muscle

Median nerve

Median cubital vein

Basilic vein

Brachialis muscle

Medial supracondylar ridge

Ulnar nerve

Triceps muscle, long head

Triceps tendon

Cephalic vein

Brachioradialis muscle

Radial nerve

Brachialis tendon

Extensor carpi radialis longus muscle

Lateral supracondylar ridge

Olecranon fossa & posterior fat pad

Triceps muscle

Biceps tendon

Biceps muscle

Median nerve

Median cubital vein

Basilic vein

Brachialis muscle

Medial supracondylar ridge

Ulnar nerve

Triceps muscle, long head

Triceps tendon

Cephalic vein

Brachioradialis muscle

Radial nerve

Brachialis tendon

Extensor carpi radialis longus muscle

Lateral supracondylar ridge

Olecranon fossa & posterior fat pad

Triceps muscle

(Top) This image is located at the superior aspect of the elbow. The olecranon fossa contains the posterior fat pad. **(Bottom)** The biceps is now almost entirely tendinous.

Shoulder

I

AXIAL T1 MR, RIGHT ARM

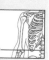

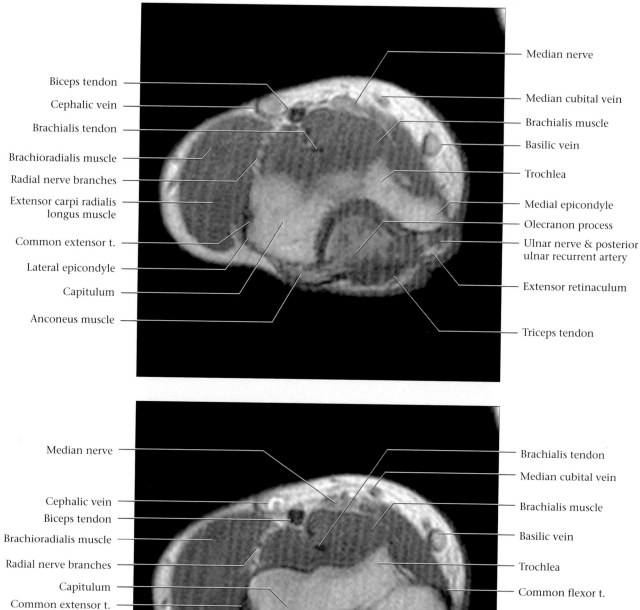

Top image labels:
- Biceps tendon
- Cephalic vein
- Brachialis tendon
- Brachioradialis muscle
- Radial nerve branches
- Extensor carpi radialis longus muscle
- Common extensor t.
- Lateral epicondyle
- Capitulum
- Anconeus muscle
- Median nerve
- Median cubital vein
- Brachialis muscle
- Basilic vein
- Trochlea
- Medial epicondyle
- Olecranon process
- Ulnar nerve & posterior ulnar recurrent artery
- Extensor retinaculum
- Triceps tendon

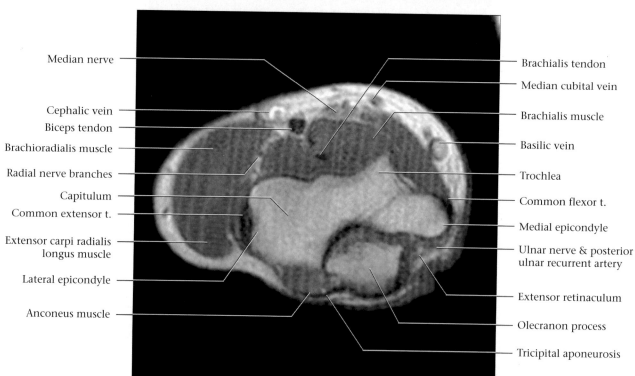

Bottom image labels:
- Median nerve
- Cephalic vein
- Biceps tendon
- Brachioradialis muscle
- Radial nerve branches
- Capitulum
- Common extensor t.
- Extensor carpi radialis longus muscle
- Lateral epicondyle
- Anconeus muscle
- Brachialis tendon
- Median cubital vein
- Brachialis muscle
- Basilic vein
- Trochlea
- Common flexor t.
- Medial epicondyle
- Ulnar nerve & posterior ulnar recurrent artery
- Extensor retinaculum
- Olecranon process
- Tricipital aponeurosis

(Top) The ulnar nerve has passed behind the medial epicondyle. **(Bottom)** The anconeus muscle arises from the lateral epicondyle.

ARM OVERVIEW

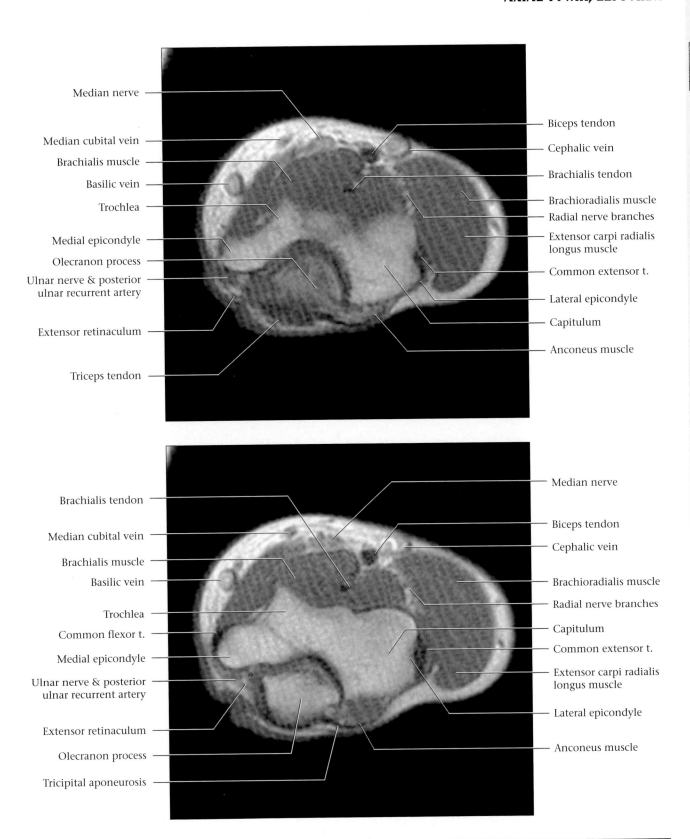

(Top) The ulnar nerve has passed behind the medial epicondyle. **(Bottom)** The anconeus muscle arises from the lateral epicondyle.

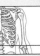
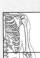

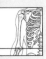

AXIAL T1 MR, RIGHT ARM

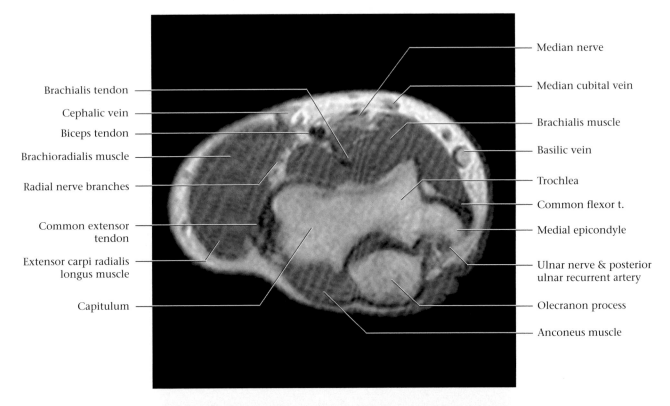

Brachialis tendon

Cephalic vein

Biceps tendon

Brachioradialis muscle

Radial nerve branches

Common extensor tendon

Extensor carpi radialis longus muscle

Capitulum

Median nerve

Median cubital vein

Brachialis muscle

Basilic vein

Trochlea

Common flexor t.

Medial epicondyle

Ulnar nerve & posterior ulnar recurrent artery

Olecranon process

Anconeus muscle

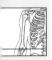

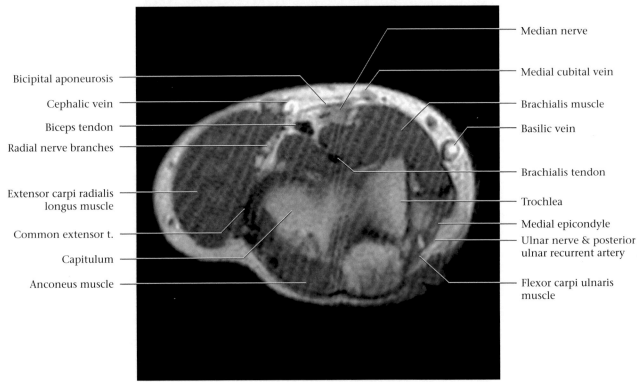

Bicipital aponeurosis

Cephalic vein

Biceps tendon

Radial nerve branches

Extensor carpi radialis longus muscle

Common extensor t.

Capitulum

Anconeus muscle

Median nerve

Medial cubital vein

Brachialis muscle

Basilic vein

Brachialis tendon

Trochlea

Medial epicondyle

Ulnar nerve & posterior ulnar recurrent artery

Flexor carpi ulnaris muscle

(Top) The bicipital aponeurosis or lacertus fibrosis has originated from the medial side of the biceps tendon.
(Bottom) The brachialis tendon is nearing the insertion on the ulnar tuberosity.

ARM OVERVIEW

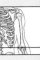

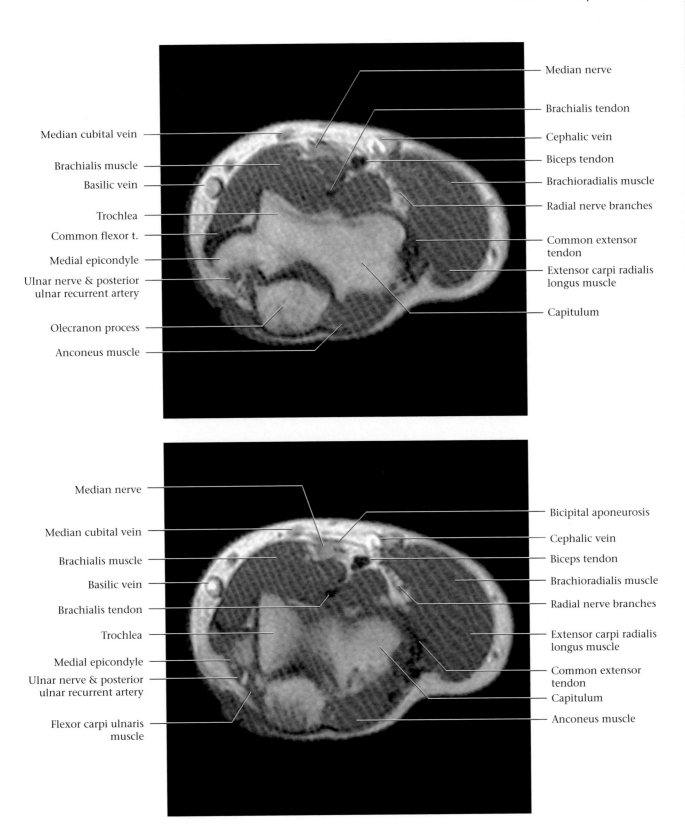

Median cubital vein

Brachialis muscle

Basilic vein

Trochlea

Common flexor t.

Medial epicondyle

Ulnar nerve & posterior
ulnar recurrent artery

Olecranon process

Anconeus muscle

Median nerve

Brachialis tendon

Cephalic vein

Biceps tendon

Brachioradialis muscle

Radial nerve branches

Common extensor
tendon

Extensor carpi radialis
longus muscle

Capitulum

Median nerve

Median cubital vein

Brachialis muscle

Basilic vein

Brachialis tendon

Trochlea

Medial epicondyle

Ulnar nerve & posterior
ulnar recurrent artery

Flexor carpi ulnaris
muscle

Bicipital aponeurosis

Cephalic vein

Biceps tendon

Brachioradialis muscle

Radial nerve branches

Extensor carpi radialis
longus muscle

Common extensor
tendon

Capitulum

Anconeus muscle

(Top) The bicipital aponeurosis or lacertus fibrosis has originated from the medial side of the biceps tendon.
(Bottom) The brachialis tendon is nearing the insertion on the ulnar tuberosity.

Shoulder

I

175

AXIAL T1 MR, RIGHT ARM

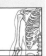

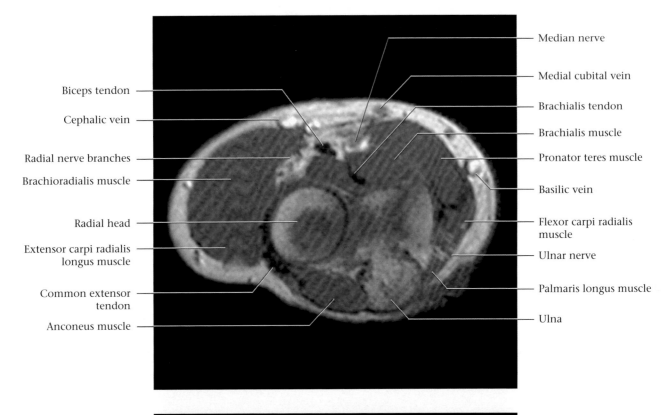

Biceps tendon

Cephalic vein

Radial nerve branches

Brachioradialis muscle

Radial head

Extensor carpi radialis longus muscle

Common extensor tendon

Anconeus muscle

Median nerve

Medial cubital vein

Brachialis tendon

Brachialis muscle

Pronator teres muscle

Basilic vein

Flexor carpi radialis muscle

Ulnar nerve

Palmaris longus muscle

Ulna

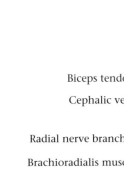

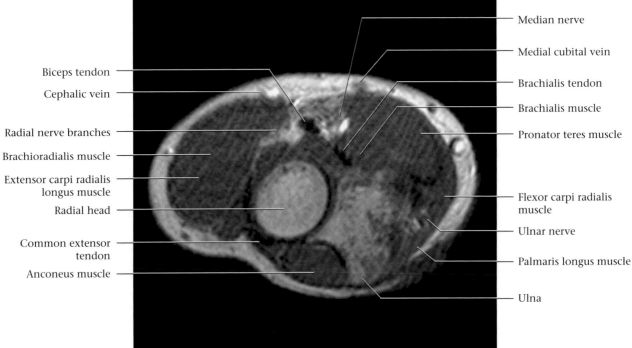

Biceps tendon

Cephalic vein

Radial nerve branches

Brachioradialis muscle

Extensor carpi radialis longus muscle

Radial head

Common extensor tendon

Anconeus muscle

Median nerve

Medial cubital vein

Brachialis tendon

Brachialis muscle

Pronator teres muscle

Flexor carpi radialis muscle

Ulnar nerve

Palmaris longus muscle

Ulna

(Top) The radial head is coming into view. The biceps tendon is coursing deep in the antecubital fossa. **(Bottom)** The majority of the muscle mass at the lateral aspect of the elbow consists of the brachioradialis and extensor carpi radialis longus muscles.

ARM OVERVIEW

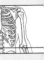

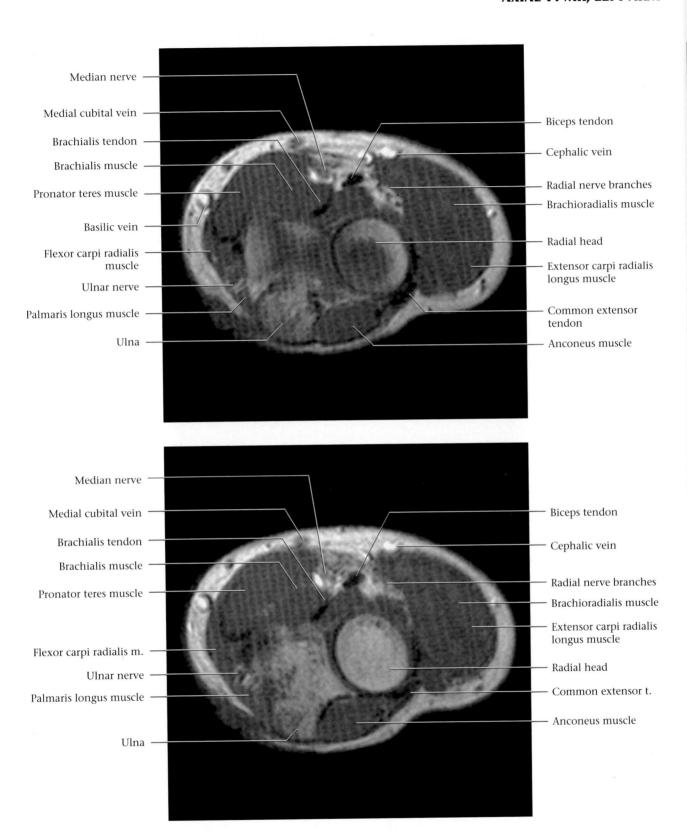

Median nerve

Medial cubital vein

Brachialis tendon

Brachialis muscle

Pronator teres muscle

Basilic vein

Flexor carpi radialis
muscle

Ulnar nerve

Palmaris longus muscle

Ulna

Biceps tendon

Cephalic vein

Radial nerve branches

Brachioradialis muscle

Radial head

Extensor carpi radialis
longus muscle

Common extensor
tendon

Anconeus muscle

Median nerve

Medial cubital vein

Brachialis tendon

Brachialis muscle

Pronator teres muscle

Flexor carpi radialis m.

Ulnar nerve

Palmaris longus muscle

Ulna

Biceps tendon

Cephalic vein

Radial nerve branches

Brachioradialis muscle

Extensor carpi radialis
longus muscle

Radial head

Common extensor t.

Anconeus muscle

(Top) The radial head is coming into view. The biceps tendon is coursing deep in the antecubital fossa. **(Bottom)** The majority of the muscle mass at the lateral aspect of the elbow consists of the brachioradialis and extensor carpi radialis longus muscles.

Shoulder

I

177

ARM OVERVIEW

CORONAL T1 MR, RIGHT ARM

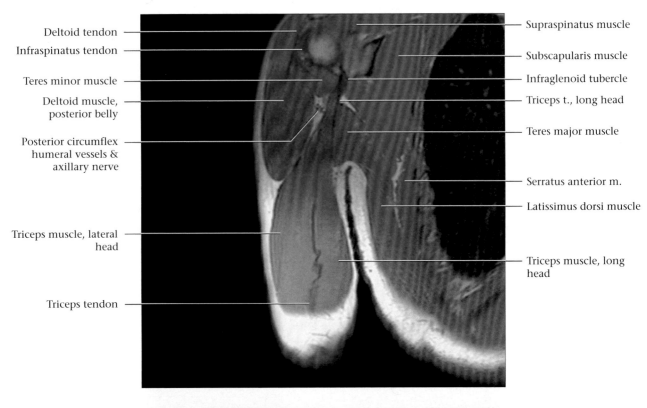

Deltoid tendon — Supraspinatus muscle

Infraspinatus tendon — Subscapularis muscle

Teres minor muscle — Infraglenoid tubercle

Deltoid muscle, posterior belly — Triceps t., long head

Posterior circumflex humeral vessels & axillary nerve — Teres major muscle

— Serratus anterior m.

— Latissimus dorsi muscle

Triceps muscle, lateral head — Triceps muscle, long head

Triceps tendon

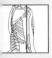

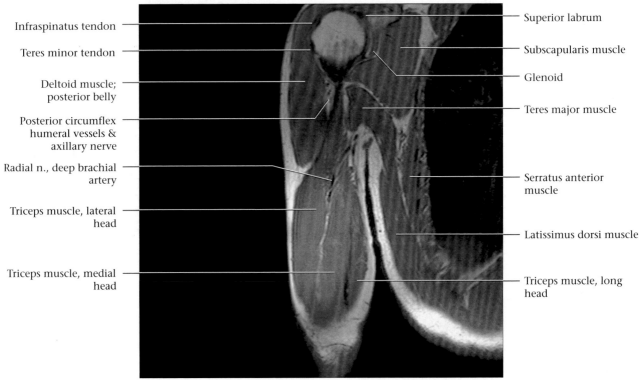

Infraspinatus tendon — Superior labrum

Teres minor tendon — Subscapularis muscle

Deltoid muscle; posterior belly — Glenoid

Posterior circumflex humeral vessels & axillary nerve — Teres major muscle

Radial n., deep brachial artery — Serratus anterior muscle

Triceps muscle, lateral head — Latissimus dorsi muscle

Triceps muscle, medial head — Triceps muscle, long head

(Top) First in series of sequential coronal T1 MR images of the right arm displayed posterior to anterior. Images were acquired at 3T. The long head of the triceps originates from the infraglenoid tubercle of the scapula. **(Bottom)** The muscle mass of the posterior arm consists of the three heads of the triceps muscle.

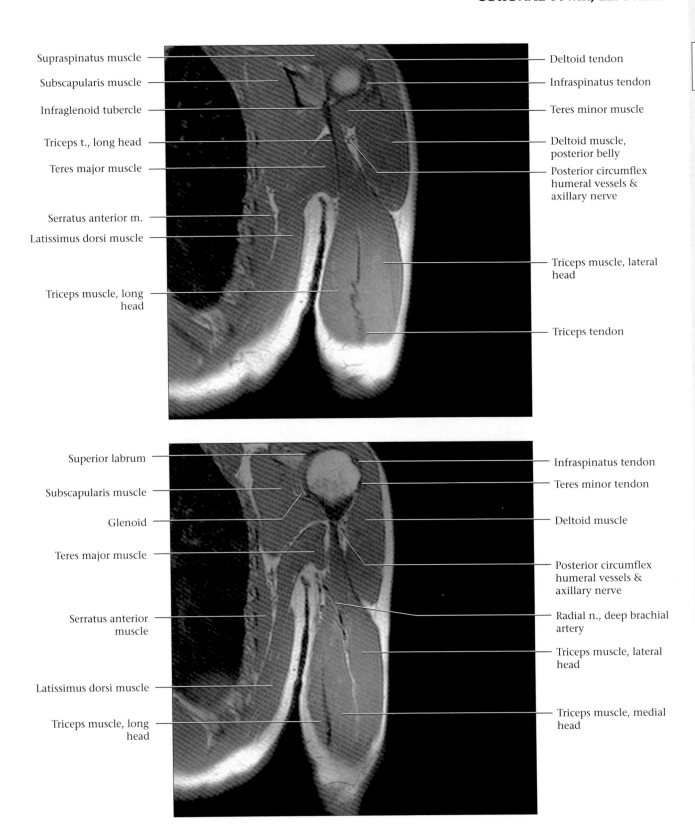

Supraspinatus muscle — Deltoid tendon

Subscapularis muscle — Infraspinatus tendon

Infraglenoid tubercle — Teres minor muscle

Triceps t., long head — Deltoid muscle, posterior belly

Teres major muscle — Posterior circumflex humeral vessels & axillary nerve

Serratus anterior m. —

Latissimus dorsi muscle —

— Triceps muscle, lateral head

Triceps muscle, long head — — Triceps tendon

Superior labrum — Infraspinatus tendon

— Teres minor tendon

Subscapularis muscle —

Glenoid — Deltoid muscle

Teres major muscle —

— Posterior circumflex humeral vessels & axillary nerve

Serratus anterior muscle — — Radial n., deep brachial artery

— Triceps muscle, lateral head

Latissimus dorsi muscle —

Triceps muscle, long head — — Triceps muscle, medial head

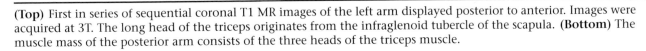

(Top) First in series of sequential coronal T1 MR images of the left arm displayed posterior to anterior. Images were acquired at 3T. The long head of the triceps originates from the infraglenoid tubercle of the scapula. **(Bottom)** The muscle mass of the posterior arm consists of the three heads of the triceps muscle.

CORONAL T1 MR, RIGHT ARM

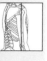

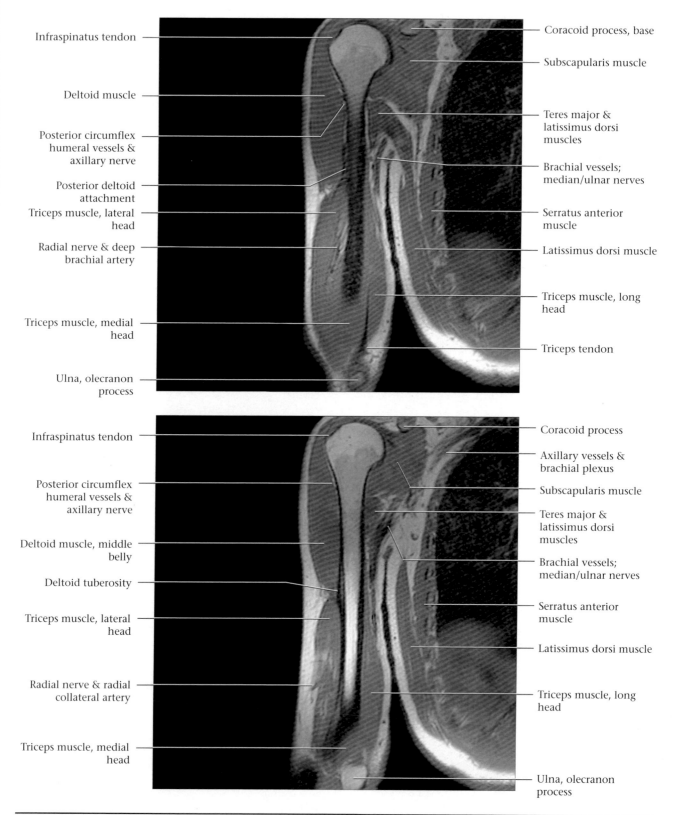

Infraspinatus tendon

Deltoid muscle

Posterior circumflex humeral vessels & axillary nerve

Posterior deltoid attachment

Triceps muscle, lateral head

Radial nerve & deep brachial artery

Triceps muscle, medial head

Ulna, olecranon process

Coracoid process, base

Subscapularis muscle

Teres major & latissimus dorsi muscles

Brachial vessels; median/ulnar nerves

Serratus anterior muscle

Latissimus dorsi muscle

Triceps muscle, long head

Triceps tendon

Infraspinatus tendon

Posterior circumflex humeral vessels & axillary nerve

Deltoid muscle, middle belly

Deltoid tuberosity

Triceps muscle, lateral head

Radial nerve & radial collateral artery

Triceps muscle, medial head

Coracoid process

Axillary vessels & brachial plexus

Subscapularis muscle

Teres major & latissimus dorsi muscles

Brachial vessels; median/ulnar nerves

Serratus anterior muscle

Latissimus dorsi muscle

Triceps muscle, long head

Ulna, olecranon process

(Top) The teres major and latissimus dorsi muscle course anteriorly to insert on the anterior humeral cortex.
(Bottom) The deltoid muscle tapers distally at the attachment to the deltoid tuberosity.

ARM OVERVIEW

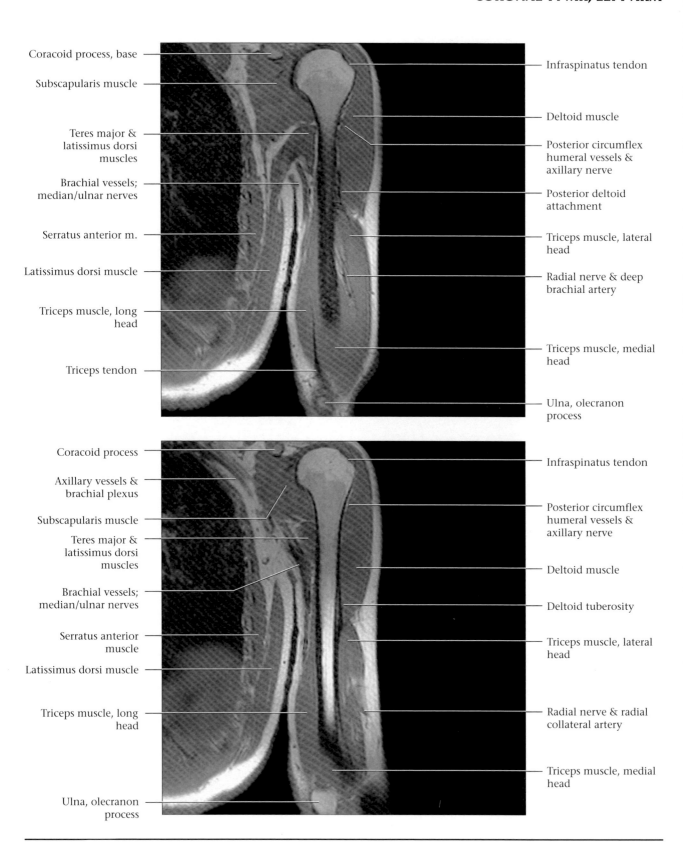

Top image labels (left side):
- Coracoid process, base
- Subscapularis muscle
- Teres major & latissimus dorsi muscles
- Brachial vessels; median/ulnar nerves
- Serratus anterior m.
- Latissimus dorsi muscle
- Triceps muscle, long head
- Triceps tendon

Top image labels (right side):
- Infraspinatus tendon
- Deltoid muscle
- Posterior circumflex humeral vessels & axillary nerve
- Posterior deltoid attachment
- Triceps muscle, lateral head
- Radial nerve & deep brachial artery
- Triceps muscle, medial head
- Ulna, olecranon process

Bottom image labels (left side):
- Coracoid process
- Axillary vessels & brachial plexus
- Subscapularis muscle
- Teres major & latissimus dorsi muscles
- Brachial vessels; median/ulnar nerves
- Serratus anterior muscle
- Latissimus dorsi muscle
- Triceps muscle, long head
- Ulna, olecranon process

Bottom image labels (right side):
- Infraspinatus tendon
- Posterior circumflex humeral vessels & axillary nerve
- Deltoid muscle
- Deltoid tuberosity
- Triceps muscle, lateral head
- Radial nerve & radial collateral artery
- Triceps muscle, medial head

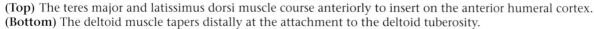

(Top) The teres major and latissimus dorsi muscle course anteriorly to insert on the anterior humeral cortex.
(Bottom) The deltoid muscle tapers distally at the attachment to the deltoid tuberosity.

Shoulder

I

181

ARM OVERVIEW

CORONAL T1 MR, RIGHT ARM

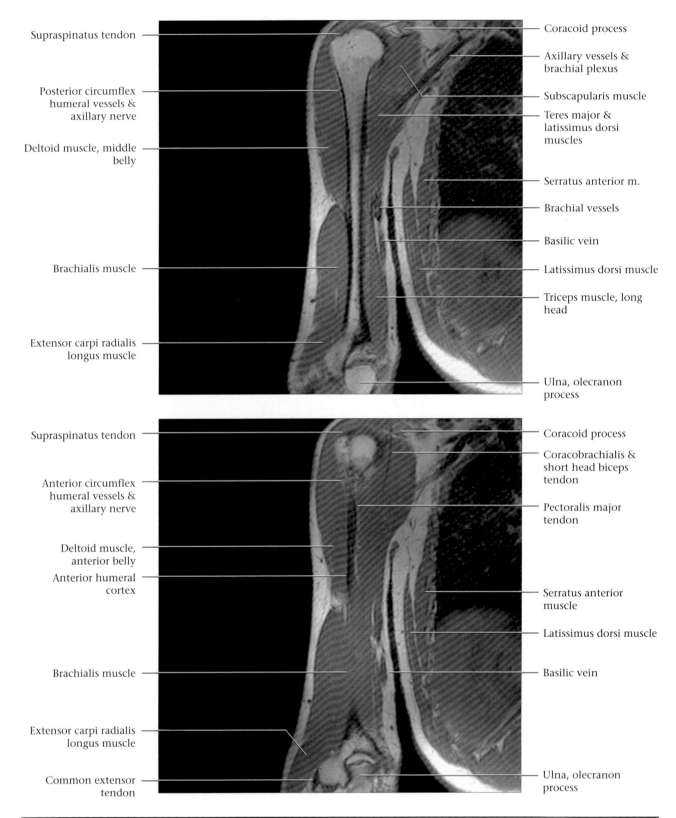

Supraspinatus tendon

Posterior circumflex humeral vessels & axillary nerve

Deltoid muscle, middle belly

Brachialis muscle

Extensor carpi radialis longus muscle

Coracoid process

Axillary vessels & brachial plexus

Subscapularis muscle

Teres major & latissimus dorsi muscles

Serratus anterior m.

Brachial vessels

Basilic vein

Latissimus dorsi muscle

Triceps muscle, long head

Ulna, olecranon process

Supraspinatus tendon

Anterior circumflex humeral vessels & axillary nerve

Deltoid muscle, anterior belly

Anterior humeral cortex

Brachialis muscle

Extensor carpi radialis longus muscle

Common extensor tendon

Coracoid process

Coracobrachialis & short head biceps tendon

Pectoralis major tendon

Serratus anterior muscle

Latissimus dorsi muscle

Basilic vein

Ulna, olecranon process

(Top) The brachialis muscle originates from the distal half of the anterior humeral cortex. **(Bottom)** The coracobrachialis and biceps short head originate from the coracoid process.

ARM OVERVIEW

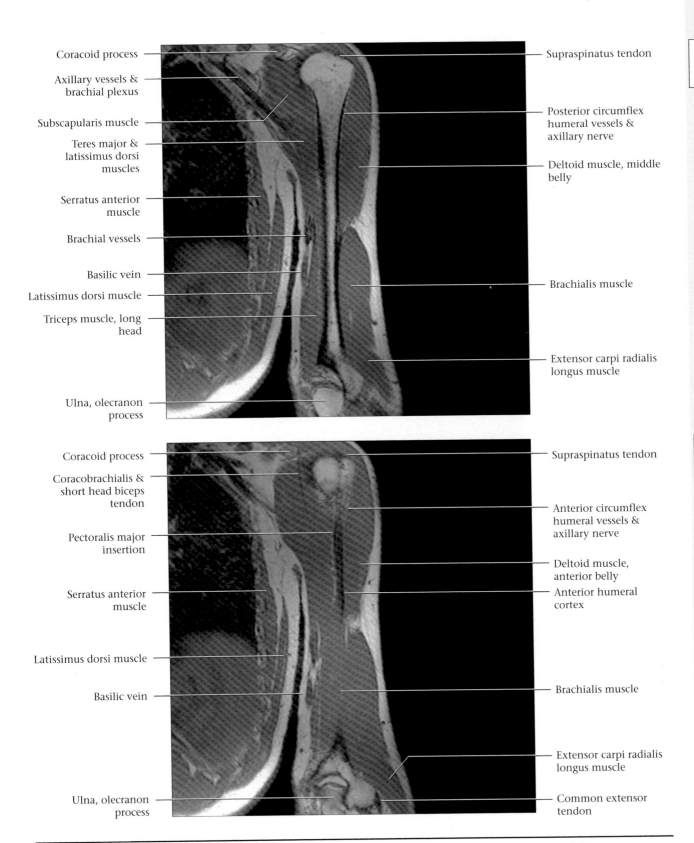

Coracoid process

Axillary vessels & brachial plexus

Subscapularis muscle

Teres major & latissimus dorsi muscles

Serratus anterior muscle

Brachial vessels

Basilic vein

Latissimus dorsi muscle

Triceps muscle, long head

Ulna, olecranon process

Supraspinatus tendon

Posterior circumflex humeral vessels & axillary nerve

Deltoid muscle, middle belly

Brachialis muscle

Extensor carpi radialis longus muscle

Coracoid process

Coracobrachialis & short head biceps tendon

Pectoralis major insertion

Serratus anterior muscle

Latissimus dorsi muscle

Basilic vein

Ulna, olecranon process

Supraspinatus tendon

Anterior circumflex humeral vessels & axillary nerve

Deltoid muscle, anterior belly

Anterior humeral cortex

Brachialis muscle

Extensor carpi radialis longus muscle

Common extensor tendon

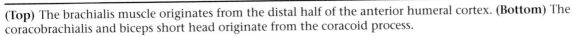

(Top) The brachialis muscle originates from the distal half of the anterior humeral cortex. **(Bottom)** The coracobrachialis and biceps short head originate from the coracoid process.

CORONAL T1 MR, RIGHT ARM

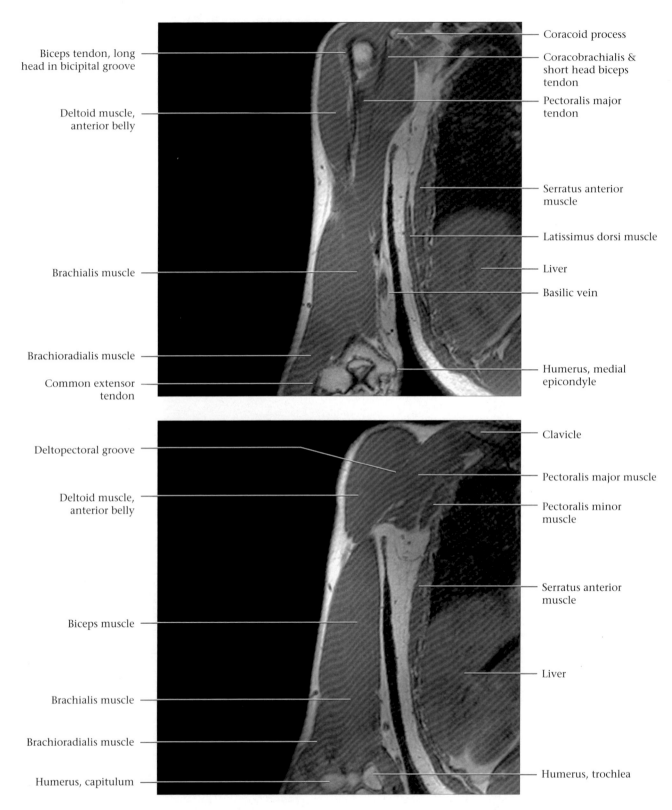

Biceps tendon, long head in bicipital groove

Deltoid muscle, anterior belly

Brachialis muscle

Brachioradialis muscle

Common extensor tendon

Coracoid process

Coracobrachialis & short head biceps tendon

Pectoralis major tendon

Serratus anterior muscle

Latissimus dorsi muscle

Liver

Basilic vein

Humerus, medial epicondyle

Deltopectoral groove

Deltoid muscle, anterior belly

Biceps muscle

Brachialis muscle

Brachioradialis muscle

Humerus, capitulum

Clavicle

Pectoralis major muscle

Pectoralis minor muscle

Serratus anterior muscle

Liver

Humerus, trochlea

(Top) The long head of the biceps tendon traverses the bicipital groove. The biceps long head and short head fuse at the upper humeral level. **(Bottom)** The most anterior image shows the deltoid muscle at the shoulder level and the biceps muscle along the length of the upper arm.

ARM OVERVIEW

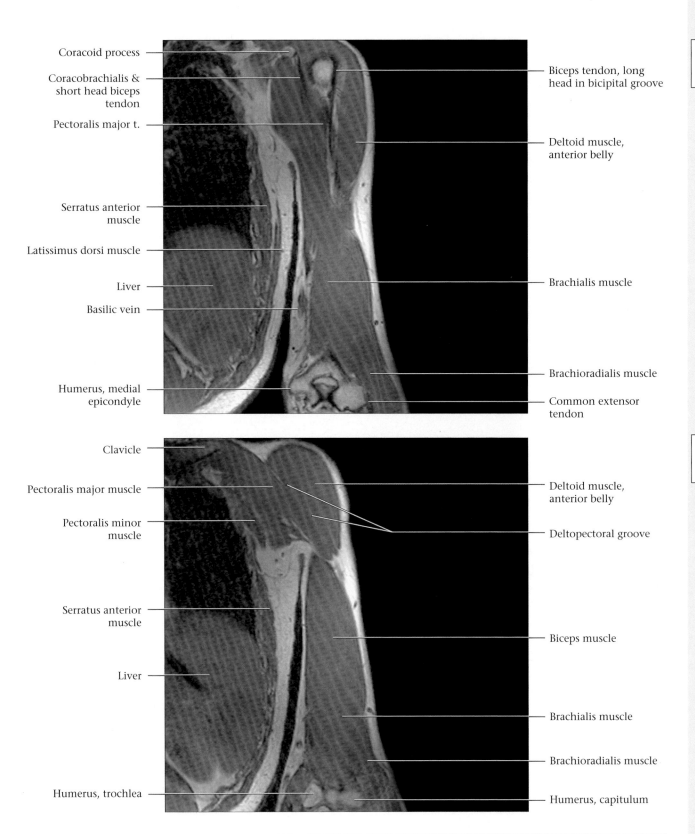

Top image labels (left side):
- Coracoid process
- Coracobrachialis & short head biceps tendon
- Pectoralis major t.
- Serratus anterior muscle
- Latissimus dorsi muscle
- Liver
- Basilic vein
- Humerus, medial epicondyle

Top image labels (right side):
- Biceps tendon, long head in bicipital groove
- Deltoid muscle, anterior belly
- Brachialis muscle
- Brachioradialis muscle
- Common extensor tendon

Bottom image labels (left side):
- Clavicle
- Pectoralis major muscle
- Pectoralis minor muscle
- Serratus anterior muscle
- Liver
- Humerus, trochlea

Bottom image labels (right side):
- Deltoid muscle, anterior belly
- Deltopectoral groove
- Biceps muscle
- Brachialis muscle
- Brachioradialis muscle
- Humerus, capitulum

(Top) The long head of the biceps tendon traverses the bicipital groove. The biceps long head and short head fuse at the upper humeral level. (Bottom) The most anterior image shows the deltoid muscle at the shoulder level and the biceps muscle along the length of the upper arm.

Shoulder

I

185

SAGITTAL T1 MR, RIGHT ARM

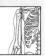

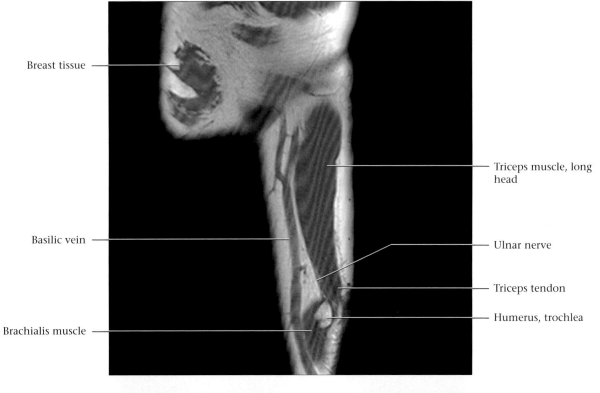

Breast tissue

Triceps muscle, long head

Basilic vein

Ulnar nerve

Triceps tendon

Humerus, trochlea

Brachialis muscle

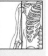

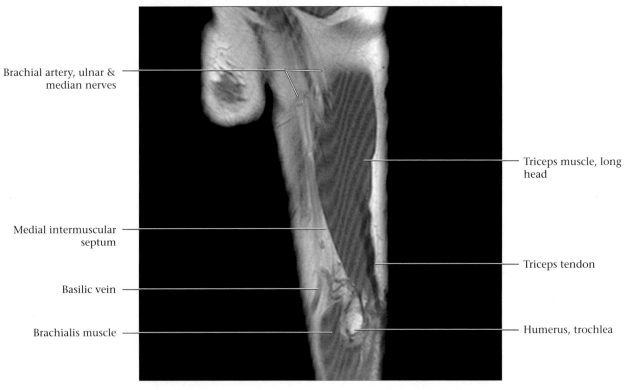

Brachial artery, ulnar & median nerves

Triceps muscle, long head

Medial intermuscular septum

Triceps tendon

Basilic vein

Brachialis muscle

Humerus, trochlea

(Top) First of eight sequential sagittal T1 MR images of the right arm displayed medial to lateral. Images were acquired at 3T. The basilic vein courses distally down the medial arm. **(Bottom)** The medial intermuscular septum separates the anterior compartment from the triceps muscle in the posterior compartment.

ARM OVERVIEW

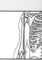

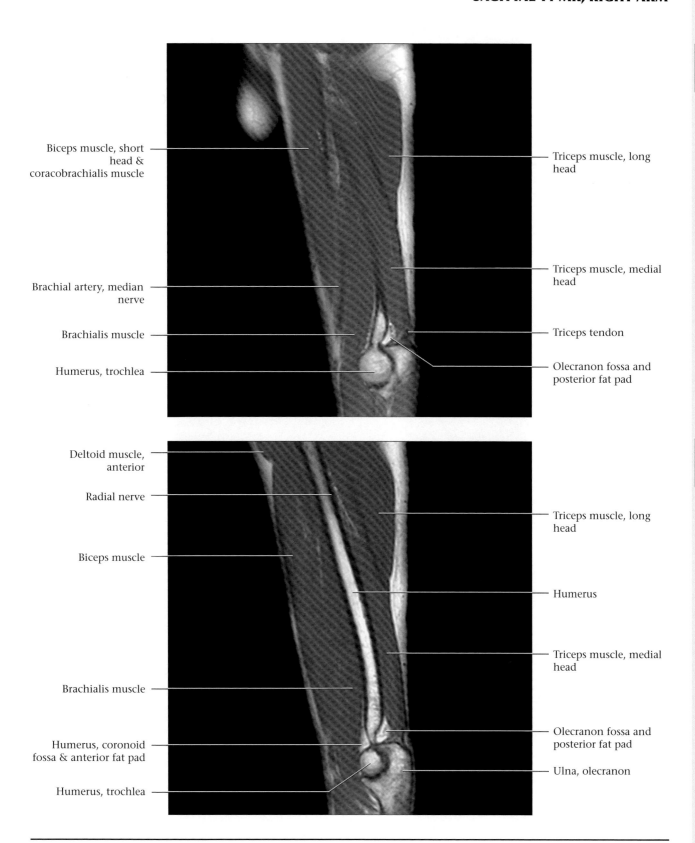

Biceps muscle, short head & coracobrachialis muscle

Triceps muscle, long head

Brachial artery, median nerve

Triceps muscle, medial head

Brachialis muscle

Triceps tendon

Humerus, trochlea

Olecranon fossa and posterior fat pad

Deltoid muscle, anterior

Radial nerve

Triceps muscle, long head

Biceps muscle

Humerus

Triceps muscle, medial head

Brachialis muscle

Olecranon fossa and posterior fat pad

Humerus, coronoid fossa & anterior fat pad

Ulna, olecranon

Humerus, trochlea

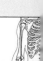

(**Top**) The triceps medial head lies deep to the long and lateral heads. (**Bottom**) The brachialis muscle originates from the anterior humeral cortex and inserts on the ulnar tuberosity.

ARM OVERVIEW

SAGITTAL T1 MR, RIGHT ARM

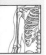

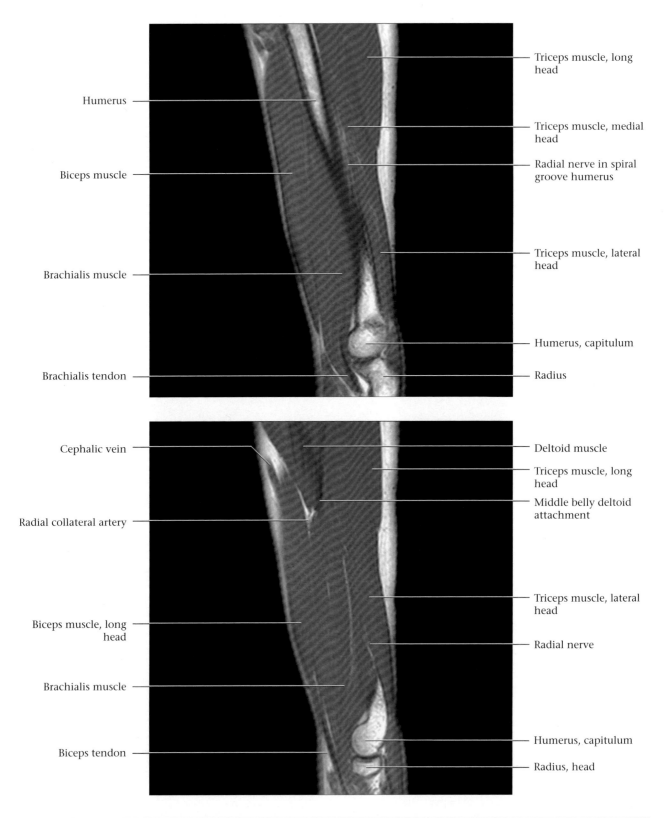

Humerus

Biceps muscle

Brachialis muscle

Brachialis tendon

Triceps muscle, long head

Triceps muscle, medial head

Radial nerve in spiral groove humerus

Triceps muscle, lateral head

Humerus, capitulum

Radius

Cephalic vein

Radial collateral artery

Biceps muscle, long head

Brachialis muscle

Biceps tendon

Deltoid muscle

Triceps muscle, long head

Middle belly deltoid attachment

Triceps muscle, lateral head

Radial nerve

Humerus, capitulum

Radius, head

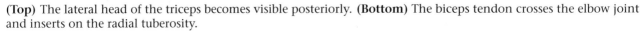

(Top) The lateral head of the triceps becomes visible posteriorly. **(Bottom)** The biceps tendon crosses the elbow joint and inserts on the radial tuberosity.

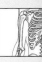

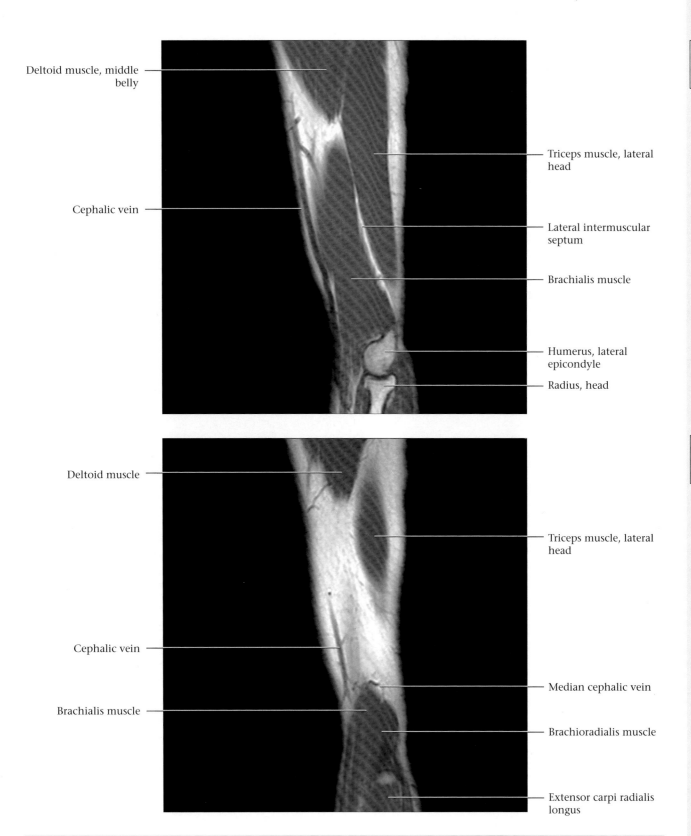

Deltoid muscle, middle belly

Cephalic vein

Triceps muscle, lateral head

Lateral intermuscular septum

Brachialis muscle

Humerus, lateral epicondyle

Radius, head

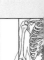

Deltoid muscle

Cephalic vein

Brachialis muscle

Triceps muscle, lateral head

Median cephalic vein

Brachioradialis muscle

Extensor carpi radialis longus

(Top) The cephalic vein is located in the subcutaneous fat of the anterolateral arm. The lateral intermuscular septum separates the anterior from posterior compartment. **(Bottom)** The extensor carpi radialis longus originates from the lateral epicondyle of the humerus.

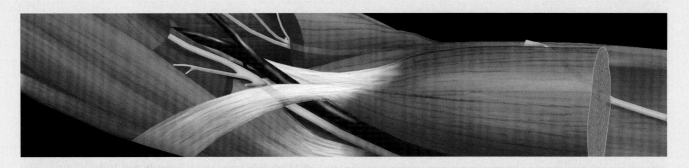

SECTION II: Elbow

Gross Anatomy

Joint

- Complex joint composed of humerus, ulna, & radius
- Has three articulations
  - **Humero-ulnar articulation**
    - Composed of trochlea of humerus and trochlear notch of ulna
    - Hinge joint, allowing flexion and extension
    - Osseous configuration provides medial-lateral stability between 0° and 30° flexion
  - **Humero-radial articulation**
    - Composed of capitellum & radial head
    - Allows both hinge and pivot motion
    - No inherent osseous stability
  - **Proximal radio-ulnar joint**
    - Composed of the radial head and the sigmoid notch of the proximal ulna
    - Pivot joint, allowing the radial head to rotate as forearm supinates and pronates
    - Stability is provided by the anular ligament, holding the head within the notch
  - Congruity of articulating surfaces varies with position of both elbow and forearm: Greatest congruity when elbow flexed 90° and forearm midway between supination and pronation
- **Joint capsule**
  - Encloses all three articulations
  - Posterior attachments: Humerus proximal to olecranon fossa and capitellum, olecranon process anterior to triceps tendon
  - Anterior attachments: Humerus proximal to coronoid and radial fossae, coronoid process, anular ligament
  - Anterior and posterior fat pads are intracapsular but extra-synovial
- **Motion of the elbow joint**
  - **Flexion**
    - Brachialis muscle: Originates at anterior surface of humerus and inserts on anterior tuberosity of ulna
    - Biceps brachii muscle: Originates at shoulder and inserts on radial tuberosity
    - Brachioradialis muscle: Originates from lateral supracondylar ridge of humerus and inserts on lateral side of the distal radius
    - Pronator teres muscle: Originates from medial epicondyle and coronoid process of ulna and inserts on lateral side of mid-shaft of the radius
  - **Extension**
    - Triceps muscle: Originates from shoulder and proximal humerus and inserts on olecranon
    - Anconeus muscle: Originates from posterior aspect of lateral epicondyle & inserts on lateral aspect of ulna and olecranon (also abducts ulna during pronation)
- **Motion of the proximal radio-ulnar joint**
  - **Supination**
    - Biceps brachii muscle (see above)
    - Supinator muscle: Originates from lateral epicondyle and supinator crest of ulna and inserts on lateral side of proximal shaft of radius
  - **Pronation**
    - Pronator teres muscle (see above)
    - Pronator quadratus muscle: Located in distal forearm, originates on distal ulna and inserts on distal radius

Ligaments

- **Lateral**
  - **Radial collateral ligament**
    - Restrains against varus stress
    - Originates on lateral epicondyle and distally blends with the anular ligament
  - **Lateral ulnar collateral ligament**
    - Restrains against posterolateral instability
    - Originates on lateral epicondyle, just posterior to radial collateral ligament
    - Courses posteromedially behind the radial neck to insert on the supinator crest on radial side of proximal ulna
- **Medial**
  - **Medial (also called ulnar) collateral ligament**
    - Restrains against valgus stress
    - Fan-shaped, extending from medial epicondyle to ulna
    - Has three components: Anterior band (functionally most important), posterior band, transverse band
- **Ligaments of the proximal radio-ulnar joint**
  - **Anular ligament:** Attached to anterior and posterior aspects of radial notch of ulna, forming a collar around the radial head
  - **Quadrate ligament:** Thin fibrous band extending from radial neck to ulna, distal to anular ligament

Tendons

- Several flexor and extensor muscles of forearm arise from the medial and lateral epicondyles of humerus
  - **Common flexor tendon**
    - Arises from medial epicondyle
    - Superficial to medial collateral ligament
    - Composed of the flexor-pronator group: Flexor carpi radialis, flexor carpi ulnaris, flexor digitorum superficialis, pronator teres, palmaris longus
  - **Common extensor tendon**
    - Arises from lateral epicondyle
    - Superficial to radial collateral ligament
    - Composed of the extensor-supinator group: Extensor carpi radialis brevis, extensor carpi radialis longus, extensor digiti minimi, extensor digitorum communis

Bursae

- **Posterior**
  - **Subcutaneous olecranon bursa:** Located subcutaneously, superficial to olecranon process
  - **Subtendinous olecranon bursa:** Located between the triceps tendon and the olecranon
- **Anterior**
  - **Bicipitoradial bursa:** Located between the biceps tendon and the radial tuberosity
- **Lateral**
  - **Radioulnar bursa:** Located between the extensor digitorum and radiohumeral joint

Nerves

- **Radial nerve**

- o Arises from posterior cord of the brachial plexus (C5-8, T1)
- o Spirals posterolaterally around the humerus with the deep brachial artery
  - ▪ Gives off posterior cutaneous nerve of forearm, which passes posterior to lateral condyle and supplies posterior forearm
- o Located anterolateral, between the brachialis and brachioradialis
- o Supplies triceps, anconeus, brachioradialis, and lateral portion of the brachialis
- o Gives articular branches to the elbow joint
- o Divides into deep and superficial branches at lateral epicondyle
- o **Deep branch**
  - ▪ Purely motor
  - ▪ Supplies extensor carpi radialis brevis and supinator muscles
  - ▪ Pierces supinator muscle and winds around lateral aspect of radial neck
  - ▪ Exits supinator muscle in posterior compartment of forearm as the posterior interosseous nerve
  - ▪ Posterior interosseous nerve supplies extensor muscles of posterior compartment of forearm
  - ▪ Posterior interosseous nerve syndrome: Compression of deep branch by arcade of Frohse (superficial proximal margin of the supinator)
- o **Superficial branch**
  - ▪ Purely sensory
  - ▪ Located in the anterolateral aspect of the forearm superficial to the supinator and pronator teres muscles (see "Forearm Overview" section)
- • **Median nerve**
  - o Arises from both the medial and lateral cords of the brachial plexus (C6-8, T1)
  - o Located in the cubital fossa, deep to the biceps aponeurosis
  - o Gives articular branches to the elbow joint
  - o Enters forearm by passing between heads of pronator teres, and located in forearm between flexor digitorum superficialis and profundus muscles
  - o May get compressed by the biceps aponeurosis or by either head of pronator teres
  - o Supplies the pronator teres, pronator quadratus, and flexors of the anterior compartment of the forearm (except flexor carpi ulnaris and medial half of flexor digitorum profundus, supplied by ulnar nerve)
  - o **Anterior interosseous nerve**
    - ▪ Arises from median nerve at level of pronator teres
    - ▪ Located in forearm, anterior to interosseous membrane, between flexor pollicis longus and flexor digitorum profundus
    - ▪ Supplies flexor pollicis longus, pronator quadratus, and lateral half of flexor digitorum profundus
    - ▪ Kiloh-Nevin syndrome: Compression of anterior interosseous nerve by ulnar head of pronator teres
- • **Ulnar nerve**
  - o Arises from medial cord of brachial plexus (C8, T1)
  - o Located posteromedially, deep to the triceps muscles in the distal arm
  - o Passes posterior to medial epicondyle in cubital tunnel

- ▪ **Cubital tunnel:** Fibro-osseous tunnel formed by medial epicondyle and cubital retinaculum ("arcuate ligament of Osborn")
- ▪ Cubital tunnel syndrome: Pain and weakness of 4th and 5th fingers due to compression of ulnar nerve in cubital tunnel
- o May sublux anterior to medial epicondyle in about 15% of people, usually during flexion
- o Gives articular branches to the elbow joint
- o Continues into forearm by dividing into superficial & deep heads of flexor carpi ulnaris
- o Supplies flexor carpi ulnaris and medial half of the flexor digitorum profundus
- • **Musculocutaneous nerve**
  - o Arises from the lateral cord of the brachial plexus (C5,6,7)
  - o Lies between the brachialis and biceps brachii muscles and supplies both
  - o Gives articular branches to the elbow joint
  - o Becomes superficial at elbow joint, continuing laterally as lateral cutaneous nerve of forearm which innervates skin of lateral side of forearm
- • **Medial cutaneous nerve of the forearm**
  - o Accompanies basilic vein in the arm
  - o Located superficially at elbow, anterior to medial epicondyle
  - o Supplies sensation to posteromedial forearm

Vessels
- • **Brachial artery**
  - o Continuation of the axillary artery
  - o Located in the cubital fossa, medial to the biceps tendon and deep to the biceps aponeurosis
  - o Accompanies median nerve
  - o Has several branches in the arm
    - ▪ Deep brachial: Descends posterolaterally with radial nerve, has branches anterior and posterior to lateral condyle forming an anastomosis
    - ▪ Superior ulnar collateral: Arises medially and descends with ulnar nerve posterior to medial condyle, forms an anastomosis with branches of ulnar artery
    - ▪ Inferior ulnar collateral: Arises distal to superior ulnar collateral artery, descends anterior to medial condyle, forming an anastomosis with branches of ulnar artery
  - o Divides into radial artery and ulnar artery at level of radial neck
- • **Cephalic vein**
  - o Lies lateral to biceps
- • **Basilic vein**
  - o Lies medial to biceps

Imaging Anatomy

Overview
- • Radiographs
  - o AP view
    - ▪ Full extension and supination
    - ▪ Medial condyle is larger than lateral
    - ▪ Lucency in distal humerus due to the olecranon and coronoid fossae

ELBOW OVERVIEW

- **Carrying angle**: Intersection of longitudinal axes of humerus and ulna, 154-178°
- **Humeral angle**: Intersection of longitudinal axis of humerus and a line tangential to articular surfaces of trochlea and capitellum, 72-95°
- **Ulnar angle**: Intersection of longitudinal axis of ulna and a line tangential to articular surfaces of trochlea and capitellum, 72-99°
  - Lateral view
    - 90° flexion
    - Lucent anterior fat pad is visible, posterior is not unless there is a joint effusion
    - Supinator line: Thin lucency of fat superficial to supinator muscle, parallels proximal radial shaft, displaced by radial head fracture or joint effusion
    - **Anterior humeral line**: Drawn along anterior cortex of humerus, intersects middle third of capitellum
  - **Radiocapitellar line**: Radial head intersects capitellum on every view
  - Normal variants
    - **Supracondylar (avian) spur**: Bony spur 5 cm proximal to medial epicondyle, present in 1-3% of population, usually asymptomatic
    - **Ligament of Struthers**: Accessory origin of pronator teres arising from supracondylar spur, may compress median nerve
    - **Os supratrochleare**: Accessory ossicle in olecranon fossa, may mimic loose body
    - **Patella cubiti**: Sesamoid in distal triceps tendon
- MR imaging
  - Trochlea and capitellum are rotated 30° anteriorly relative to humerus
  - Synovial recesses: Best appreciated when joint is distended by effusion or contrast
    - Olecranon recess: Largest, has superior, medial, and lateral portions around the olecranon process
    - Anterior humeral recess: Proximal to coronoid fossa
    - Anular recess: Surrounds radial neck
    - Ulnar collateral ligament recess: Deep to the ligament
    - Radial collateral ligament recess: Deep to the ligament
  - Synovial folds: Also called synovial fringe
    - Project into the joint
    - Best appreciated with joint effusion or contrast
    - Common locations: Radiocapitellar joint (meniscus-like), olecranon recess

Anatomy-Based Imaging Issues

Imaging Recommendations
- Radiographs
  - Standard projections: AP, oblique, lateral
  - Supplemental views
    - Radial head: Elbow flexed 90°, X-ray beam angled 45°, demonstrates radial head and neck

- Flexed ("ulnar sulcus"): Elbow flexed with hand on shoulder, shoulder and elbow in same plane, X-ray beam straight down, demonstrates olecranon process en face, medial and lateral epicondyles, and ulnar sulcus
- MR imaging
  - Elbow may be scanned at patient's side or **"superman" position** (patient prone, arm straight out over head)
  - Axial, sagittal, coronal planes
  - T1-weighted and proton density with or without fat suppression
  - Supplemental imaging
    - Coronal plane with 20° postero-inferior tilt: Better demonstrates medial collateral and lateral ulnar collateral ligaments
    - **FABS**: Flexed (elbow), **AB**ducted (arm), **S**upinated (forearm), the superman position with elbow flexed, excellent demonstration of distal biceps tendon and insertion
    - MR arthrography: Useful for evaluation of stability of capitellar osteochondral fracture and integrity of medial collateral ligament

Imaging Pitfalls
- Radiographs
  - Lucency of radial tuberosity: Mimics lytic lesion
  - Irregular ossification of capitellar and trochlear epiphyses: Mimics osteochondral fracture
  - Lucent notch in radial metaphysis: Mimics fracture or lesion
  - Incomplete union of ossification centers: Mimics fracture
- MR imaging
  - **Pseudodefect of the capitellum**
    - Normal groove between the capitellum and lateral condyle
    - Located on posterolateral aspect of capitellum
    - Mimics an osteochondral fracture on coronal and sagittal images
  - **Pseudodefect of the trochlear groove**
    - Normal notch on both the medial and lateral sides of the trochlear notch of ulna, at junction of olecranon and coronoid
    - Mimics fracture on sagittal images through medial or lateral side of ulna
    - Not present on midline sagittal images
  - **Transverse trochlear ridge**
    - Normal bony ridge running transverse across trochlear notch of ulna, at junction of olecranon and coronoid
    - May be incomplete across
    - Has no overlying articular cartilage
    - Mimics intra-articular osteophyte or post-traumatic deformity on sagittal images

Selected References

1. Rosenberg ZS et al: MR features of nerve disorders at the elbow. Magn Reson Imaging Clin N Am. 5(3):545-65, 1997
2. Rosenberg ZS et al: MR imaging of normal variants and interpretation pitfalls of the elbow. Magn Reson Imaging Clin N Am. 5(3):481-99, 1997

ELBOW OVERVIEW

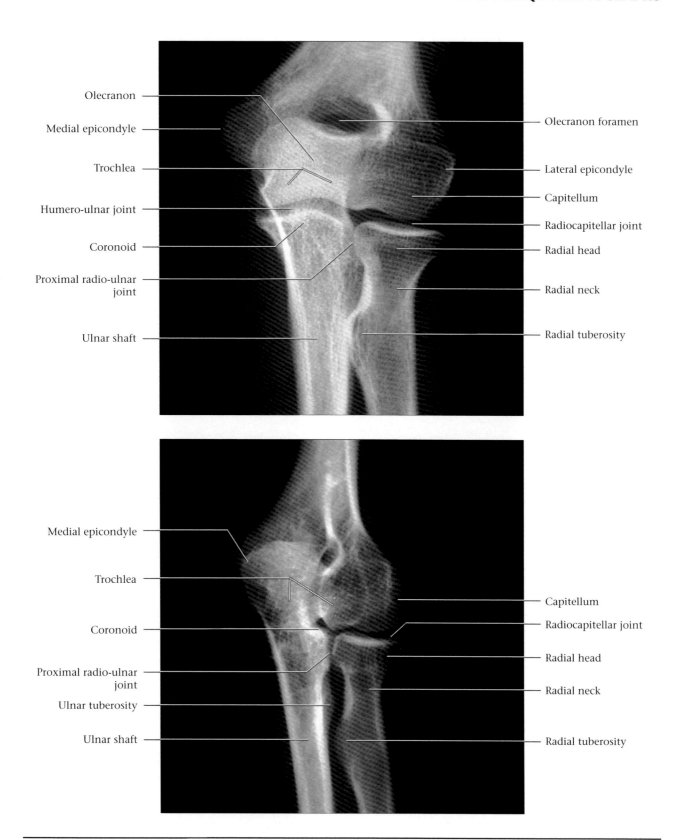

Olecranon

Medial epicondyle

Trochlea

Humero-ulnar joint

Coronoid

Proximal radio-ulnar joint

Ulnar shaft

Olecranon foramen

Lateral epicondyle

Capitellum

Radiocapitellar joint

Radial head

Radial neck

Radial tuberosity

Medial epicondyle

Trochlea

Coronoid

Proximal radio-ulnar joint

Ulnar tuberosity

Ulnar shaft

Capitellum

Radiocapitellar joint

Radial head

Radial neck

Radial tuberosity

(Top) AP view of the elbow. This person has an olecranon foramen, a normal variation in which there is a hole in the cortex between the olecranon fossa and coronoid fossa. **(Bottom)** External oblique view. The radius and ulna are no longer overlapped, and both the radial and ulnar tuberosities are well seen.

Elbow

II

ELBOW OVERVIEW

LATERAL & RADIAL HEAD RADIOGRAPHS

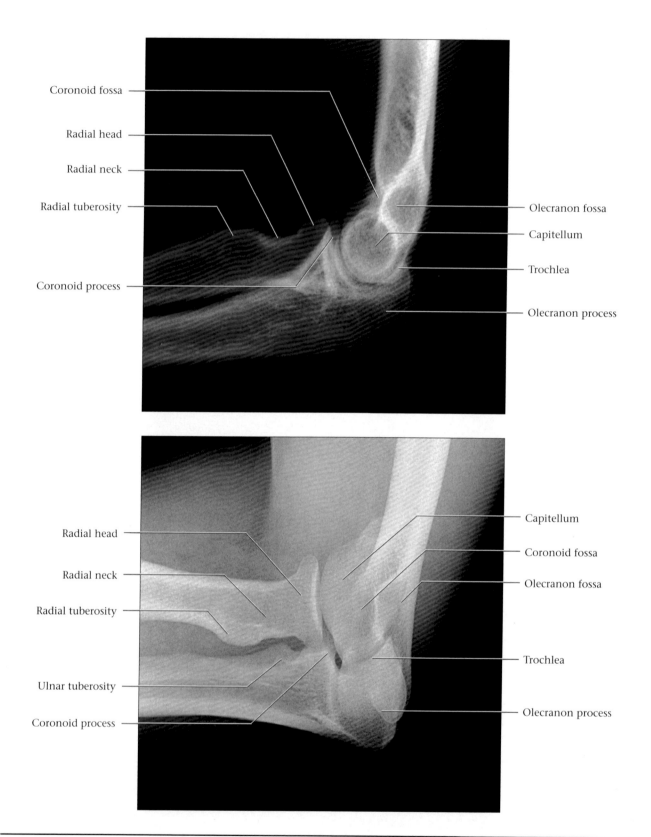

(Top) Lateral radiograph. The capitellum and trochlea are superimposed on each other. The head of the radius should always intersect the capitellum (radiocapitellar line) and a line drawn along the anterior cortex of the humerus should always intersect the middle of the capitellum (anterior humeral line). **(Bottom)** Radial head view. A lateral view with the X-ray beam angled transversely. The radial head is better seen than on a conventional lateral because the head is not overlapping the coronoid. This view is useful for the evaluation of a suspected radial head fracture.

ELBOW OVERVIEW

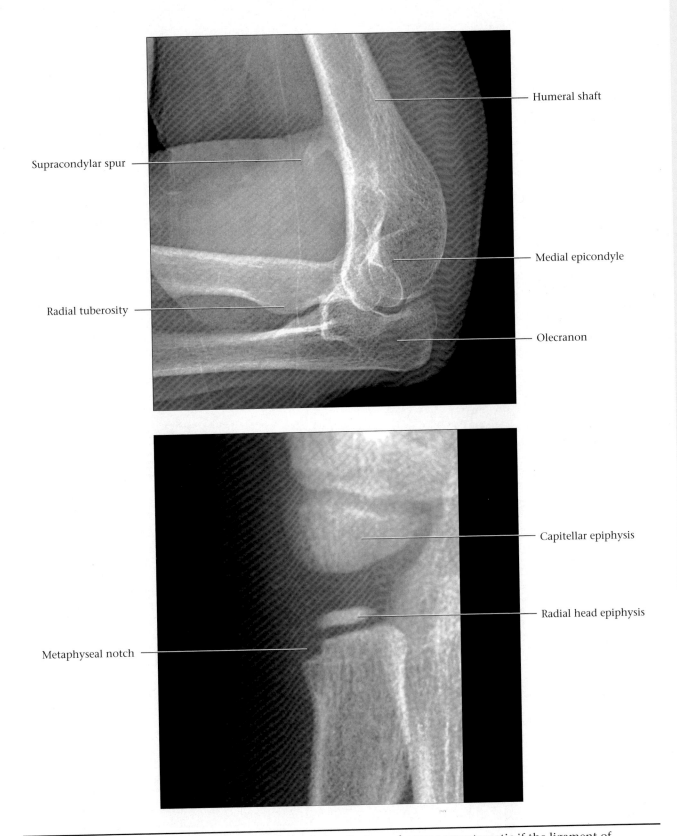

Humeral shaft

Supracondylar spur

Medial epicondyle

Radial tuberosity

Olecranon

Capitellar epiphysis

Radial head epiphysis

Metaphyseal notch

(Top) The supracondylar (avian) spur is a normal variation that may become symptomatic if the ligament of Struthers, which connects it to the medial epicondyle, compresses the median nerve. **(Bottom)** The metaphyseal notch is a normal variant in children which fills in as the bone matures and the physis closes (courtesy of Richard Shore, MD).

GRAPHIC, JOINT CAPSULE: ANTERIOR VIEW

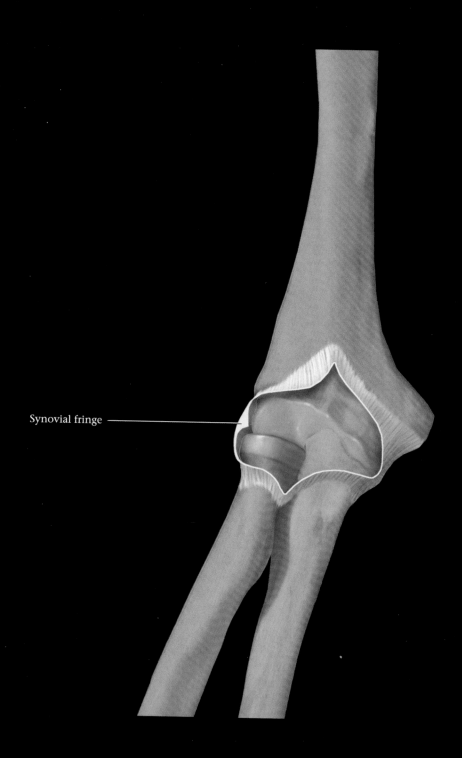

Synovial fringe

The anterior aspect of the joint capsule has been removed, showing the outline of its osseous attachments. Notice the focal meniscus-like thickening of the capsule at the radiocapitellar joint, called the synovial fringe.

GRAPHIC, JOINT CAPSULE: LATERAL VIEW

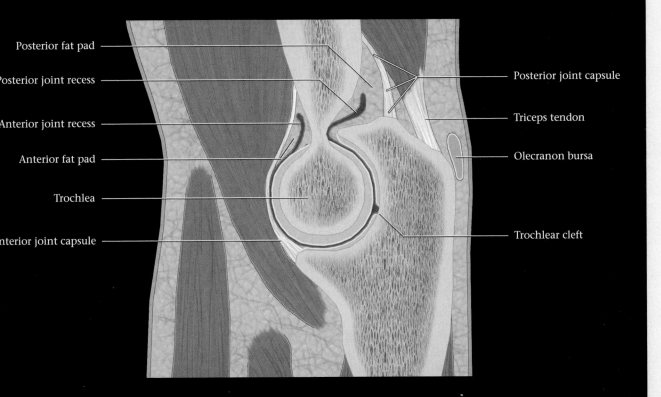

Posterior fat pad

Posterior joint recess

Anterior joint recess

Anterior fat pad

Trochlea

Anterior joint capsule

Posterior joint capsule

Triceps tendon

Olecranon bursa

Trochlear cleft

The anterior and posterior fat pads are intracapsular but extra-synovial. They may be pushed outward by a joint effusion. Note the trochlear cleft which is the border of the olecranon and coronoid and is not covered by articular cartilage; it may mimic a loose body or be seen as a pseudodefect.

GRAPHIC, JOINT CAPSULE: POSTERIOR VIEW

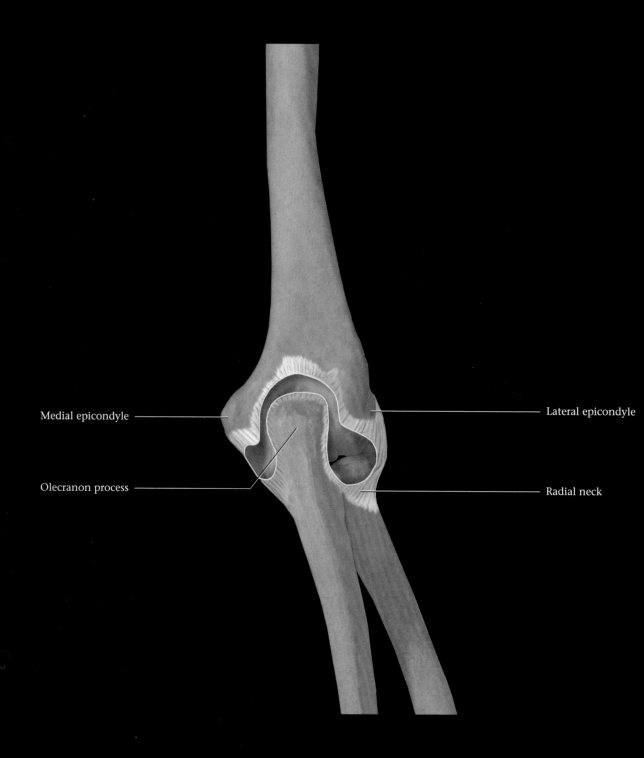

Medial epicondyle

Lateral epicondyle

Olecranon process

Radial neck

The posterior aspect of the joint capsule has been removed to show the outline of its posterior osseous attachment.

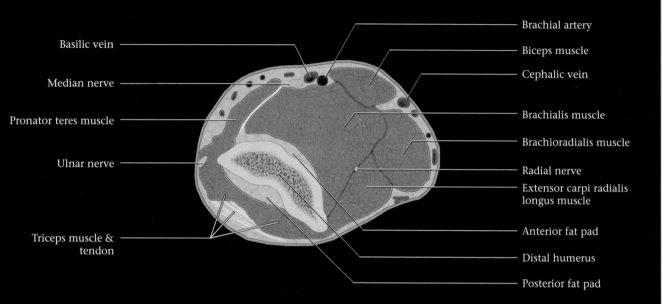

Basilic vein

Median nerve

Pronator teres muscle

Ulnar nerve

Triceps muscle & tendon

Brachial artery

Biceps muscle

Cephalic vein

Brachialis muscle

Brachioradialis muscle

Radial nerve

Extensor carpi radialis longus muscle

Anterior fat pad

Distal humerus

Posterior fat pad

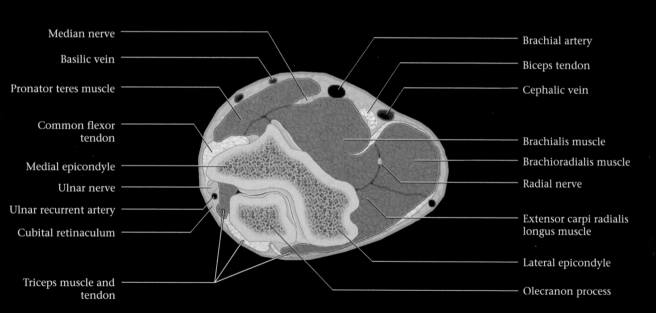

Median nerve

Basilic vein

Pronator teres muscle

Common flexor tendon

Medial epicondyle

Ulnar nerve

Ulnar recurrent artery

Cubital retinaculum

Triceps muscle and tendon

Brachial artery

Biceps tendon

Cephalic vein

Brachialis muscle

Brachioradialis muscle

Radial nerve

Extensor carpi radialis longus muscle

Lateral epicondyle

Olecranon process

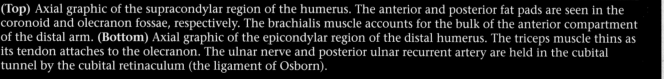

(Top) Axial graphic of the supracondylar region of the humerus. The anterior and posterior fat pads are seen in the coronoid and olecranon fossae, respectively. The brachialis muscle accounts for the bulk of the anterior compartment of the distal arm. **(Bottom)** Axial graphic of the epicondylar region of the distal humerus. The triceps muscle thins as its tendon attaches to the olecranon. The ulnar nerve and posterior ulnar recurrent artery are held in the cubital tunnel by the cubital retinaculum (the ligament of Osborn).

ELBOW OVERVIEW

GRAPHICS, AXIAL ELBOW

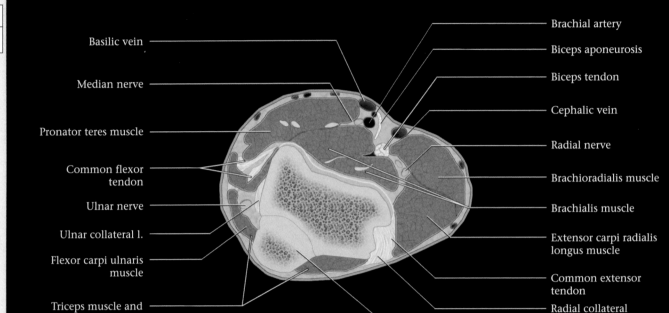

Basilic vein

Median nerve

Pronator teres muscle

Common flexor tendon

Ulnar nerve

Ulnar collateral l.

Flexor carpi ulnaris muscle

Triceps muscle and tendon

Brachial artery

Biceps aponeurosis

Biceps tendon

Cephalic vein

Radial nerve

Brachioradialis muscle

Brachialis muscle

Extensor carpi radialis longus muscle

Common extensor tendon

Radial collateral ligament

Olecranon process

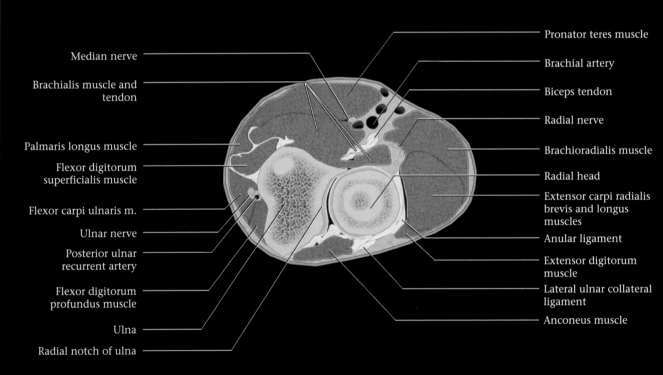

Median nerve

Brachialis muscle and tendon

Palmaris longus muscle

Flexor digitorum superficialis muscle

Flexor carpi ulnaris m.

Ulnar nerve

Posterior ulnar recurrent artery

Flexor digitorum profundus muscle

Ulna

Radial notch of ulna

Pronator teres muscle

Brachial artery

Biceps tendon

Radial nerve

Brachioradialis muscle

Radial head

Extensor carpi radialis brevis and longus muscles

Anular ligament

Extensor digitorum muscle

Lateral ulnar collateral ligament

Anconeus muscle

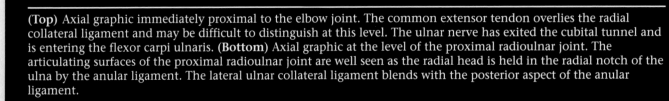

(Top) Axial graphic immediately proximal to the elbow joint. The common extensor tendon overlies the radial collateral ligament and may be difficult to distinguish at this level. The ulnar nerve has exited the cubital tunnel and is entering the flexor carpi ulnaris. **(Bottom)** Axial graphic at the level of the proximal radioulnar joint. The articulating surfaces of the proximal radioulnar joint are well seen as the radial head is held in the radial notch of the ulna by the anular ligament. The lateral ulnar collateral ligament blends with the posterior aspect of the anular ligament.

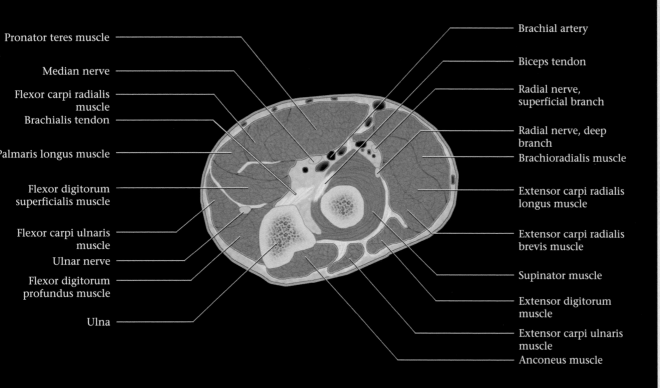

Pronator teres muscle

Median nerve

Flexor carpi radialis muscle

Brachialis tendon

Palmaris longus muscle

Flexor digitorum superficialis muscle

Flexor carpi ulnaris muscle

Ulnar nerve

Flexor digitorum profundus muscle

Ulna

Brachial artery

Biceps tendon

Radial nerve, superficial branch

Radial nerve, deep branch

Brachioradialis muscle

Extensor carpi radialis longus muscle

Extensor carpi radialis brevis muscle

Supinator muscle

Extensor digitorum muscle

Extensor carpi ulnaris muscle

Anconeus muscle

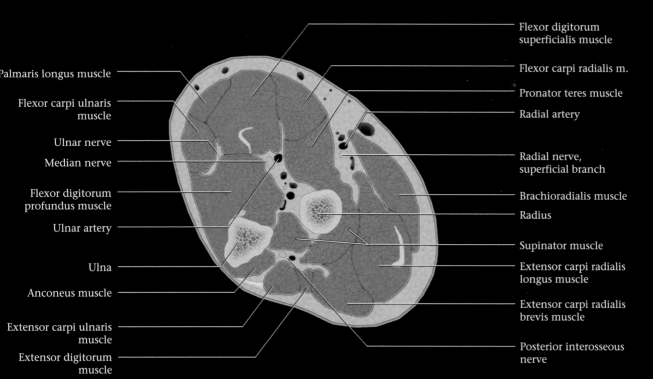

Palmaris longus muscle

Flexor carpi ulnaris muscle

Ulnar nerve

Median nerve

Flexor digitorum profundus muscle

Ulnar artery

Ulna

Anconeus muscle

Extensor carpi ulnaris muscle

Extensor digitorum muscle

Flexor digitorum superficialis muscle

Flexor carpi radialis m.

Pronator teres muscle

Radial artery

Radial nerve, superficial branch

Brachioradialis muscle

Radius

Supinator muscle

Extensor carpi radialis longus muscle

Extensor carpi radialis brevis muscle

Posterior interosseous nerve

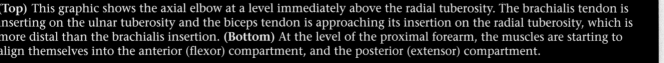

(Top) This graphic shows the axial elbow at a level immediately above the radial tuberosity. The brachialis tendon is inserting on the ulnar tuberosity and the biceps tendon is approaching its insertion on the radial tuberosity, which is more distal than the brachialis insertion. (Bottom) At the level of the proximal forearm, the muscles are starting to align themselves into the anterior (flexor) compartment, and the posterior (extensor) compartment.

GRAPHIC, ARTERIES AROUND ELBOW

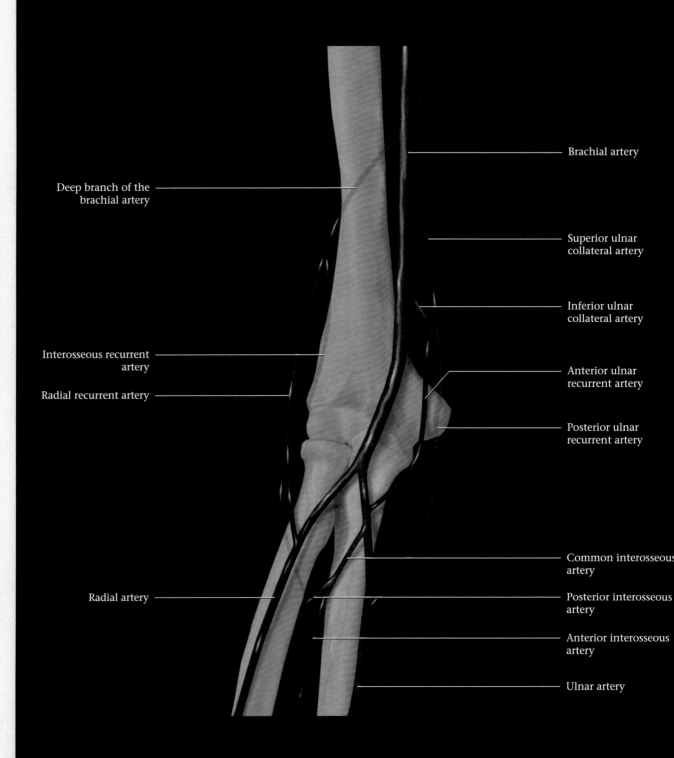

Deep branch of the brachial artery

Interosseous recurrent artery

Radial recurrent artery

Radial artery

Brachial artery

Superior ulnar collateral artery

Inferior ulnar collateral artery

Anterior ulnar recurrent artery

Posterior ulnar recurrent artery

Common interosseous artery

Posterior interosseous artery

Anterior interosseous artery

Ulnar artery

The brachial artery, the major artery of the arm, is a direct continuation of the axillary artery. It gives off several branches in the arm which form anastomoses medially and laterally with branches from the ulnar and radial arteries, respectively, which are themselves terminal branches of the brachial artery.

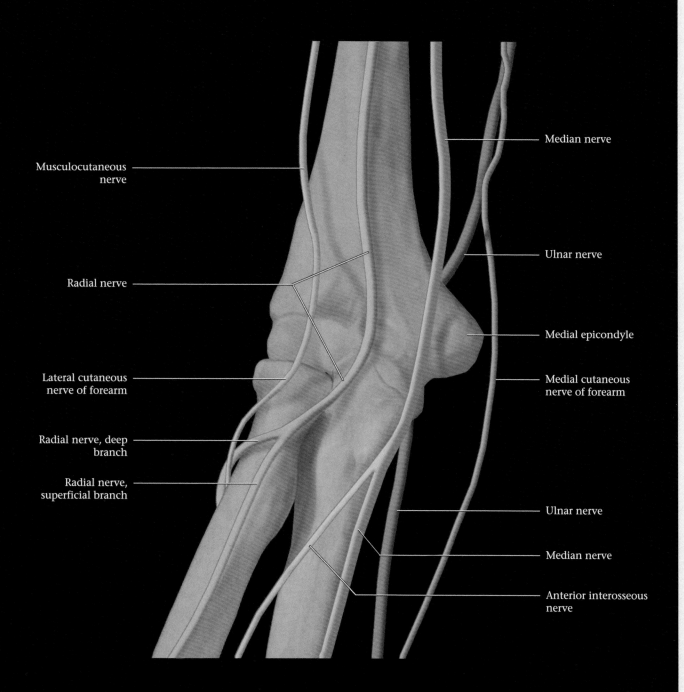

Musculocutaneous nerve

Median nerve

Radial nerve

Ulnar nerve

Medial epicondyle

Lateral cutaneous nerve of forearm

Medial cutaneous nerve of forearm

Radial nerve, deep branch

Radial nerve, superficial branch

Ulnar nerve

Median nerve

Anterior interosseous nerve

The nerves of the elbow region and their major branches are shown. The lateral cutaneous nerve of the forearm is a continuation of the musculocutaneous nerve of the arm. The deep branch of the radial nerve winds around the radial neck through the supinator muscle to become the posterior interosseous nerve of the forearm. The ulnar nerve is located posterior to the medial epicondyle and enters the forearm by passing between the superficial and deep heads of the flexor carpi ulnaris muscle. The anterior interosseous nerve is a branch of the median nerve, originating between the pronator teres muscle proximally and the biceps aponeurosis distally.

GRAPHIC, CUBITAL FOSSA

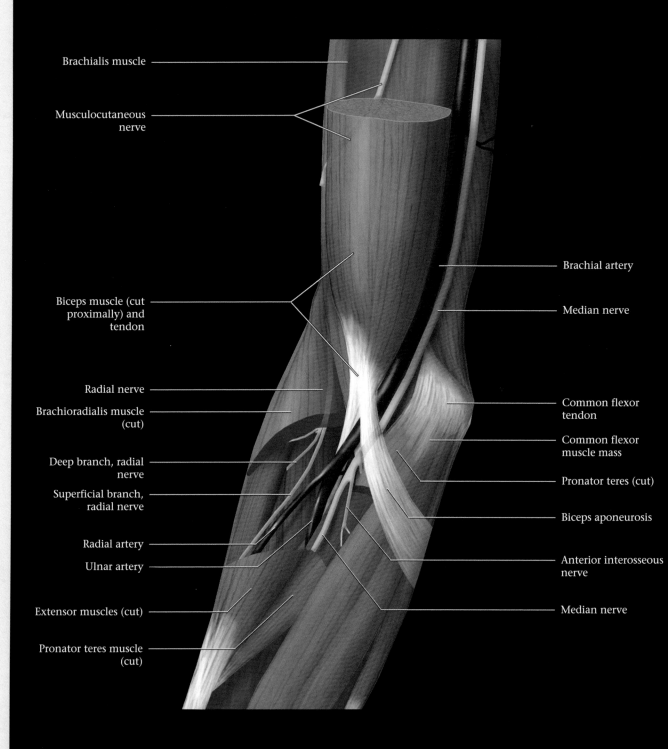

Brachialis muscle

Musculocutaneous nerve

Biceps muscle (cut proximally) and tendon

Radial nerve

Brachioradialis muscle (cut)

Deep branch, radial nerve

Superficial branch, radial nerve

Radial artery

Ulnar artery

Extensor muscles (cut)

Pronator teres muscle (cut)

Brachial artery

Median nerve

Common flexor tendon

Common flexor muscle mass

Pronator teres (cut)

Biceps aponeurosis

Anterior interosseous nerve

Median nerve

Anterior view of the cubital fossa shows the median nerve and brachial artery passing underneath the the biceps aponeurosis. The anterior interosseous nerve arises from the median nerve as the median nerve passes between the two heads of the pronator teres muscle. The radial nerve, deep to the brachioradialis muscle, is seen dividing into superficial and deep branches.

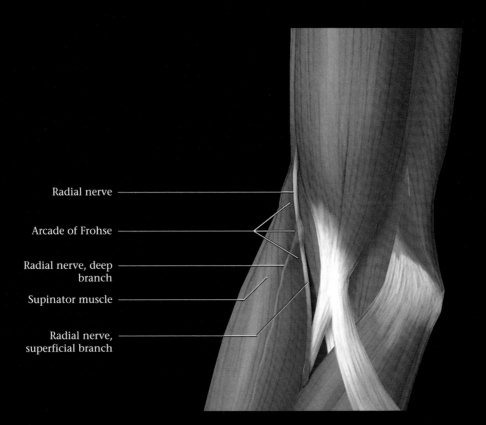

Radial nerve

Arcade of Frohse

Radial nerve, deep branch

Supinator muscle

Radial nerve, superficial branch

The radial nerve and/or its deep branch may be impinged by the arcade of Frohse, the superior edge of the supinator muscle.

GRAPHIC, MEDIAN NERVE ENTRAPMENT

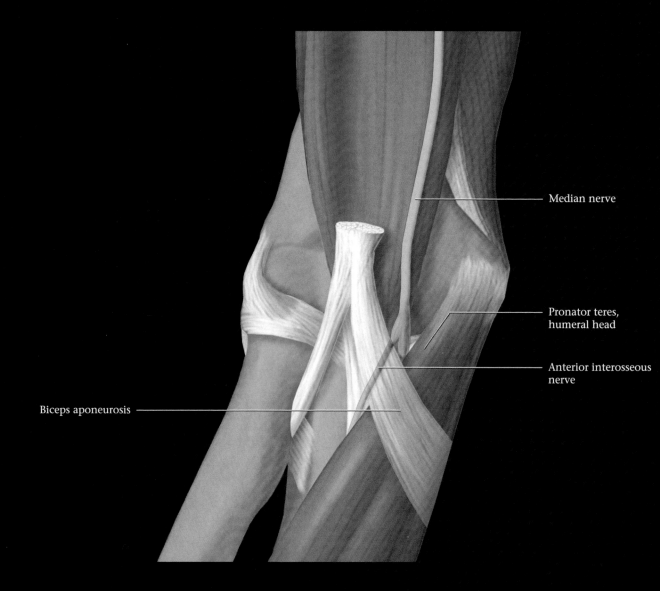

Median nerve

Pronator teres, humeral head

Anterior interosseous nerve

Biceps aponeurosis

The median nerve may be entrapped between the two heads of the pronator teres muscle or by the overlying biceps aponeurosis. The anterior interosseous branch of the median nerve may also be compressed by the overlying bicipital aponeurosis.

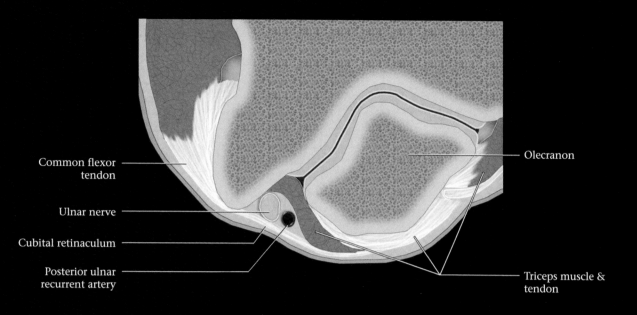

Common flexor tendon

Ulnar nerve

Cubital retinaculum

Posterior ulnar recurrent artery

Olecranon

Triceps muscle & tendon

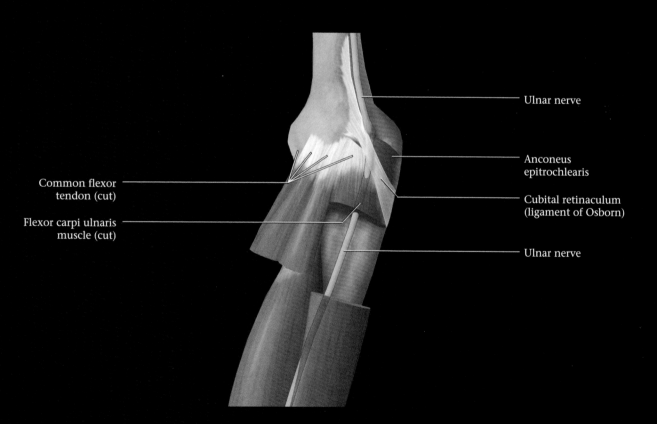

Ulnar nerve

Anconeus epitrochlearis

Cubital retinaculum (ligament of Osborn)

Ulnar nerve

Common flexor tendon (cut)

Flexor carpi ulnaris muscle (cut)

(Top) Axial graphic of the cubital tunnel. The ulnar nerve may be compressed within the cubital tunnel ("cubital tunnel syndrome") by a mass, post-traumatic osseous deformity, or aneurysm of the recurrent ulnar artery. The ulnar nerve may also be subluxed out of the cubital tunnel by the adjacent medial head of the triceps. **(Bottom)** Medial graphic of the cubital tunnel. The anconeus epitrochlearis is an inconstant accessory muscle that is deep to the ulnar nerve and may compress the nerve against the cubital retinaculum.

AXIAL T1 MR, RIGHT ELBOW

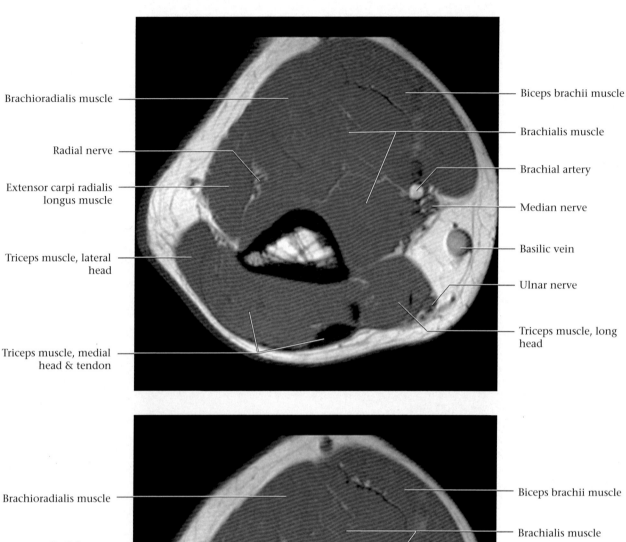

Brachioradialis muscle

Radial nerve

Extensor carpi radialis longus muscle

Triceps muscle, lateral head

Triceps muscle, medial head & tendon

Biceps brachii muscle

Brachialis muscle

Brachial artery

Median nerve

Basilic vein

Ulnar nerve

Triceps muscle, long head

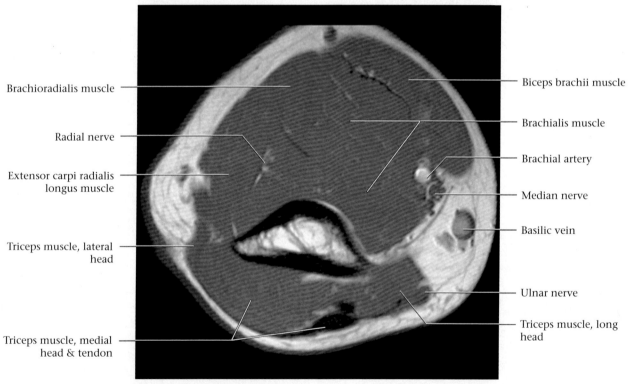

Brachioradialis muscle

Radial nerve

Extensor carpi radialis longus muscle

Triceps muscle, lateral head

Triceps muscle, medial head & tendon

Biceps brachii muscle

Brachialis muscle

Brachial artery

Median nerve

Basilic vein

Ulnar nerve

Triceps muscle, long head

(Top) Axial T1 MR series through the elbow, proximal to distal. In this proximal image, the radial, ulnar, and median nerves are visibile. The three heads of the triceps occupy the entire posterior compartment. **(Bottom)** The brachialis muscle accounts for most of the bulk in the anterior compartment.

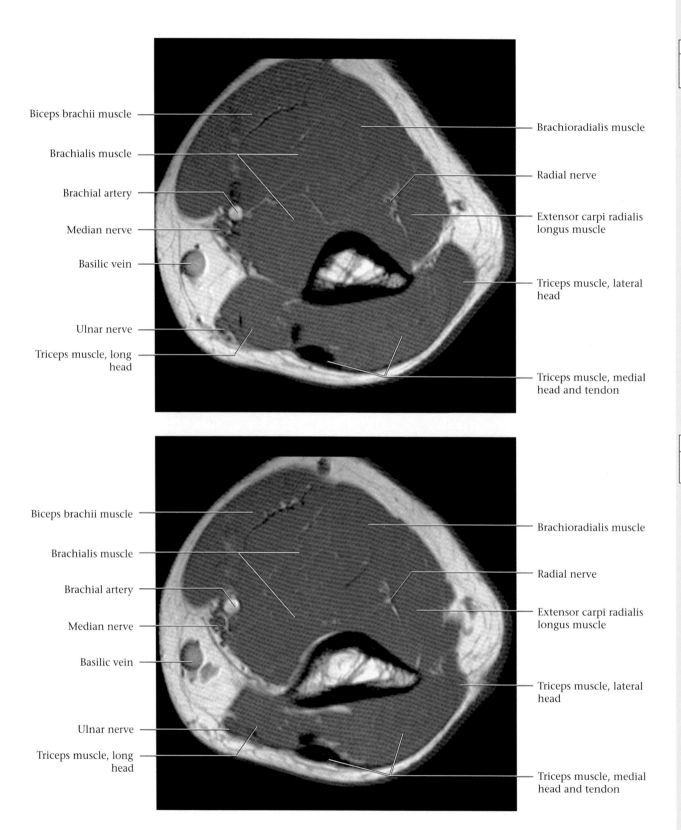

Biceps brachii muscle

Brachialis muscle

Brachial artery

Median nerve

Basilic vein

Ulnar nerve

Triceps muscle, long head

Brachioradialis muscle

Radial nerve

Extensor carpi radialis longus muscle

Triceps muscle, lateral head

Triceps muscle, medial head and tendon

Biceps brachii muscle

Brachialis muscle

Brachial artery

Median nerve

Basilic vein

Ulnar nerve

Triceps muscle, long head

Brachioradialis muscle

Radial nerve

Extensor carpi radialis longus muscle

Triceps muscle, lateral head

Triceps muscle, medial head and tendon

(Top) Axial T1 MR series through the elbow, proximal to distal. In this proximal image, the radial, ulnar, and median nerves are visibile. The three heads of the triceps occupy the entire posterior compartment. **(Bottom)** The brachialis muscle accounts for most of the bulk in the anterior compartment.

AXIAL T1 MR, RIGHT ELBOW

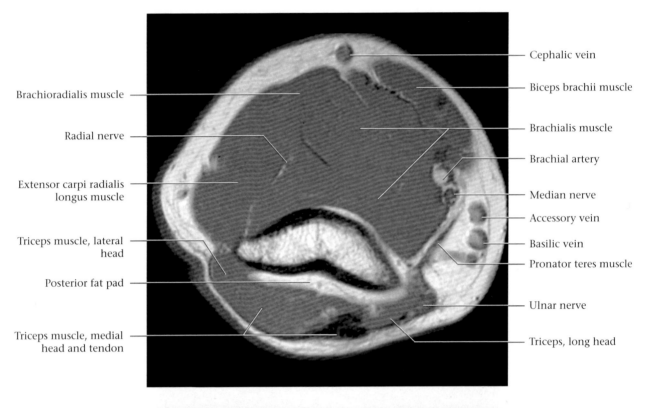

Brachioradialis muscle

Radial nerve

Extensor carpi radialis
longus muscle

Triceps muscle, lateral
head

Posterior fat pad

Triceps muscle, medial
head and tendon

Cephalic vein

Biceps brachii muscle

Brachialis muscle

Brachial artery

Median nerve

Accessory vein

Basilic vein

Pronator teres muscle

Ulnar nerve

Triceps, long head

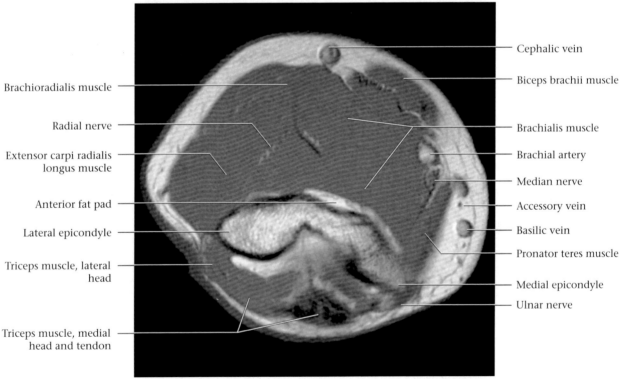

Brachioradialis muscle

Radial nerve

Extensor carpi radialis
longus muscle

Anterior fat pad

Lateral epicondyle

Triceps muscle, lateral
head

Triceps muscle, medial
head and tendon

Cephalic vein

Biceps brachii muscle

Brachialis muscle

Brachial artery

Median nerve

Accessory vein

Basilic vein

Pronator teres muscle

Medial epicondyle

Ulnar nerve

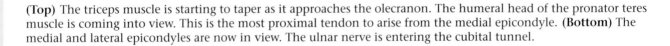

(Top) The triceps muscle is starting to taper as it approaches the olecranon. The humeral head of the pronator teres muscle is coming into view. This is the most proximal tendon to arise from the medial epicondyle. **(Bottom)** The medial and lateral epicondyles are now in view. The ulnar nerve is entering the cubital tunnel.

AXIAL T1 MR, LEFT ELBOW

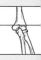

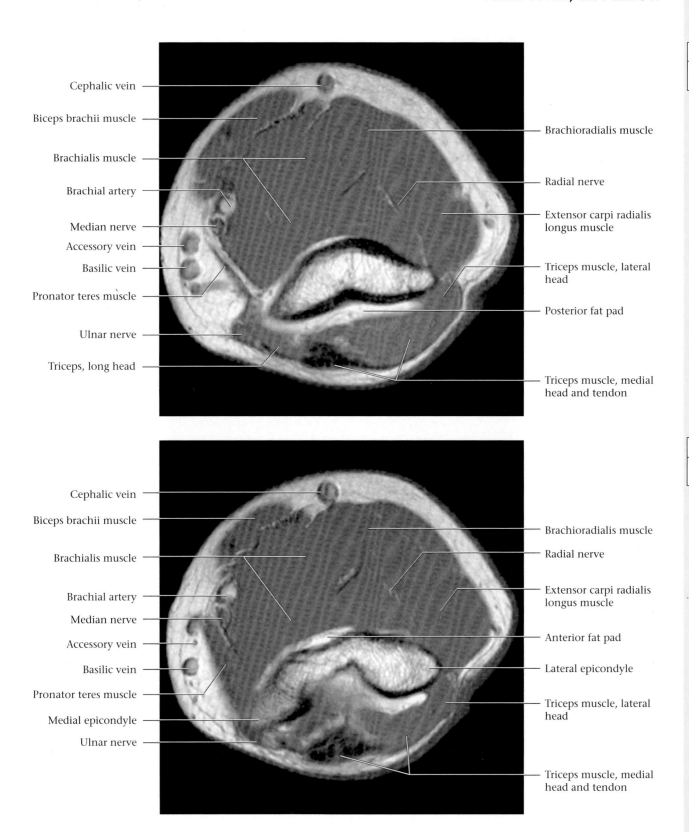

Cephalic vein

Biceps brachii muscle

Brachialis muscle

Brachial artery

Median nerve

Accessory vein

Basilic vein

Pronator teres muscle

Ulnar nerve

Triceps, long head

Brachioradialis muscle

Radial nerve

Extensor carpi radialis longus muscle

Triceps muscle, lateral head

Posterior fat pad

Triceps muscle, medial head and tendon

Cephalic vein

Biceps brachii muscle

Brachialis muscle

Brachial artery

Median nerve

Accessory vein

Basilic vein

Pronator teres muscle

Medial epicondyle

Ulnar nerve

Brachioradialis muscle

Radial nerve

Extensor carpi radialis longus muscle

Anterior fat pad

Lateral epicondyle

Triceps muscle, lateral head

Triceps muscle, medial head and tendon

(Top) The triceps muscle is starting to taper as it approaches the olecranon. The humeral head of the pronator teres muscle is coming into view. This is the most proximal tendon to arise from the medial epicondyle. **(Bottom)** The medial and lateral epicondyles are now in view. The ulnar nerve is entering the cubital tunnel.

Elbow

II

AXIAL T1 MR, RIGHT ELBOW

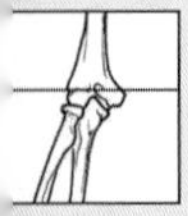

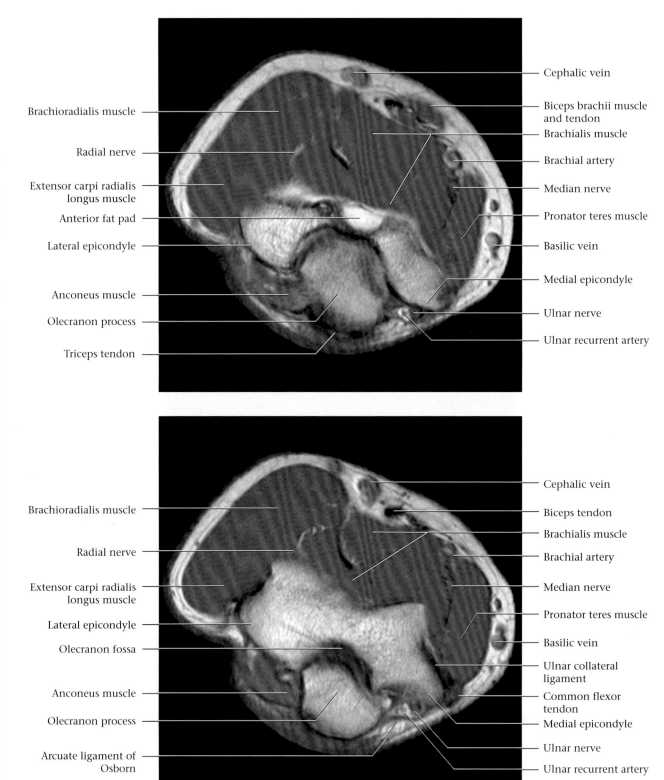

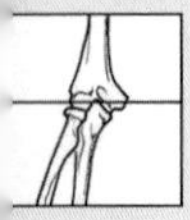

Top image labels (left side):
- Brachioradialis muscle
- Radial nerve
- Extensor carpi radialis longus muscle
- Anterior fat pad
- Lateral epicondyle
- Anconeus muscle
- Olecranon process
- Triceps tendon

Top image labels (right side):
- Cephalic vein
- Biceps brachii muscle and tendon
- Brachialis muscle
- Brachial artery
- Median nerve
- Pronator teres muscle
- Basilic vein
- Medial epicondyle
- Ulnar nerve
- Ulnar recurrent artery

Bottom image labels (left side):
- Brachioradialis muscle
- Radial nerve
- Extensor carpi radialis longus muscle
- Lateral epicondyle
- Olecranon fossa
- Anconeus muscle
- Olecranon process
- Arcuate ligament of Osborn

Bottom image labels (right side):
- Cephalic vein
- Biceps tendon
- Brachialis muscle
- Brachial artery
- Median nerve
- Pronator teres muscle
- Basilic vein
- Ulnar collateral ligament
- Common flexor tendon
- Medial epicondyle
- Ulnar nerve
- Ulnar recurrent artery

(Top) The triceps tendon is inserting on the olecranon process. The biceps brachii muscle is tapering to its distal tendon. **(Bottom)** The ulnar nerve is in the cubital tunnel, accompanied by the posterior ulnar recurrent artery.

ELBOW OVERVIEW

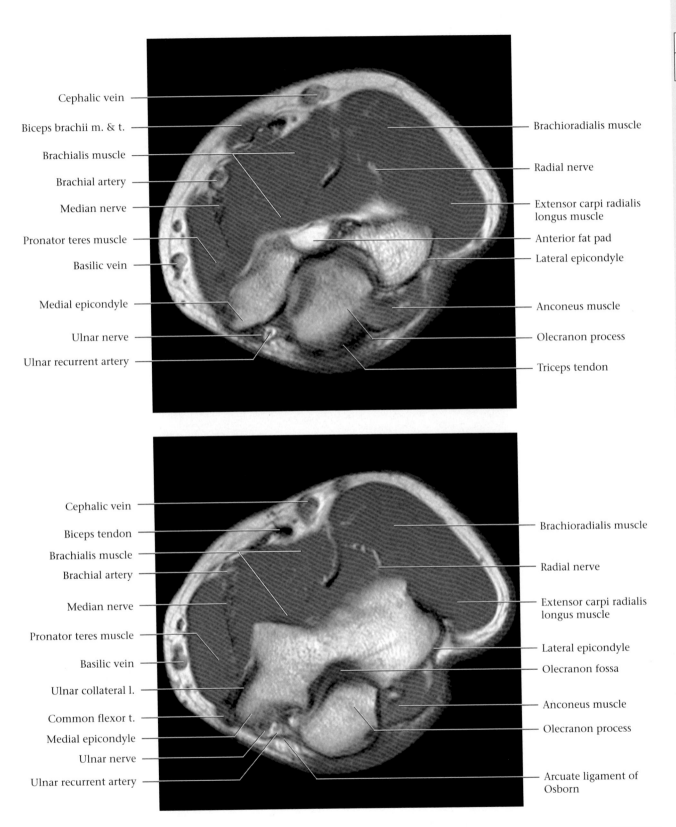

AXIAL T1 MR, LEFT ELBOW

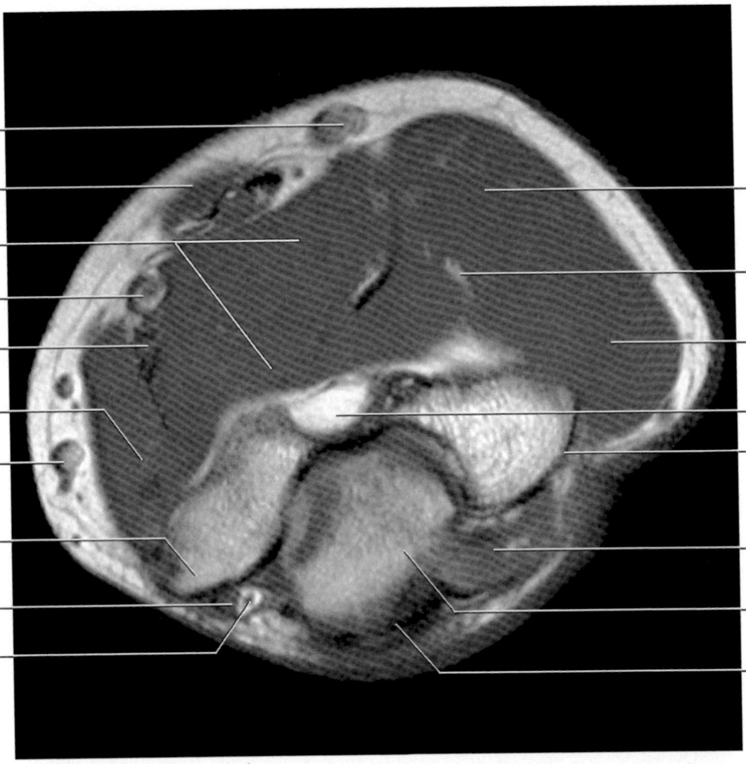
Cephalic vein
Biceps brachii m. & t.
Brachialis muscle
Brachial artery
Median nerve
Pronator teres muscle
Basilic vein
Medial epicondyle
Ulnar nerve
Ulnar recurrent artery
Brachioradialis muscle
Radial nerve
Extensor carpi radialis longus muscle
Anterior fat pad
Lateral epicondyle
Anconeus muscle
Olecranon process
Triceps tendon

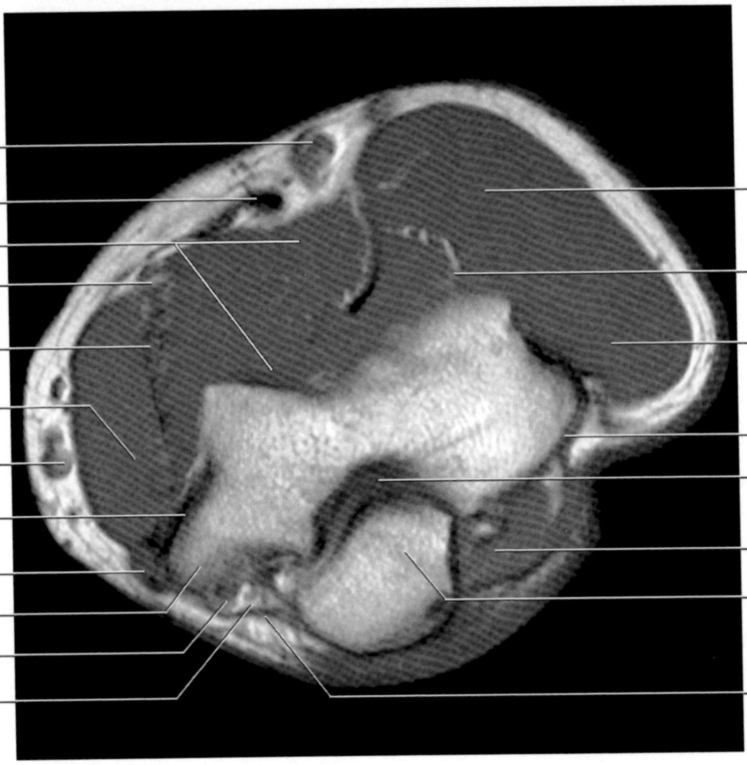
Cephalic vein
Biceps tendon
Brachialis muscle
Brachial artery
Median nerve
Pronator teres muscle
Basilic vein
Ulnar collateral l.
Common flexor t.
Medial epicondyle
Ulnar nerve
Ulnar recurrent artery
Brachioradialis muscle
Radial nerve
Extensor carpi radialis longus muscle
Lateral epicondyle
Olecranon fossa
Anconeus muscle
Olecranon process
Arcuate ligament of Osborn

(Top) The triceps tendon is inserting on the olecranon process. The biceps brachii muscle is tapering to its distal tendon. **(Bottom)** The ulnar nerve is in the cubital tunnel, accompanied by the posterior ulnar recurrent artery.

AXIAL T1 MR, RIGHT ELBOW

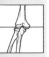

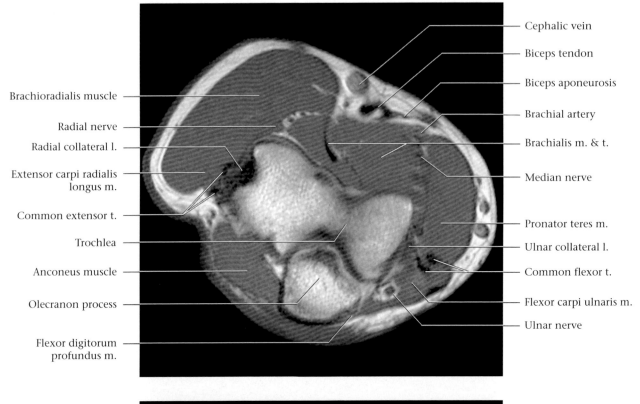

Brachioradialis muscle

Radial nerve

Radial collateral l.

Extensor carpi radialis longus m.

Common extensor t.

Trochlea

Anconeus muscle

Olecranon process

Flexor digitorum profundus m.

Cephalic vein

Biceps tendon

Biceps aponeurosis

Brachial artery

Brachialis m. & t.

Median nerve

Pronator teres m.

Ulnar collateral l.

Common flexor t.

Flexor carpi ulnaris m.

Ulnar nerve

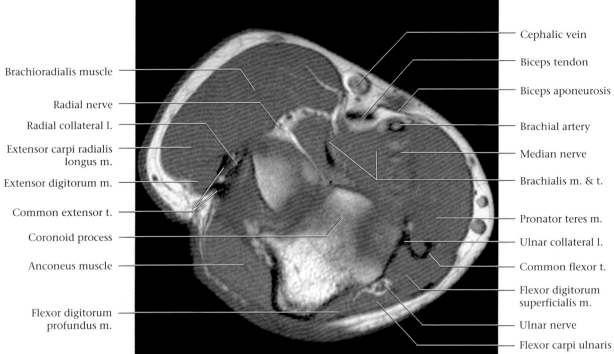

Brachioradialis muscle

Radial nerve

Radial collateral l.

Extensor carpi radialis longus m.

Extensor digitorum m.

Common extensor t.

Coronoid process

Anconeus muscle

Flexor digitorum profundus m.

Cephalic vein

Biceps tendon

Biceps aponeurosis

Brachial artery

Median nerve

Brachialis m. & t.

Pronator teres m.

Ulnar collateral l.

Common flexor t.

Flexor digitorum superficialis m.

Ulnar nerve

Flexor carpi ulnaris

(Top) The ulnar nerve has passed through the cubital tunnel and is now entering the flexor carpi ulnaris muscle. **(Bottom)** The flexor digitorum profundus muscle is now visible, arising from the medial side of the olecranon. The biceps aponeurosis extends from the biceps tendon to the superficial surface of the common flexor mass.

AXIAL T1 MR, LEFT ELBOW

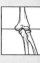

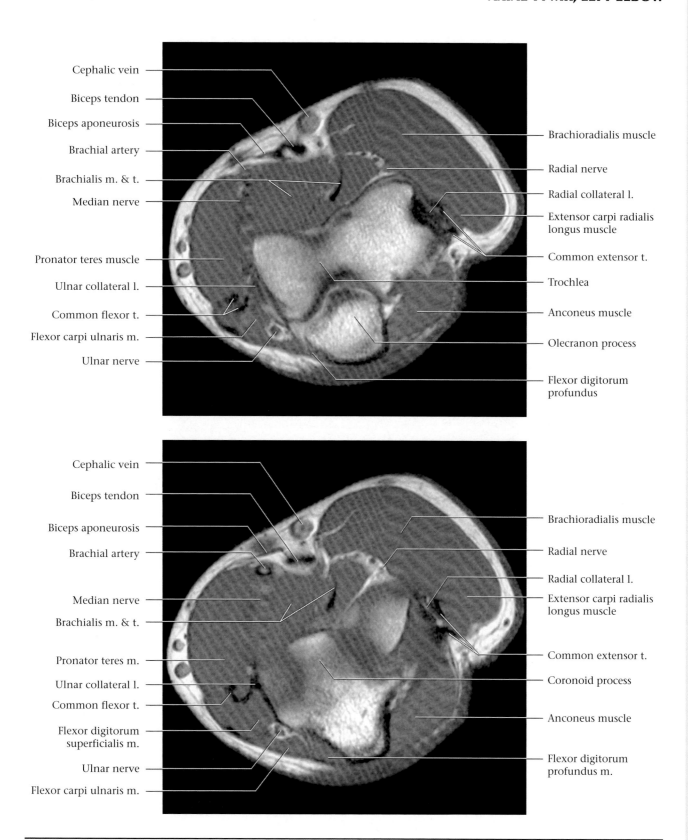

Cephalic vein

Biceps tendon

Biceps aponeurosis

Brachial artery

Brachialis m. & t.

Median nerve

Pronator teres muscle

Ulnar collateral l.

Common flexor t.

Flexor carpi ulnaris m.

Ulnar nerve

Brachioradialis muscle

Radial nerve

Radial collateral l.

Extensor carpi radialis longus muscle

Common extensor t.

Trochlea

Anconeus muscle

Olecranon process

Flexor digitorum profundus

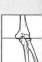

Cephalic vein

Biceps tendon

Biceps aponeurosis

Brachial artery

Median nerve

Brachialis m. & t.

Pronator teres m.

Ulnar collateral l.

Common flexor t.

Flexor digitorum superficialis m.

Ulnar nerve

Flexor carpi ulnaris m.

Brachioradialis muscle

Radial nerve

Radial collateral l.

Extensor carpi radialis longus muscle

Common extensor t.

Coronoid process

Anconeus muscle

Flexor digitorum profundus m.

(Top) The ulnar nerve has passed through the cubital tunnel and is now entering the flexor carpi ulnaris muscle. **(Bottom)** The flexor digitorum profundus muscle is now visible, arising from the medial side of the olecranon. The biceps aponeurosis extends from the biceps tendon to the superficial surface of the common flexor mass.

AXIAL T1 MR, RIGHT ELBOW

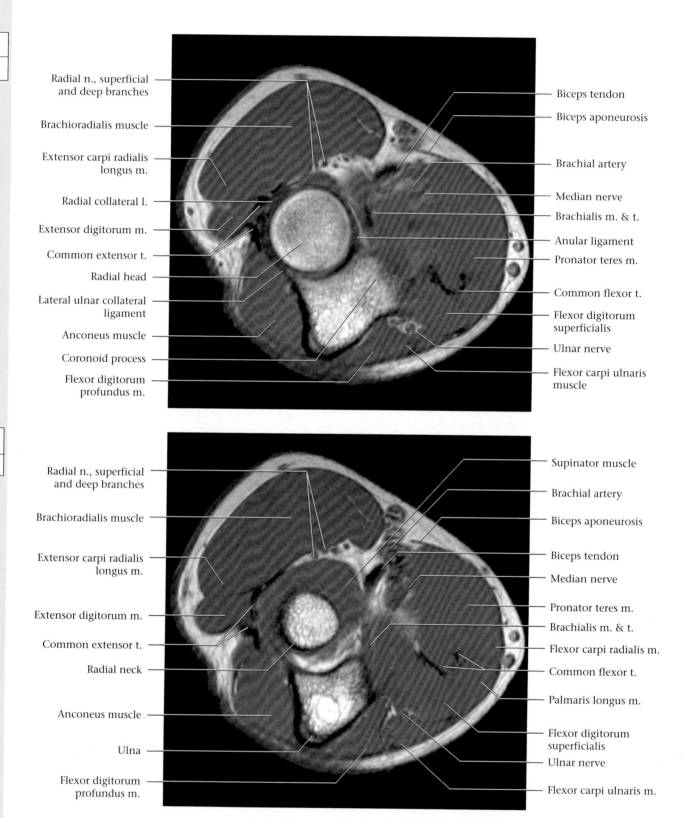

(Top) Labels (left, top to bottom): Radial n., superficial and deep branches; Brachioradialis muscle; Extensor carpi radialis longus m.; Radial collateral l.; Extensor digitorum m.; Common extensor t.; Radial head; Lateral ulnar collateral ligament; Anconeus muscle; Coronoid process; Flexor digitorum profundus m.

Labels (right, top to bottom): Biceps tendon; Biceps aponeurosis; Brachial artery; Median nerve; Brachialis m. & t.; Anular ligament; Pronator teres m.; Common flexor t.; Flexor digitorum superficialis; Ulnar nerve; Flexor carpi ulnaris muscle.

(Bottom) Labels (left, top to bottom): Radial n., superficial and deep branches; Brachioradialis muscle; Extensor carpi radialis longus m.; Extensor digitorum m.; Common extensor t.; Radial neck; Anconeus muscle; Ulna; Flexor digitorum profundus m.

Labels (right, top to bottom): Supinator muscle; Brachial artery; Biceps aponeurosis; Biceps tendon; Median nerve; Pronator teres m.; Brachialis m. & t.; Flexor carpi radialis m.; Common flexor t.; Palmaris longus m.; Flexor digitorum superficialis; Ulnar nerve; Flexor carpi ulnaris m.

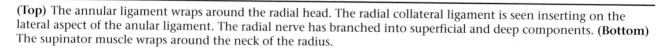

(Top) The annular ligament wraps around the radial head. The radial collateral ligament is seen inserting on the lateral aspect of the anular ligament. The radial nerve has branched into superficial and deep components. **(Bottom)** The supinator muscle wraps around the neck of the radius.

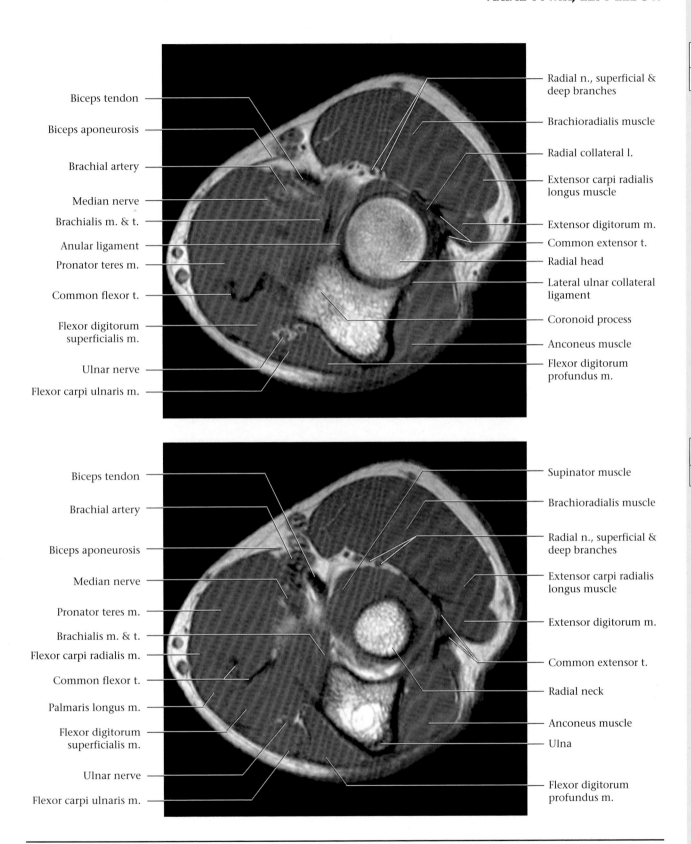

Biceps tendon

Biceps aponeurosis

Brachial artery

Median nerve

Brachialis m. & t.

Anular ligament

Pronator teres m.

Common flexor t.

Flexor digitorum
superficialis m.

Ulnar nerve

Flexor carpi ulnaris m.

Radial n., superficial &
deep branches

Brachioradialis muscle

Radial collateral l.

Extensor carpi radialis
longus muscle

Extensor digitorum m.

Common extensor t.

Radial head

Lateral ulnar collateral
ligament

Coronoid process

Anconeus muscle

Flexor digitorum
profundus m.

Biceps tendon

Brachial artery

Biceps aponeurosis

Median nerve

Pronator teres m.

Brachialis m. & t.

Flexor carpi radialis m.

Common flexor t.

Palmaris longus m.

Flexor digitorum
superficialis m.

Ulnar nerve

Flexor carpi ulnaris m.

Supinator muscle

Brachioradialis muscle

Radial n., superficial &
deep branches

Extensor carpi radialis
longus muscle

Extensor digitorum m.

Common extensor t.

Radial neck

Anconeus muscle

Ulna

Flexor digitorum
profundus m.

(Top) The annular ligament wraps around the radial head. The radial collateral ligament is seen inserting on the lateral aspect of the anular ligament. The radial nerve has branched into superficial and deep components. **(Bottom)** The supinator muscle wraps around the neck of the radius.

AXIAL T1 MR, RIGHT ELBOW

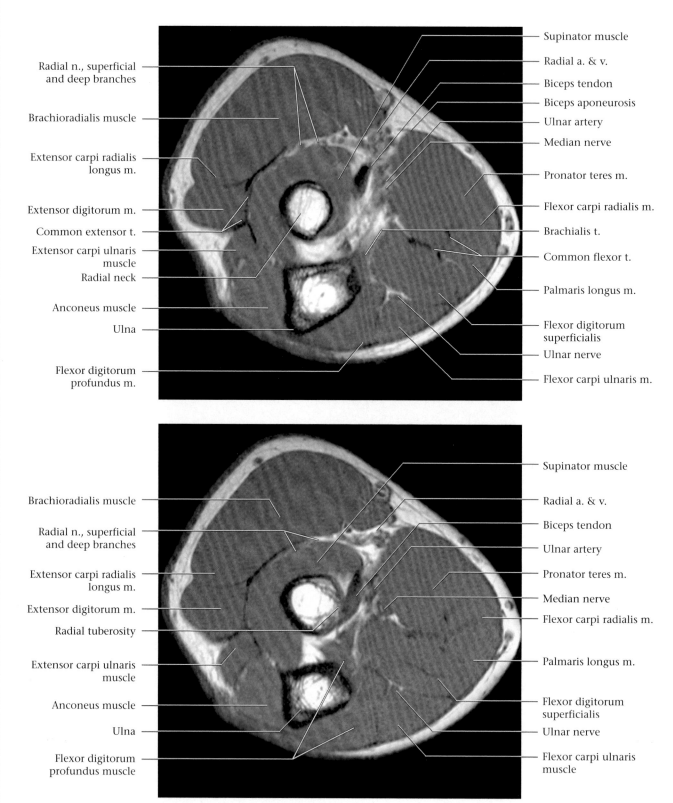

Radial n., superficial and deep branches

Brachioradialis muscle

Extensor carpi radialis longus m.

Extensor digitorum m.

Common extensor t.

Extensor carpi ulnaris muscle

Radial neck

Anconeus muscle

Ulna

Flexor digitorum profundus m.

Supinator muscle

Radial a. & v.

Biceps tendon

Biceps aponeurosis

Ulnar artery

Median nerve

Pronator teres m.

Flexor carpi radialis m.

Brachialis t.

Common flexor t.

Palmaris longus m.

Flexor digitorum superficialis

Ulnar nerve

Flexor carpi ulnaris m.

Brachioradialis muscle

Radial n., superficial and deep branches

Extensor carpi radialis longus m.

Extensor digitorum m.

Radial tuberosity

Extensor carpi ulnaris muscle

Anconeus muscle

Ulna

Flexor digitorum profundus muscle

Supinator muscle

Radial a. & v.

Biceps tendon

Ulnar artery

Pronator teres m.

Median nerve

Flexor carpi radialis m.

Palmaris longus m.

Flexor digitorum superficialis

Ulnar nerve

Flexor carpi ulnaris muscle

(Top) The brachialis tendon is seen inserting on the ulnar tuberosity. The brachial artery has divided into radial and ulnar branches. **(Bottom)** The biceps tendon is seen inserting on the radial tuberosity. The deep branch of the radial nerve is starting to enter the supinator muscle on its way to the posterior compartment of the forearm.

ELBOW OVERVIEW

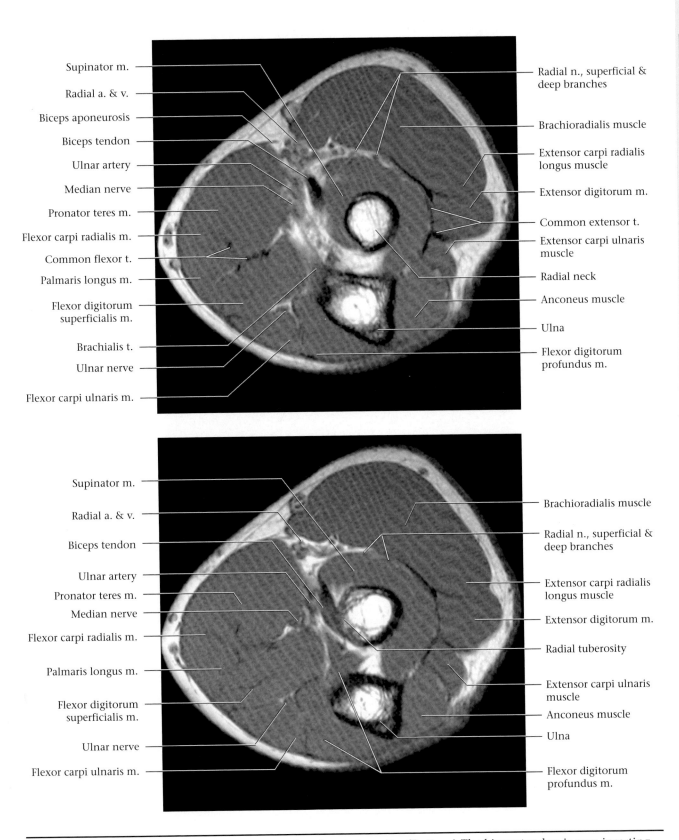

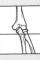

(Top) The brachialis tendon is seen inserting on the ulnar tuberosity. **(Bottom)** The biceps tendon is seen inserting on the radial tuberosity. The deep branch of the radial nerve is starting to enter the supinator muscle on its way to the posterior compartment of the forearm.

AXIAL T1 MR, RIGHT ELBOW

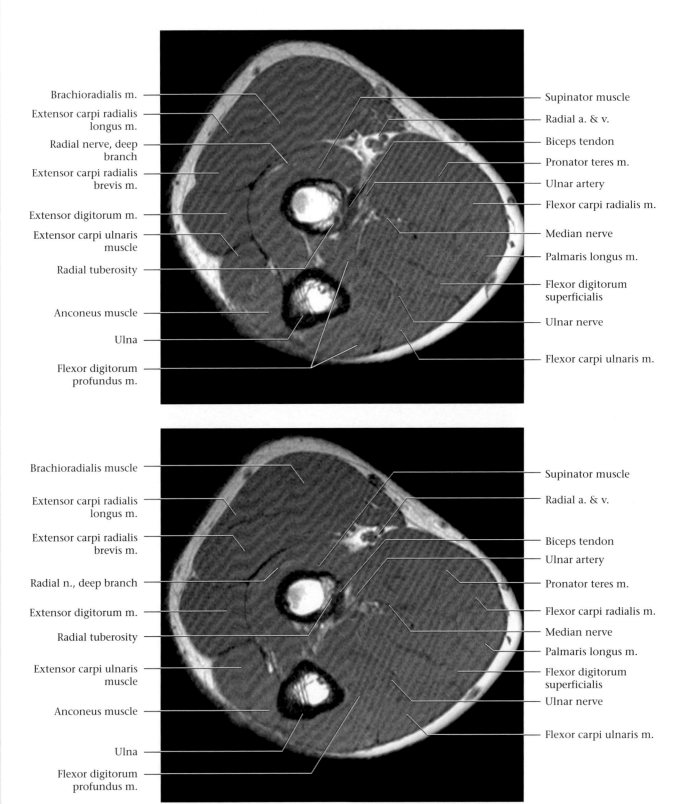

Brachioradialis m.

Extensor carpi radialis longus m.

Radial nerve, deep branch

Extensor carpi radialis brevis m.

Extensor digitorum m.

Extensor carpi ulnaris muscle

Radial tuberosity

Anconeus muscle

Ulna

Flexor digitorum profundus m.

Supinator muscle

Radial a. & v.

Biceps tendon

Pronator teres m.

Ulnar artery

Flexor carpi radialis m.

Median nerve

Palmaris longus m.

Flexor digitorum superficialis

Ulnar nerve

Flexor carpi ulnaris m.

Brachioradialis muscle

Extensor carpi radialis longus m.

Extensor carpi radialis brevis m.

Radial n., deep branch

Extensor digitorum m.

Radial tuberosity

Extensor carpi ulnaris muscle

Anconeus muscle

Ulna

Flexor digitorum profundus m.

Supinator muscle

Radial a. & v.

Biceps tendon

Ulnar artery

Pronator teres m.

Flexor carpi radialis m.

Median nerve

Palmaris longus m.

Flexor digitorum superficialis

Ulnar nerve

Flexor carpi ulnaris m.

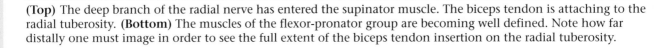

(Top) The deep branch of the radial nerve has entered the supinator muscle. The biceps tendon is attaching to the radial tuberosity. **(Bottom)** The muscles of the flexor-pronator group are becoming well defined. Note how far distally one must image in order to see the full extent of the biceps tendon insertion on the radial tuberosity.

Elbow

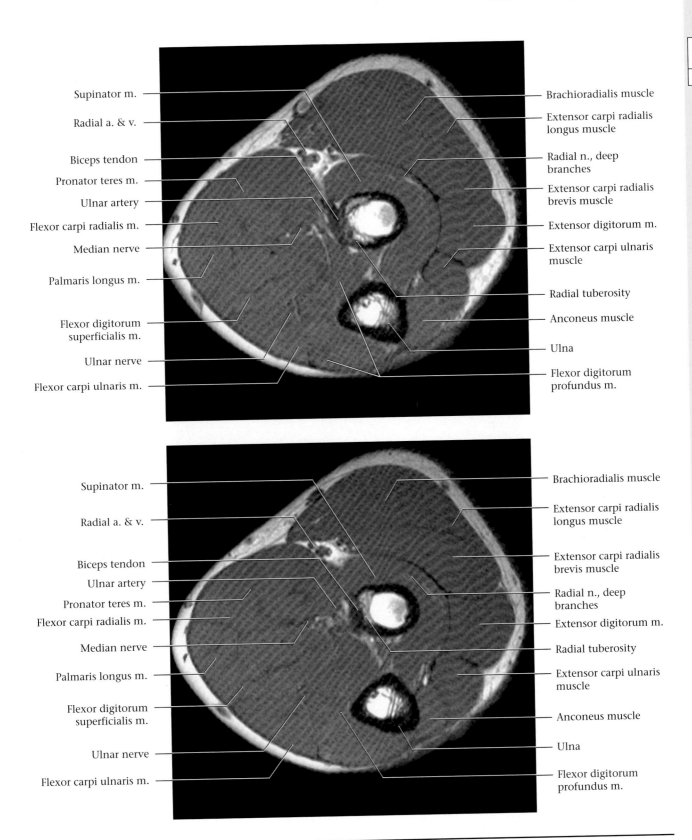

Supinator m.

Radial a. & v.

Biceps tendon

Pronator teres m.

Ulnar artery

Flexor carpi radialis m.

Median nerve

Palmaris longus m.

Flexor digitorum
superficialis m.

Ulnar nerve

Flexor carpi ulnaris m.

Brachioradialis muscle

Extensor carpi radialis
longus muscle

Radial n., deep
branches

Extensor carpi radialis
brevis muscle

Extensor digitorum m.

Extensor carpi ulnaris
muscle

Radial tuberosity

Anconeus muscle

Ulna

Flexor digitorum
profundus m.

Supinator m.

Radial a. & v.

Biceps tendon

Ulnar artery

Pronator teres m.

Flexor carpi radialis m.

Median nerve

Palmaris longus m.

Flexor digitorum
superficialis m.

Ulnar nerve

Flexor carpi ulnaris m.

Brachioradialis muscle

Extensor carpi radialis
longus muscle

Extensor carpi radialis
brevis muscle

Radial n., deep
branches

Extensor digitorum m.

Radial tuberosity

Extensor carpi ulnaris
muscle

Anconeus muscle

Ulna

Flexor digitorum
profundus m.

(Top) The deep branch of the radial nerve has entered the supinator muscle. The biceps tendon is attaching to the radial tuberosity. **(Bottom)** The muscles of the flexor-pronator group are becoming well defined. Note how far distally one must image in order to see elbe full extent of the biceps tendon insertion on the radial tuberosity.

Elbow

II

33

CORONAL T1 MR, RIGHT ELBOW

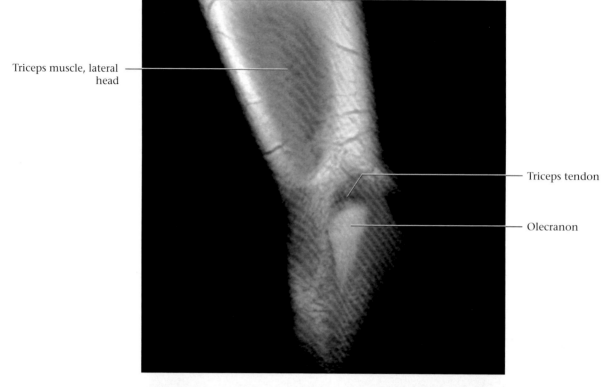

Triceps muscle, lateral head

Triceps tendon

Olecranon

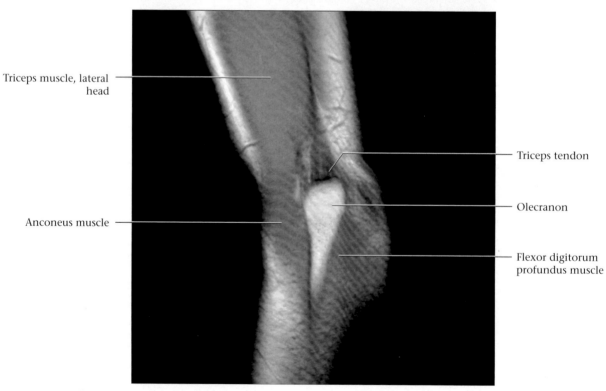

Triceps muscle, lateral head

Anconeus muscle

Triceps tendon

Olecranon

Flexor digitorum profundus muscle

(Top) Series of coronal images, from posterior to anterior. At the extreme posterior aspect of the arm, the olecranon process is just coming into view. **(Bottom)** The triceps tendon is inserting on the olecranon.

ELBOW OVERVIEW

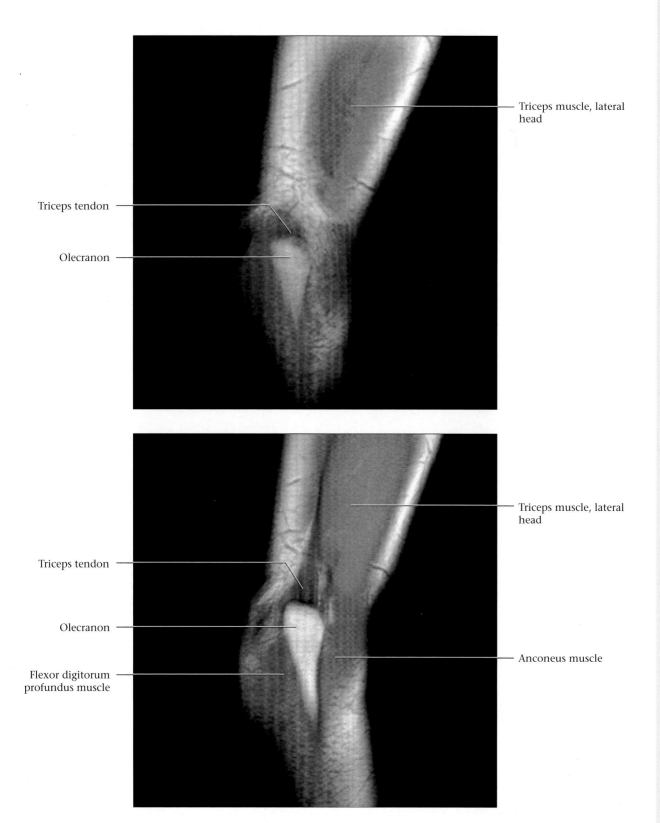

Triceps muscle, lateral head

Triceps tendon

Olecranon

Triceps muscle, lateral head

Triceps tendon

Olecranon

Anconeus muscle

Flexor digitorum profundus muscle

(Top) Series of coronal images, from posterior to anterior. At the extreme posterior aspect of the arm, the olecranon process is just coming into view. **(Bottom)** The triceps tendon is inserting on the olecranon.

CORONAL T1 MR, RIGHT ELBOW

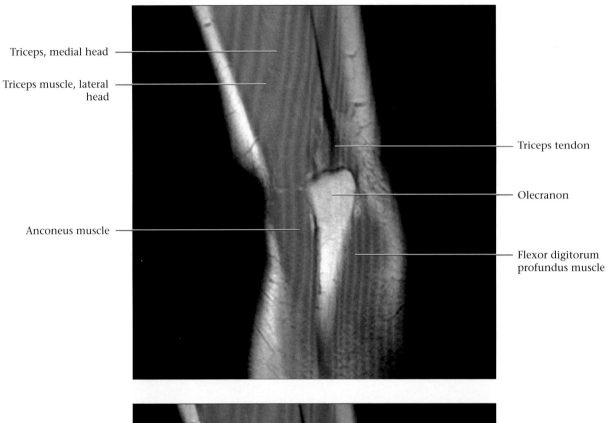

Triceps, medial head

Triceps muscle, lateral head

Anconeus muscle

Triceps tendon

Olecranon

Flexor digitorum profundus muscle

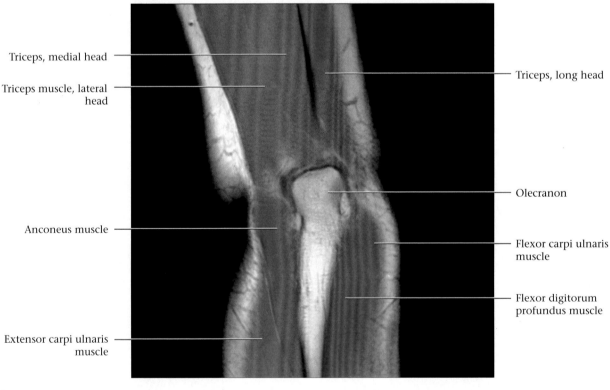

Triceps, medial head

Triceps muscle, lateral head

Anconeus muscle

Extensor carpi ulnaris muscle

Triceps, long head

Olecranon

Flexor carpi ulnaris muscle

Flexor digitorum profundus muscle

(Top) The anconeus and flexor digitorum profundus muscles are now better seen. **(Bottom)** The flexor carpi ulnaris and extensor carpi ulnaris tendons are now coming into view.

ELBOW OVERVIEW

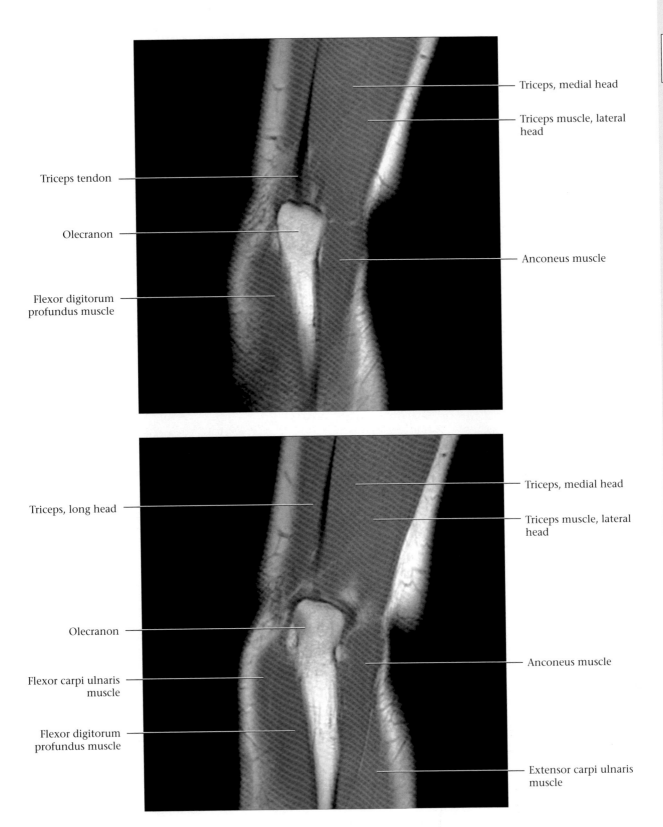

Triceps, medial head

Triceps muscle, lateral head

Triceps tendon

Olecranon

Anconeus muscle

Flexor digitorum profundus muscle

Triceps, medial head

Triceps muscle, lateral head

Triceps, long head

Olecranon

Anconeus muscle

Flexor carpi ulnaris muscle

Flexor digitorum profundus muscle

Extensor carpi ulnaris muscle

(Top) The anconeus and flexor digitorum profundus muscles are now better seen. **(Bottom)** The flexor carpi ulnaris and extensor carpi ulnaris tendons are now coming into view.

ELBOW OVERVIEW

CORONAL T1 MR, RIGHT ELBOW

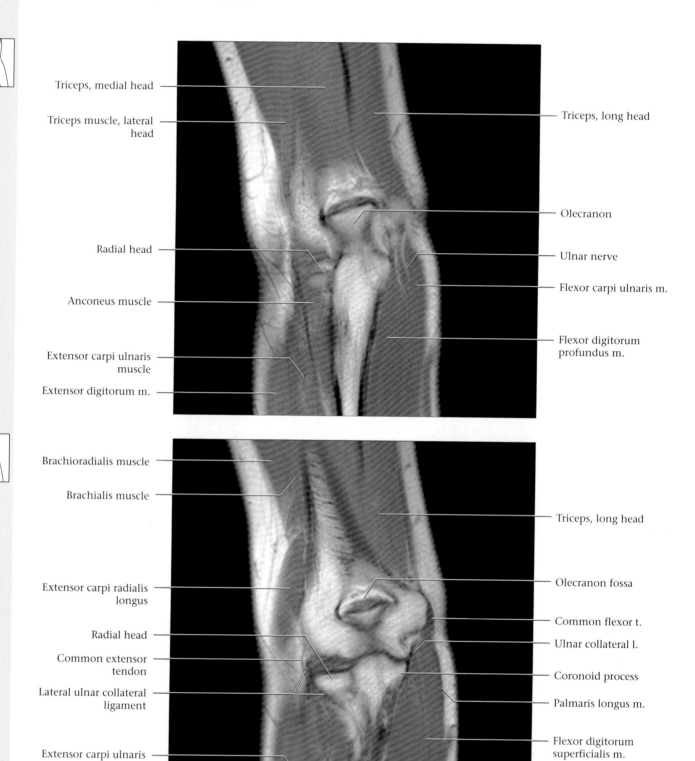

Triceps, medial head

Triceps muscle, lateral head

Radial head

Anconeus muscle

Extensor carpi ulnaris muscle

Extensor digitorum m.

Triceps, long head

Olecranon

Ulnar nerve

Flexor carpi ulnaris m.

Flexor digitorum profundus m.

Brachioradialis muscle

Brachialis muscle

Extensor carpi radialis longus

Radial head

Common extensor tendon

Lateral ulnar collateral ligament

Extensor carpi ulnaris muscle

Extensor digitorum m.

Triceps, long head

Olecranon fossa

Common flexor t.

Ulnar collateral l.

Coronoid process

Palmaris longus m.

Flexor digitorum superficialis m.

Flexor digitorum profundus m.

(Top) The ulnar nerve is seen passing behind the medial epicondyle (epicondyle not in this image). **(Bottom)** The lateral ulnar collateral ligament runs like a sling behind the radial neck to prevent posterolateral instability.

ELBOW OVERVIEW

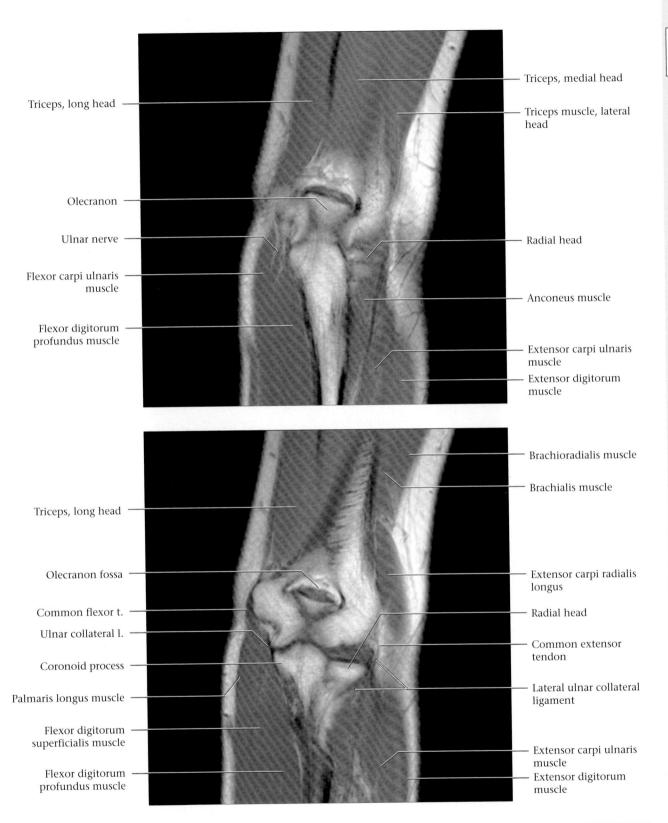

Triceps, long head

Olecranon

Ulnar nerve

Flexor carpi ulnaris muscle

Flexor digitorum profundus muscle

Triceps, medial head

Triceps muscle, lateral head

Radial head

Anconeus muscle

Extensor carpi ulnaris muscle

Extensor digitorum muscle

Triceps, long head

Olecranon fossa

Common flexor t.

Ulnar collateral l.

Coronoid process

Palmaris longus muscle

Flexor digitorum superficialis muscle

Flexor digitorum profundus muscle

Brachioradialis muscle

Brachialis muscle

Extensor carpi radialis longus

Radial head

Common extensor tendon

Lateral ulnar collateral ligament

Extensor carpi ulnaris muscle

Extensor digitorum muscle

(Top) The ulnar nerve is seen passing behind the medial epicondyle (epicondyle not in this image). **(Bottom)** The lateral ulnar collateral ligament runs like a sling behind the radial neck to prevent posterolateral instability.

ELBOW OVERVIEW

CORONAL T1 MR, RIGHT ELBOW

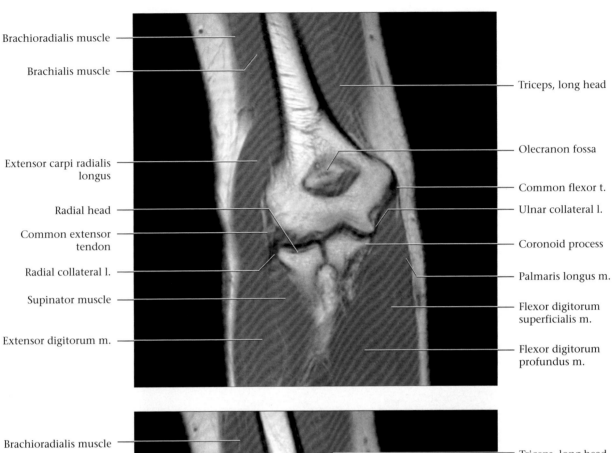

Brachioradialis muscle

Brachialis muscle

Extensor carpi radialis longus

Radial head

Common extensor tendon

Radial collateral l.

Supinator muscle

Extensor digitorum m.

Triceps, long head

Olecranon fossa

Common flexor t.

Ulnar collateral l.

Coronoid process

Palmaris longus m.

Flexor digitorum superficialis m.

Flexor digitorum profundus m.

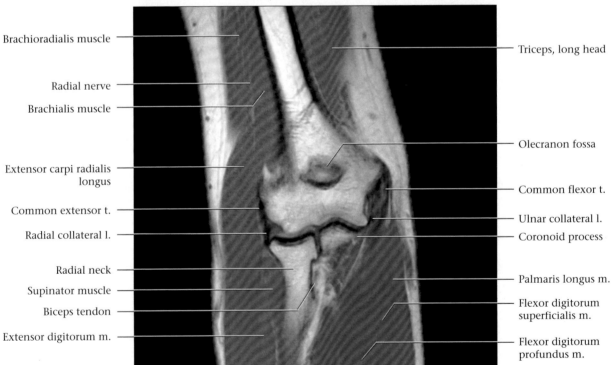

Brachioradialis muscle

Radial nerve

Brachialis muscle

Extensor carpi radialis longus

Common extensor t.

Radial collateral l.

Radial neck

Supinator muscle

Biceps tendon

Extensor digitorum m.

Triceps, long head

Olecranon fossa

Common flexor t.

Ulnar collateral l.

Coronoid process

Palmaris longus m.

Flexor digitorum superficialis m.

Flexor digitorum profundus m.

(Top) The common extensor tendon is long and thin, while the common flexor tendon is short and broad. **(Bottom)** The radial nerve courses between the brachialis and brachioradialis muscles. The distal biceps tendon is approaching its insertion on the radial tuberosity.

Elbow

II

40

ELBOW OVERVIEW

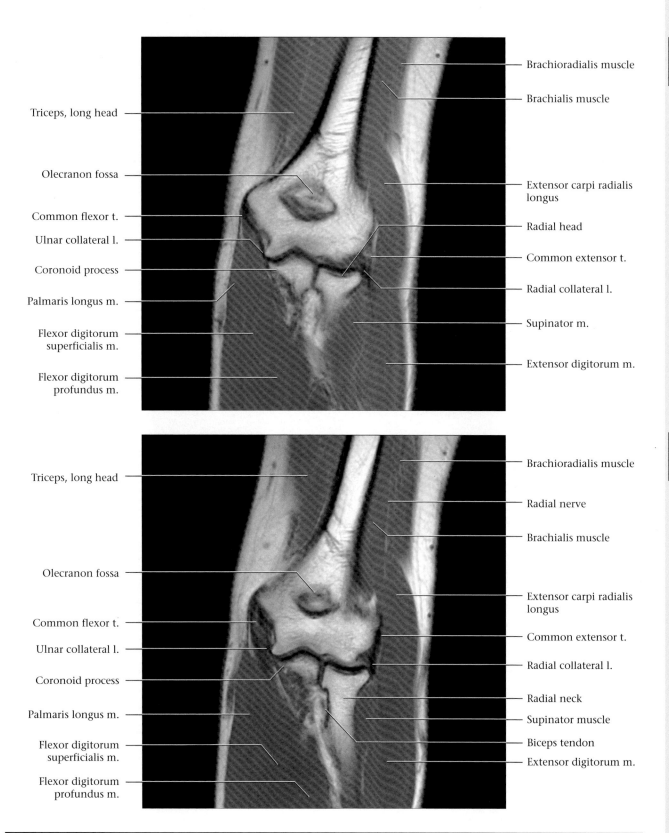

Triceps, long head

Olecranon fossa

Common flexor t.

Ulnar collateral l.

Coronoid process

Palmaris longus m.

Flexor digitorum superficialis m.

Flexor digitorum profundus m.

Brachioradialis muscle

Brachialis muscle

Extensor carpi radialis longus

Radial head

Common extensor t.

Radial collateral l.

Supinator m.

Extensor digitorum m.

Triceps, long head

Olecranon fossa

Common flexor t.

Ulnar collateral l.

Coronoid process

Palmaris longus m.

Flexor digitorum superficialis m.

Flexor digitorum profundus m.

Brachioradialis muscle

Radial nerve

Brachialis muscle

Extensor carpi radialis longus

Common extensor t.

Radial collateral l.

Radial neck

Supinator muscle

Biceps tendon

Extensor digitorum m.

(Top) The common extensor tendon is long and thin, while the common flexor tendon is short and broad. (Bottom) The radial nerve courses between the brachialis and brachioradialis muscles. The distal biceps tendon is approaching its insertion on the radial tuberosity.

CORONAL T1 MR, RIGHT ELBOW

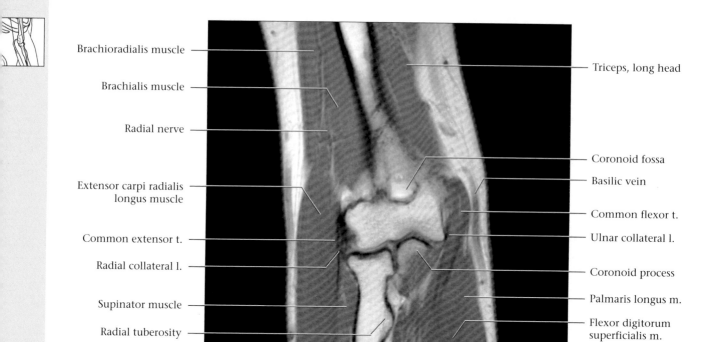

Brachioradialis muscle

Brachialis muscle

Radial nerve

Extensor carpi radialis longus muscle

Common extensor t.

Radial collateral l.

Supinator muscle

Radial tuberosity

Extensor digitorum m.

Triceps, long head

Coronoid fossa

Basilic vein

Common flexor t.

Ulnar collateral l.

Coronoid process

Palmaris longus m.

Flexor digitorum superficialis m.

Flexor digitorum profundus m.

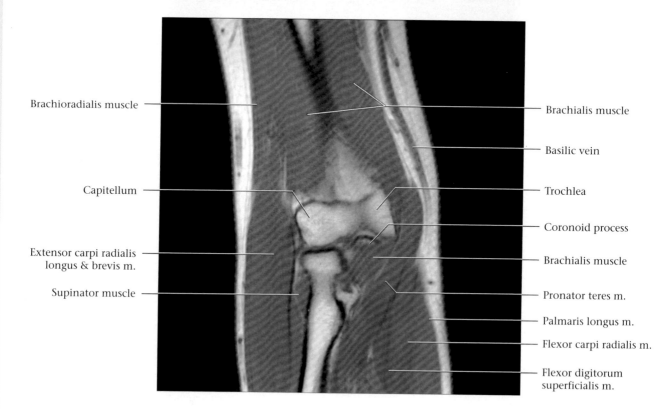

Brachioradialis muscle

Capitellum

Extensor carpi radialis longus & brevis m.

Supinator muscle

Brachialis muscle

Basilic vein

Trochlea

Coronoid process

Brachialis muscle

Pronator teres m.

Palmaris longus m.

Flexor carpi radialis m.

Flexor digitorum superficialis m.

(Top) The profile of the radial tuberosity is well seen. **(Bottom)** The brachialis muscle is draping over the anterior aspect of the humeral shaft.

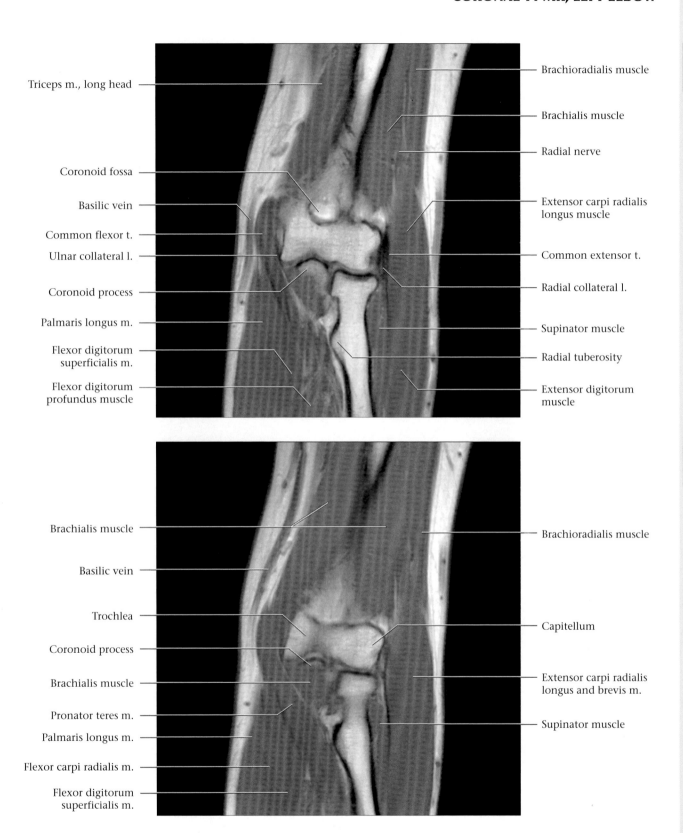

Triceps m., long head

Coronoid fossa

Basilic vein

Common flexor t.

Ulnar collateral l.

Coronoid process

Palmaris longus m.

Flexor digitorum superficialis m.

Flexor digitorum profundus muscle

Brachioradialis muscle

Brachialis muscle

Radial nerve

Extensor carpi radialis longus muscle

Common extensor t.

Radial collateral l.

Supinator muscle

Radial tuberosity

Extensor digitorum muscle

Brachialis muscle

Basilic vein

Trochlea

Coronoid process

Brachialis muscle

Pronator teres m.

Palmaris longus m.

Flexor carpi radialis m.

Flexor digitorum superficialis m.

Brachioradialis muscle

Capitellum

Extensor carpi radialis longus and brevis m.

Supinator muscle

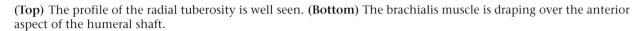

(Top) The profile of the radial tuberosity is well seen. **(Bottom)** The brachialis muscle is draping over the anterior aspect of the humeral shaft.

Elbow

II

43

CORONAL T1 MR, RIGHT ELBOW

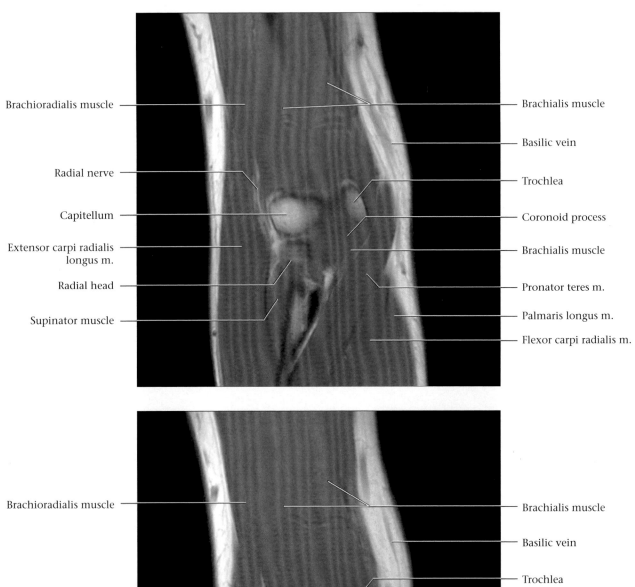

Brachioradialis muscle — Brachialis muscle

Radial nerve — Basilic vein

Capitellum — Trochlea

Extensor carpi radialis longus m. — Coronoid process

Radial head — Brachialis muscle

Supinator muscle — Pronator teres m.

Palmaris longus m.

Flexor carpi radialis m.

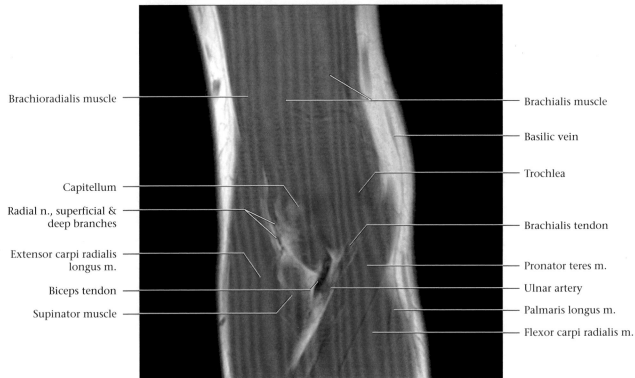

Brachioradialis muscle — Brachialis muscle

Basilic vein

Capitellum — Trochlea

Radial n., superficial & deep branches — Brachialis tendon

Extensor carpi radialis longus m. — Pronator teres m.

Biceps tendon — Ulnar artery

Supinator muscle — Palmaris longus m.

Flexor carpi radialis m.

(Top) The pronator teres muscle wraps around the anterior aspect of the forearm. (Bottom) The biceps and brachialis tendons are visualized as they dive toward their insertions. The radial nerve has split into its superficial and deep branches.

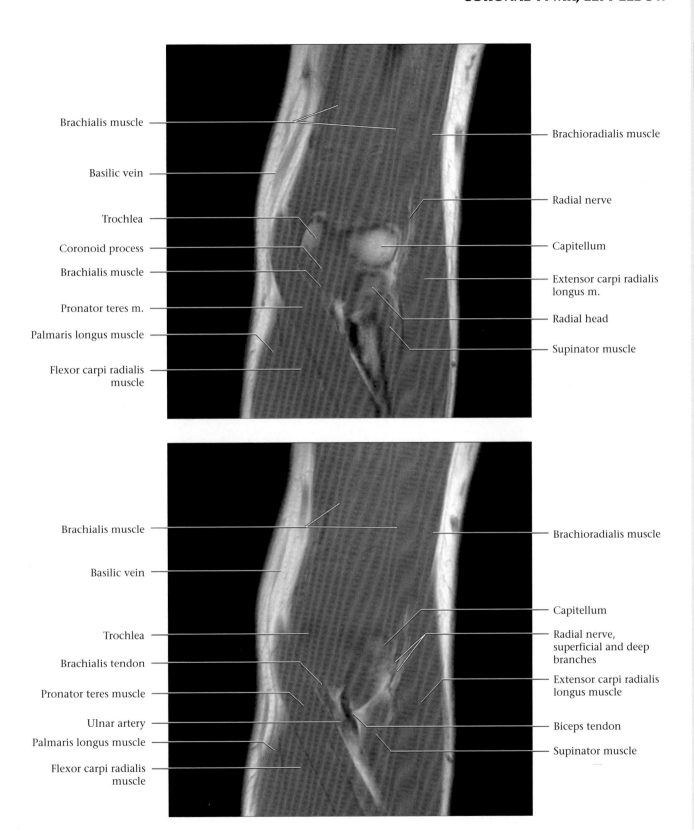

(Top) The pronator teres muscle wraps around the anterior aspect of the forearm. (Bottom) The biceps and brachialis tendons are visualized as they dive toward their insertions. The radial nerve has split into its superficial and deep branches.

CORONAL T1 MR, RIGHT ELBOW

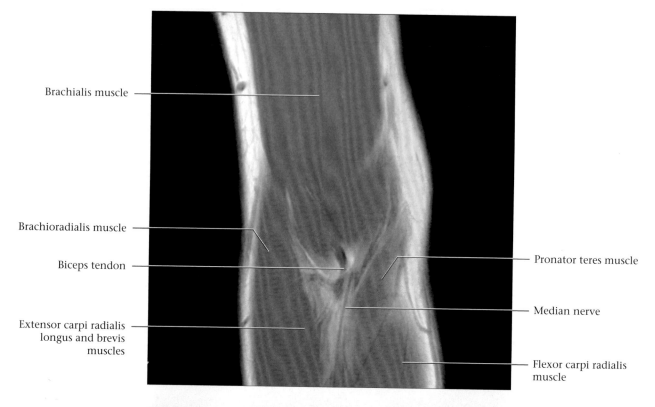

Brachialis muscle —

Brachioradialis muscle —

Biceps tendon —

— Pronator teres muscle

— Median nerve

Extensor carpi radialis longus and brevis muscles —

— Flexor carpi radialis muscle

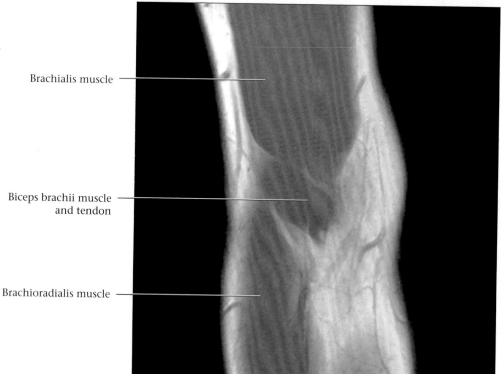

Brachialis muscle —

Biceps brachii muscle and tendon —

Brachioradialis muscle —

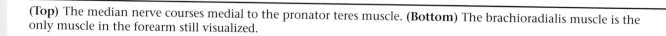

(Top) The median nerve courses medial to the pronator teres muscle. (Bottom) The brachioradialis muscle is the only muscle in the forearm still visualized.

ELBOW OVERVIEW

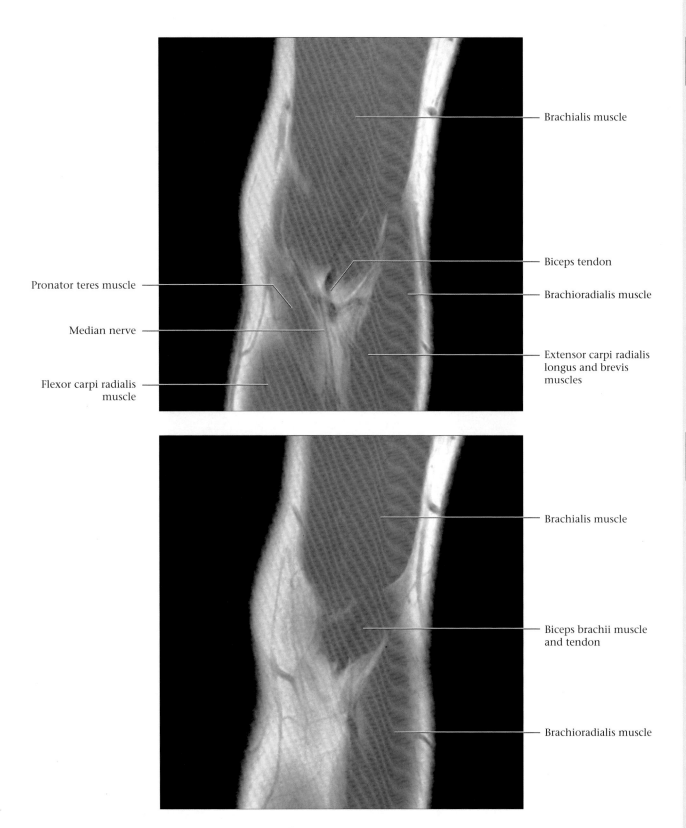

Brachialis muscle

Biceps tendon

Pronator teres muscle

Brachioradialis muscle

Median nerve

Extensor carpi radialis longus and brevis muscles

Flexor carpi radialis muscle

Brachialis muscle

Biceps brachii muscle and tendon

Brachioradialis muscle

(Top) The median nerve courses medial to the pronator teres muscle. **(Bottom)** The brachioradialis muscle is the only muscle in the forearm still visualized.

CORONAL T1 MR, RIGHT ELBOW

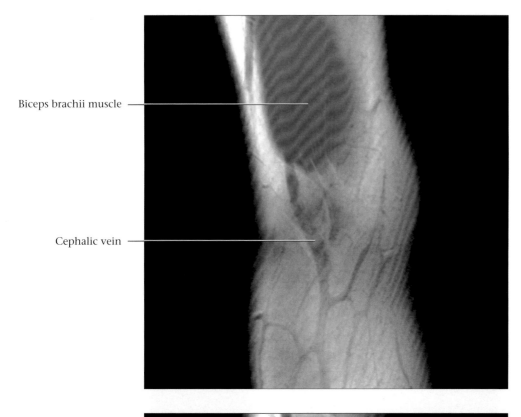

Biceps brachii muscle

Cephalic vein

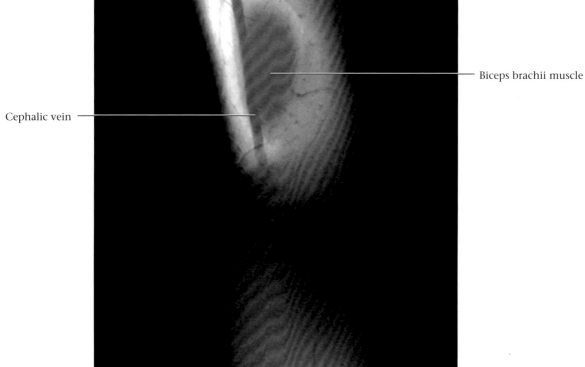

Cephalic vein

Biceps brachii muscle

(Top) The biceps brachii muscle is the only muscle still visualized. (Bottom) Just below the subcutaneous fat, the cephalic vein and biceps muscle are still seen.

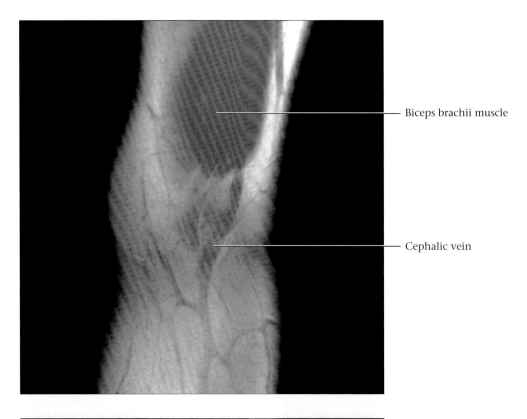

Biceps brachii muscle

Cephalic vein

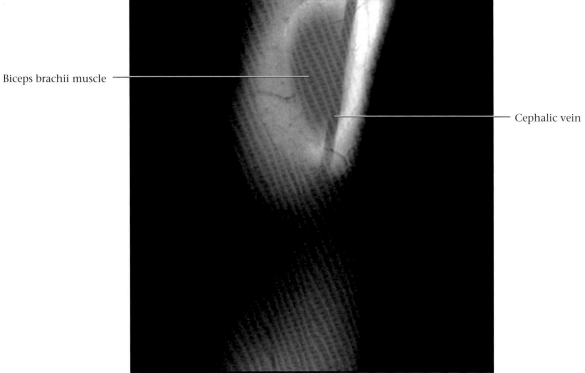

Biceps brachii muscle

Cephalic vein

(Top) The biceps brachii muscle is the only muscle still visualized. (Bottom) Just below the subcutaneous fat, the cephalic vein and biceps muscle are still seen.

SAGITTAL T1 MR, LEFT ELBOW

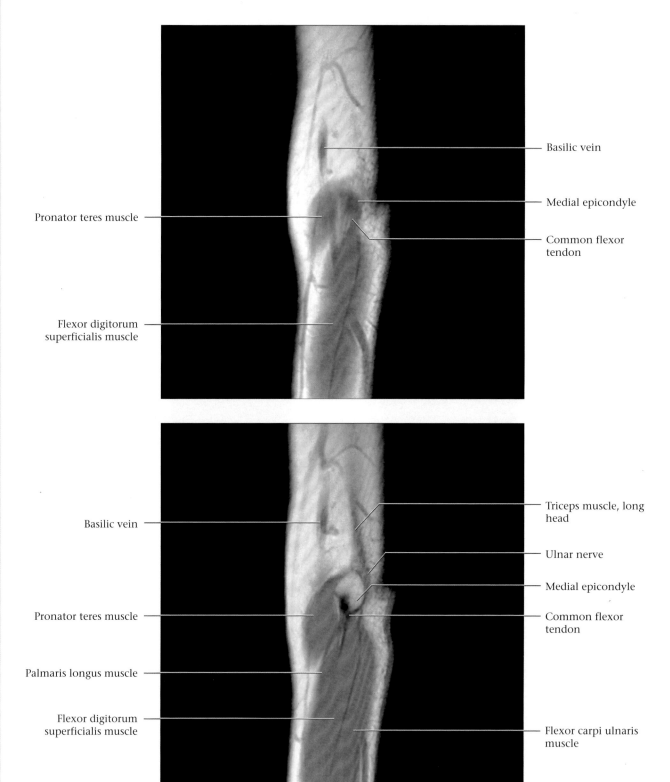

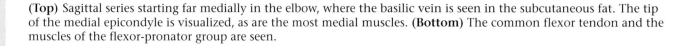

(Top) Sagittal series starting far medially in the elbow, where the basilic vein is seen in the subcutaneous fat. The tip of the medial epicondyle is visualized, as are the most medial muscles. **(Bottom)** The common flexor tendon and the muscles of the flexor-pronator group are seen.

SAGITTAL T1 MR, LEFT ELBOW

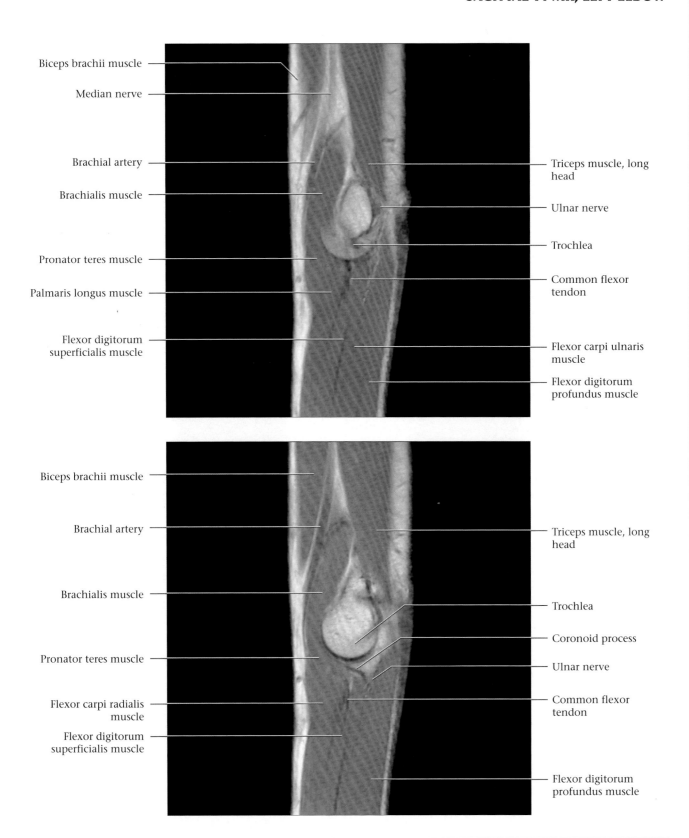
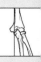

Biceps brachii muscle

Median nerve

Brachial artery

Brachialis muscle

Pronator teres muscle

Palmaris longus muscle

Flexor digitorum superficialis muscle

Triceps muscle, long head

Ulnar nerve

Trochlea

Common flexor tendon

Flexor carpi ulnaris muscle

Flexor digitorum profundus muscle

Biceps brachii muscle

Brachial artery

Brachialis muscle

Pronator teres muscle

Flexor carpi radialis muscle

Flexor digitorum superficialis muscle

Triceps muscle, long head

Trochlea

Coronoid process

Ulnar nerve

Common flexor tendon

Flexor digitorum profundus muscle

(Top) The structures of the anterior compartment of the arm are now coming into view. **(Bottom)** The coronoid process of the ulna is coming into view. The biceps brachii muscle is seen anteriorly in the arm.

Elbow

II

51

SAGITTAL T1 MR, LEFT ELBOW

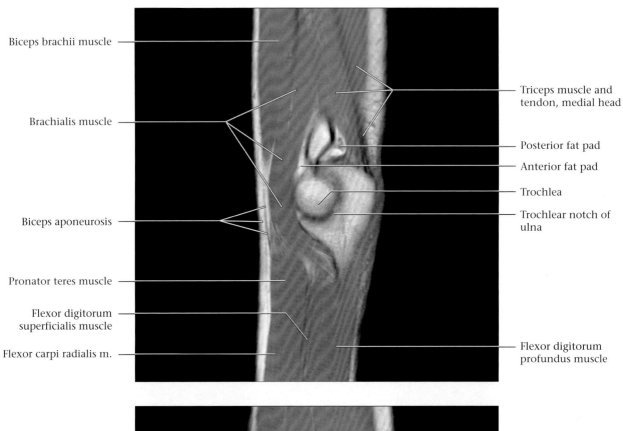

Biceps brachii muscle

Brachialis muscle

Biceps aponeurosis

Pronator teres muscle

Flexor digitorum superficialis muscle

Flexor carpi radialis m.

Triceps muscle and tendon, medial head

Posterior fat pad

Anterior fat pad

Trochlea

Trochlear notch of ulna

Flexor digitorum profundus muscle

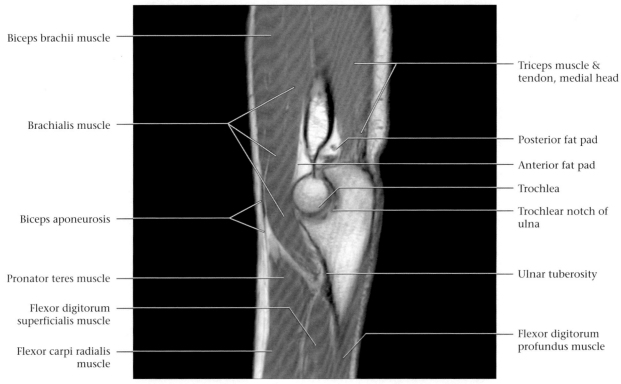

Biceps brachii muscle

Brachialis muscle

Biceps aponeurosis

Pronator teres muscle

Flexor digitorum superficialis muscle

Flexor carpi radialis muscle

Triceps muscle & tendon, medial head

Posterior fat pad

Anterior fat pad

Trochlea

Trochlear notch of ulna

Ulnar tuberosity

Flexor digitorum profundus muscle

(Top) The triceps tendon is seen inserting on the olecranon process of the ulna. Notice that the triceps muscle itself also inserts on the olecranon. **(Bottom)** The distal aspect of the brachialis muscle is seen diving toward its insertion on the ulnar tuberosity. The biceps aponeurosis is seen in cross section, anterior to the brachialis.

SAGITTAL T1 MR, LEFT ELBOW

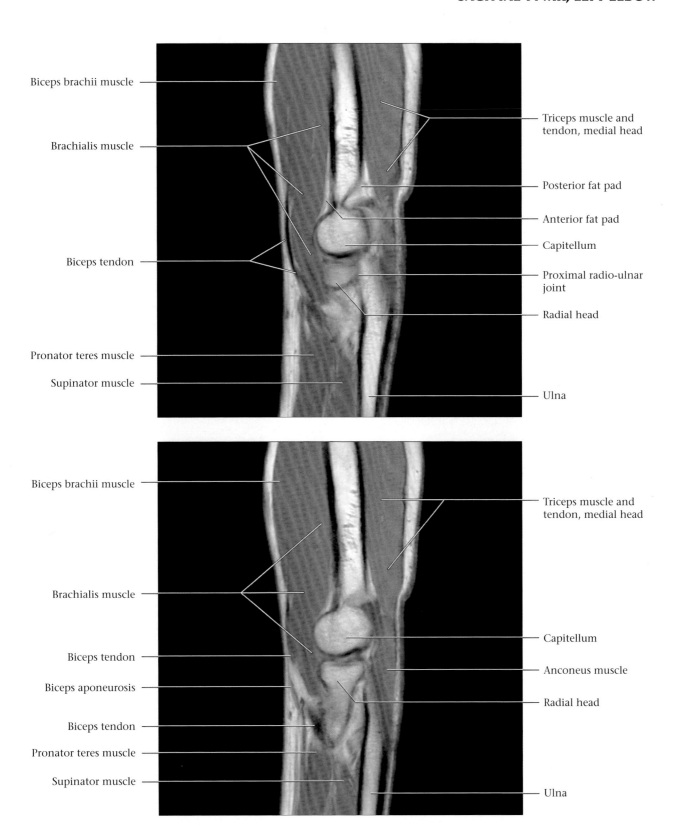

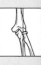

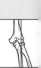

Biceps brachii muscle

Brachialis muscle

Biceps tendon

Pronator teres muscle

Supinator muscle

Triceps muscle and tendon, medial head

Posterior fat pad

Anterior fat pad

Capitellum

Proximal radio-ulnar joint

Radial head

Ulna

Biceps brachii muscle

Brachialis muscle

Biceps tendon

Biceps aponeurosis

Biceps tendon

Pronator teres muscle

Supinator muscle

Triceps muscle and tendon, medial head

Capitellum

Anconeus muscle

Radial head

Ulna

(Top) The biceps tendon is now seen, diving toward the insertion on the radial tuberosity. **(Bottom)** The anconeus muscle is now visible as the image passes lateral to the olecranon.

SAGITTAL T1 MR, LEFT ELBOW

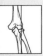

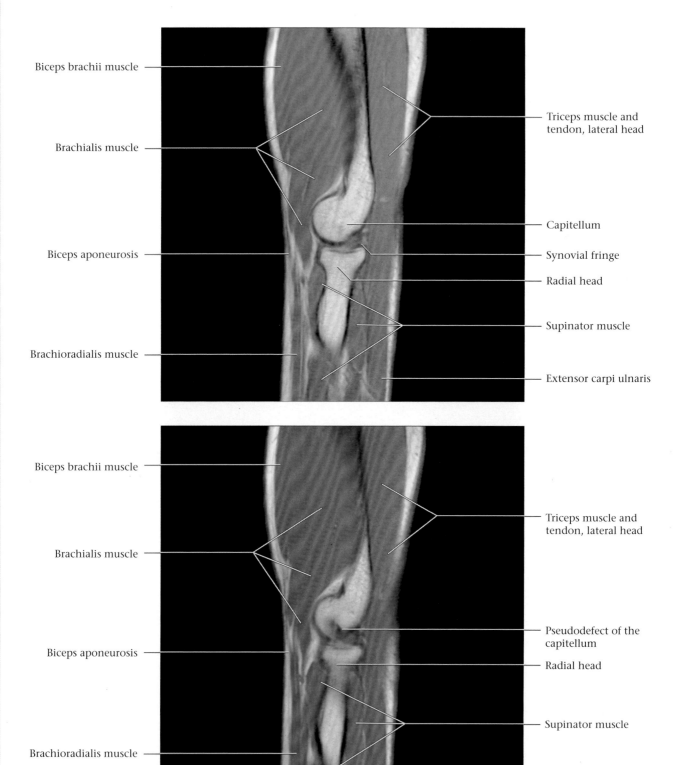

Biceps brachii muscle

Brachialis muscle

Biceps aponeurosis

Brachioradialis muscle

Triceps muscle and tendon, lateral head

Capitellum

Synovial fringe

Radial head

Supinator muscle

Extensor carpi ulnaris

Biceps brachii muscle

Brachialis muscle

Biceps aponeurosis

Brachioradialis muscle

Triceps muscle and tendon, lateral head

Pseudodefect of the capitellum

Radial head

Supinator muscle

Extensor carpi ulnaris muscle

(Top) The brachioradialis muscle is seen anteriorly. A fold of synovium, called the synovial fringe or plica, projects into the radio-capitellar joint. **(Bottom)** The pseudodefect of the capitellum, located in the posterior aspect of the capitellum, is a groove between the capitellum and lateral epicondyle, mimicking an osteochondral defect.

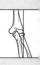

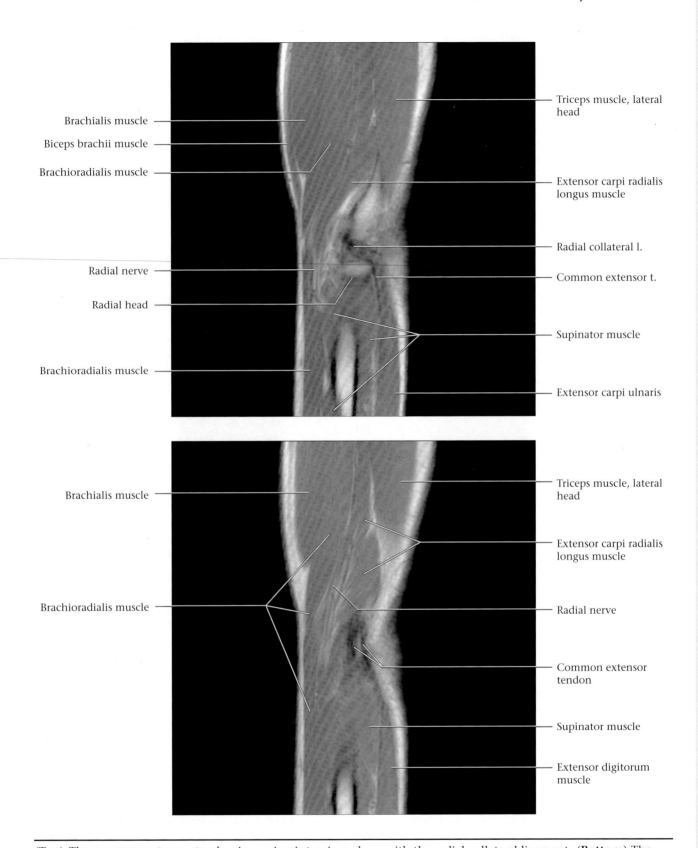

Brachialis muscle

Biceps brachii muscle

Brachioradialis muscle

Radial nerve

Radial head

Brachioradialis muscle

Triceps muscle, lateral head

Extensor carpi radialis longus muscle

Radial collateral l.

Common extensor t.

Supinator muscle

Extensor carpi ulnaris

Brachialis muscle

Brachioradialis muscle

Triceps muscle, lateral head

Extensor carpi radialis longus muscle

Radial nerve

Common extensor tendon

Supinator muscle

Extensor digitorum muscle

(Top) The common extensor tendon is coming into view, along with the radial collateral ligament. **(Bottom)** The common extensor tendon is now well seen. The brachioradialis muscle sweeps forward and becomes the most lateral muscle of the forearm.

MUSCLES AND TENDONS

Gross Anatomy

Overview
- Elbow is divided into 4 compartments: Anterior, posterior, medial, lateral

Compartments
- Anterior
  - Contains elbow flexors
  - **Biceps brachii**
    - Origin: Supraglenoid tubercle (long head), coracoid process (short head)
    - Insertion: Radial tuberosity
    - Innervation: Musculocutaneous nerve
    - Action: Elbow flexion, forearm supination
    - **Lacertus fibrosus (biceps aponeurosis):** Connects distal biceps tendon to fascia overlying common flexor mass
    - Lacertus fibrosus may compress underlying median nerve
    - Lacertus fibrosus can prevent retraction of ruptured biceps tendon
  - **Brachialis**
    - Origin: Anterior surface of humerus
    - Insertion: Ulnar tuberosity
    - Innervation: Musculocutaneous nerve
    - Action: Elbow flexion
    - Lies deep to biceps brachii
- Posterior
  - Contains elbow extensors
  - **Triceps**
    - Origin: Infraglenoid tubercle (long head), posterior humerus proximal to radial groove (lateral head), posterior humerus distal to radial groove (medial head)
    - Insertion: Olecranon process
    - Innervation: Radial nerve
    - Action: Elbow extension
  - **Anconeus**
    - Origin: Lateral epicondyle
    - Insertion: Lateral portion of olecranon, posterior aspect of ulna
    - Innervation: Radial nerve
    - Action: Elbow extension, abduction of ulna during pronation
  - **Anconeus epitrochlearis**
    - Accessory muscle
    - Anatomically inconstant, present in up to 1/3 of population
    - Origin: Medial epicondyle
    - Insertion: Medial portion of olecranon
    - Action: Elbow extension
    - Courses through cubital tunnel, posteromedial to ulnar nerve
    - May protect ulnar nerve from direct trauma, but may also compress it causing cubital tunnel syndrome
- Lateral
  - Contains the extensor-supinator group and one elbow flexor
  - **Brachioradialis**
    - Origin: Superior aspect of lateral supracondylar ridge
    - Insertion: Lateral side of distal radius
    - Innervation: Radial nerve (usually only supplies extensors)
    - Action: Elbow flexion
    - Only elbow flexor in lateral compartment
  - **Extensor carpi radialis longus**
    - Origin: Inferior aspect of lateral supracondylar ridge (may blend with origin of brachioradialis)
    - Insertion: Dorsum of base of second metacarpal
    - Innervation: Radial nerve
    - Action: Extends and abducts wrist
  - **Common extensor tendon**
    - Conjoined tendon of extensor carpi radialis brevis, extensor digitorum, extensor digiti minimi, extensor carpi ulnaris
    - Origin: Anterior aspect of lateral epicondyle and lateral supracondylar ridge
    - Insertion: See following individual muscles listed
  - **Extensor carpi radialis brevis**
    - Origin: Common extensor tendon and radial collateral ligament
    - Insertion: Dorsum of base of third metacarpal
    - Innervation: Deep branch of radial nerve
    - Action: Extends and abducts wrist
  - **Extensor digitorum**
    - Origin: Common extensor tendon, intermuscular septum
    - Insertion: Dorsum of 2nd-5th fingers
    - Innervation: Posterior interosseous branch of radial nerve
    - Action: Extends fingers at metacarpophalangeal and interphalangeal joints, extends wrist
  - **Extensor digiti minimi**
    - Origin: Common extensor tendon
    - Insertion: Dorsum of 5th finger
    - Innervation: Posterior interosseous branch of radial nerve
    - Action: Extends 5th finger
  - **Extensor carpi ulnaris**
    - Origin: Common extensor tendon and posterior aspect of ulna
    - Insertion: Dorsum of 5th metacarpal
    - Innervation: Posterior interosseous branch of radial nerve
    - Action: Extends and adducts wrist
  - **Supinator**
    - Has two heads of origin
    - Origin of humeral head: Lateral epicondyle, radial collateral ligament, anular ligament
    - Origin of ulnar head: Supinator fossa of ulna (anterior) and supinator crest of ulna (posterior)
    - Insertion: Lateral side of proximal radial shaft
    - Innervation: Deep branch of radial nerve
    - Action: Supinates forearm
- Medial
  - Contains the flexor-pronator group
  - **Common flexor tendon**
    - Conjoined tendon of flexor carpi radialis, flexor carpi ulnaris, flexor digitorum superficialis (also called sublimis), palmaris longus, pronator teres
    - Origin: Medial epicondyle and medial supracondylar ridge
    - Insertion: See individual muscles listed below

MUSCLES AND TENDONS

○ **Flexor carpi radialis**
  ▪ Origin: Common flexor tendon
  ▪ Insertion: Volar aspect of base of 2nd metacarpal
  ▪ Innervation: Median nerve
  ▪ Action: Flexes and abducts wrist, weak flexor of elbow
○ **Flexor carpi ulnaris**
  ▪ Has two heads
  ▪ Origin of humeral head: Common flexor tendon
  ▪ Origin of ulnar head: Medial aspect of olecranon and posterior aspect of ulna
  ▪ Insertion: Pisiform, hook of Hamate, base of 5th metacarpal
  ▪ Innervation: Ulnar nerve
  ▪ Action: Flexes and adducts wrist
○ **Flexor digitorum superficialis**
  ▪ Has two heads
  ▪ Origin of humero-ulnar head: Common flexor tendon, ulnar collateral ligament, coronoid process
  ▪ Origin of radial head: Anterior aspect of proximal radius
  ▪ Insertion: Volar aspect of middle phalanges of 2nd-5th fingers
  ▪ Innervation: Median nerve
  ▪ Action: Flexes the proximal interphalangeal joints, weak flexor of metacarpophalangeal and wrist joints
○ **Palmaris longus**
  ▪ Origin: Common flexor tendon
  ▪ Insertion: Palmer aponeurosis of hand
  ▪ Innervation: Median nerve
  ▪ Action: Flexes wrist
○ **Pronator teres**
  ▪ Has two heads
  ▪ Origin of humeral head: Common flexor tendon
  ▪ Origin of ulnar head: Coronoid process
  ▪ Insertion: Lateral aspect of mid shaft of radius
  ▪ Innervation: Median nerve
  ▪ Action: Pronates forearm, flexes elbow

Imaging Anatomy

Overview
- **Common extensor tendon**
  ○ Longer and thinner than common flexor tendon
  ○ May be hard to distinguish from underlying radial collateral ligament
- Triceps tendon
  ○ May look wavy on sagittal images with full elbow extension
- **Bicipitoradial bursa**
  ○ Located between distal biceps tendon and radial tuberosity
  ○ Reduces friction on biceps tendon during pronation
  ○ Has inverted tear-drop shape

Anatomy-Based Imaging Issues

Imaging Recommendations
- **Distal biceps tendon**

○ Hard to visualize longitudinally in standard sagittal plane
○ **FABS view**
  ▪ **F**lexed (elbow), **AB**ducted (arm), **S**upinated (forearm)
  ▪ Patient in superman position with arm flexed
  ▪ Allows full longitudinal visualization of biceps tendon and insertion on radial tuberosity
  ▪ Obtain scout images in plane coronal to patient's body (will be sagittal to flexed elbow)
  ▪ Plot images perpendicular to radius (coronal to humerus)
  ▪ Also shows longitudinal extent of brachialis tendon
- Snapping triceps tendon
  ○ Medial head snaps over medial epicondyle during elbow flexion
  ○ May cause ulnar nerve to dislocate anteriorly during flexion
  ○ Must image in axial plane in both extension and flexion
  ○ Dynamic scanning can be performed sonographically as elbow flexes and extends

Selected References

1. Giuffre BM et al: Optimal positioning for MRI of the distal biceps brachii tendon: flexed abducted supinated view. AJR Am J Roentgenol. 182(4):944-6, 2004
2. Skaf AY et al: Bicipitoradial bursitis: MR imaging findings in eight patients and anatomic data from contrast material opacification of bursae followed by routine radiography and MR imaging in cadavers. Radiology. 212(1):111-6, 1999
3. Cotten A et al: Normal Anatomy of the Elbow on Conventional MR Imaging and MR Arthrography. Semin Musculoskelet Radiol. 2(2):133-140, 1998
4. Spinner RJ et al: Snapping of the medial head of the triceps and recurrent dislocation of the ulnar nerve. Anatomical and dynamic factors. J Bone Joint Surg Am. 80(2):239-47, 1998

Elbow

II

57

GRAPHIC, BICEPS TENDON AND APONEUROSIS

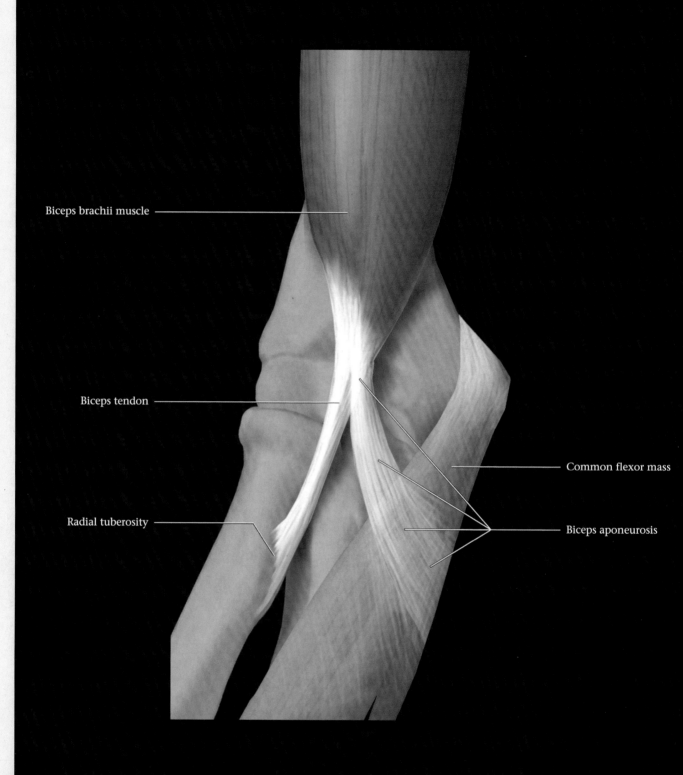

Biceps brachii muscle

Biceps tendon

Radial tuberosity

Common flexor mass

Biceps aponeurosis

The biceps aponeurosis, also called the lacertus fibrosus, is a thin sheet of fascia that connects the biceps tendon to the superficial fascia of the common flexor mass. It prevents a ruptured biceps tendon from retracting proximally.

Elbow

II

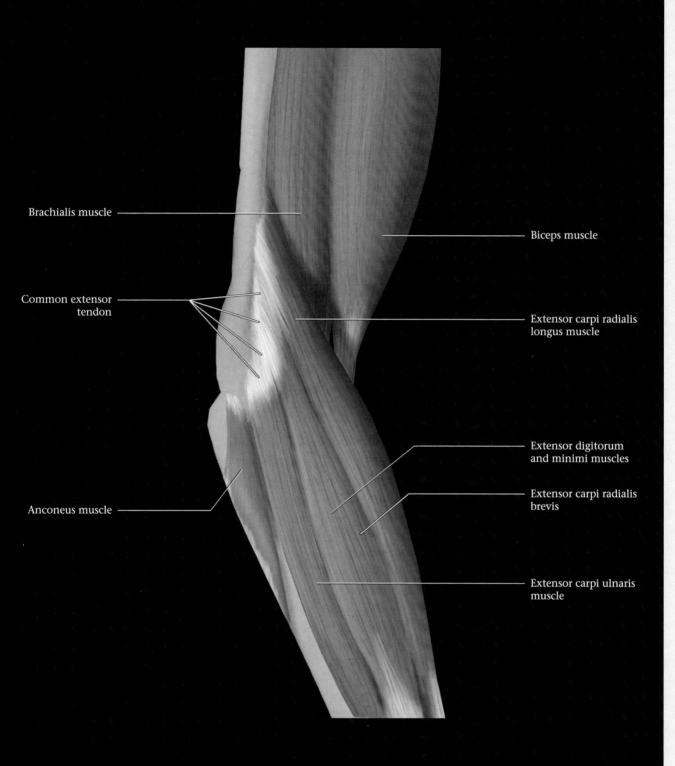

Brachialis muscle

Biceps muscle

Common extensor tendon

Extensor carpi radialis longus muscle

Extensor digitorum and minimi muscles

Extensor carpi radialis brevis

Anconeus muscle

Extensor carpi ulnaris muscle

A side view of the lateral aspect of the elbow shows the extensor-supinator group and its common extensor tendon, attaching to the lateral epicondyle and supracondylar aspect of the humerus. The common extensor tendon is comprised of the extensor carpi radialis brevis, extensor digitorum, extensor digiti minimi, and extensor carpi ulnaris.

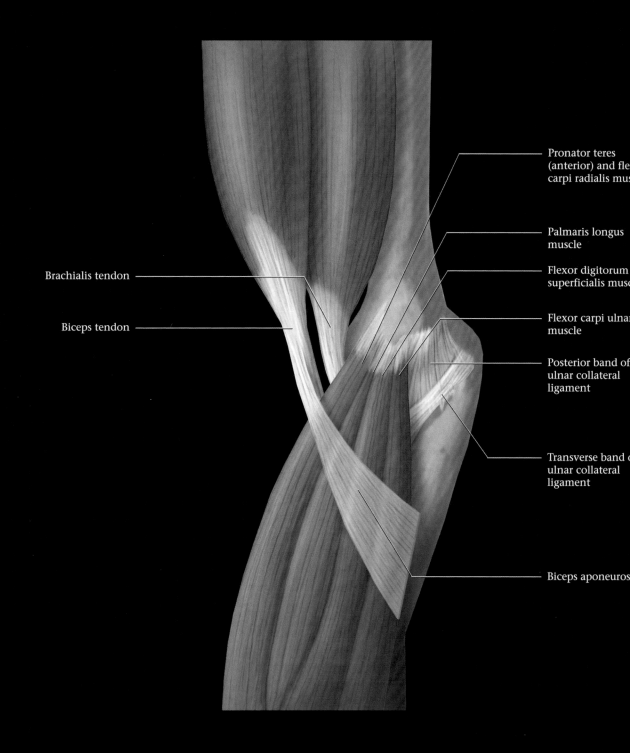

Pronator teres (anterior) and fle[...] carpi radialis mus[...]

Palmaris longus muscle

Flexor digitorum superficialis mus[...]

Flexor carpi ulna[...] muscle

Posterior band of ulnar collateral ligament

Transverse band [...] ulnar collateral ligament

Biceps aponeuros[...]

Brachialis tendon

Biceps tendon

A side view of the medial aspect of the elbow shows the flexor-pronator group and its common flexor tendon, attaching to the medial epicondyle. The anterior band of the ulnar collateral ligament is deep to the common tendon. The biceps aponeurosis blends with the anterior aspect of the common flexor mass. The flexor digitorum profundus (not shown) arises from the proximal humerus, posterior and deep to the flexor carpi ulnaris, and doe[...] not act on the elbow and is not part of the flexor-pronator group.

MUSCLES AND TENDONS

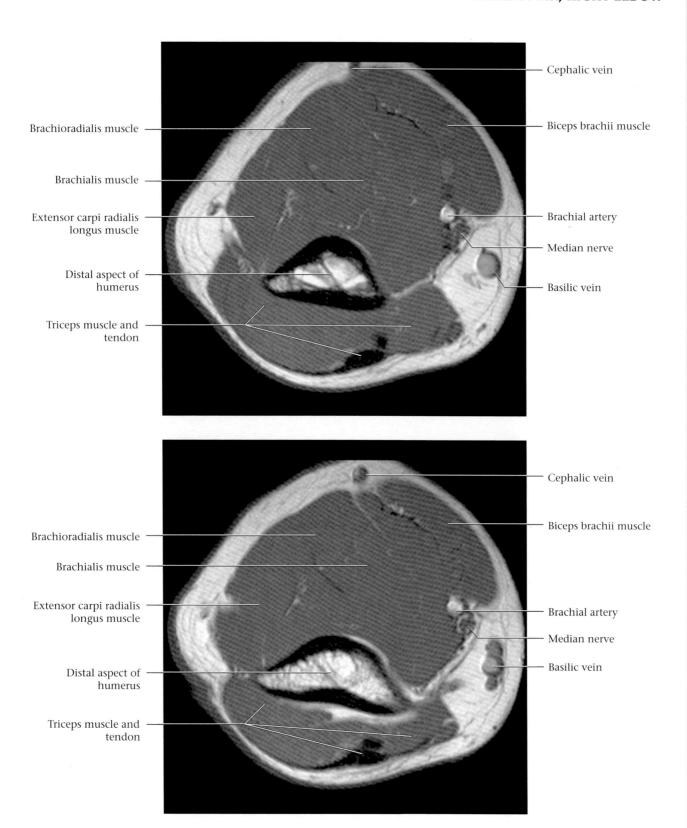

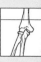

(Top) First of fourteen axial images in the distal aspect of the arm, the triceps muscle accounts for the entire posterior compartment, and the brachialis muscle accounts for most of the anterior compartment. **(Bottom)** At the supracondylar level of the humerus, the triceps muscle is starting to thin out.

AXIAL T1 MR, RIGHT ELBOW

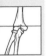

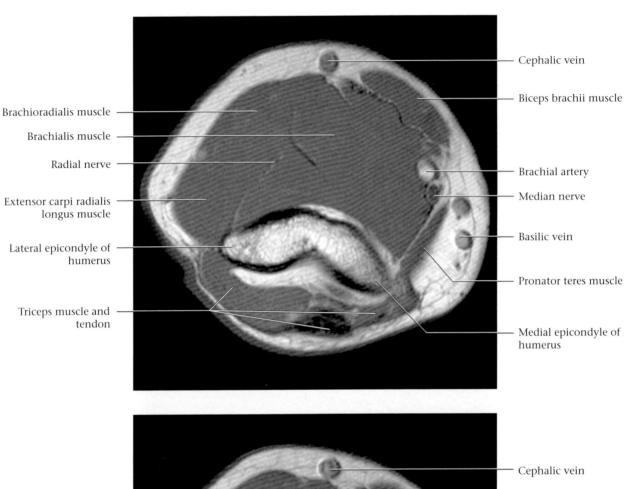

Brachioradialis muscle

Brachialis muscle

Radial nerve

Extensor carpi radialis longus muscle

Lateral epicondyle of humerus

Triceps muscle and tendon

Cephalic vein

Biceps brachii muscle

Brachial artery

Median nerve

Basilic vein

Pronator teres muscle

Medial epicondyle of humerus

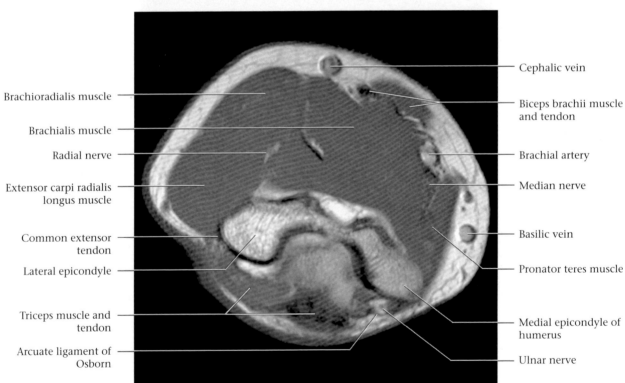

Brachioradialis muscle

Brachialis muscle

Radial nerve

Extensor carpi radialis longus muscle

Common extensor tendon

Lateral epicondyle

Triceps muscle and tendon

Arcuate ligament of Osborn

Cephalic vein

Biceps brachii muscle and tendon

Brachial artery

Median nerve

Basilic vein

Pronator teres muscle

Medial epicondyle of humerus

Ulnar nerve

(Top) At the level of the superior aspect of the epicondyles, the pronator teres muscle origin is now visualized. **(Bottom)** The lateral head of the triceps is still present, adjacent to the olecranon process. The small ulnar nerve is well seen in the cubital tunnel, surrounded by high signal intensity fat and enclosed by the arcuate ligament.

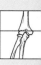

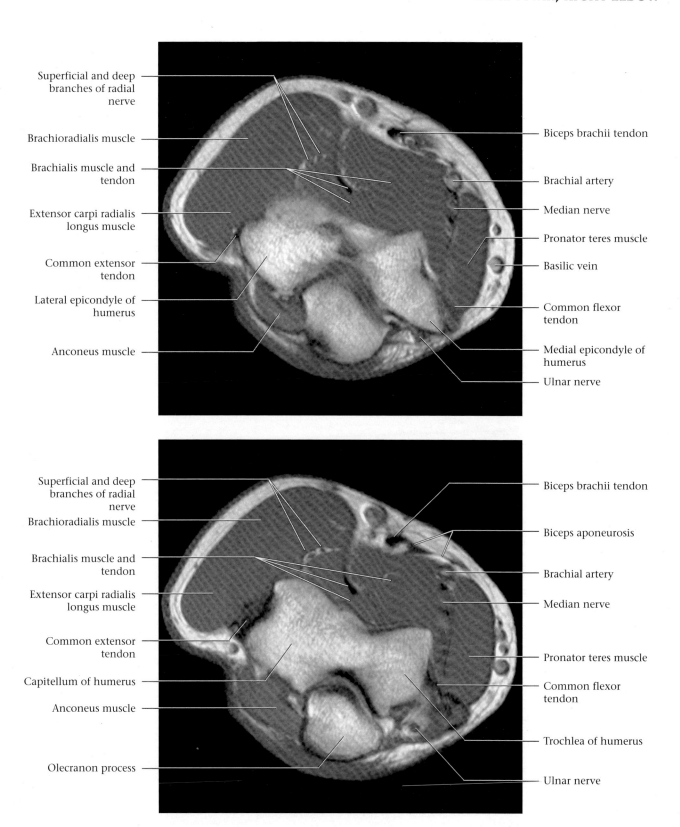

Superficial and deep branches of radial nerve

Brachioradialis muscle

Brachialis muscle and tendon

Extensor carpi radialis longus muscle

Common extensor tendon

Lateral epicondyle of humerus

Anconeus muscle

Biceps brachii tendon

Brachial artery

Median nerve

Pronator teres muscle

Basilic vein

Common flexor tendon

Medial epicondyle of humerus

Ulnar nerve

Superficial and deep branches of radial nerve

Brachioradialis muscle

Brachialis muscle and tendon

Extensor carpi radialis longus muscle

Common extensor tendon

Capitellum of humerus

Anconeus muscle

Olecranon process

Biceps brachii tendon

Biceps aponeurosis

Brachial artery

Median nerve

Pronator teres muscle

Common flexor tendon

Trochlea of humerus

Ulnar nerve

(Top) The anconeus muscle is now visible between the olecranon and lateral epicondyle. The biceps brachii muscle has tapered to its distal tendon, and the common extensor and flexor tendons are visible at their attachments to the condyles. The radial nerve has split into its superficial and deep branches. **(Bottom)** The thin biceps aponeurosis ("lacertus fibrosus") can be seen arising from the distal biceps tendon and heading medially toward the pronator teres of the common flexor muscle group.

Elbow

II

MUSCLES AND TENDONS

AXIAL T1 MR, RIGHT ELBOW

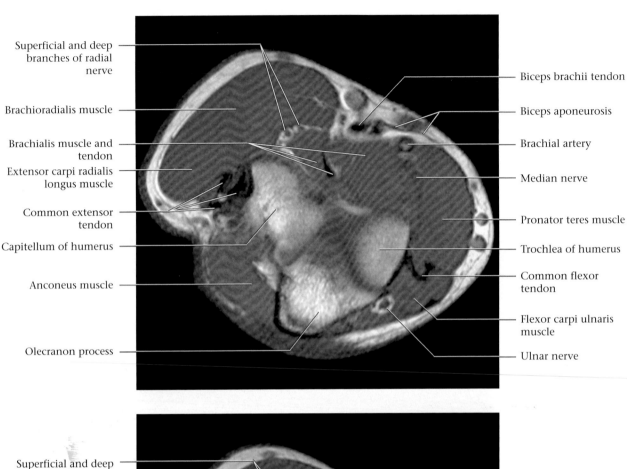

Superficial and deep branches of radial nerve

Brachioradialis muscle

Brachialis muscle and tendon

Extensor carpi radialis longus muscle

Common extensor tendon

Capitellum of humerus

Anconeus muscle

Olecranon process

Biceps brachii tendon

Biceps aponeurosis

Brachial artery

Median nerve

Pronator teres muscle

Trochlea of humerus

Common flexor tendon

Flexor carpi ulnaris muscle

Ulnar nerve

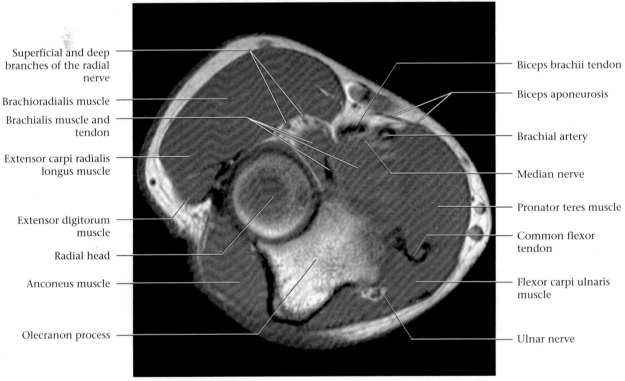

Superficial and deep branches of the radial nerve

Brachioradialis muscle

Brachialis muscle and tendon

Extensor carpi radialis longus muscle

Extensor digitorum muscle

Radial head

Anconeus muscle

Olecranon process

Biceps brachii tendon

Biceps aponeurosis

Brachial artery

Median nerve

Pronator teres muscle

Common flexor tendon

Flexor carpi ulnaris muscle

Ulnar nerve

(Top) The ulnar nerve has passed through the cubital tunnel and is now entering the forearm between the two heads of the flexor carpi ulnaris muscle. The common extensor tendon is starting to divide into its individual components. **(Bottom)** The brachialis muscle is tapering as its tendon heads toward its insertion on the ulnar tuberosity.

MUSCLES AND TENDONS

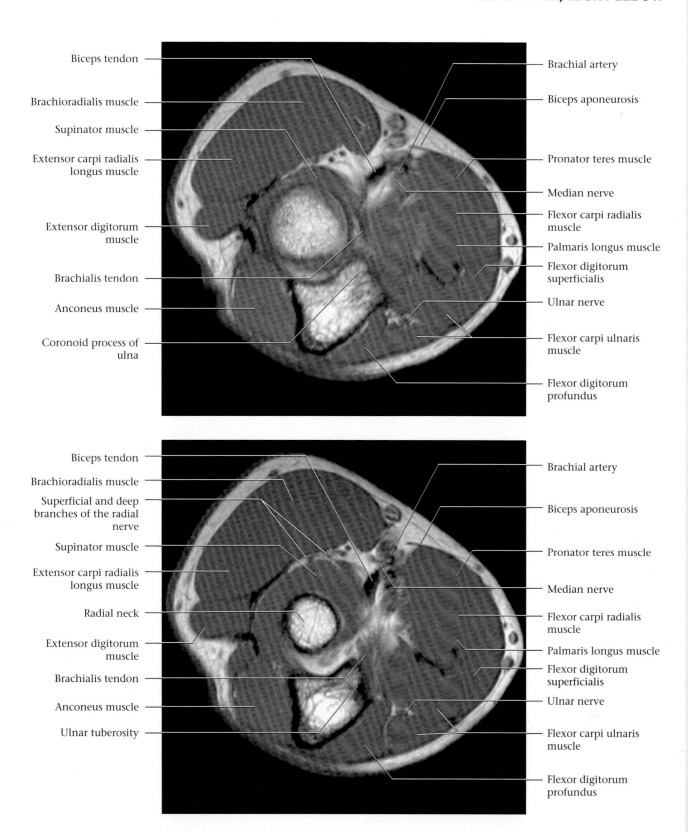

Biceps tendon

Brachioradialis muscle

Supinator muscle

Extensor carpi radialis longus muscle

Extensor digitorum muscle

Brachialis tendon

Anconeus muscle

Coronoid process of ulna

Brachial artery

Biceps aponeurosis

Pronator teres muscle

Median nerve

Flexor carpi radialis muscle

Palmaris longus muscle

Flexor digitorum superficialis

Ulnar nerve

Flexor carpi ulnaris muscle

Flexor digitorum profundus

Biceps tendon

Brachioradialis muscle

Superficial and deep branches of the radial nerve

Supinator muscle

Extensor carpi radialis longus muscle

Radial neck

Extensor digitorum muscle

Brachialis tendon

Anconeus muscle

Ulnar tuberosity

Brachial artery

Biceps aponeurosis

Pronator teres muscle

Median nerve

Flexor carpi radialis muscle

Palmaris longus muscle

Flexor digitorum superficialis

Ulnar nerve

Flexor carpi ulnaris muscle

Flexor digitorum profundus

(Top) The components of the common flexor mass are becoming visible, as the biceps aponeurosis blends with the anterior surface. The proximal aspect of the supinator muscle is also becoming visible around the radial head and neck. **(Bottom)** The brachialis tendon inserts on the ulnar tuberosity. The supinator muscle is now well seen extending around the radial neck, with the superficial and deep branches of the radial nerve on its anterior aspect. The ulnar nerve lies between the superficial and deep heads of the flexor carpi ulnaris muscle.

MUSCLES AND TENDONS

AXIAL T1 MR, RIGHT ELBOW

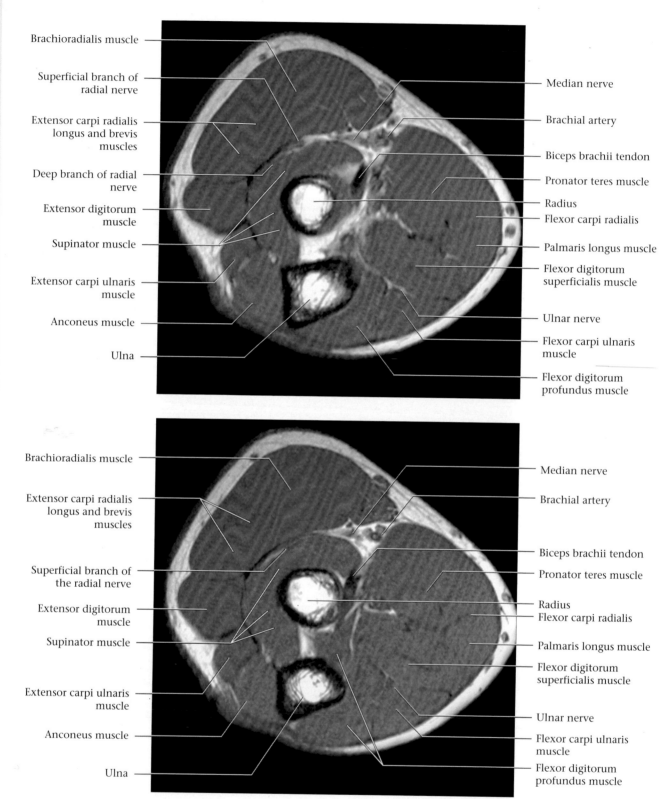

Brachioradialis muscle —

Superficial branch of radial nerve —

Extensor carpi radialis longus and brevis muscles —

Deep branch of radial nerve —

Extensor digitorum muscle —

Supinator muscle —

Extensor carpi ulnaris muscle —

Anconeus muscle —

Ulna —

— **Median nerve**

— **Brachial artery**

— **Biceps brachii tendon**

— **Pronator teres muscle**

— **Radius**

— **Flexor carpi radialis**

— **Palmaris longus muscle**

— **Flexor digitorum superficialis muscle**

— **Ulnar nerve**

— **Flexor carpi ulnaris muscle**

— **Flexor digitorum profundus muscle**

Brachioradialis muscle —

Extensor carpi radialis longus and brevis muscles —

Superficial branch of the radial nerve —

Extensor digitorum muscle —

Supinator muscle —

Extensor carpi ulnaris muscle —

Anconeus muscle —

Ulna —

— **Median nerve**

— **Brachial artery**

— **Biceps brachii tendon**

— **Pronator teres muscle**

— **Radius**

— **Flexor carpi radialis**

— **Palmaris longus muscle**

— **Flexor digitorum superficialis muscle**

— **Ulnar nerve**

— **Flexor carpi ulnaris muscle**

— **Flexor digitorum profundus muscle**

(Top) The deep branch of the radial nerve starts to enter the anterior aspect of the supinator muscle, where it will exit posteriorly as the posterior interosseous nerve. The distal biceps tendon nears its insertion on the radial tuberosity. **(Bottom)** The biceps tendon inserts on the radial tuberosity. The deep branch of the radial nerve is not well appreciated on this image.

MUSCLES AND TENDONS

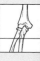

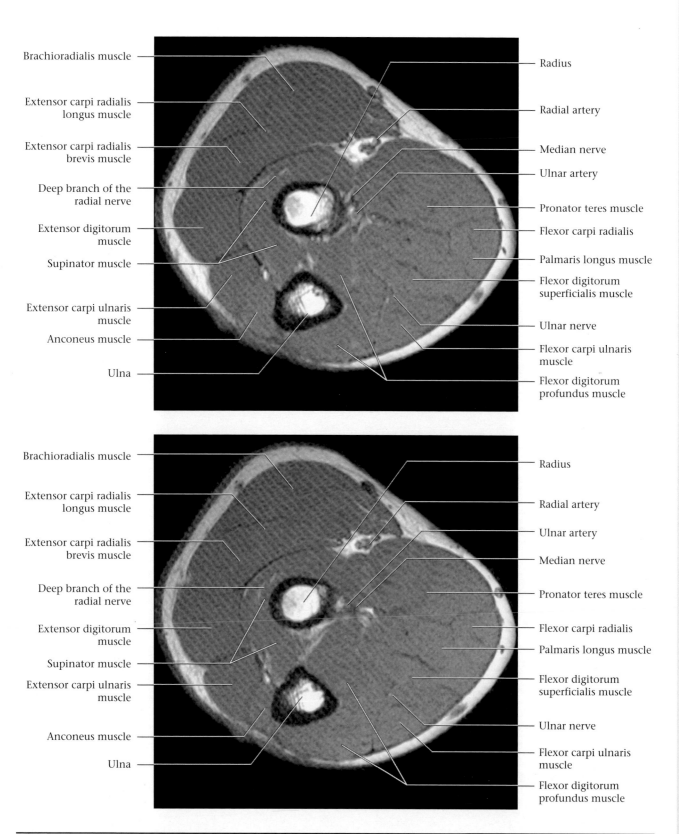

Brachioradialis muscle — Radius

Extensor carpi radialis longus muscle — Radial artery

Extensor carpi radialis brevis muscle — Median nerve

Deep branch of the radial nerve — Ulnar artery

Extensor digitorum muscle — Pronator teres muscle

Supinator muscle — Flexor carpi radialis

— Palmaris longus muscle

Extensor carpi ulnaris muscle — Flexor digitorum superficialis muscle

Anconeus muscle — Ulnar nerve

Ulna — Flexor carpi ulnaris muscle

— Flexor digitorum profundus muscle

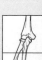

Brachioradialis muscle — Radius

Extensor carpi radialis longus muscle — Radial artery

Extensor carpi radialis brevis muscle — Ulnar artery

— Median nerve

Deep branch of the radial nerve — Pronator teres muscle

Extensor digitorum muscle — Flexor carpi radialis

Supinator muscle — Palmaris longus muscle

Extensor carpi ulnaris muscle — Flexor digitorum superficialis muscle

Anconeus muscle — Ulnar nerve

Ulna — Flexor carpi ulnaris muscle

— Flexor digitorum profundus muscle

(Top) The deep branch of the radial nerve is visualized within the supinator muscle, but the superficial branch is not well seen on this image. The individual components of the flexor-pronator group are now well delineated. **(Bottom)** The components of the extensor group are now starting to be delineated.

Elbow

II

MUSCLES AND TENDONS

CORONAL T1 MR, LEFT ELBOW

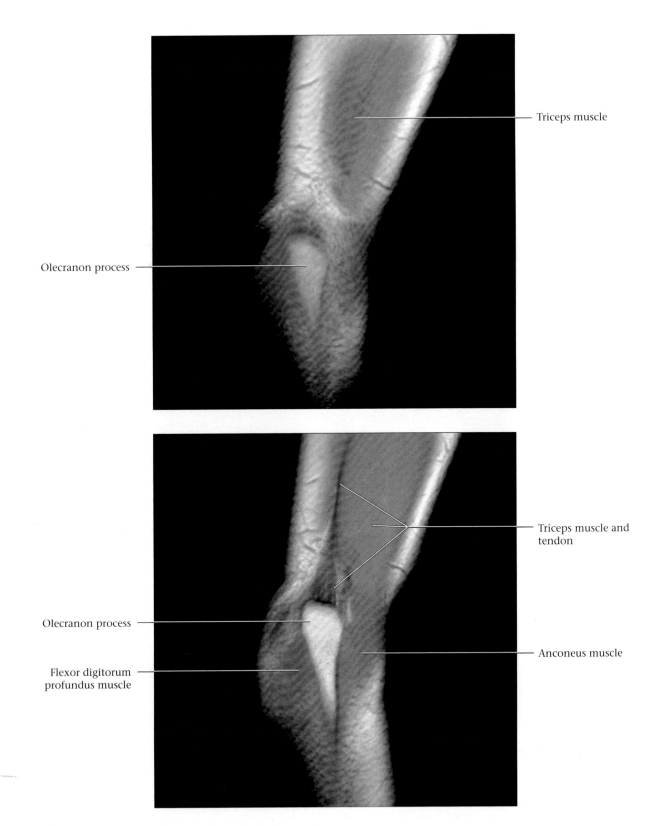

Triceps muscle

Olecranon process

Triceps muscle and tendon

Olecranon process

Anconeus muscle

Flexor digitorum profundus muscle

(Top) First of twelve coronal images at the posterior aspect of the elbow, the triceps muscle and olecranon process are seen. The triceps tendon is not yet visualized. **(Bottom)** The triceps tendon is now seen attaching to the olecranon. The posterior aspects of the anconeus on the lateral side and flexor digitorum profundus on the medial side are also now coming into view.

MUSCLES AND TENDONS

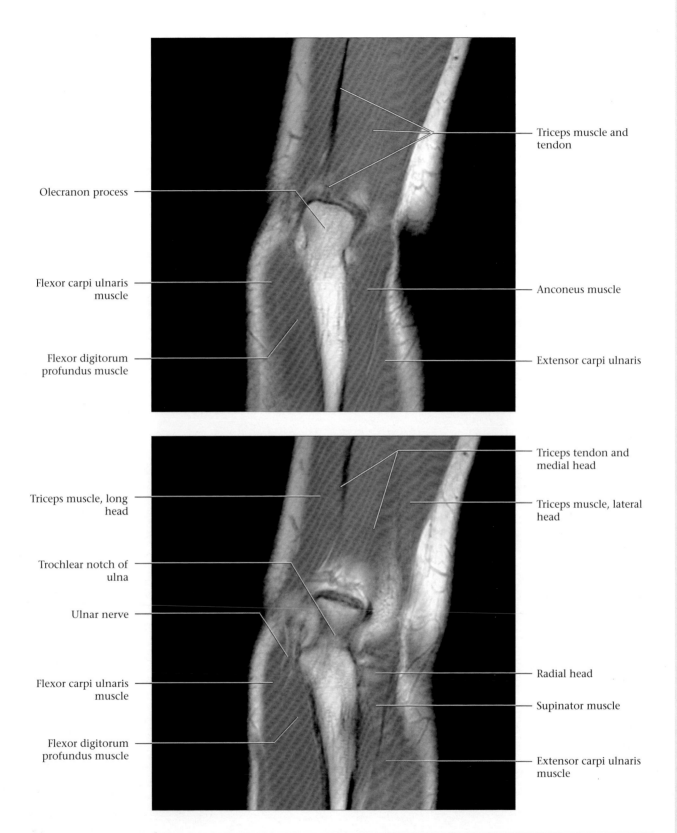

Triceps muscle and tendon

Olecranon process

Flexor carpi ulnaris muscle

Anconeus muscle

Flexor digitorum profundus muscle

Extensor carpi ulnaris

Triceps tendon and medial head

Triceps muscle, long head

Triceps muscle, lateral head

Trochlear notch of ulna

Ulnar nerve

Flexor carpi ulnaris muscle

Radial head

Supinator muscle

Flexor digitorum profundus muscle

Extensor carpi ulnaris muscle

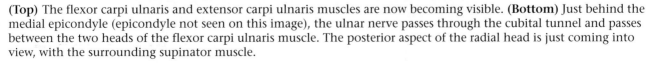

(Top) The flexor carpi ulnaris and extensor carpi ulnaris muscles are now becoming visible. **(Bottom)** Just behind the medial epicondyle (epicondyle not seen on this image), the ulnar nerve passes through the cubital tunnel and passes between the two heads of the flexor carpi ulnaris muscle. The posterior aspect of the radial head is just coming into view, with the surrounding supinator muscle.

MUSCLES AND TENDONS

CORONAL T1 MR, LEFT ELBOW

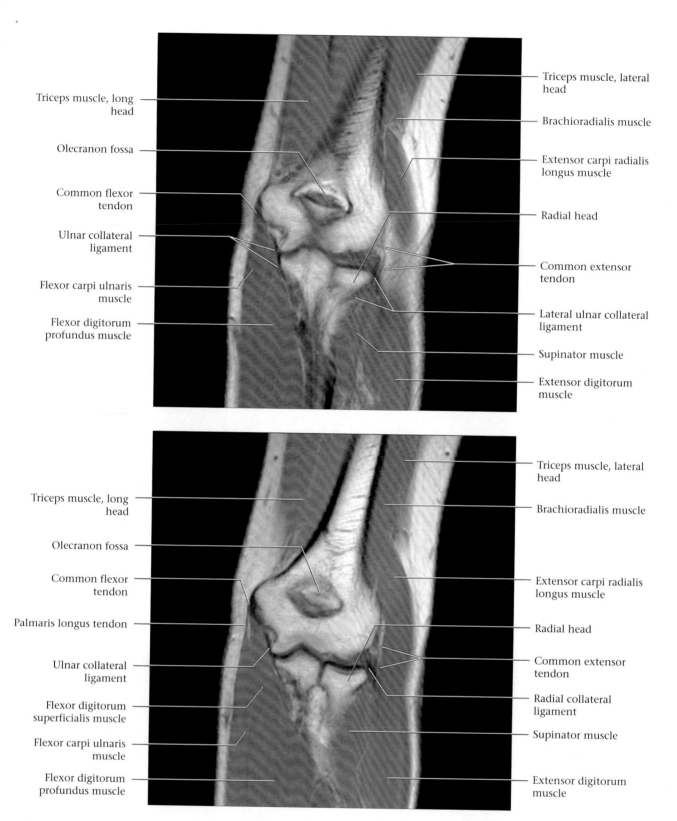

Triceps muscle, long head

Olecranon fossa

Common flexor tendon

Ulnar collateral ligament

Flexor carpi ulnaris muscle

Flexor digitorum profundus muscle

Triceps muscle, lateral head

Brachioradialis muscle

Extensor carpi radialis longus muscle

Radial head

Common extensor tendon

Lateral ulnar collateral ligament

Supinator muscle

Extensor digitorum muscle

Triceps muscle, long head

Olecranon fossa

Common flexor tendon

Palmaris longus tendon

Ulnar collateral ligament

Flexor digitorum superficialis muscle

Flexor carpi ulnaris muscle

Flexor digitorum profundus muscle

Triceps muscle, lateral head

Brachioradialis muscle

Extensor carpi radialis longus muscle

Radial head

Common extensor tendon

Radial collateral ligament

Supinator muscle

Extensor digitorum muscle

(Top) The posterior aspect of the common extensor tendon is seen superficial to the lateral ulnar collateral ligament. The lateral ulnar collateral ligament is seen winding posterior to the radius towards its attachment on the ulna. The common flexor tendon is shorter and broader than the common extensor tendon, and is seen attaching to the medial epicondyle. **(Bottom)** The common extensor tendon is now better visualized, superficial to the radial collateral ligament. The palmaris longus component of the common flexor tendon is also seen, with the ulnar collateral ligament deep to the common flexor muscle group.

Elbow

II

70

MUSCLES AND TENDONS

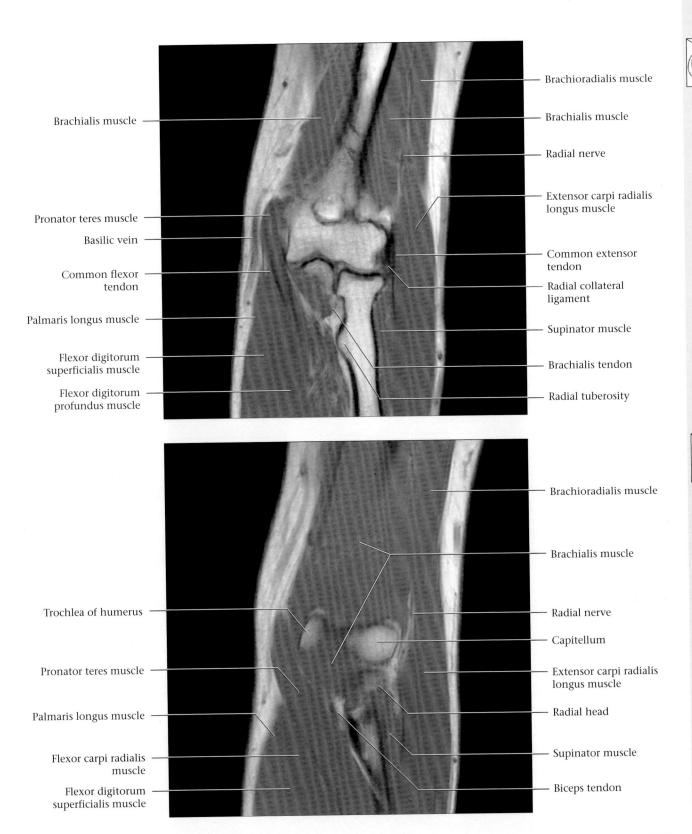

Brachioradialis muscle

Brachialis muscle

Brachialis muscle

Radial nerve

Pronator teres muscle

Extensor carpi radialis
longus muscle

Basilic vein

Common flexor
tendon

Common extensor
tendon

Radial collateral
ligament

Palmaris longus muscle

Supinator muscle

Flexor digitorum
superficialis muscle

Brachialis tendon

Flexor digitorum
profundus muscle

Radial tuberosity

Brachioradialis muscle

Brachialis muscle

Trochlea of humerus

Radial nerve

Capitellum

Pronator teres muscle

Extensor carpi radialis
longus muscle

Palmaris longus muscle

Radial head

Flexor carpi radialis
muscle

Supinator muscle

Flexor digitorum
superficialis muscle

Biceps tendon

(Top) The radial nerve can be seen running between the brachioradialis and brachialis muscles. The brachialis tendon approaches its insertion on the ulnar tuberosity. **(Bottom)** The distal biceps tendon is visualized, proximal to its insertion on the radial tuberosity. The course of the pronator teres muscle is well seen, extending from the medial side of the humerus to the proximal shaft of the radius.

MUSCLES AND TENDONS

CORONAL T1 MR, LEFT ELBOW

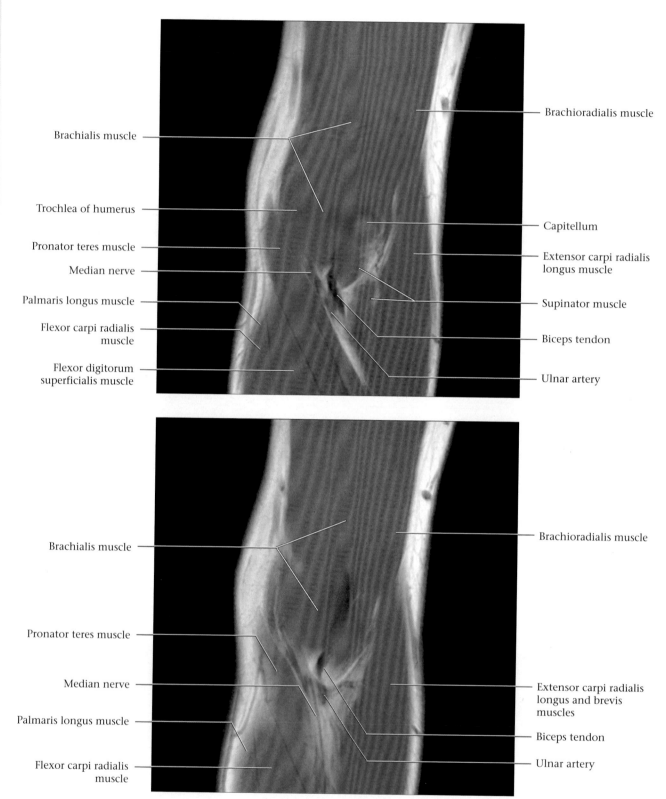

Brachialis muscle

Trochlea of humerus

Pronator teres muscle

Median nerve

Palmaris longus muscle

Flexor carpi radialis muscle

Flexor digitorum superficialis muscle

Brachioradialis muscle

Capitellum

Extensor carpi radialis longus muscle

Supinator muscle

Biceps tendon

Ulnar artery

Brachialis muscle

Pronator teres muscle

Median nerve

Palmaris longus muscle

Flexor carpi radialis muscle

Brachioradialis muscle

Extensor carpi radialis longus and brevis muscles

Biceps tendon

Ulnar artery

(Top) The median nerve and ulnar artery are coming into view, adjacent to the biceps tendon. **(Bottom)** The longitudinal extent of the median nerve is well seen.

MUSCLES AND TENDONS

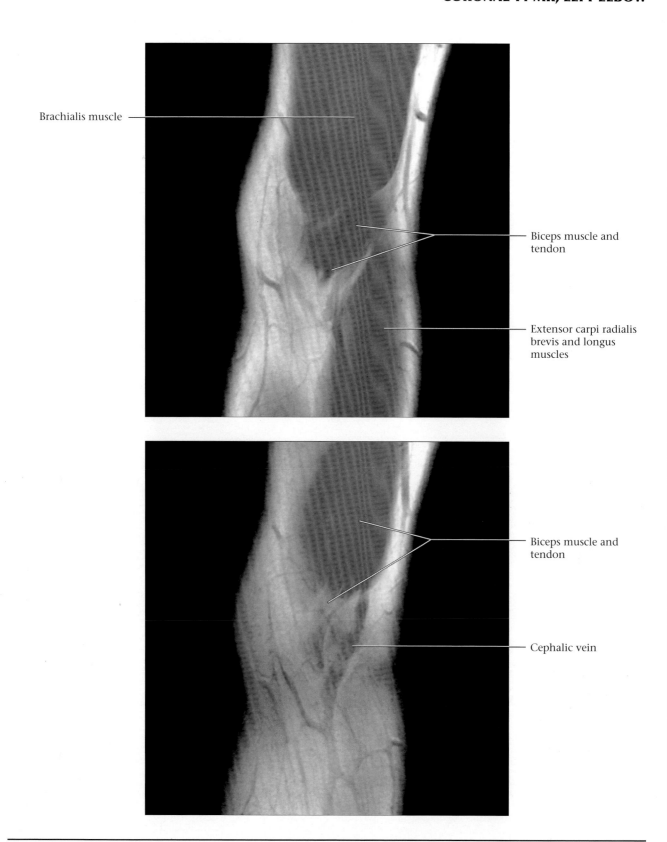

Brachialis muscle

Biceps muscle and tendon

Extensor carpi radialis brevis and longus muscles

Biceps muscle and tendon

Cephalic vein

(Top) The biceps muscle is now coming into view. **(Bottom)** The only muscle seen at the most extreme anterior of the elbow is the biceps.

SAGITTAL T1 MR, LEFT ELBOW

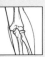

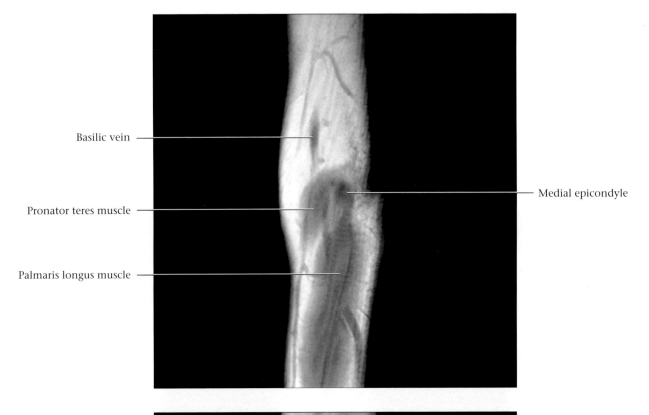

Basilic vein

Pronator teres muscle

Palmaris longus muscle

Medial epicondyle

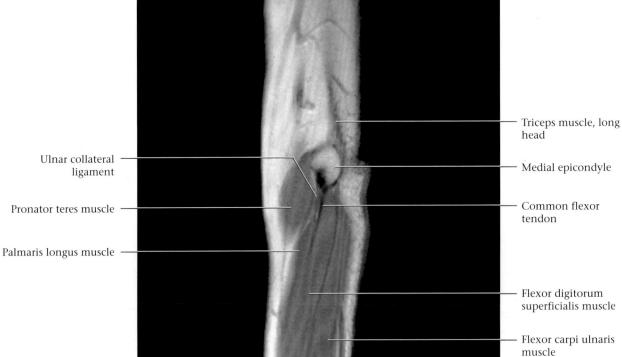

Ulnar collateral ligament

Pronator teres muscle

Palmaris longus muscle

Triceps muscle, long head

Medial epicondyle

Common flexor tendon

Flexor digitorum superficialis muscle

Flexor carpi ulnaris muscle

(Top) First of twelve sagittal images. Only the extreme tip of the medial epicondyle is visible in this medial section. The pronator teres and palmaris longus muscles are the most medially located and are just coming into view. **(Bottom)** The medial epicondyle is now better seen, with the attachments of the ulnar collateral ligament and common flexor tendon.

MUSCLES AND TENDONS

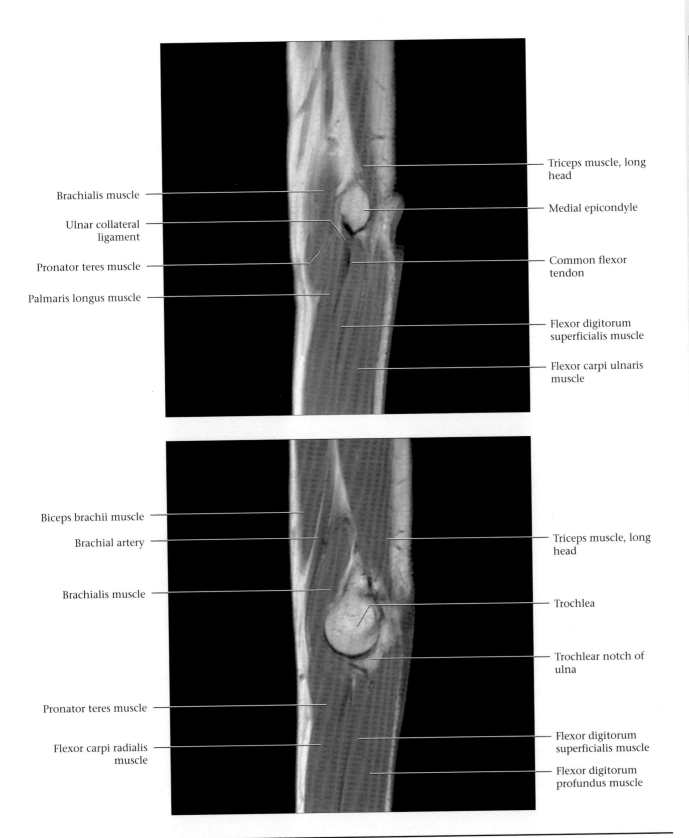
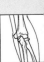

Top image labels:

Brachialis muscle

Ulnar collateral ligament

Pronator teres muscle

Palmaris longus muscle

Triceps muscle, long head

Medial epicondyle

Common flexor tendon

Flexor digitorum superficialis muscle

Flexor carpi ulnaris muscle

Bottom image labels:

Biceps brachii muscle

Brachial artery

Brachialis muscle

Pronator teres muscle

Flexor carpi radialis muscle

Triceps muscle, long head

Trochlea

Trochlear notch of ulna

Flexor digitorum superficialis muscle

Flexor digitorum profundus muscle

(Top) The brachialis muscle is now coming into view. **(Bottom)** The brachialis muscle is now better seen and the more superficial biceps brachii muscle is coming into view, with the brachial artery in between them.

MUSCLES AND TENDONS

SAGITTAL T1 MR, LEFT ELBOW

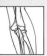

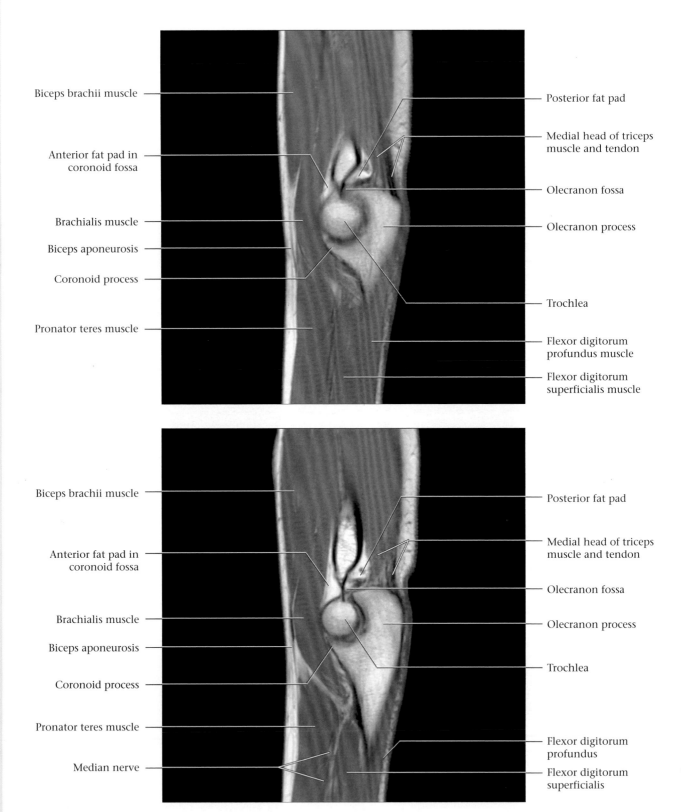

Biceps brachii muscle — | — Posterior fat pad

Anterior fat pad in coronoid fossa — | — Medial head of triceps muscle and tendon

— Olecranon fossa

Brachialis muscle — | — Olecranon process

Biceps aponeurosis —

Coronoid process —

— Trochlea

Pronator teres muscle — | — Flexor digitorum profundus muscle

— Flexor digitorum superficialis muscle

Biceps brachii muscle — | — Posterior fat pad

Anterior fat pad in coronoid fossa — | — Medial head of triceps muscle and tendon

— Olecranon fossa

Brachialis muscle — | — Olecranon process

Biceps aponeurosis —

Coronoid process —

— Trochlea

Pronator teres muscle — | — Flexor digitorum profundus

Median nerve — | — Flexor digitorum superficialis

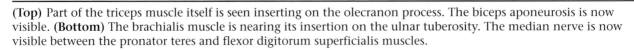

(Top) Part of the triceps muscle itself is seen inserting on the olecranon process. The biceps aponeurosis is now visible. **(Bottom)** The brachialis muscle is nearing its insertion on the ulnar tuberosity. The median nerve is now visible between the pronator teres and flexor digitorum superficialis teuscles.

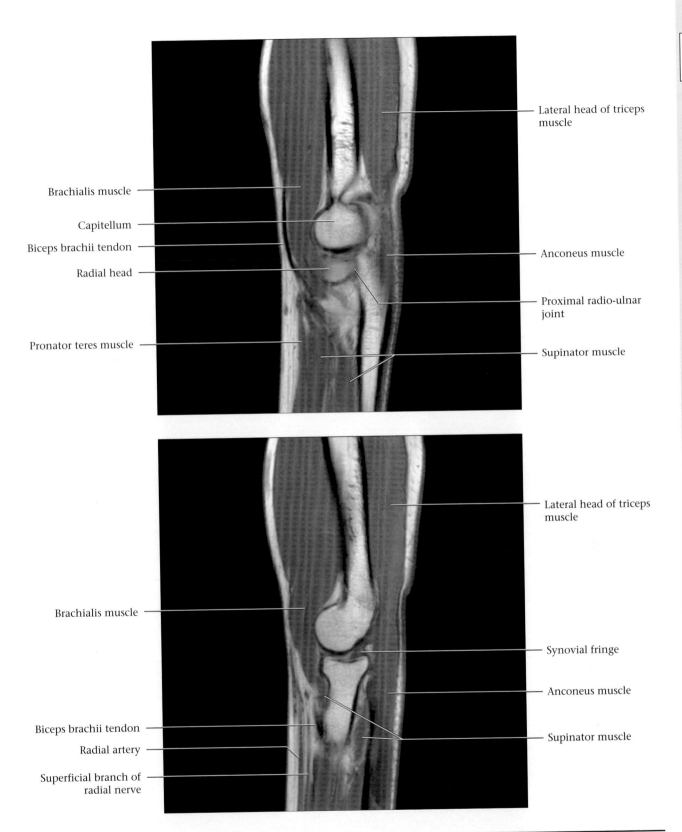

Lateral head of triceps muscle

Brachialis muscle

Capitellum

Biceps brachii tendon

Radial head

Anconeus muscle

Proximal radio-ulnar joint

Pronator teres muscle

Supinator muscle

Lateral head of triceps muscle

Brachialis muscle

Synovial fringe

Anconeus muscle

Biceps brachii tendon

Radial artery

Supinator muscle

Superficial branch of radial nerve

(Top) The radial head and proximal radio-ulnar joint are coming into view. The distal biceps tendon is diving toward its insertion on the radial tuberosity. **(Bottom)** The biceps tendon is seen attaching to the radial tuberosity. A synovial fringe, also called a synovial plica, is a meniscus-shaped ten-folding of the joint capsule.

Elbow

II

MUSCLES AND TENDONS

SAGITTAL T1 MR, LEFT ELBOW

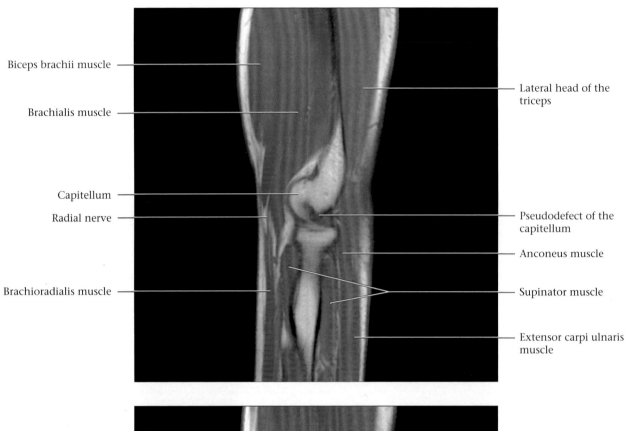

Biceps brachii muscle

Brachialis muscle

Capitellum

Radial nerve

Brachioradialis muscle

Lateral head of the triceps

Pseudodefect of the capitellum

Anconeus muscle

Supinator muscle

Extensor carpi ulnaris muscle

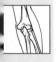

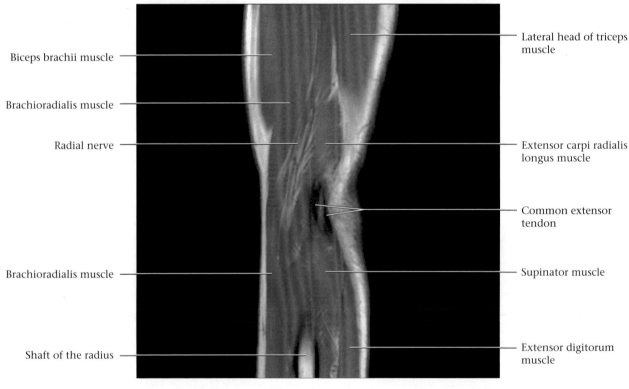

Biceps brachii muscle

Brachioradialis muscle

Radial nerve

Brachioradialis muscle

Shaft of the radius

Lateral head of triceps muscle

Extensor carpi radialis longus muscle

Common extensor tendon

Supinator muscle

Extensor digitorum muscle

(Top) The pseudodefect of the capitellum is seen at the posterior aspect of the capitellum, representing a normal groove between the round capitellum and lateral condyle. (Bottom) The common extensor tendon is inserting at the tip of the lateral epicondyle.

MUSCLES AND TENDONS

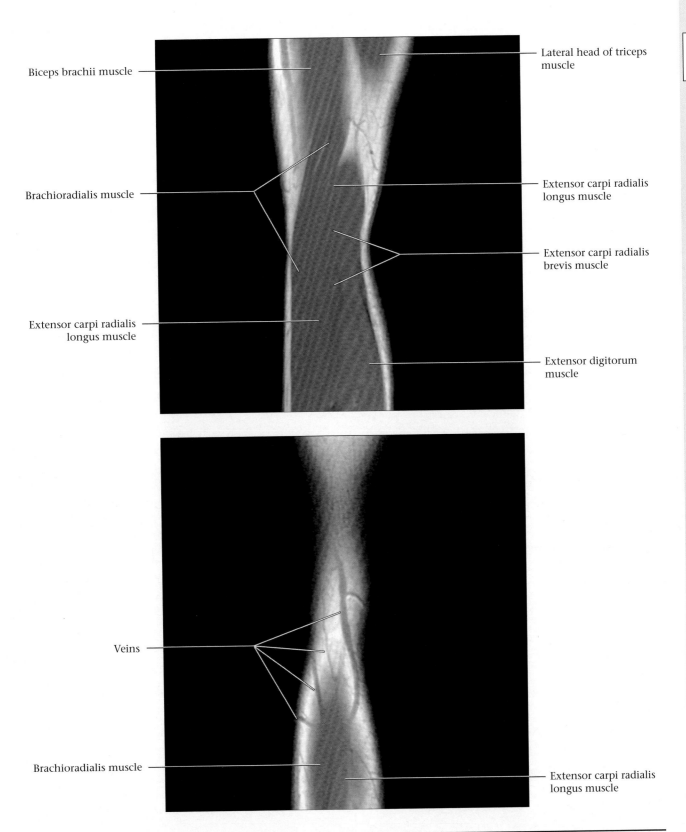

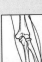

Biceps brachii muscle

Brachioradialis muscle

Extensor carpi radialis longus muscle

Lateral head of triceps muscle

Extensor carpi radialis longus muscle

Extensor carpi radialis brevis muscle

Extensor digitorum muscle

Veins

Brachioradialis muscle

Extensor carpi radialis longus muscle

(Top) Along the far lateral aspect of the elbow, the muscles of the extensor group are visualized, forming the fleshy lateral aspect of the forearm. **(Bottom)** Coming out of the lateral muscles into the subcutaneous fat, numerous veins are seen.

MUSCLES AND TENDONS

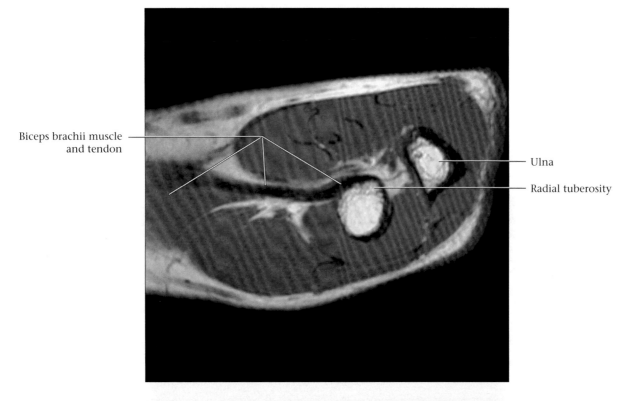

Biceps brachii muscle and tendon

Ulna

Radial tuberosity

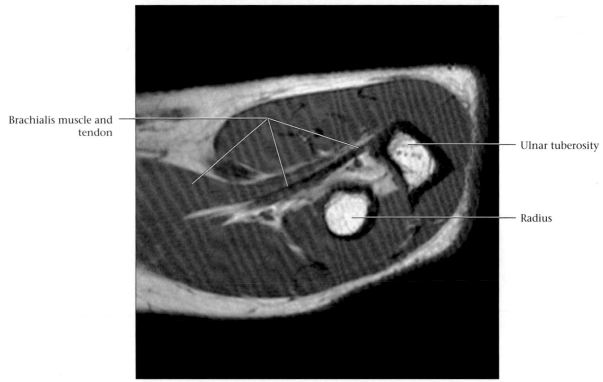

Brachialis muscle and tendon

Ulnar tuberosity

Radius

(Top) Imaging transverse to the forearm in the FABS position shows the full longitudinal extent of the distal biceps tendon inserting on the radial tuberosity. **(Bottom)** Imaging transverse to the forearm in the FABS position also shows the full longitudinal extent of the brachialis tendon inserting on the ulnar tuberosity.

MUSCLES AND TENDONS

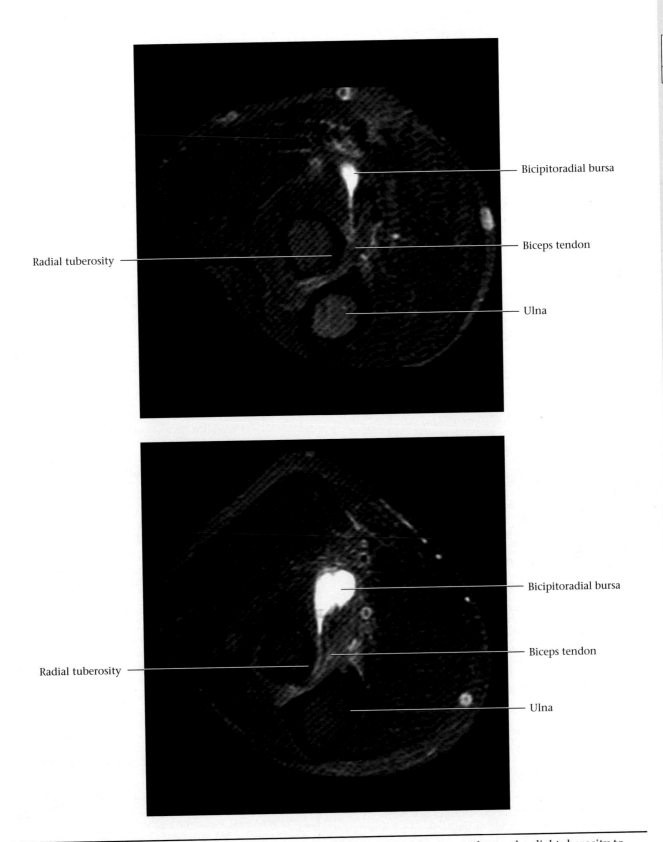

Bicipitoradial bursa

Biceps tendon

Radial tuberosity

Ulna

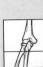

Bicipitoradial bursa

Radial tuberosity

Biceps tendon

Ulna

(Top) The bicipitoradial bursa is tear-drop shaped and located between the biceps tendon and radial tuberosity to protect the tendon during pronation. **(Bottom)** In a different patient, the bicipitoradial bursa is more distended but still tear-drop shaped. The biceps tendon is mildly tendinotic, manifest by swelling and signal alteration.

LIGAMENTS

Terminology

Abbreviations
- Ulnar collateral ligament (UCL)
- Radial collateral ligament (RCL)

Definitions
- Elbow ligaments are intrinsic ligaments: Thickenings of the joint capsule

Imaging Anatomy

Lateral Side of Elbow Joint
- **Lateral collateral ligament complex**
  - **Radial collateral ligament**
    - Triangular shaped
    - Apex is on the lateral epicondyle
    - Base blends with anular ligament around radial head
    - Lies deep to overlying common extensor tendon
    - Provides origin for the superficial head of supinator muscle
  - **Lateral UCL**
    - Thin ligament
    - Provides restraint to posterolateral instability of radial head
    - Origin: Lateral epicondyle, blending with posterior aspect of origin of RCL
    - Insertion: Supinator crest of lateral side of proximal ulna
    - Courses posterior to radial head, partially blending with anular ligament
  - **Anular ligament**
    - Attached to anterior and posterior aspects of radial notch of ulna
    - Forms a ring or collar around radial head
    - Anterior attachment becomes taut in supination
    - Posterior attachment becomes taut in extreme pronation
    - Provides origin for superficial head of supinator muscle
  - **Accessory lateral collateral ligament**
    - Anatomically inconstant
    - Origin: Anterior inferior aspect of anular ligament
    - Insertion: Supinator crest of ulna, blending with insertion of lateral UCL
    - Stabilizes anular ligament during varus stress

Medial Side of Elbow Joint
- **Ulnar (medial) collateral ligament**
  - Restraint against valgus stress
  - Triangular shaped
  - Origin: Inferior surface of medial epicondyle
  - Insertion: Coronoid and olecranon portions of ulna
  - Composed of three bands
    - Anterior: Functionally most important, extends from medial epicondyle of humerus to sublime tubercle of coronoid process
    - Posterior: Functionally less important but maintains reciprocal tautness with anterior band, extends from medial epicondyle to olecranon
    - Transverse: Functionally unimportant, forms base of triangle between anterior and posterior bands
  - Lies deep to common flexor tendon

Proximal Radio-Ulnar Joint
- Anular ligament: See prior
- **Quadrate ligament**
  - Thin fibrous band
  - Origin: Lateral side of ulna, distal to radial notch
  - Insertion: Medial side of radial neck, distal to anular ligament
  - Stabilizes proximal radio-ulnar joint in full supination
- **Oblique cord**
  - Anatomically inconstant
  - Origin: Lateral side of ulna, distal to tuberosity
  - Insertion: Medial side of radius, distal to tuberosity

Anatomy-Based Imaging Issues

Radial Collateral Ligament
- Seen best on coronal images
- Low signal intensity structure, may be difficult to distinguish from overlying common extensor tendon
- Meniscus-like synovial fold may project from its deep surface into the radiocapitellar joint

Lateral UCL
- Difficult to visualize because of thin size and oblique course
  - Improved visualization with
    - Thin section coronal plane
    - Oblique coronal plane
    - MR-arthrography

Ulnar Collateral Ligament
- Anterior band is routinely visualized on coronal images, other bands are not
- Coronal images: Inverted triangle appearance
  - Broad proximal aspect attaching to undersurface of medial condyle
    - May have intermediate signal intensity
  - Thin distal aspect attaching to sublime tubercle of coronoid process, flush with edge of coronoid
    - Uniformly low signal intensity
- Usually separated from overlying common flexor tendon by deep fascial fat
- Improved visualization with oblique coronal plane
- May require MR-arthrography to visualize partial tear of deep distal aspect ("T" sign)

Anular Ligament
- Best visualized on axial images at level of radial head

Selected References

1. Cotten A et al: Collateral ligaments of the elbow: conventional MR imaging and MR arthrography with coronal oblique plane and elbow flexion. Radiology. 204(3):806-12, 1997
2. Morrey BF et al: Functional anatomy of the ligaments of the elbow. Clin Orthop Relat Res. (201):84-90, 1985

LIGAMENTS

GRAPHICS, RADIAL COLLATERAL LIGAMENT COMPLEX

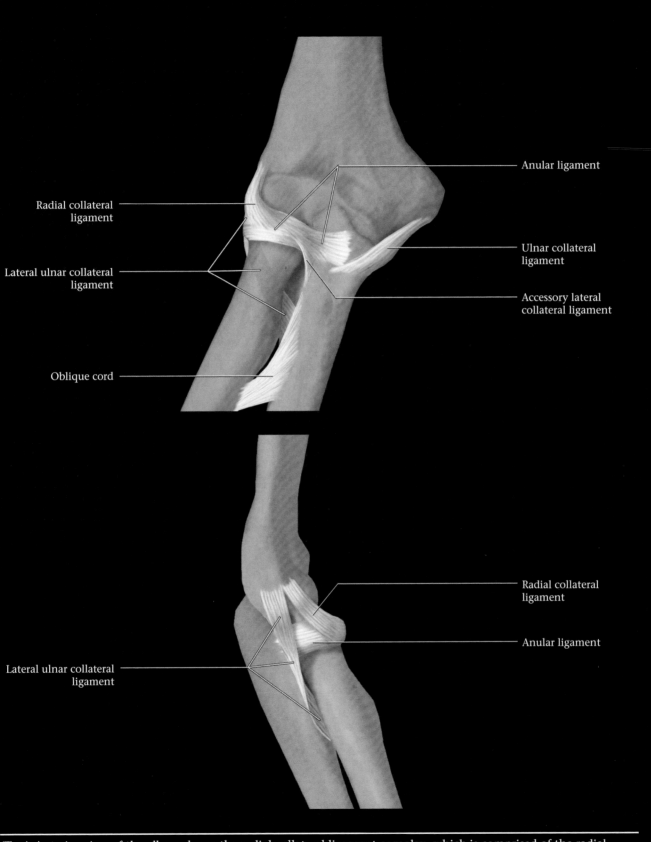

Radial collateral ligament

Lateral ulnar collateral ligament

Oblique cord

Anular ligament

Ulnar collateral ligament

Accessory lateral collateral ligament

Lateral ulnar collateral ligament

Radial collateral ligament

Anular ligament

(Top) Anterior view of the elbow shows the radial collateral ligament complex, which is comprised of the radial collateral ligament (provides varus stability), the lateral ulnar collateral ligament (provides posterolateral stability), the anular ligament (holds the radial head against the radial notch of the ulna), and the accessory lateral collateral ligament (reinforces the anular ligament). The oblique cord is part of the proximal radioulnar joint. **(Bottom)** Lateral view shows the posterior course of the lateral ulnar collateral ligament. It blends with the anular ligament as it passes behind the radial head.

LIGAMENTS

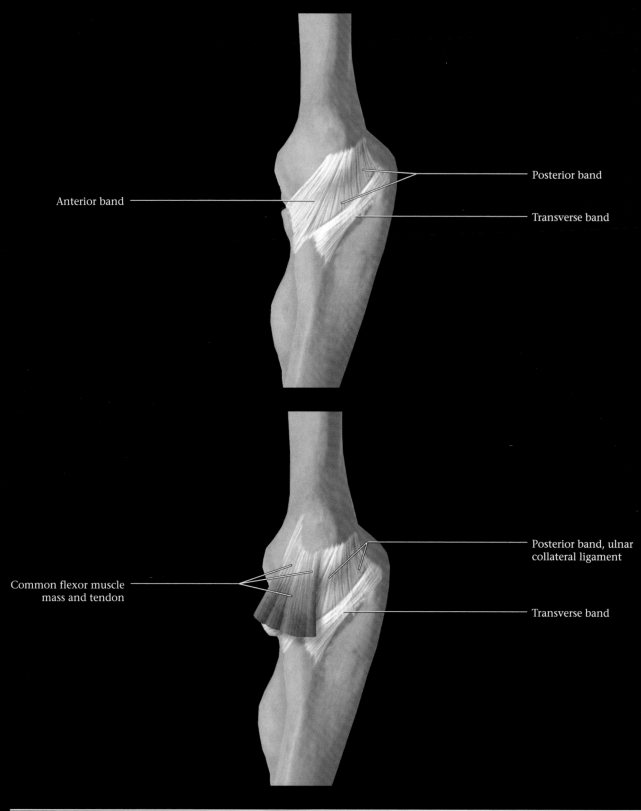

(Top) Side view of the medial aspect of the elbow shows the three components of the ulnar collateral ligament: The anterior band, posterior band, and transverse band. **(Bottom)** The common flexor tendon overlies the anterior band of the ulnar collateral ligament.

GRAPHIC, CORONAL VIEW OF LIGAMENTS AND TENDONS

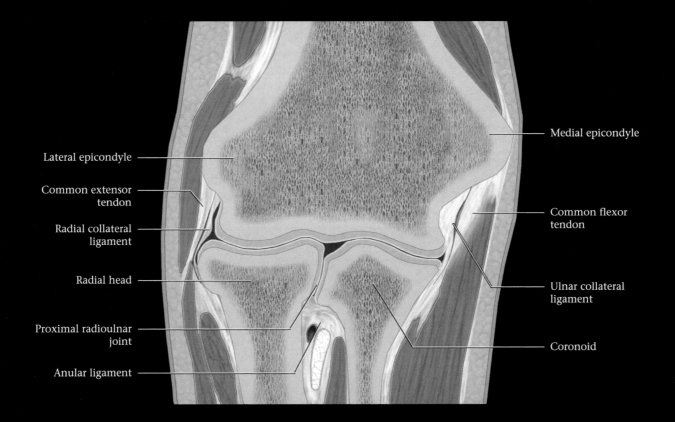

Lateral epicondyle

Common extensor tendon

Radial collateral ligament

Radial head

Proximal radioulnar joint

Anular ligament

Medial epicondyle

Common flexor tendon

Ulnar collateral ligament

Coronoid

Coronal section through the level of the epicondyles shows the collateral ligaments deep to the common tendon groups. Although the radial collateral ligament is shown, the section is too anterior to show the ulnar lateral collateral ligament, which originates just posterior to the radial collateral.

LIGAMENTS

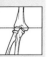

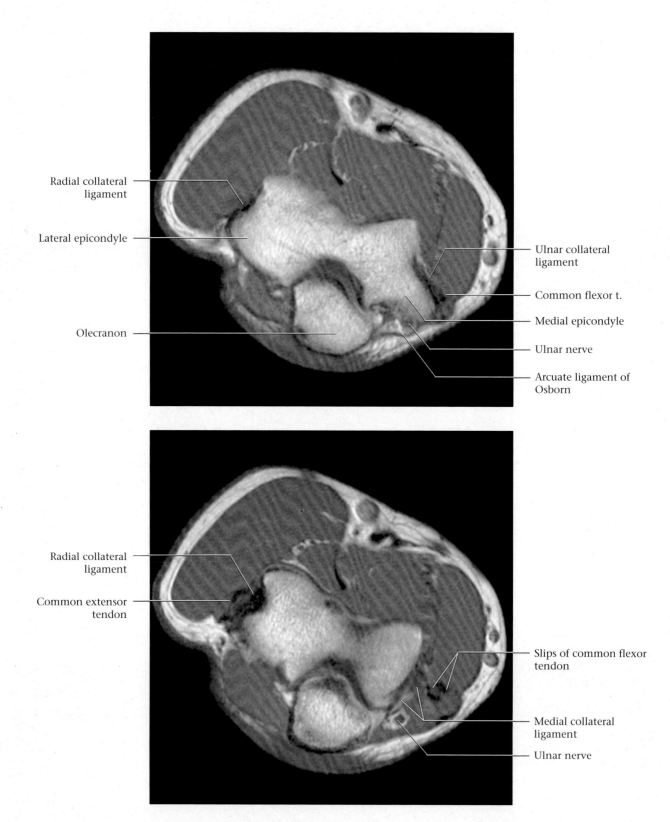

Radial collateral ligament

Lateral epicondyle

Olecranon

Ulnar collateral ligament

Common flexor t.

Medial epicondyle

Ulnar nerve

Arcuate ligament of Osborn

Radial collateral ligament

Common extensor tendon

Slips of common flexor tendon

Medial collateral ligament

Ulnar nerve

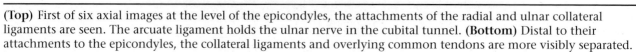

(Top) First of six axial images at the level of the epicondyles, the attachments of the radial and ulnar collateral ligaments are seen. The arcuate ligament holds the ulnar nerve in the cubital tunnel. **(Bottom)** Distal to their attachments to the epicondyles, the collateral ligaments and overlying common tendons are more visibly separated.

LIGAMENTS

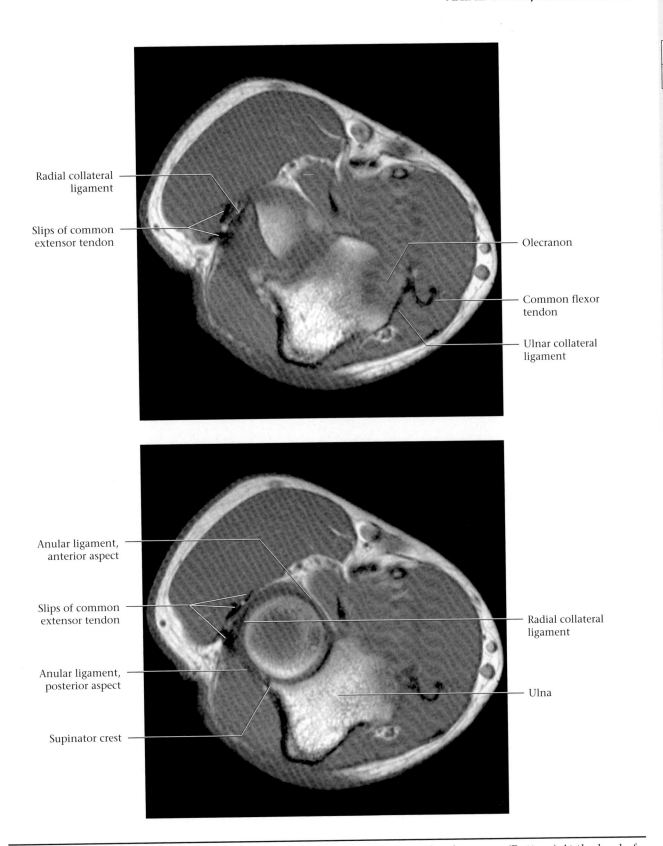

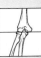

(Top) The anterior band of the ulnar collateral ligament is seen attaching to the olecranon. **(Bottom)** At the level of the radial head, the radial collateral ligament blends with the anular ligament.

AXIAL T1 MR, RIGHT ELBOW

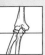

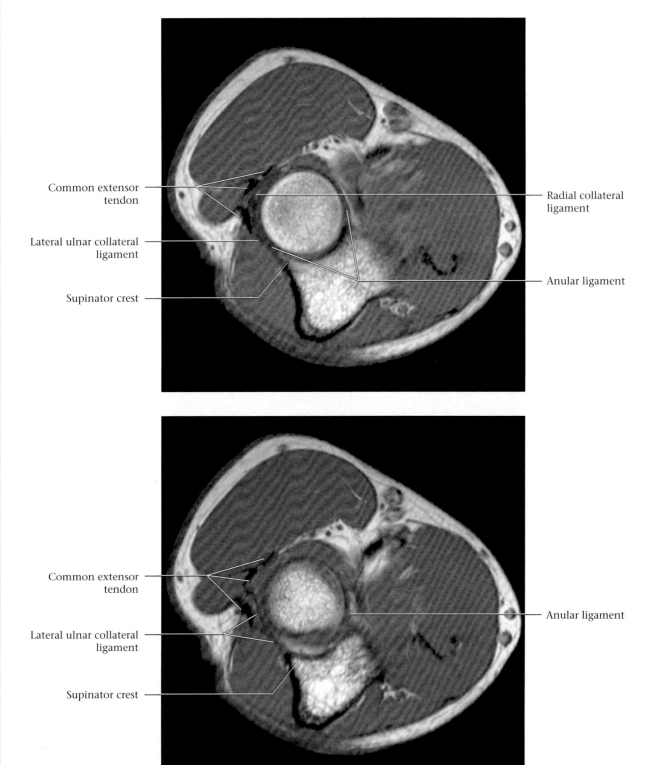

Common extensor tendon

Radial collateral ligament

Lateral ulnar collateral ligament

Anular ligament

Supinator crest

Common extensor tendon

Anular ligament

Lateral ulnar collateral ligament

Supinator crest

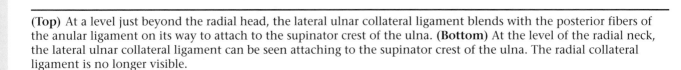

(Top) At a level just beyond the radial head, the lateral ulnar collateral ligament blends with the posterior fibers of the anular ligament on its way to attach to the supinator crest of the ulna. **(Bottom)** At the level of the radial neck, the lateral ulnar collateral ligament can be seen attaching to the supinator crest of the ulna. The radial collateral ligament is no longer visible.

LIGAMENTS

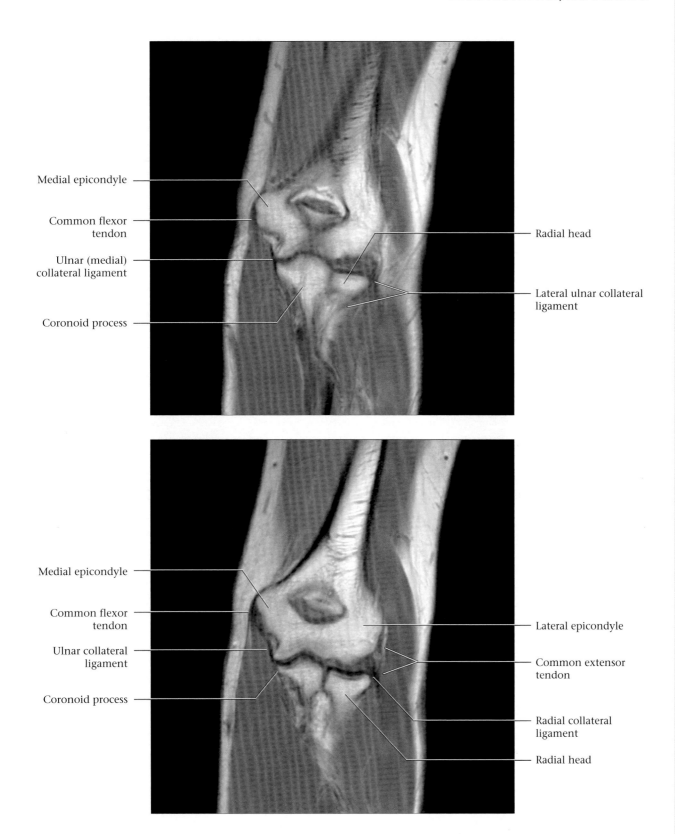

Medial epicondyle

Common flexor tendon

Ulnar (medial) collateral ligament

Coronoid process

Radial head

Lateral ulnar collateral ligament

Medial epicondyle

Common flexor tendon

Ulnar collateral ligament

Coronoid process

Lateral epicondyle

Common extensor tendon

Radial collateral ligament

Radial head

(Top) First of four coronal images. This section is located posteriorly within the elbow joint. The lateral ulnar collateral ligament is a thin band, seen at the level of the posterior aspect of the radial head. It extends from its origin posterior to the origin of the radial collateral ligament, posterior to the radial head & neck, to insert on the supinator crest of the ulna. **(Bottom)** At a coronal image midway through the radial head (anterior to the prior image), the radial collateral ligament is seen, deep to the common extensor tendon. The ulnar collateral ligament extends from the undersurface of the medial epicondyle to the coronoid process of the ulna, also well seen at this level.

CORONAL T1 MR, LEFT ELBOW

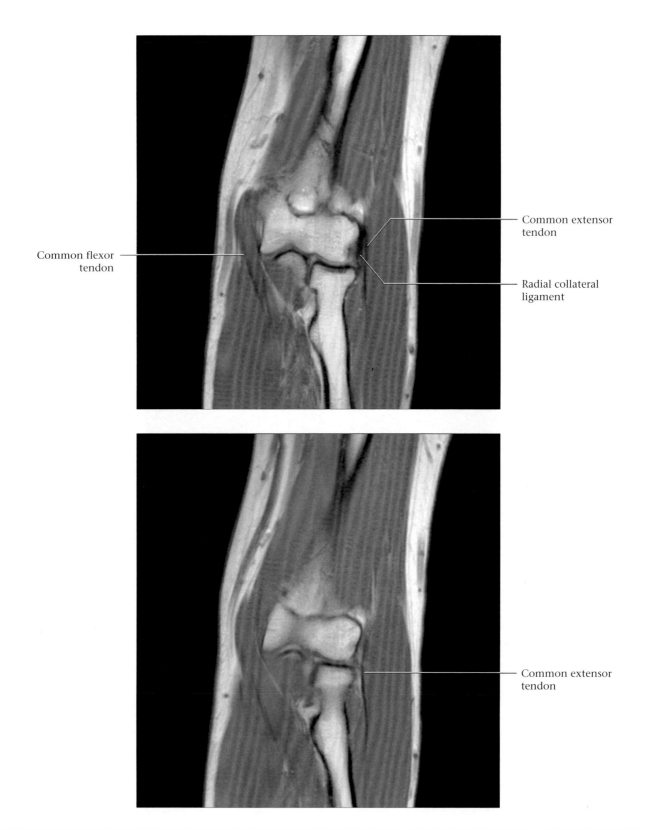

Common flexor tendon

Common extensor tendon

Radial collateral ligament

Common extensor tendon

(Top) At a level through the extreme anterior aspect of the coronoid, the ulnar collateral ligament is no longer seen. The radial collateral ligament is seen deep to the common extensor tendon. **(Bottom)** Further anteriorly, the collateral ligaments are no longer seen.

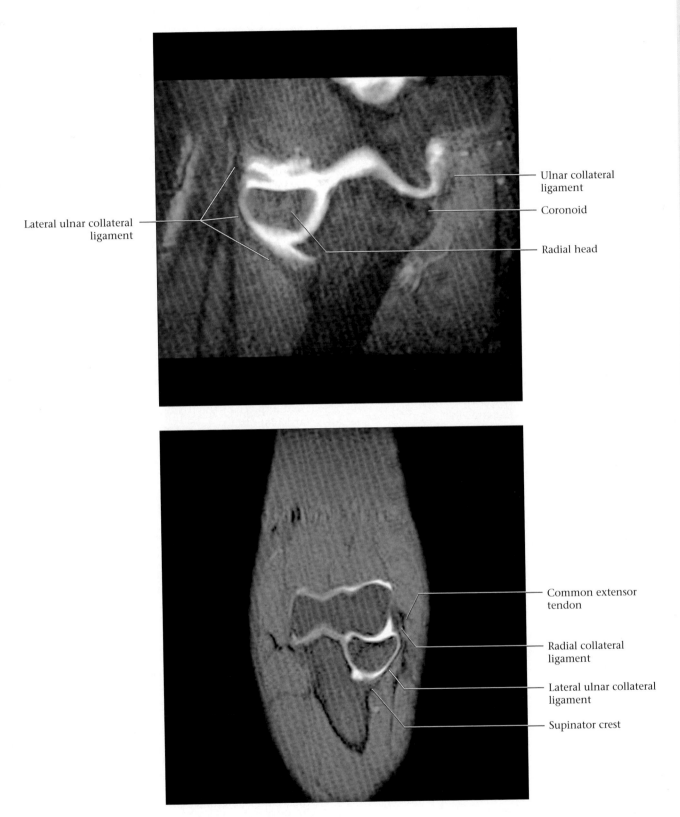

Lateral ulnar collateral ligament

Ulnar collateral ligament

Coronoid

Radial head

Common extensor tendon

Radial collateral ligament

Lateral ulnar collateral ligament

Supinator crest

(Top) Fat-suppressed T1 weighted coronal MR-arthrogram located posteriorly within the joint shows the lateral ulnar collateral ligament sweeping around the radial head and neck (neck not seen). The contrast also outlines the articular surface of the ulnar collateral ligament, which is frayed in this case. **(Bottom)** Fat-suppressed T1 weighted coronal MR-arthrogram at the same location in a different patient. The distal aspect of the lateral ulnar collateral ligament is seen inserting on the supinator crest of the ulna. The proximal aspect is partially volumed with the posterior aspect of the radial collateral ligament.

Elbow

II

FOREARM OVERVIEW

Gross Anatomy

Osseous Anatomy
- **Radius**
  - Laterally located
  - Shorter than ulna
  - Wider distally
  - Head
    - Disc shaped
    - Covered with articular cartilage along superior surface and circumference
    - Articulates with capitellum of elbow joint and ulnar notch of proximal radioulnar joint
  - Neck
    - Attachment of joint capsule
    - Angled 15° with shaft of radius
  - Radial tuberosity
    - At junction of neck and shaft
    - Insertion of biceps brachii tendon
  - Shaft
    - Medial surface: Sharp and straight, attachment site of interosseous membrane
    - Lateral surface: Rounded and convex lateral, with pronator tubercle at apex
    - **Anterior oblique line**: Ridge on anterior surface extending from radial tuberosity (proximal medial) to pronator tubercle (distal lateral)
    - Proximal 75% of shaft is concave anterior
    - Distal 25% of shaft is flat and wide
    - Styloid process: Most distal extent of radius
    - **Dorsal ("Lister") tubercle**: On dorsum of distal aspect, separates second and third extensor compartments, is origin of some extrinsic ligaments of wrist
    - **Ulnar notch**: Medial distal aspect, articulates with distal ulna
    - Distal articular surface articulates with carpus via scaphoid fossa and lunate fossa
- **Ulna**
  - Located medially
  - Longer than radius
  - Wider proximally
  - Olecranon process: Most proximal extent
  - **Coronoid process**
    - Anterior projection of proximal shaft
    - **Ulnar tuberosity**: Anterior inferior aspect, insertion of brachialis tendon
  - **Trochlear notch**
    - Formed by coronoid and olecranon processes
    - Articulates with trochlea of humerus
    - Transverse trochlear ridge: Demarcates junction of olecranon and coronoid (see "Elbow Overview" section)
    - Trochlear grooves: normal grooves on either side of trochlear notch (see "Elbow overview" section)
  - **Radial notch**
    - Lateral aspect of coronoid process
    - Articulates with radial head
  - **Supinator fossa**
    - Depression on lateral side of shaft, just below radial notch
    - Gives clearance to radial tuberosity during pronation/supination
    - Origin of ulnar head of supinator muscle
  - **Supinator crest**
    - Posterior aspect of supinator fossa
    - Origin of ulnar head of supinator muscle
    - Insertion of lateral ulnar collateral ligament
  - Shaft: Has three surfaces
    - Lateral: Flat and sharp, attachment site of interosseous membrane
    - Posterior: Rounded ridge, dividing line between extensors (lateral) and flexors (medial)
    - Anterior: Rounded, covered by flexor digitorum profundus origin
  - Distal
    - Small styloid process medially
    - Small round head: Articulates with ulnar notch of distal radius
    - Does not articulate with carpus

Articulations
- **Proximal radioulnar joint**
  - Pivot joint
  - Disc-shaped radial head and radial notch of ulna
  - Held in place by annular ligament
  - Enclosed within elbow joint capsule
  - Communicates with elbow joint
- **Distal radioulnar joint**
  - Pivot joint
  - Ulnar head and ulnar notch of radius
  - Held in place by the triangular fibrocartilage (articular disc)
  - Synovial joint with its own capsule
  - Does not normally communicate with radiocarpal joint
- Motions
  - Supination
    - Principal muscles: Biceps brachii, supinator
  - Pronation
    - Principal muscles: Pronator teres, pronator quadratus

Interosseous Fibrous Attachments
- **Anular ligament**: Holds radial head in radial notch of proximal radioulnar joint
- **Quadrate ligament**: Thin fibrous band connecting radial neck to ulna, distal to anular ligament
- **Oblique cord**
  - Anatomically inconstant
  - Unknown functional significance, if any
  - Extends from inferior aspect of ulnar tuberosity to inferior aspect of radial tuberosity
- **Interosseous membrane**
  - Thin, broad sheet of fibrous tissue
  - Connects medial side of radius to lateral side of ulna
  - Begins 2-3 cm distal to radial tuberosity
  - Provides attachment for deep muscles of forearm (see below)
  - Fibers course inferomedially
    - Transfers load from distal radius to ulna, and from there up to humerus and shoulder
    - Fibers are taut in mid-prone position (the usual position of function)
- **Triangular fibrocartilage** (articular disc): Holds ulnar head in ulna notch of distal radioulnar joint
- **Extensor retinaculum**

- ○ Dorsum of distal forearm and wrist
- ○ Origin: Distal radius
- ○ Insertion: Ulnar styloid, triquetrum, pisiform
- ○ Has deep slips that form the 6 extensor tendon compartments of distal forearm and wrist
  - ▪ 1st extensor compartment: Abductor pollicis longus, extensor pollicis brevis
  - ▪ 2nd extensor compartment: Extensor carpi radialis longus and brevis
  - ▪ 3rd extensor compartment: Extensor pollicis longus
  - ▪ 4th extensor compartment: Extensor digitorum, extensor indicis
  - ▪ 5th extensor compartment: Extensor digiti minimi
  - ▪ 6th extensor compartment: Extensor carpi ulnaris
- ○ Prevents bowstringing of extensor tendons

Muscles

- • **Anterior compartment**
  - ○ Has 8 flexor muscles, in three groups
- • Anterior compartment: **Superficial group**
  - ○ Flexor carpi radialis, flexor carpi ulnaris, pronator teres, palmaris longus
  - ○ Originate from common flexor tendon of elbow (see "Muscles and Tendons" section)
- • Anterior compartment: **Intermediate group**
  - ○ Flexor digitorum superficialis
  - ○ Originates from common flexor tendon of elbow (see "Muscles and Tendons" section)
- • Anterior compartment: **Deep group**
  - ○ Flexor digitorum profundus
    - ▪ Origin: Proximal 75% of anterior and medial surfaces of ulna and adjacent interosseous membrane
    - ▪ Insertion: Base of the 2nd-5th distal phalanges
    - ▪ Innervation: Ulnar nerve for 4th and 5th fingers, anterior interosseous nerve of median nerve for 2nd and 3rd fingers
    - ▪ Actions: Flexion of distal and proximal interphalangeal joints, metacarpophalangeal joints, wrist joint
  - ○ Flexor pollicis longus
    - ▪ Lies lateral to flexor digitorum profundus
    - ▪ Origin: Anterior surface of radius (distal to anterior oblique line), lateral aspect of interosseous membrane
    - ▪ Insertion: Palmer aspect of base of distal phalanx of thumb
    - ▪ Innervation: Anterior interosseous nerve of median nerve
    - ▪ Action: Flexion of interphalangeal joint of thumb, 1st metacarpophalangeal joint, carpometacarpal joint, and wrist joint
  - ○ Pronator quadratus
    - ▪ Deepest muscle of anterior forearm
    - ▪ Origin: Distal 25% of anterior surface of ulna
    - ▪ Insertion: Distal 25% of anterior surface of radius
    - ▪ Innervation: Anterior interosseous nerve of median nerve
    - ▪ Action: Pronation of forearm, holds distal radius and ulna together
- • **Posterior compartment**
  - ○ Has 9 extensor muscles, in two groups

- • Posterior compartment: **Superficial group**
  - ○ Extensor carpi radialis brevis, extensor carpi ulnaris, extensor digitorum, extensor digiti minimi
    - ▪ Originate from common extensor tendon of elbow (see "Muscles and Tendons" section)
  - ○ Extensor carpi radialis longus
    - ▪ Arises from lateral supracondylar ridge humerus (see "Muscles and Tendons" section)
- • Posterior compartment: **Deep group**
  - ○ Abductor pollicis longus
    - ▪ Origin: Posterior surfaces of radius, ulna, and interosseous membrane
    - ▪ Insertion: Posterior surface of base of 1st metacarpal
    - ▪ Innervation: Posterior interosseous nerve
    - ▪ Action: Abducts and extends thumb at metacarpophalangeal joint
    - ▪ Distal tendon forms anterior (volar) aspect of anatomic snuff box of wrist
  - ○ Extensor pollicis brevis
    - ▪ Origin: Posterior surface of radius and interosseous membrane
    - ▪ Insertion: Posterior surface of base of 1st proximal phalanx
    - ▪ Innervation: Posterior interosseous nerve
    - ▪ Action: Extends thumb at carpometacarpal and metacarpophalangeal joints
    - ▪ Distal tendon forms anterior (volar) aspect of anatomic snuff box of wrist
  - ○ Extensor pollicis longus
    - ▪ Origin: Posterior surface of ulna and interosseous membrane
    - ▪ Insertion: Posterior surface of base of 1st distal phalanx
    - ▪ Innervation: Posterior interosseous nerve
    - ▪ Action: Extends interphalangeal joint of thumb and 1st metacarpophalangeal joint
    - ▪ Distal tendon forms posterior (dorsal) aspect of anatomic snuff box of wrist
  - ○ Extensor indicis
    - ▪ Origin: Posterior surface of ulna and interosseous membrane
    - ▪ Insertion: Extensor hood expansion of 2nd finger
    - ▪ Innervation: Posterior interosseous nerve
    - ▪ Action: Extends 2nd metacarpophalangeal joint

Nerves

- • **Anterior compartment**
  - ○ **Median nerve**
    - ▪ Principal nerve of anterior compartment
    - ▪ Supplies: Pronator teres, flexor carpi radialis, palmaris longus, flexor digitorum superficialis
    - ▪ Enters forearm from cubital fossa by passing between the humeral and ulnar heads of pronator teres
    - ▪ Courses distally, attached to deep surface of flexor digitorum superficialis muscle by a fascial sheath
    - ▪ Pronator syndrome: Compression of median nerve as it passes between pronator heads and under flexor digitorum superficialis
    - ▪ At wrist, emerges from lateral side of flexor digitorum superficialis and is deep to palmaris longus tendon and flexor retinaculum

FOREARM OVERVIEW

- o **Anterior interosseous nerve**
  - Arises from median nerve at level of pronator teres
  - Courses distally along anterior surface of interosseous membrane
  - Accompanied by interosseous branch of ulnar artery
  - Lies between flexor digitorum profundus and flexor pollicis longus
  - Ends at pronator quadratus muscle, giving articular branches to wrist joint and the palmar cutaneous branch (superficial to flexor retinaculum)
  - Supplies: Flexor pollicis longus, pronator quadratus, lateral half of flexor digitorum profundus
  - Kiloh-Nevin syndrome: Compression of anterior interosseus nerve, most often due to fibrous bands
- o **Ulnar nerve**
  - After passing behind medial epicondyle, enters forearm by passing between humeral and ulnar heads of flexor carpi ulnaris
  - Courses distally between flexor carpi ulnaris and flexor digitorum profundus
  - Distally, becomes superficial and passes into wrist superficial to flexor retinaculum
  - Supplies: Flexor carpi ulnaris, medial half of flexor digitorum profundus
  - Palmer cutaneous branch: Arises in middle of forearm and supplies skin over medial side of palm
  - Dorsal cutaneous branch: Arises distally between ulna and flexor carpi ulnaris to supply dorsal surface of medial side of hand
- o **Superficial branch of radial nerve**
  - Direct continuation of radial nerve after deep branch has split off at level of lateral epicondyle
  - Courses distally, deep to brachioradialis
  - In distal forearm passes into posterior compartment
  - Gives terminal branches to supply skin of lateral 2/3 of dorsum of wrist, hand, and lateral 2 1/2 fingers
- o **Lateral cutaneous nerve**
  - Continuation of musculocutaneous nerve of elbow
  - Supplies skin of lateral aspect of forearm
- o **Medial cutaneous nerve**
  - Arises from medial cord of brachial plexus (C8, T1)
  - Accompanies basilic vein in arm
  - Anterior to medial epicondyle
  - Supplies skin of posteromedial forearm
- **Posterior compartment**
  - o **Posterior interosseous nerve**
    - Purely motor
    - Continuation of deep branch of radial nerve after deep branch passes through supinator muscle to reach posterior compartment
    - Lies on posterior surface of interosseous membrane, deep to extensor pollicis longus
    - Accompanied by posterior interosseous artery

- Supplies: Extensor digitorum, extensor digiti minimi, extensor indicis, extensor carpi ulnaris, abductor pollicis longus, extensor pollicis brevis, extensor pollicis longus
- Terminates in articular branches to wrist joint
- Posterior osseous nerve syndrome: Compression of deep branch of radial nerve as it enters supinator muscle

Arteries
- **Brachial artery** divides into radial artery and ulnar artery in cubital fossa
- **Radial artery**
  - o Medial to distal biceps tendon
  - o Covered by brachioradialis muscle
  - o Distally, leaves forearm and moves laterally, crossing floor of anatomical snuff box
  - o Terminates in deep palmar arch of hand
  - o Radial recurrent artery
    - Runs proximally along lateral side of elbow to form anastomosis with branches of deep brachial artery
  - o Muscular branches to lateral side of forearm
  - o Distal anastomotic branches: Palmar carpal arch, superficial palmar arch, dorsal carpal arch
- **Ulnar artery**
  - o Proximally, deep to pronator teres
  - o Distally, lies on flexor digitorum profundus and is lateral to ulnar nerve
  - o Anterior and posterior ulnar recurrent arteries: Form anastomosis around medial side of elbow with branches of brachial artery
  - o Common interosseous artery: Arises in distal aspect of cubital fossa
    - Anterior interosseous artery: Runs distally on interosseous membrane and ends in dorsal carpal arch
    - Posterior interosseous artery: Enters posterior compartment proximal to interosseous membrane, between supinator and abductor pollicis longus, supplies posterior muscles
  - o Muscular branches to medial side of forearm
  - o Distal anastomotic branches: palmar carpal arch, dorsal carpal arch

Anatomy-Based Imaging Issues

Anomalous Muscles
- Duplicate muscles, accessory muscles, anomalous origins and insertions
  - o Commonly involve palmaris longus, flexor carpi ulnaris, abductor digiti minimi, flexor digiti minimi
    - May present clinically as mass: Has signal characteristics and appearance of muscle
    - May present clinically due to compression of adjacent nerve

Selected References

1. Hodler J et al: Magnetic resonance imaging of the forearm: cross-sectional anatomy in a cadaveric model. Invest Radiol. 33(1):6-11, 1998

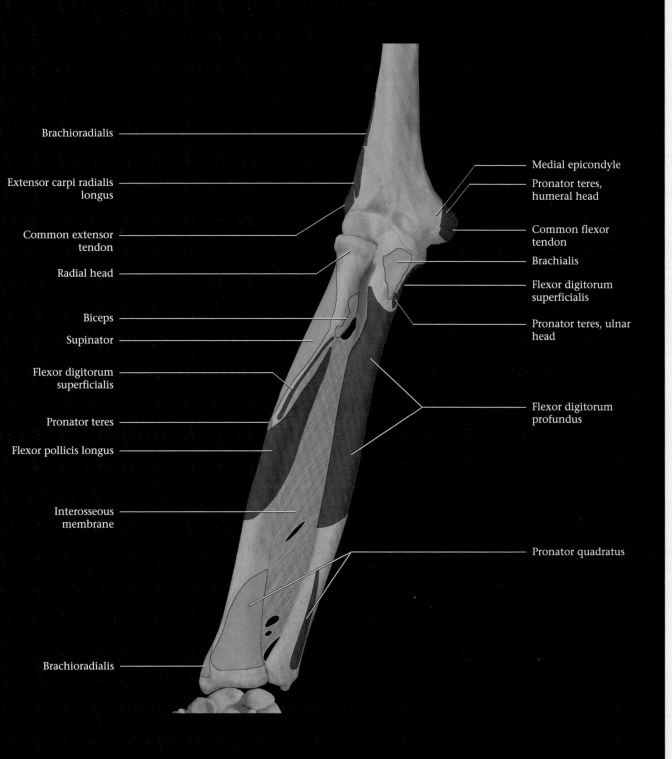

Brachioradialis

Extensor carpi radialis longus

Common extensor tendon

Radial head

Biceps

Supinator

Flexor digitorum superficialis

Pronator teres

Flexor pollicis longus

Interosseous membrane

Brachioradialis

Medial epicondyle

Pronator teres, humeral head

Common flexor tendon

Brachialis

Flexor digitorum superficialis

Pronator teres, ulnar head

Flexor digitorum profundus

Pronator quadratus

Origins are in red, insertions in blue. Note that no muscles originate from the anterior surface of the interosseous membrane.

GRAPHIC, POSTERIOR VIEW OF FOREARM: ORIGINS & INSERTIONS

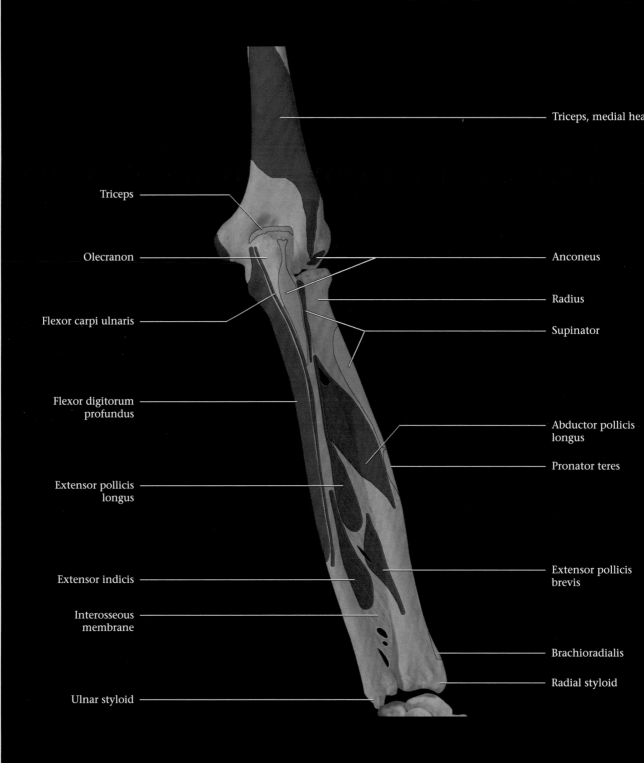

Triceps, medial hea

Triceps

Olecranon

Anconeus

Radius

Flexor carpi ulnaris

Supinator

Flexor digitorum
profundus

Abductor pollicis
longus

Pronator teres

Extensor pollicis
longus

Extensor indicis

Extensor pollicis
brevis

Interosseous
membrane

Brachioradialis

Radial styloid

Ulnar styloid

Origins are in red, insertions in blue. Notice that several muscles take origin partially from the posterior surface of the interosseous membrane.

FOREARM OVERVIEW

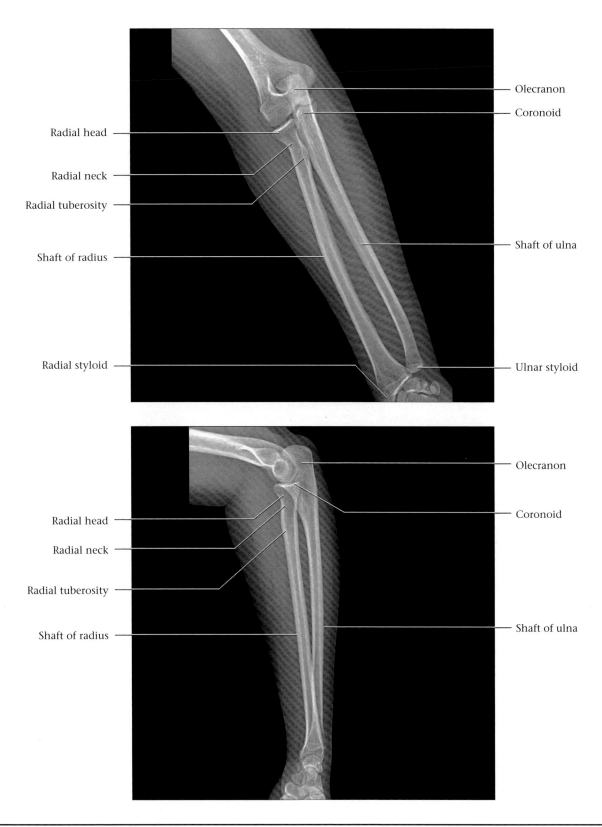

Radial head

Radial neck

Radial tuberosity

Shaft of radius

Radial styloid

Olecranon

Coronoid

Shaft of ulna

Ulnar styloid

Radial head

Radial neck

Radial tuberosity

Shaft of radius

Olecranon

Coronoid

Shaft of ulna

(Top) AP radiograph shows normal mild bowing of the radius and ulna. (Bottom) Lateral radiograph shows no bowing of the radius and ulna. The distal aspects of the radius and ulna should overlap at the distal radioulnar joint.

FOREARM OVERVIEW

AXIAL T1 MR, RIGHT FOREARM

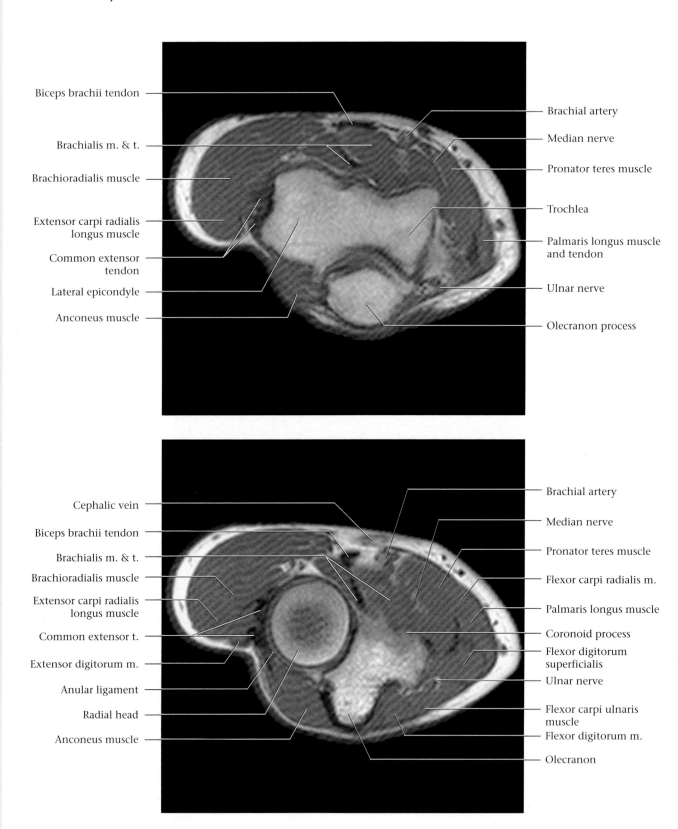

Biceps brachii tendon

Brachialis m. & t.

Brachioradialis muscle

Extensor carpi radialis longus muscle

Common extensor tendon

Lateral epicondyle

Anconeus muscle

Brachial artery

Median nerve

Pronator teres muscle

Trochlea

Palmaris longus muscle and tendon

Ulnar nerve

Olecranon process

Cephalic vein

Biceps brachii tendon

Brachialis m. & t.

Brachioradialis muscle

Extensor carpi radialis longus muscle

Common extensor t.

Extensor digitorum m.

Anular ligament

Radial head

Anconeus muscle

Brachial artery

Median nerve

Pronator teres muscle

Flexor carpi radialis m.

Palmaris longus muscle

Coronoid process

Flexor digitorum superficialis

Ulnar nerve

Flexor carpi ulnaris muscle

Flexor digitorum m.

Olecranon

(Top) Axial series through the forearm, proximal to distal. The proximal aspects of the flexor-pronator group and the extensor group are seen. **(Bottom)** At the level of the proximal radioulnar joint, there is a combination of muscles that act on the elbow, wrist and hand.

FOREARM OVERVIEW

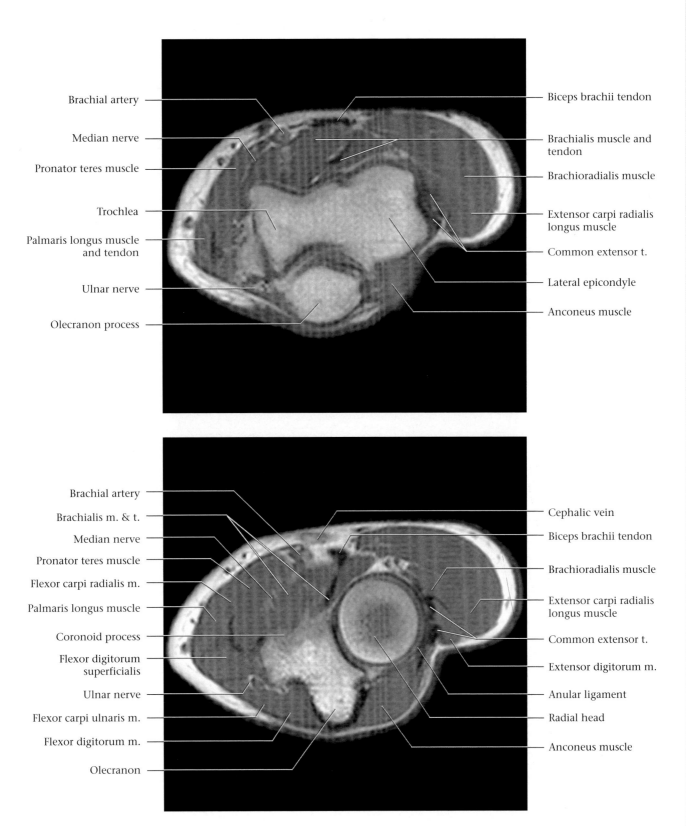

Top image labels (left): Brachial artery, Median nerve, Pronator teres muscle, Trochlea, Palmaris longus muscle and tendon, Ulnar nerve, Olecranon process

Top image labels (right): Biceps brachii tendon, Brachialis muscle and tendon, Brachioradialis muscle, Extensor carpi radialis longus muscle, Common extensor t., Lateral epicondyle, Anconeus muscle

Bottom image labels (left): Brachial artery, Brachialis m. & t., Median nerve, Pronator teres muscle, Flexor carpi radialis m., Palmaris longus muscle, Coronoid process, Flexor digitorum superficialis, Ulnar nerve, Flexor carpi ulnaris m., Flexor digitorum m., Olecranon

Bottom image labels (right): Cephalic vein, Biceps brachii tendon, Brachioradialis muscle, Extensor carpi radialis longus muscle, Common extensor t., Extensor digitorum m., Anular ligament, Radial head, Anconeus muscle

(Top) Axial series through the forearm, proximal to distal. The proximal aspects of the flexor-pronator group and the extensor group are seen. **(Bottom)** At the level of the proximal radioulnar joint, there is a combination of muscles that act on the elbow, wrist and hand.

AXIAL T1 MR, RIGHT FOREARM

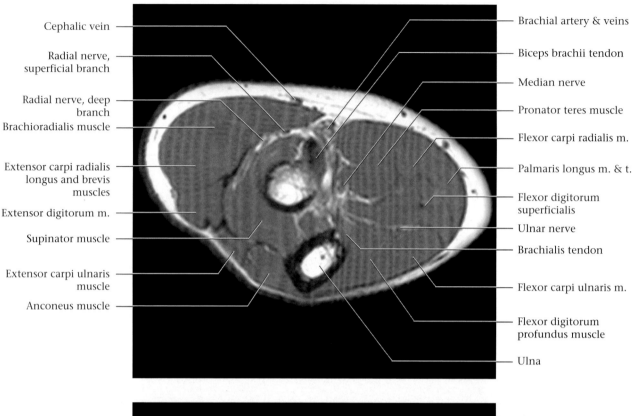

Cephalic vein

Radial nerve, superficial branch

Radial nerve, deep branch

Brachioradialis muscle

Extensor carpi radialis longus and brevis muscles

Extensor digitorum m.

Supinator muscle

Extensor carpi ulnaris muscle

Anconeus muscle

Brachial artery & veins

Biceps brachii tendon

Median nerve

Pronator teres muscle

Flexor carpi radialis m.

Palmaris longus m. & t.

Flexor digitorum superficialis

Ulnar nerve

Brachialis tendon

Flexor carpi ulnaris m.

Flexor digitorum profundus muscle

Ulna

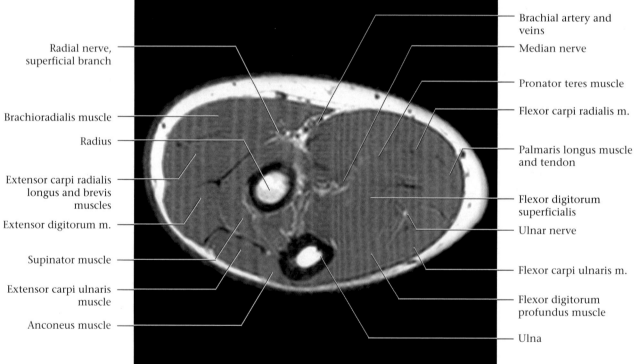

Radial nerve, superficial branch

Brachioradialis muscle

Radius

Extensor carpi radialis longus and brevis muscles

Extensor digitorum m.

Supinator muscle

Extensor carpi ulnaris muscle

Anconeus muscle

Brachial artery and veins

Median nerve

Pronator teres muscle

Flexor carpi radialis m.

Palmaris longus muscle and tendon

Flexor digitorum superficialis

Ulnar nerve

Flexor carpi ulnaris m.

Flexor digitorum profundus muscle

Ulna

(Top) The flexor muscles are grouped anteriorly, and the extensors posteriorly. **(Bottom)** The deep branch of the radial nerve has entered the supinator muscle on its way toward the posterior compartment of the forearm and is not discernible.

FOREARM OVERVIEW

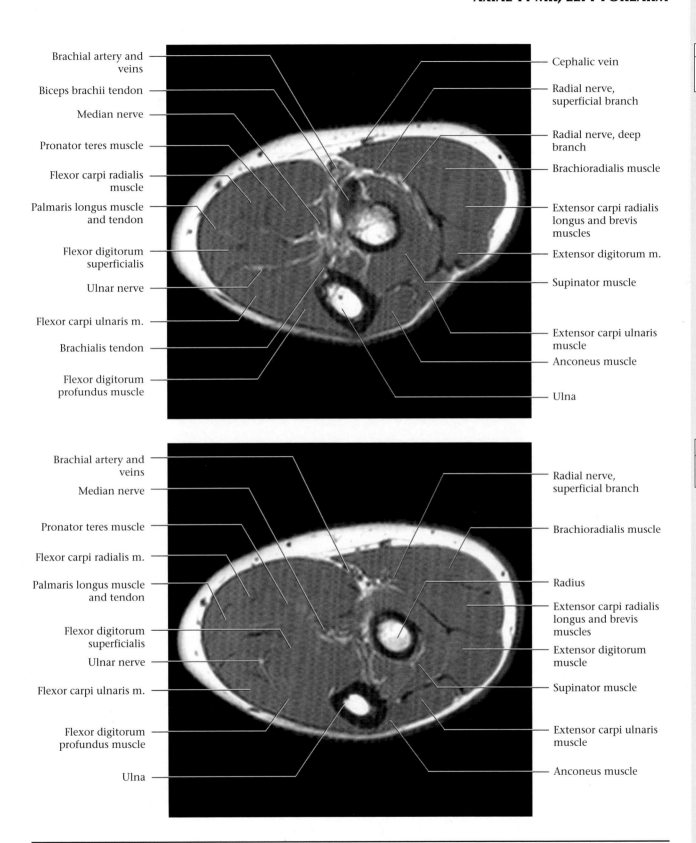

Brachial artery and veins

Biceps brachii tendon

Median nerve

Pronator teres muscle

Flexor carpi radialis muscle

Palmaris longus muscle and tendon

Flexor digitorum superficialis

Ulnar nerve

Flexor carpi ulnaris m.

Brachialis tendon

Flexor digitorum profundus muscle

Cephalic vein

Radial nerve, superficial branch

Radial nerve, deep branch

Brachioradialis muscle

Extensor carpi radialis longus and brevis muscles

Extensor digitorum m.

Supinator muscle

Extensor carpi ulnaris muscle

Anconeus muscle

Ulna

Brachial artery and veins

Median nerve

Pronator teres muscle

Flexor carpi radialis m.

Palmaris longus muscle and tendon

Flexor digitorum superficialis

Ulnar nerve

Flexor carpi ulnaris m.

Flexor digitorum profundus muscle

Ulna

Radial nerve, superficial branch

Brachioradialis muscle

Radius

Extensor carpi radialis longus and brevis muscles

Extensor digitorum muscle

Supinator muscle

Extensor carpi ulnaris muscle

Anconeus muscle

(Top) The flexor muscles are grouped anteriorly, and the extensors posteriorly. (Bottom) The deep branch of the radial nerve has entered the supinator muscle on its way toward the posterior compartment of the forearm and is not discernible.

Elbow

II

101

FOREARM OVERVIEW

AXIAL T1 MR, RIGHT FOREARM

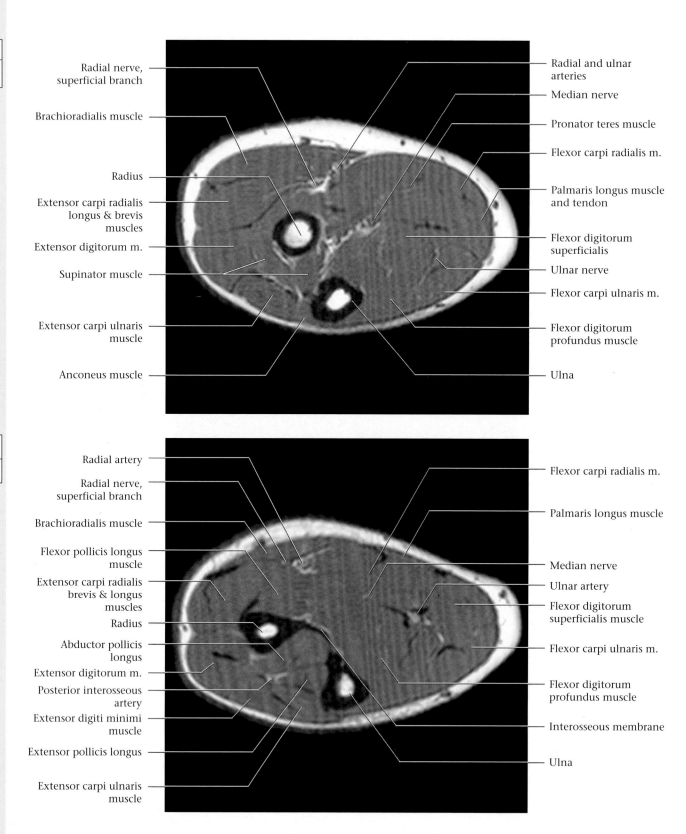

Radial nerve, superficial branch

Brachioradialis muscle

Radius

Extensor carpi radialis longus & brevis muscles

Extensor digitorum m.

Supinator muscle

Extensor carpi ulnaris muscle

Anconeus muscle

Radial and ulnar arteries

Median nerve

Pronator teres muscle

Flexor carpi radialis m.

Palmaris longus muscle and tendon

Flexor digitorum superficialis

Ulnar nerve

Flexor carpi ulnaris m.

Flexor digitorum profundus muscle

Ulna

Radial artery

Radial nerve, superficial branch

Brachioradialis muscle

Flexor pollicis longus muscle

Extensor carpi radialis brevis & longus muscles

Radius

Abductor pollicis longus

Extensor digitorum m.

Posterior interosseous artery

Extensor digiti minimi muscle

Extensor pollicis longus

Extensor carpi ulnaris muscle

Flexor carpi radialis m.

Palmaris longus muscle

Median nerve

Ulnar artery

Flexor digitorum superficialis muscle

Flexor carpi ulnaris m.

Flexor digitorum profundus muscle

Interosseous membrane

Ulna

(Top) Just distal to the radial tuberosity, the supinator muscle is still visible wrapping around the proximal shaft of the radius. **(Bottom)** The interosseous membrane is now visible, helping to separate the anterior and posterior compartments.

AXIAL T1 MR, LEFT FOREARM

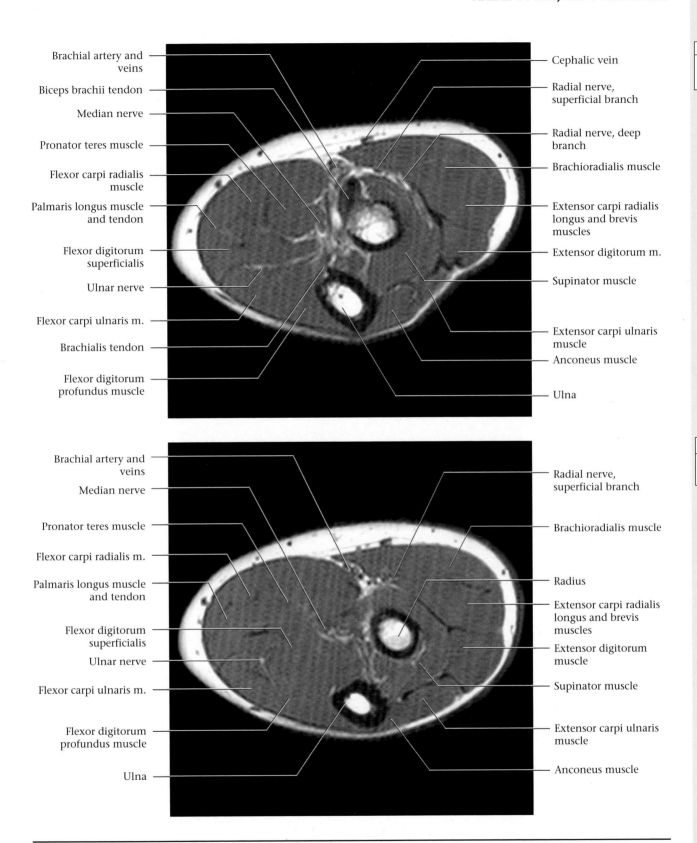

Brachial artery and veins

Biceps brachii tendon

Median nerve

Pronator teres muscle

Flexor carpi radialis muscle

Palmaris longus muscle and tendon

Flexor digitorum superficialis

Ulnar nerve

Flexor carpi ulnaris m.

Brachialis tendon

Flexor digitorum profundus muscle

Cephalic vein

Radial nerve, superficial branch

Radial nerve, deep branch

Brachioradialis muscle

Extensor carpi radialis longus and brevis muscles

Extensor digitorum m.

Supinator muscle

Extensor carpi ulnaris muscle

Anconeus muscle

Ulna

Brachial artery and veins

Median nerve

Pronator teres muscle

Flexor carpi radialis m.

Palmaris longus muscle and tendon

Flexor digitorum superficialis

Ulnar nerve

Flexor carpi ulnaris m.

Flexor digitorum profundus muscle

Ulna

Radial nerve, superficial branch

Brachioradialis muscle

Radius

Extensor carpi radialis longus and brevis muscles

Extensor digitorum muscle

Supinator muscle

Extensor carpi ulnaris muscle

Anconeus muscle

(Top) The flexor muscles are grouped anteriorly, and the extensors posteriorly. **(Bottom)** The deep branch of the radial nerve has entered the supinator muscle on its way toward the posterior compartment of the forearm and is not discernible.

FOREARM OVERVIEW

AXIAL T1 MR, RIGHT FOREARM

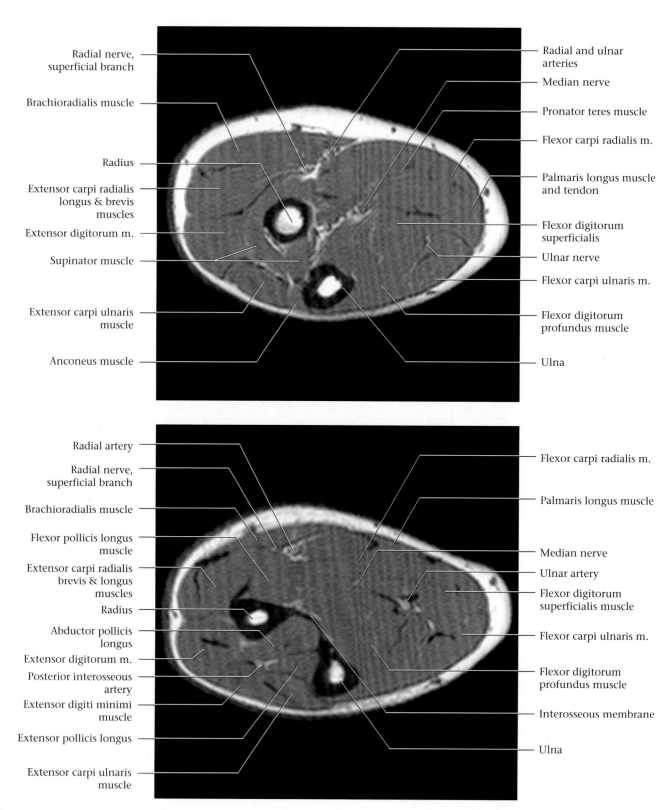

Radial nerve, superficial branch

Brachioradialis muscle

Radius

Extensor carpi radialis longus & brevis muscles

Extensor digitorum m.

Supinator muscle

Extensor carpi ulnaris muscle

Anconeus muscle

Radial and ulnar arteries

Median nerve

Pronator teres muscle

Flexor carpi radialis m.

Palmaris longus muscle and tendon

Flexor digitorum superficialis

Ulnar nerve

Flexor carpi ulnaris m.

Flexor digitorum profundus muscle

Ulna

Radial artery

Radial nerve, superficial branch

Brachioradialis muscle

Flexor pollicis longus muscle

Extensor carpi radialis brevis & longus muscles

Radius

Abductor pollicis longus

Extensor digitorum m.

Posterior interosseous artery

Extensor digiti minimi muscle

Extensor pollicis longus

Extensor carpi ulnaris muscle

Flexor carpi radialis m.

Palmaris longus muscle

Median nerve

Ulnar artery

Flexor digitorum superficialis muscle

Flexor carpi ulnaris m.

Flexor digitorum profundus muscle

Interosseous membrane

Ulna

(Top) Just distal to the radial tuberosity, the supinator muscle is still visible wrapping around the proximal shaft of the radius. **(Bottom)** The interosseous membrane is now visible, helping to separate the anterior and posterior compartments.

FOREARM OVERVIEW

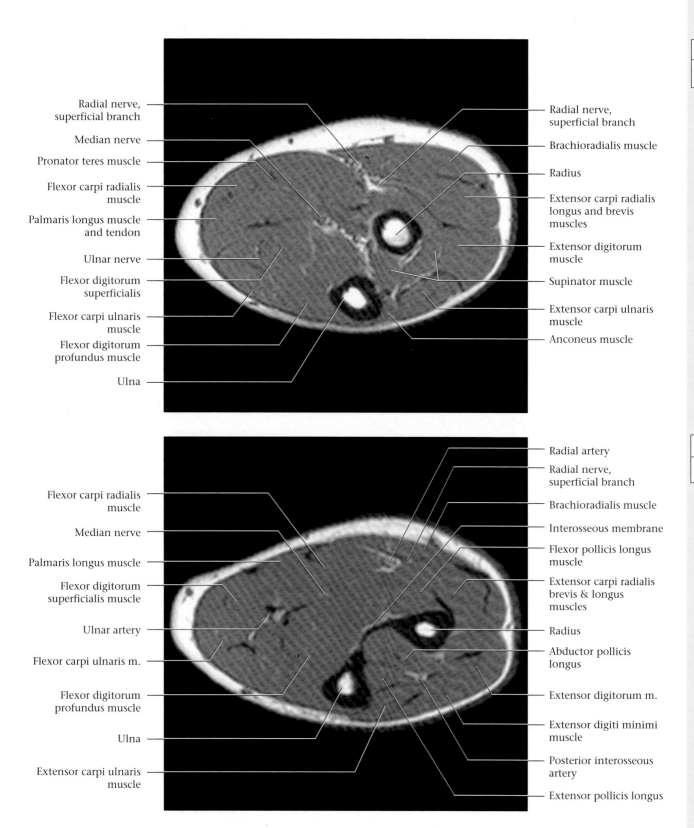

Radial nerve, superficial branch

Median nerve

Pronator teres muscle

Flexor carpi radialis muscle

Palmaris longus muscle and tendon

Ulnar nerve

Flexor digitorum superficialis

Flexor carpi ulnaris muscle

Flexor digitorum profundus muscle

Ulna

Radial nerve, superficial branch

Brachioradialis muscle

Radius

Extensor carpi radialis longus and brevis muscles

Extensor digitorum muscle

Supinator muscle

Extensor carpi ulnaris muscle

Anconeus muscle

Flexor carpi radialis muscle

Median nerve

Palmaris longus muscle

Flexor digitorum superficialis muscle

Ulnar artery

Flexor carpi ulnaris m.

Flexor digitorum profundus muscle

Ulna

Extensor carpi ulnaris muscle

Radial artery

Radial nerve, superficial branch

Brachioradialis muscle

Interosseous membrane

Flexor pollicis longus muscle

Extensor carpi radialis brevis & longus muscles

Radius

Abductor pollicis longus

Extensor digitorum m.

Extensor digiti minimi muscle

Posterior interosseous artery

Extensor pollicis longus

(Top) Just distal to the radial tuberosity, the supinator muscle is still visible wrapping around the proximal shaft of the radius. **(Bottom)** The interosseous membrane is now visible, helping to separate the anterior and posterior compartments.

AXIAL T1 MR, RIGHT FOREARM

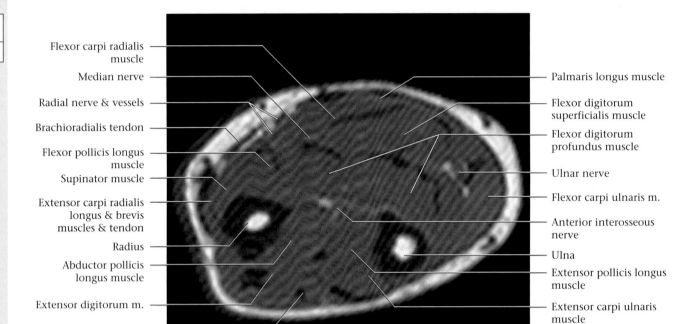

Flexor carpi radialis muscle

Median nerve

Radial nerve & vessels

Brachioradialis tendon

Flexor pollicis longus muscle

Supinator muscle

Extensor carpi radialis longus & brevis muscles & tendon

Radius

Abductor pollicis longus muscle

Extensor digitorum m.

Extensor digiti minimi muscle

Palmaris longus muscle

Flexor digitorum superficialis muscle

Flexor digitorum profundus muscle

Ulnar nerve

Flexor carpi ulnaris m.

Anterior interosseous nerve

Ulna

Extensor pollicis longus muscle

Extensor carpi ulnaris muscle

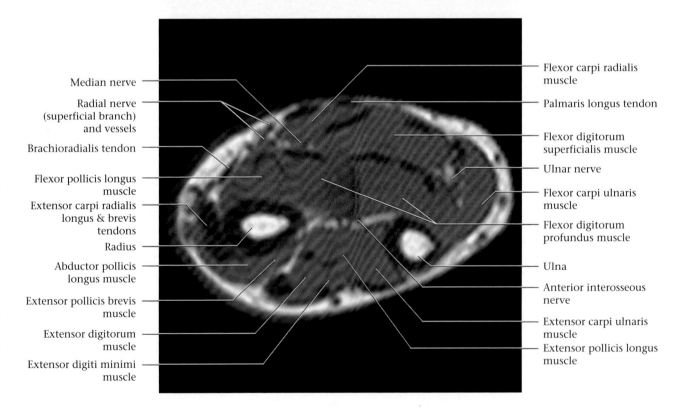

Median nerve

Radial nerve (superficial branch) and vessels

Brachioradialis tendon

Flexor pollicis longus muscle

Extensor carpi radialis longus & brevis tendons

Radius

Abductor pollicis longus muscle

Extensor pollicis brevis muscle

Extensor digitorum muscle

Extensor digiti minimi muscle

Flexor carpi radialis muscle

Palmaris longus tendon

Flexor digitorum superficialis muscle

Ulnar nerve

Flexor carpi ulnaris muscle

Flexor digitorum profundus muscle

Ulna

Anterior interosseous nerve

Extensor carpi ulnaris muscle

Extensor pollicis longus muscle

(Top) The interosseous membrane is not as prominent in this image as the previous one. The ulnar nerve and median nerve are located in the intermuscular septum between the deep flexors (flexor digitorum and flexor pollicis longus) and the more superficial flexors of the anterior compartment. **(Bottom)** The anterior interosseous nerve and accompanying vessels are well seen anterior to the interosseous membrane.

FOREARM OVERVIEW

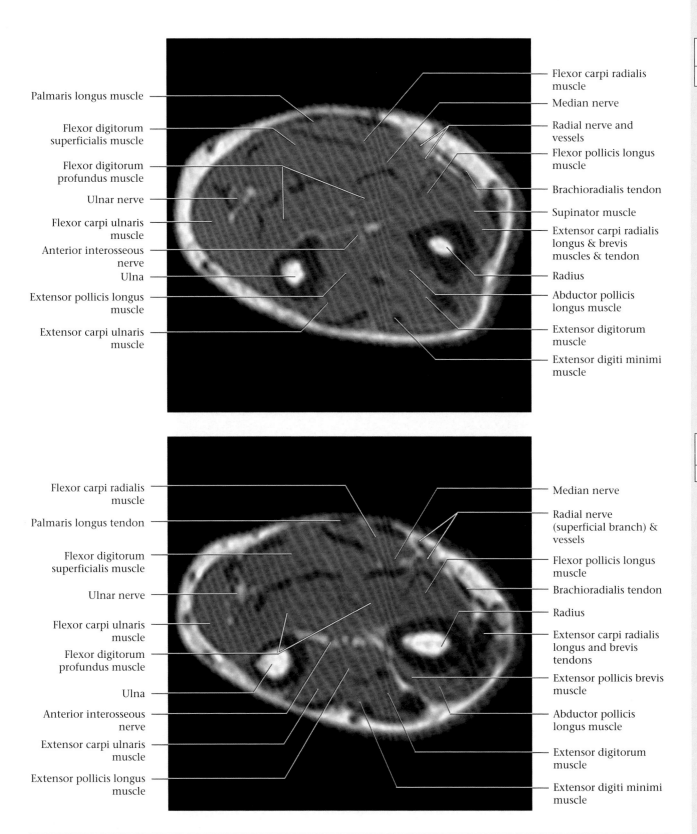

Top image labels (left):
- Palmaris longus muscle
- Flexor digitorum superficialis muscle
- Flexor digitorum profundus muscle
- Ulnar nerve
- Flexor carpi ulnaris muscle
- Anterior interosseous nerve
- Ulna
- Extensor pollicis longus muscle
- Extensor carpi ulnaris muscle

Top image labels (right):
- Flexor carpi radialis muscle
- Median nerve
- Radial nerve and vessels
- Flexor pollicis longus muscle
- Brachioradialis tendon
- Supinator muscle
- Extensor carpi radialis longus & brevis muscles & tendon
- Radius
- Abductor pollicis longus muscle
- Extensor digitorum muscle
- Extensor digiti minimi muscle

Bottom image labels (left):
- Flexor carpi radialis muscle
- Palmaris longus tendon
- Flexor digitorum superficialis muscle
- Ulnar nerve
- Flexor carpi ulnaris muscle
- Flexor digitorum profundus muscle
- Ulna
- Anterior interosseous nerve
- Extensor carpi ulnaris muscle
- Extensor pollicis longus muscle

Bottom image labels (right):
- Median nerve
- Radial nerve (superficial branch) & vessels
- Flexor pollicis longus muscle
- Brachioradialis tendon
- Radius
- Extensor carpi radialis longus and brevis tendons
- Extensor pollicis brevis muscle
- Abductor pollicis longus muscle
- Extensor digitorum muscle
- Extensor digiti minimi muscle

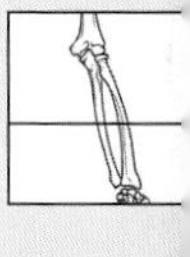

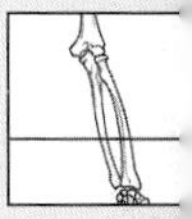

(Top) The interosseous membrane is not as prominent in this image as the previous one. The ulnar nerve and median nerve are located in the intermuscular septum between the deep flexors (flexor digitorum and flexor pollicis longus) and the more superficial flexors of the anterior compartment. **(Bottom)** The anterior interosseous nerve and accompanying vessels are well seen anterior to the interosseous membrane.

AXIAL T1 MR, RIGHT FOREARM

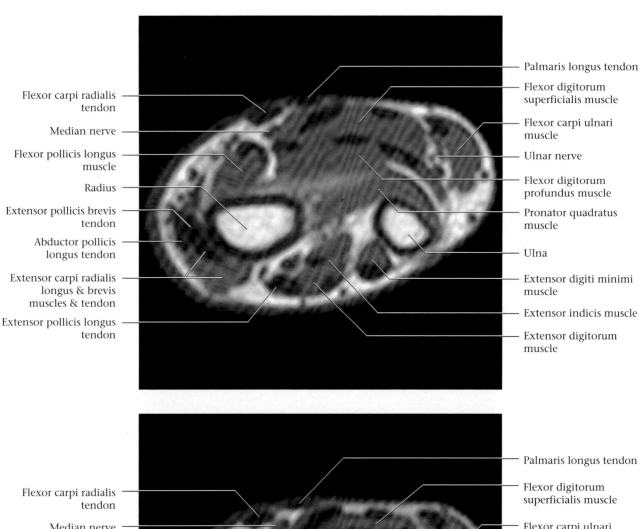

Flexor carpi radialis tendon
Median nerve
Flexor pollicis longus muscle
Radius
Extensor pollicis brevis tendon
Abductor pollicis longus tendon
Extensor carpi radialis longus & brevis muscles & tendon
Extensor pollicis longus tendon

Palmaris longus tendon
Flexor digitorum superficialis muscle
Flexor carpi ulnari muscle
Ulnar nerve
Flexor digitorum profundus muscle
Pronator quadratus muscle
Ulna
Extensor digiti minimi muscle
Extensor indicis muscle
Extensor digitorum muscle

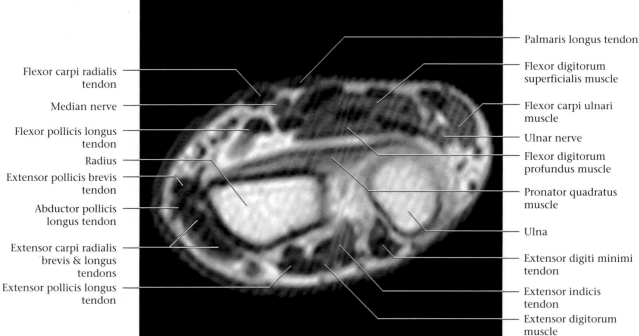

Flexor carpi radialis tendon
Median nerve
Flexor pollicis longus tendon
Radius
Extensor pollicis brevis tendon
Abductor pollicis longus tendon
Extensor carpi radialis brevis & longus tendons
Extensor pollicis longus tendon

Palmaris longus tendon
Flexor digitorum superficialis muscle
Flexor carpi ulnari muscle
Ulnar nerve
Flexor digitorum profundus muscle
Pronator quadratus muscle
Ulna
Extensor digiti minimi tendon
Extensor indicis tendon
Extensor digitorum muscle

(Top) The tendons of the abductor pollicis longus and extensor pollicis brevis cross superficial and anterior to the tendons of the extensor carpi radialis brevis and longus. At this level of the distal forearm, the pronator quadratus is now visible. **(Bottom)** The extensor tendons are starting to align themselves into the six extensor compartments of the wrist.

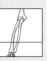

AXIAL, T1 MR LEFT FOREARM

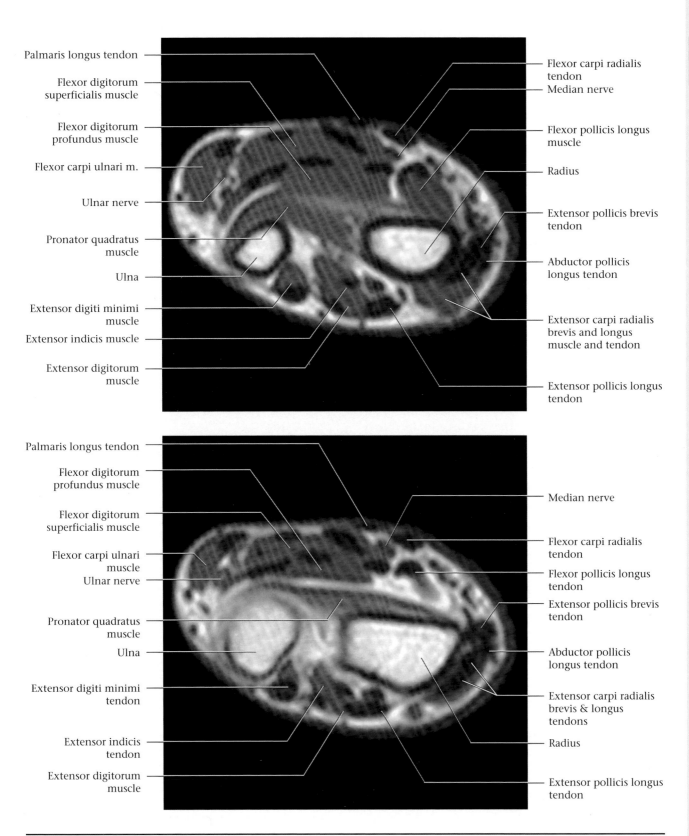

Top image labels:

Left side:
- Palmaris longus tendon
- Flexor digitorum superficialis muscle
- Flexor digitorum profundus muscle
- Flexor carpi ulnari m.
- Ulnar nerve
- Pronator quadratus muscle
- Ulna
- Extensor digiti minimi muscle
- Extensor indicis muscle
- Extensor digitorum muscle

Right side:
- Flexor carpi radialis tendon
- Median nerve
- Flexor pollicis longus muscle
- Radius
- Extensor pollicis brevis tendon
- Abductor pollicis longus tendon
- Extensor carpi radialis brevis and longus muscle and tendon
- Extensor pollicis longus tendon

Bottom image labels:

Left side:
- Palmaris longus tendon
- Flexor digitorum profundus muscle
- Flexor digitorum superficialis muscle
- Flexor carpi ulnari muscle
- Ulnar nerve
- Pronator quadratus muscle
- Ulna
- Extensor digiti minimi tendon
- Extensor indicis tendon
- Extensor digitorum muscle

Right side:
- Median nerve
- Flexor carpi radialis tendon
- Flexor pollicis longus tendon
- Extensor pollicis brevis tendon
- Abductor pollicis longus tendon
- Extensor carpi radialis brevis & longus tendons
- Radius
- Extensor pollicis longus tendon

(Top) The tendons of the abductor pollicis longus and extensor pollicis brevis cross superficial and anterior to the tendons of the extensor carpi radialis brevis and longus. At this level of the distal forearm, the pronator quadratus is now visible. **(Bottom)** The extensor tendons are starting to align themselves into the six extensor compartments of the wrist.

Elbow

II

107

AXIAL T1 MR, RIGHT FOREARM

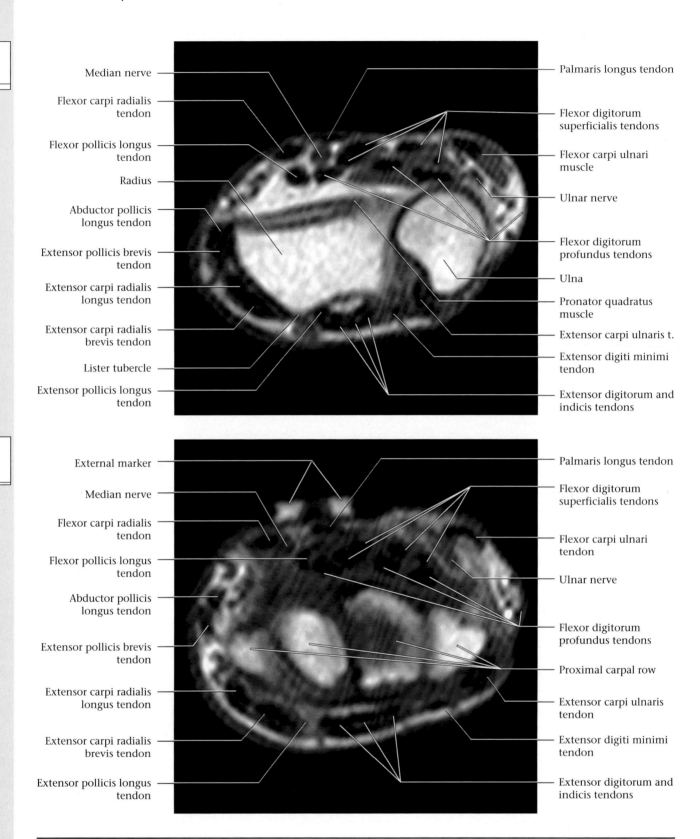

Median nerve

Flexor carpi radialis tendon

Flexor pollicis longus tendon

Radius

Abductor pollicis longus tendon

Extensor pollicis brevis tendon

Extensor carpi radialis longus tendon

Extensor carpi radialis brevis tendon

Lister tubercle

Extensor pollicis longus tendon

Palmaris longus tendon

Flexor digitorum superficialis tendons

Flexor carpi ulnari muscle

Ulnar nerve

Flexor digitorum profundus tendons

Ulna

Pronator quadratus muscle

Extensor carpi ulnaris t.

Extensor digiti minimi tendon

Extensor digitorum and indicis tendons

External marker

Median nerve

Flexor carpi radialis tendon

Flexor pollicis longus tendon

Abductor pollicis longus tendon

Extensor pollicis brevis tendon

Extensor carpi radialis longus tendon

Extensor carpi radialis brevis tendon

Extensor pollicis longus tendon

Palmaris longus tendon

Flexor digitorum superficialis tendons

Flexor carpi ulnari tendon

Ulnar nerve

Flexor digitorum profundus tendons

Proximal carpal row

Extensor carpi ulnaris tendon

Extensor digiti minimi tendon

Extensor digitorum and indicis tendons

(Top) The wrist is supinated. The six extensor compartments are visualized. **(Bottom)** The tendons of the forearm muscles have now passed into the wrist.

FOREARM OVERVIEW

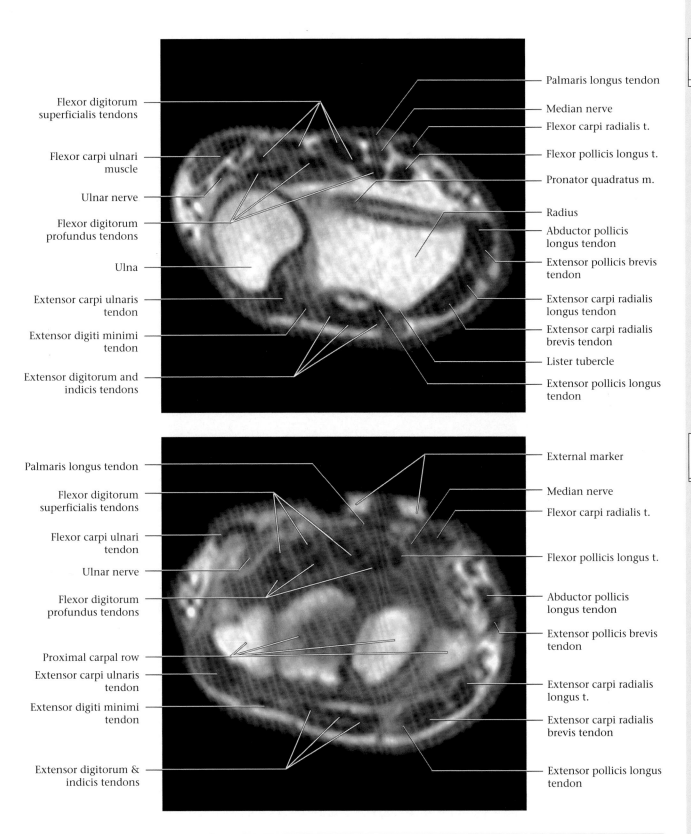

Flexor digitorum superficialis tendons

Flexor carpi ulnari muscle

Ulnar nerve

Flexor digitorum profundus tendons

Ulna

Extensor carpi ulnaris tendon

Extensor digiti minimi tendon

Extensor digitorum and indicis tendons

Palmaris longus tendon

Median nerve

Flexor carpi radialis t.

Flexor pollicis longus t.

Pronator quadratus m.

Radius

Abductor pollicis longus tendon

Extensor pollicis brevis tendon

Extensor carpi radialis longus tendon

Extensor carpi radialis brevis tendon

Lister tubercle

Extensor pollicis longus tendon

Palmaris longus tendon

Flexor digitorum superficialis tendons

Flexor carpi ulnari tendon

Ulnar nerve

Flexor digitorum profundus tendons

Proximal carpal row

Extensor carpi ulnaris tendon

Extensor digiti minimi tendon

Extensor digitorum & indicis tendons

External marker

Median nerve

Flexor carpi radialis t.

Flexor pollicis longus t.

Abductor pollicis longus tendon

Extensor pollicis brevis tendon

Extensor carpi radialis longus t.

Extensor carpi radialis brevis tendon

Extensor pollicis longus tendon

(Top) The wrist is supinated. The six extensor compartments are visualized. **(Bottom)** The tendons of the forearm muscles have now passed into the wrist.

CORONAL T1 MR, RIGHT FOREARM

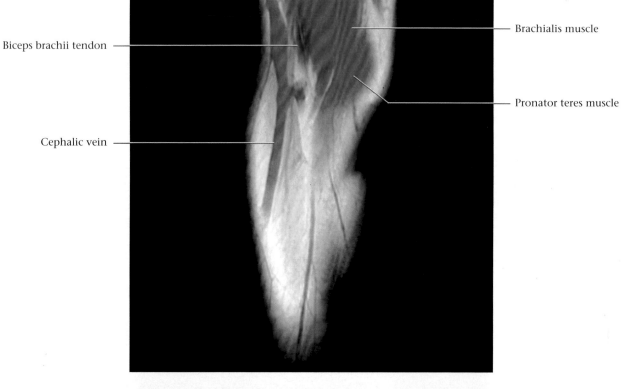

Biceps brachii tendon —

Cephalic vein —

— Brachialis muscle

— Pronator teres muscle

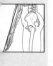

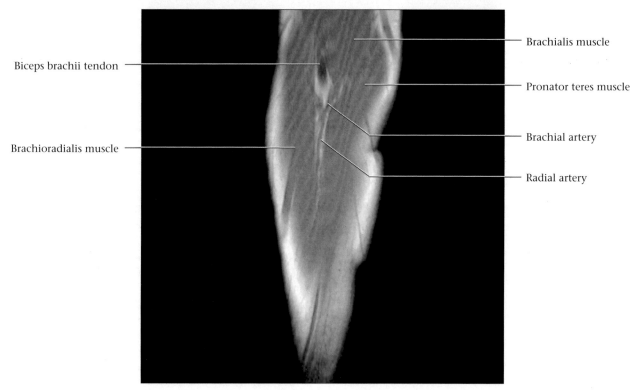

Biceps brachii tendon —

Brachioradialis muscle —

— Brachialis muscle

— Pronator teres muscle

— Brachial artery

— Radial artery

(Top) Coronal series of the forearm, anterior to posterior. The muscles about the elbow are seen at this extremely anterior location. (Bottom) The brachial artery has divided into the radial artery (seen) and the ulnar artery (not seen in this image).

FOREARM OVERVIEW

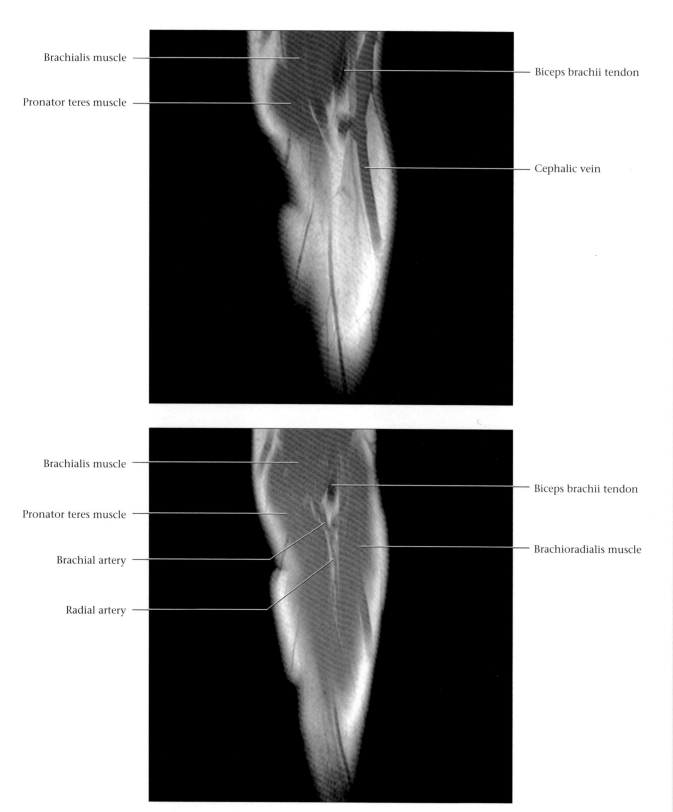

Brachialis muscle — Biceps brachii tendon

Pronator teres muscle — Cephalic vein

Brachialis muscle — Biceps brachii tendon

Pronator teres muscle — Brachioradialis muscle

Brachial artery

Radial artery

(Top) Coronal series of the forearm, anterior to posterior. The muscles about the elbow are seen at this extremely anterior location. (Bottom) The brachial artery has divided into the radial artery (seen) and the ulnar artery (not seen in this image).

CORONAL T1 MR, RIGHT FOREARM

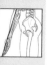

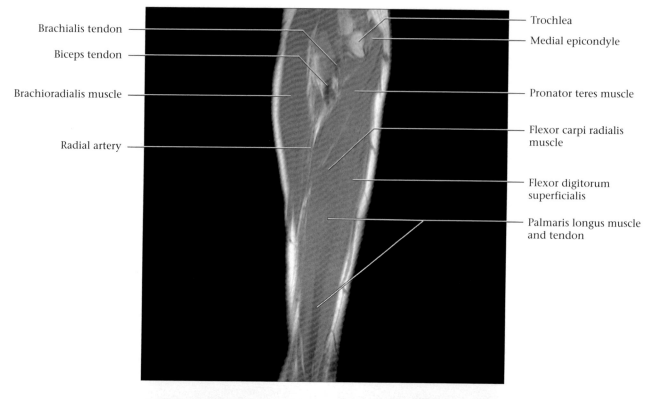

Brachialis tendon

Biceps tendon

Brachioradialis muscle

Radial artery

Trochlea

Medial epicondyle

Pronator teres muscle

Flexor carpi radialis muscle

Flexor digitorum superficialis

Palmaris longus muscle and tendon

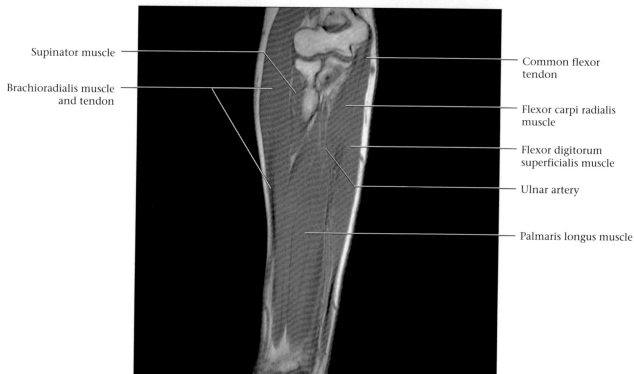

Supinator muscle

Brachioradialis muscle and tendon

Common flexor tendon

Flexor carpi radialis muscle

Flexor digitorum superficialis muscle

Ulnar artery

Palmaris longus muscle

(Top) The pronator teres sweeps from the medial epicondyle to the proximal radius. Note the brachialis tendon located medial to the biceps tendon. **(Bottom)** The brachioradialis muscle is the most lateral of all the forearm muscles.

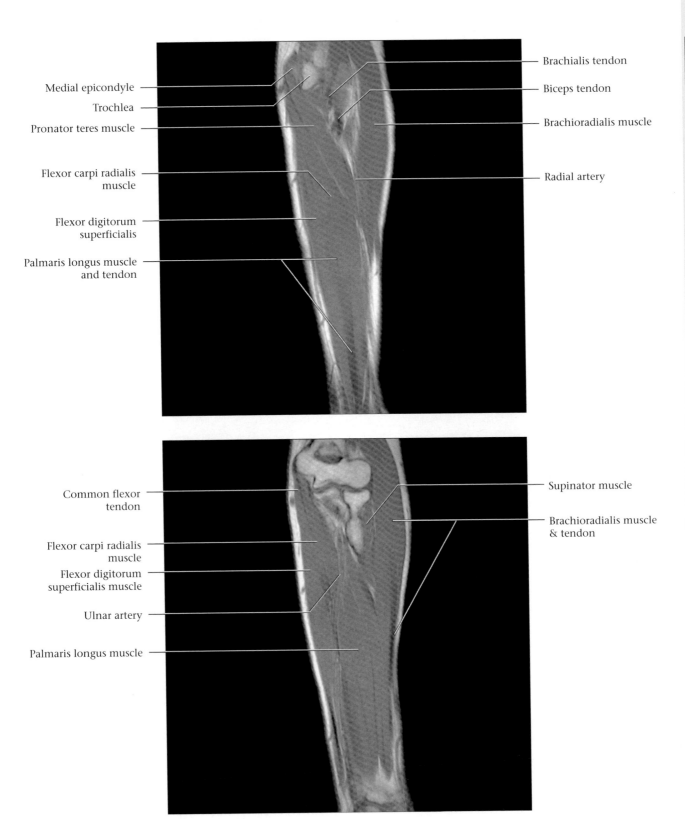

Medial epicondyle

Trochlea

Pronator teres muscle

Flexor carpi radialis muscle

Flexor digitorum superficialis

Palmaris longus muscle and tendon

Brachialis tendon

Biceps tendon

Brachioradialis muscle

Radial artery

Common flexor tendon

Flexor carpi radialis muscle

Flexor digitorum superficialis muscle

Ulnar artery

Palmaris longus muscle

Supinator muscle

Brachioradialis muscle & tendon

(Top) The pronator teres sweeps from the medial epicondyle to the proximal radius. Note the brachialis tendon located medial to the biceps tendon. **(Bottom)** The brachioradialis muscle is the most lateral of all the forearm muscles.

Elbow

II

CORONAL T1 MR, RIGHT FOREARM

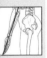

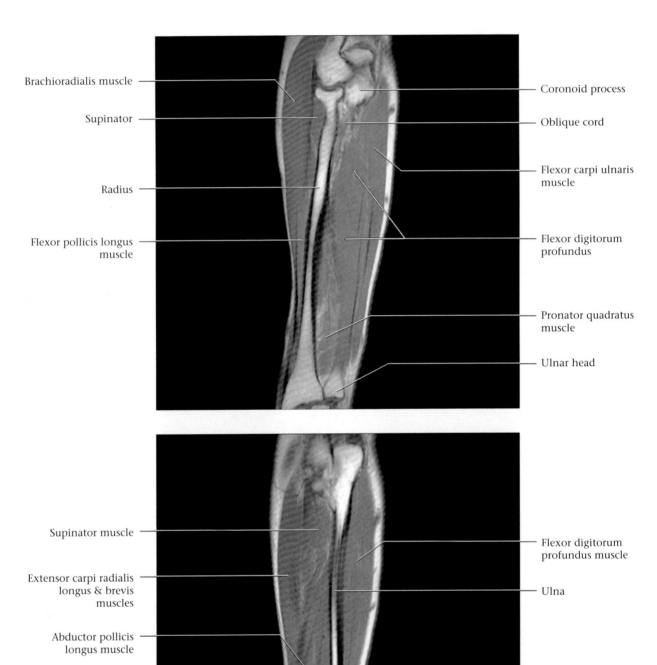

Brachioradialis muscle

Supinator

Radius

Flexor pollicis longus muscle

Coronoid process

Oblique cord

Flexor carpi ulnaris muscle

Flexor digitorum profundus

Pronator quadratus muscle

Ulnar head

Supinator muscle

Extensor carpi radialis longus & brevis muscles

Abductor pollicis longus muscle

Extensor pollicis brevis muscle

Flexor digitorum profundus muscle

Ulna

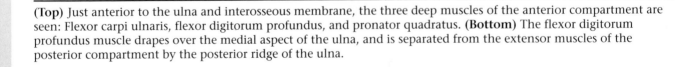

(Top) Just anterior to the ulna and interosseous membrane, the three deep muscles of the anterior compartment are seen: Flexor carpi ulnaris, flexor digitorum profundus, and pronator quadratus. **(Bottom)** The flexor digitorum profundus muscle drapes over the medial aspect of the ulna, and is separated from the extensor muscles of the posterior compartment by the posterior ridge of the ulna.

FOREARM OVERVIEW

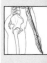

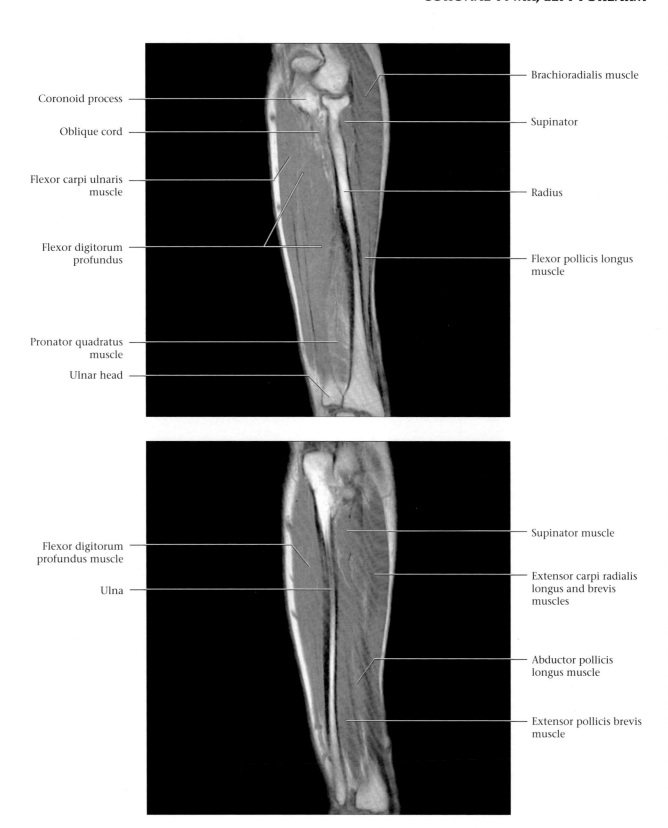

Coronoid process

Oblique cord

Flexor carpi ulnaris muscle

Flexor digitorum profundus

Pronator quadratus muscle

Ulnar head

Brachioradialis muscle

Supinator

Radius

Flexor pollicis longus muscle

Flexor digitorum profundus muscle

Ulna

Supinator muscle

Extensor carpi radialis longus and brevis muscles

Abductor pollicis longus muscle

Extensor pollicis brevis muscle

(Top) Just anterior to the ulna and interosseous membrane, the three deep muscles of the anterior compartment are seen: Flexor carpi ulnaris, flexor digitorum profundus, and pronator quadratus. **(Bottom)** The flexor digitorum profundus muscle drapes over the medial aspect of the ulna, and is separated from the extensor muscles of the posterior compartment by the posterior ridge of the ulna.

FOREARM OVERVIEW

CORONAL T1 MR, RIGHT FOREARM

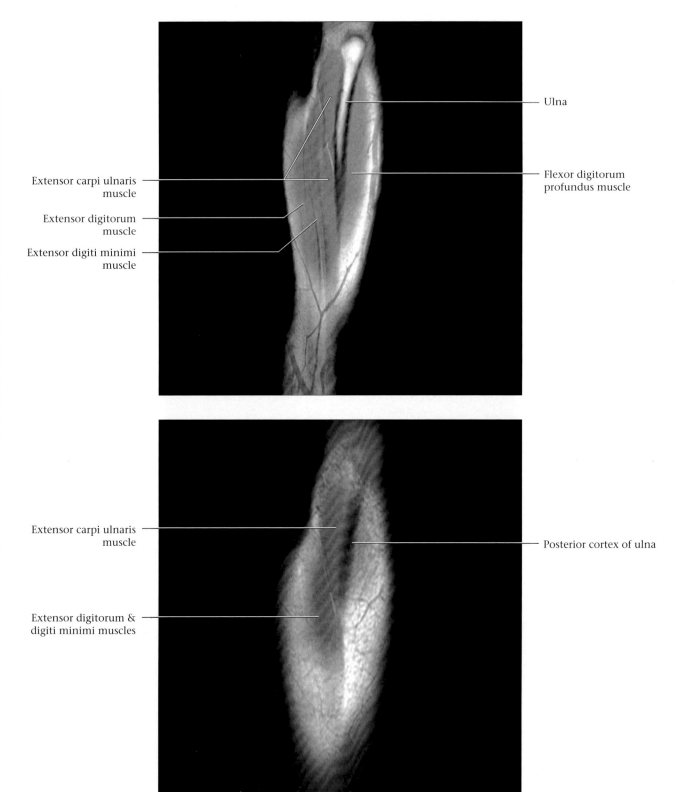

Ulna

Flexor digitorum profundus muscle

Extensor carpi ulnaris muscle

Extensor digitorum muscle

Extensor digiti minimi muscle

Extensor carpi ulnaris muscle

Posterior cortex of ulna

Extensor digitorum & digiti minimi muscles

(Top) The extensor carpi ulnaris muscle is the most medial muscle of the posterior compartment. **(Bottom)** The extensor carpi ulnaris and extensor digitorum and digiti minimi muscles are the most superficial muscles of the posterior (extensor) compartment.

CORONAL T1 MR, LEFT FOREARM

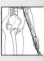

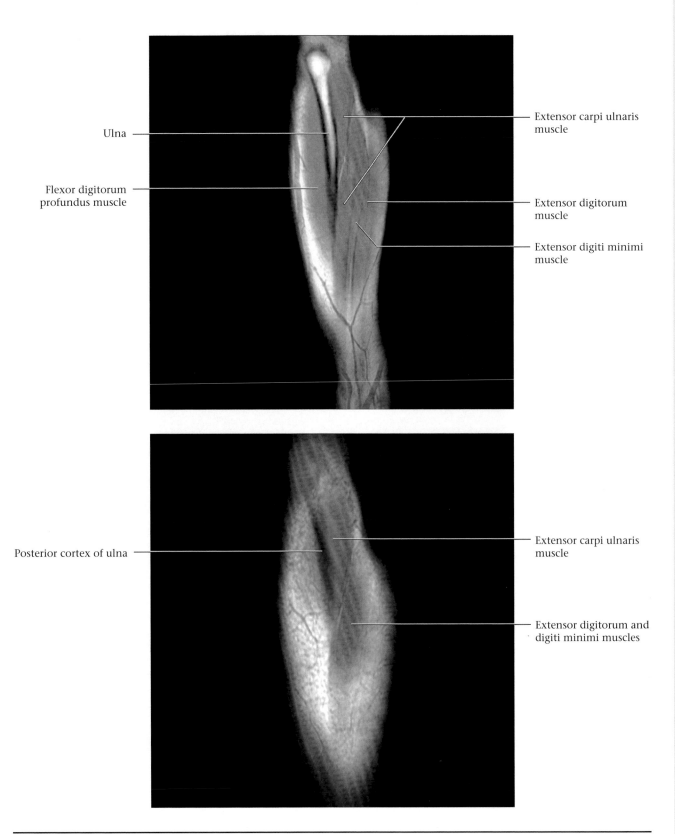

Ulna

Flexor digitorum profundus muscle

Extensor carpi ulnaris muscle

Extensor digitorum muscle

Extensor digiti minimi muscle

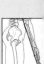

Posterior cortex of ulna

Extensor carpi ulnaris muscle

Extensor digitorum and digiti minimi muscles

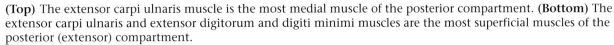

(Top) The extensor carpi ulnaris muscle is the most medial muscle of the posterior compartment. **(Bottom)** The extensor carpi ulnaris and extensor digitorum and digiti minimi muscles are the most superficial muscles of the posterior (extensor) compartment.

SAGITTAL T1 MR, LEFT FOREARM

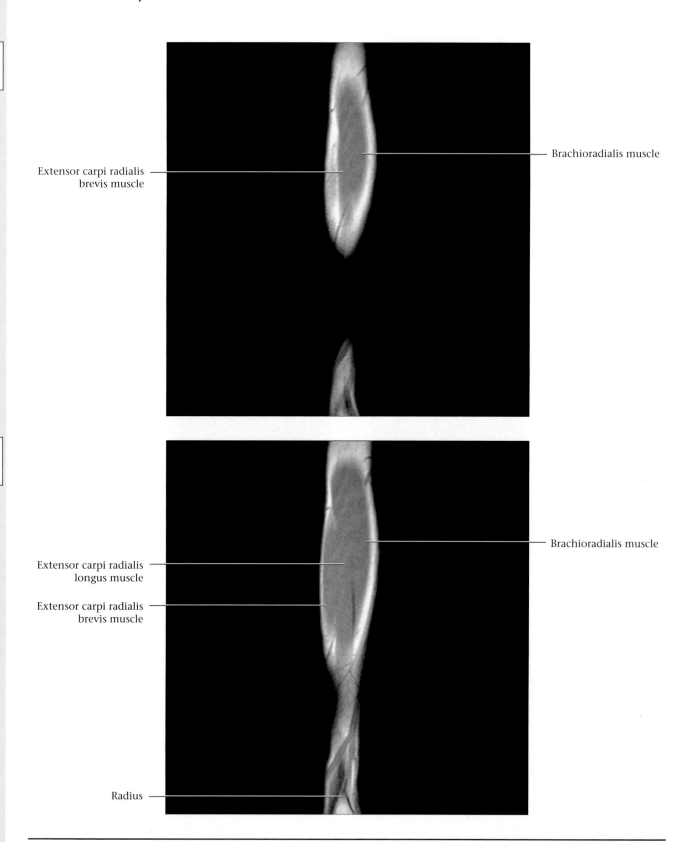

Extensor carpi radialis brevis muscle

Brachioradialis muscle

Extensor carpi radialis longus muscle

Extensor carpi radialis brevis muscle

Brachioradialis muscle

Radius

(Top) Sagittal series of the forearm, lateral to medial. At the extreme lateral aspect of the forearm, only the brachioradialis muscle anteriorly and the extensor carpi radialis brevis muscle posteriorly are visualized. (Bottom) The extensor carpi radialis longus muscle is now visible, anterior to the brevis muscle.

FOREARM OVERVIEW

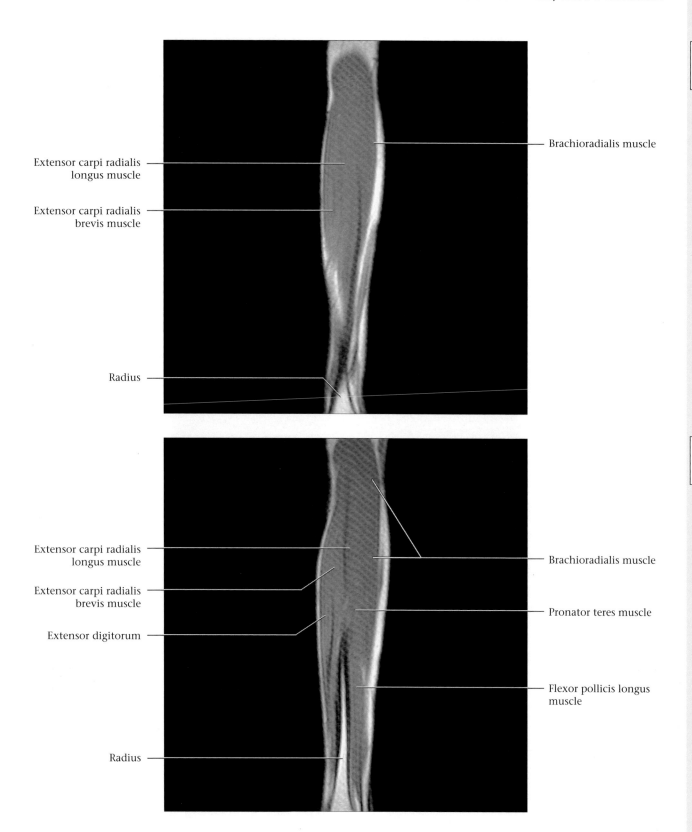

Extensor carpi radialis longus muscle

Extensor carpi radialis brevis muscle

Radius

Brachioradialis muscle

Extensor carpi radialis longus muscle

Extensor carpi radialis brevis muscle

Extensor digitorum

Radius

Brachioradialis muscle

Pronator teres muscle

Flexor pollicis longus muscle

(Top) The brachioradialis tendon will insert on the distal aspect of the radius, while the tendons of the extensor carpi radialis longus and brevis will pass into the wrist via the 2nd extensor compartment. **(Bottom)** The brachioradialis muscle is a flexor of the elbow, the pronator teres is a rotator of the radioulnar joints, and the other muscles seen in this image act on the wrist or fingers.

Elbow

II

119

SAGITTAL T1 MR, LEFT FOREARM

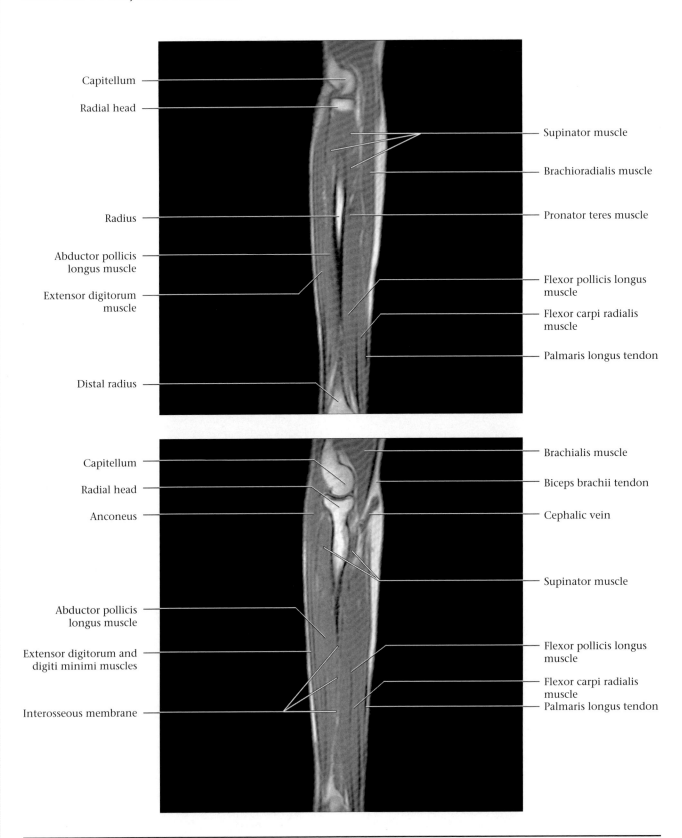

Capitellum

Radial head

Supinator muscle

Brachioradialis muscle

Radius

Pronator teres muscle

Abductor pollicis longus muscle

Extensor digitorum muscle

Flexor pollicis longus muscle

Flexor carpi radialis muscle

Palmaris longus tendon

Distal radius

Capitellum

Brachialis muscle

Radial head

Biceps brachii tendon

Anconeus

Cephalic vein

Supinator muscle

Abductor pollicis longus muscle

Extensor digitorum and digiti minimi muscles

Flexor pollicis longus muscle

Flexor carpi radialis muscle

Interosseous membrane

Palmaris longus tendon

(Top) The palmaris longus muscle has a long tendon in the extreme anterior aspect of the forearm. This tendon is often harvested for surgical grafts. **(Bottom)** The thin cross section of the interosseous membrane is seen, dividing the forearm into anterior (flexor) and posterior (extensor) compartments.

FOREARM OVERVIEW

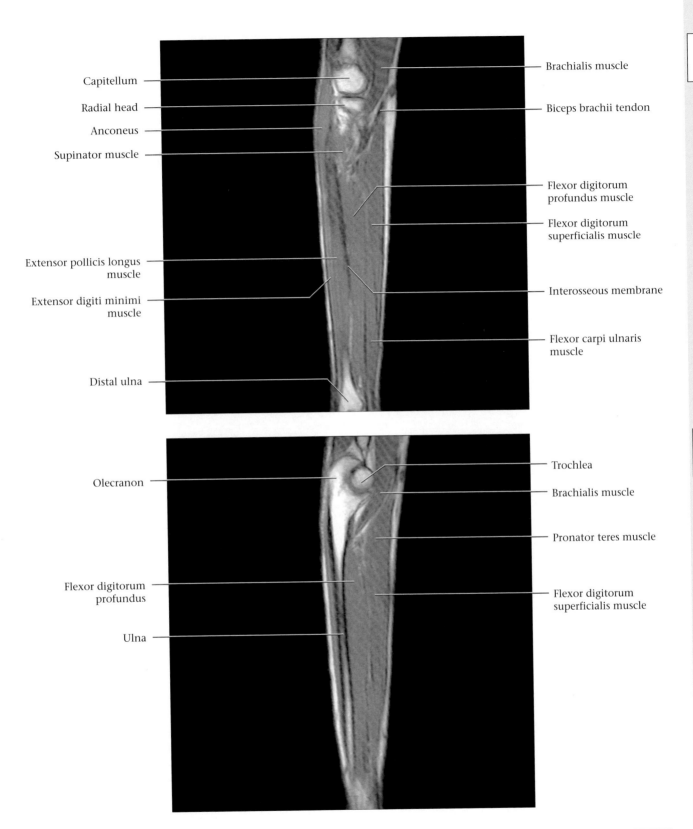

Capitellum

Radial head

Anconeus

Supinator muscle

Extensor pollicis longus muscle

Extensor digiti minimi muscle

Distal ulna

Brachialis muscle

Biceps brachii tendon

Flexor digitorum profundus muscle

Flexor digitorum superficialis muscle

Interosseous membrane

Flexor carpi ulnaris muscle

Olecranon

Flexor digitorum profundus

Ulna

Trochlea

Brachialis muscle

Pronator teres muscle

Flexor digitorum superficialis muscle

(Top) The flexor digitorum profundus is the deepest and largest muscle of the anterior compartment. **(Bottom)** The pronator teres muscle is seen in cross section as it courses obliquely across the proximal aspect of the forearm from its humero-ulnar origins to its radial insertion.

Elbow

II

SAGITTAL T1 MR, LEFT FOREARM

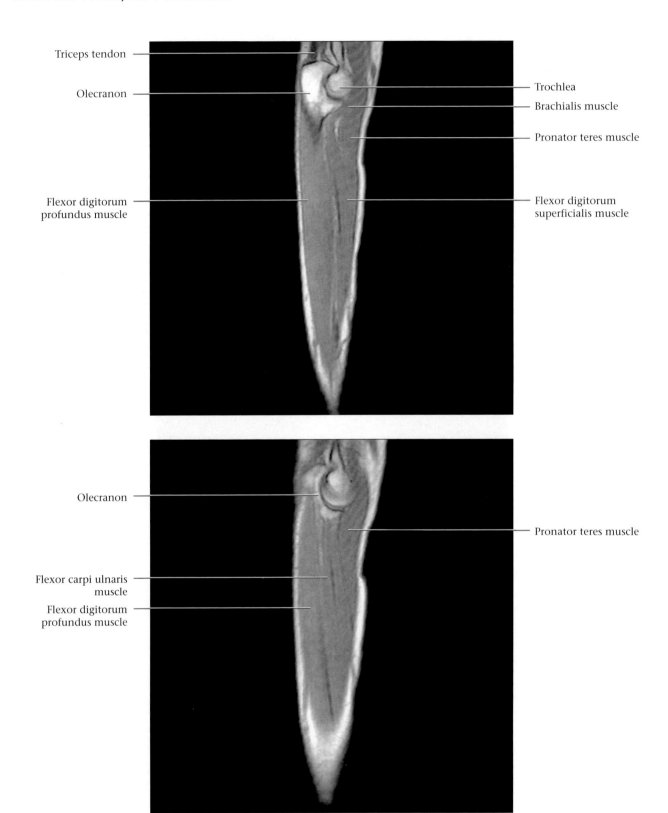

Triceps tendon

Olecranon

Flexor digitorum profundus muscle

Trochlea

Brachialis muscle

Pronator teres muscle

Flexor digitorum superficialis muscle

Olecranon

Flexor carpi ulnaris muscle

Flexor digitorum profundus muscle

Pronator teres muscle

(Top) Medial to the posterior ridge of the ulna, all the muscles are flexors. **(Bottom)** The flexor digitorum profundus muscle drapes over the medial side of the ulna, and is therefore both anterior and medial to the ulnar shaft.

FOREARM OVERVIEW

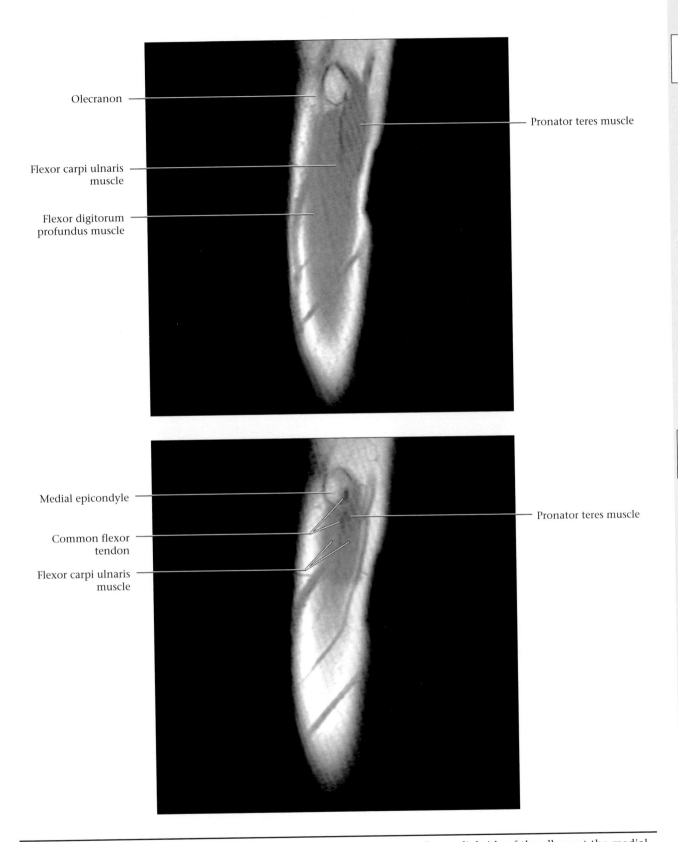

Olecranon

Flexor carpi ulnaris muscle

Flexor digitorum profundus muscle

Pronator teres muscle

Medial epicondyle

Common flexor tendon

Flexor carpi ulnaris muscle

Pronator teres muscle

(Top) The pronator teres muscle, seen here in cross section, originates on the medial side of the elbow at the medial epicondyle and proximal ulna, and sweeps anterior and distal across the forearm to insert on the mid-shaft of the radius. **(Bottom)** The flexor carpi ulnaris muscle is the most medial of the forearm muscles.

Elbow

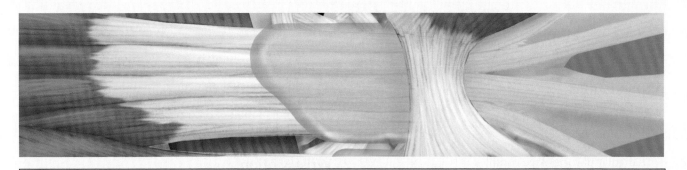

SECTION III: Wrist

WRIST OVERVIEW

Terminology

Abbreviations

- Carpometacarpal (CMC)
- Distal radioulnar joint (DRUJ)
- Metacarpal (MC)
- Triangular fibrocartilage (TFC)
- Triangular fibrocartilage complex (TFCC)
- Abductor pollicis longus (APL)
- Abductor pollicis brevis (APB)
- Extensor carpi radialis brevis (ECRB)
- Extensor carpi radialis longus (ECRL)
- Extensor carpi ulnaris (ECU)
- Extensor digitorum (ED)
- Extensor pollicis brevis (EPB)
- Extensor pollicis longus (EPL)
- Extensor indicis (EI)
- Extensor digiti minimi (EDM)
- Flexor carpi radialis (FCR)
- Flexor carpi ulnaris (FCU)
- Flexor digitorum profundus (FDP)
- Flexor digitorum superficialis (FDS)
- Flexor pollicis longus (FPL)
- Palmaris brevis (PB)
- Palmaris longus (PL)
- Pronator quadratus (PQ)
- Pronator teres (PT)
- Gadolinium (Gd)
- Normal saline (NS)
- Range of motion (ROM)

Definitions

- Volar = palmar
- Ulnar = medial
- Radial = lateral

Gross Anatomy

Overview

- Wrist joint refers to complex articulations including distal radioulnar joint, radiocarpal, pisotriquetral, midcarpal, 1st CMC, 2nd-5th CMC joints & attendant ligamentous & tendinous attachments

Joints

- Distal (inferior) radioulnar: Pivot joint; ROM: Distal radius rotates around distal ulna; radius & ulna are parallel in full supination
- Radiocarpal: Ellipsoid joint created by proximal carpal row articulating with distal radius & ulna; ROM: Flexion, extension, abduction, adduction, circumduction, no rotation
- Pisotriquetral: Gliding joint created by pisiform & triquetrum; discretely separate from radiocarpal joint in 10-25%; ROM: Minimal
- Midcarpal: Gliding joint created by articulation of proximal & distal carpal rows; ROM: Some extension, abduction, minimal rotation
- Intercarpal: Gliding joints created by interface of individual carpal bones; ROM: Complex
- Carpometacarpal

- First CMC (thumb base): Saddle joint, highly mobile; ROM: Flexion, extension, abduction, adduction, circumduction, rotation, opposition
- Intermetacarpals 2nd-5th: Gliding joints; ROM: Limited mobility of 2nd & 3rd CMC, increasing mobility of 4th & 5th CMC
- See "Osseous Structures" section

Wrist Motion

- **Tendon contribution** to motion
  - Flexion: FCU, FCR, PL, APL (FDS & FDP may assist when fingers are in full extension)
  - Extension: ECRL, ERCB, ECU (ED & EPL may assist when fingers in clenched fist)
  - Radial deviation (wrist abduction): APL, EPB with contribution by FCR, ECRL, ERCB, EPL
  - Ulnar deviation (wrist adduction): FCU, ECU
  - Pronation: PQ, PT
  - Supination: Supinator, biceps brachii

Nerves of Wrist Joint

- Three major nerves serve wrist region
- **Median**
  - Origin: Brachial plexus lateral & medial cords
  - Course in wrist: Deep to flexor retinaculum, superficial to FDS/FDP, lateral in carpal tunnel
  - Supplies: PT, FCR, PL, FDS
  - Branch: **Anterior interosseous**
    - Course in wrist: Distal interosseous membrane between FPL & FDP to terminate in PQ & radiocarpal joint
    - Supplies: Radial 1/2 of FDP, FPL, PQ
- **Ulnar**
  - Origin: Brachial plexus medial cord
  - Course in wrist: Medial to ulnar artery, superficial to flexor retinaculum, deep to PB; bifurcates in Guyon canal
  - Supplies: FCU, ulnar 1/2 of FDP
- **Radial**
  - Origin: Brachial plexus posterior cord; multiple branches; terminates in superficial & deep branches
  - **Superficial** branch course in the wrist: Passes under brachioradialis tendon into dorsal wrist & divides
    - **Lateral** branch: Supplies radial wrist & thumb skin
    - **Medial** branch: Supplies dorsal wrist skin; divides to dorsal digital nerves
  - **Deep** branch course in the wrist: Enters supinator muscle ventrally; exits distally & posteriorly as **posterior interosseous** nerve
    - Supplies ECRB, supinator, ED, EDM, ECU, EPL, APL, EI
- See "Neurovascular Structures" section

Vessels of Wrist Joint

- Supplied by three major arteries
  - **Radial**: Terminal branch of brachial artery
  - **Ulnar**: Terminal branch of brachial artery
  - **Common interosseous**: Branch of ulnar artery
    - Branches into **anterior** & **posterior** interosseous arteries
- Vessels create three major volar arches & one major dorsal arch
- See "Neurovascular Structures" section

WRIST OVERVIEW

Imaging Anatomy

Osseous Structures

- **Distal radius:** Articulates with scaphoid, lunate & ulna; structure: Scaphoid & lunate fossae; radial styloid; Lister tubercle - dorsal prominence; sigmoid notch - medial concavity for ulna
- **Distal ulna:** Articulates with radius, articular disc (TFC); structure: Head - distal & lateral ulna, articulates with radius; ulnar styloid; ulnar fossa - base of styloid
  - Ulnar variance refers to length of distal ulna relative to distal radius; ulnar minus: Ulna > 2 mm shorter than radius; ulnar plus: ulna longer than radius
- **Proximal carpal row:** Scaphoid, lunate, triquetrum, pisiform
  - **Scaphoid:** Articulates with radius, lunate, capitate, trapezium, trapezoid; structure: Waist - mid portion of carpal; tuberosity - distal volar prominence
  - **Lunate:** Articulates with scaphoid, radius, articular disc (TFC), triquetrum, capitate; structure: Lunar or half-moon shape; concavity directed distally
  - **Triquetrum:** Articulates with articular disc (TFC), lunate, pisiform, hamate; structure: Triangular shape
  - **Pisiform:** Articulates with triquetrum; structure: Sesamoid-like; FCU attaches & continues distally as pisohamate & pisometacarpal ligaments
- **Distal carpal row:** Trapezium, trapezoid, capitate, hamate
  - **Trapezium** (greater multangular): Articulates with 1st, 2nd MCs, scaphoid, trapezoid; structure: Saddle shape: Link between carpals & thumb
  - **Trapezoid** (lesser multangular): Articulates with trapezium, scaphoid, capitate, 2nd MC; structure: Wedge shape
  - **Capitate:** Articulates with scaphoid, lunate, hamate, trapezoid, 2nd, 3rd MCs; structure: Head - proximal rounded portion; neck (or waist) - narrowed mid portion; body - bulky distal portion
  - **Hamate:** Articulates with triquetrum, capitate, 4th, 5th MCs; structure: Wedge shape; hook (hamulus) - prominent volar projection
- See "Osseous Structures" section

Ligaments

- **Extrinsic** (connect radius, ulna to carpals or carpals to MC) or **intrinsic** (interconnect carpals)
- Major wrist stabilizers: Volar ligaments
- Summary by location
  - **Volar radiocarpal:** Radioscaphocapitate, long radiolunate, radioscapholunate, short radiolunate
  - **Ulnocarpal:** Ulnolunate, ulnotriquetral; ulnocapitate
  - **Dorsal radiocarpal:** Dorsal radiocarpal, dorsal intercarpal, dorsal scaphotriquetral
  - **Volar midcarpal:** Scaphotrapeziotrapezoid, scaphocapitate, triquetrocapitate, triquetrohamate
  - **Proximal interosseous:** Scapholunate, lunotriquetral
  - **Distal interosseous:** Trapeziotrapezoid, trapeziocapitate, capitohamate
  - **Distal radioulnar:** Dorsal radioulnar, volar (palmar) radioulnar, articular disc (TFC)
- See "Ligaments" section

Muscles & Tendons

- Muscles acting on the wrist joint or tendons crossing the wrist joints (listed by action on the wrist)
- **Flexors, deep**
  - **Flexor digitorum profundus:** Origin ulna, insertion index, middle, ring & little finger distal phalangeal bases
  - **Flexor pollicis longus:** Origin radius, interosseous membrane & coronoid process ulna, insertion thumb distal phalangeal base
  - **Pronator quadratus:** Origin ulna & aponeurosis, insertion distal radius
- **Flexors, superficial**
  - **Flexor carpi radialis:** Origin medial epicondyle, insertion 2nd MC base with slip to 3rd MC
  - **Palmaris longus:** Origin medial epicondyle, insertion superficial flexor retinaculum & palmar aponeurosis
  - **Flexor carpi ulnaris:** Origin (humeral head) medial epicondyle & (ulnar head) medial olecranon/proximal ulna, insertion pisiform & flexor retinaculum
  - **Flexor digitorum superficialis:** Origin (humeroulnar head) medial epicondyle & coronoid process of ulna & (radial head) anterior radius, insertion index through little finger middle phalangeal bases
- **Extensors, deep**
  - **Abductor pollicis longus:** Origin ulna, insertion radial 1st MC base with slips to trapezium & APB
  - **Extensor pollicis brevis:** Origin radius, insertion thumb proximal phalangeal base
  - **Extensor pollicis longus:** Origin mid ulna, insertion thumb distal phalangeal base
  - **Extensor indicis** (proprius): Origin mid ulna, insertion joins with ulnar side of ED tendon inserting into 2nd digit extensor hood
- **Extensors, superficial**
  - **Brachioradialis:** Origin proximal humerus, insertion radial styloid base
  - **Extensor carpi radialis longus:** Origin lateral supracondylar ridge of humerus, insertion dorsal radial 2nd MC base
  - **Extensor carpi radialis brevis:** Origin lateral humeral epicondyle, insertion dorsal radial 3rd MC base
  - **Extensor digitorum** (communis): Origin lateral humeral epicondyle, insertion into middle & distal phalanges
  - **Extensor digiti minimi** [Ex digiti quinti (V) proprius]: Origin common extensor tendon of lateral humeral epicondyle, insertion extensor hood little finger
  - **Extensor carpi ulnaris:** Origin common extensor tendon of lateral humeral epicondyle, insertion 5th MC base
- **Thenar**
  - **Abductor pollicis brevis:** Origin flexor retinaculum, scaphoid tuberosity & trapezium ridge, insertion thumb proximal phalanx
  - **Opponens pollicis:** Origin trapezium & flexor retinaculum, insertion 1st MC

- ○ **Flexor pollicis brevis:** Superficial origin flexor retinaculum & trapezium, deep origin trapezoid & capitate, insertion thumb proximal phalanx
- ○ **Adductor pollicis:** Origin capitate, 2nd & 3rd MC bases, insertion ulnar thumb proximal phalanx
- **Hypothenar**
  - ○ **Palmaris brevis:** Origin flexor retinaculum & palmar aponeurosis, insertion skin of palm
  - ○ **Adductor digiti minimi:** Origin pisiform & FCU, insertion little finger proximal phalanx
  - ○ **Flexor digiti minimi brevis:** Origin hamate hook & flexor retinaculum, insertion ulnar little finger proximal phalanx
  - ○ **Opponens digiti minimi:** Origin hamate hook & flexor retinaculum, insertion 5th MC
- See "Tendons" section

Retinacula

- **Flexor retinaculum**
  - ○ Superficial (volar carpal ligament or ligamentum carpi palmare): Attached to styloid processes of ulna & radius; merges with deep component distally
  - ○ Deep (transverse carpal ligament or ligamentum flexorum): Attached to pisiform & hook of hamate medially, scaphoid & trapezium laterally
- **Extensor retinaculum**
  - ○ Attaches to ulnar styloid process, triquetrum & pisiform medially, crosses obliquely to attach Lister tubercle & radial styloid process laterally
    - ▪ Sends septae to radius creating compartments for extensor tendons
  - ○ Compartment contents: 1) APL, EPB; 2) ECRL, ECRB; 3) EPL; 4) ED, EI; 5) EDM; 6) ECU
- See "Tendons" section

Anatomic Spaces

- **Anatomic snuffbox**
  - ○ **Margins:** Distal radius (proximal margin), EPL (dorsal margin), APL & EPB (volar margin) convergence of APL/EPB just distal to 1st CMC (distal margin); snuffbox base formed by radial styloid, scaphoid, trapezium & 1st CMC
  - ○ **Contents:** Cephalic vein, radial nerve, (superficial branch), radial artery
- **Carpal tunnel**
  - ○ **Margins:** Carpals (dorsal margin), flexor retinaculum (volar margin); pisiform & hook of the hamate (medial margin), scaphoid & trapezium (lateral margin), radiocarpal joint (proximal margin) & MC base (distal margin)
  - ○ **Contents:** FDS, FDP, FPL, median nerve
- **Guyon canal**
  - ○ **Margins:** Superficial flexor retinaculum (volar carpal ligament or ligamentum carpi palmare) [ventral margin], pisiform & FCU [medial margin], deep flexor retinaculum (transverse carpal ligament or ligamentum flexorum) [lateral & dorsal margin]
  - ○ **Contents:** Ulnar artery & vein, ulnar nerve
- See "Tendons" and "Neurovascular Structures" sections

Anatomy-Based Imaging Issues

Imaging Recommendations

- Radiography: For alignment, joint space width, mineralization, range of motion
- Arthrography: For intrinsic ligaments & TFC integrity
  - ○ Injectate: Undiluted iodinated contrast
  - ○ Volumes: Midcarpal: 4-5 cc; radiocarpal: 2-3 cc; DRUJ: 1 cc
- CT: Acquire thin section (0.5-1 mm) with 2D and 3D reformation; for alignment, cortical integrity
- CT arthrography: Used if unable to undergo MR
  - ○ Injectate: Iodinated contrast: NS (1:2-3)
- MR: Dedicated coils, 8-10 cm field of view, thin sections essential for imaging small, complex wrist anatomy
  - ○ T1: Single plane; for anatomy, marrow, spaces
  - ○ Inversion recovery: Coronal plane; for marrow contusion, soft tissue masses, fluid collections
    - ▪ Limitations: Poor spatial resolution
  - ○ GRE (T2*): Coronal plane; for ligaments, articular cartilage
    - ▪ Limitations: Magic angle effect, susceptibility artifact
  - ○ PD/T2 (w/ or w/o fat suppression): Axial plane; marrow, cartilage, ligaments, fluid collections
  - ○ Intravenous Gd/T1 w/fat suppression: For suspected masses, inflammation, infections
  - ○ Structures best visualized (by plane)
    - ▪ Coronal: Osseous structures, alignment, intrinsic & extrinsic ligaments, TFCC
    - ▪ Axial: Tendons, neurovascular structures, DRUJ, pisotriquetral joint
    - ▪ Sagittal: Alignment, cross section ligaments, pisotriquetral joint
- MR arthrography
  - ○ Injectate: Gd: Fluid mix (1:100-200); fluid: NS/iodinated contrast (50:50); allows for diagnostic/CT arthrography
- Ultrasound: Dynamic evaluation of tendons, ligaments, neurovascular structures

Imaging Pitfalls

- Many tendon variations include split or duplicated tendons
- Small amount extensor tendon sheath fluid is common (particularly ECRB & ECRL); should not be mistaken for tenosynovitis
- TFCC attachments may mimic tears: Radial attachments to hyaline cartilage rather than cortex; ulnar attachment to ulna fossa often intermediate signal due to magic angle or volume averaging
  - ○ Articular disc may develop asymptomatic attritional tears
- Scapholunate & lunotriquetral ligaments may attach to articular cartilage rather than cortex
- Malpositioning: Ulnar or radial deviation may create apparent instability patterns
- Magic angle effect: Organized fibers (t. or l.) crossing at 55° to main magnetic field may have intermediate signal on short TE imaging (T1, PD, GRE)
  - ○ Examples: ECU crossing dorsum of ulna; EPL crossing dorsal wrist obliquely

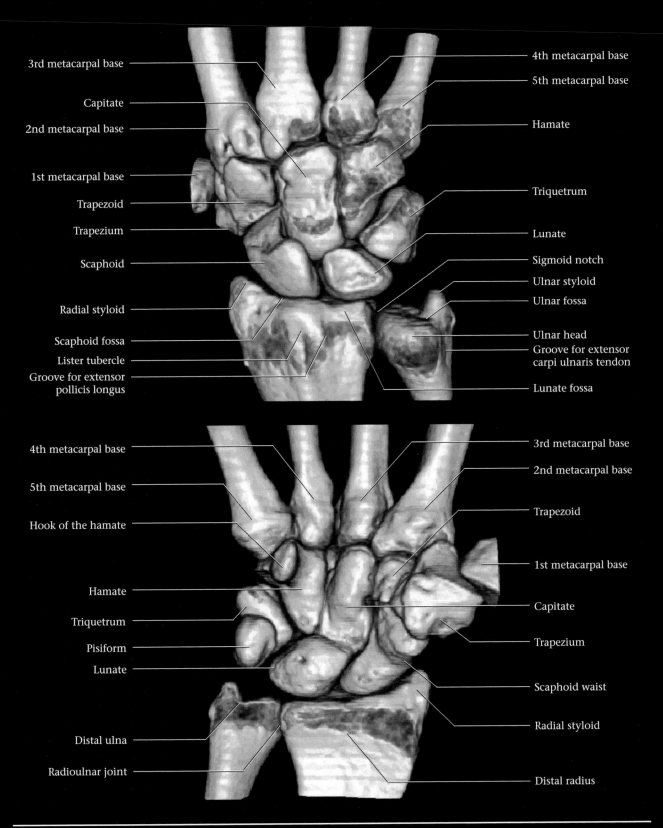

3rd metacarpal base

Capitate

2nd metacarpal base

1st metacarpal base

Trapezoid

Trapezium

Scaphoid

Radial styloid

Scaphoid fossa

Lister tubercle

Groove for extensor pollicis longus

4th metacarpal base

5th metacarpal base

Hamate

Triquetrum

Lunate

Sigmoid notch

Ulnar styloid

Ulnar fossa

Ulnar head

Groove for extensor carpi ulnaris tendon

Lunate fossa

4th metacarpal base

5th metacarpal base

Hook of the hamate

Hamate

Triquetrum

Pisiform

Lunate

Distal ulna

Radioulnar joint

3rd metacarpal base

2nd metacarpal base

Trapezoid

1st metacarpal base

Capitate

Trapezium

Scaphoid waist

Radial styloid

Distal radius

(Top) 3D surface rendering, dorsal wrist, positioned in pronation. **(Bottom)** Volar wrist, positioned in pronation.

WRIST OVERVIEW

RADIOGRAPHS, PA & LATERAL

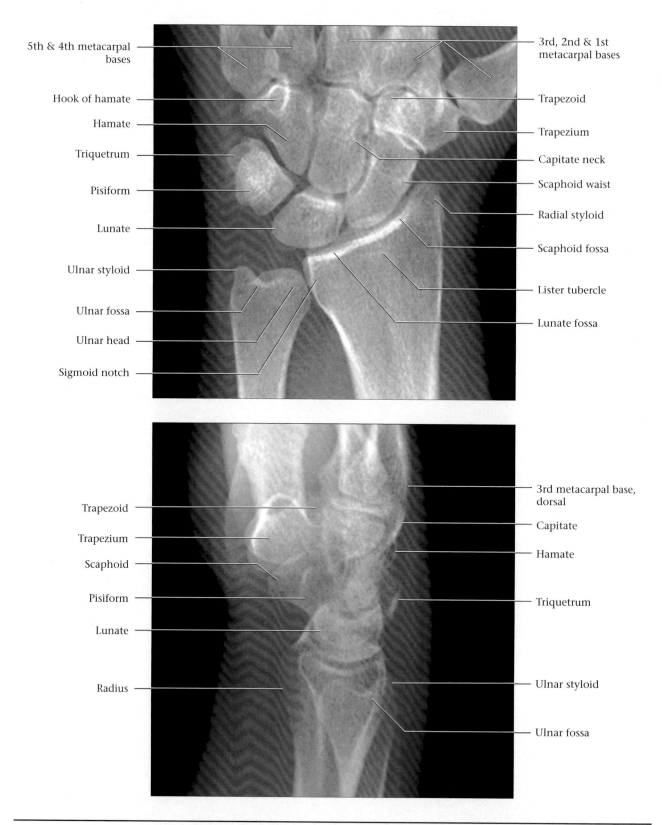

5th & 4th metacarpal bases

Hook of hamate

Hamate

Triquetrum

Pisiform

Lunate

Ulnar styloid

Ulnar fossa

Ulnar head

Sigmoid notch

3rd, 2nd & 1st metacarpal bases

Trapezoid

Trapezium

Capitate neck

Scaphoid waist

Radial styloid

Scaphoid fossa

Lister tubercle

Lunate fossa

Trapezoid

Trapezium

Scaphoid

Pisiform

Lunate

Radius

3rd metacarpal base, dorsal

Capitate

Hamate

Triquetrum

Ulnar styloid

Ulnar fossa

(Top) PA radiograph of the wrist. Image is obtained at zero-rotation by positioning patient at 90 degrees abduction of shoulder & 90 degree flexion of elbow. **(Bottom)** Lateral radiograph obtained in zero-rotation position. Note the position of the pisiform overlying the mid waist of the scaphoid indicates a properly positioned lateral. Image is obtained with the wrist resting on the film cassette with the shoulder at 90 degrees abduction & the elbow at 90 degree flexion.

WRIST OVERVIEW

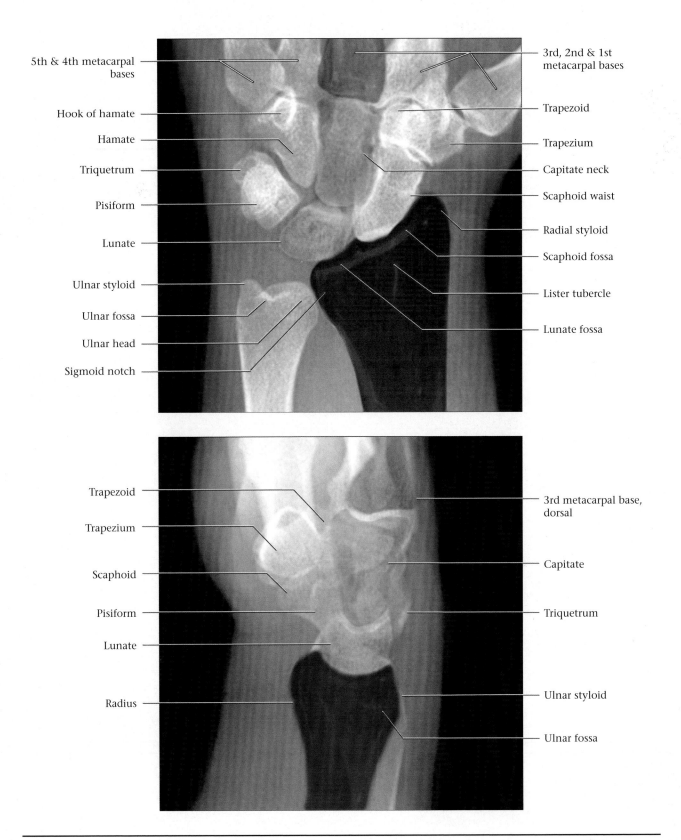

5th & 4th metacarpal bases

Hook of hamate

Hamate

Triquetrum

Pisiform

Lunate

Ulnar styloid

Ulnar fossa

Ulnar head

Sigmoid notch

3rd, 2nd & 1st metacarpal bases

Trapezoid

Trapezium

Capitate neck

Scaphoid waist

Radial styloid

Scaphoid fossa

Lister tubercle

Lunate fossa

Trapezoid

Trapezium

Scaphoid

Pisiform

Lunate

Radius

3rd metacarpal base, dorsal

Capitate

Triquetrum

Ulnar styloid

Ulnar fossa

(Top) PA radiograph of the wrist. Color-coded to facilitate key structure identification. Third metacarpal: Magenta; capitate: Blue; lunate: Yellow; radius: Red. **(Bottom)** Lateral radiograph obtained in zero-rotation position. Color-coded to facilitate key structure identification. Third metacarpal: Magenta; capitate: Blue; lunate: Yellow; radius: Red.

GRAPHICS, DORSAL & VOLAR LIGAMENTS

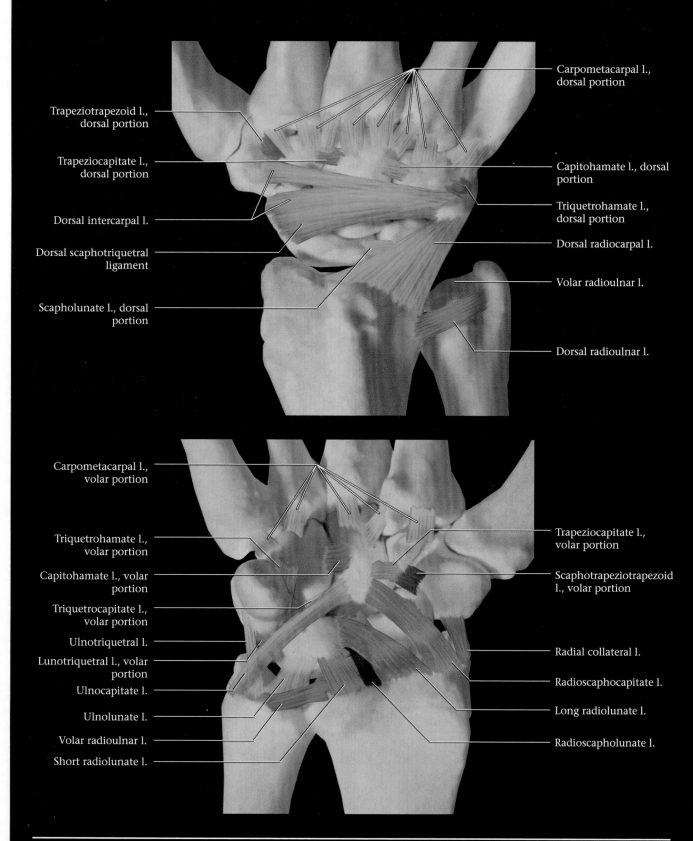

Carpometacarpal l., dorsal portion

Trapeziotrapezoid l., dorsal portion

Trapeziocapitate l., dorsal portion

Dorsal intercarpal l.

Dorsal scaphotriquetral ligament

Scapholunate l., dorsal portion

Capitohamate l., dorsal portion

Triquetrohamate l., dorsal portion

Dorsal radiocarpal l.

Volar radioulnar l.

Dorsal radioulnar l.

Carpometacarpal l., volar portion

Triquetrohamate l., volar portion

Capitohamate l., volar portion

Triquetrocapitate l., volar portion

Ulnotriquetral l.

Lunotriquetral l., volar portion

Ulnocapitate l.

Ulnolunate l.

Volar radioulnar l.

Short radiolunate l.

Trapeziocapitate l., volar portion

Scaphotrapeziotrapezoid l., volar portion

Radial collateral l.

Radioscaphocapitate l.

Long radiolunate l.

Radioscapholunate l.

(Top) Intrinsic and extrinsic ligaments of dorsal wrist by location. Dorsal radiocarpal: Dorsal radiocarpal, dorsal scaphotriquetral, dorsal intercarpal. Proximal interosseous: Scapholunate, lunotriquetral. Distal interosseous: Trapeziotrapezoid, trapeziocapitate, capitohamate. Distal radioulnar volar & dorsal ligaments. **(Bottom)** Extrinsic and intrinsic ligaments of the volar wrist by location. Volar radiocarpal: Radioscaphocapitate, long radiolunate, radioscapholunate, short radiolunate. Ulnocarpal: Ulnolunate, ulnotriquetral, ulnocapitate. Volar midcarpal: Scaphotrapeziotrapezoid, scaphocapitate, triquetrocapitate, triquetrohamate. Proximal interosseous: Scapholunate, lunotriquetral. Distal interosseous: Trapeziotrapezoid, trapeziocapitate, capitohamate. Distal radioulnar volar & dorsal ligaments.

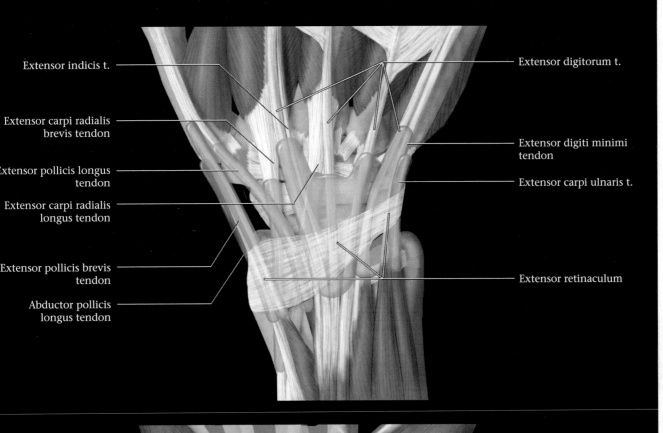

Extensor indicis t.

Extensor carpi radialis brevis tendon

Extensor pollicis longus tendon

Extensor carpi radialis longus tendon

Extensor pollicis brevis tendon

Abductor pollicis longus tendon

Extensor digitorum t.

Extensor digiti minimi tendon

Extensor carpi ulnaris t.

Extensor retinaculum

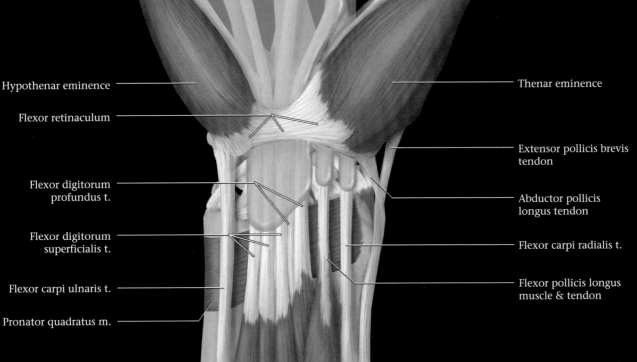

Hypothenar eminence

Flexor retinaculum

Flexor digitorum profundus t.

Flexor digitorum superficialis t.

Flexor carpi ulnaris t.

Pronator quadratus m.

Thenar eminence

Extensor pollicis brevis tendon

Abductor pollicis longus tendon

Flexor carpi radialis t.

Flexor pollicis longus muscle & tendon

(Top) Tendons and retinaculum of the dorsal wrist. The extensor retinaculum attaches to the triquetrum and pisiform medially, crossing obliquely to attach to Lister tubercle and the radial styloid laterally, creating a series of compartments which separate the various tendons and their associated sheaths. Extensor tendons are enclosed in individual tenosynovial sheaths as they pass under the extensor retinaculum. **(Bottom)** Tendons and retinaculum of the volar wrist. The flexor retinaculum spans the palmar arch, attaching to the radial and ulnar styloid processes. The thenar eminence musculature includes abductor pollicis brevis, opponens pollicis, flexor pollicis brevis and adductor pollicis. The hypothenar musculature includes palmaris brevis, adductor digiti minimi, flexor digiti minimi brevis and opponens digiti minimi.

GRAPHICS, DORSAL & VOLAR ARTERIES & VEINS

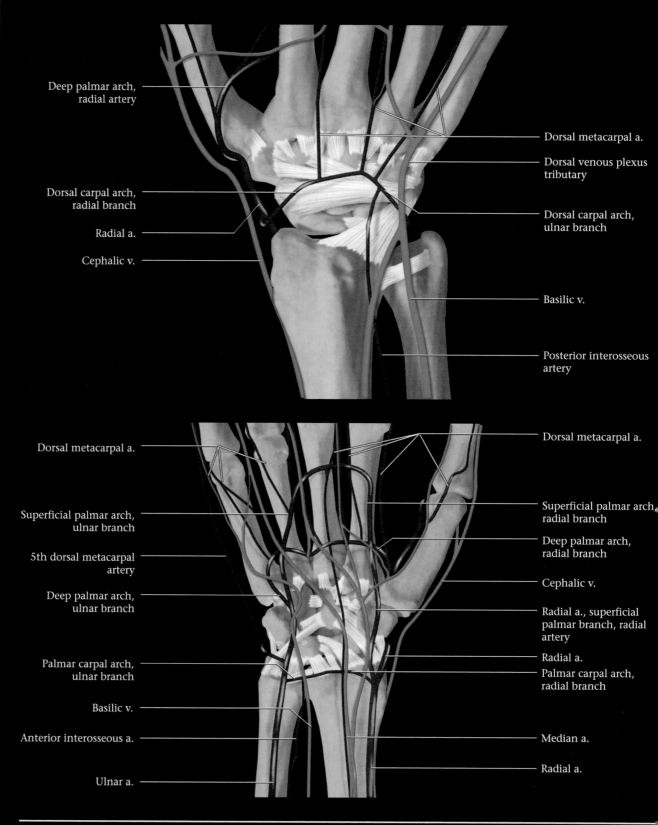

Deep palmar arch, radial artery

Dorsal metacarpal a.

Dorsal venous plexus tributary

Dorsal carpal arch, radial branch

Radial a.

Cephalic v.

Dorsal carpal arch, ulnar branch

Basilic v.

Posterior interosseous artery

Dorsal metacarpal a.

Dorsal metacarpal a.

Superficial palmar arch, ulnar branch

5th dorsal metacarpal artery

Deep palmar arch, ulnar branch

Palmar carpal arch, ulnar branch

Basilic v.

Anterior interosseous a.

Ulnar a.

Superficial palmar arch, radial branch

Deep palmar arch, radial branch

Cephalic v.

Radial a., superficial palmar branch, radial artery

Radial a.

Palmar carpal arch, radial branch

Median a.

Radial a.

(Top) Vasculature of the dorsal wrist. The dorsal carpal arch supplies the distal radius, distal carpal row and lateral proximal carpal row. The venous plexus drains into two main venous systems, the cephalic and basilic, with multiple anastomotic communications. **(Bottom)** Vasculature of the ovolar wrist. Three major arterial arches are contributed to by the radial, ulnar and interosseous arteries: Palmar (volar) carpal, deep and superficial palmar arches. A dorsal venous plexus drains into the cephalic and basilic veins.

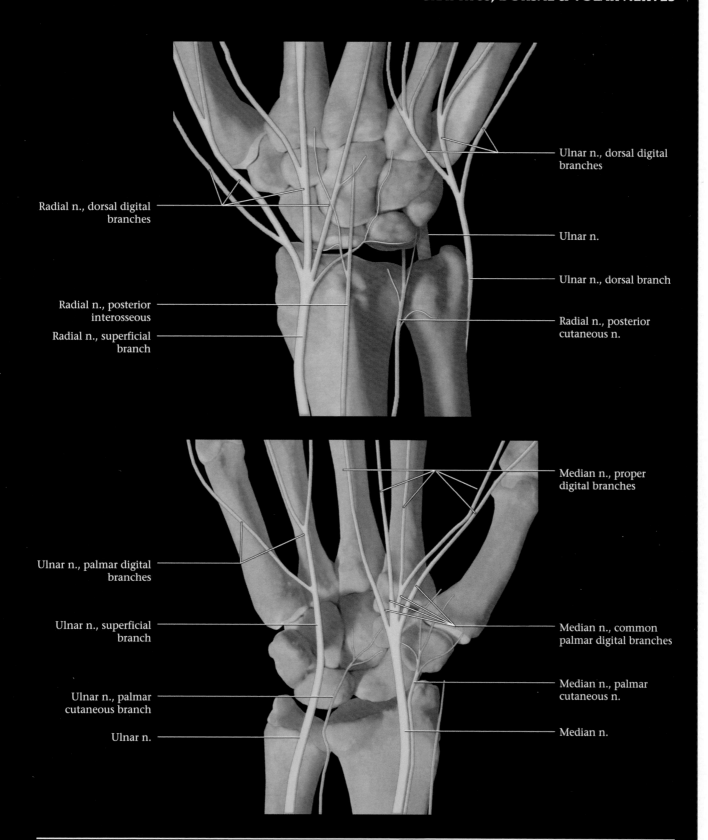

Radial n., dorsal digital branches

Radial n., posterior interosseous

Radial n., superficial branch

Ulnar n., dorsal digital branches

Ulnar n.

Ulnar n., dorsal branch

Radial n., posterior cutaneous n.

Ulnar n., palmar digital branches

Ulnar n., superficial branch

Ulnar n., palmar cutaneous branch

Ulnar n.

Median n., proper digital branches

Median n., common palmar digital branches

Median n., palmar cutaneous n.

Median n.

(Top) Nerves of the dorsal wrist. The radial nerve branches in the forearm with the superficial, posterior cutaneous & posterior interosseous branches serving the wrist and hand. The ulnar nerve provides branches to dorsal and volar wrist. **(Bottom)** Nerves of the volar wrist. The ulnar nerve provides motor and sensory branches to the ulnar aspect of the wrist. The median nerve passes through the carpal tunnel, with several branches serving the palmar & radial aspects of the wrist and hand.

AXIAL T1 MR, RIGHT WRIST

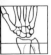

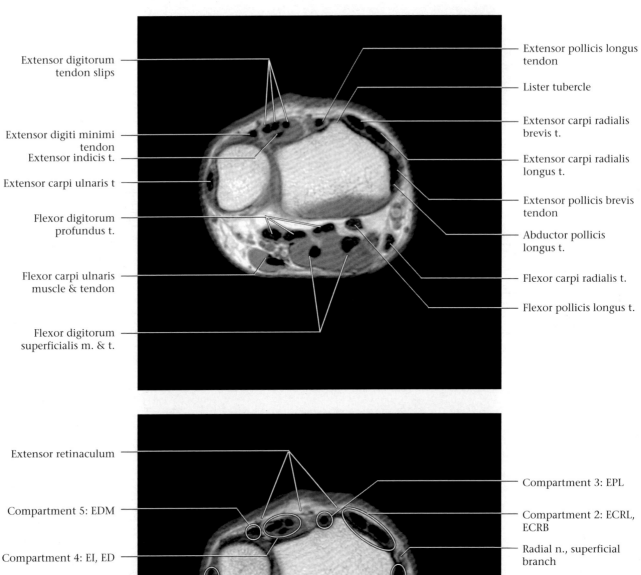

Extensor digitorum tendon slips

Extensor digiti minimi tendon
Extensor indicis t.

Extensor carpi ulnaris t

Flexor digitorum profundus t.

Flexor carpi ulnaris muscle & tendon

Flexor digitorum superficialis m. & t.

Extensor pollicis longus tendon

Lister tubercle

Extensor carpi radialis brevis t.

Extensor carpi radialis longus t.

Extensor pollicis brevis tendon

Abductor pollicis longus t.

Flexor carpi radialis t.

Flexor pollicis longus t.

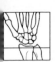

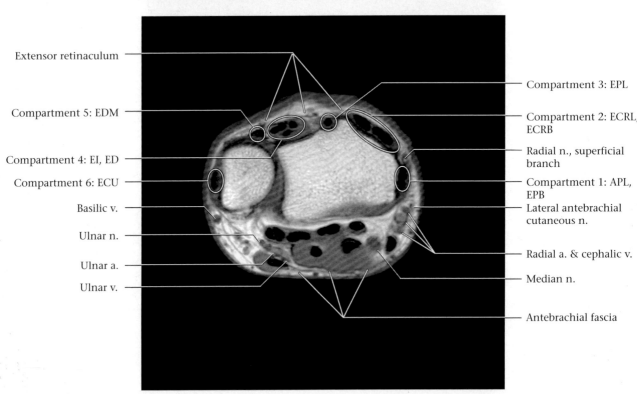

Extensor retinaculum

Compartment 5: EDM

Compartment 4: EI, ED

Compartment 6: ECU

Basilic v.

Ulnar n.

Ulnar a.

Ulnar v.

Compartment 3: EPL

Compartment 2: ECRL, ECRB

Radial n., superficial branch

Compartment 1: APL, EPB

Lateral antebrachial cutaneous n.

Radial a. & cephalic v.

Median n.

Antebrachial fascia

(Top) First of eighteen sequential T1 axial images of right wrist, from proximal to distal, displays tendons & musculature at Lister tubercle. **(Bottom)** Slightly distal, at level of ulnar head & distal radius, neurovascular structures & fascia are annotated. The extensor retinaculum creates six separate tunnels or compartments as it attaches to underlying bone. Each compartment contains one or more tendons as follows: 1) Abductor pollicis longus, extensor pollicis brevis; 2) Extensor carpi radialis longus & brevis; 3) Extensor pollicis longus; 4) Extensor indicis, extensor digitorum; 5) Extensor digiti minimi; 6) Extensor carpi ulnaris.

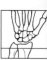

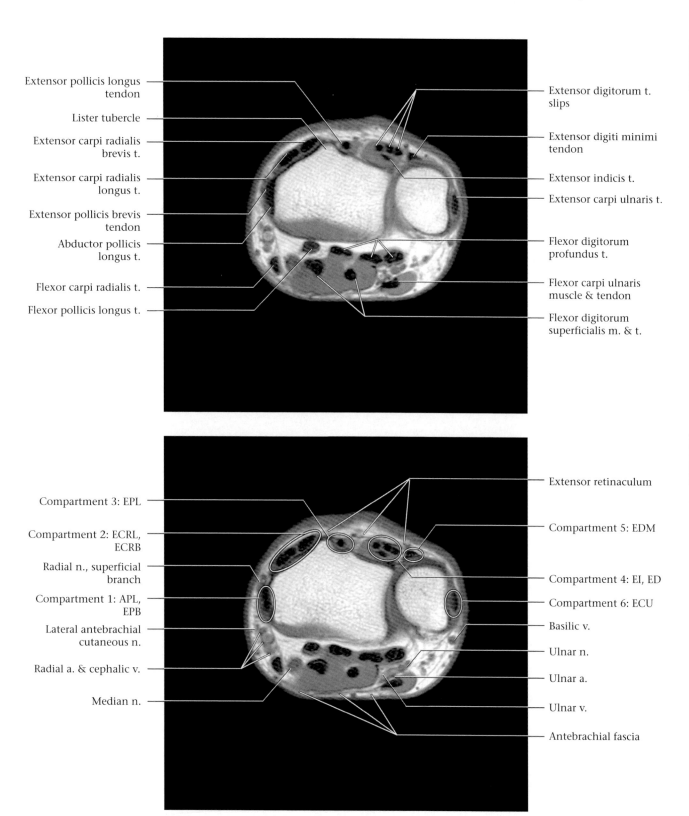

Extensor pollicis longus tendon

Lister tubercle

Extensor carpi radialis brevis t.

Extensor carpi radialis longus t.

Extensor pollicis brevis tendon

Abductor pollicis longus t.

Flexor carpi radialis t.

Flexor pollicis longus t.

Extensor digitorum t. slips

Extensor digiti minimi tendon

Extensor indicis t.

Extensor carpi ulnaris t.

Flexor digitorum profundus t.

Flexor carpi ulnaris muscle & tendon

Flexor digitorum superficialis m. & t.

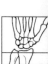

Compartment 3: EPL

Compartment 2: ECRL, ECRB

Radial n., superficial branch

Compartment 1: APL, EPB

Lateral antebrachial cutaneous n.

Radial a. & cephalic v.

Median n.

Extensor retinaculum

Compartment 5: EDM

Compartment 4: EI, ED

Compartment 6: ECU

Basilic v.

Ulnar n.

Ulnar a.

Ulnar v.

Antebrachial fascia

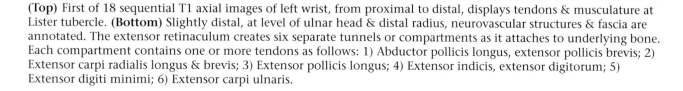

(Top) First of 18 sequential T1 axial images of left wrist, from proximal to distal, displays tendons & musculature at Lister tubercle. **(Bottom)** Slightly distal, at level of ulnar head & distal radius, neurovascular structures & fascia are annotated. The extensor retinaculum creates six separate tunnels or compartments as it attaches to underlying bone. Each compartment contains one or more tendons as follows: 1) Abductor pollicis longus, extensor pollicis brevis; 2) Extensor carpi radialis longus & brevis; 3) Extensor pollicis longus; 4) Extensor indicis, extensor digitorum; 5) Extensor digiti minimi; 6) Extensor carpi ulnaris.

AXIAL T1 MR, RIGHT WRIST

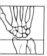

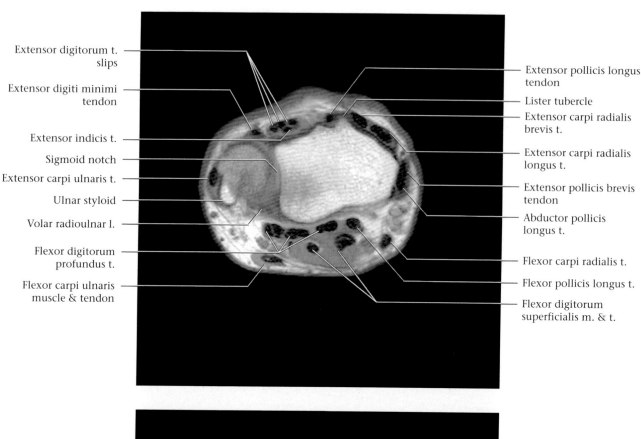

Extensor digitorum t. slips

Extensor digiti minimi tendon

Extensor indicis t.

Sigmoid notch

Extensor carpi ulnaris t.

Ulnar styloid

Volar radioulnar l.

Flexor digitorum profundus t.

Flexor carpi ulnaris muscle & tendon

Extensor pollicis longus tendon

Lister tubercle

Extensor carpi radialis brevis t.

Extensor carpi radialis longus t.

Extensor pollicis brevis tendon

Abductor pollicis longus t.

Flexor carpi radialis t.

Flexor pollicis longus t.

Flexor digitorum superficialis m. & t.

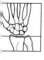

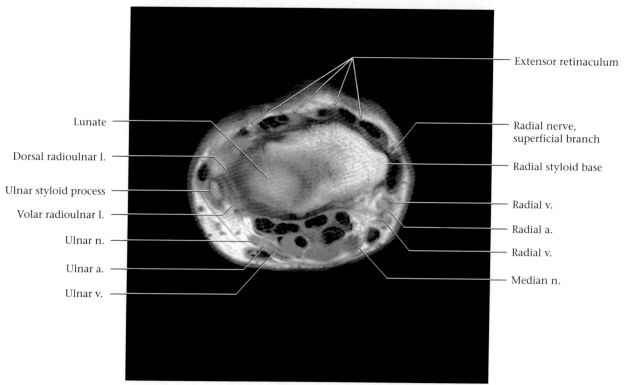

Lunate

Dorsal radioulnar l.

Ulnar styloid process

Volar radioulnar l.

Ulnar n.

Ulnar a.

Ulnar v.

Extensor retinaculum

Radial nerve, superficial branch

Radial styloid base

Radial v.

Radial a.

Radial v.

Median n.

(Top) Extensor tendons are tethered by extensor retinaculum. Extensor pollicis longus tendon lies within a dorsal osseous groove ulnar to Lister tubercle. Flexor musculotendinous junctions are visualized proximal to carpal tunnel. Palmaris longus tendon is absent as it is in approximately 10% of the general population. **(Bottom)** Extensor retinaculum is identifiable at ulnar styloid tip & radial styloid base. Median & ulnar nerves are readily visualized as is superficial branch of radial nerve.

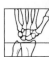

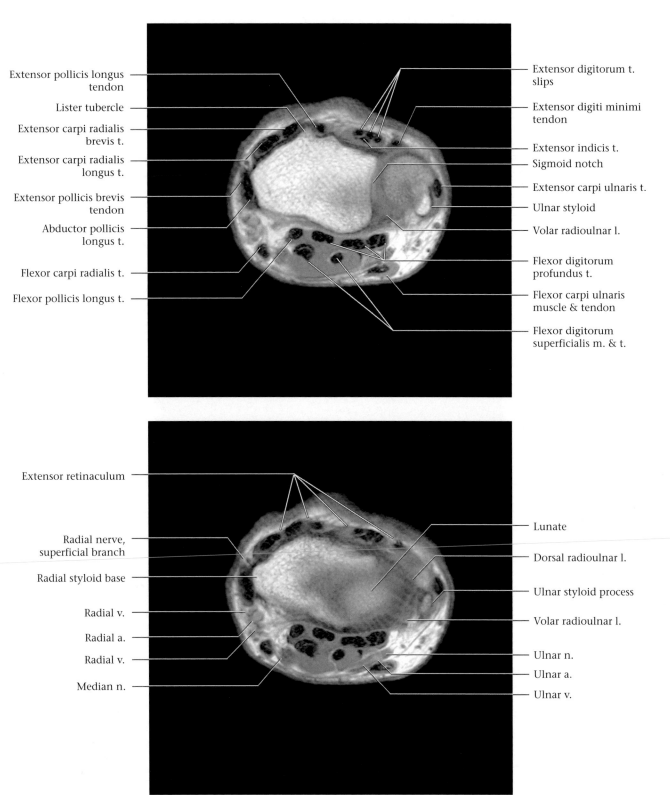

Extensor pollicis longus tendon

Lister tubercle

Extensor carpi radialis brevis t.

Extensor carpi radialis longus t.

Extensor pollicis brevis tendon

Abductor pollicis longus t.

Flexor carpi radialis t.

Flexor pollicis longus t.

Extensor digitorum t. slips

Extensor digiti minimi tendon

Extensor indicis t.

Sigmoid notch

Extensor carpi ulnaris t.

Ulnar styloid

Volar radioulnar l.

Flexor digitorum profundus t.

Flexor carpi ulnaris muscle & tendon

Flexor digitorum superficialis m. & t.

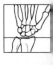

Extensor retinaculum

Radial nerve, superficial branch

Radial styloid base

Radial v.

Radial a.

Radial v.

Median n.

Lunate

Dorsal radioulnar l.

Ulnar styloid process

Volar radioulnar l.

Ulnar n.

Ulnar a.

Ulnar v.

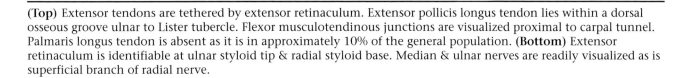

(Top) Extensor tendons are tethered by extensor retinaculum. Extensor pollicis longus tendon lies within a dorsal osseous groove ulnar to Lister tubercle. Flexor musculotendinous junctions are visualized proximal to carpal tunnel. Palmaris longus tendon is absent as it is in approximately 10% of the general population. **(Bottom)** Extensor retinaculum is identifiable at ulnar styloid tip & radial styloid base. Median & ulnar nerves are readily visualized as is superficial branch of radial nerve.

AXIAL T1 MR, RIGHT WRIST

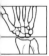

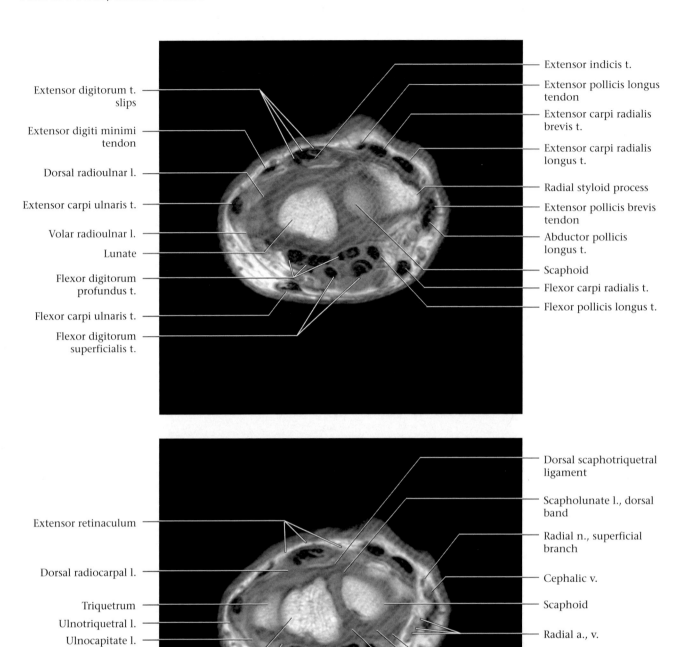

Extensor digitorum t. slips

Extensor digiti minimi tendon

Dorsal radioulnar l.

Extensor carpi ulnaris t.

Volar radioulnar l.

Lunate

Flexor digitorum profundus t.

Flexor carpi ulnaris t.

Flexor digitorum superficialis t.

Extensor indicis t.

Extensor pollicis longus tendon

Extensor carpi radialis brevis t.

Extensor carpi radialis longus t.

Radial styloid process

Extensor pollicis brevis tendon

Abductor pollicis longus t.

Scaphoid

Flexor carpi radialis t.

Flexor pollicis longus t.

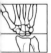

Extensor retinaculum

Dorsal radiocarpal l.

Triquetrum

Ulnotriquetral l.

Ulnocapitate l.

Lunate

Ulnolunate l.

Ulnar n.

Ulnar a., v.

Dorsal scaphotriquetral ligament

Scapholunate l., dorsal band

Radial n., superficial branch

Cephalic v.

Scaphoid

Radial a., v.

Radioscaphocapitate l.

Long radiolunate l.

Scapholunate l., volar band

Median n.

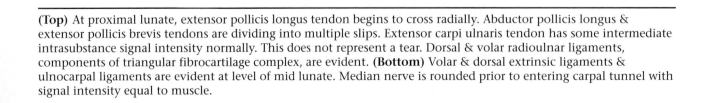

(Top) At proximal lunate, extensor pollicis longus tendon begins to cross radially. Abductor pollicis longus & extensor pollicis brevis tendons are dividing into multiple slips. Extensor carpi ulnaris tendon has some intermediate intrasubstance signal intensity normally. This does not represent a tear. Dorsal & volar radioulnar ligaments, components of triangular fibrocartilage complex, are evident. **(Bottom)** Volar & dorsal extrinsic ligaments & ulnocarpal ligaments are evident at level of mid lunate. Median nerve is rounded prior to entering carpal tunnel with signal intensity equal to muscle.

AXIAL T1 MR, LEFT WRIST

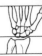

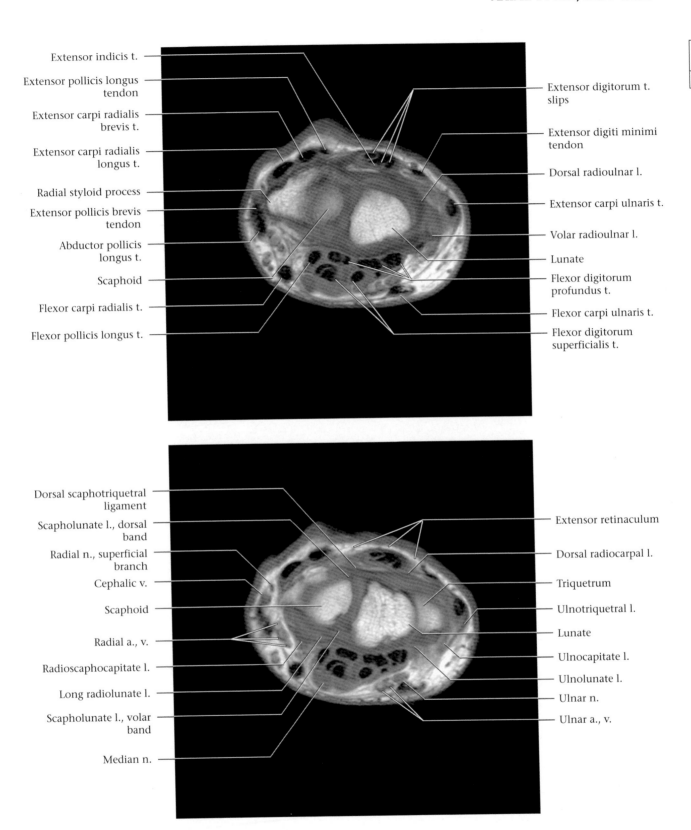

Extensor indicis t.

Extensor pollicis longus tendon

Extensor carpi radialis brevis t.

Extensor carpi radialis longus t.

Radial styloid process

Extensor pollicis brevis tendon

Abductor pollicis longus t.

Scaphoid

Flexor carpi radialis t.

Flexor pollicis longus t.

Extensor digitorum t. slips

Extensor digiti minimi tendon

Dorsal radioulnar l.

Extensor carpi ulnaris t.

Volar radioulnar l.

Lunate

Flexor digitorum profundus t.

Flexor carpi ulnaris t.

Flexor digitorum superficialis t.

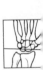

Dorsal scaphotriquetral ligament

Scapholunate l., dorsal band

Radial n., superficial branch

Cephalic v.

Scaphoid

Radial a., v.

Radioscaphocapitate l.

Long radiolunate l.

Scapholunate l., volar band

Median n.

Extensor retinaculum

Dorsal radiocarpal l.

Triquetrum

Ulnotriquetral l.

Lunate

Ulnocapitate l.

Ulnolunate l.

Ulnar n.

Ulnar a., v.

(Top) At proximal lunate, extensor pollicis longus tendon begins to cross radially. Abductor pollicis longus & extensor pollicis brevis tendons are dividing into multiple slips. Extensor carpi ulnaris tendon has some intermediate intrasubstance signal intensity normally. This does not represent a tear. Dorsal & volar radioulnar ligaments, components of triangular fibrocartilage complex, are evident. **(Bottom)** Volar & dorsal extrinsic ligaments & ulnocarpal ligaments are evident at level of mid lunate. Median nerve is rounded prior to entering carpal tunnel with signal intensity equal to muscle.

AXIAL T1 MR, RIGHT WRIST

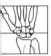

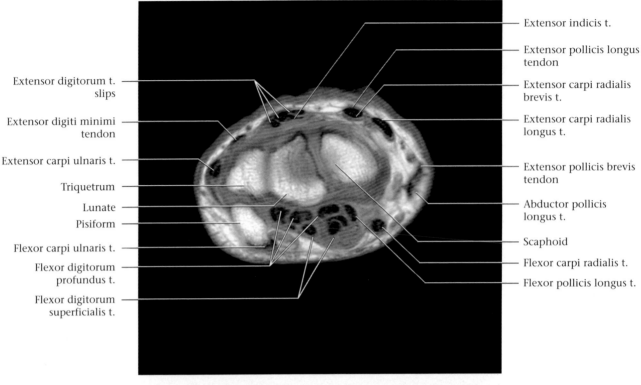

Extensor digitorum t. slips

Extensor digiti minimi tendon

Extensor carpi ulnaris t.

Triquetrum

Lunate

Pisiform

Flexor carpi ulnaris t.

Flexor digitorum profundus t.

Flexor digitorum superficialis t.

Extensor indicis t.

Extensor pollicis longus tendon

Extensor carpi radialis brevis t.

Extensor carpi radialis longus t.

Extensor pollicis brevis tendon

Abductor pollicis longus t.

Scaphoid

Flexor carpi radialis t.

Flexor pollicis longus t.

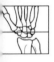

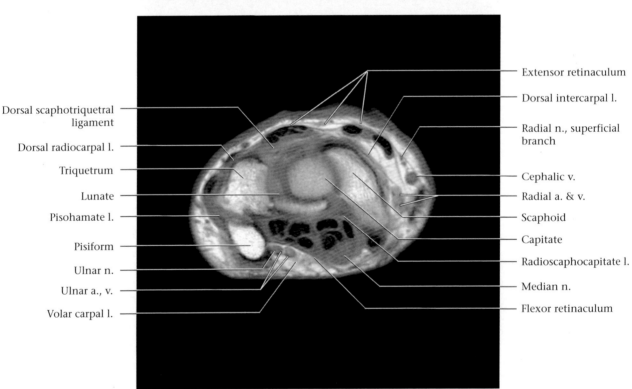

Dorsal scaphotriquetral ligament

Dorsal radiocarpal l.

Triquetrum

Lunate

Pisohamate l.

Pisiform

Ulnar n.

Ulnar a., v.

Volar carpal l.

Extensor retinaculum

Dorsal intercarpal l.

Radial n., superficial branch

Cephalic v.

Radial a. & v.

Scaphoid

Capitate

Radioscaphocapitate l.

Median n.

Flexor retinaculum

(Top) Slightly more distal, at level of distal lunate & proximal pisiform, extensor pollicis longus tendon is not easily identified as a separate structure as it crosses dorsal to extensor carpi radialis brevis tendon. **(Bottom)** Extensor retinaculum distal fibers are visualized at level of lunocapitate articulation. Extrinsic dorsal & volar ligaments are apparent as components of capsule. Median nerve remains rounded as it enters proximal carpal tunnel. Guyon canal is bordered by pisiform, deep & superficial bands of flexor retinaculum, transverse carpal ligament proximally & volar carpal ligament.

WRIST OVERVIEW

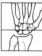

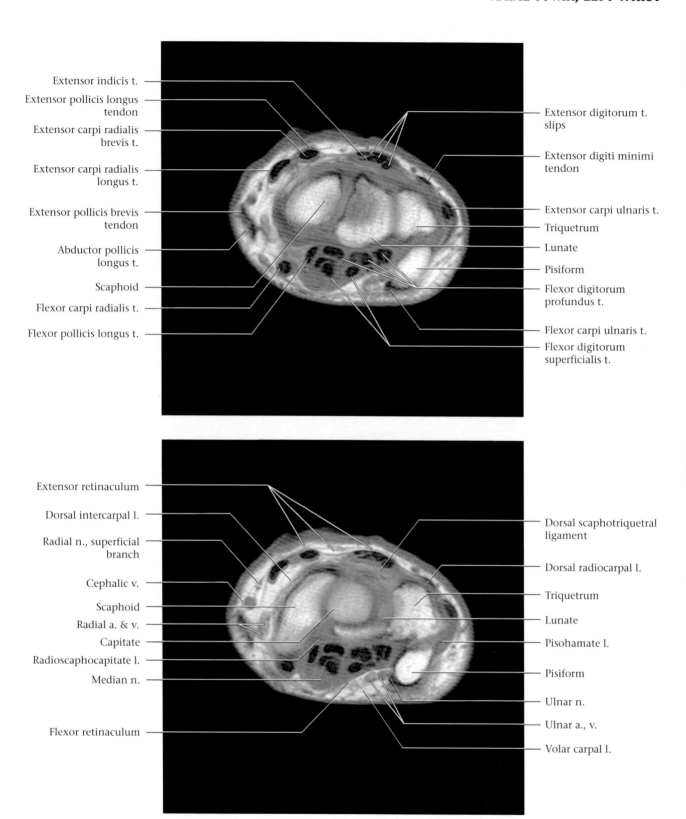

Top image labels (left side):
- Extensor indicis t.
- Extensor pollicis longus tendon
- Extensor carpi radialis brevis t.
- Extensor carpi radialis longus t.
- Extensor pollicis brevis tendon
- Abductor pollicis longus t.
- Scaphoid
- Flexor carpi radialis t.
- Flexor pollicis longus t.

Top image labels (right side):
- Extensor digitorum t. slips
- Extensor digiti minimi tendon
- Extensor carpi ulnaris t.
- Triquetrum
- Lunate
- Pisiform
- Flexor digitorum profundus t.
- Flexor carpi ulnaris t.
- Flexor digitorum superficialis t.

Bottom image labels (left side):
- Extensor retinaculum
- Dorsal intercarpal l.
- Radial n., superficial branch
- Cephalic v.
- Scaphoid
- Radial a. & v.
- Capitate
- Radioscaphocapitate l.
- Median n.
- Flexor retinaculum

Bottom image labels (right side):
- Dorsal scaphotriquetral ligament
- Dorsal radiocarpal l.
- Triquetrum
- Lunate
- Pisohamate l.
- Pisiform
- Ulnar n.
- Ulnar a., v.
- Volar carpal l.

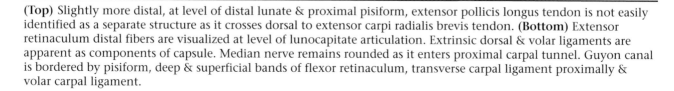

(Top) Slightly more distal, at level of distal lunate & proximal pisiform, extensor pollicis longus tendon is not easily identified as a separate structure as it crosses dorsal to extensor carpi radialis brevis tendon. **(Bottom)** Extensor retinaculum distal fibers are visualized at level of lunocapitate articulation. Extrinsic dorsal & volar ligaments are apparent as components of capsule. Median nerve remains rounded as it enters proximal carpal tunnel. Guyon canal is bordered by pisiform, deep & superficial bands of flexor retinaculum, transverse carpal ligament proximally & volar carpal ligament.

AXIAL T1 MR, RIGHT WRIST

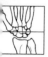

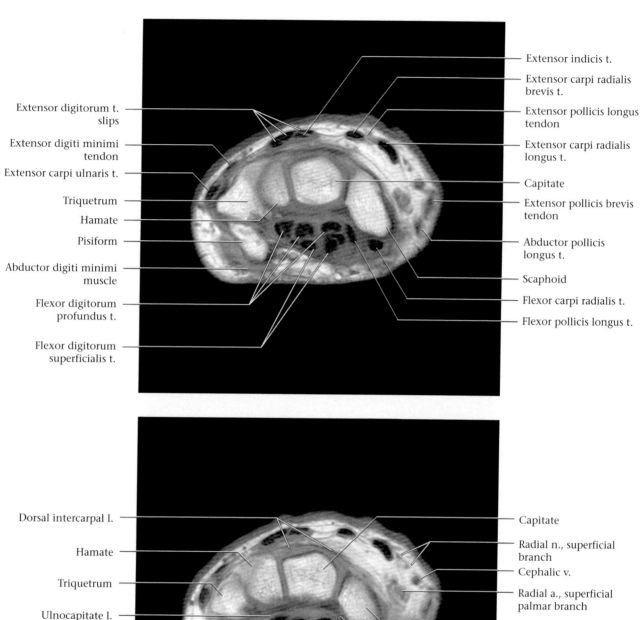

Extensor digitorum t. slips

Extensor digiti minimi tendon

Extensor carpi ulnaris t.

Triquetrum

Hamate

Pisiform

Abductor digiti minimi muscle

Flexor digitorum profundus t.

Flexor digitorum superficialis t.

Extensor indicis t.

Extensor carpi radialis brevis t.

Extensor pollicis longus tendon

Extensor carpi radialis longus t.

Capitate

Extensor pollicis brevis tendon

Abductor pollicis longus t.

Scaphoid

Flexor carpi radialis t.

Flexor pollicis longus t.

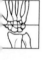

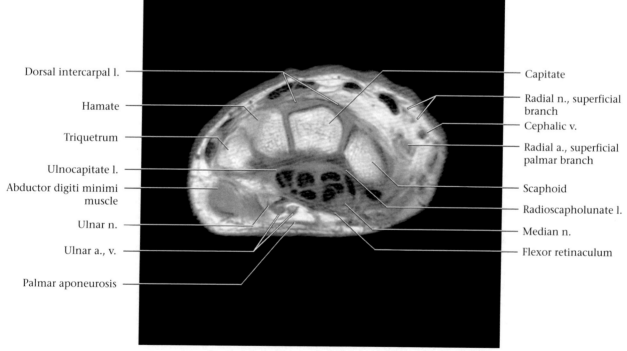

Dorsal intercarpal l.

Hamate

Triquetrum

Ulnocapitate l.

Abductor digiti minimi muscle

Ulnar n.

Ulnar a., v.

Palmar aponeurosis

Capitate

Radial n., superficial branch

Cephalic v.

Radial a., superficial palmar branch

Scaphoid

Radioscapholunate l.

Median n.

Flexor retinaculum

(Top) At distal pisotriquetral articulation, Guyon canal is located radial to pisiform & contains ulnar nerve, artery & vein. Extensor pollicis longus tendon crosses dorsal to extensor carpi radialis brevis tendon & its obliquity makes it difficult to distinguish as a separate tendon. **(Bottom)** At the level of distal triquetrum & distal pole of scaphoid, ulnar nerve branches into deep & superficial branches. Note beginning of thenar & hypothenar muscles which originate from flexor retinaculum.

WRIST OVERVIEW

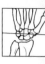

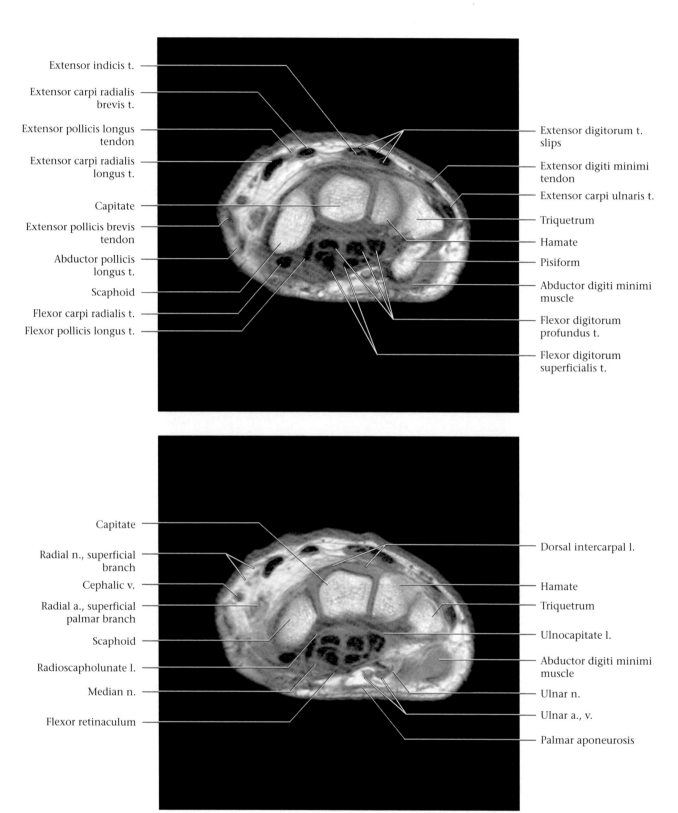

Extensor indicis t.

Extensor carpi radialis brevis t.

Extensor pollicis longus tendon

Extensor carpi radialis longus t.

Capitate

Extensor pollicis brevis tendon

Abductor pollicis longus t.

Scaphoid

Flexor carpi radialis t.

Flexor pollicis longus t.

Extensor digitorum t. slips

Extensor digiti minimi tendon

Extensor carpi ulnaris t.

Triquetrum

Hamate

Pisiform

Abductor digiti minimi muscle

Flexor digitorum profundus t.

Flexor digitorum superficialis t.

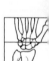

Capitate

Radial n., superficial branch

Cephalic v.

Radial a., superficial palmar branch

Scaphoid

Radioscapholunate l.

Median n.

Flexor retinaculum

Dorsal intercarpal l.

Hamate

Triquetrum

Ulnocapitate l.

Abductor digiti minimi muscle

Ulnar n.

Ulnar a., v.

Palmar aponeurosis

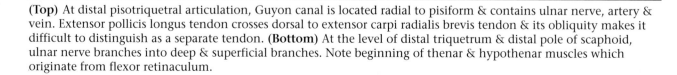

(Top) At distal pisotriquetral articulation, Guyon canal is located radial to pisiform & contains ulnar nerve, artery & vein. Extensor pollicis longus tendon crosses dorsal to extensor carpi radialis brevis tendon & its obliquity makes it difficult to distinguish as a separate tendon. **(Bottom)** At the level of distal triquetrum & distal pole of scaphoid, ulnar nerve branches into deep & superficial branches. Note beginning of thenar & hypothenar muscles which originate from flexor retinaculum.

WRIST OVERVIEW

AXIAL T1 MR, RIGHT WRIST

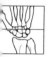

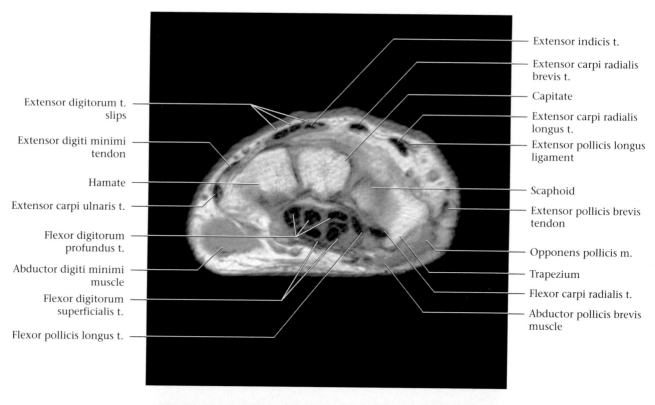

Extensor indicis t.

Extensor carpi radialis brevis t.

Capitate

Extensor carpi radialis longus t.

Extensor pollicis longus ligament

Scaphoid

Extensor pollicis brevis tendon

Opponens pollicis m.

Trapezium

Flexor carpi radialis t.

Abductor pollicis brevis muscle

Extensor digitorum t. slips

Extensor digiti minimi tendon

Hamate

Extensor carpi ulnaris t.

Flexor digitorum profundus t.

Abductor digiti minimi muscle

Flexor digitorum superficialis t.

Flexor pollicis longus t.

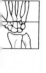

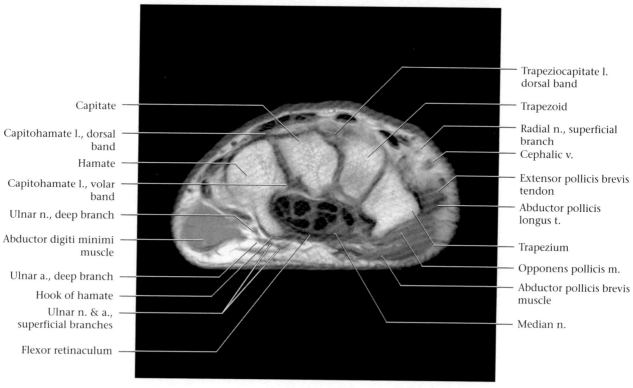

Trapeziocapitate l. dorsal band

Trapezoid

Radial n., superficial branch

Cephalic v.

Extensor pollicis brevis tendon

Abductor pollicis longus t.

Trapezium

Opponens pollicis m.

Abductor pollicis brevis muscle

Median n.

Capitate

Capitohamate l., dorsal band

Hamate

Capitohamate l., volar band

Ulnar n., deep branch

Abductor digiti minimi muscle

Ulnar a., deep branch

Hook of hamate

Ulnar n. & a., superficial branches

Flexor retinaculum

(Top) Hamate body (proximal to hook) & scaphotrapeziotrapezoid articulation correspond to mid-level carpal tunnel. EPL tendon intersects dorsally with ECRL tendon. The median nerve is slightly flattened. **(Bottom)** At hook of hamate & trapezium tubercle, ulnar nerve branches into deep & superficial branches with deep branch passing dorsal & ulnar to hamate hook. Portions of volar & dorsal interosseous ligaments are visualized.

WRIST OVERVIEW

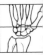

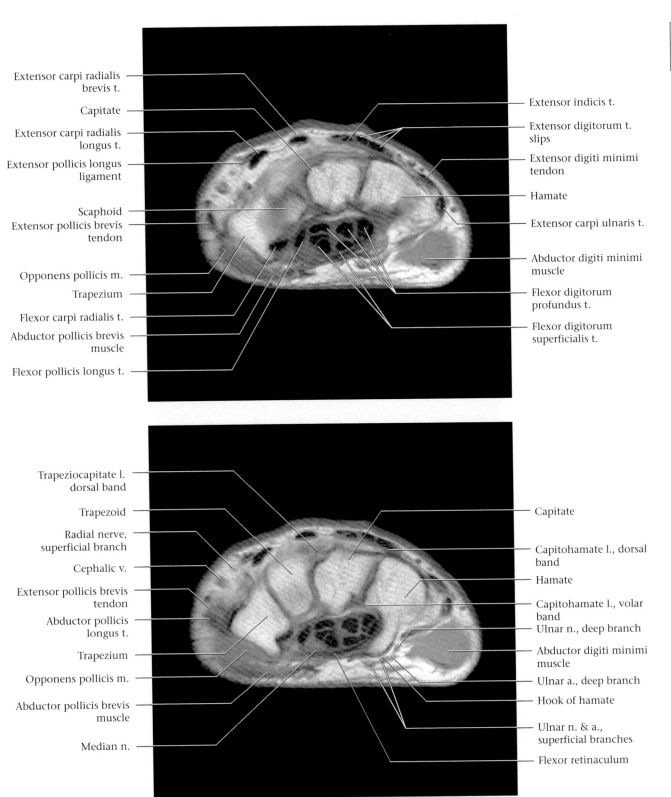

Extensor carpi radialis brevis t.

Capitate

Extensor carpi radialis longus t.

Extensor pollicis longus ligament

Scaphoid

Extensor pollicis brevis tendon

Opponens pollicis m.

Trapezium

Flexor carpi radialis t.

Abductor pollicis brevis muscle

Flexor pollicis longus t.

Extensor indicis t.

Extensor digitorum t. slips

Extensor digiti minimi tendon

Hamate

Extensor carpi ulnaris t.

Abductor digiti minimi muscle

Flexor digitorum profundus t.

Flexor digitorum superficialis t.

Trapeziocapitate l. dorsal band

Trapezoid

Radial nerve, superficial branch

Cephalic v.

Extensor pollicis brevis tendon

Abductor pollicis longus t.

Trapezium

Opponens pollicis m.

Abductor pollicis brevis muscle

Median n.

Capitate

Capitohamate l., dorsal band

Hamate

Capitohamate l., volar band

Ulnar n., deep branch

Abductor digiti minimi muscle

Ulnar a., deep branch

Hook of hamate

Ulnar n. & a., superficial branches

Flexor retinaculum

(Top) Hamate body (proximal to hook) & scaphotrapeziotrapezoid articulation correspond to mid-level carpal tunnel. EPL tendon intersects dorsally with ECRL tendon. The median nerve is slightly flattened. **(Bottom)** At hook of hamate & trapezium tubercle, ulnar nerve branches into deep & superficial branches with deep branch passing dorsal & ulnar to hamate hook. Portions of volar & dorsal interosseous ligaments are visualized.

AXIAL T1 MR, RIGHT WRIST

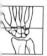

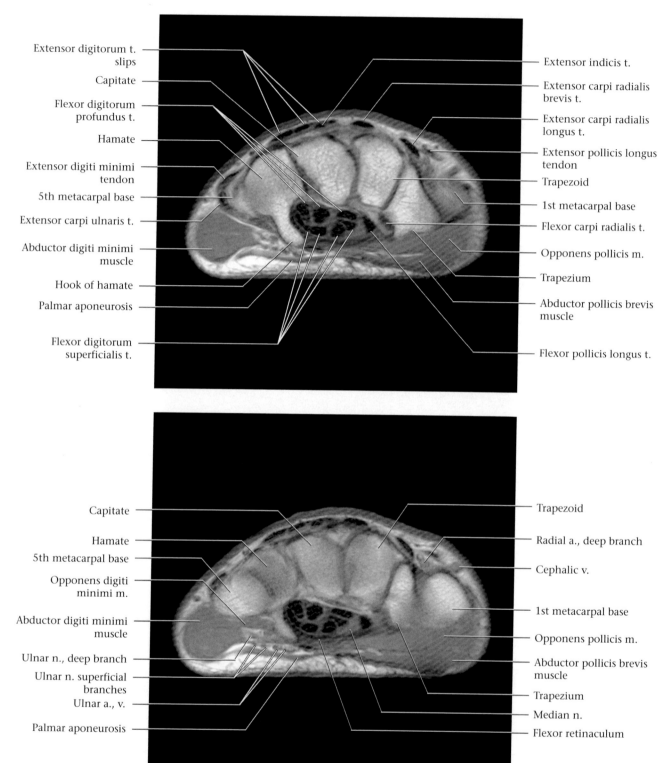

Extensor digitorum t. slips

Capitate

Flexor digitorum profundus t.

Hamate

Extensor digiti minimi tendon

5th metacarpal base

Extensor carpi ulnaris t.

Abductor digiti minimi muscle

Hook of hamate

Palmar aponeurosis

Flexor digitorum superficialis t.

Extensor indicis t.

Extensor carpi radialis brevis t.

Extensor carpi radialis longus t.

Extensor pollicis longus tendon

Trapezoid

1st metacarpal base

Flexor carpi radialis t.

Opponens pollicis m.

Trapezium

Abductor pollicis brevis muscle

Flexor pollicis longus t.

Capitate

Hamate

5th metacarpal base

Opponens digiti minimi m.

Abductor digiti minimi muscle

Ulnar n., deep branch

Ulnar n. superficial branches

Ulnar a., v.

Palmar aponeurosis

Trapezoid

Radial a., deep branch

Cephalic v.

1st metacarpal base

Opponens pollicis m.

Abductor pollicis brevis muscle

Trapezium

Median n.

Flexor retinaculum

(Top) At distal hook of hamate, flexor digitorum tendons pass through carpal tunnel with two most superficial tendons extending to long & ring fingers, two intermediate tendons to index & small fingers & profundus tendons comprising deep layer. **(Bottom)** Distal carpal tunnel contents are passing through narrowest portion of carpal tunnel at level of carpometacarpal articulations. Ulnar nerve deep branches pass dorsal & distal to hook of hamate. Ulnar nerve superficial branches continue distally into palm. A portion of deep palmar arch (radial artery, deep branch) is visualized. However, major dorsal & volar vascular arches are typically not readily visualized.

AXIAL T1 MR, LEFT WRIST

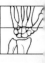

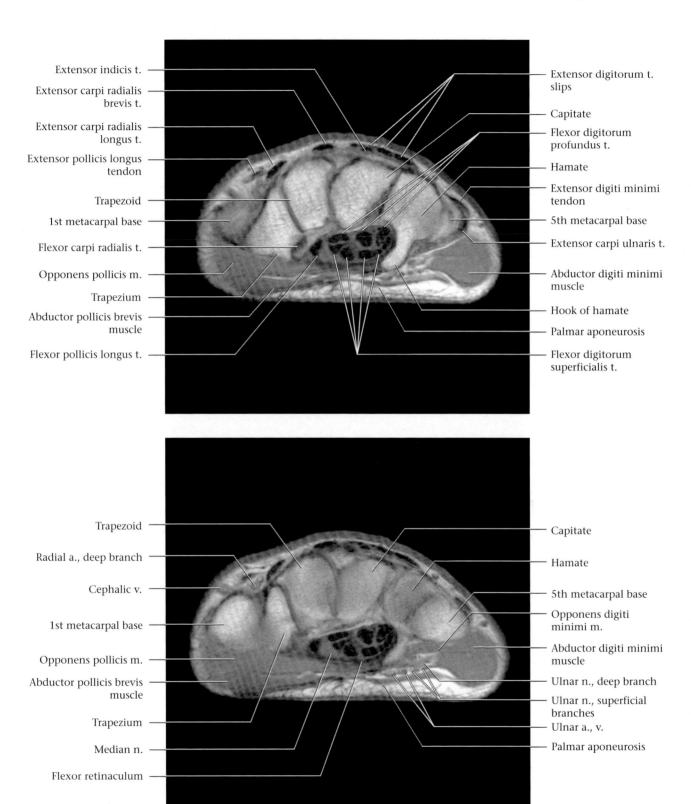

Extensor indicis t.

Extensor carpi radialis brevis t.

Extensor carpi radialis longus t.

Extensor pollicis longus tendon

Trapezoid

1st metacarpal base

Flexor carpi radialis t.

Opponens pollicis m.

Trapezium

Abductor pollicis brevis muscle

Flexor pollicis longus t.

Extensor digitorum t. slips

Capitate

Flexor digitorum profundus t.

Hamate

Extensor digiti minimi tendon

5th metacarpal base

Extensor carpi ulnaris t.

Abductor digiti minimi muscle

Hook of hamate

Palmar aponeurosis

Flexor digitorum superficialis t.

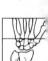

Trapezoid

Radial a., deep branch

Cephalic v.

1st metacarpal base

Opponens pollicis m.

Abductor pollicis brevis muscle

Trapezium

Median n.

Flexor retinaculum

Capitate

Hamate

5th metacarpal base

Opponens digiti minimi m.

Abductor digiti minimi muscle

Ulnar n., deep branch

Ulnar n., superficial branches

Ulnar a., v.

Palmar aponeurosis

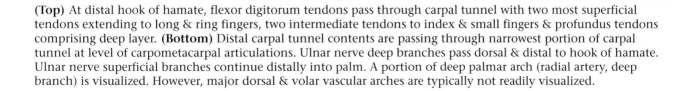

(Top) At distal hook of hamate, flexor digitorum tendons pass through carpal tunnel with two most superficial tendons extending to long & ring fingers, two intermediate tendons to index & small fingers & profundus tendons comprising deep layer. **(Bottom)** Distal carpal tunnel contents are passing through narrowest portion of carpal tunnel at level of carpometacarpal articulations. Ulnar nerve deep branches pass dorsal & distal to hook of hamate. Ulnar nerve superficial branches continue distally into palm. A portion of deep palmar arch (radial artery, deep branch) is visualized. However, major dorsal & volar vascular arches are typically not readily visualized.

AXIAL T1 MR, RIGHT WRIST

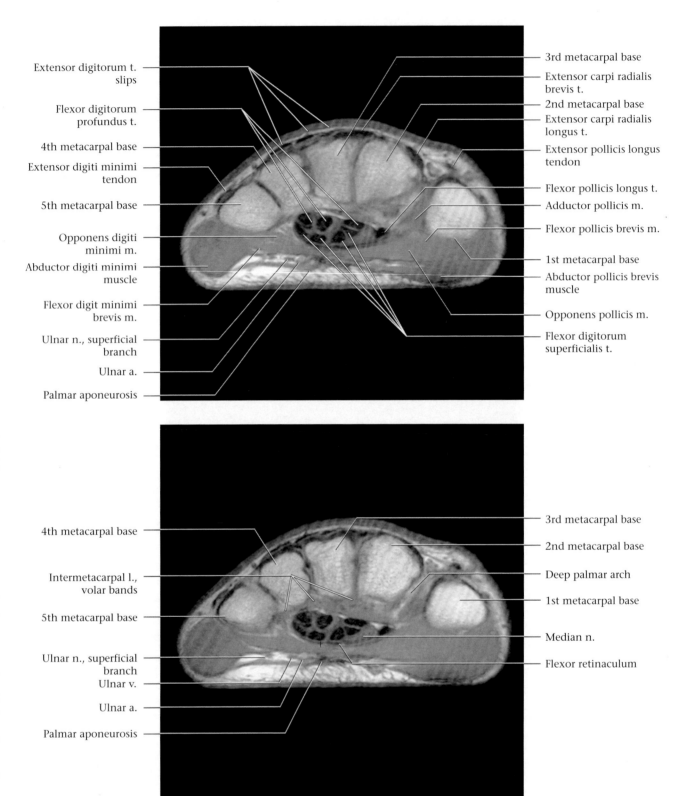

Extensor digitorum t. slips

Flexor digitorum profundus t.

4th metacarpal base

Extensor digiti minimi tendon

5th metacarpal base

Opponens digiti minimi m.

Abductor digiti minimi muscle

Flexor digit minimi brevis m.

Ulnar n., superficial branch

Ulnar a.

Palmar aponeurosis

3rd metacarpal base

Extensor carpi radialis brevis t.

2nd metacarpal base

Extensor carpi radialis longus t.

Extensor pollicis longus tendon

Flexor pollicis longus t.

Adductor pollicis m.

Flexor pollicis brevis m.

1st metacarpal base

Abductor pollicis brevis muscle

Opponens pollicis m.

Flexor digitorum superficialis t.

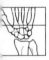

4th metacarpal base

Intermetacarpal l., volar bands

5th metacarpal base

Ulnar n., superficial branch

Ulnar v.

Ulnar a.

Palmar aponeurosis

3rd metacarpal base

2nd metacarpal base

Deep palmar arch

1st metacarpal base

Median n.

Flexor retinaculum

(Top) Thenar & hypothenar musculature is well-developed at carpometacarpal articulation. Extensor pollicis longus tendon now becomes evident again as its course becomes more perpendicular to axial plane. Extensor digitorum tendons are becoming flattened near insertion sites. **(Bottom)** At distal flexor retinaculum & metacarpal bases, the carpal tunnel ends with median nerve branching into muscular branches & digital nerves. Ulnar nerve, superficial branch, remains evident. A small portion of radial contribution to deep palmar arch is seen between 1st & 2nd metacarpal bases.

AXIAL T1 MR, LEFT WRIST

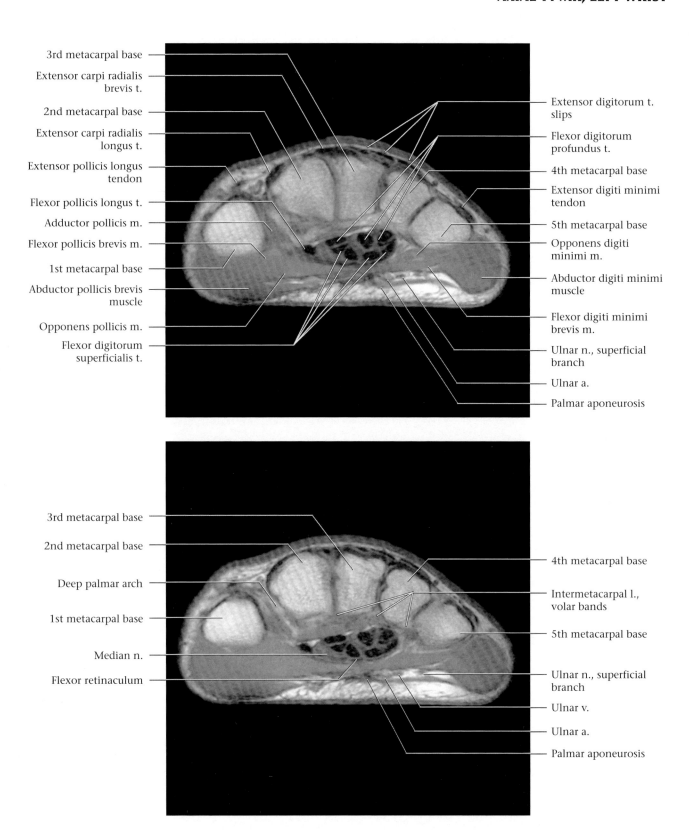

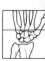

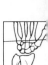

Top image labels (left):
- 3rd metacarpal base
- Extensor carpi radialis brevis t.
- 2nd metacarpal base
- Extensor carpi radialis longus t.
- Extensor pollicis longus tendon
- Flexor pollicis longus t.
- Adductor pollicis m.
- Flexor pollicis brevis m.
- 1st metacarpal base
- Abductor pollicis brevis muscle
- Opponens pollicis m.
- Flexor digitorum superficialis t.

Top image labels (right):
- Extensor digitorum t. slips
- Flexor digitorum profundus t.
- 4th metacarpal base
- Extensor digiti minimi tendon
- 5th metacarpal base
- Opponens digiti minimi m.
- Abductor digiti minimi muscle
- Flexor digiti minimi brevis m.
- Ulnar n., superficial branch
- Ulnar a.
- Palmar aponeurosis

Bottom image labels (left):
- 3rd metacarpal base
- 2nd metacarpal base
- Deep palmar arch
- 1st metacarpal base
- Median n.
- Flexor retinaculum

Bottom image labels (right):
- 4th metacarpal base
- Intermetacarpal l., volar bands
- 5th metacarpal base
- Ulnar n., superficial branch
- Ulnar v.
- Ulnar a.
- Palmar aponeurosis

(Top) Thenar & hypothenar musculature is well-developed at carpometacarpal articulation. Extensor pollicis longus tendon now becomes evident again as its course becomes more perpendicular to axial plane. Extensor digitorum tendons are becoming flattened near insertion sites. **(Bottom)** At distal flexor retinaculum & metacarpal bases, the carpal tunnel ends with median nerve branching into muscular branches & digital nerves. Ulnar nerve, superficial branch, remains evident. A small portion of radial contribution to deep palmar arch is seen between 1st & 2nd metacarpal bases.

AXIAL T1 MR, RIGHT WRIST

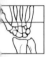

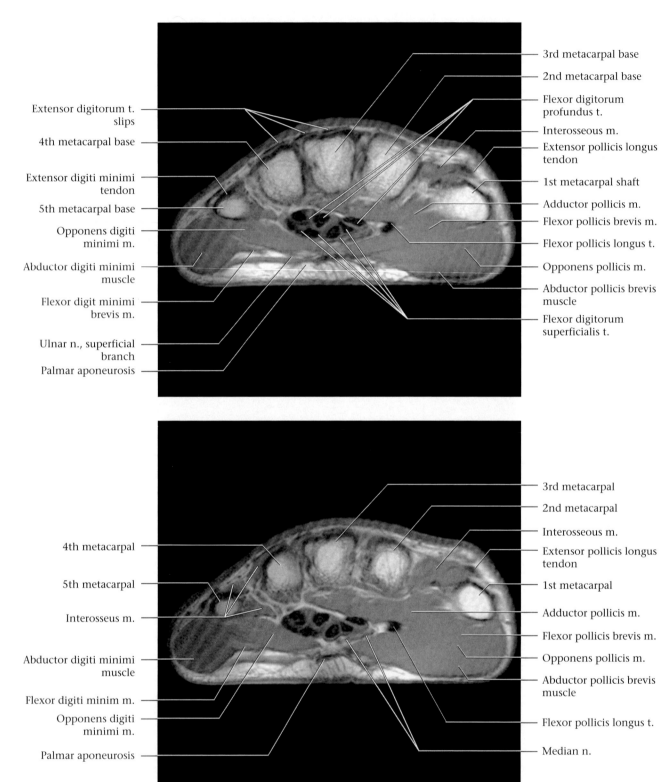

Extensor digitorum t. slips

4th metacarpal base

Extensor digiti minimi tendon

5th metacarpal base

Opponens digiti minimi m.

Abductor digiti minimi muscle

Flexor digit minimi brevis m.

Ulnar n., superficial branch

Palmar aponeurosis

3rd metacarpal base

2nd metacarpal base

Flexor digitorum profundus t.

Interosseous m.

Extensor pollicis longus tendon

1st metacarpal shaft

Adductor pollicis m.

Flexor pollicis brevis m.

Flexor pollicis longus t.

Opponens pollicis m.

Abductor pollicis brevis muscle

Flexor digitorum superficialis t.

4th metacarpal

5th metacarpal

Interosseus m.

Abductor digiti minimi muscle

Flexor digiti minim m.

Opponens digiti minimi m.

Palmar aponeurosis

3rd metacarpal

2nd metacarpal

Interosseous m.

Extensor pollicis longus tendon

1st metacarpal

Adductor pollicis m.

Flexor pollicis brevis m.

Opponens pollicis m.

Abductor pollicis brevis muscle

Flexor pollicis longus t.

Median n.

(Top) Metacarpal bases mark transition from wrist into hand. Extensor digitorum tendons flatten & spread across dorsum of metacarpal bases. **(Bottom)** Interosseous musculature is evident at metacarpal bases. Thenar & hypothenar musculature is well-developed. Distal branches of radial & ulnar nerves are not discernible, but median nerve branches are visible.

WRIST OVERVIEW

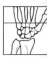

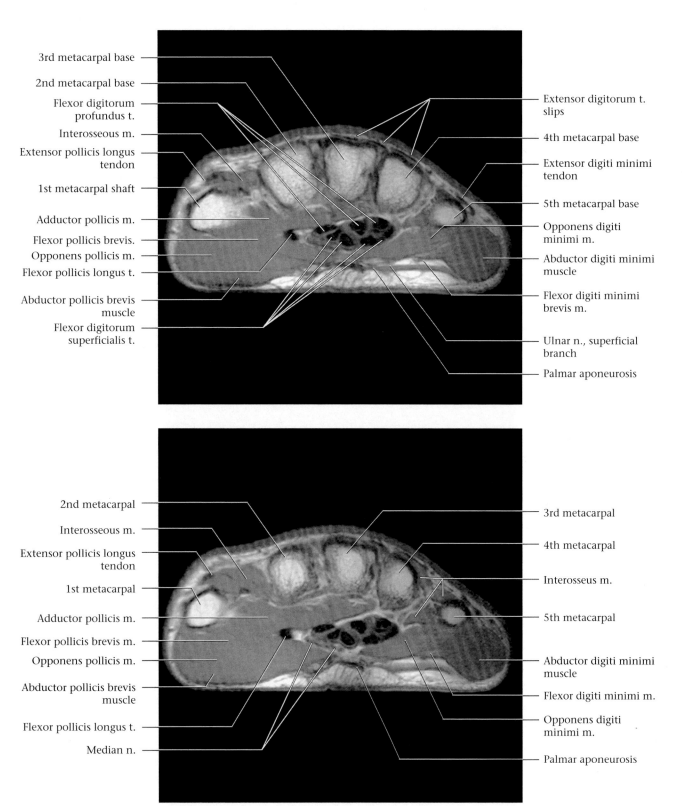

3rd metacarpal base

2nd metacarpal base

Flexor digitorum profundus t.

Interosseous m.

Extensor pollicis longus tendon

1st metacarpal shaft

Adductor pollicis m.

Flexor pollicis brevis.

Opponens pollicis m.

Flexor pollicis longus t.

Abductor pollicis brevis muscle

Flexor digitorum superficialis t.

Extensor digitorum t. slips

4th metacarpal base

Extensor digiti minimi tendon

5th metacarpal base

Opponens digiti minimi m.

Abductor digiti minimi muscle

Flexor digiti minimi brevis m.

Ulnar n., superficial branch

Palmar aponeurosis

2nd metacarpal

Interosseous m.

Extensor pollicis longus tendon

1st metacarpal

Adductor pollicis m.

Flexor pollicis brevis m.

Opponens pollicis m.

Abductor pollicis brevis muscle

Flexor pollicis longus t.

Median n.

3rd metacarpal

4th metacarpal

Interosseus m.

5th metacarpal

Abductor digiti minimi muscle

Flexor digiti minimi m.

Opponens digiti minimi m.

Palmar aponeurosis

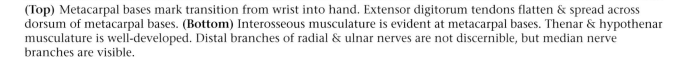

(Top) Metacarpal bases mark transition from wrist into hand. Extensor digitorum tendons flatten & spread across dorsum of metacarpal bases. **(Bottom)** Interosseous musculature is evident at metacarpal bases. Thenar & hypothenar musculature is well-developed. Distal branches of radial & ulnar nerves are not discernible, but median nerve branches are visible.

CORONAL T1 MR, RIGHT WRIST

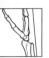

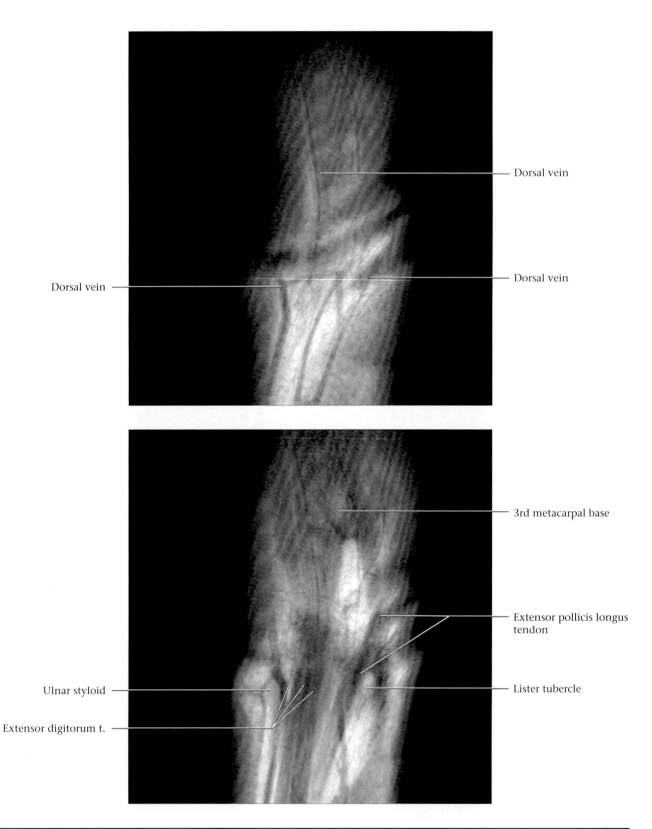

Dorsal vein

Dorsal vein

Dorsal vein

3rd metacarpal base

Extensor pollicis longus tendon

Ulnar styloid

Lister tubercle

Extensor digitorum t.

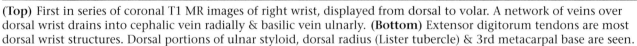

(Top) First in series of coronal T1 MR images of right wrist, displayed from dorsal to volar. A network of veins over dorsal wrist drains into cephalic vein radially & basilic vein ulnarly. **(Bottom)** Extensor digitorum tendons are most dorsal wrist structures. Dorsal portions of ulnar styloid, dorsal radius (Lister tubercle) & 3rd metacarpal base are seen.

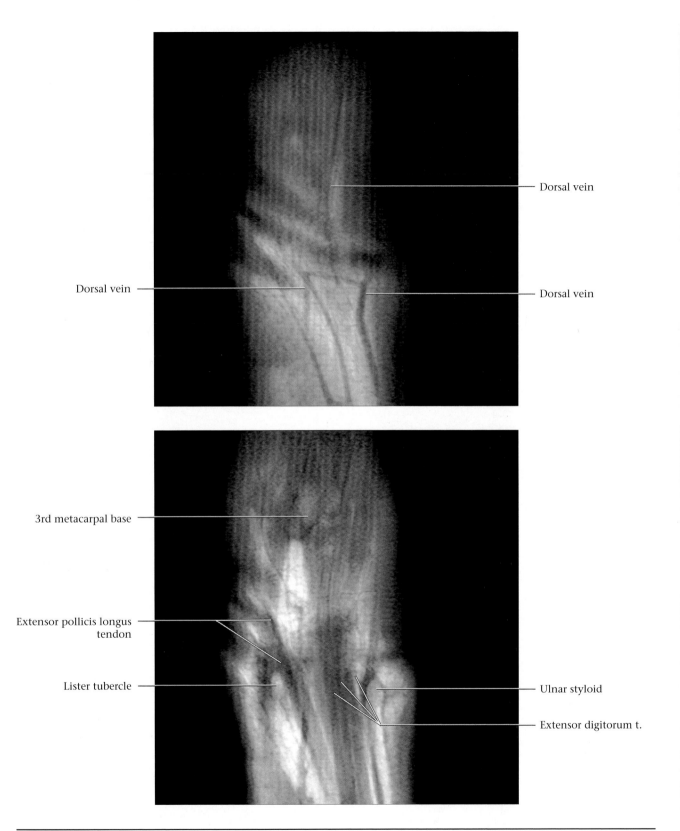

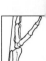

Dorsal vein

Dorsal vein — — **Dorsal vein**

3rd metacarpal base

Extensor pollicis longus tendon

Lister tubercle

Ulnar styloid

Extensor digitorum t.

(Top) First in series of coronal T1 MR images of right wrist, displayed from dorsal to volar. A network of veins over dorsal wrist drains into cephalic vein radially & basilic vein ulnarly. **(Bottom)** Extensor digitorum tendons are most dorsal wrist structures. Dorsal portions of ulnar styloid, dorsal radius (Lister tubercle) & 3rd metacarpal base are seen.

CORONAL T1 MR, RIGHT WRIST

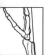

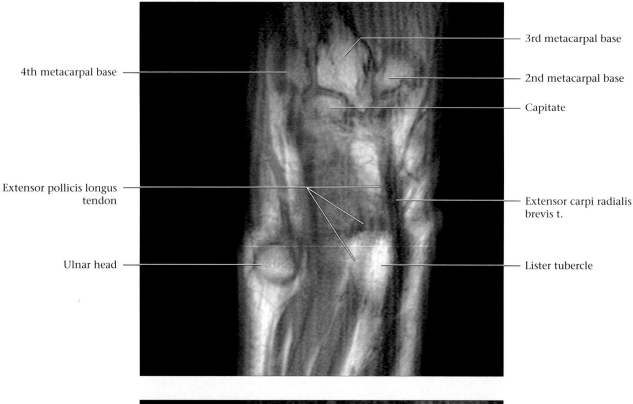

4th metacarpal base —

Extensor pollicis longus tendon —

Ulnar head —

— 3rd metacarpal base

— 2nd metacarpal base

— Capitate

— Extensor carpi radialis brevis t.

— Lister tubercle

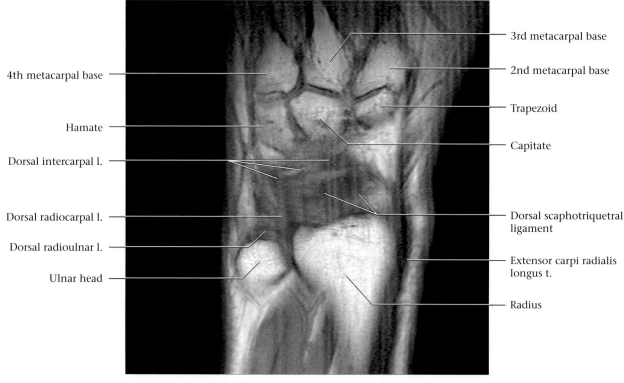

4th metacarpal base —

Hamate —

Dorsal intercarpal l. —

Dorsal radiocarpal l. —

Dorsal radioulnar l. —

Ulnar head —

— 3rd metacarpal base

— 2nd metacarpal base

— Trapezoid

— Capitate

— Dorsal scaphotriquetral ligament

— Extensor carpi radialis longus t.

— Radius

(Top) Lister tubercle & ulnar head are dorsally positioned with extensor pollicis longus tendon passing ulnar to tubercle in a shallow groove & coursing radially over extensor carpi radialis (ECR) tendon. ECR passes radial to tubercle. **(Bottom)** Dorsal extrinsic & intrinsic ligaments are visualized as thin low signal intensity bands coursing horizontally across wrist. Though many of these small, thin ligaments may be difficult to identify as discrete structures, dorsal intercarpal & dorsal radiocarpal ligaments are routinely seen.

CORONAL T1 MR, LEFT WRIST

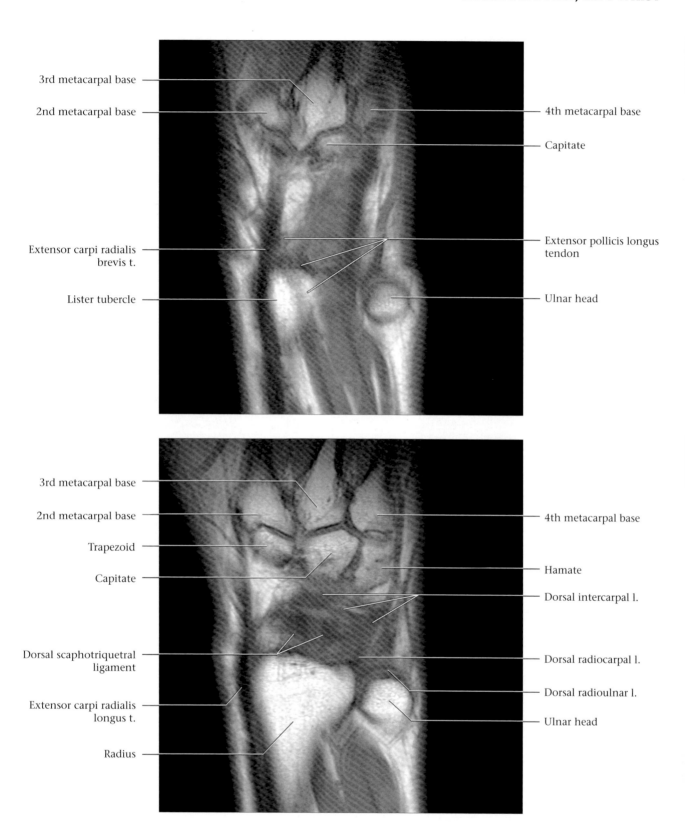

3rd metacarpal base

2nd metacarpal base

4th metacarpal base

Capitate

Extensor carpi radialis brevis t.

Extensor pollicis longus tendon

Lister tubercle

Ulnar head

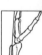

3rd metacarpal base

2nd metacarpal base

Trapezoid

Capitate

4th metacarpal base

Hamate

Dorsal intercarpal l.

Dorsal scaphotriquetral ligament

Dorsal radiocarpal l.

Dorsal radioulnar l.

Extensor carpi radialis longus t.

Ulnar head

Radius

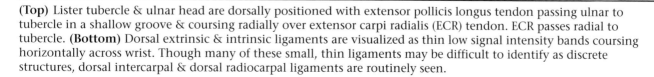

(Top) Lister tubercle & ulnar head are dorsally positioned with extensor pollicis longus tendon passing ulnar to tubercle in a shallow groove & coursing radially over extensor carpi radialis (ECR) tendon. ECR passes radial to tubercle. **(Bottom)** Dorsal extrinsic & intrinsic ligaments are visualized as thin low signal intensity bands coursing horizontally across wrist. Though many of these small, thin ligaments may be difficult to identify as discrete structures, dorsal intercarpal & dorsal radiocarpal ligaments are routinely seen.

Wrist

III

CORONAL T1 MR, RIGHT WRIST

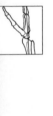

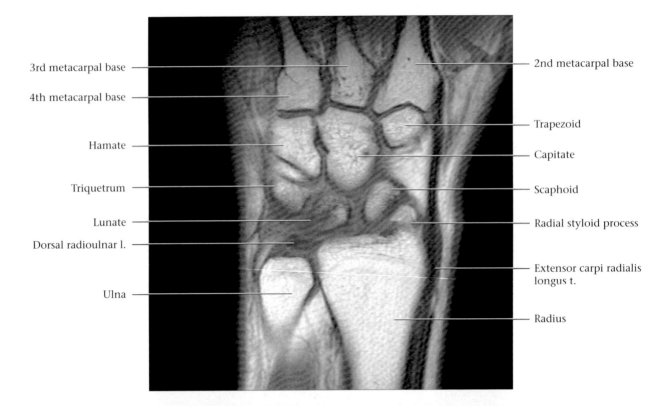

3rd metacarpal base

4th metacarpal base

Hamate

Triquetrum

Lunate

Dorsal radioulnar l.

Ulna

2nd metacarpal base

Trapezoid

Capitate

Scaphoid

Radial styloid process

Extensor carpi radialis longus t.

Radius

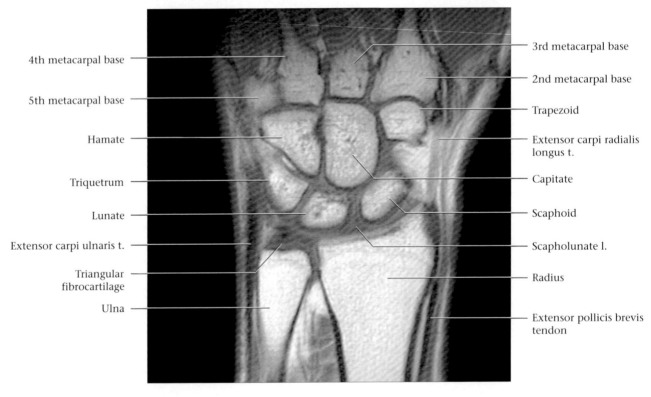

4th metacarpal base

5th metacarpal base

Hamate

Triquetrum

Lunate

Extensor carpi ulnaris t.

Triangular fibrocartilage

Ulna

3rd metacarpal base

2nd metacarpal base

Trapezoid

Extensor carpi radialis longus t.

Capitate

Scaphoid

Scapholunate l.

Radius

Extensor pollicis brevis tendon

(Top) Slightly volar to the dorsal ligaments, the dorsal radioulnar ligament, a component of triangular fibrocartilage complex is evident as are dorsal proximal & distal row carpi. Extensor carpi radialis tendon courses distally to attach to 2nd metacarpal base. **(Bottom)** Ulnar head is seated in sigmoid notch of distal radius. Triangular fibrocartilage articular disc is readily visualized. Extensor carpi ulnaris (ECU) tendon passes dorsally in ECU ulnar groove. Small intrinsic carpal row ligaments, scapholunate & lunotriquetral, are present but poorly seen on T1 imaging.

CORONAL T1 MR, LEFT WRIST

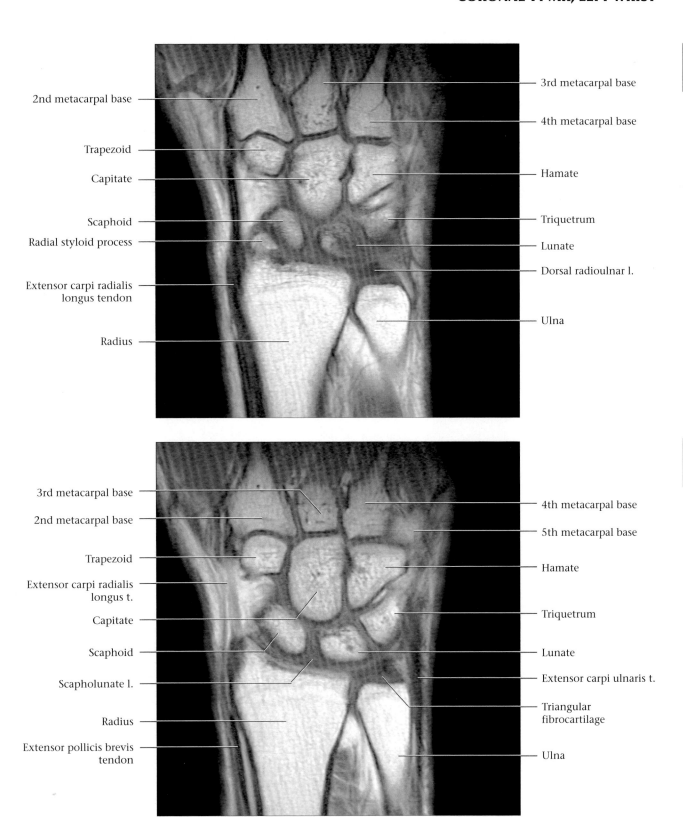

Top image labels:
- 2nd metacarpal base
- Trapezoid
- Capitate
- Scaphoid
- Radial styloid process
- Extensor carpi radialis longus tendon
- Radius
- 3rd metacarpal base
- 4th metacarpal base
- Hamate
- Triquetrum
- Lunate
- Dorsal radioulnar l.
- Ulna

Bottom image labels:
- 3rd metacarpal base
- 2nd metacarpal base
- Trapezoid
- Extensor carpi radialis longus t.
- Capitate
- Scaphoid
- Scapholunate l.
- Radius
- Extensor pollicis brevis tendon
- 4th metacarpal base
- 5th metacarpal base
- Hamate
- Triquetrum
- Lunate
- Extensor carpi ulnaris t.
- Triangular fibrocartilage
- Ulna

(Top) Slightly volar to the dorsal ligaments, the dorsal radioulnar ligament, a component of triangular fibrocartilage complex is evident as are dorsal proximal & distal row carpi. Extensor carpi radialis tendon courses distally to attach to 2nd metacarpal base. **(Bottom)** Ulnar head is seated in sigmoid notch of distal radius. Triangular fibrocartilage articular disc is readily visualized. Extensor carpi ulnaris (ECU) tendon passes dorsally in ECU ulnar groove. Small intrinsic carpal row ligaments, scapholunate & lunotriquetral, are present but poorly seen on T1 imaging.

Wrist

III

CORONAL T1 MR, RIGHT WRIST

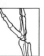

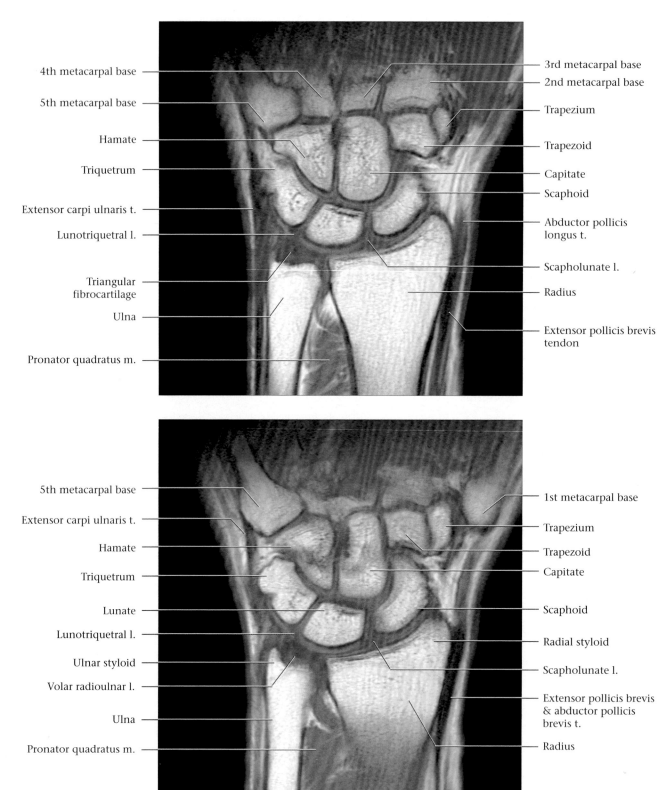

4th metacarpal base

5th metacarpal base

Hamate

Triquetrum

Extensor carpi ulnaris t.

Lunotriquetral l.

Triangular fibrocartilage

Ulna

Pronator quadratus m.

3rd metacarpal base

2nd metacarpal base

Trapezium

Trapezoid

Capitate

Scaphoid

Abductor pollicis longus t.

Scapholunate l.

Radius

Extensor pollicis brevis tendon

5th metacarpal base

Extensor carpi ulnaris t.

Hamate

Triquetrum

Lunate

Lunotriquetral l.

Ulnar styloid

Volar radioulnar l.

Ulna

Pronator quadratus m.

1st metacarpal base

Trapezium

Trapezoid

Capitate

Scaphoid

Radial styloid

Scapholunate l.

Extensor pollicis brevis & abductor pollicis brevis t.

Radius

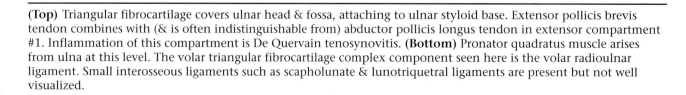

(Top) Triangular fibrocartilage covers ulnar head & fossa, attaching to ulnar styloid base. Extensor pollicis brevis tendon combines with (& is often indistinguishable from) abductor pollicis longus tendon in extensor compartment #1. Inflammation of this compartment is De Quervain tenosynovitis. **(Bottom)** Pronator quadratus muscle arises from ulna at this level. The volar triangular fibrocartilage complex component seen here is the volar radioulnar ligament. Small interosseous ligaments such as scapholunate & lunotriquetral ligaments are present but not well visualized.

CORONAL T1 MR, LEFT WRIST

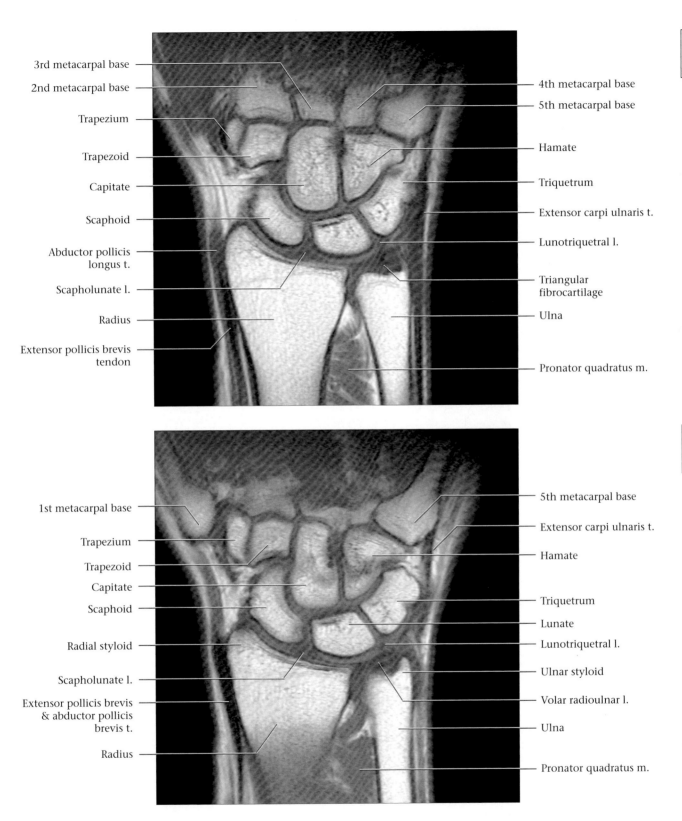

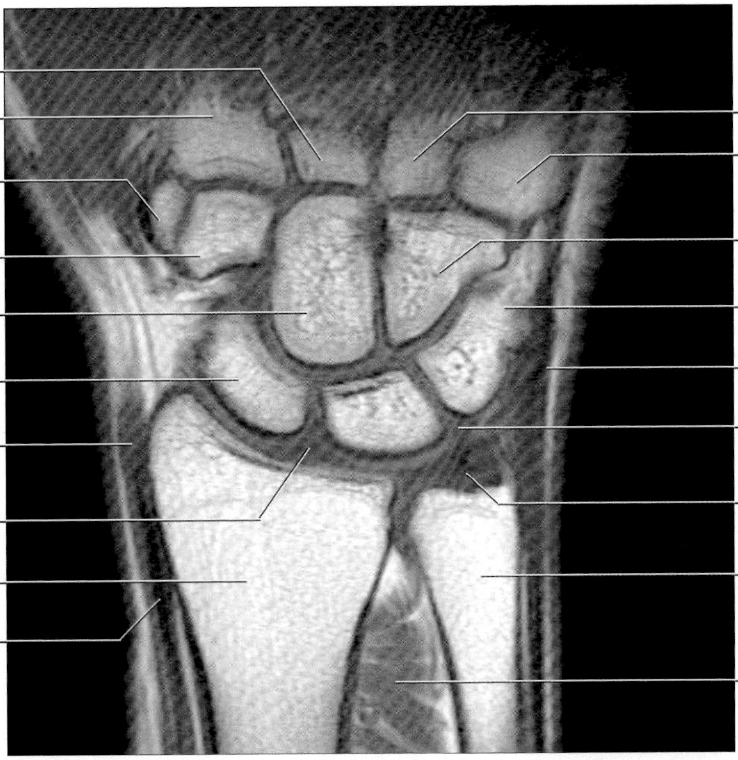
3rd metacarpal base
2nd metacarpal base
Trapezium
Trapezoid
Capitate
Scaphoid
Abductor pollicis longus t.
Scapholunate l.
Radius
Extensor pollicis brevis tendon
4th metacarpal base
5th metacarpal base
Hamate
Triquetrum
Extensor carpi ulnaris t.
Lunotriquetral l.
Triangular fibrocartilage
Ulna
Pronator quadratus m.

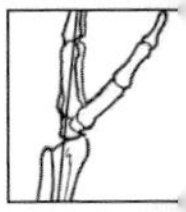

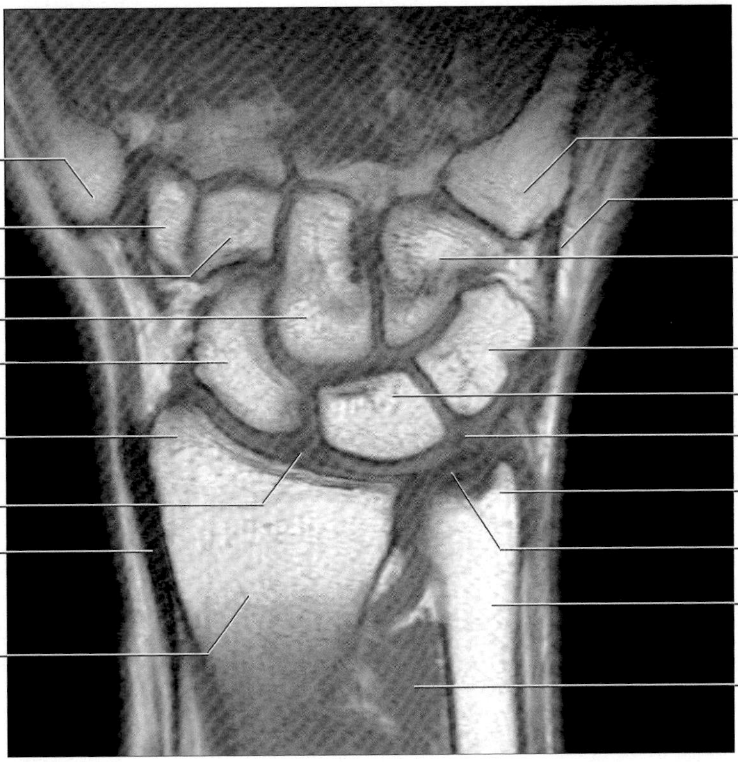
1st metacarpal base
Trapezium
Trapezoid
Capitate
Scaphoid
Radial styloid
Scapholunate l.
Extensor pollicis brevis & abductor pollicis brevis t.
Radius
5th metacarpal base
Extensor carpi ulnaris t.
Hamate
Triquetrum
Lunate
Lunotriquetral l.
Ulnar styloid
Volar radioulnar l.
Ulna
Pronator quadratus m.

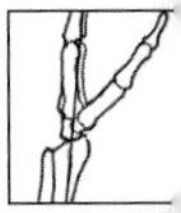

(Top) Triangular fibrocartilage covers ulnar head & fossa, attaching to ulnar styloid base. Extensor pollicis brevis tendon combines with (& is often indistinguishable from) abductor pollicis longus tendon in extensor compartment #1. Inflammation of this compartment is De Quervain tenosynovitis. **(Bottom)** Pronator quadratus muscle arises from ulna at this level. The volar triangular fibrocartilage complex component seen here is the volar radioulnar ligament. Small interosseous ligaments such as scapholunate & lunotriquetral ligaments are present but not well visualized.

CORONAL T1 MR, RIGHT WRIST

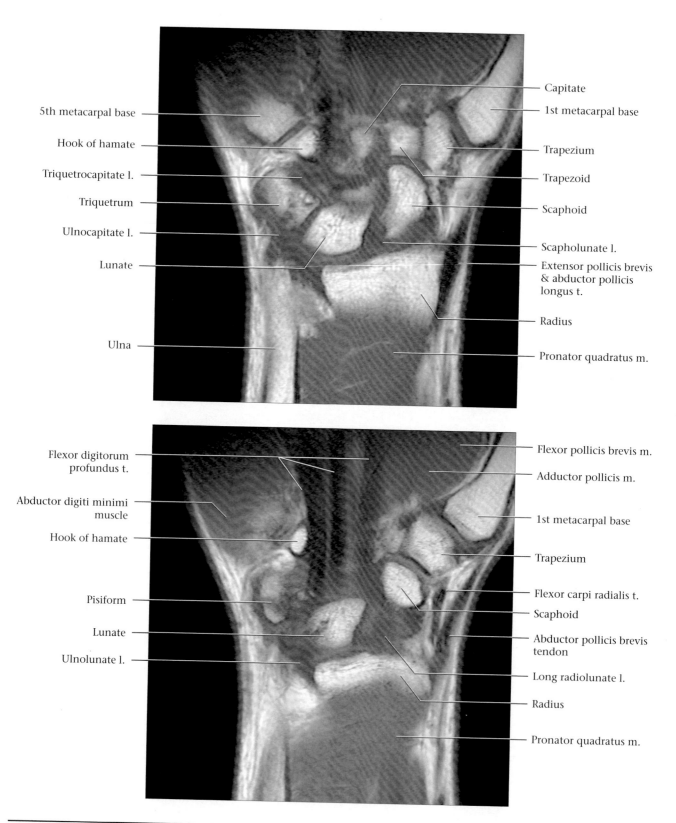

Top image labels (left): 5th metacarpal base, Hook of hamate, Triquetrocapitate l., Triquetrum, Ulnocapitate l., Lunate, Ulna

Top image labels (right): Capitate, 1st metacarpal base, Trapezium, Trapezoid, Scaphoid, Scapholunate l., Extensor pollicis brevis & abductor pollicis longus t., Radius, Pronator quadratus m.

Bottom image labels (left): Flexor digitorum profundus t., Abductor digiti minimi muscle, Hook of hamate, Pisiform, Lunate, Ulnolunate l.

Bottom image labels (right): Flexor pollicis brevis m., Adductor pollicis m., 1st metacarpal base, Trapezium, Flexor carpi radialis t., Scaphoid, Abductor pollicis brevis tendon, Long radiolunate l., Radius, Pronator quadratus m.

(Top) At level of dorsal pisotriquetral joint & base of scaphoid tubercle, portions of volar ligaments are noted including ulnocapitate & triquetrocapitate ligaments. Extensor pollicis brevis & abductor pollicis longus tendons pass through snuffbox region of wrist. The hook of the hamate is evident. **(Bottom)** At level of volar side of pisotriquetral joint & scaphoid tubercle, pronator quadratus muscle belly is visualized. Flexor digitorum profundus tendons pass through dorsal carpal tunnel.

WRIST OVERVIEW

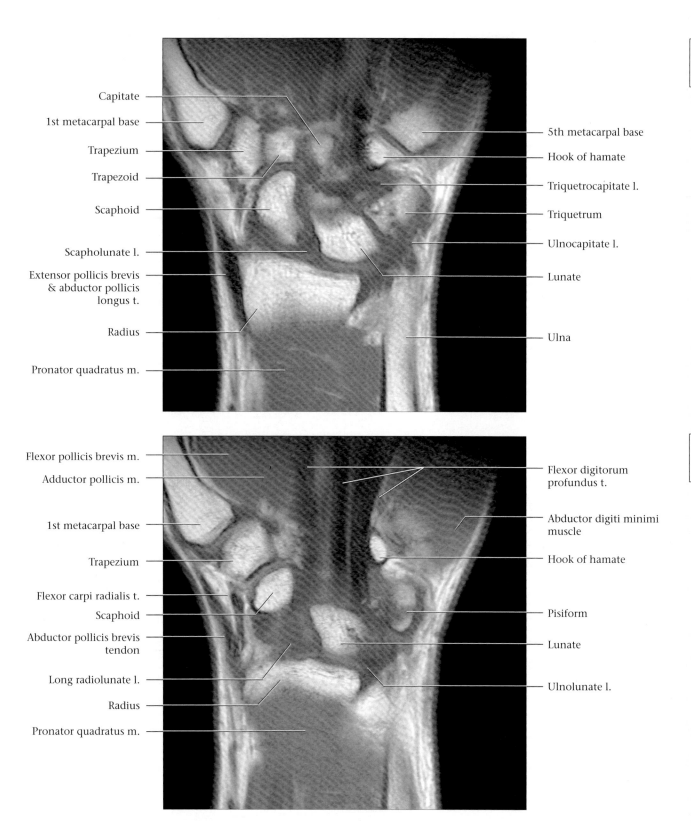

Capitate

1st metacarpal base

Trapezium

Trapezoid

Scaphoid

Scapholunate l.

Extensor pollicis brevis
& abductor pollicis
longus t.

Radius

Pronator quadratus m.

5th metacarpal base

Hook of hamate

Triquetrocapitate l.

Triquetrum

Ulnocapitate l.

Lunate

Ulna

Flexor pollicis brevis m.

Adductor pollicis m.

1st metacarpal base

Trapezium

Flexor carpi radialis t.

Scaphoid

Abductor pollicis brevis
tendon

Long radiolunate l.

Radius

Pronator quadratus m.

Flexor digitorum
profundus t.

Abductor digiti minimi
muscle

Hook of hamate

Pisiform

Lunate

Ulnolunate l.

(Top) At level of dorsal pisotriquetral joint & base of scaphoid tubercle, portions of volar ligaments are noted including ulnocapitate & triquetrocapitate ligaments. Extensor pollicis brevis & abductor pollicis longus tendons pass through snuffbox region of wrist. The hook of the hamate is evident. (Bottom) At level of volar side of pisotriquetral joint & scaphoid tubercle, pronator quadratus muscle belly is visualized. Flexor digitorum profundus tendons pass through dorsal carpal tunnel.

Wrist

III

CORONAL T1 MR, RIGHT WRIST

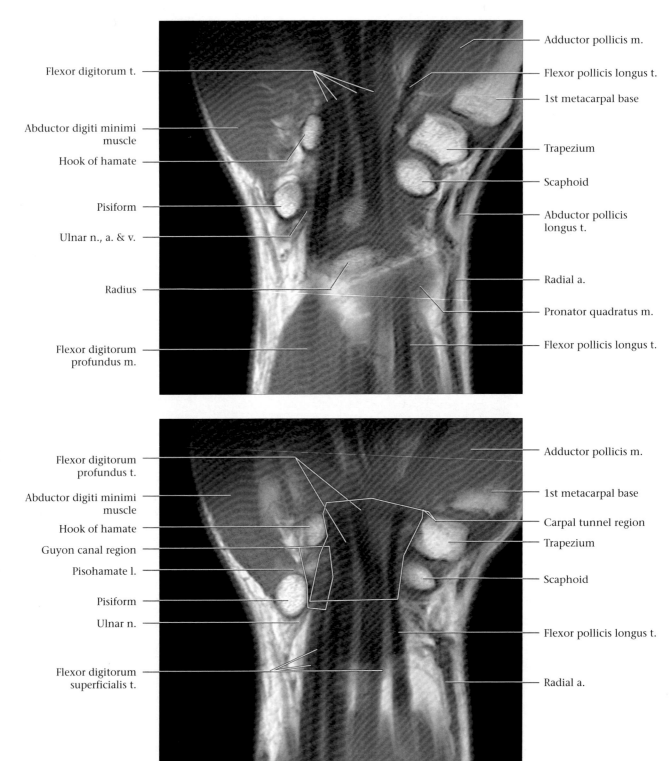

Top image labels (left):
- Flexor digitorum t.
- Abductor digiti minimi muscle
- Hook of hamate
- Pisiform
- Ulnar n., a. & v.
- Radius
- Flexor digitorum profundus m.

Top image labels (right):
- Adductor pollicis m.
- Flexor pollicis longus t.
- 1st metacarpal base
- Trapezium
- Scaphoid
- Abductor pollicis longus t.
- Radial a.
- Pronator quadratus m.
- Flexor pollicis longus t.

Bottom image labels (left):
- Flexor digitorum profundus t.
- Abductor digiti minimi muscle
- Hook of hamate
- Guyon canal region
- Pisohamate l.
- Pisiform
- Ulnar n.
- Flexor digitorum superficialis t.

Bottom image labels (right):
- Adductor pollicis m.
- 1st metacarpal base
- Carpal tunnel region
- Trapezium
- Scaphoid
- Flexor pollicis longus t.
- Radial a.

(Top) Volar to radius & ulna, flexor digitorum profundus & superficialis tendons pass dorsal (deep) to flexor retinaculum. Radial & ulnar arteries are visualized in proximal wrist but rapidly branch into smaller vessels which may not be evident on routine MR imaging. **(Bottom)** Guyon canal region is defined by pisiform & deep & superficial components of medial flexor retinaculum. It contains ulnar nerve, artery & veins as well as fat. Carpal tunnel region is dorsal (deep) to Guyon canal & contains flexor digitorum profundus & superficialis tendons, flexor pollicis longus tendon & median nerve.

CORONAL T1 MR, LEFT WRIST

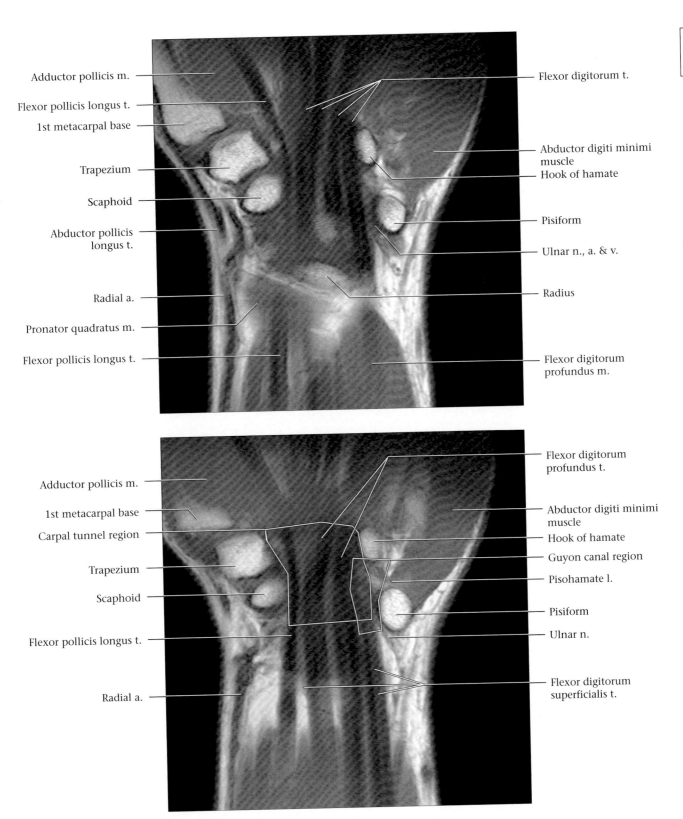

Adductor pollicis m.

Flexor pollicis longus t.

1st metacarpal base

Trapezium

Scaphoid

Abductor pollicis longus t.

Radial a.

Pronator quadratus m.

Flexor pollicis longus t.

Flexor digitorum t.

Abductor digiti minimi muscle

Hook of hamate

Pisiform

Ulnar n., a. & v.

Radius

Flexor digitorum profundus m.

Adductor pollicis m.

1st metacarpal base

Carpal tunnel region

Trapezium

Scaphoid

Flexor pollicis longus t.

Radial a.

Flexor digitorum profundus t.

Abductor digiti minimi muscle

Hook of hamate

Guyon canal region

Pisohamate l.

Pisiform

Ulnar n.

Flexor digitorum superficialis t.

(Top) Volar to radius & ulna, flexor digitorum profundus & superficialis tendons pass dorsal (deep) to flexor retinaculum. Radial & ulnar arteries are visualized in proximal wrist but rapidly branch into smaller vessels which may not be evident on routine MR imaging. **(Bottom)** Guyon canal region is defined by pisiform & deep & superficial components of medial flexor retinaculum. It contains ulnar nerve, artery & veins as well as fat. Carpal tunnel region is dorsal (deep) to Guyon canal & contains flexor digitorum profundus & superficialis tendons, flexor pollicis longus tendon & median nerve.

CORONAL T1 MR, RIGHT WRIST

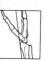

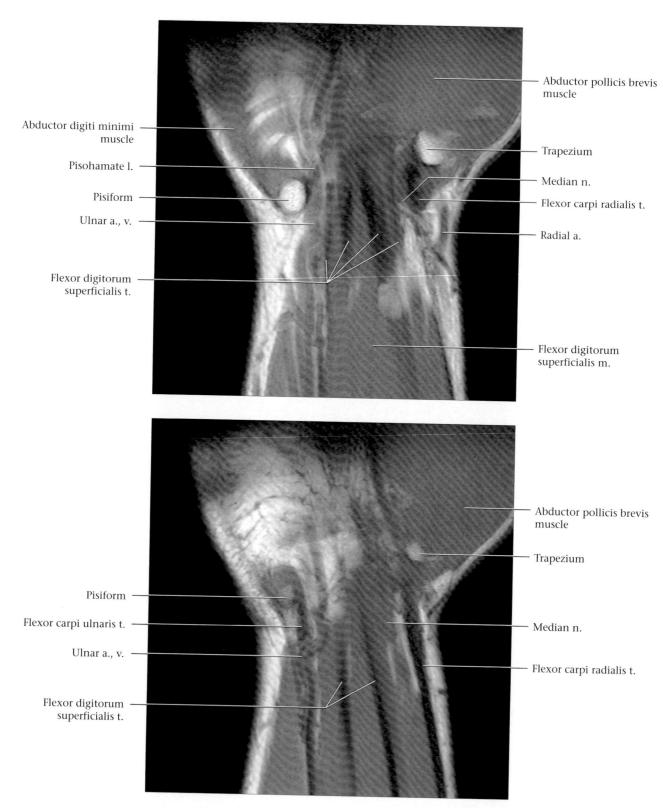

Abductor pollicis brevis muscle

Abductor digiti minimi muscle

Trapezium

Pisohamate l.

Median n.

Pisiform

Flexor carpi radialis t.

Ulnar a., v.

Radial a.

Flexor digitorum superficialis t.

Flexor digitorum superficialis m.

Abductor pollicis brevis muscle

Trapezium

Pisiform

Flexor carpi ulnaris t.

Median n.

Ulnar a., v.

Flexor carpi radialis t.

Flexor digitorum superficialis t.

(Top) Small slips of flexor retinaculum pass horizontally from scaphoid toward hamate & pisiform. The flexor digitorum superficialis tendons are just dorsal to flexor retinaculum. Ulnar nerve is ulnar to ulnar artery & vein as it passes through Guyon canal. (Bottom) Median nerve is superficial & radial in carpal tunnel & is typically isointense to muscle, which may make it difficult to distinguish on T1 imaging.

WRIST OVERVIEW

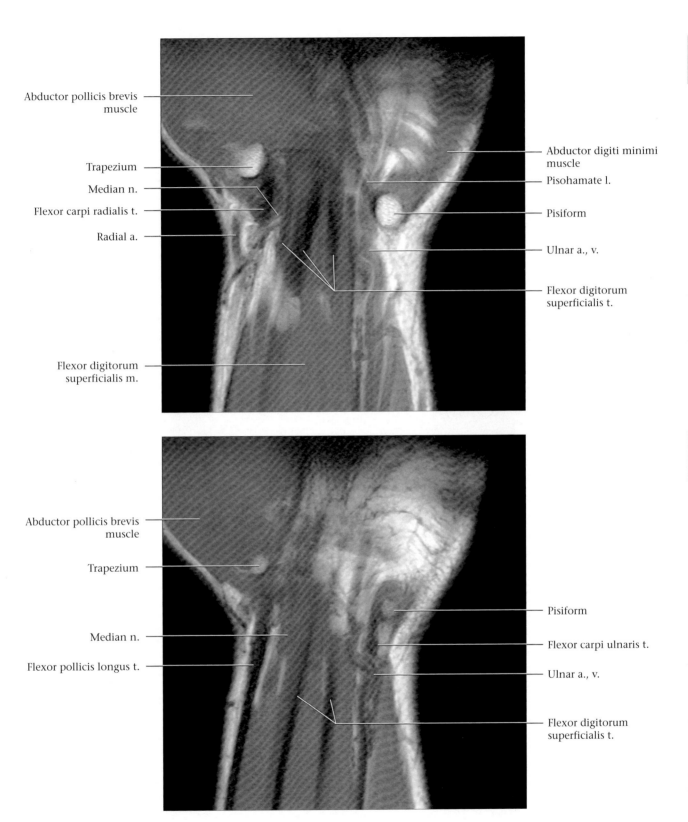

Abductor pollicis brevis muscle

Trapezium

Median n.

Flexor carpi radialis t.

Radial a.

Flexor digitorum superficialis m.

Abductor digiti minimi muscle

Pisohamate l.

Pisiform

Ulnar a., v.

Flexor digitorum superficialis t.

Abductor pollicis brevis muscle

Trapezium

Median n.

Flexor pollicis longus t.

Pisiform

Flexor carpi ulnaris t.

Ulnar a., v.

Flexor digitorum superficialis t.

(Top) Small slips of flexor retinaculum pass horizontally from scaphoid toward hamate & pisiform. The flexor digitorum superficialis tendons are just dorsal to flexor retinaculum. Ulnar nerve is ulnar to ulnar artery & vein as it passes through Guyon canal. **(Bottom)** Median nerve is superficial & radial in carpal tunnel & is typically isointense to muscle, which may make it difficult to distinguish on T1 imaging.

CORONAL T1 MR, RIGHT WRIST

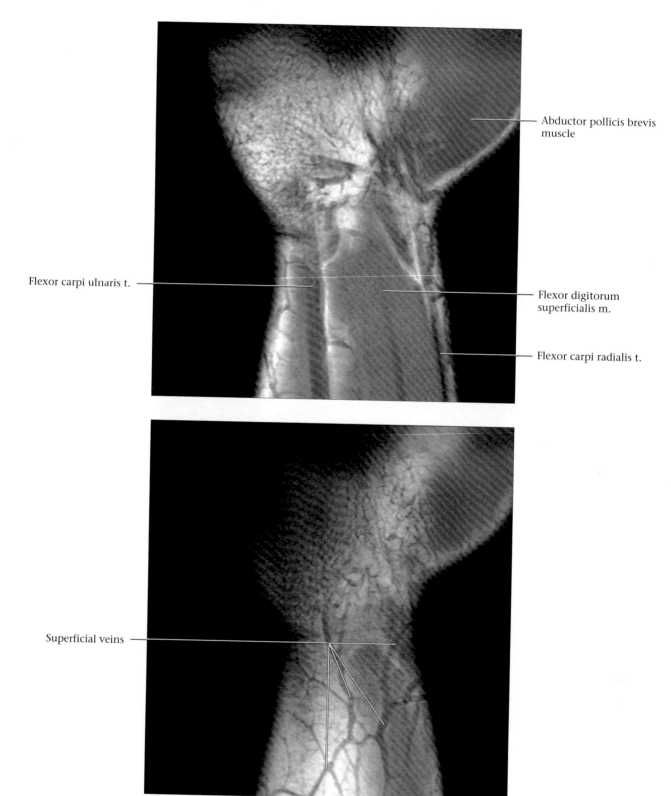

Abductor pollicis brevis muscle

Flexor carpi ulnaris t.

Flexor digitorum superficialis m.

Flexor carpi radialis t.

Superficial veins

(Top) Volar musculature of distal forearm & thenar eminence is readily seen. **(Bottom)** A network of veins over volar wrist drains into cephalic vein radially & basilic vein ulnarly.

WRIST OVERVIEW

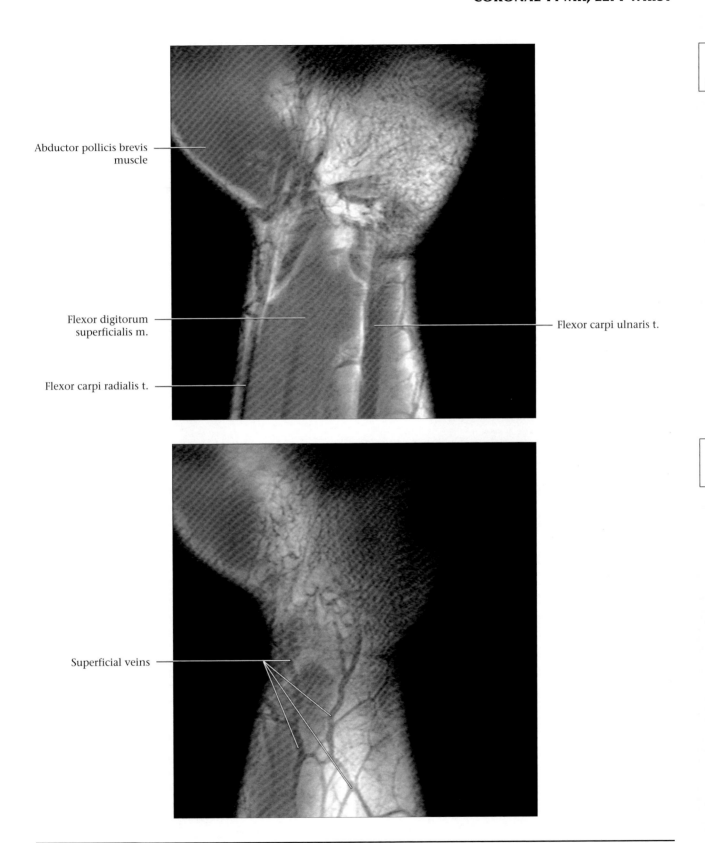

Abductor pollicis brevis muscle

Flexor digitorum superficialis m.

Flexor carpi radialis t.

Flexor carpi ulnaris t.

Superficial veins

(Top) Volar musculature of distal forearm & thenar eminence is readily seen. **(Bottom)** A network of veins over volar wrist drains into cephalic vein radially & basilic vein ulnarly.

SAGITTAL T1 MR, WRIST

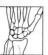

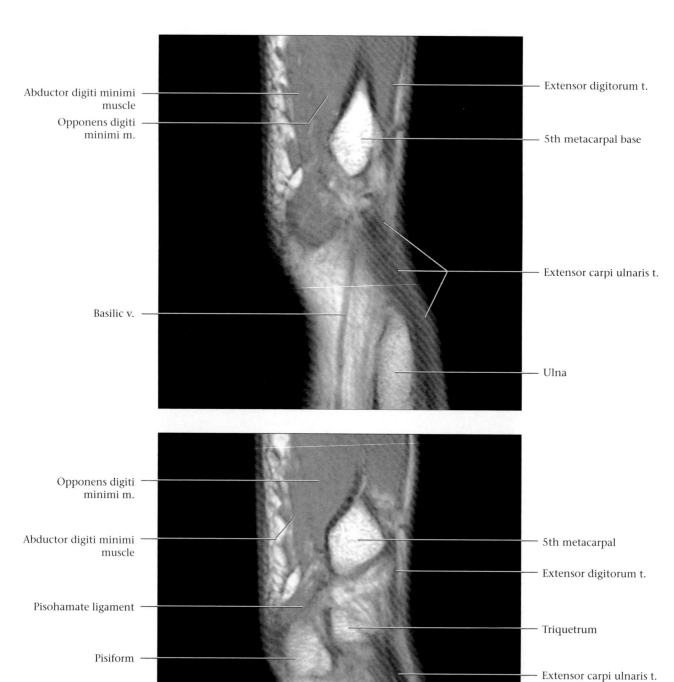

Abductor digiti minimi muscle

Opponens digiti minimi m.

Basilic v.

Extensor digitorum t.

5th metacarpal base

Extensor carpi ulnaris t.

Ulna

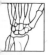

Opponens digiti minimi m.

Abductor digiti minimi muscle

Pisohamate ligament

Pisiform

5th metacarpal

Extensor digitorum t.

Triquetrum

Extensor carpi ulnaris t.

Ulnar styloid process

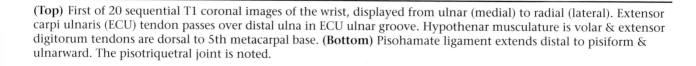

(Top) First of 20 sequential T1 coronal images of the wrist, displayed from ulnar (medial) to radial (lateral). Extensor carpi ulnaris (ECU) tendon passes over distal ulna in ECU ulnar groove. Hypothenar musculature is volar & extensor digitorum tendons are dorsal to 5th metacarpal base. **(Bottom)** Pisohamate ligament extends distal to pisiform & ulnarward. The pisotriquetral joint is noted.

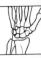

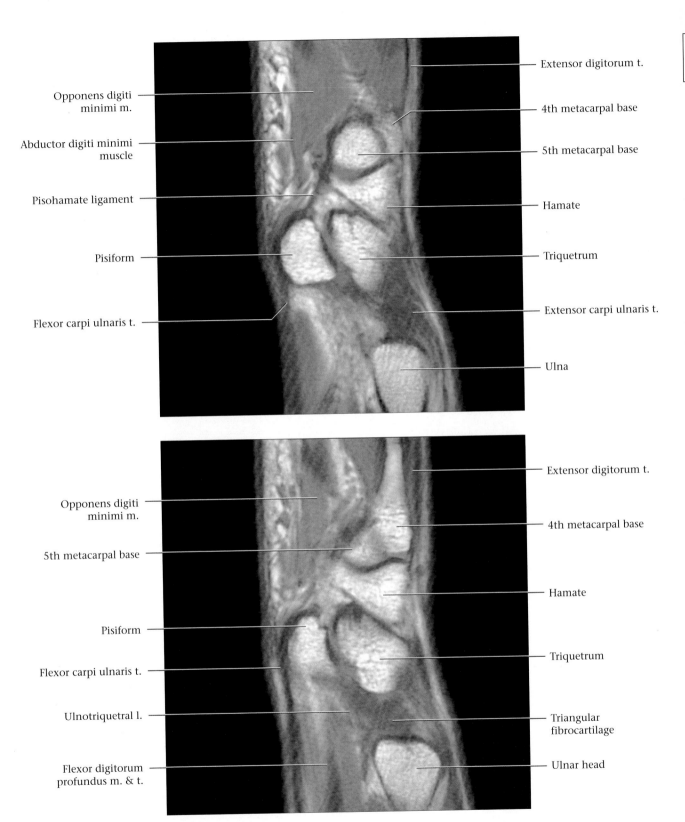

(Top) Pisotriquetral joint is readily evident as is pisohamate ligament. Hypothenar musculature is less robust near its origin from flexor retinaculum. **(Bottom)** Flexor carpi ulnaris tendon inserts on pisiform. Ulnotriquetral ligament arises from volar radioulnar ligament, inserting on volar triquetrum.

Wrist

47

SAGITTAL T1 MR, WRIST

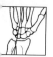

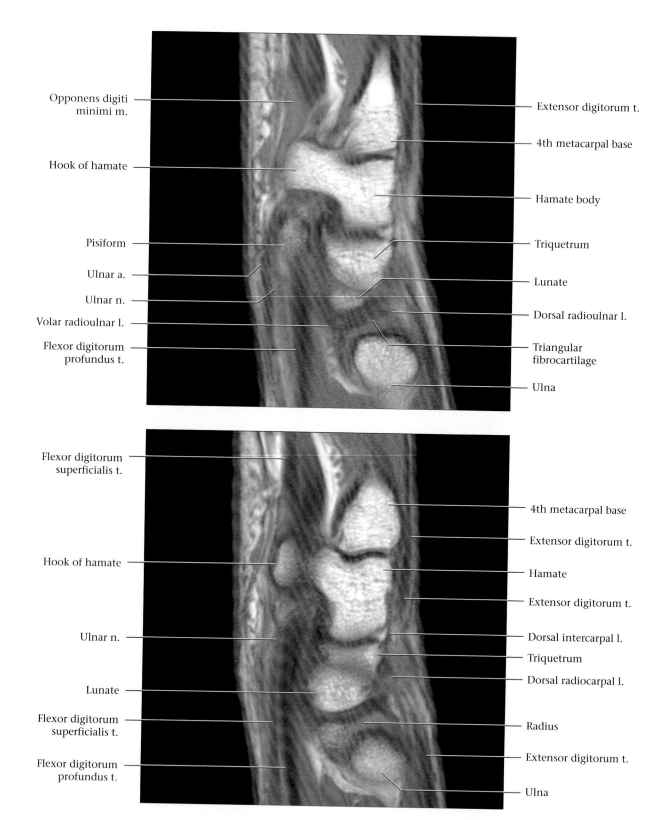

Opponens digiti minimi m.

Hook of hamate

Pisiform

Ulnar a.

Ulnar n.

Volar radioulnar l.

Flexor digitorum profundus t.

Extensor digitorum t.

4th metacarpal base

Hamate body

Triquetrum

Lunate

Dorsal radioulnar l.

Triangular fibrocartilage

Ulna

Flexor digitorum superficialis t.

Hook of hamate

Ulnar n.

Lunate

Flexor digitorum superficialis t.

Flexor digitorum profundus t.

4th metacarpal base

Extensor digitorum t.

Hamate

Extensor digitorum t.

Dorsal intercarpal l.

Triquetrum

Dorsal radiocarpal l.

Radius

Extensor digitorum t.

Ulna

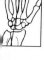

(Top) Ulnar nerve & artery pass lateral & distal to pisiform within Guyon canal. Hook of hamate is prominent. Triangular fibrocartilage (TFC) is visualized as a low signal intensity disc interposed between ulnar head & triquetrum. Volar & dorsal radioulnar ligaments combine with TFC & adjacent structures to form triangular fibrocartilage complex. (Bottom) Intrinsic & extrinsic ligaments may be difficult to identify as individual structures, particularly in the absence of joint distension. Ligaments are labeled where visible or in the region of an expected ligament. Dorsal intercarpal ligament is a key dorsal wrist stabilizer but is visualized in only limited fashion.

WRIST OVERVIEW

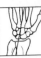

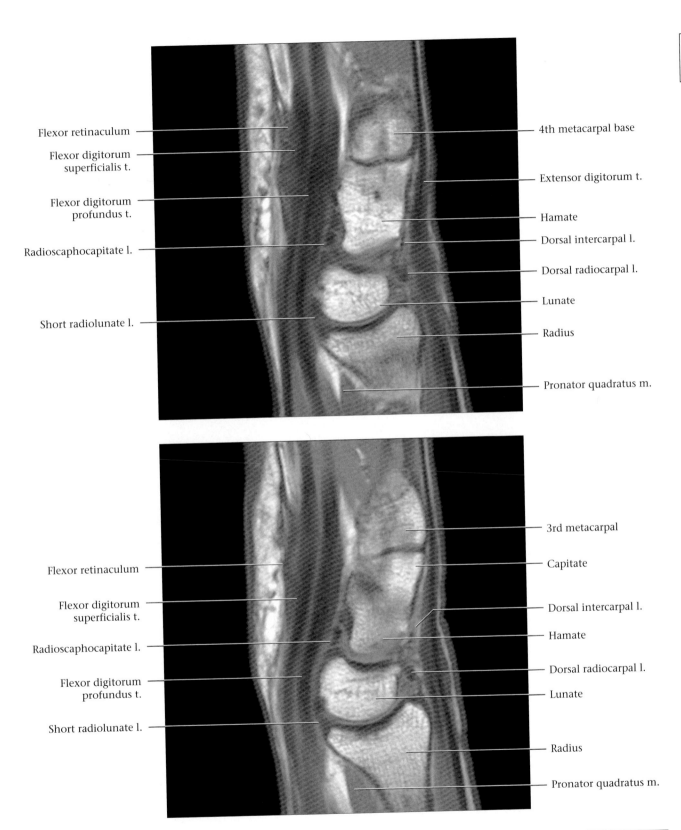

Top image labels (left):
- Flexor retinaculum
- Flexor digitorum superficialis t.
- Flexor digitorum profundus t.
- Radioscaphocapitate l.
- Short radiolunate l.

Top image labels (right):
- 4th metacarpal base
- Extensor digitorum t.
- Hamate
- Dorsal intercarpal l.
- Dorsal radiocarpal l.
- Lunate
- Radius
- Pronator quadratus m.

Bottom image labels (left):
- Flexor retinaculum
- Flexor digitorum superficialis t.
- Radioscaphocapitate l.
- Flexor digitorum profundus t.
- Short radiolunate l.

Bottom image labels (right):
- 3rd metacarpal
- Capitate
- Dorsal intercarpal l.
- Hamate
- Dorsal radiocarpal l.
- Lunate
- Radius
- Pronator quadratus m.

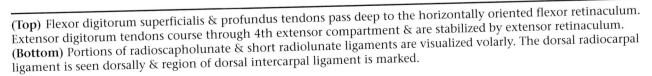

(Top) Flexor digitorum superficialis & profundus tendons pass deep to the horizontally oriented flexor retinaculum. Extensor digitorum tendons course through 4th extensor compartment & are stabilized by extensor retinaculum. **(Bottom)** Portions of radioscapholunate & short radiolunate ligaments are visualized volarly. The dorsal radiocarpal ligament is seen dorsally & region of dorsal intercarpal ligament is marked.

SAGITTAL T1 MR, WRIST

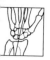

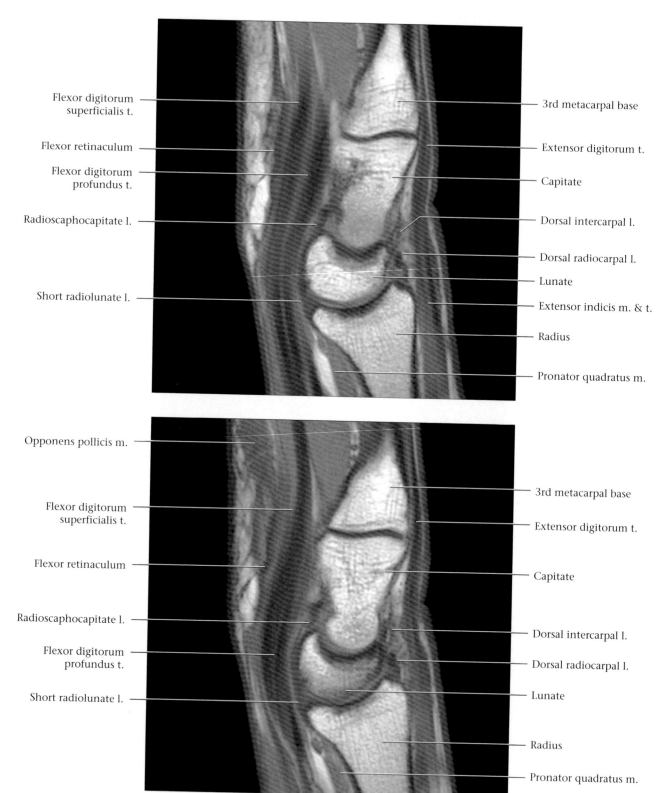

Flexor digitorum superficialis t.

Flexor retinaculum

Flexor digitorum profundus t.

Radioscaphocapitate l.

Short radiolunate l.

3rd metacarpal base

Extensor digitorum t.

Capitate

Dorsal intercarpal l.

Dorsal radiocarpal l.

Lunate

Extensor indicis m. & t.

Radius

Pronator quadratus m.

Opponens pollicis m.

Flexor digitorum superficialis t.

Flexor retinaculum

Radioscaphocapitate l.

Flexor digitorum profundus t.

Short radiolunate l.

3rd metacarpal base

Extensor digitorum t.

Capitate

Dorsal intercarpal l.

Dorsal radiocarpal l.

Lunate

Radius

Pronator quadratus m.

(Top) Third metacarpal base, capitate, lunate & lunate fossa of radius align, creating a stable central axis of wrist. **(Bottom)** Extensor indicis tendon is radial-most tendon in 4th extensor compartment. Opponens pollicis tendon originates from flexor retinaculum at this level.

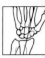

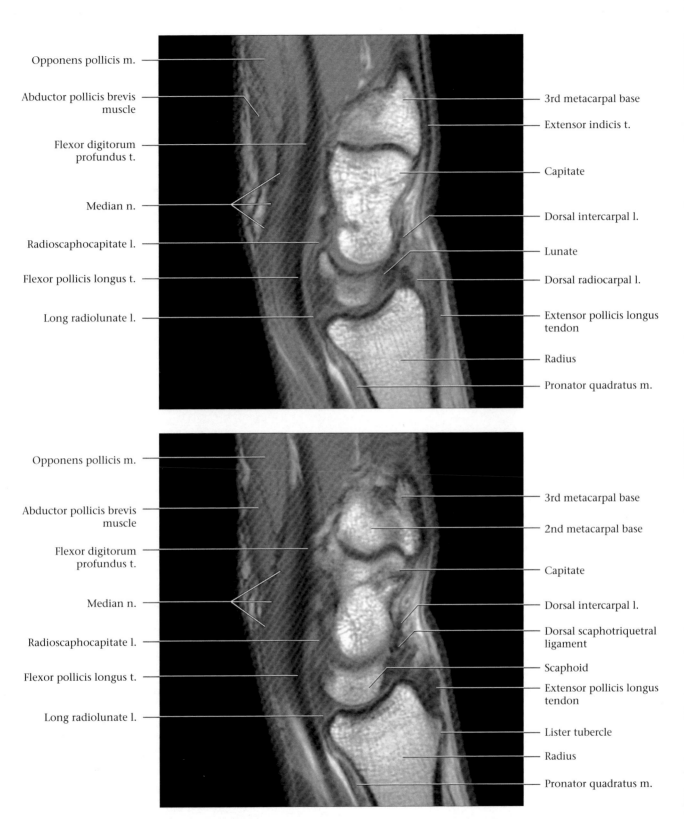

Opponens pollicis m.

Abductor pollicis brevis muscle

Flexor digitorum profundus t.

Median n.

Radioscaphocapitate l.

Flexor pollicis longus t.

Long radiolunate l.

3rd metacarpal base

Extensor indicis t.

Capitate

Dorsal intercarpal l.

Lunate

Dorsal radiocarpal l.

Extensor pollicis longus tendon

Radius

Pronator quadratus m.

Opponens pollicis m.

Abductor pollicis brevis muscle

Flexor digitorum profundus t.

Median n.

Radioscaphocapitate l.

Flexor pollicis longus t.

Long radiolunate l.

3rd metacarpal base

2nd metacarpal base

Capitate

Dorsal intercarpal l.

Dorsal scaphotriquetral ligament

Scaphoid

Extensor pollicis longus tendon

Lister tubercle

Radius

Pronator quadratus m.

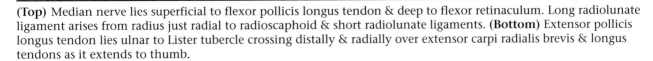

(Top) Median nerve lies superficial to flexor pollicis longus tendon & deep to flexor retinaculum. Long radiolunate ligament arises from radius just radial to radioscaphoid & short radiolunate ligaments. **(Bottom)** Extensor pollicis longus tendon lies ulnar to Lister tubercle crossing distally & radially over extensor carpi radialis brevis & longus tendons as it extends to thumb.

SAGITTAL T1 MR, WRIST

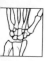

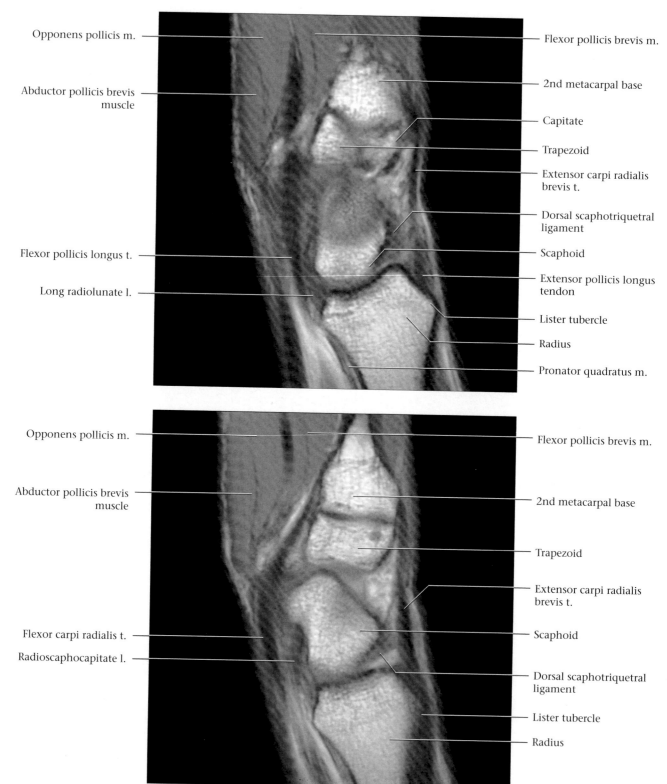

Opponens pollicis m.

Flexor pollicis brevis m.

Abductor pollicis brevis muscle

2nd metacarpal base

Capitate

Trapezoid

Extensor carpi radialis brevis t.

Dorsal scaphotriquetral ligament

Flexor pollicis longus t.

Scaphoid

Long radiolunate l.

Extensor pollicis longus tendon

Lister tubercle

Radius

Pronator quadratus m.

Opponens pollicis m.

Flexor pollicis brevis m.

Abductor pollicis brevis muscle

2nd metacarpal base

Trapezoid

Extensor carpi radialis brevis t.

Flexor carpi radialis t.

Scaphoid

Radioscaphocapitate l.

Dorsal scaphotriquetral ligament

Lister tubercle

Radius

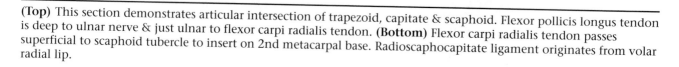

(Top) This section demonstrates articular intersection of trapezoid, capitate & scaphoid. Flexor pollicis longus tendon is deep to ulnar nerve & just ulnar to flexor carpi radialis tendon. **(Bottom)** Flexor carpi radialis tendon passes superficial to scaphoid tubercle to insert on 2nd metacarpal base. Radioscaphocapitate ligament originates from volar radial lip.

WRIST OVERVIEW

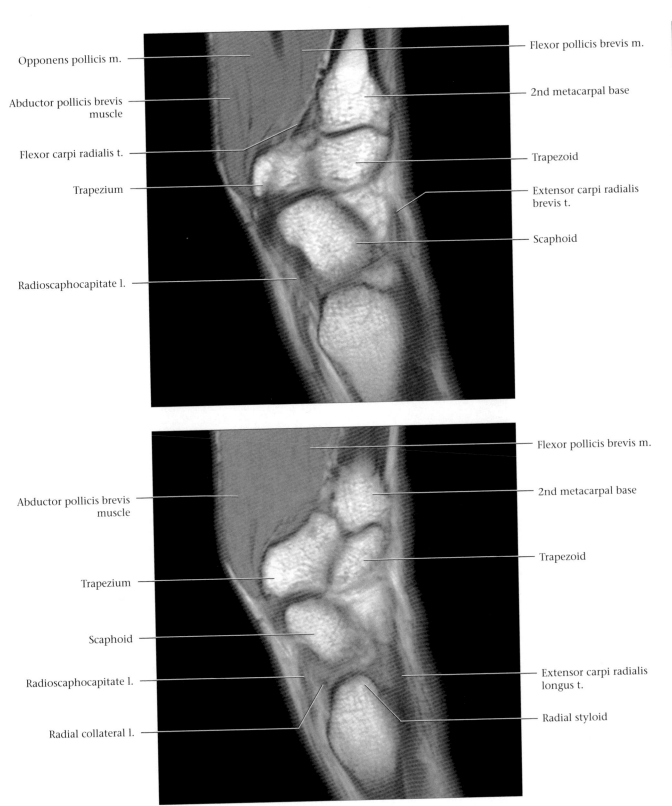

Opponens pollicis m.

Abductor pollicis brevis muscle

Flexor carpi radialis t.

Trapezium

Radioscaphocapitate l.

Flexor pollicis brevis m.

2nd metacarpal base

Trapezoid

Extensor carpi radialis brevis t.

Scaphoid

Abductor pollicis brevis muscle

Trapezium

Scaphoid

Radioscaphocapitate l.

Radial collateral l.

Flexor pollicis brevis m.

2nd metacarpal base

Trapezoid

Extensor carpi radialis longus t.

Radial styloid

(Top) Flexor carpi radialis tendon passes superficial to scaphoid tubercle to insert on 2nd metacarpal base. Extensor carpi radialis brevis tendon crosses dorsum of wrist to insert on dorsal 3rd metacarpal base. **(Bottom)** Radial-most component of radioscaphocapitate ligament is sometimes called radial collateral ligament. Extensor carpi radialis longus tendon crosses dorsum of wrist to insert on 2nd metacarpal base.

WRIST OVERVIEW

SAGITTAL T1 MR, WRIST

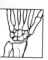

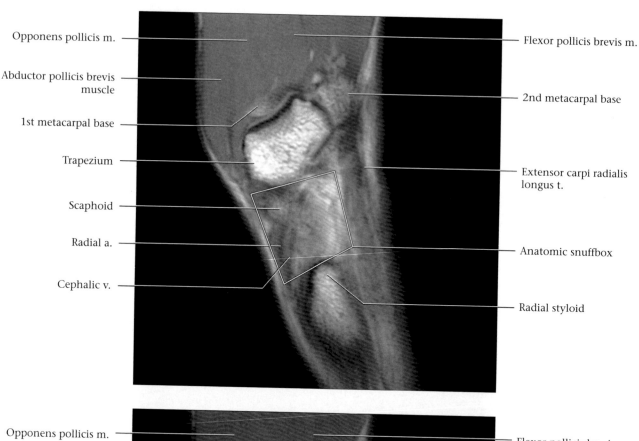

Opponens pollicis m.

Abductor pollicis brevis muscle

1st metacarpal base

Trapezium

Scaphoid

Radial a.

Cephalic v.

Flexor pollicis brevis m.

2nd metacarpal base

Extensor carpi radialis longus t.

Anatomic snuffbox

Radial styloid

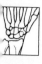

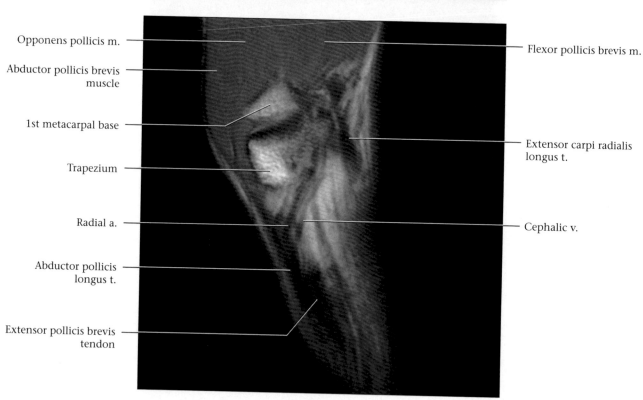

Opponens pollicis m.

Abductor pollicis brevis muscle

1st metacarpal base

Trapezium

Radial a.

Abductor pollicis longus t.

Extensor pollicis brevis tendon

Flexor pollicis brevis m.

Extensor carpi radialis longus t.

Cephalic v.

(Top) Radial artery, superficial radial nerve & cephalic vein pass through anatomic snuff box which is bounded by trapezium, scaphoid, & radial styloid. Abductor pollicis longus & extensor pollicis brevis tendons form volar margin of snuffbox & extensor pollicis longus tendon forms dorsal margin. **(Bottom)** Abductor pollicis longus & extensor pollicis brevis tendons form distal margin of snuffbox as they convergence just distal to 1st carpometacarpal joint.

SAGITTAL T1 MR, WRIST

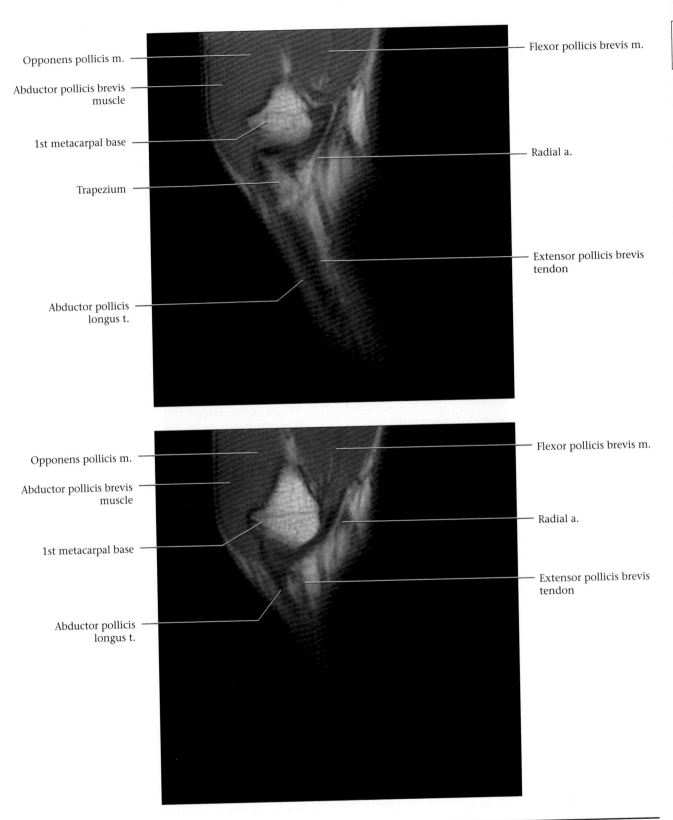

Opponens pollicis m.

Abductor pollicis brevis
muscle

1st metacarpal base

Trapezium

Abductor pollicis
longus t.

Flexor pollicis brevis m.

Radial a.

Extensor pollicis brevis
tendon

Opponens pollicis m.

Abductor pollicis brevis
muscle

1st metacarpal base

Abductor pollicis
longus t.

Flexor pollicis brevis m.

Radial a.

Extensor pollicis brevis
tendon

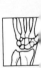

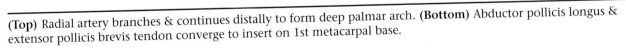

(Top) Radial artery branches & continues distally to form deep palmar arch. **(Bottom)** Abductor pollicis longus & extensor pollicis brevis tendon converge to insert on 1st metacarpal base.

OSSEOUS STRUCTURES

Terminology

Abbreviations

- Abductor pollicis longus (APL)
- Carpometacarpal (CMC)
- Distal radioulnar joint (DRUJ)
- Extensor pollicis brevis (EPB)
- Field of view (FOV)
- Flexor carpi ulnaris (FCU)
- Flexor retinaculum (FR)
- Metacarpal (MC)
- Opponens digiti minimi (ODM)
- Radioscapholunate ligament (RSC)
- Triangular fibrocartilage (TFC)
- Triangular fibrocartilage complex (TFCC)
- Volar intercalated segment instability (VISI)

Definitions

- Intercalated = interposed
- Palmar = volar
- Radial = lateral
- Ulnar = medial
- Wrist abduction = radial flexion
- Wrist adduction = ulnar flexion

Imaging Anatomy

Osseous Anatomy

- Eight carpals with 6 main surfaces (except pisiform)
  - **Dorsal & volar**: Non-articular; roughened surfaces for ligament attachments; dorsal surface broader than volar (except scaphoid & lunate)
  - **Proximal & distal**: Proximal surface convex, distal surface concave; covered with articular cartilage
  - **Medial & lateral**: Covered with articular cartilage
- **Proximal carpal row**
  - **Scaphoid (carpal navicular)**: Largest proximal carpal bone
    - Articulates with radius, trapezium, trapezoid, lunate, capitate
    - Key contours: Tuberosity - distal volar prominence; waist (ridge) - mid lateral portion, location for vascular channels & ligament attachments; proximal pole - proximal to waist; distal pole - distal to waist
    - Variants: Bipartite scaphoid with ossicles separated at waist
  - **Lunate**
    - Articulates with radius, capitate, hamate, triquetrum, scaphoid, TFC
    - Key contours: Volar > dorsal height
    - Variants: Type I (34.5%) - no articulation with hamate; type II (65.5%) - facet articulates with hamate
  - **Triquetrum**
    - Articulates with pisiform, lunate, hamate, TFC
    - Key contours: Ovoid facet articulates with pisiform
    - Dorsal & volar ligament attachments equally strong (unlike other carpals); dorsal ligaments converge on triquetrum, may avulse bone fragment with forceful wrist flexion

- **Pisiform**: Only carpal with tendon attachment (FCU)
  - Articulates with triquetrum
  - Key contours: Ovoid articular facet
  - Sesamoid-like with FCU inserting & continuing on as pisohamate & pisometacarpal ligaments
- **Distal carpal row**
  - **Trapezium (greater multangular)**: Saddle-shaped
    - Articulates with scaphoid, 1st & 2nd MCs, trapezoid
    - Key contours: Groove for FCR; volar tubercle (ridge) - attachment for FR, intrinsic & extrinsic ligaments
    - Key link between carpals & 1st MC
  - **Trapezoid (lesser multangular)**
    - Articulates with scaphoid, 2nd MC, trapezium, capitate
    - Key contours: Articular facets
    - Variants: Small facet articulates with 3rd MC (33%)
  - **Capitate**: Largest carpal bone
    - Articulates with scaphoid, lunate, 2nd, 3rd & 4th MCs, trapezoid, hamate
    - Key contours: Head - proximal portion; neck - constricted region just distal to head; body - distal portion; volar surface near neck attachment of deltoid volar carpal ligaments
    - Variants: Small facet for 4th MC (85%); multiple ossification centers
  - **Hamate**: Wedge-shaped
    - Articulates with lunate, 4th & 5th MCs, triquetrum, capitate
    - Key contours: Articular facet winds around waist, facilitates triquetral motion on volar hamate; hook (hamulus) of hamate - volar distal projection attachment for FR, pisohamate ligament & ODM
    - Variants: Hypoplastic hamate hook; hook as separate ossicle
- **Distal radius**
  - Articulates with scaphoid, lunate, & ulna
  - Key contours: Lister tubercle - dorsal ridge; scaphoid & lunate fossa - concavities articulate with proximal scaphoid & lunate; radial styloid - lateral distal prominence; sigmoid notch (fossa, ulnar notch) - medial concavity articulates with ulnar head; lateral parallel grooves for EPB & APL; dorsal grooves for extensor compartments
- **Distal ulna**
  - Articulates with radius, scaphoid & TFC
  - Key contours: Head - smooth, rounded distal articular surface; fovea (fossa) - concavity at base of styloid for attachment of TFCC; styloid - medial distal prominence; dorsal groove for ECU
- **Wrist variants**
  - Osseous coalitions: May be fibrous, cartilaginous or osseous; lunotriquetral most common
  - Ossicles: Common about wrist; rounded & well-corticated; can be mistaken for loose bodies or fractures
    - Lunula: Between TFC & triquetrum, may fuse to ulnar styloid; may be difficult to distinguish from prior ulnar styloid avulsion

- Os styloideum: Dorsal between 2nd & 3rd MC bases; known as carpal boss if fused with 3rd MC
    - Os hamuli: Ossicle at tip of hamate hook
    - Epilunate: Dorsal to lunate
- **Vascular channels**
    - Small, discretely defined channels are entry points of nutrient vessels; may mimic erosions
    - Vessels enter along ligament & capsule attachments, at non-articular bone surfaces without cartilage cover
- **Cartilage surfaces**
    - Hyaline cartilage (1.0-1.5 mm) lines all gliding surfaces; visible on distal radius, ulnar head & carpal surfaces
    - May be difficult to distinguish from adjacent joint fluid on routine imaging
- **Synovial surfaces**
    - Covers all wrist joint surfaces
    - Typically not visualized on routine imaging; may enhance with intravenous gadolinium

Compartments

- Wrist is multiple articulations organized into compartments by ligamentous attachments
    - Distal (inferior) radioulnar margins: Distal radioulnar articulation, capsule, TFCC
    - Radiocarpal margins: Distal radius, TFCC, proximal margin of proximal carpal row, radial collateral ligament; communicates with pisotriquetral joint in ~ 80%
    - Midcarpal margins: Distal margin of proximal carpal row, intercarpal articulations of distal carpal row, communicates with common carpometacarpal joint
    - Pisotriquetral margins: Pisiform, triquetrum
    - Common carpometacarpal margins: Space between 2nd-5th MC bases; space between hamate, 4th & 5th MCs is occasionally separate compartment
    - First carpometacarpal margins: Trapezium, 1st MC base
- Individual compartments can be injected to evaluate integrity (see: "Ligaments" section)

Carpal Alignment

- **Normal forces across wrist**: Axial compression by forearm muscles
    - **Axial compression** of forearm muscles is borne along long axis of radius, lunate & capitate
        - Distal radial volar tilt: Displaces lunate volarly
        - Lunate: Shorter dorsally; tends to rotate dorsally
        - Scaphoid: Tends to volarflex
        - Triquetrum: Glides along volar hamate; tends to dorsiflex
        - Scapholunate & lunotriquetral ligaments stabilize carpal tendency to flex volarly or dorsally
    - **Distal radius** angulation tends to direct carpals volarly & ulnarly
        - Extrinsic volar & dorsal radiocarpal ligaments stabilize carpal tendency to tilt or translate
- **Functional organization theories**
    - **Row concept**: Carpals function as proximal & distal row; scaphoid bridges two rows
        - Proximal carpals intercalated between radius & distal carpals with no tendon attachments

- **Columnar concept**: Carpals function in three columns
    - **Radial**: Mobile column comprised of radius, scaphoid, trapezium, trapezoid; **central**: Flex/extend column comprised of radius, lunate, capitate; **ulnar**: Rotational column comprised of triquetrum & hamate
    - **Ring concept**: Carpals function as ring with mobile proximal carpal row & rigid distal carpal row; ring disruption = instability
- **Alignment varies with wrist position**
- **Neutral alignment**
    - Defined as long axes of radius, lunate, & capitate
- **Dorsiflexion**
    - Occurs primarily across midcarpal row
    - Lunate & capitate dorsiflexed; pisiform pulled proximally by FCU
    - Muscle pull is asymmetric resulting in dorsiflexion being slightly radially deviated
- **Volarflexion**
    - Occurs primarily at radiocarpal joint
    - Lunate & capitate volarflexed
    - Muscle pull is asymmetric resulting in volarflexion being slightly ulnar deviated
- **Wrist abduction (radial flexion or deviation)**
    - Scaphoid flexes volarly around RSC (sling) ligament, becoming foreshortened; trapeziotrapezoid complex rides dorsal to scaphoid distal pole; lunate flexes volarly, becoming triangular; triquetrum volarflexes, moving proximal to hamate; pisiform pulled distally by pisohamate & pisotriquetral ligaments; capitate body slightly dorsiflexed
- **Wrist adduction (ulnar flexion or deviation)**
    - Triquetrum glides distally & volarly along hamate into dorsiflexion, slightly overlapping hamate; lunate dorsiflexes, becoming trapezoidal; scaphoid pulled into longitudinal attitude; capitate is slightly volarflexed
- **Rotation**
    - Radius rotates around ulna; pronation: Ulna slightly dorsal to radius; supination: Ulna slightly volar

Radiographic Analysis

- Measurements may be used to evaluate & describe wrist alignment or malalignment due to arthropathies, trauma, congenital deformities
- **Posteroanterior radiograph measurements**
    - **Radial tilt** (radial inclination, radial deviation, ulnar inclination, radial angle)
        - Tangent to radial styloid & ulnar radius intersects line drawn perpendicular to ulnar long axis (nl: $21° \pm 3.6°$)
    - **Carpal arcs**
        - **Arcs of Gilula**: Arcs outlining 1) proximal margin, proximal carpal row; 2) distal margin, proximal carpal row; 3) proximal margin, distal carpal row; should be smooth & parallel
        - **Greater & lesser arcs**: Lesser arc – circumscribe joints around lunate; greater arc - crosses mid or proximal portions of scaphoid, capitate, hamate & triquetrum

OSSEOUS STRUCTURES

- **Vulnerable zone:** Region encompassed between greater & lesser arcs as well as scaphoid & trapezium; majority of wrist fractures & ligamentous injuries occur in vulnerable zone
- ○ **Carpometacarpal joint alignment**
  - CMC joints 2-5 are parallel & create a contour reminiscent of an "M"; clenched fist views disrupt this smooth line on radiograph
- ○ **Ulnar variance** (radioulnar index)
  - Comparison of distal radius cortex (ulnar aspect) to distal ulna cortex (radial aspect)
  - Ulnar neutral: Ulna, no more than 2 mm shorter than radius; ulnar minus: Ulna > 2 mm shorter than radius, associated with Kienbock disease; ulnar plus: Ulna longer than radius, associated with ulnolunate impaction syndrome & TFC tears
- ○ **Carpal angle**
  - Angle formed by lines drawn tangent to proximal scaphoid/lunate & proximal triquetrum/lunate (nl: 130°)
- ○ **Carpal height ratio**
  - Carpal height: Distance from 3rd MC base to distal radial articular surface
  - Carpal height ratio: Ratio of carpal height/3rd MC shaft length (nl: 0.54)
  - Can also be measured as a ratio of carpal height/capitate length (nl: 1.57 ± .05)
- ○ **Carpal height index**
  - Ratio of carpal height ratio dominant hand/carpal height vs. ratio non-dominant hand (nl: 1.0 ± 0.15)
- ○ **Ulnar head inclination**
  - Intersection of lines drawn parallel to ulna long axis & along ulnar head articular surface facing sigmoid notch; compare injured to non-injured wrist (nl: 11-27°)
- ○ **Radioulnar angle**
  - Intersection of lines drawn along ulnar head articular surface facing sigmoid notch & along radial & ulnar distal radius joint; compare injured to non-injured wrist (n: 90-111°)
- ○ **Lunate overhang**
  - Width of lunate compared to radial lunate fossa (nl: < 50% of lunate "overhangs" ulnar edge of radius)
- **Lateral radiograph measurements**
  - ○ **Volar tilt** (volar angle, dorsal tilt, palmar tilt, palmar slope)
    - Line drawn tangent to anterior & posterior radial margins intersects line drawn perpendicular to radius long axis (nl: 10-12°)
  - ○ **Carpal axes**
    - Radius: Line through long axis of radius, from midpoint of bone at 2 & 5 cm proximal to radiocarpal joint
    - Lunate: Line perpendicular to line drawn between two distal poles
    - Capitate: Line vertical through head & body or tangent to dorsal 3rd MC
    - Scaphoid: Line drawn between palmar proximal & distal margins
    - Triquetrum: Line drawn through proximal & distal poles

- ○ **Carpal angles**
  - Radiolunate: < 15°
  - Scapholunate: 30-60°
  - Capitolunate: 0-30°
  - Lunotriquetral: 14-16°
- **Distal radioulnar alignment**
  - ○ Assessment with radiography limited to gross malalignment; more subtle subluxation best defined by axial imaging (CT/MR)
  - ○ All methods have some limitations; comparison with unaffected side may be useful
  - ○ **Radioulnar ratio:** Identify center of ulnar head (C); draw line from volar (A) to dorsal (B) margins of sigmoid notch (line AB); drop perpendicular from ulnar head center (C) to margin line (D); ratio = AD/AB (nl pronation: 0.6 ± 0.05; neutral: 0.5 ± 0.04; supination: 0.37 ± 0.09)

Anatomy-Based Imaging Issues

Imaging Recommendations

- **Radiographic evaluation**
  - ○ Basic survey
    - PA, lateral, semipronated oblique
  - ○ Range of motion & alignment
    - Ulnar & radial deviation, dorsiflexion, volarflexion, clenched fist
  - ○ Other views for fractures, arthritis, foreign bodies
    - Scaphoid view, semisupinated oblique, carpal tunnel, carpal bridge
- **CT evaluation**
  - ○ Thin section imaging (0.5 mm), small FOV, multiplanar reformations
  - ○ Positioning
    - Routine: Palm on table, forearm aligned perpendicular to gantry
    - Scaphoid imaging: Palm on table with long axis of scaphoid parallel to gantry
  - ○ Addition of arthrography may improve cartilage & ligament evaluation
- **MR evaluation**
  - ○ Meticulous positioning with wrist in neutral alignment as near center of magnetic field as possible; 8-12 cm FOV; dedicated coils
  - ○ Ideal positioning with patient prone, wrist pronated above head ("Superman" position)
  - ○ Cortices uniformly low signal intensity; marrow spaces intermediate signal intensity, interspersed with trabeculae
  - ○ Marrow edema may be readily apparent on fluid sensitive sequences
  - ○ GRE (T2) imaging commonly used for ligament evaluation but susceptible to field inhomogeneity caused by trabeculae; underestimates edema

Imaging Pitfalls

- Alignment analysis on MR may be problematic
  - ○ Patient in "Superman" position may have wrist in slight ulnar deviation; results in lunate volar angulation which may mimic VISI
  - ○ Pronated wrist: Ulna appears dorsally subluxated
- Vascular channels are not erosions

OSSEOUS STRUCTURES

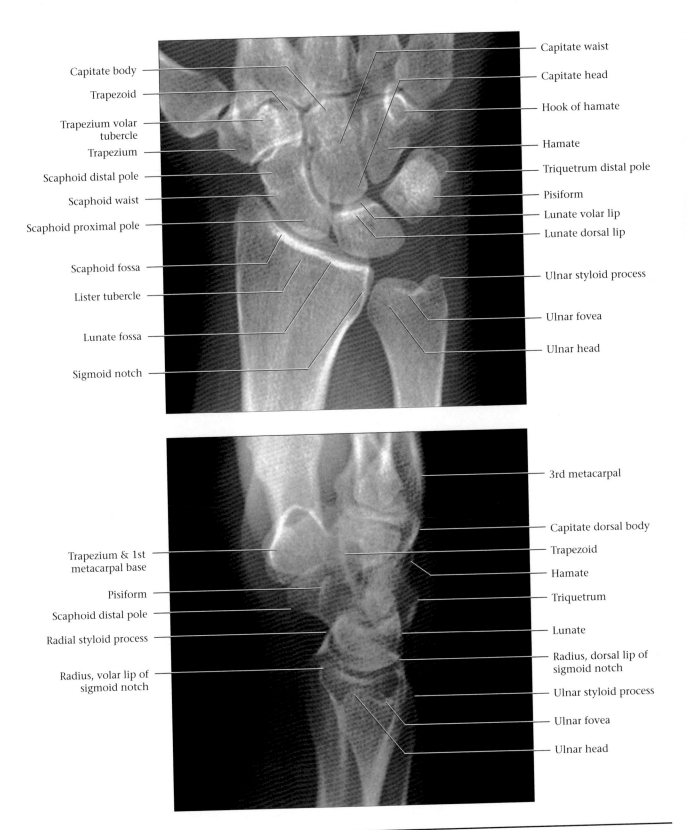

Capitate body

Trapezoid

Trapezium volar tubercle

Trapezium

Scaphoid distal pole

Scaphoid waist

Scaphoid proximal pole

Scaphoid fossa

Lister tubercle

Lunate fossa

Sigmoid notch

Capitate waist

Capitate head

Hook of hamate

Hamate

Triquetrum distal pole

Pisiform

Lunate volar lip

Lunate dorsal lip

Ulnar styloid process

Ulnar fovea

Ulnar head

Trapezium & 1st metacarpal base

Pisiform

Scaphoid distal pole

Radial styloid process

Radius, volar lip of sigmoid notch

3rd metacarpal

Capitate dorsal body

Trapezoid

Hamate

Triquetrum

Lunate

Radius, dorsal lip of sigmoid notch

Ulnar styloid process

Ulnar fovea

Ulnar head

(Top) Zero-rotation PA radiograph. Image obtained by positioning patient at 90° abduction of shoulder & 90° flexion of elbow. Hand prone on cassette. Beam perpendicular to cassette & centered on capitate head. **(Bottom)** Zero-rotation lateral radiograph. Image obtained with similar shoulder & elbow positioning. Hand lateral with ulnar side on cassette. Beam perpendicular to cassette & centered on capitate head. Note that in this ideal lateral, there is slight dorsal placement of the ulna relative to the radius. This positioning allows evaluation of the coaxial arrangement of the radius, lunate, capitate, and 3rd metacarpal.

OSSEOUS STRUCTURES

RADIOGRAPHS, DORSIFLEXION & VOLARFLEXION

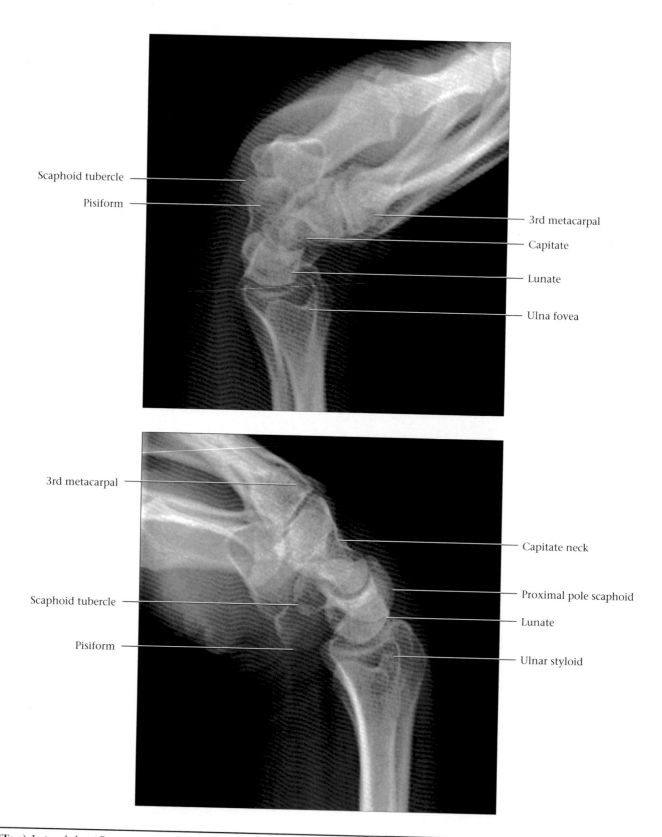

Scaphoid tubercle
Pisiform
3rd metacarpal
Capitate
Lunate
Ulna fovea

3rd metacarpal
Scaphoid tubercle
Pisiform
Capitate neck
Proximal pole scaphoid
Lunate
Ulnar styloid

(**Top**) Lateral dorsiflexion. Wrist placed in neutral lateral on cassette & maximally dorsiflexed. Center beam perpendicular to cassette & centered on scaphoid waist. (**Bottom**) Lateral volarflexion. Wrist placed in neutral lateral on cassette & maximally volarflexed. Center beam perpendicular to cassette & centered on scaphoid waist.

OSSEOUS STRUCTURES

RADIOGRAPHS, SEMIPRONATED & SEMISUPINATED

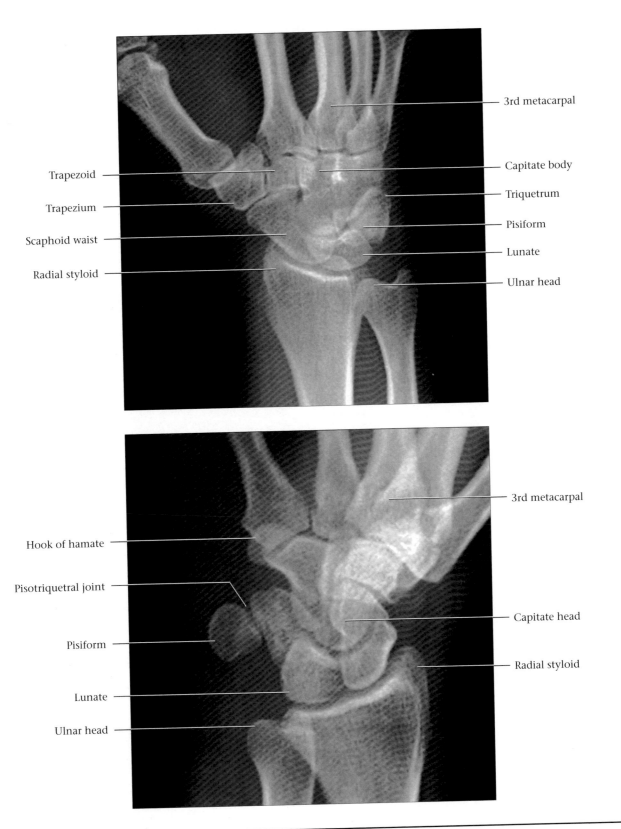

Trapezoid — Capitate body
Trapezium — 3rd metacarpal
Scaphoid waist — Triquetrum
Radial styloid — Pisiform
— Lunate
— Ulnar head

Hook of hamate — 3rd metacarpal
Pisotriquetral joint
Pisiform — Capitate head
Lunate — Radial styloid
Ulnar head

(Top) PA semipronated oblique. Radial hand raised 45° from cassette without flexion or extension. Beam perpendicular to cassette & centered on capitate head. **(Bottom)** Semisupinated oblique. Ulnar wrist placed with 30-45° supination from neutral lateral position. Center beam perpendicular to cassette & centered on capitate head. The supinated oblique is ideal for evaluation of the hook of hamate, pisiform, or triquetral fractures.

OSSEOUS STRUCTURES

RADIOGRAPHS, RADIAL & ULNAR DEVIATION

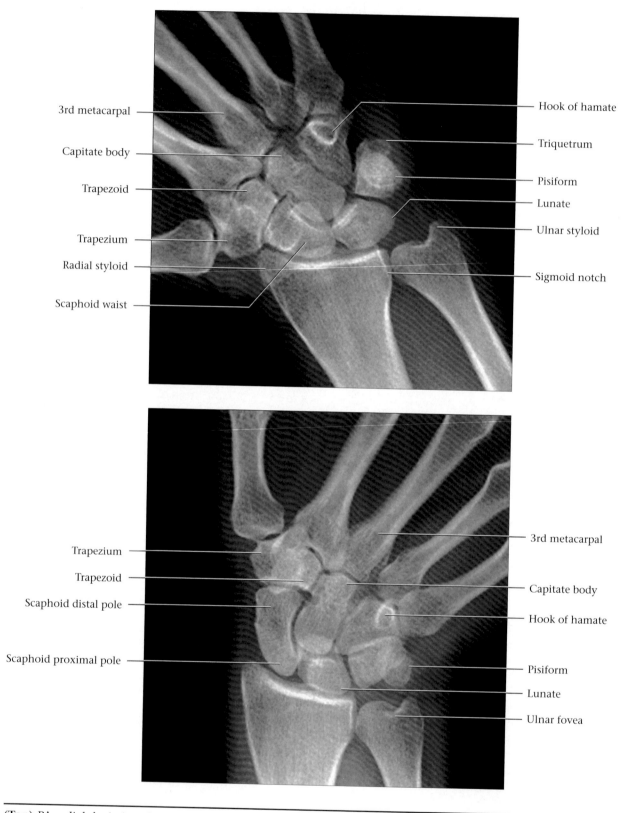

(Top) PA radial deviation. Positioned palm flat on cassette, wrist in maximum abduction without flexion or extension. Beam perpendicular to cassette & centered on capitate head. Note the "target sign" of the volarflexed scaphoid, making evaluation of the waist for fracture quite difficult. (Bottom) PA ulnar deviation. Positioned palm flat on cassette, wrist in maximum abduction without flexion or extension. Beam perpendicular to cassette & centered on capitate head. Note that ulnar deviation elongates the scaphoid, and is ideal for evaluation for scaphoid waist fracture.

OSSEOUS STRUCTURES

RADIOGRAPHS, SCAPHOID & CLENCHED FIST VIEWS

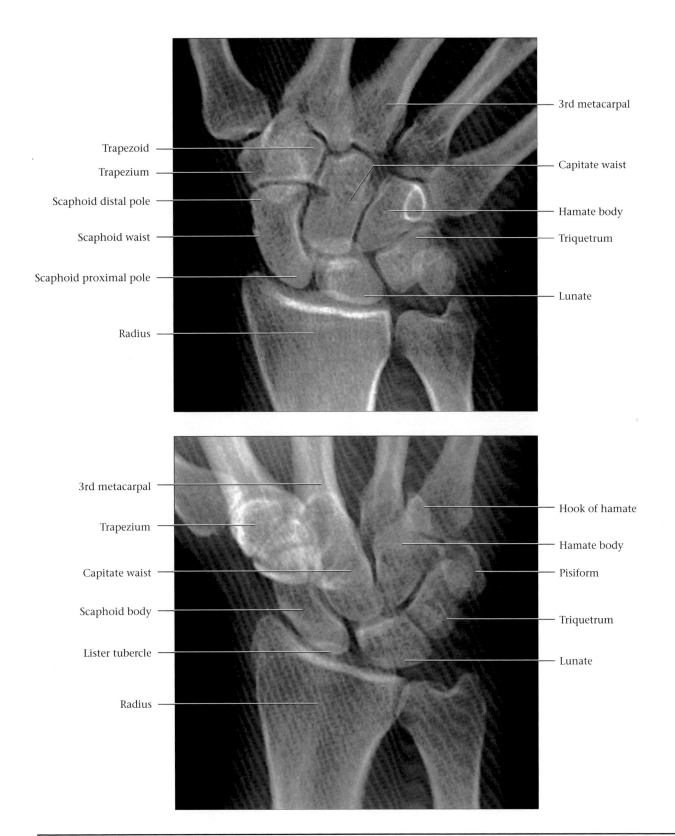

(Top) Scaphoid view. Radial wrist raised 30° off cassette with slight ulnar deviation. Beam angulated 35° toward elbow & centered on scaphoid waist. **(Bottom)** Clenched fist. Wrist placed prone (or supine) on cassette & hand is clenched tightly. Center beam perpendicular to cassette & centered on capitate head.

OSSEOUS STRUCTURES

RADIOGRAPHS, CARPAL TUNNEL & BRIDGE

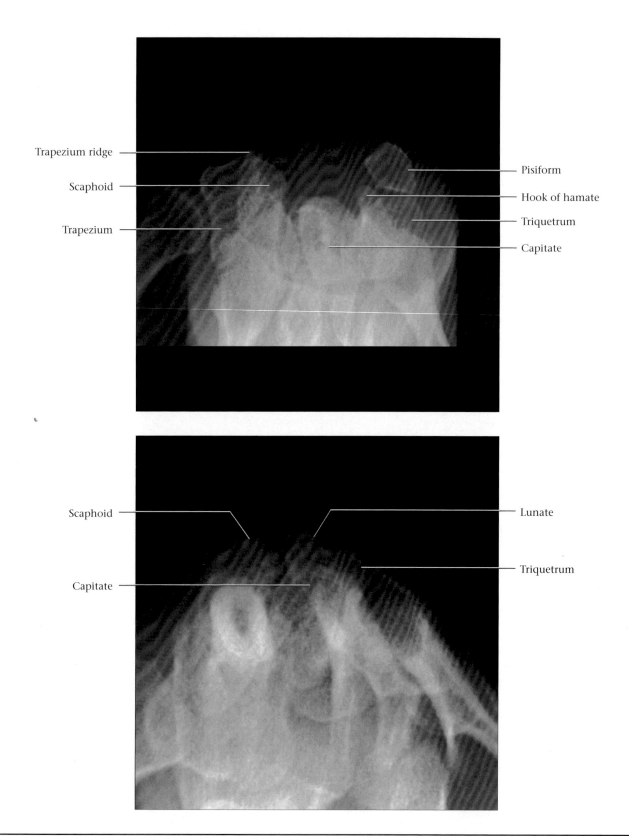

Trapezium ridge

Scaphoid

Trapezium

Pisiform

Hook of hamate

Triquetrum

Capitate

Scaphoid

Capitate

Lunate

Triquetrum

(Top) Carpal tunnel view. Hand placed on cassette palm down & maximally dorsiflexed. Center beam directly tangent to palmar wrist & centered on center of carpal tunnel. **(Bottom)** Carpal bridge view. Dorsal forearm on cassette with wrist maximally flexed. Beam angled 45° tangent to & centered on dorsal wrist center.

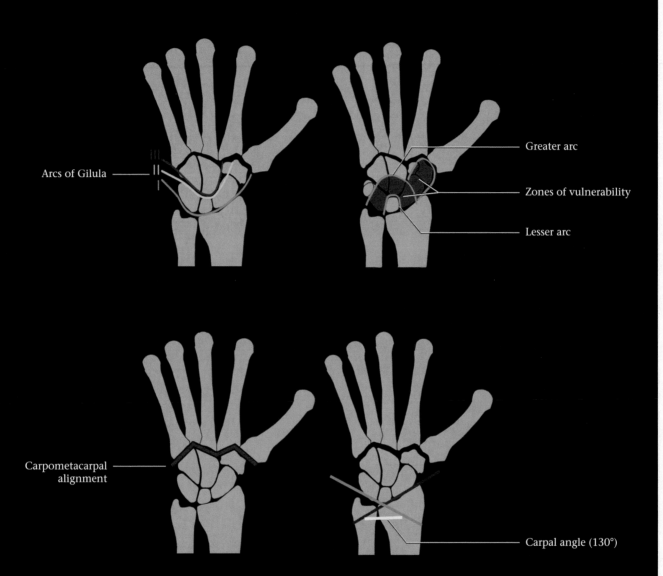

Images clockwise from upper left: Arcs of Gilula outline three smooth curves paralleling articular surfaces. Disruption of these smooth flowing arcs is an indication of trauma or carpal malalignment. Second image: Greater & lesser arcs describe joints around lunate (lesser arc) & mid scaphoid, capitate, hamate & triquetrum. Vulnerable zone is the area encompassed by greater, lesser arcs, scaphoid & trapezium; region where majority of fractures occur. Third image: Carpometacarpal alignment on PA wrist creates an "M". Disruption of contour suggests joint injury. Fourth image: Carpal angle evaluates developing carpal collapse related to arthritis or trauma.

GRAPHICS, PA RADIOGRAPHIC MEASUREMENTS

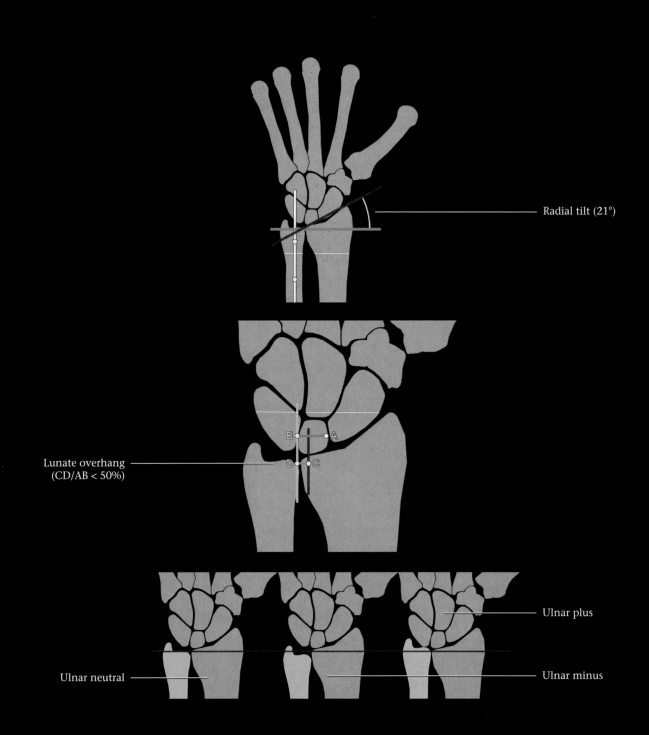

Radial tilt (21°)

Lunate overhang
(CD/AB < 50%)

Ulnar plus

Ulnar neutral

Ulnar minus

First image: Radial tilt (inclination) measures normal distal radius angulation & may be disrupted in fractures. Normal tilt is 21° (range 16-28°). Second iamge: Ulnar carpal translation measures lunate overhang. AB is width of lunate & CD is overhang of medial lunate relative to sigmoid notch. Normal ratio is CD/AB < 50%, i.e., at least 50% of the lunate articular surface should articulate with the radius on a PA radiograph. Third image: Ulnar variance is measured as the length of distal ulna compared to distal radius. Ulnar neutral requires the ulna to be equal in length to the radius, or no more than 2 mm shorter. Ulnar minus occurs when the ulna is greater than 2 mm shorter than the radius. Ulnar plus variance occurs when the ulna is longer than the radius.

OSSEOUS STRUCTURES

GRAPHICS, PA & LATERAL RADIOGRAPHIC MEASUREMENTS

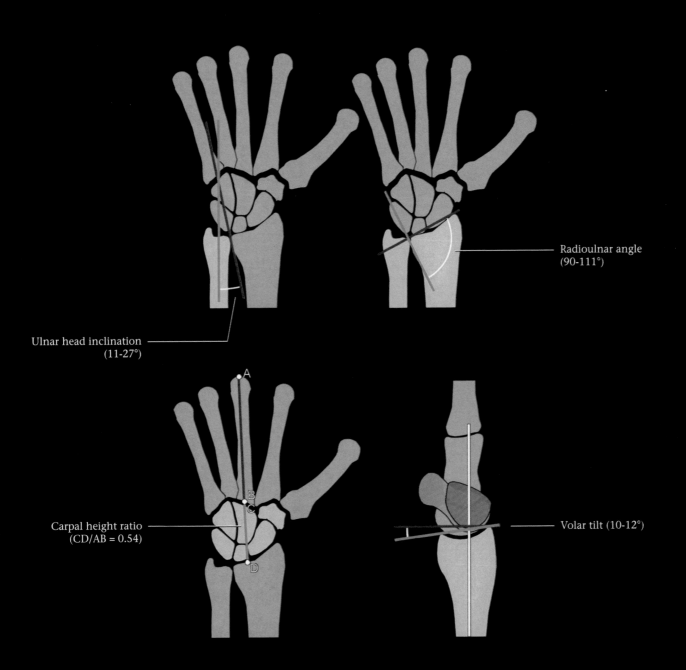

Radioulnar angle
(90-111°)

Ulnar head inclination
(11-27°)

A

B
C

D

Carpal height ratio
(CD/AB = 0.54)

Volar tilt (10-12°)

Ulnar head inclination assists in evaluating distal radioulnar joint injury. Radioulnar angle evaluates radiocarpal injury & carpal malalignment. Carpal height ratio measures CD/AB is normally 0.54 & assists in evaluating of carpal collapse in arthropathies. Volar tilt measures normal radius volar angulation & may be disrupted in trauma.

GRAPHICS, LATERAL CARPAL AXES

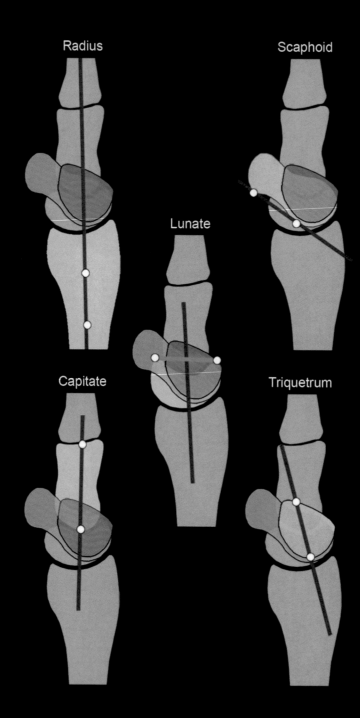

Radius

Scaphoid

Lunate

Capitate

Triquetrum

Ideal points of carpal axis measurement to allow accurate evaluation of carpal alignment. On the graphic, the bone in which the axis is being drawn is colored yellow.

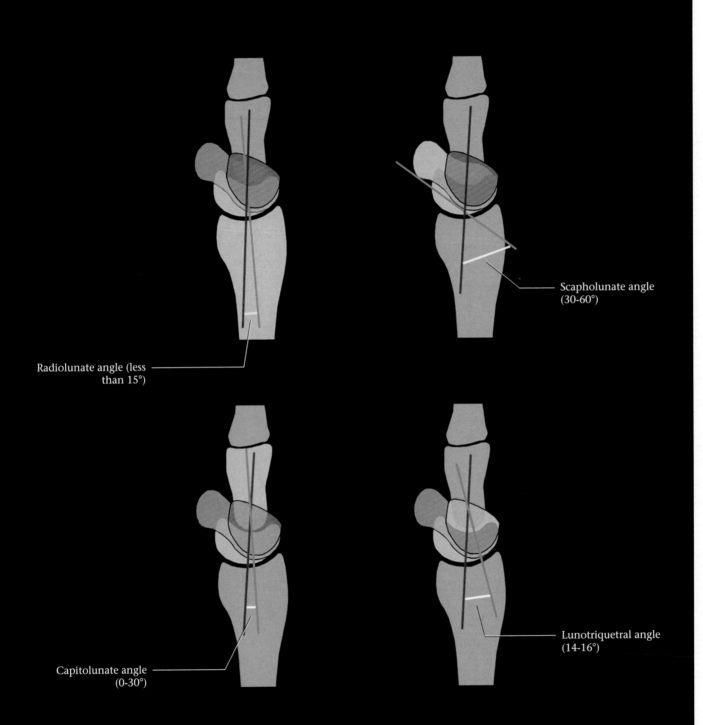

Scapholunate angle
(30-60°)

Radiolunate angle (less
than 15°)

Capitolunate angle
(0-30°)

Lunotriquetral angle
(14-16°)

Carpal alignment. Disruption is indicative of carpal instability and/or trauma. In the graphic, the lunate axis is colored red, and the axis against which it is being measured is blue.

OSSEOUS STRUCTURES

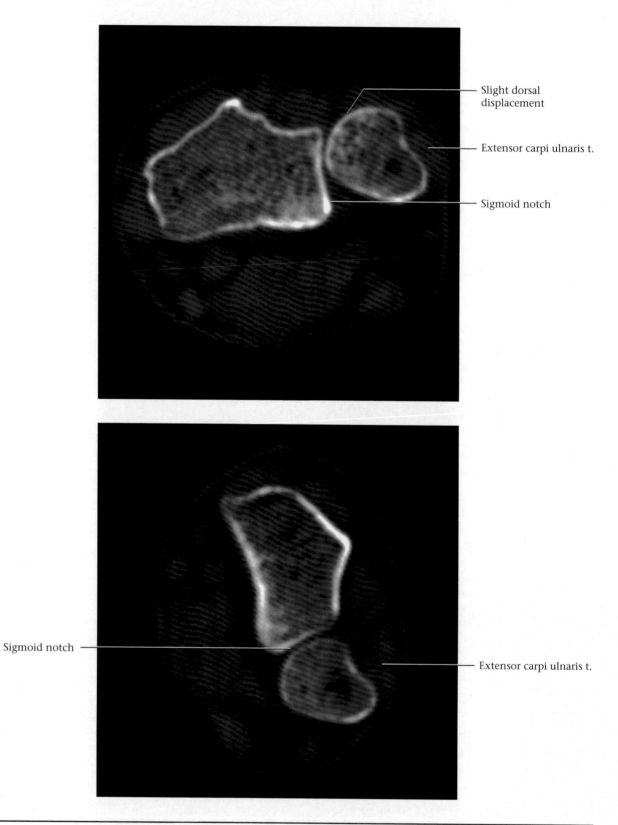

Slight dorsal displacement

Extensor carpi ulnaris t.

Sigmoid notch

Sigmoid notch

Extensor carpi ulnaris t.

(Top) Full pronation. Placing wrist in full pronation results in slight dorsal displacement of ulna in sigmoid notch. ECU is seated within ulnar groove. Radius rotates around ulna. **(Bottom)** Neutral. Placing wrist in neutral rotation allows distal ulna to be fully seated in radial sigmoid notch. ECU is seated within ulnar groove.

OSSEOUS STRUCTURES

SUPINATED & PRONATED AXIAL CT, DISTAL RADIOULNAR JOINT ALIGNMENT

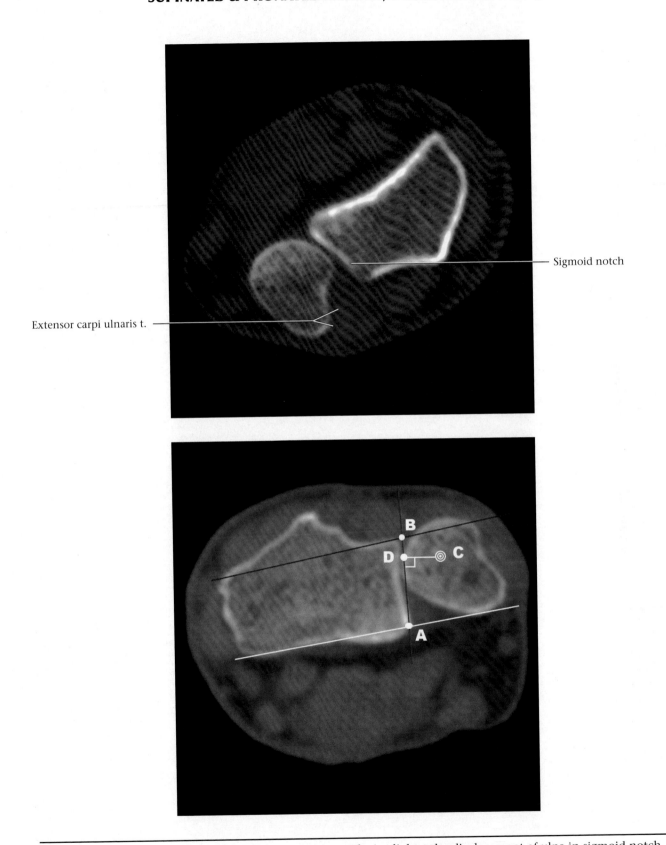

Sigmoid notch

Extensor carpi ulnaris t.

(Top) Full supination. Placing wrist in full supination results in slight volar displacement of ulna in sigmoid notch. ECU is draped over medial rim of ulnar groove. Radius rotates around ulna. **(Bottom)** Radioulnar ratio is used for evaluation of subtle subluxation. Identify ulnar head center & draw perpendicular to line drawn across margins of sigmoid notch. AD/AB: Radioulnar ratio. Normal ratio depends on patient position.

3D RECONSTRUCTION CT, DORSAL & VOLAR WRIST

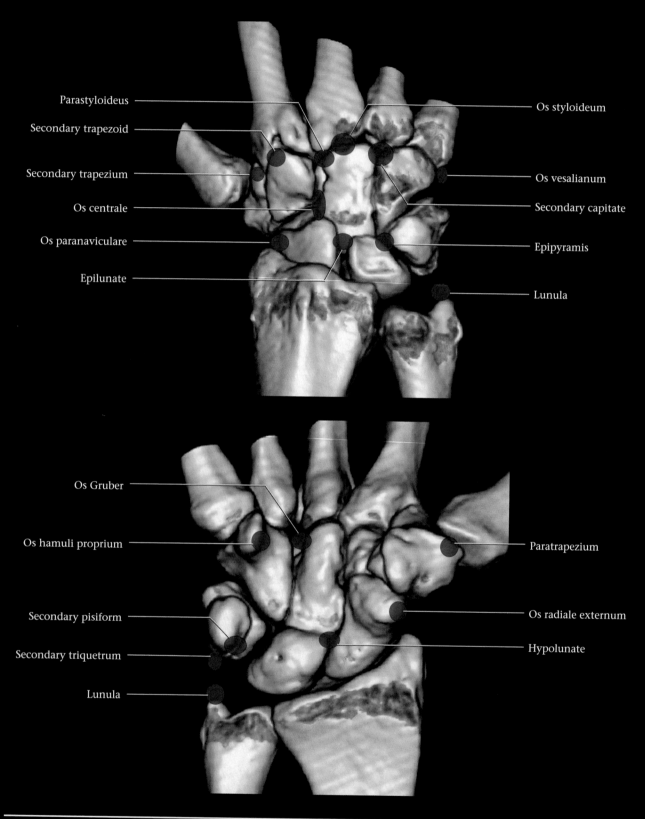

Parastyloideus

Secondary trapezoid

Secondary trapezium

Os centrale

Os paranaviculare

Epilunate

Os styloideum

Os vesalianum

Secondary capitate

Epipyramis

Lunula

Os Gruber

Os hamuli proprium

Secondary pisiform

Secondary triquetrum

Lunula

Paratrapezium

Os radiale externum

Hypolunate

(Top) Dorsal accessory ossicles. **(Bottom)** Volar accessory ossicles. Accessory ossicles are common & may mimic fractures.

3D RECONSTRUCTION CT, VOLAR OBLIQUE WRIST

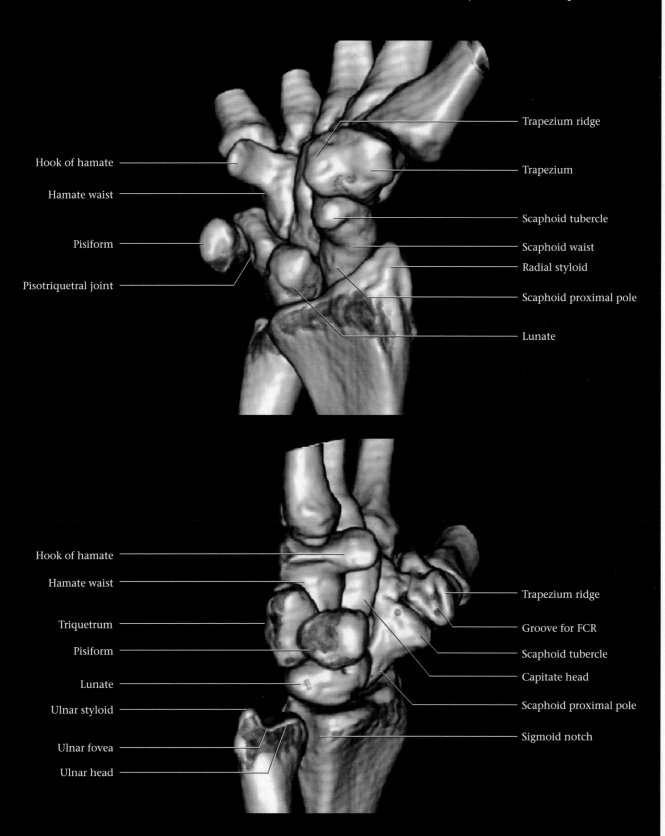

Trapezium ridge

Hook of hamate

Trapezium

Hamate waist

Scaphoid tubercle

Pisiform

Scaphoid waist

Radial styloid

Pisotriquetral joint

Scaphoid proximal pole

Lunate

Hook of hamate

Hamate waist

Trapezium ridge

Triquetrum

Groove for FCR

Pisiform

Scaphoid tubercle

Lunate

Capitate head

Ulnar styloid

Scaphoid proximal pole

Ulnar fovea

Sigmoid notch

Ulnar head

(Top) 3D reconstruction CT demonstrates key osseous contours & relationships. **(Bottom)** With rotational manipulation of imaging data, structures can be viewed in multiple planes.

OSSEOUS STRUCTURES

GRAPHIC & PA RADIOGRAPH, WRIST COMPARTMENTS

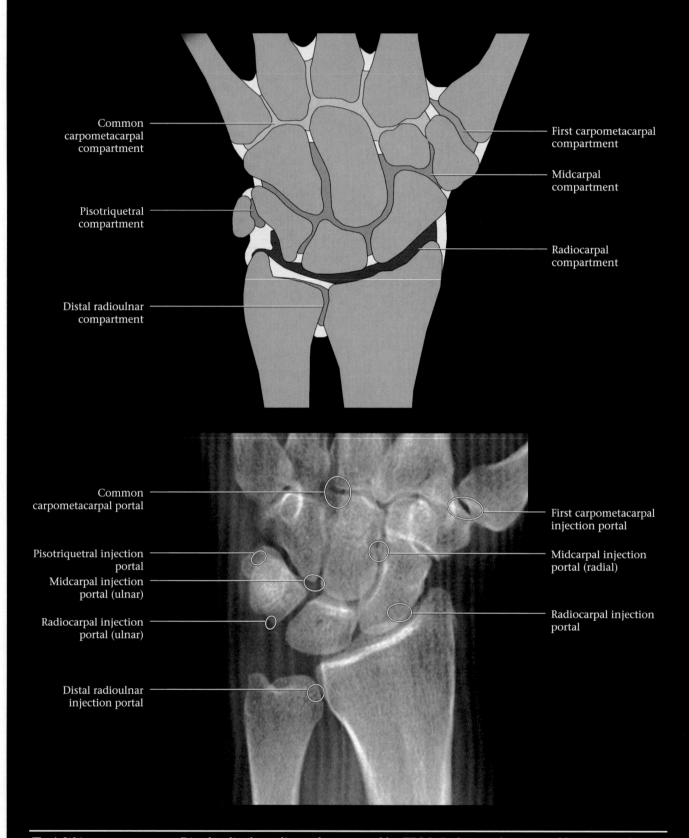

Common carpometacarpal compartment

First carpometacarpal compartment

Midcarpal compartment

Pisotriquetral compartment

Radiocarpal compartment

Distal radioulnar compartment

Common carpometacarpal portal

First carpometacarpal injection portal

Pisotriquetral injection portal

Midcarpal injection portal (radial)

Midcarpal injection portal (ulnar)

Radiocarpal injection portal (ulnar)

Radiocarpal injection portal

Distal radioulnar injection portal

(Top) Wrist compartments: Distal radioulnar, discretely separated by TFCC. Radiocarpal, separated by proximal scapholunate & lunotriquetral ligaments as well as TFCC. Pisotriquetral, separated from radiocarpal in 20%. Midcarpal, separated by scapholunate & lunotriquetral ligaments, typically communicates with carpometacarpal joint. First carpometacarpal separated from common carpometacarpal by trapeziometacarpal ligament. **(Bottom)** Arthrography can be accomplished by placing needle tip at indicated points for injection of contrast agent. Joint volumes: Distal radioulnar, 1-2 cc; radiocarpal, 2-3 cc; midcarpal, 3-5 cc (common carpometacarpal joint often fills simultaneously); pisotriquetral, 1-2 cc; first carpometacarpal, 1-2 cc.

OSSEOUS STRUCTURES

CORONAL T1 & GRE MR, BONE & CARTILAGE STRUCTURE

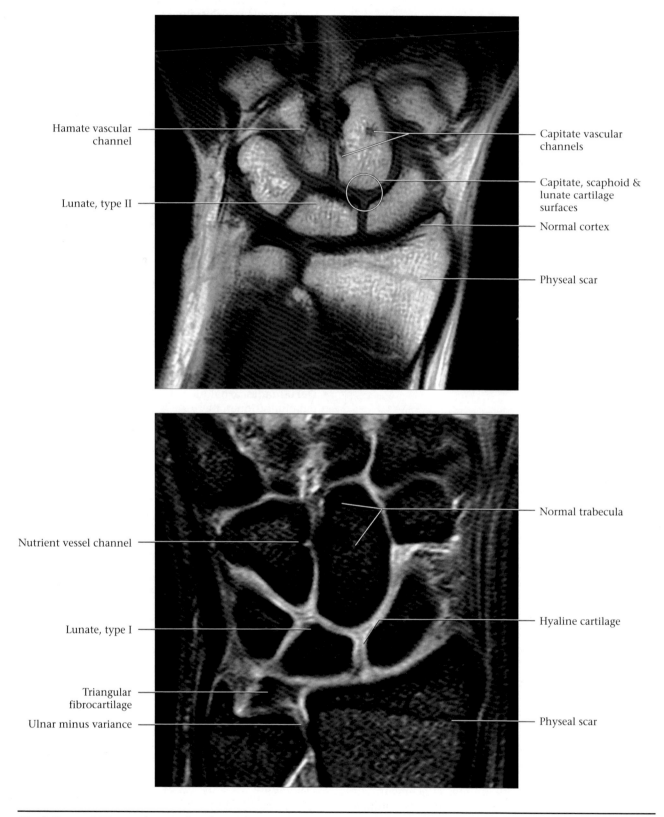

Hamate vascular channel

Lunate, type II

Capitate vascular channels

Capitate, scaphoid & lunate cartilage surfaces

Normal cortex

Physeal scar

Nutrient vessel channel

Lunate, type I

Triangular fibrocartilage

Ulnar minus variance

Normal trabecula

Hyaline cartilage

Physeal scar

(Top) Coronal T1 reveals vascular channels at capitate waist & dorsal hamate. Cortical margins are thin, low signal intensity but trabecular pattern is clearly evident as fine meshwork. This meshwork creates field inhomogeneity in GRE imaging. Cartilage surfaces are present but visualized in slimited fashion in non-contrast imaging. Note type II lunate with facet articulating with hamate. **(Bottom)** Coronal GRE (1.5 tesla) reveals normal trabecular pattern with low signal intensity cortices. Cartilage is well seen in gradient sequences as a high signal structure. Note ulnar minus variance with compensatory thickening of triangular fibrocartilage. Type I lunate is present. Field inhomogeneity in this sequence may obscure intraosseous edema.

LIGAMENTS

Terminology

Abbreviations

- Carpometacarpal (CMC)
- Dorsal radiocarpal (DRC)
- Dorsal radioulnar (DRU)
- Extensor carpi radialis longus (ECRL)
- Extensor carpi ulnaris (ECU)
- Field of view (FOV)
- Flexor carpi ulnaris (FCU)
- Gadolinium (Gd)
- Long radiolunate ligament (LRL)
- Lunotriquetral (LT)
- Metacarpal (MC)
- Normal saline (NS)
- Radioscaphocapitate ligament (RSC)
- Range of motion (ROM)
- Scapholunate (SL)
- Scaphotrapezium-trapezoid (STT)
- Short radiolunate ligament (SRL)
- Triangular fibrocartilage (TFC)
- Triangular fibrocartilage complex (TFCC)
- Triquetrocapitate (TC)
- Ulnocapitate (UC)
- Ulnolunate (UL)
- Ulnotriquetral (UT)
- Volar radioulnar (VRU)

Definitions

- Intrinsic ligaments: Connect carpals to carpals
- Extrinsic ligaments: Connect radius/ulna to carpals; carpals to metacarpals

Imaging Anatomy

Overview

- Terminology
  - Ligament terminology variable in literature
  - Ligament names, where controversial, are based on anatomic dissection studies (Berger, 1997) with alternate terms in parentheses
- Generalizations
  - Ligaments run obliquely; from periphery to midline; from proximal to distal
  - Volar ligaments are key stabilizers; dorsal ligaments, less crucial
  - Capitate & lunate have most ligament attachments
  - Triquetrum is ulnar anchor for capsular ligaments
  - All adjacent carpals have interosseous ligaments: Medial/lateral, distal/proximal (except lunate & capitate - no proximal/distal ligament)

Volar Radiocarpal Ligaments

- **Radioscaphocapitate** (sling, radiocapitate)
  - **Origin**: Distal radius, radial styloid; **course**: Passes across scaphoid waist with minimal attachment; **insertion**: Capitate body (10% of fibers); arcs around distal lunate, interdigitates with UC & TC to form **arcuate ligament**
    - **Radial collateral**: Radial-most fibers of RSC; existence as separate ligament debated
  - **Action**: Constrains radiocarpal pronation, ulnocarpal translocation; stabilizes distal scaphoid pole; creates sling for scaphoid
- **Long radiolunate** (volar radiolunotriquetral, volar radiotriquetral ligament)
  - **Origin**: Radius ulnar to RSC; **course**: Passes volar to scaphoid & SL ligament; **insertion**: Volar lunate rim; continues to triquetrum
  - **Action**: Constrains ulnar translocation & distal translation of lunate; creates sling for lunate
  - May appear as two separate ligaments: Radiolunate & lunotriquetral
- **Radioscapholunate** (ligament of Testut; intra-articular fat pad)
  - **Origin**: Volar radius ulnar to LRL; **insertion**: Proximal scaphoid, lunate & SL ligament
  - **Action**: Mechanoreceptor of SL relationship
  - Not true ligament: Contains fat, arterioles, venules & small nerves
- **Short radiolunate**
  - **Origin**: Volar radius ulnar to LRL; **insertion**: Volar lunate (radial 2/3)
  - **Action**: Stabilizes lunate; facilitates motion in flexion/extension
- **Arcuate ("V" ligament)**: Confluence of ligaments on volar capitate including RSC, UC & TC

Dorsal Radiocarpal Ligament

- **Dorsal radiocarpal** (dorsal radiotriquetral; dorsal radiolunotriquetral)
  - **Origin**: Broad attachment to dorsal radius from Lister tubercle to sigmoid notch; **insertion**: Dorsal lunate & triquetrum
  - **Action**: Reinforces dorsal LT ligament; constrains ulnar translocation of carpals; creates dorsal sling for triquetrum

Volar Midcarpal Ligaments

- **Scaphotrapezium-trapezoid**
  - **Origin**: Scaphoid tubercle; **insertion**: Volar trapezium; few fibers to trapezoid
  - **Action**: Maintains scaphoid in volarflexion; stabilizes scaphoid, trapezium & trapezoid
- **Scaphocapitate**
  - **Origin**: Volar scaphoid distal pole; **insertion**: Volar capitate body
  - **Action**: Stabilizer of scaphoid; balances volar flexion tendency of STT ligament
- **Triquetrocapitate**
  - **Origin**: Volar triquetrum; **insertion**: Volar capitate body
  - **Action**: Midcarpal stabilization
- **Triquetrohamate**
  - **Origin**: Volar triquetrum; **insertion**: Volar hamate body at hook base
  - **Action**: Midcarpal stabilization
- **Pisohamate**
  - **Origin**: Volar pisiform; **insertion**: Hook of hamate
  - **Action**: Transmits pull of FCU on pisiform to carpals; considered a prolongation of FCU
- **Deltoid**: Confluence of scaphocapitate & triquetrocapitate ligaments; parallels arcuate ligament

LIGAMENTS

Dorsal Midcarpal Ligaments
- **Dorsal intercarpal**
  - **Origin**: Dorsal triquetrum, interdigitating with DRC ligament; **insertion**: Scaphoid & dorsal trapezoid
  - **Action**: Envelops radial artery in anatomic snuffbox; constrains midcarpal rotation; acts as labrum to capitate head & proximal hamate
- **Dorsal scaphotriquetral**
  - **Origin**: Scaphoid, extending dorsal & distal to SL/LT ligaments; **insertion**: Dorsal triquetrum
  - **Action**: Stabilizes SL/LT ligaments; labrum for capitate head & hamate proximal pole

Proximal Interosseous Ligaments
- **Scapholunate**
  - **Origin/insertion**: Ulnar scaphoid to radial lunate; hyaline cartilage attachment
  - **Action**: Dorsal portion resists volar-dorsal translation; volar portion limits flexion/extension rotation; proximal accommodates compression & shear forces across radiocarpal joint
  - U-shaped ligament with dorsal, proximal & volar components
    - Dorsal component thicker (5 mm) than volar (1-2 mm); functionally more important than proximal portion
    - Proximal component is meniscus-like avascular fibrocartilage; triangular shape
  - Attritional tears with age
- **Lunotriquetral**
  - **Origin/insertion**: Ulnar lunate to radial triquetrum; hyaline cartilage attachment
  - **Action**: Volar portion limits translation of lunate & triquetrum; dorsal portion stabilizes joint
  - U-shaped ligament with dorsal, proximal & volar components
    - Volar component thicker (2.3 mm) than dorsal (1 mm); functionally more important than proximal portion
    - Proximal component is meniscus-like avascular fibrocartilage; triangular shape
  - Attritional tears with age

Distal Interosseous Ligaments
- **Trapeziotrapezoid**
  - Dorsal & volar components: Thickness 2 mm; forms floor of ECRL tendon sheath
  - **Action**: Stabilizes distal carpals; maintains carpal arch
- **Trapeziocapitate**
  - Dorsal, volar & deep components: Thickness 1-2 mm; deep portion connects dorsal trapezoid to volar capitate
  - **Action**: Stabilizes distal carpals; maintains carpal arch
- **Capitohamate**
  - Dorsal, volar & deep components: Thickness 1-2 mm; volar aspect contiguous with volar ligaments, contributing to ligamentous ring of carpal tunnel
  - **Action**: Stabilizes distal carpals; maintains carpal arch

Carpometacarpal Ligaments
- **Pisometacarpal**
  - **Origin**: Volar pisiform; **insertion**: Volar 5th MC
  - **Action**: Transmits pull of FCU on pisiform to metacarpals; considered a prolongation of FCU
- **Carpometacarpal ligaments of thumb**
  - **Origin**: Dorsal, lateral & radial trapezium; **insertion**: Dorsal, volar & lateral thumb MC base
  - **Action**: Stabilizes highly mobile thumb base
- **Dorsal carpometacarpal**
  - **Origin**: Adjacent carpals give 2-3 ligament slips each; **insertion**: 2nd-5th dorsal MC bases
  - **Action**: Stabilizes CMC joints sliding motion
- **Volar carpometacarpal**
  - **Origin**: Adjacent carpals give 1-2 ligament slips each; **insertion**: 2nd-5th dorsal MC bases
  - **Action**: Stabilizes CMC joints sliding motion

Distal Radioulnar Ligaments
- **Dorsal radioulnar**
  - **Origin**: Dorsal sigmoid notch, bone attachment; **insertion**: Dorsal fibers form ECU sheath & attach to styloid process; volar fibers attach to ulnar fovea
  - **Action**: Stabilizes distal ulna, preventing volar subluxation during supination
- **Volar radioulnar**
  - **Origin**: Volar sigmoid notch, bone attachment; **insertion**: Ulnar fovea; joins with volar fibers of DRU & creates a "ring" (apparent on MR)
  - **Action**: Serves as base for UL & UT ligament origins; stabilizes distal ulna, preventing dorsal subluxation during pronation

Ulnocarpal Structures
- **Ulnolunate**
  - **Origin**: Arises from VRU; ulnar to SRL; **insertion**: Lunate (ulnar 1/3) adjacent to SRL
  - **Action**: Stabilizes lunate through wrist ROM
  - Arises from ligament rather than bone, reducing effect of forearm rotation to carpals
- **Ulnotriquetral**
  - **Lateral band**
    - **Origin**: Arises from VRU ulnar to UL; **insertion**: Triquetrum, medial to LT ligament
    - **Action**: Restricts & stabilizes triquetrum
  - **Medial band (ulnar collateral ligament)**
    - **Origin**: Arises from DRU at its insertion on ulnar styloid; **insertion**: Lateral triquetrum
    - **Action**: Forms floor of ECU tendon sheath; constrains distal translation of triquetrum
    - Actual existence of ulnar collateral ligament is debated
  - Arises from ligament rather than bone, reducing effects of forearm rotation on carpals
  - Lateral & medial bands separate just distal to prestyloid recess; lead to pisotriquetral joint (in 90%)
- **Ulnocapitate**
  - **Origin**: Ulnar fovea, bone attachment; **insertion**: Fibers interdigitate with volar LT ligament; continue distally to capitate; blend with RSC to form arcuate ligament

- o **Action**: Reinforces ulnocarpal joint capsule & LT joint; anchors carpals to ulna; creates volar sling for triquetrum
- **Ulnocarpal meniscal homologue**
  - o Capsular thickening, triangular shape; variably present
  - o Lies distal to ulnar TFC & ulnar styloid tip; between DRU & radial volar ECU tendon sheath; separated from TFC by prestyloid recess opening
- **Triangular fibrocartilage (articular disc)**
  - o **Origin**: Arises from radial sigmoid notch, attaching to hyaline cartilage; **insertion**: Ulnar fovea & styloid tip
  - o Variable thickness proportional to ulnar length (thicker with ulnar minus, thinner with ulnar plus); ulnar portion 2-3x thicker than radial
  - o Ulnar portion is vascularized; radial & central portions are not
  - o Attritional tears with age
- **Triangular fibrocartilage complex**
  - o Complex includes articular disc, DRU, VRU, UL, UT & ECU tendon sheath
  - o **Action**: Transmits portion of axial load from ulnar carpals to distal ulna; stabilizer of DRU joint; stabilizer of ulnar carpals

Recesses

- May be seen arthrographically &/or arthroscopically
- **Interligamentous sulcus**: Arthroscopic landmark; separates RSC from LRL allowing motion between these ligaments on radial & ulnar deviation
- **Space of Poirier**: Area of weakness in volar capsule accessed via interligamentous sulcus; located just proximal to deltoid ligament; volar lunate dislocation can occur here.
- **RSC ligament region**: Space between volar scaphoid proximal pole & RSC deep surface
- **Prestyloid recess**: Located at apex of DRU & VRU ligaments just distal to ulnar fovea; lined with synovium; variably communicates with ulnar styloid tip
- **Dorsal transverse recess**: Arises between dorsal capitate head/neck, hamate & dorsal midcarpal joint capsule, dorsal distal scaphoid
- **Ulnar recess**: Arises medial to triquetrohamate articulation
- **Radial recess**: Arises lateral to STT & palmar recess anterior to capitate

Anatomy-Based Imaging Issues

Imaging Recommendations

- **MR appearance**
  - o Extrinsic ligaments: Low signal or striated bands on all sequences
  - o Interosseous ligaments: Low signal bands; variably visualized, especially in midcarpal & distal rows; deep components tend to be thick, short ligaments
    - Scapholunate/lunotriquetral ligaments: Dorsal & volar contours band-like with proximal (central) portion triangular in shape

- Normal signal varies from uniform low to striated intermediate signal; may be amorphous in proximal portion
- Attach to cartilage rather than bone; should not be mistaken for a tear
- Visualized on coronal & axial; important to scrutinize axial imaging as disruption of dorsal, volar components correlates with instability
- o TFCC: Low signal intensity articular disc attaches to cartilage along sigmoid notch
- **Arthrography**
  - o Good evaluation for integrity of SL, LT & TFC; limited for extrinsic ligaments
  - o Injections spaced to allow contrast resorption one compartment before 2nd injected
    - Radiocarpal joint injected first (most likely to document with single injection); if no tear, wait 30-60 minutes & proceed sequentially with DRU & midcarpal injections
  - o Digital subtraction allows dynamic evaluation of ligament status & sequential compartment injection without delay
  - o Injectate: Iodinated contrast (180-300 mg I/ml); volumes: Midcarpal, 4-5 cc; radiocarpal, 2-3 cc; DRU, 1-2 cc; pisotriquetral, 1-2 cc
- **MR imaging**
  - o GRE (T2) imaging maximizes visualization of ligaments in absence of intra-articular fluid
  - o Coronal: SL, LT, TFCC, extrinsic ligaments
  - o Axial: TFCC, dorsal & volar SL/LT, extrinsic ligaments
  - o Sagittal: Extrinsic ligaments
  - o **MR arthrography**: Injectate: 1/200 NS:Gd; volumes as noted above
- **CT imaging**
  - o Ligaments not seen in absence of contrast; **CT arthrography** allows evaluation of ligament integrity; diagnostic efficacy equal to MR
  - o Injectate: 1:1 NS:iodinated contrast; allows standard arthrography & CT arthrography
- **Ultrasound**
  - o Described for evaluation of extrinsic ligament tears; performed with stand-off pad; 10-12 MHz transducer; highly operator-dependent

Imaging Pitfalls

- Attritional tears/fenestrations: TFC, SL, LT
- Ligament attachments to cartilage rather than bone mimics tears (e.g., TFC, SL, LT)
- Satisfaction of search: If intrinsic ligament tear seen, examine extrinsic ligaments carefully for accompanying abnormalities

Selected References

1. Theumann NH et al: Extrinsic carpal ligaments: normal MR arthrographic appearance in cadavers. Radiology. 226(1):171-9, 2003
2. Berger RA: The ligaments of the wrist. A current overview of anatomy with considerations of their potential functions. Hand Clin. 13(1):63-82, 1997

LIGAMENTS

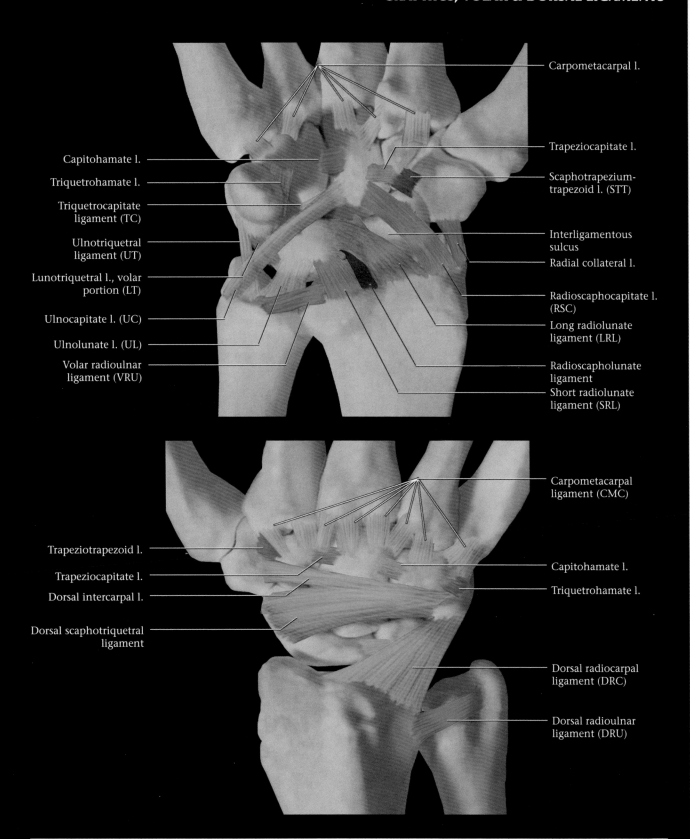

Carpometacarpal l.

Trapeziocapitate l.

Scaphotrapezium-
trapezoid l. (STT)

Interligamentous
sulcus

Radial collateral l.

Radioscaphocapitate l.
(RSC)

Long radiolunate
ligament (LRL)

Radioscapholunate
ligament

Short radiolunate
ligament (SRL)

Capitohamate l.

Triquetrohamate l.

Triquetrocapitate
ligament (TC)

Ulnotriquetral
ligament (UT)

Lunotriquetral l., volar
portion (LT)

Ulnocapitate l. (UC)

Ulnolunate l. (UL)

Volar radioulnar
ligament (VRU)

Carpometacarpal
ligament (CMC)

Capitohamate l.

Triquetrohamate l.

Dorsal radiocarpal
ligament (DRC)

Dorsal radioulnar
ligament (DRU)

Trapeziotrapezoid l.

Trapeziocapitate l.

Dorsal intercarpal l.

Dorsal scaphotriquetral
ligament

(Top) Volar intrinsic & extrinsic ligaments. Extrinsic ligaments connect carpals to bones of forearm (radius & ulna) & hand (metacarpals) & are often capsular. Intrinsic ligaments connect carpals to carpals. Abbreviations on the graphics are those used in the introductory text. Note that the arcuate ligament (not labeled) is formed by interdigitating fibers of the radioscaphocapitate, ulnocapitate & triquetrocapitate. Note that the deltoid ligament, running parallel to the arcuate ligament, lies deep to these structures and is not shown here. **(Bottom)** Dorsal ligaments stabilize & restrict motion but are less critical to stability of wrist structures than volar ligaments.

AXIAL GRE MR ARTHROGRAM, INTRINSIC & EXTRINSIC LIGAMENTS

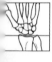

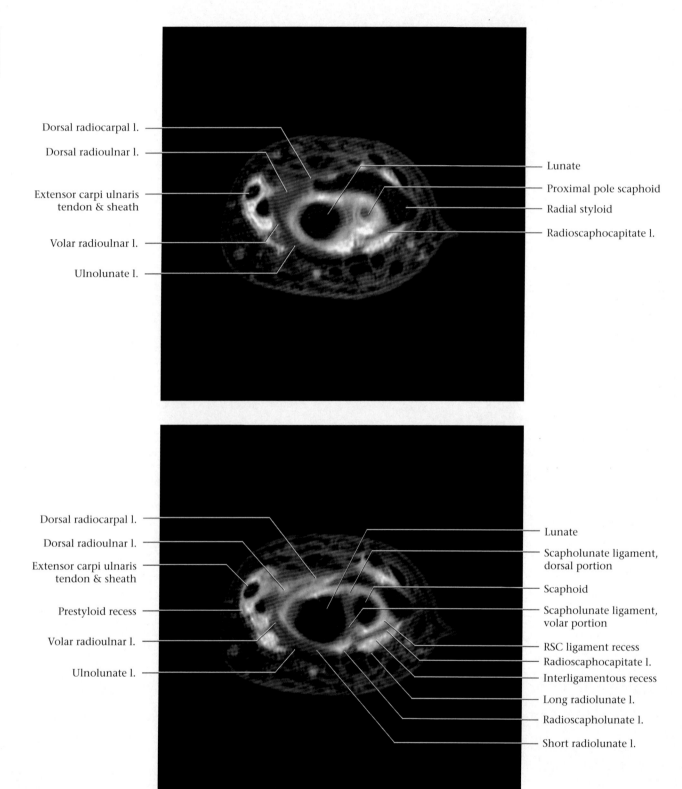

Dorsal radiocarpal l.

Dorsal radioulnar l.

Extensor carpi ulnaris tendon & sheath

Volar radioulnar l.

Ulnolunate l.

Lunate

Proximal pole scaphoid

Radial styloid

Radioscaphocapitate l.

Dorsal radiocarpal l.

Dorsal radioulnar l.

Extensor carpi ulnaris tendon & sheath

Prestyloid recess

Volar radioulnar l.

Ulnolunate l.

Lunate

Scapholunate ligament, dorsal portion

Scaphoid

Scapholunate ligament, volar portion

RSC ligament recess

Radioscaphocapitate l.

Interligamentous recess

Long radiolunate l.

Radioscapholunate l.

Short radiolunate l.

(Top) First of twelve axial GRE images from MR arthrogram (proximal to distal). Joint distention accentuates volar & dorsal ligaments & associated recesses. Radiocarpal compartment may communicate with ECU tendon sheath, as with this normal individual. **(Bottom)** Key ligaments appear as low signal intensity on all MR sequences. Interligamentous recess is a key arthroscopic recess as it leads to space of Poirier. Prestyloid recess is interposed between TFCC & meniscal homologue.

LIGAMENTS

AXIAL GRE MR ARTHROGRAM, INTRINSIC & EXTRINSIC LIGAMENTS

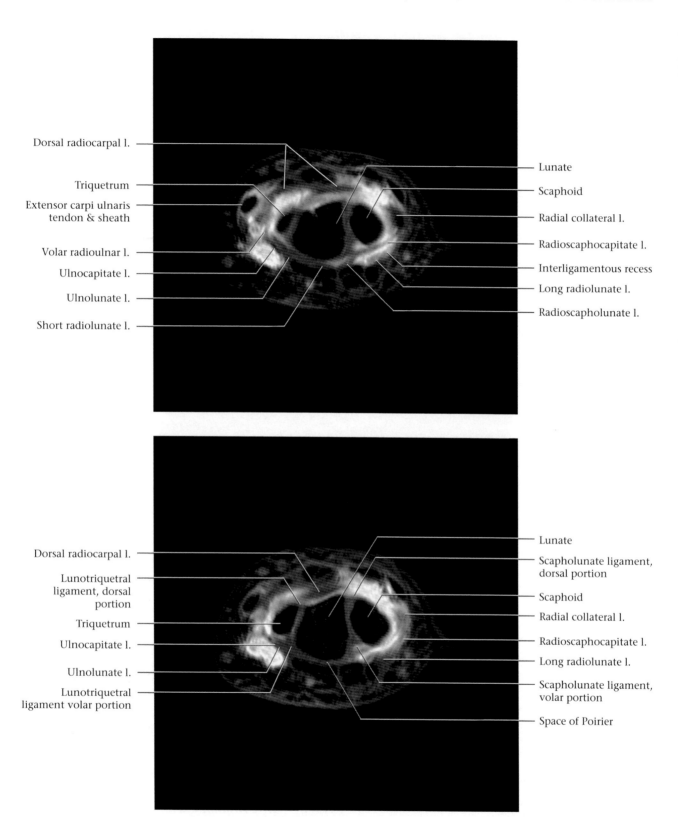

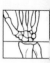

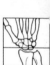

(Top) Dorsal radiocarpal ligament is primary proximal dorsal stabilizer, spanning medial dorsal radial cortex & sweeping distally to dorsal triquetrum. Volar stabilizers include radioscaphocapitate, long & short radiolunate & ulnocarpal ligaments. **(Bottom)** Radioscaphocapitate & ulnocapitate ligaments insert on volar capitate, creating the arcuate or "V" ligaments, leaving volar lunate vulnerable in space of Poirier.

AXIAL GRE MR ARTHROGRAM, INTRINSIC & EXTRINSIC LIGAMENTS

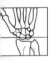

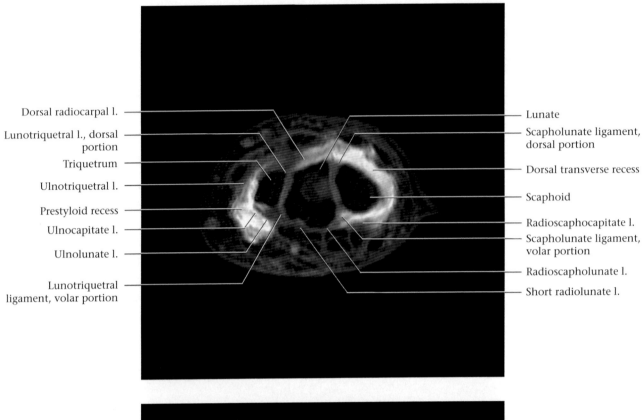

Dorsal radiocarpal l.
Lunotriquetral l., dorsal portion
Triquetrum
Ulnotriquetral l.
Prestyloid recess
Ulnocapitate l.
Ulnolunate l.
Lunotriquetral ligament, volar portion

Lunate
Scapholunate ligament, dorsal portion
Dorsal transverse recess
Scaphoid
Radioscaphocapitate l.
Scapholunate ligament, volar portion
Radioscapholunate l.
Short radiolunate l.

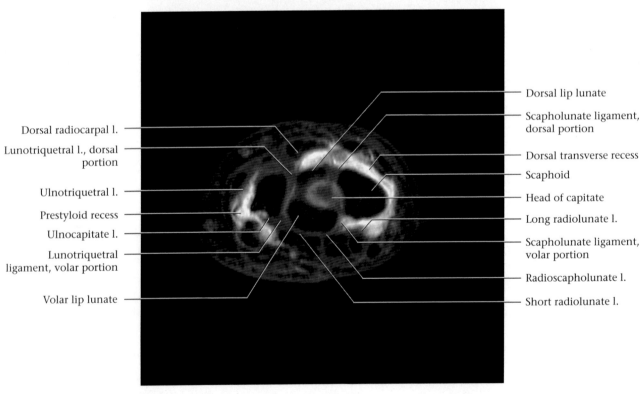

Dorsal radiocarpal l.
Lunotriquetral l., dorsal portion
Ulnotriquetral l.
Prestyloid recess
Ulnocapitate l.
Lunotriquetral ligament, volar portion
Volar lip lunate

Dorsal lip lunate
Scapholunate ligament, dorsal portion
Dorsal transverse recess
Scaphoid
Head of capitate
Long radiolunate l.
Scapholunate ligament, volar portion
Radioscapholunate l.
Short radiolunate l.

(Top) Proximal row carpal ligaments are U-shaped with dorsal, volar & proximal portions. Prestyloid & dorsal transverse recesses are evident. **(Bottom)** Extrinsic ligaments serve as capsular reinforcements.

AXIAL GRE MR ARTHROGRAM, INTRINSIC & EXTRINSIC LIGAMENTS

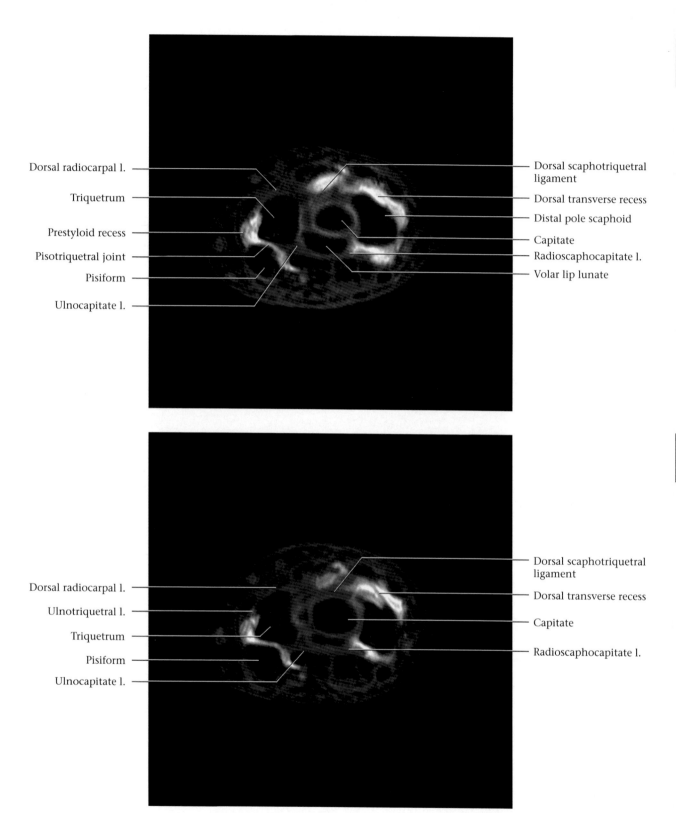
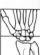
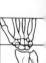

Dorsal radiocarpal l.

Triquetrum

Prestyloid recess

Pisotriquetral joint

Pisiform

Ulnocapitate l.

Dorsal scaphotriquetral ligament

Dorsal transverse recess

Distal pole scaphoid

Capitate

Radioscaphocapitate l.

Volar lip lunate

Dorsal radiocarpal l.

Ulnotriquetral l.

Triquetrum

Pisiform

Ulnocapitate l.

Dorsal scaphotriquetral ligament

Dorsal transverse recess

Capitate

Radioscaphocapitate l.

(Top) At the level of the junction of proximal and distal carpal rows, the dorsal & volar ligaments become less numerous. Radioscaphocapitate & ulnocapitate ligaments create arcuate or "V" ligament volarly. Dorsal scaphotriquetral ligament fibers span dorsal proximal carpal row. **(Bottom)** Ulnotriquetral ligament may be seen as two bands. Medial band forms ECU tendon sheath floor & is sometimes referred to as ulnar collateral ligament.

LIGAMENTS

AXIAL GRE MR ARTHROGRAM, INTRINSIC & EXTRINSIC LIGAMENTS

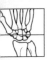

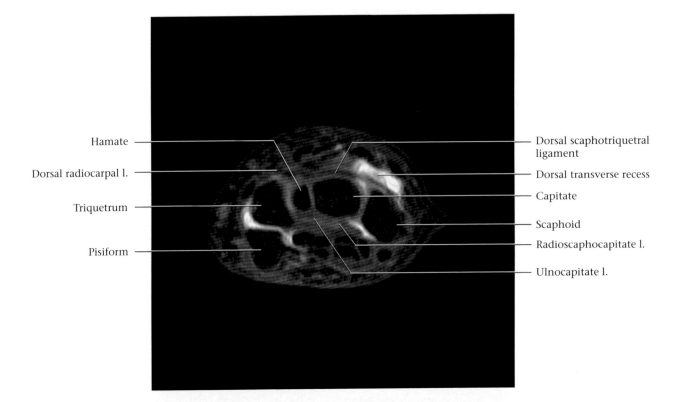

Hamate — — Dorsal scaphotriquetral ligament

Dorsal radiocarpal l. — — Dorsal transverse recess

Triquetrum — — Capitate

Pisiform — — Scaphoid

— Radioscaphocapitate l.

— Ulnocapitate l.

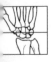

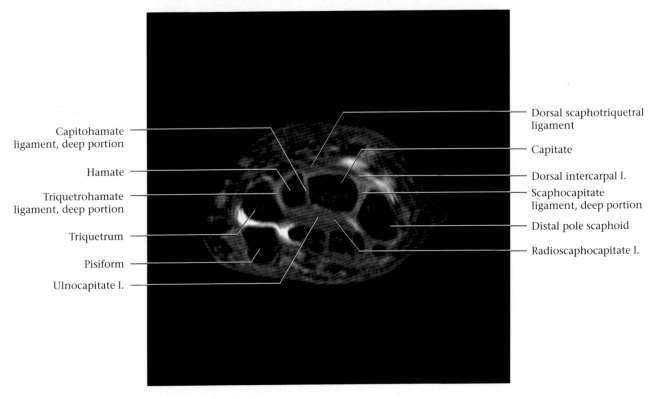

Capitohamate ligament, deep portion — — Dorsal scaphotriquetral ligament

Hamate — — Capitate

Triquetrohamate ligament, deep portion — — Dorsal intercarpal l.

— Scaphocapitate ligament, deep portion

Triquetrum — — Distal pole scaphoid

Pisiform — — Radioscaphocapitate l.

Ulnocapitate l. —

(Top) Volar extrinsic ligaments form the carpal tunnel floor. Small interosseous ligaments are present between all carpals, proximally, distally, medially & laterally (except lunate-capitate relation, where there are no proximal-distal ligaments). **(Bottom)** Dorsal intercarpal ligament arises distal to scaphotriquetral ligament, spanning scaphoid & trapezoid (radially) to triquetrum (ulnarly).

LIGAMENTS

AXIAL GRE MR ARTHROGRAM, INTRINSIC & EXTRINSIC LIGAMENTS

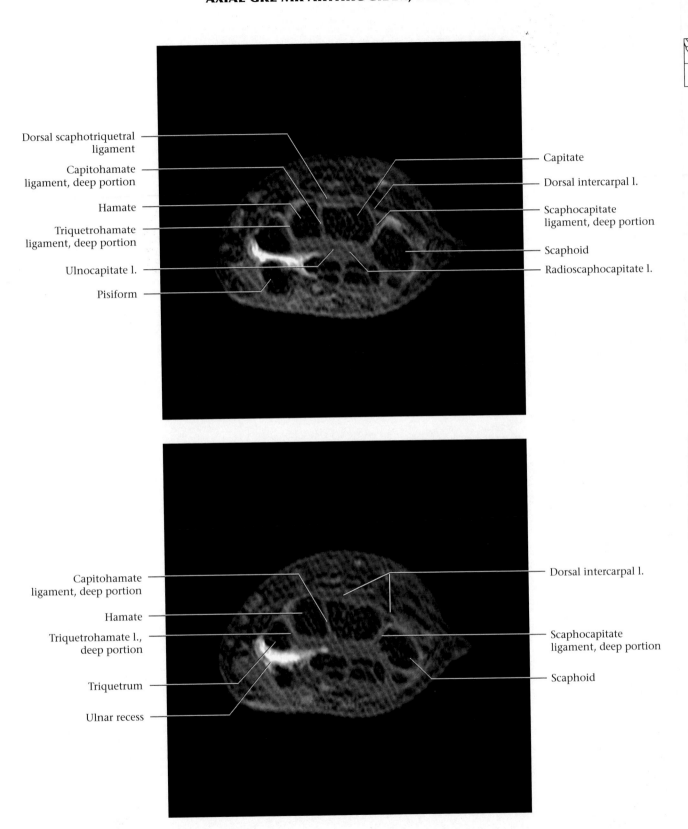

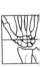

Dorsal scaphotriquetral ligament

Capitohamate ligament, deep portion

Hamate

Triquetrohamate ligament, deep portion

Ulnocapitate l.

Pisiform

Capitate

Dorsal intercarpal l.

Scaphocapitate ligament, deep portion

Scaphoid

Radioscaphocapitate l.

Capitohamate ligament, deep portion

Hamate

Triquetrohamate l., deep portion

Triquetrum

Ulnar recess

Dorsal intercarpal l.

Scaphocapitate ligament, deep portion

Scaphoid

(Top) Interosseous ligaments are present but poorly visualized without joint distention. **(Bottom)** Dorsal intercarpal ligament serves as dorsal distal stabilizing ligament, blending with dorsal scaphotriquetral ligament at triquetrum. Ulnar recess is medial to triquetrohamate articulation.

LIGAMENTS

GRAPHICS & CORONAL GRE MR, SCAPHOLUNATE & LUNOTRIQUETRAL LIGAMENTS

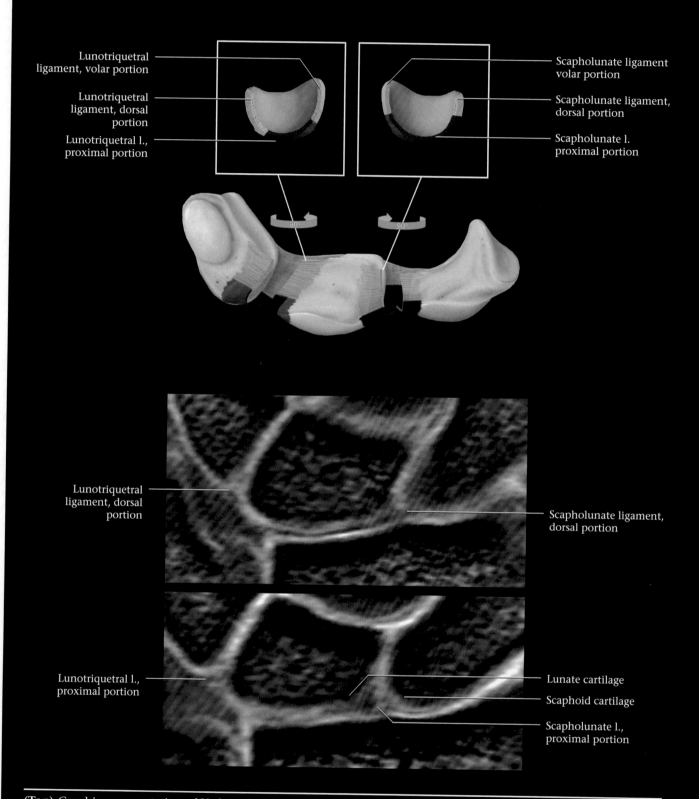

Lunotriquetral ligament, volar portion

Lunotriquetral ligament, dorsal portion

Lunotriquetral l., proximal portion

Scapholunate ligament volar portion

Scapholunate ligament, dorsal portion

Scapholunate l. proximal portion

Lunotriquetral ligament, dorsal portion

Scapholunate ligament, dorsal portion

Lunotriquetral l., proximal portion

Lunate cartilage

Scaphoid cartilage

Scapholunate l., proximal portion

(Top) Graphic representation of U-shaped scapholunate & lunotriquetral ligaments reveals volar portion, thicker in lunotriquetral than scapholunate; proximal portion & dorsal portion, thicker in scapholunate than lunotriquetral ligament. Volar (blue) and part of proximal portions (red) are depicted as cut in this graphic. **(Bottom)** Two coronal GRE images, located dorsal and mid section, coned down to demonstrate the interosseous ligaments. Note that the thick dorsal portion of scapholunate ligament is readily seen on the upper image while the thinner dorsal portion of lunotriquetral ligament is less well visualized. Proximal portions of both scapholunate & lunotriquetral ligaments are triangular in shape (lower image).

LIGAMENTS

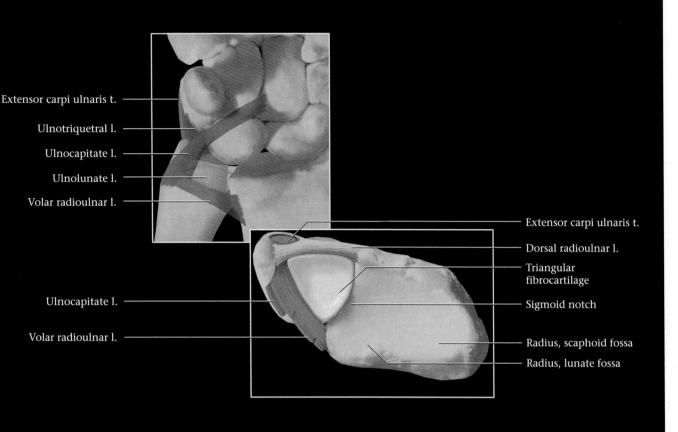

Extensor carpi ulnaris t.
Ulnotriquetral l.
Ulnocapitate l.
Ulnolunate l.
Volar radioulnar l.

Extensor carpi ulnaris t.
Dorsal radioulnar l.
Triangular fibrocartilage
Ulnocapitate l.
Sigmoid notch
Volar radioulnar l.
Radius, scaphoid fossa
Radius, lunate fossa

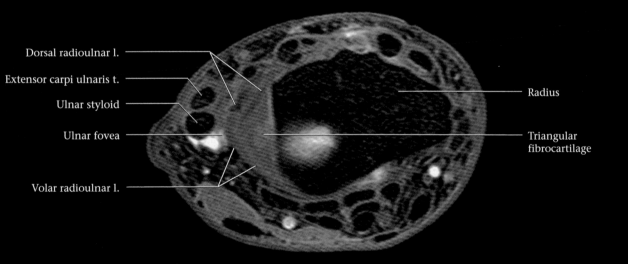

Dorsal radioulnar l.
Extensor carpi ulnaris t.
Ulnar styloid
Ulnar fovea
Radius
Triangular fibrocartilage
Volar radioulnar l.

(**Top**) Volar & intra-articular graphics of ulnocarpal structures. Triangular fibrocartilage (central) is surrounded by dorsal & volar radioulnar ligaments (periphery). Fibers of dorsal radioulnar ligament contribute to ECU sheath. Triangular fibrocartilage complex includes these structures as well as ulnolunate & ulnotriquetral ligaments.
(**Bottom**) Axial GRE MR through the radiocarpal joint shows the dorsal & volar radioulnar ligaments meeting at the ulnar fovea, creating a semicircular contour of ligaments surrounding the central triangular fibrocartilage.

CORONAL GRE & T1 FS MR ARTHROGRAM, TFCC

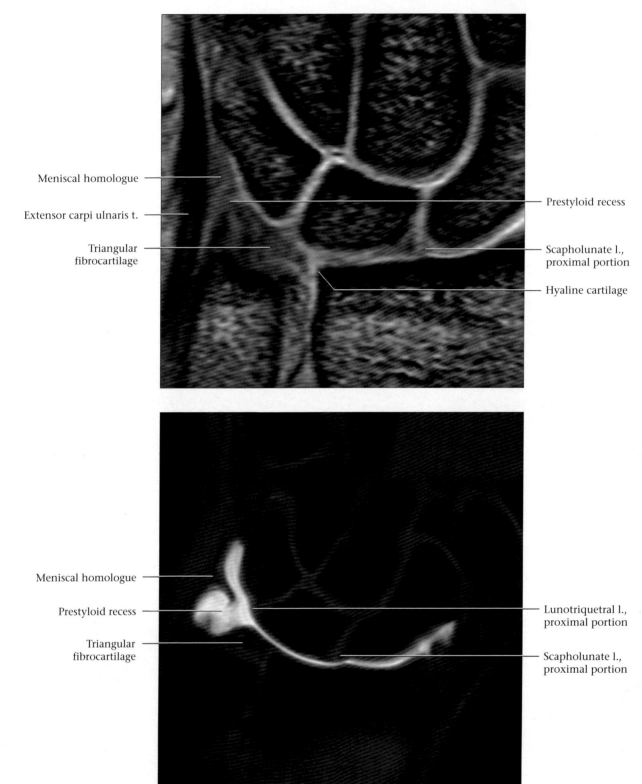

Meniscal homologue

Extensor carpi ulnaris t.

Triangular fibrocartilage

Prestyloid recess

Scapholunate l., proximal portion

Hyaline cartilage

Meniscal homologue

Prestyloid recess

Triangular fibrocartilage

Lunotriquetral l., proximal portion

Scapholunate l., proximal portion

(Top) Coronal view of triangular fibrocartilage demonstrates normal fibrocartilage attachment to hyaline cartilage of radial sigmoid notch. Linear signal in extensor carpi ulnaris tendon is normal. Meniscal homologue represents a capsular thickening that is variably visualized & is separated from triangular fibrocartilage by the prestyloid recess. **(Bottom)** Coronal T1 fat suppressed radiocarpal arthrogram image accentuates meniscal homologue. Triangular fibrocartilage, scapholunate & lunotriquetral ligaments are intact.

LIGAMENTS

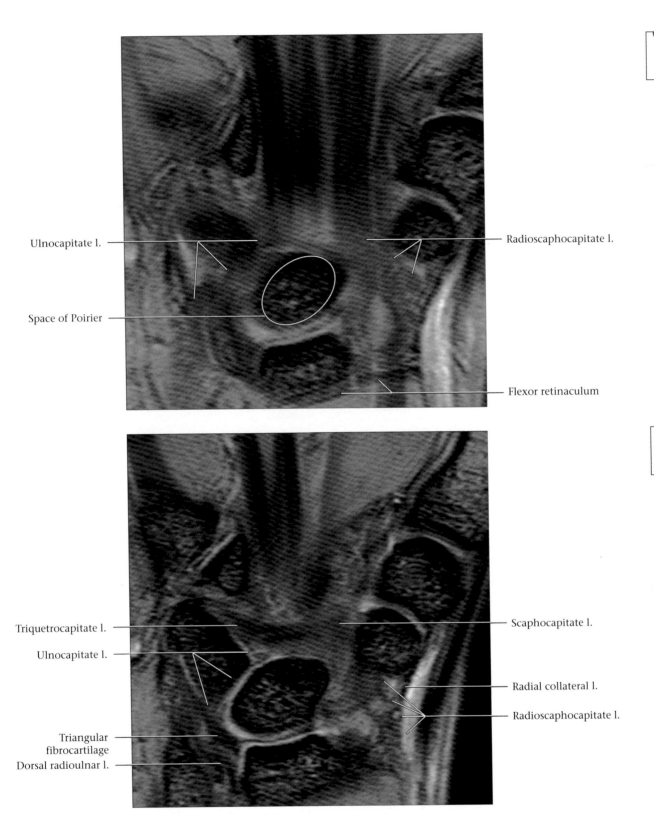

Ulnocapitate l.

Space of Poirier

Radioscaphocapitate l.

Flexor retinaculum

Triquetrocapitate l.

Ulnocapitate l.

Scaphocapitate l.

Radial collateral l.

Radioscaphocapitate l.

Triangular fibrocartilage

Dorsal radioulnar l.

(Top) First of eight selected coronal GRE images (from volar to dorsal). Radioscaphocapitate & ulnocapitate ligaments blend with triquetrocapitate ligaments to create arcuate (inverted "V") ligament. Lunate is immediately proximal to this confluence of ligaments which creates a vulnerable place in volar capsule, the space of Poirier. **(Bottom)** Ligaments are often wispy, thin, striated structures as demonstrated by the radioscaphocapitate & ulnocapitate ligaments in this image. Ligaments may blend together, making identification of individual ligaments more challenging.

Wrist

III

89

CORONAL GRE MR, INTRINSIC LIGAMENTS

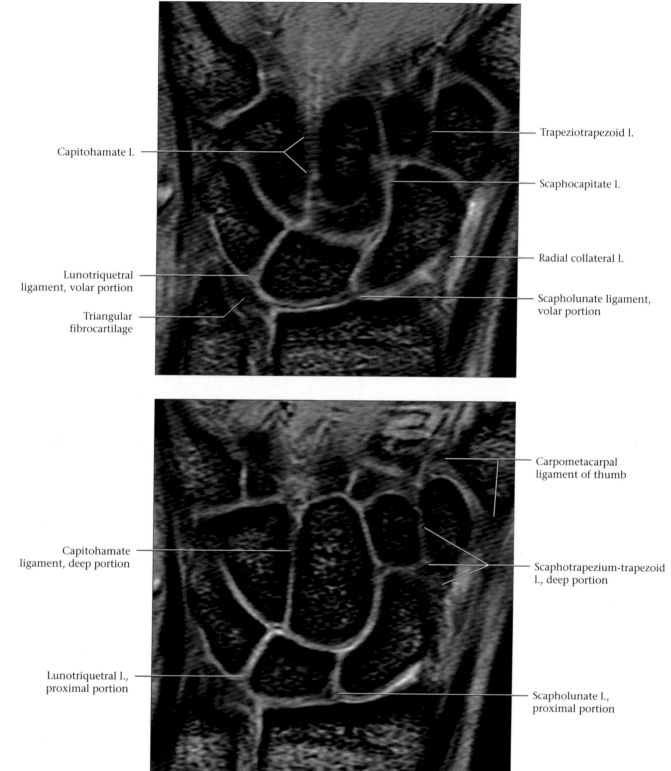

Capitohamate l. — Trapeziotrapezoid l.

— Scaphocapitate l.

— Radial collateral l.

Lunotriquetral ligament, volar portion — Scapholunate ligament, volar portion

Triangular fibrocartilage

Carpometacarpal ligament of thumb

Capitohamate ligament, deep portion — Scaphotrapezium-trapezoid l., deep portion

Lunotriquetral l., proximal portion — Scapholunate l., proximal portion

(Top) Triangular fibrocartilage shows intermediate signal intensity. Proximal carpal row interosseous ligaments are low signal dorsally & volarly with low to intermediate signal in proximal portion. **(Bottom)** Proximal portions of lunotriquetral & scapholunate ligaments are triangular in shape & may be heterogeneous. Interosseous ligaments in distal carpal row have not only volar & dorsal portions but deep thick bands which contribute to stability.

LIGAMENTS

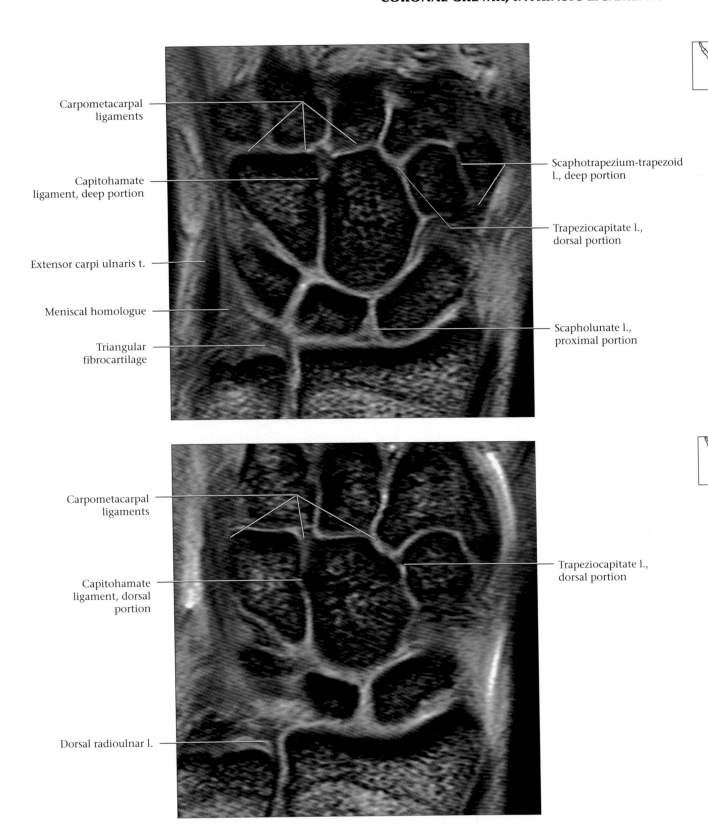

Carpometacarpal ligaments

Capitohamate ligament, deep portion

Extensor carpi ulnaris t.

Meniscal homologue

Triangular fibrocartilage

Scaphotrapezium-trapezoid l., deep portion

Trapeziocapitate l., dorsal portion

Scapholunate l., proximal portion

Carpometacarpal ligaments

Capitohamate ligament, dorsal portion

Dorsal radioulnar l.

Trapeziocapitate l., dorsal portion

(Top) Triangular fibrocartilage, scapholunate & lunotriquetral ligaments attach to hyaline cartilage covering sigmoid notch, scaphoid, lunate & triquetrum respectively & create a region of intermediate signal between ligaments & adjacent bone. This should not be mistaken for a tear. **(Bottom)** Carpometacarpal & interosseous ligaments are visualized dorsally.

CORONAL GRE MR, EXTRINSIC LIGAMENTS

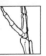

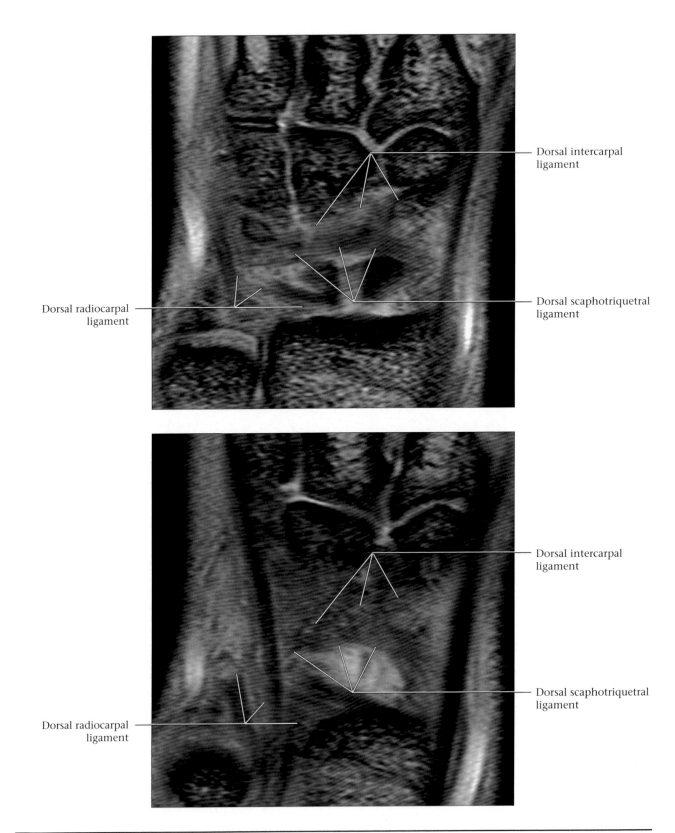

Dorsal intercarpal ligament

Dorsal radiocarpal ligament

Dorsal scaphotriquetral ligament

Dorsal intercarpal ligament

Dorsal scaphotriquetral ligament

Dorsal radiocarpal ligament

(Top) Dorsal stabilizing ligaments include dorsal radiocarpal, scaphotriquetral & intercarpal ligaments. **(Bottom)** The triquetrum serves as an anchor point for the major dorsal midcarpal ligaments.

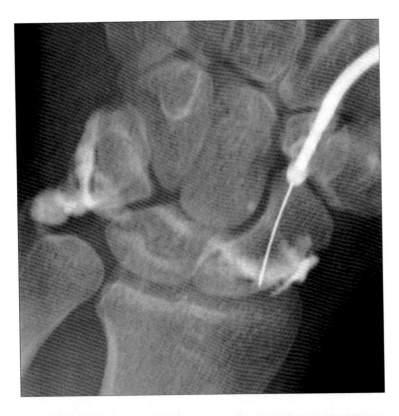

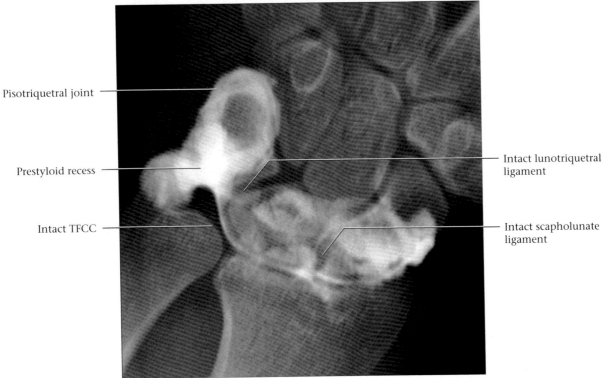

Pisotriquetral joint

Prestyloid recess

Intact TFCC

Intact lunotriquetral ligament

Intact scapholunate ligament

(Top) Radiocarpal arthrogram. Injection performed from dorsal approach with 2-3 ccs contrast introduced. **(Bottom)** Intact radiocarpal compartment with contrast filling pisotriquetral joint via prestyloid recess. Triangular fibrocartilage distal surface is outlined. Scapholunate & lunotriquetral ligaments are intact, with no evidence of spill into midcarpal compartment.

LIGAMENTS

PA RADIOGRAPH ARTHROGRAM, DISTAL RADIOULNAR COMPARTMENT

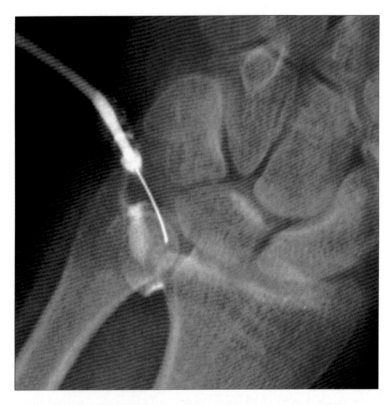

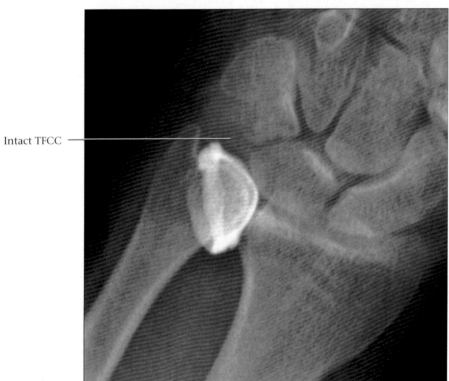

Intact TFCC

(Top) Distal radioulnar joint injection, performed 60 minutes after radiocarpal compartment injection. 1 cc of contrast was instilled. **(Bottom)** Normal distal radioulnar joint with cap-like filling of capsule, outlines TFCC undersurface.

LIGAMENTS

PA RADIOGRAPH ARTHROGRAM, MID CARPAL COMPARTMENT

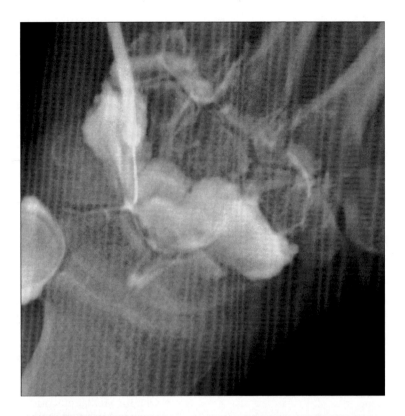

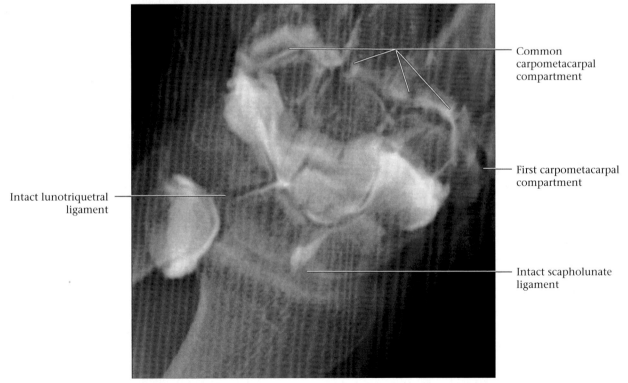

Common carpometacarpal compartment

First carpometacarpal compartment

Intact lunotriquetral ligament

Intact scapholunate ligament

(Top) Midcarpal compartment injection, performed immediately after distal radioulnar compartment injection. The needle is placed at the "4 corners", the junction of lunate, triquetrum, hamate, and capitate. 4 ccs of contrast are instilled. **(Bottom)** Contrast fills the midcarpal & common carpometacarpal compartments. The first carpometacarpal compartment remains separate. Note contrast extending into scapholunate & lunotriquetral joints without passing into radiocarpal compartment, indicating intact scapholunate & lunotriquetral ligaments.

Terminology

Abbreviations

- Abductor pollicis brevis (APB)
- Abductor pollicis longus (APL)
- Adductor digiti minimi (ADM)
- Adductor pollicis (AP)
- Carpal tunnel (CT)
- Carpal tunnel syndrome (CTS)
- Carpometacarpal (CMC)
- Extensor carpi radialis brevis (ECRB)
- Extensor carpi radialis longus (ECRL)
- Extensor carpi ulnaris (ECU)
- Extensor digitorum (ED)
- Extensor digiti minimi (EDM)
- Extensor indicis (EI)
- Extensor pollicis brevis (EPB)
- Extensor pollicis longus (EPL)
- Flexor carpi radialis (FCR)
- Flexor carpi ulnaris (FCU)
- Flexor digitorum (FD)
- Flexor digitorum profundus (FDP)
- Flexor digitorum superficialis (FDS)
- Flexor pollicis brevis (FPB)
- Flexor pollicis longus (FPL)
- Flexor retinaculum (FR)
- Interphalangeal (IP)
- Metacarpal (MC)
- Metacarpophalangeal (MCP)
- Palmaris longus (PL)
- Pronator quadratus (PQ)
- Proximal interphalangeal (PIP)

Definitions

- Palmar = volar
- Ulnar = medial
- Radial = lateral
- Wrist abduction = radial flexion
- Wrist adduction = ulnar flexion

Imaging Anatomy

Flexors

- **Deep flexor group**
  - **Flexor digitorum profundus**
    - **Origin**: Proximal ulna; **course**: Splits into 4 tendons proximal to PQ, passing through CT, deep to FR & FDS tendons; **insertion**: Index, middle, ring & little finger distal phalangeal bases
    - **Action**: Flexes distal phalanges; flexes other phalanges & hand with continued action
    - **Innervation**: Median, anterior interosseous, ulnar nerve
    - **Variants**: Duplicated slips
  - **Flexor pollicis longus**
    - **Origin**: Radius, interosseous membrane, coronoid process; **course**: Passes deep to FR between FPB & AP; **insertion**: Thumb distal phalangeal base
    - **Action**: Flexes thumb IP; flexes thumb MCP with continued action
    - **Innervation**: Median nerve, anterior interosseous
    - **Variant**: Additional slip to index finger

- **Pronator quadratus**
  - **Origin**: Medial distal volar ulna; **course**: Passes medial to lateral; **insertion**: Lateral distal dorsal radius
  - **Action**: Pronates hand
  - **Innervation**: Median nerve, anterior interosseous
  - **Variants**: May split into 2 or 3 layers; additional proximal or distal attachments
- **Superficial**
  - **Flexor carpi radialis**
    - **Origin**: Medial epicondyle/common flexor tendon; **course**: Thin tendon passes through canal in lateral FR across volar trapezium groove; **insertion**: 2nd MC base; slip to 3rd MC base
    - **Action**: Flexes hand at wrist; abducts wrist
    - **Innervation**: Median nerve
    - **Variants**: May attach to trapezium &/or 4th MC
  - **Palmaris longus**
    - **Origin**: Medial epicondyle/common flexor tendon; **course**: Thin tendon passes superficial to FR; **insertion**: Volar distal FR & aponeurosis
    - **Action**: Flexes hand at wrist
    - **Innervation**: Median nerve
    - **Variants**: Absent in 10%; duplicated; complete or partial insertion on antebrachial fascia, FCU tendon, pisiform, or scaphoid; short tendon with low lying muscle belly may compress median n.
  - **Flexor carpi ulnaris**
    - **Origin**: Medial epicondyle/common flexor tendon (humeral head) & medial proximal ulna (ulnar head); **course**: Runs medial to the ulnar neurovascular bundle; **insertion**: Pisiform (continuing distally as pisohamate & pisometacarpal ligaments)
    - **Action**: Flexes hand; adducts wrist
    - **Innervation**: Ulnar nerve
  - **Flexor digitorum superficialis**
    - **Origin**: Medial epicondyle/common flexor tendon & ulnar coronoid process (humeroulnar head); volar proximal radius (radial head); **course**: Divides into superficial (tendons to middle & ring fingers) & deep (tendons to index & little fingers); passes deep to FR with superficial tendons volar to deep tendons; **insertion**: Middle phalanges of index, middle, ring & little fingers
    - **Action**: Flexes PIP & MCP joints of index, middle, ring & little fingers
    - **Innervation**: Median nerve
    - **Variants**: Absent little finger slip; accessory slips to index & middle fingers; distal muscle belly along proximal phalanges may mimic mass

Extensors

- **Deep**
  - **Abductor pollicis longus**
    - **Origin**: Dorsal lateral ulna, dorsal mid radius; **course**: Passes obliquely distal & lateral; crossing over ECRB & ECRL, passing (with EPB) into extensor compartment #1; **insertion**: 1st MC radial base with slips to trapezium & APB
    - **Action**: Abducts & extends thumb; abducts wrist; flexes wrist minimally

Wrist

- **Innervation**: Deep radial nerve, posterior interosseous branch
- **Variants**: Multiple slips; insert on trapezium or FR
- APL & EPB intersect ECRB & ECRL just proximal to extensor retinaculum; may impinge at musculotendinous intersection
  - ○ Extensor pollicis brevis
    - **Origin**: Dorsal mid radius; **course**: Medial & contiguous with APL; crossing over ECRB & ECRL to enter extensor compartment #1 with APL; **insertion**: Thumb proximal phalangeal base
    - **Action**: Extends thumb MCP; extends 1st MC at CMC with continued action; abducts wrist
    - **Innervation**: Deep radial nerve, posterior interosseous branch
    - **Variants**: May be absent; fused with EPL
  - ○ Extensor pollicis longus
    - **Origin**: Dorsal mid ulna; **course**: Passes into wrist under extensor retinaculum in compartment #3; crosses lateral & superficial to ECRL & ECRB at 45°; **insertion**: Thumb distal phalanx base
    - **Action**: Extends thumb tip; extends thumb proximal phalanx & 1st MC by continued action
    - **Innervation**: Deep radial nerve, posterior interosseous branch
    - **Variant**: Fused with EPB
  - ○ Extensor indicis (proprius)
    - **Origin**: Dorsal mid ulna & interosseous membrane; **course**: Passes under extensor retinaculum in compartment #4, running deep & medial to ED; joins tendon slip near ulnar index finger; **insertion**: Extensor hood of index finger
    - **Action**: Extends & adducts index finger
    - **Innervation**: Deep radial nerve, posterior interosseous branch
    - **Variants**: Duplicated muscle; slip to middle finger
- **Superficial**
  - ○ Extensor carpi radialis longus
    - **Origin**: Lateral epicondyle/common extensor tendon; **course**: Proximal to carpus, crosses beneath APL & EPB; passes deep to extensor retinaculum in compartment #2; **insertion**: Dorsal radial 2nd MC
    - **Action**: Extends & abducts hand at wrist
    - **Innervation**: Radial nerve
    - **Variants**: Multiple tendons, insert on 2nd, 3rd, or 4th MC
  - ○ Extensor carpi radialis brevis
    - **Origin**: Lateral epicondyle/common extensor tendon; **course**: Passes beneath APL & EPB; passes deep to extensor retinaculum in compartment #2; **insertion**: Dorsal radial 3rd MC
    - **Action**: Extends & abducts hand at wrist
    - **Innervation**: Radial nerve
    - **Variants**: Multiple tendons, insert on 2nd, 3rd, or 4th MC
  - ○ Extensor digitorum (communis)
    - **Origin**: Lateral epicondyle/common extensor tendon; **course**: Passes distally, dividing into 4 slips; passes deep to extensor retinaculum in compartment #4; extends into index, middle, ring, little fingers; **insertion**: Middle & distal phalanges of index, middle, ring, little fingers

- **Action**: Extends index, middle, ring, little fingers; abducts index, ring & little fingers away from middle finger; extends hand at wrist with continued action
- **Innervation**: Deep radial nerve
- **Variants**: Multiple slips; insertion on thumb
  - ○ Extensor digiti minimi (extensor digiti quinti (V) proprius)
    - **Origin**: Lateral epicondyle/common extensor tendon; **course**: Passes medial to ED & lateral to ECU; passes deep to extensor retinaculum in compartment #5; **insertion**: Extensor hood of little finger proximal phalanx with slip to ring finger
    - **Action**: Extends little finger; extends hand at wrist with continued action
    - **Innervation**: Deep radial nerve
    - **Variants**: Fused with ED; absent ring finger slip
  - ○ Extensor carpi ulnaris
    - **Origin**: Common extensor tendon & dorsal ulna; **course**: Passes into wrist deep to extensor retinaculum in compartment #6; **insertion**: Dorsal ulnar 5th MC base
    - **Action**: Extends & adducts hand
    - **Innervation**: Deep radial nerve
    - **Variants**: Insertion on 4th MC

Muscles Originating at Wrist
- **Thenar**
  - ○ Abductor pollicis brevis
    - **Origin**: FR, scaphoid tuberosity, trapezium ridge; **course**: Extends laterally; **insertion**: Radial thumb proximal phalangeal base
    - **Action**: Abducts thumb at CMC & MC joints; draws thumb away from palm at right angle
    - **Innervation**: Median nerve
    - **Variants**: Absent or duplicated tendon slips
  - ○ Opponens pollicis
    - **Origin**: FR, trapezium ridge; **course**: Deep to APB; **insertion**: Radial thumb MC
    - **Action**: Abducts, flexes & rotates 1st MC; draws thumbs across palm
    - **Innervation**: Median nerve
  - ○ Flexor pollicis brevis
    - Consists of superficial (larger & lateral) & deep (smaller & medial) components
    - **Origin**: Superficial-distal FR & trapezium tubercle; deep-trapezoid & capitate; **course**: Located medial & distal to APB; **insertion**: Common tendon inserts on radial thumb proximal phalangeal base
    - **Action**: Flexes thumb proximal phalanx; medially rotates thumb MC
    - **Innervation**: Superficial-median n.; deep-ulnar n.
  - ○ Adductor pollicis
    - **Origin**: Oblique head-capitate, 2nd & 3rd MC bases, FCR tendon sheath; transverse head-3rd MC; **course**: Oblique-passes obliquely distally & converges to tendon (which contains sesamoid); transverse-fibers converge laterally; **insertion**: Oblique & transverse-ulnar thumb proximal phalangeal base
    - **Action**: Abducts thumb proximal phalanx toward palm

TENDONS

- **Innervation**: Ulnar nerve
- **Hypothenar**
  - **Palmar brevis**
    - **Origin**: FR & palmar aponeurosis; **insertion**: Skin of ulnar palm
    - **Action**: Draws skin of ulnarward palm toward middle
    - **Innervation**: Ulnar nerve, superficial branch
  - **Abductor digiti minimi**
    - **Origin**: Pisiform & FCU tendon; **insertion**: Ulnar little finger proximal phalangeal base
    - **Action**: Abducts little finger away from ring finger; flexes proximal phalanx
    - **Innervation**: Ulnar nerve, deep branch
  - **Flexor digiti minimi brevis**
    - **Origin**: Hook of hamate & FR; **insertion**: Ulnar little finger proximal phalangeal base
    - **Action**: Flexes little finger at MCP
    - **Innervation**: Ulnar nerve, deep branch
    - **Variant**: Anomalous origin may compress ulnar nerve
  - **Opponens digiti minimi**
    - **Origin**: Hook of hamate & FR; **insertion**: Length of 5th MC
    - **Action**: Abducts, flexes & laterally rotates 5th MC
    - **Innervation**: Ulnar nerve, deep branch

Anomalous Muscles

- May present as a soft tissue mass; may create neural compression
- **Accessory palmaris longus**: Superficial to FD tendons, medial to FCR
- **Extensor digitorum manus brevis**: Arises from distal radius or dorsal radiocarpal ligament; inserts on 2nd MC
  - May be tender or present as mass
- **Extensor carpi radialis intermedius**: Arises from humerus or as accessory slip from ECRB or ECRL; inserts on 2nd &/or 3rd MC
- **Extensor carpi radialis accessory**: Arises from humerus or ECRL; inserts 1st MC, APB, or 1st dorsal interosseous
- **Accessory extensor pollicis longus**: Located in #3 extensor compartment may be tender & mimic mass
- **Accessory abductor digiti minimi**: Arises from FR or PL; inserts on ADM. May compress ulnar or median n.
- **Lumbrical** muscles: Arise from FD tendons distal to carpal tunnel but may arise proximally within carpal tunnel causing CTS

Fascia & Retinacula

- **Flexor retinaculum**
  - **Superficial (volar carpal ligament or ligamentum carpi palmare) portion**
    - Thickened distal antebrachial fascia combined with transverse fibrous bundles
    - Attaches at ulnar styloid process & radial styloid process; blends distally with FR
    - Creates roof of Guyon canal; ulnar nerve, artery & veins run deep to fascial layer but superficial to FR
  - **Flexor retinaculum (transverse ligament or ligamentum flexorum)**

- Attaches at pisiform, hook of hamate, scaphoid tuberosity, trapezium palmar surface & ridge; deep surface of palmar aponeurosis
- Creates carpal tunnel containing median nerve, FDS, FDP & FPL; creates tunnel for FCR across trapezium
- Hypothenar & thenar musculature arise from FR
- Carpal tunnel release typically divides FR ulnarly near hook of hamate attachment

- **Extensor retinaculum (dorsal carpal ligament)**
  - Thickened distal antebrachial fascia combined with transverse fibrous bundles
  - Attaches to ulnar styloid process, medial margin of pisiform & triquetrum, lateral radius margin
  - Attaches to dorsal radial ridges, creating fibro-osseous compartments (referred to by number)
    - #1 - APL, EPB; #2 - ECRL, ECRB; #3 - EPL; #4 - ED, EI; #5 - EDM; #6 - ECU

Tendon Sheaths

- Wrist & hand synovial tendon sheaths are specialized bursae; tubular with visceral & parietal layers; intervening potential space contains minimal fluid & small blood vessels normally; fills with fluid when inflamed
- **Flexor sheaths**
  - **Common flexor tendon sheath** (ulnar bursa) encases FDS, FDP; arises 2.5 cm proximal to FR; index, middle & ring sheaths terminate in palm, little finger sheath at distal phalanx
  - **Flexor pollicis longus tendon sheath** (radial bursa) encases FPL; arises 2.5 cm proximal to FR; terminates at thumb distal phalanx
- **Extensor sheaths**
  - Six discrete tendon sheaths encase tendons of six extensor compartments; arise proximal to extensor retinaculum; terminate adjacent to dorsal MC base/shaft

Anatomic Snuffbox

- **Margins**: Distal radius (proximal margin), EPL (dorsal margin), APL & EPB (volar margin), APL & EPB converge just distal to 1st CMC (distal margin), scaphoid, trapezium, 1st CMC & radial styloid (deep margin)
- **Contents**: Cephalic vein, radial nerve, radial artery

Anatomy-Based Imaging Issues

Imaging Issues

- Many variations of flexor & extensor muscles & tendons
- Multiple tendon slips can mimic longitudinal tendon tears (e.g., APL)
- Magic angle effect: Collagen bundle orientation so that images obtained 55° to main magnetic field may yield intermediate signal rather than expected low signal intensity (especially in short TE imaging - T1, proton density or GRE) (e.g., ECU, EPL)
- Small amount of fluid common in tendon sheath (e.g., ECRB, ECRL, ECU)

TENDONS

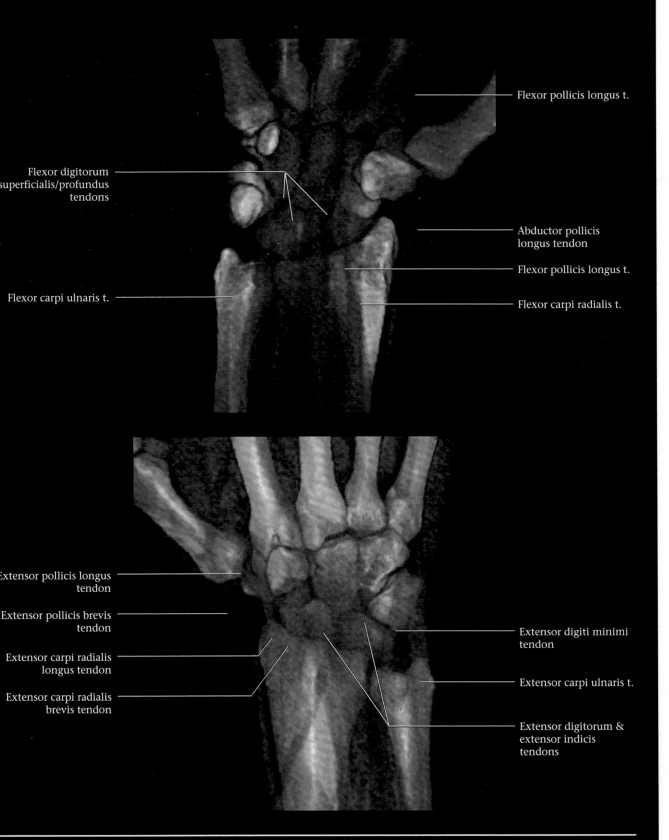

Flexor pollicis longus t.

Flexor digitorum superficialis/profundus tendons

Abductor pollicis longus tendon

Flexor pollicis longus t.

Flexor carpi ulnaris t.

Flexor carpi radialis t.

Extensor pollicis longus tendon

Extensor pollicis brevis tendon

Extensor carpi radialis longus tendon

Extensor carpi radialis brevis tendon

Extensor digiti minimi tendon

Extensor carpi ulnaris t.

Extensor digitorum & extensor indicis tendons

(Top) 3D reconstruction with soft tissue overlay reveals volar tendons extending from forearm into wrist & hand. (Bottom) Dorsal tendons are similarly displayed.

TENDONS

GRAPHICS, VOLAR & DORSAL TENDONS

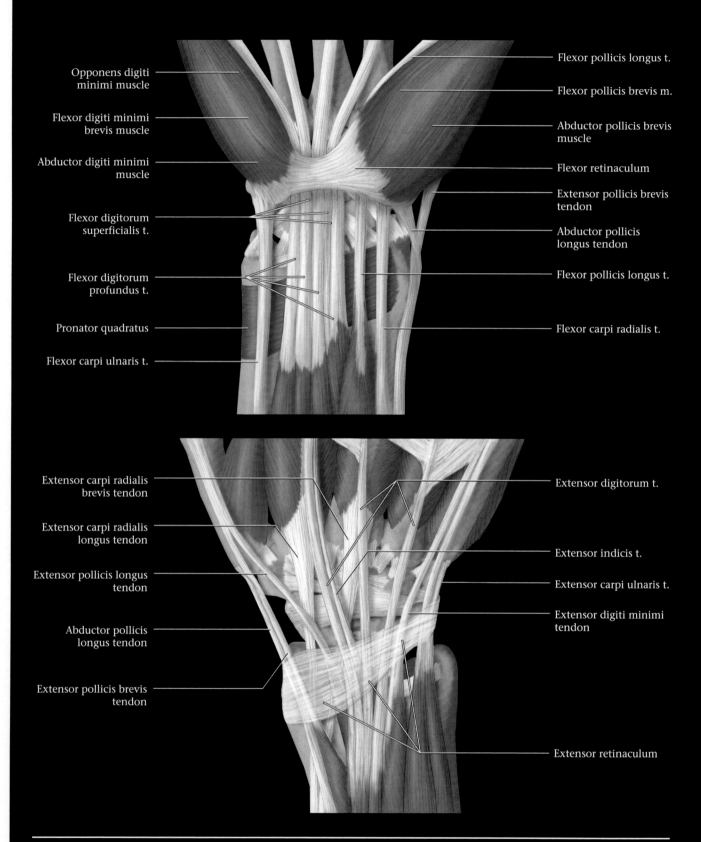

Opponens digiti minimi muscle

Flexor digiti minimi brevis muscle

Abductor digiti minimi muscle

Flexor digitorum superficialis t.

Flexor digitorum profundus t.

Pronator quadratus

Flexor carpi ulnaris t.

Flexor pollicis longus t.

Flexor pollicis brevis m.

Abductor pollicis brevis muscle

Flexor retinaculum

Extensor pollicis brevis tendon

Abductor pollicis longus tendon

Flexor pollicis longus t.

Flexor carpi radialis t.

Extensor carpi radialis brevis tendon

Extensor carpi radialis longus tendon

Extensor pollicis longus tendon

Abductor pollicis longus tendon

Extensor pollicis brevis tendon

Extensor digitorum t.

Extensor indicis t.

Extensor carpi ulnaris t.

Extensor digiti minimi tendon

Extensor retinaculum

(Top) Volar muscles & tendons are displayed with their relation to flexor retinaculum. Note muscles of thenar & hypothenar eminences arise from the retinaculum itself. Flexor digitorum & flexor pollicis longus tendons pass deep to retinaculum while flexor carpi radialis is lateral but within fibers of lateral retinaculum. **(Bottom)** Dorsal extensor tendons pass deep to extensor retinaculum, separated into six compartments by fibrous attachments of retinaculum to underlying bone. Compartment contents: #1 - APL, EPB; #2 - ECRL, ECRB; #3 - EPL; #4 - ED, EI; #5 - EDM; #6 - ECU.

GRAPHICS, VOLAR & DORSAL TENDONS SHEATHS

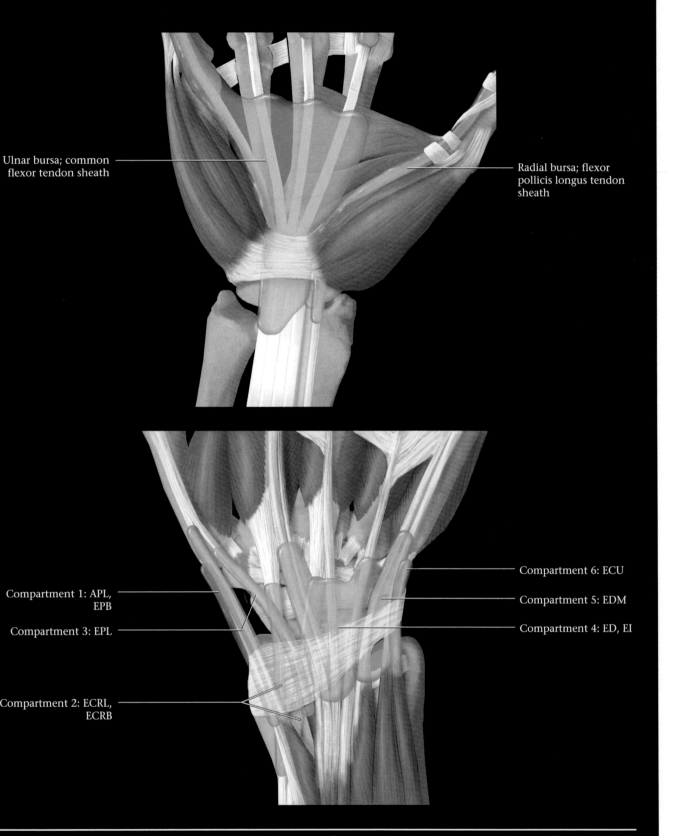

Ulnar bursa; common flexor tendon sheath

Radial bursa; flexor pollicis longus tendon sheath

Compartment 6: ECU

Compartment 1: APL, EPB

Compartment 5: EDM

Compartment 3: EPL

Compartment 4: ED, EI

Compartment 2: ECRL, ECRB

(Top) Volar bursae include ulnar & radial sheaths. Common flexor tendon sheath encases index, middle, ring & little finger tendons, beginning proximal to flexor retinaculum & extending distally to midshaft metacarpals. Sheath also extends distally to little finger distal phalanx. Flexor pollicis longus has a separate sheath. **(Bottom)** Separate tendon sheaths enclose dorsal extensor tendons in compartments 1-6 individually.

GRAPHIC & AXIAL T1 MR, PROXIMAL WRIST

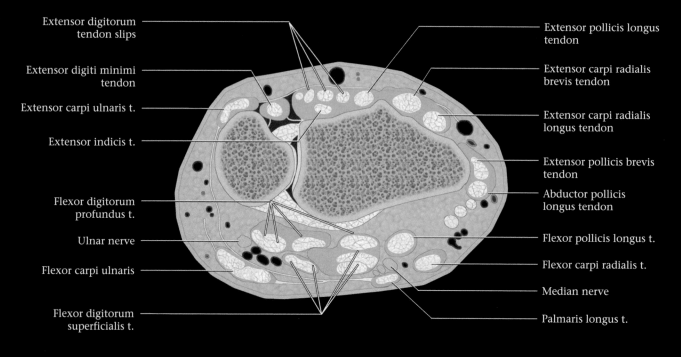

Extensor digitorum tendon slips

Extensor digiti minimi tendon

Extensor carpi ulnaris t.

Extensor indicis t.

Flexor digitorum profundus t.

Ulnar nerve

Flexor carpi ulnaris

Flexor digitorum superficialis t.

Extensor pollicis longus tendon

Extensor carpi radialis brevis tendon

Extensor carpi radialis longus tendon

Extensor pollicis brevis tendon

Abductor pollicis longus tendon

Flexor pollicis longus t.

Flexor carpi radialis t.

Median nerve

Palmaris longus t.

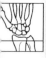

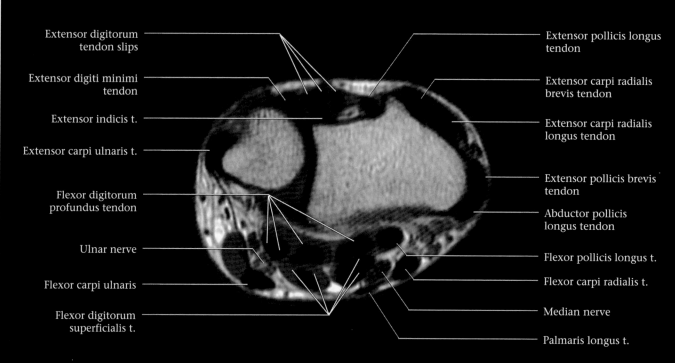

Extensor digitorum tendon slips

Extensor digiti minimi tendon

Extensor indicis t.

Extensor carpi ulnaris t.

Flexor digitorum profundus tendon

Ulnar nerve

Flexor carpi ulnaris

Flexor digitorum superficialis t.

Extensor pollicis longus tendon

Extensor carpi radialis brevis tendon

Extensor carpi radialis longus tendon

Extensor pollicis brevis tendon

Abductor pollicis longus tendon

Flexor pollicis longus t.

Flexor carpi radialis t.

Median nerve

Palmaris longus t.

(Top) Graphic representation of tendons in proximal wrist. Extensor tendons are deep to extensor retinaculum while flexor tendons are proximal to flexor retinaculum at this level in the wrist. **(Bottom)** Corresponding axial MR demonstrates uniform low signal intensity of tendons. Extensor retinaculum is present but thin & indiscernible.

TENDONS

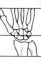

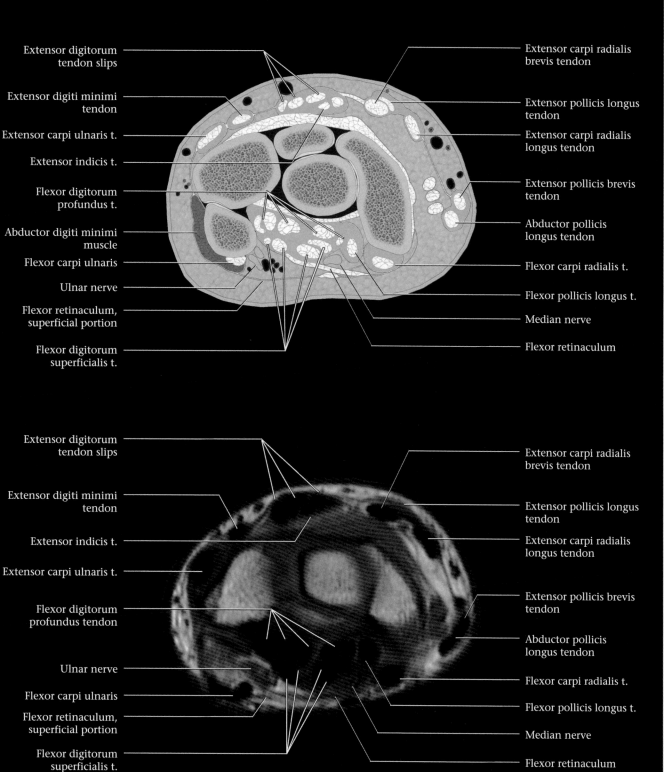

Extensor digitorum tendon slips

Extensor digiti minimi tendon

Extensor carpi ulnaris t.

Extensor indicis t.

Flexor digitorum profundus t.

Abductor digiti minimi muscle

Flexor carpi ulnaris

Ulnar nerve

Flexor retinaculum, superficial portion

Flexor digitorum superficialis t.

Extensor carpi radialis brevis tendon

Extensor pollicis longus tendon

Extensor carpi radialis longus tendon

Extensor pollicis brevis tendon

Abductor pollicis longus tendon

Flexor carpi radialis t.

Flexor pollicis longus t.

Median nerve

Flexor retinaculum

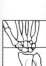

Extensor digitorum tendon slips

Extensor digiti minimi tendon

Extensor indicis t.

Extensor carpi ulnaris t.

Flexor digitorum profundus tendon

Ulnar nerve

Flexor carpi ulnaris

Flexor retinaculum, superficial portion

Flexor digitorum superficialis t.

Extensor carpi radialis brevis tendon

Extensor pollicis longus tendon

Extensor carpi radialis longus tendon

Extensor pollicis brevis tendon

Abductor pollicis longus tendon

Flexor carpi radialis t.

Flexor pollicis longus t.

Median nerve

Flexor retinaculum

(Top) Graphic representation of tendons in carpal tunnel. Flexor digitorum profundus tendons are ordered with little, ring, middle & index tendons side by side (ulnar to radial). Flexor digitorum superficialis tendons are organized with two deep tendons going to middle & ring fingers & two superficial tendons extending to little & index fingers. Extensor pollicis longus tendon is crossing superficial to extensor carpi radialis brevis tendon. **(Bottom)** Corresponding axial MR of tendons in carpal tunnel. Note magic angle effect on EPL as it crosses over ECRB. Tendon is angled 55° to main magnetic field resulting in loss of normal low signal.

TENDONS

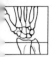

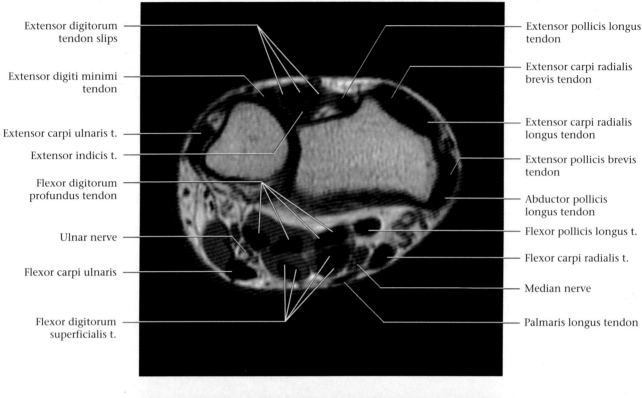

Extensor digitorum tendon slips

Extensor digiti minimi tendon

Extensor carpi ulnaris t.

Extensor indicis t.

Flexor digitorum profundus tendon

Ulnar nerve

Flexor carpi ulnaris

Flexor digitorum superficialis t.

Extensor pollicis longus tendon

Extensor carpi radialis brevis tendon

Extensor carpi radialis longus tendon

Extensor pollicis brevis tendon

Abductor pollicis longus tendon

Flexor pollicis longus t.

Flexor carpi radialis t.

Median nerve

Palmaris longus tendon

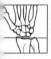

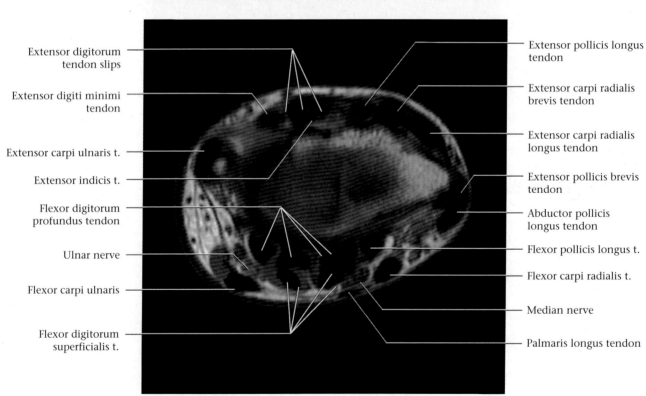

Extensor digitorum tendon slips

Extensor digiti minimi tendon

Extensor carpi ulnaris t.

Extensor indicis t.

Flexor digitorum profundus tendon

Ulnar nerve

Flexor carpi ulnaris

Flexor digitorum superficialis t.

Extensor pollicis longus tendon

Extensor carpi radialis brevis tendon

Extensor carpi radialis longus tendon

Extensor pollicis brevis tendon

Abductor pollicis longus tendon

Flexor pollicis longus t.

Flexor carpi radialis t.

Median nerve

Palmaris longus tendon

(Top) First of six selected axial MR images (from proximal to distal) demonstrate tendon course & relationship to surrounding osseous structures. **(Bottom)** Extensor retinaculum secures various extensor tendons into six discrete compartments.

AXIAL T1 MR, MID WRIST

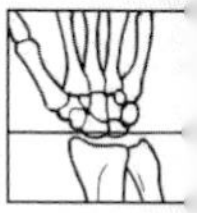

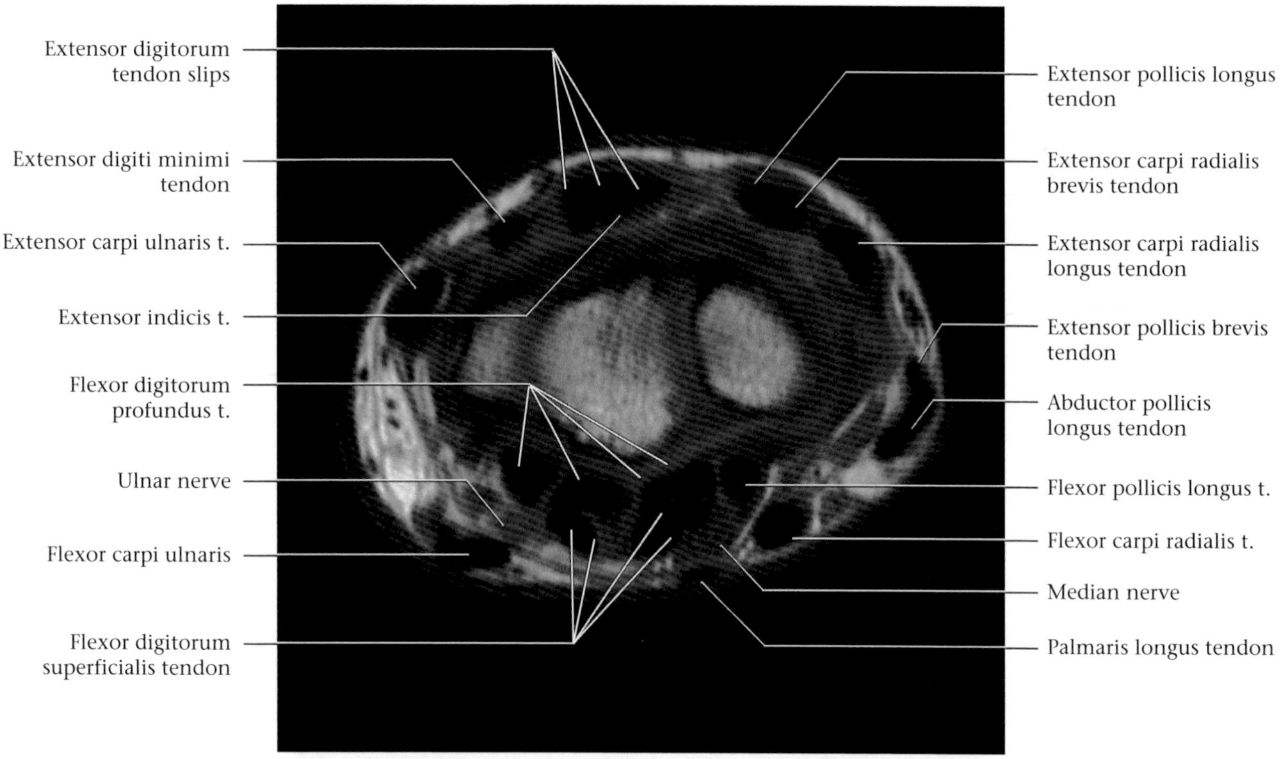
Extensor digitorum tendon slips
Extensor digiti minimi tendon
Extensor carpi ulnaris t.
Extensor indicis t.
Flexor digitorum profundus t.
Ulnar nerve
Flexor carpi ulnaris
Flexor digitorum superficialis tendon
Extensor pollicis longus tendon
Extensor carpi radialis brevis tendon
Extensor carpi radialis longus tendon
Extensor pollicis brevis tendon
Abductor pollicis longus tendon
Flexor pollicis longus t.
Flexor carpi radialis t.
Median nerve
Palmaris longus tendon

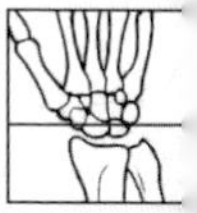

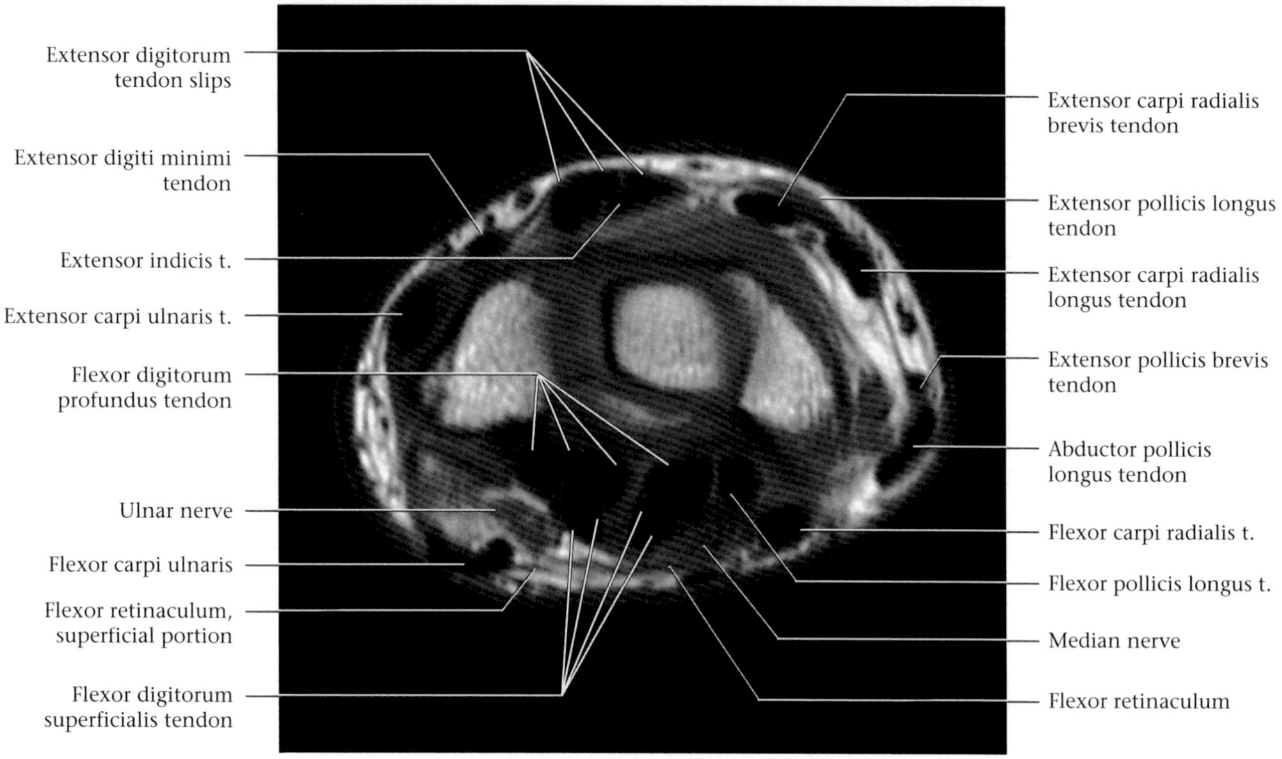
Extensor digitorum tendon slips
Extensor digiti minimi tendon
Extensor indicis t.
Extensor carpi ulnaris t.
Flexor digitorum profundus tendon
Ulnar nerve
Flexor carpi ulnaris
Flexor retinaculum, superficial portion
Flexor digitorum superficialis tendon
Extensor carpi radialis brevis tendon
Extensor pollicis longus tendon
Extensor carpi radialis longus tendon
Extensor pollicis brevis tendon
Abductor pollicis longus tendon
Flexor carpi radialis t.
Flexor pollicis longus t.
Median nerve
Flexor retinaculum

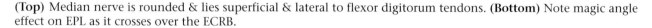

(Top) Median nerve is rounded & lies superficial & lateral to flexor digitorum tendons. **(Bottom)** Note magic angle effect on EPL as it crosses over the ECRB.

AXIAL T1 MR, MID WRIST

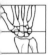

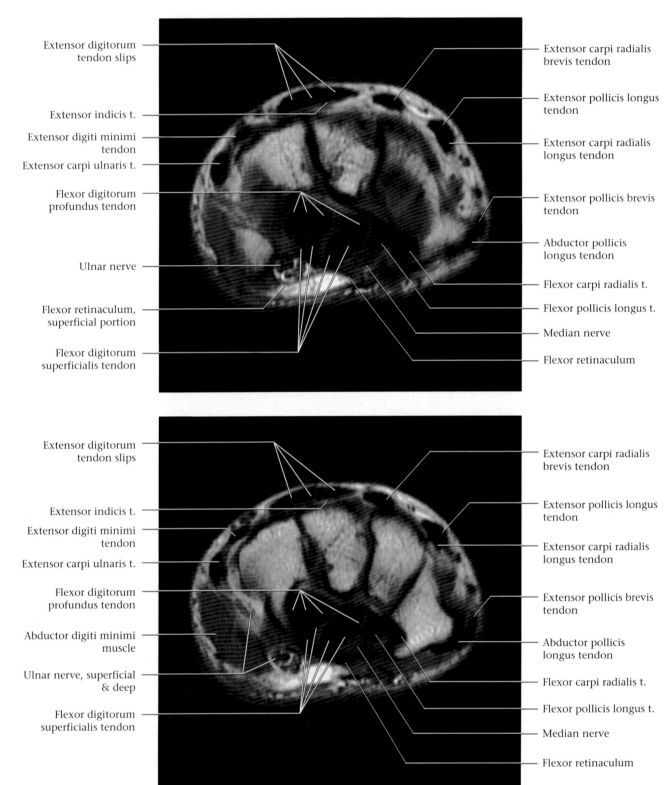

Extensor digitorum tendon slips

Extensor indicis t.

Extensor digiti minimi tendon

Extensor carpi ulnaris t.

Flexor digitorum profundus tendon

Ulnar nerve

Flexor retinaculum, superficial portion

Flexor digitorum superficialis tendon

Extensor carpi radialis brevis tendon

Extensor pollicis longus tendon

Extensor carpi radialis longus tendon

Extensor pollicis brevis tendon

Abductor pollicis longus tendon

Flexor carpi radialis t.

Flexor pollicis longus t.

Median nerve

Flexor retinaculum

Extensor digitorum tendon slips

Extensor indicis t.

Extensor digiti minimi tendon

Extensor carpi ulnaris t.

Flexor digitorum profundus tendon

Abductor digiti minimi muscle

Ulnar nerve, superficial & deep

Flexor digitorum superficialis tendon

Extensor carpi radialis brevis tendon

Extensor pollicis longus tendon

Extensor carpi radialis longus tendon

Extensor pollicis brevis tendon

Abductor pollicis longus tendon

Flexor carpi radialis t.

Flexor pollicis longus t.

Median nerve

Flexor retinaculum

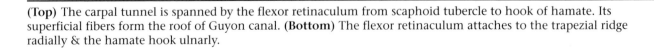

(Top) The carpal tunnel is spanned by the flexor retinaculum from scaphoid tubercle to hook of hamate. Its superficial fibers form the roof of Guyon canal. **(Bottom)** The flexor retinaculum attaches to the trapezial ridge radially & the hamate hook ulnarly.

TENDONS

3D RECONSTRUCTION CT & AXIAL T1 MR, ANATOMIC SNUFFBOX

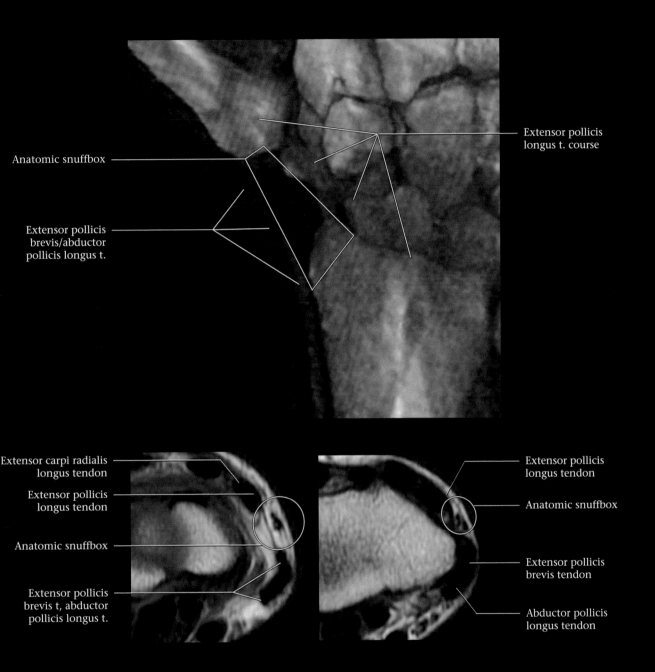

Extensor pollicis longus t. course

Anatomic snuffbox

Extensor pollicis brevis/abductor pollicis longus t.

Extensor carpi radialis longus tendon

Extensor pollicis longus tendon

Anatomic snuffbox

Extensor pollicis brevis t, abductor pollicis longus t.

Extensor pollicis longus tendon

Anatomic snuffbox

Extensor pollicis brevis tendon

Abductor pollicis longus tendon

3D reconstruction CT with soft tissue overlay delineates margins of anatomic snuffbox with EPL crossing from medial to lateral over ECRB & ECRL forming dorsal margin, while APL & EPB form volar margin. Radial nerve, superficial branch, as well as arterial & venous branches pass through snuffbox. MR images demonstrate snuffbox in axial plane.

3D RECONSTRUCTION CT & AXIAL T1 MR, INTERSECTION ANATOMY

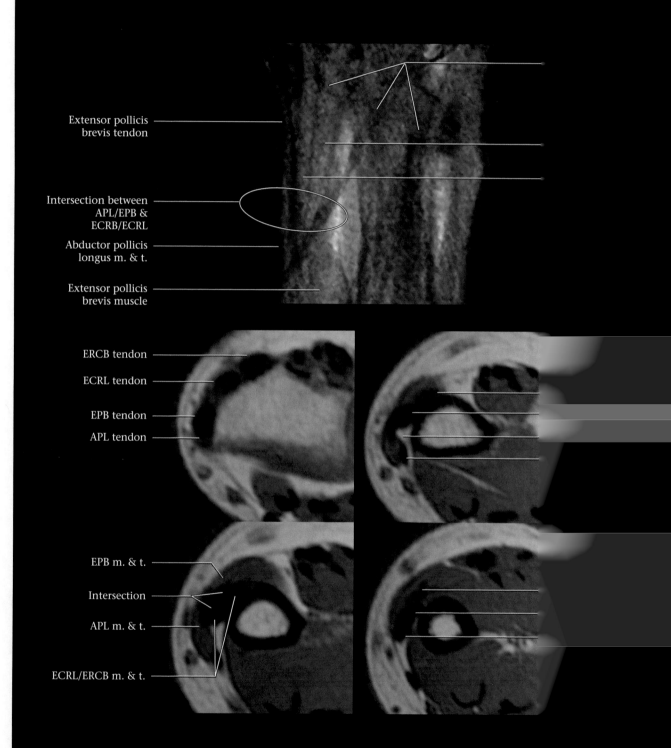

Extensor pollicis
brevis tendon

Intersection between
APL/EPB &
ECRB/ECRL

Abductor pollicis
longus m. & t.

Extensor pollicis
brevis muscle

ERCB tendon

ECRL tendon

EPB tendon

APL tendon

EPB m. & t.

Intersection

APL m. & t.

ECRL/ERCB m. & t.

3D reconstruction CT with soft tissue overlay demonstrates abductor pollicis longus & extens
musculotendinous junctions sweeping distally & laterally, crossing over extensor carpi radial
tendons just proximal to extensor retinaculum. Axial MR demonstrates this complex relation
Lower right MR is in distal forearm, & shows APL & EPB to be superficial & slightly dorsal to
left & upper right MRs show APL & EPB crossing over ECRL & ECRB, to lie on lateral aspect o
is the most distal of this set, at level of Lister tubercle. The crossover is complete at this point
carnal positions, with APL & EPB located lateral to the radius & ECRL & ECRB located dorsol

TENDONS

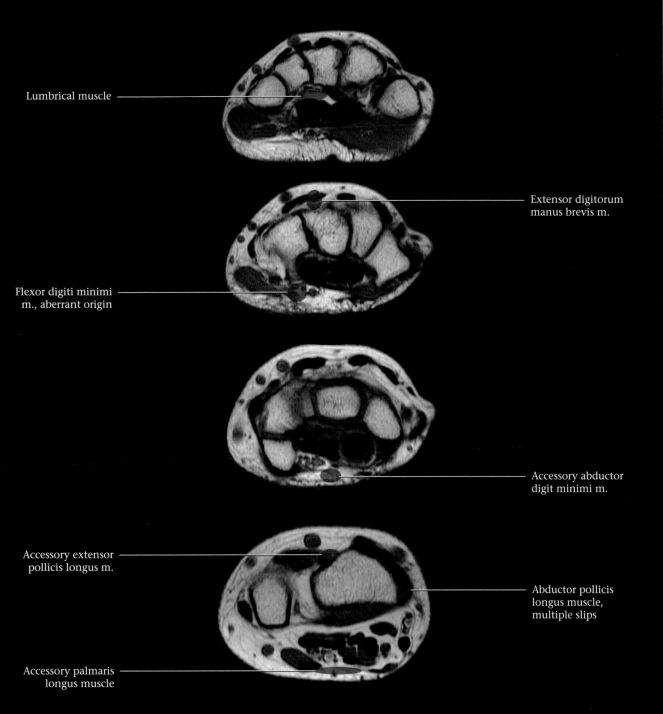

Lumbrical muscle

Extensor digitorum manus brevis m.

Flexor digiti minimi m., aberrant origin

Accessory abductor digit minimi m.

Accessory extensor pollicis longus m.

Abductor pollicis longus muscle, multiple slips

Accessory palmaris longus muscle

Anomalous muscle origins. Lumbrical muscles may arise proximally within carpal tunnel, causing carpal tunnel syndrome. Extensor digitorum manus brevis may present as tender mass. Aberrant flexor digiti minimi origin may compress ulnar nerve. Accessory abductor digiti minimi may compress ulnar or median nerve. Accessory extensor pollicis longus may present as a tender mass. Abductor pollicis longus may have multiple slips & should not be mistaken for a tear. Palmaris longus has many variants; low-lying muscle bellies or multiple slips may compress median nerve.

Wrist

III

SAGITTAL T1 MR

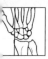

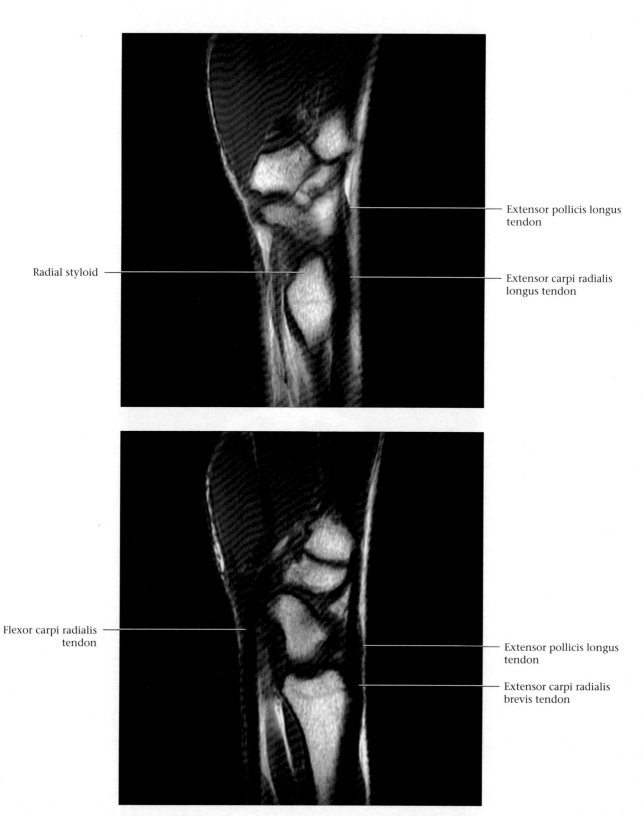

Extensor pollicis longus tendon

Radial styloid

Extensor carpi radialis longus tendon

Flexor carpi radialis tendon

Extensor pollicis longus tendon

Extensor carpi radialis brevis tendon

(Top) First of eight selected sagittal images (from radial to ulnar). Extensor carpi radialis longus extends distal to 2nd metacarpal base. Extensor pollicis longus is a thin tendon passing superficial & distal to extensor carpi radialis longus & brevis tendons. (Bottom) Flexor carpi radialis medial to scaphoid & along trapezium volar groove. Extensor carpi radialis brevis is medial to extensor carpi radialis longus & extends to 3rd metacarpal base.

TENDONS

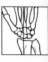

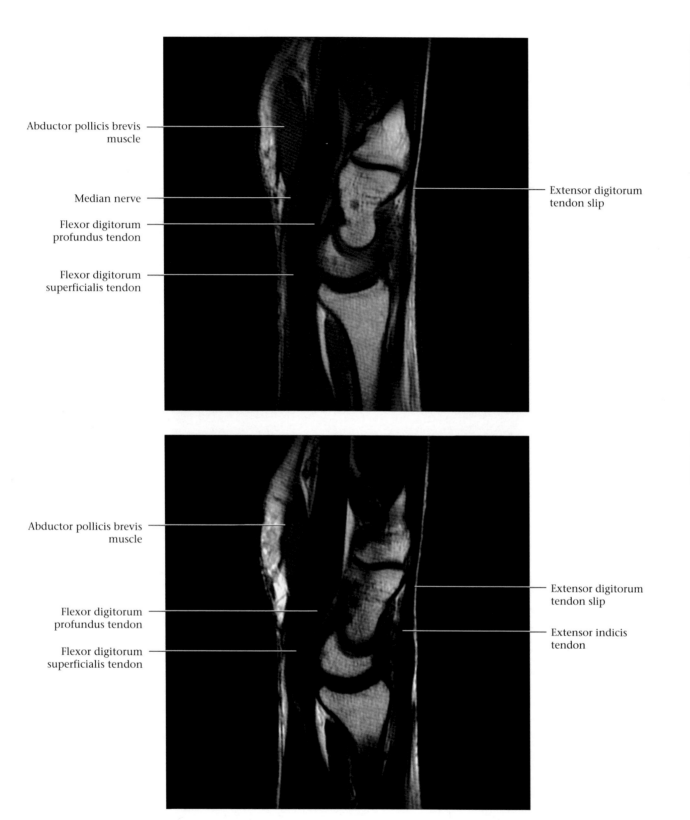

Abductor pollicis brevis muscle

Median nerve

Flexor digitorum profundus tendon

Flexor digitorum superficialis tendon

Extensor digitorum tendon slip

Abductor pollicis brevis muscle

Flexor digitorum profundus tendon

Flexor digitorum superficialis tendon

Extensor digitorum tendon slip

Extensor indicis tendon

(Top) Flexor digitorum superficialis & profundus tendons are apparent in lateral carpal tunnel. Abductor pollicis brevis muscle arises from flexor retinaculum. **(Bottom)** Slightly medially, extensor indicis tendon is deep to extensor digitorum tendon slips.

SAGITTAL T1 MR

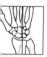

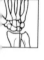

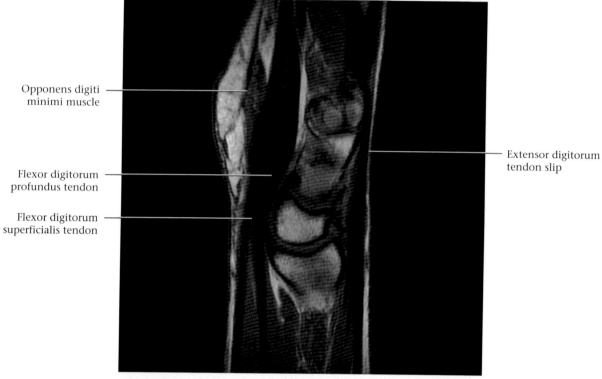

Opponens digiti minimi muscle

Flexor digitorum profundus tendon

Flexor digitorum superficialis tendon

Extensor digitorum tendon slip

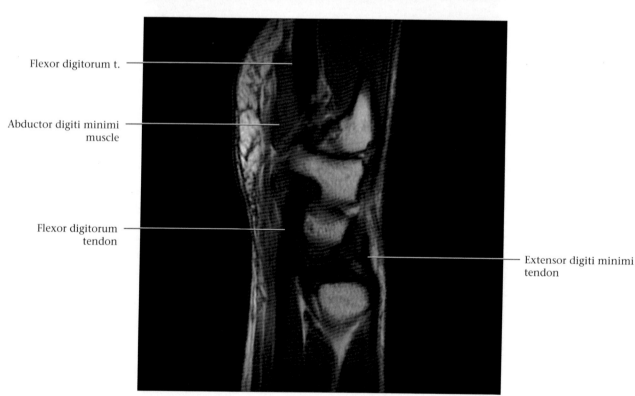

Flexor digitorum t.

Abductor digiti minimi muscle

Flexor digitorum tendon

Extensor digiti minimi tendon

(Top) Flexor tendons of ring & little finger pass deep to flexor retinaculum in medial carpal tunnel. Hypothenar muscles take rise from flexor retinaculum. (Bottom) Abductor digiti minimi arises from flexor retinaculum. Extensor digiti minimi passes through 5th extensor compartment.

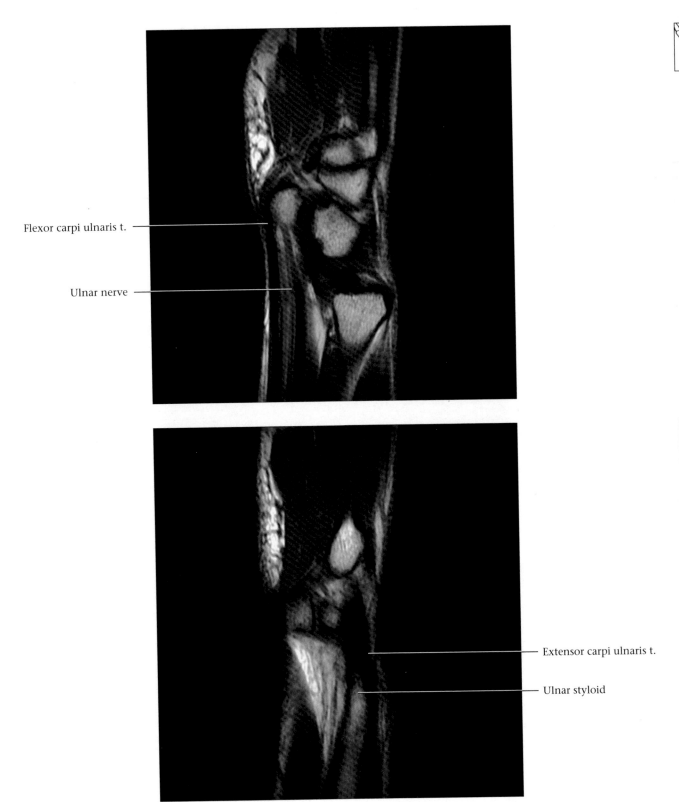

Flexor carpi ulnaris t.

Ulnar nerve

Extensor carpi ulnaris t.

Ulnar styloid

(Top) Flexor carpi ulnaris inserts on pisiform with fibers continuing distally as pisohamate & pisometacarpal ligaments. **(Bottom)** Extensor carpi ulnaris tendon passes over dorsal groove of distal ulna to insert on 5th metacarpal base.

TENDONS

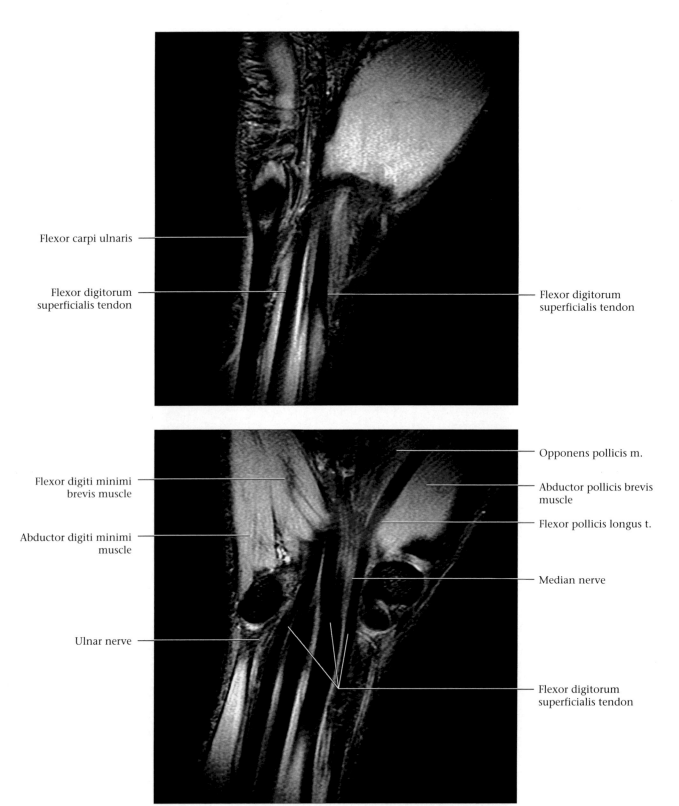

Flexor carpi ulnaris

Flexor digitorum superficialis tendon

Flexor digitorum superficialis tendon

Opponens pollicis m.

Flexor digiti minimi brevis muscle

Abductor pollicis brevis muscle

Abductor digiti minimi muscle

Flexor pollicis longus t.

Median nerve

Ulnar nerve

Flexor digitorum superficialis tendon

(Top) Series of eight selected coronal images (from volar to dorsal). Flexor carpi ulnaris inserts on pisiform while flexor digitorum superficialis tendons run deep to flexor retinaculum. **(Bottom)** Deep to flexor retinaculum, flexor digitorum profundus & superficialis tendons extend tento hand. Hypothenar musculature arises from pisiform, hook of hamate & flexor retinaculum. Thenar musculature arises from flexor retinaculum, scaphoid, trapezium & trapezoid.

Wrist

III

TENDONS

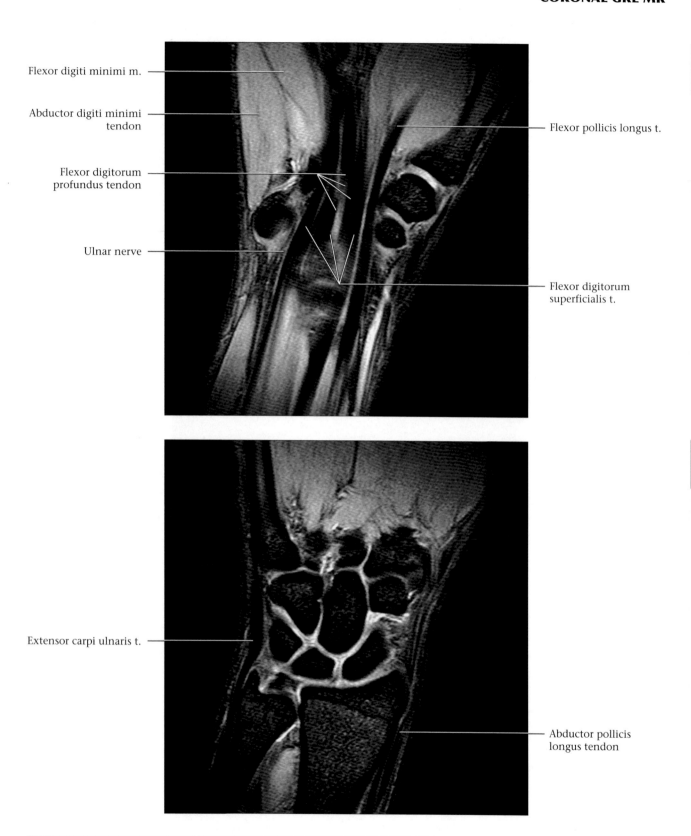

Flexor digiti minimi m.

Abductor digiti minimi tendon

Flexor digitorum profundus tendon

Ulnar nerve

Flexor pollicis longus t.

Flexor digitorum superficialis t.

Extensor carpi ulnaris t.

Abductor pollicis longus tendon

(Top) Carpal tunnel contains flexor digitorum tendons (profundus & superficialis) as well as flexor pollicis longus.
(Bottom) Extensor carpi ulnaris passes over FCU groove in distal ulna while abductor pollicis longus passes over radial styloid.

Wrist

III

CORONAL GRE MR

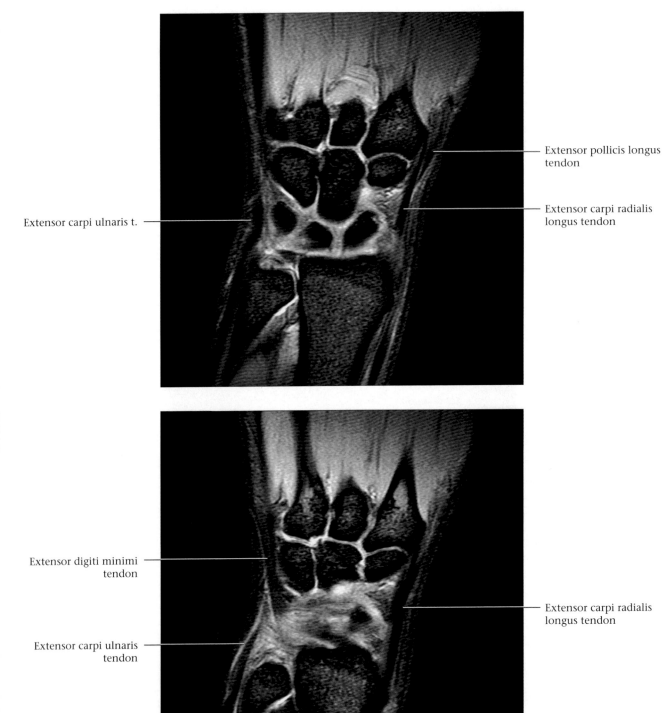

Extensor pollicis longus tendon

Extensor carpi radialis longus tendon

Extensor carpi ulnaris t.

Extensor digiti minimi tendon

Extensor carpi radialis longus tendon

Extensor carpi ulnaris tendon

(Top) Dorsally, portions of extensor tendons become visible. (Bottom) Extensor digiti minimi sweeps distally & medially to insert on little finger extensor hood. Extensor carpi radialis longus inserts on 2nd metacarpal.

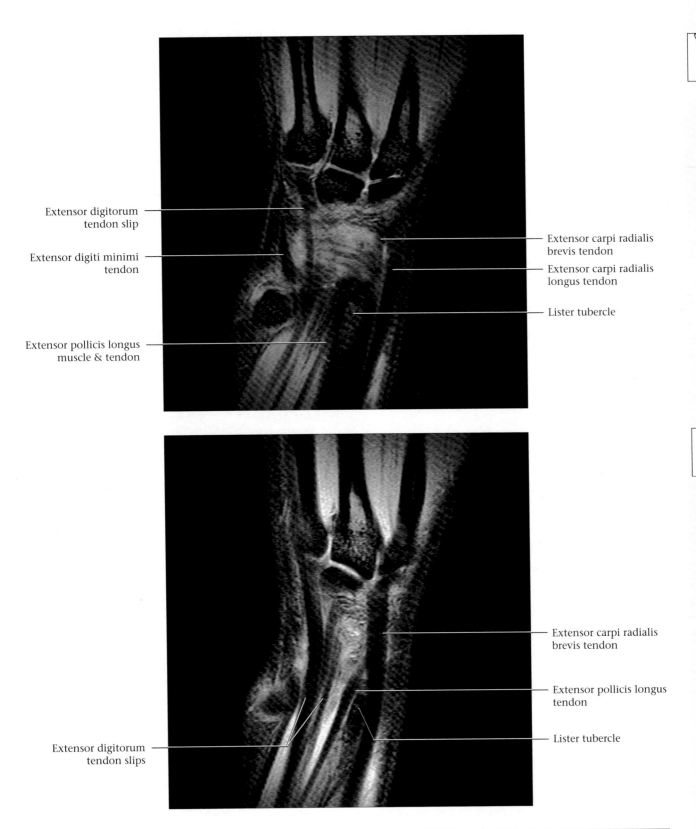

Extensor digitorum tendon slip

Extensor digiti minimi tendon

Extensor pollicis longus muscle & tendon

Extensor carpi radialis brevis tendon

Extensor carpi radialis longus tendon

Lister tubercle

Extensor carpi radialis brevis tendon

Extensor pollicis longus tendon

Lister tubercle

Extensor digitorum tendon slips

(Top) Extensor pollicis longus tendon is located medial to Lister tubercle, which separates it from extensor carpi radialis brevis at this level. Distal to the tubercle, extensor pollicis longus crosses superficial to extensor carpi radialis brevis, and courses laterally towards its insertion on the thumb. **(Bottom)** Extensor digitorum tendon slips pass through 4th compartment. Extensor carpi radialis brevis inserts on 2nd & 3rd metacarpals.

NEUROVASCULAR STRUCTURES

Terminology

Abbreviations

- Abductor digiti minimi (ADM)
- Abductor pollicis brevis (APB)
- Abductor pollicis longus (APL)
- Adductor pollicis (AP)
- Avascular necrosis (AVN)
- Carpal tunnel (CT)
- Carpal tunnel syndrome (CTS)
- Distal radioulnar joint (DRUJ)
- Extensor carpi radialis brevis (ERCB)
- Extensor digitorum (ED)
- Extensor digiti minimi (EDM)
- Extensor pollicis brevis (EPB)
- Extensor pollicis longus (EPL)
- Field of view (FOV)
- Flexor carpi radialis (FCR)
- Flexor carpi ulnaris (FCU)
- Flexor digiti minimi brevis (FDMB)
- Flexor digitorum superficial (FDS)
- Flexor pollicis brevis (FPB)
- Flexor pollicis longus (FPL)
- Flexor retinaculum (FR)
- Metacarpal (MC)
- Opponens digiti minimi (ODM)
- Opponens pollicis (OP)
- Palmaris brevis (PB)
- Palmaris longus (PL)
- Pronator quadratus (PQ)
- Pronator teres (PT)

Definitions

- Palmar = volar
- Ulnar = medial
- Radial = lateral

Imaging Anatomy

Nerves of Wrist Joint

- **Median nerve**
  - Origin: Brachial plexus-lateral & medial cords
  - Course in wrist
    - **At DRUJ:** Nerve is rounded; deep to PL, medial & superficial to FCR & FPL, lateral & superficial to FDS
    - **At level of pisiform (proximal CT):** Nerve slightly flattened; deep to FR, superficial to FPL & FDS
    - **At level of hook of hamate (distal CT):** Nerve flattened; deep to FR, superficial to FPL & FDS
  - Branches
    - **Muscular** branches near elbow; supply PT, FCR, PL, FDS
    - **Anterior interosseous** branch travels along distal volar interosseous membrane between FPL & FDP to terminate in PQ & radiocarpal joint; supplies radial ½ FDP, FPL & PQ

  - **Palmar cutaneous** branch arises proximal to carpal tunnel & remains superficial to FR; supplies palmar skin of thenar eminence; may be injured during carpal tunnel release as it is small & difficult to identify; impingement may mimic CTS
  - **Muscular** branches arise distal to CT; supplies APB, OP, FPB
  - Terminal branches to 1st-3rd **common palmar digital** & **proper digital** nerves; supply lumbricals & volar skin of fingers
  - Variants: Bifid median nerve, high bifurcation of median nerve in forearm, resulting in medial & lateral branches at wrist
- **Radial nerve**
  - Origin: Brachial plexus-posterior cord
  - Course in wrist: Branches into superficial & deep branches in distal forearm
  - Branches
    - **Superficial** branch passes under brachioradialis tendon into dorsal wrist; divides into **lateral branch** (supplies radial wrist & thumb skin) & **medial branch** (supplies mid & ulnar wrist skin); divides to **dorsal digital** nerves supplying ulnar thumb, index, middle & radial ring fingers
    - **Deep** branch enters supinator volarly; exits distally & posteriorly as **posterior interosseous** nerve; supplies ECRB, supinator, ED, EDM, ECU, EPL, APL & EI
- **Ulnar nerve**
  - Origin: Brachial plexus-medial cord
  - Course in wrist: Radial to FCU, close to ulnar artery
    - **At proximal pisiform:** Nerve proximal to bifurcation; nerve deep to FCU, ulnar to ulnar artery & veins
    - **At distal pisiform:** Nerve bifurcates into deep (motor) & superficial (sensory) branches
    - **At hook of hamate: Superficial** branches volar to hook of hamate & ADM; nerve ulnar to ulnar artery & veins; **deep** branches are dorsal & ulnar to hook of hamate, deep to ADM, superficial to pisometacarpal ligament
  - Branches
    - **Muscular** branches (near elbow); supply FCU, ulnar ½ FDP
    - **Dorsal** branch passes between FCU & ulna, divides into **dorsal digital** nerves; supplies dorsal ulnar hand sensory innervation
    - **Palmar cutaneous** branch parallels ulnar artery, perforates FR; supplies palmar ulnar hand sensory innervation
    - **Terminal** ulnar nerve crosses ulnar wrist with ulnar artery, deep to PB; divides into superficial & deep branches
    - **Superficial** branch located superficial to fascia of ADM; divides into **common** & **palmar digital** branches; supplies PB, hypothenar eminence skin & ring/little fingers
    - **Deep** branch courses sharply ulnarward over hook of hamate through pisohamate hiatus (risk for compression in this region); supplies motor innervation to ADM, FDMB, ODM, AP, 3rd & 4th lumbricals, all interossei
- **Joint innervation**

- DRUJ: Median nerve, anterior interosseous branch; radial nerve, posterior interosseous branch
  - Radiocarpal: Median nerve, anterior interosseous branch; radial nerve, posterior interosseous branch; ulnar nerve, dorsal & deep branches
  - Mid carpal: Ulnar nerve, carpal branches; median nerve; radial nerve, posterior interosseous branch
- Volar dermatomes: C6 - thumb, thenar eminence; C7 - palm, index & middle fingers; C8 - hypothenar eminence, ring & little fingers
- Dorsal dermatomes: C6 - thumb; C7 - dorsal wrist, index & middle fingers; C8 - dorsal wrist, ring & little fingers

Anatomic Spaces

- Carpal tunnel
  - Fibro-osseous tunnel bordered by carpals (dorsal), scaphoid & trapezium tubercles (lateral), hook of hamate & pisiform (medial) & FR (volar)
  - Contents: 4 FDS, 4 FDP, FPL, median nerve
  - Anatomic variants seen in 41%: Include bifid median nerve; persistent median artery; anomalous muscles including reversed palmaris longus, palmaris profundus, accessory FDS, aberrant thenar or lumbrical origins
  - Anatomic variants may result in compression in (relatively) rigid tunnel
- Guyon canal
  - Fibro-osseous triangular canal bordered by pisiform bone & pisohamate ligament (medial), hook of hamate (distal), FR (dorsal) & volar carpal ligament (volar)
  - Contents: Ulnar artery, ulnar nerve, ulnar vein, fat
  - Zones (area containing ulnar nerve, based on bifurcation): 1) nerve proximal to bifurcation; 2) ulnar nerve, deep branch (motor); 3) ulnar nerve, superficial branch (sensory)
  - Anatomic variants seen in 25%; include reversed palmaris longus, accessory ADM, accessory FCU

Vessels of Wrist Joint

- Extraosseous vascular supply
- Radial artery
  - Origin: Terminal branch of brachial artery
  - Superficial to PQ (volar & radial); continues dorsally around radial styloid process; passes deep to APL & EPB, across anatomic snuffbox & deep to EPL
  - Branches
    - Palmar carpal branch arises near distal edge of PQ; runs across palmar wrist at radiocarpal level to anastomose (variably) with ulnar artery, palmar carpal branch, & anterior interosseous branches to form palmar (volar or transverse) radiocarpal arch
    - Small dorsal branch just proximal to anatomic snuffbox passes dorsally, & remains deep to extensor compartments joining ulnar artery to form dorsal radiocarpal arch

- Superficial palmar branch continues distally, superficial to FR; passes through thenar eminence muscle to anastomose (variably) with ulnar artery to form superficial palmar arch at metacarpal base level; may give a small branch that joins ulnar artery branch to form volar intercarpal arch
- Main radial artery continues dorsal at radial styloid, deep to EPB & APL, crossing anatomic snuffbox
- Dorsal carpal branch at level of dorsal scaphoid waist joins ulnar artery, dorsal carpal branch, to create dorsal carpal (intercarpal) arch
- Main radial artery continues distal, passes between heads of 1st dorsal interosseous muscle to enter palm, joining ulnar artery, deep palmar branch, to form deep palmar arch
- Ulnar artery
  - Origin: Terminal branch of brachial artery
  - Course in wrist: Superficial to PQ (volar & ulnar); continuing between FCU & FDS tendons
  - Branches
    - Common interosseous artery branches in forearm to anterior & posterior interosseous arteries
    - Anterior interosseous artery travels volar to interosseous membrane deep to FDP & FPL; at proximal PQ gives small branch which pierces PQ & joins volar radiocarpal arch; pierces membrane, entering dorsal forearm where it anastomoses with posterior interosseous artery joining dorsal radiocarpal & intercarpal arches; median artery (branch of anterior interosseous artery) arises in forearm & may persist (accompanying median nerve) into carpal tunnel, contributing to superficial palmar arch
    - Posterior interosseous artery travels distal between deep & superficial extensors, superficial to EPB & APL to anastomose with anterior interosseous artery
    - Palmar carpal branch arises at proximal carpals, anastomoses with radial artery, palmar carpal branch, & anterior interosseous branches to form palmar (volar or transverse) radiocarpal arch
    - Dorsal carpal branch arises at pisiform, passes dorsally beneath FCU into dorsum of wrist, deep to extensor tendons, to anastomose with radial artery, dorsal carpal branch, to create dorsal carpal (intercarpal) arch
    - Deep palmar branch arises at FR; passes medially through hypothenar muscles (AP & FDMB); turns lateral into palm to anastomose with radial artery, deep palmar branch, to form deep palmar arch
    - Superficial palmar branch continues distal superficial to FR to join radial artery, superficial branch, creating superficial palmar arch
- Vascular variations: Many variations are described, particularly related to vessel contributions to vascular arches
  - Dorsal arches

NEUROVASCULAR STRUCTURES

- **Radiocarpal arch:** Present in 80%, most important for carpal vascular supply; anastomoses variable: Radial & anterior interosseous (occurs 80%); radial, ulnar & interosseous (occurs less commonly)
- **Dorsal carpal (intercarpal) arch:** Present in 99%; anastomoses variable: Radial, ulnar, & interosseous (occurs 53%); radial & ulnar (20%); radial & interosseous (20%); ulnar & interosseous (7%)
- **Basal metacarpal arch:** Complete in 27%, absent in 27%; partial (radial only) in 46%
- **Volar arches**
  - **Radiocarpal arch:** Present in 100%; anastomoses: Ulnar, radial & interosseous anastomoses (87%); radial & ulnar (13%)
  - **Intercarpal arch:** Smallest & most variable; seen in only 53%; anastomoses: Radial, ulnar & interosseous (75%); radial & ulnar (25%)
  - **Deep palmar arch:** Present in 100%; anastomoses: Radial & ulnar (97%); no anastomoses between radial & ulnar (13%): Proximal, deep & distal systems arise from this arch; volar arches are connected longitudinally by radial, ulnar & interosseous arteries & deep palmar recurrent arteries (which arise from deep palmar arch)
- **Vessel visualization** on standard multiplanar imaging at mid-carpal level
  - **Radial & ulnar a.:** 3-4 mm; typically visualized
  - **Vascular arches:** 1 mm; inconsistently visualized
  - **Multiple branches & anastomoses:** < 1 mm; rarely visualized
- **Intraosseous vascular supply**
  - **Overview**
    - Extensive volar & dorsal anastomoses typically exist
    - Vessels enter in areas without cartilaginous cover, nonarticular, at ligament or capsule attachments
    - Pitfall: Entry points of nutrient vessels should not be mistaken for erosions on MR or CT scanning
  - **Carpal vessel entry points (number of vessels) & anastomoses**
    - **Scaphoid:** Distal (at volar distal pole), laterovolar (at scaphoid waist), & dorsal (at dorsal ridge) at ligamentous attachments with rich anastomoses; 1 inconsequential proximal pole vessel enters at radioscapholunate ligament attachment (13-14% have no vessel entering proximal to scaphoid waist); proximal pole is at high risk if trauma occurs at scaphoid waist proximal to vessel entries
    - **Lunate:** Dorsal & volar (1-2) at ligamentous attachments; extensive anastomoses
    - **Triquetrum:** Dorsal (2-4 along dorsal ridge) supply 60% of carpus; volar (2-3 proximal to pisiform) supply 40%; extensive anastomoses in 86%
    - **Pisiform:** Proximal & distal poles (1-3); extensive anastomoses
    - **Trapezium:** Dorsal (1-3), volar (1-3) & lateral (5-6); anastomoses but dorsal supply dominates
    - **Trapezoid:** Dorsal (3-4) supply 70% of carpus; volar (1-2) supply 30%; no anastomoses

- **Capitate:** Dorsal (2-4) & volar (1-3); no significant anastomoses in 70%
- **Hamate:** Dorsal (3-5) supply 30% of carpus; volar (1 in hook of hamate) supplies 70%; anastomoses with dorsal in 50%
  - **Intraosseous vascular supply** correlated with clinical incidence of avascular necrosis
    - Group 1: Vessels entering from only one surface or large areas dependent on one vessel; includes scaphoid, capitate & 8% of lunates; high risk for AVN
    - Group 2: Bones with absence of internal anastomoses; hamate & trapezoid; less risk for AVN
    - Group 3: Bones with rich internal anastomoses; trapezium, triquetrum, pisiform & 92% of lunates; least risk for AVN

Anatomy-Based Imaging Issues

Imaging Recommendations

- **Neural structure** evaluation
  - Appearance: Isointense to muscle on all sequences; larger nerves may have a stippled appearance (in axial section) as longitudinally-oriented fascicles have slight increased signal intensity compared to lower signal intensity of surrounding epi/perineurium
  - Best plane for neural evaluation: Axial plane; 8-12 cm FOV
  - Sequences for neural evaluation: T1 for anatomic detail; PD or T2 fat suppression or STIR to evaluate abnormal increased signal
  - Patient positioning needs to maximize patient comfort; best with wrist in center of magnetic field; patient in prone position with hand pronated above head ("Superman") position
- **Vascular** evaluation
  - Gadolinium-enhanced MR angiography provides detail of vessels including small digital arteries; comparable to conventional angiography
    - 12-14 cm FOV to visualize multiple branches
    - Fast 3D spoiled gradient-echo sequence in combination with high quality receiver coil allows short acquisition time with adequate signal-to-noise ratio; acquire pre-injection 3D images & post-injection beginning approximately 15 seconds after injection; acquire 3-4 sequences to maximize data acquisition in arterial, capillary & venous phases
    - Limited in patients with flexion contractures, inability to remain still, physical restrictions to undergoing MR (i.e., pacemaker)
  - Gadolinium-enhanced MR facilitates evaluation of bone viability; results in sensitivity 66%, specificity 88% & accuracy 83%

Imaging Pitfalls

- Neural signal intensity is typically intermediate in spin echo imaging; with fast spin echo technique, nerves demonstrate increased signal that should not be mistaken as abnormal

NEUROVASCULAR STRUCTURES

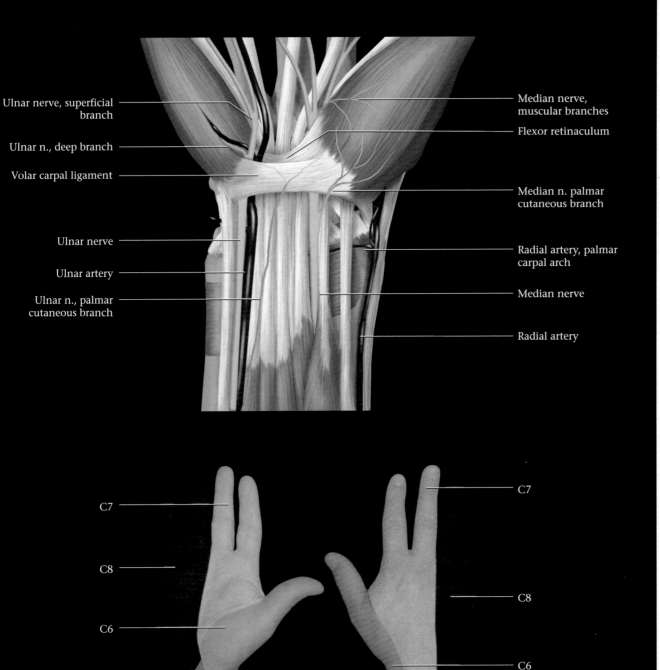

(Top) Relationship of nerves & arteries to volar carpal ligament (superficial fibers of flexor retinaculum which form roof of Guyon canal) & flexor retinaculum (which forms roof of carpal tunnel). Ulnar nerve (& accompanying artery) pass deep to volar ligament before branching into deep & superficial branches. Median nerve gives rise to palmar cutaneous nerve proximal to carpal tunnel. This branch does not enter tunnel but lies superficial to flexor retinaculum & may be injured with carpal tunnel release. (Bottom) Dermatomes of hand & wrist correlated to corresponding cervical or thoracic nerve.

NEUROVASCULAR STRUCTURES

GRAPHICS, VOLAR & DORSAL NERVES

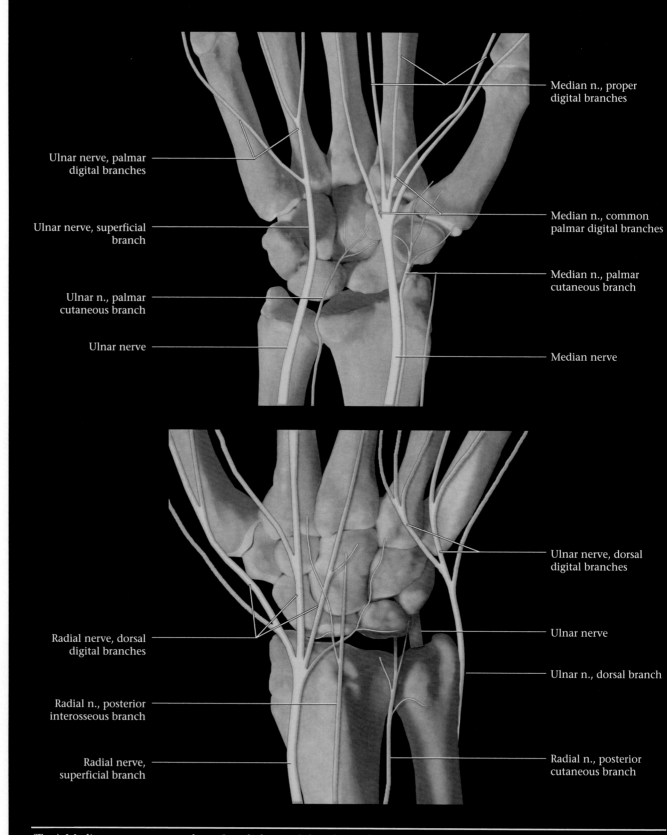

Ulnar nerve, palmar digital branches

Ulnar nerve, superficial branch

Ulnar n., palmar cutaneous branch

Ulnar nerve

Median n., proper digital branches

Median n., common palmar digital branches

Median n., palmar cutaneous branch

Median nerve

Radial nerve, dorsal digital branches

Radial n., posterior interosseous branch

Radial nerve, superficial branch

Ulnar nerve, dorsal digital branches

Ulnar nerve

Ulnar n., dorsal branch

Radial n., posterior cutaneous branch

(Top) Median nerve serves palmar & radial wrist & hand. A palmar cutaneous branch arises proximal to carpal tunnel, innervating palmar skin. Muscular branches supply thenar eminence musculature. Ulnar nerve serves palmar & ulnar wrist & hand. Deep (not shown) & superficial branches supply motor & sensory to hypothenar eminence. **(Bottom)** Ulnar nerve serves ulnar wrist & hand. A dorsal branch passes between FCU & ulna to serve dorsal ulnar wrist. Radial nerve, superficial & posterior interosseous branches, supply innervation to dorsal radial wrist & hand.

NEUROVASCULAR STRUCTURES

GRAPHIC & AXIAL T1 MR, PROXIMAL WRIST

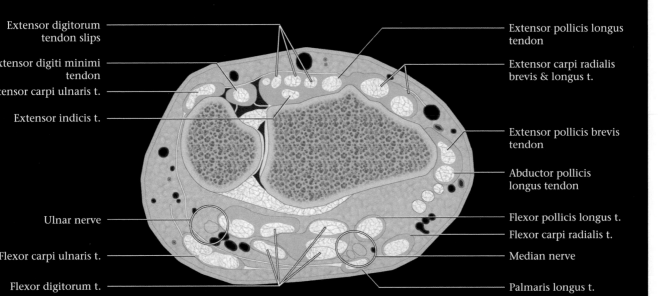

Extensor digitorum tendon slips

Extensor digiti minimi tendon

Extensor carpi ulnaris t.

Extensor indicis t.

Ulnar nerve

Flexor carpi ulnaris t.

Flexor digitorum t.

Extensor pollicis longus tendon

Extensor carpi radialis brevis & longus t.

Extensor pollicis brevis tendon

Abductor pollicis longus tendon

Flexor pollicis longus t.

Flexor carpi radialis t.

Median nerve

Palmaris longus t.

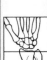

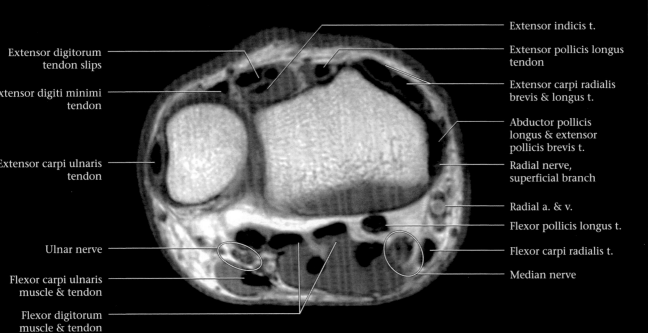

Extensor indicis t.

Extensor pollicis longus tendon

Extensor carpi radialis brevis & longus t.

Abductor pollicis longus & extensor pollicis brevis t.

Radial nerve, superficial branch

Radial a. & v.

Flexor pollicis longus t.

Flexor carpi radialis t.

Median nerve

Extensor digitorum tendon slips

Extensor digiti minimi tendon

Extensor carpi ulnaris tendon

Ulnar nerve

Flexor carpi ulnaris muscle & tendon

Flexor digitorum muscle & tendon

op) Distal radioulnar joint. Median nerve is rounded or may be bifid, lying deep to palmaris longus tendon & perficial to flexor pollicis longus tendon, lateral to flexor digitorum tendons. **(Bottom)** Ulnar artery & veins company ulnar nerve. The ulnar neurovascular bundle lies deep to flexor carpi ulnaris tendon at this level. Median rve lies radial to flexor tendons & muscles & deep to flexor carpi radialis tendon. Radial nerve lies superficial to mpartment #1 extensor tendons.

NEUROVASCULAR STRUCTURES

GRAPHIC & AXIAL T1 MR, PROXIMAL CARPAL TUNNEL

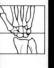

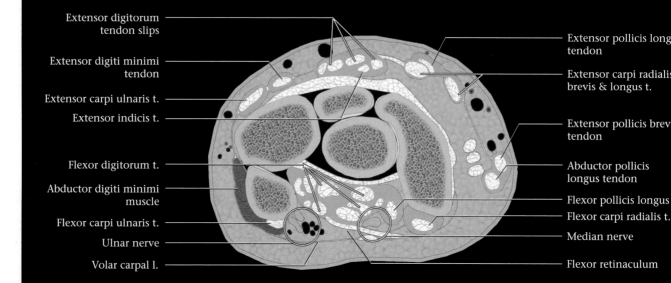

Extensor digitorum tendon slips

Extensor digiti minimi tendon

Extensor carpi ulnaris t.

Extensor indicis t.

Flexor digitorum t.

Abductor digiti minimi muscle

Flexor carpi ulnaris t.

Ulnar nerve

Volar carpal l.

Extensor pollicis long tendon

Extensor carpi radialis brevis & longus t.

Extensor pollicis brev tendon

Abductor pollicis longus tendon

Flexor pollicis longus

Flexor carpi radialis t.

Median nerve

Flexor retinaculum

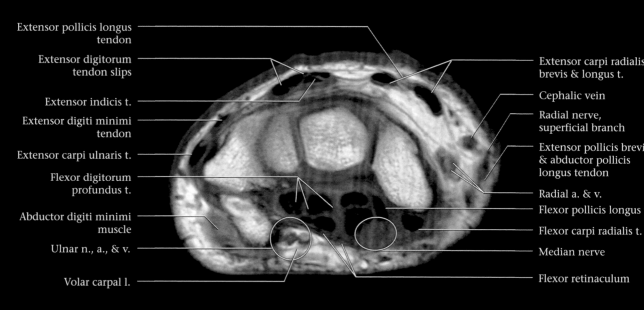

Extensor pollicis longus tendon

Extensor digitorum tendon slips

Extensor indicis t.

Extensor digiti minimi tendon

Extensor carpi ulnaris t.

Flexor digitorum profundus t.

Abductor digiti minimi muscle

Ulnar n., a., & v.

Volar carpal l.

Extensor carpi radialis brevis & longus t.

Cephalic vein

Radial nerve, superficial branch

Extensor pollicis brevi & abductor pollicis longus tendon

Radial a. & v.

Flexor pollicis longus

Flexor carpi radialis t.

Median nerve

Flexor retinaculum

(Top) Mid pisiform level. Median nerve is slightly flattened as it passes deep to flexor retinaculum but remains superficial to flexor pollicis longus tendon & radial to flexor digitorum tendons. Ulnar nerve, artery & veins lie later to pisiform & divide near pisiform into deep & superficial branches. **(Bottom)** Median nerve is slightly stippled in appearance & may remain rounded or become slightly flattened in carpal tunnel. Ulnar nerve is medial to ulnar artery which is medial to ulnar vein. Radial nerve remains dorsal & adjacent to compartment #1.

NEUROVASCULAR STRUCTURES

GRAPHIC & AXIAL T1 MR, MID CARPAL TUNNEL

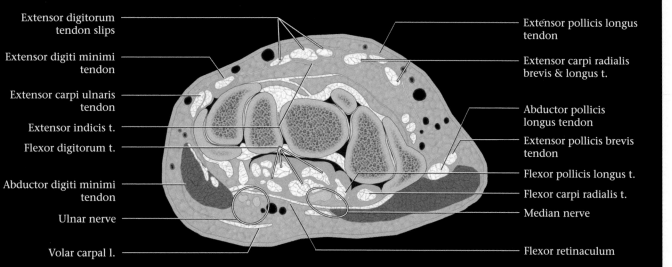

Extensor digitorum tendon slips
Extensor digiti minimi tendon
Extensor carpi ulnaris tendon
Extensor indicis t.
Flexor digitorum t.
Abductor digiti minimi tendon
Ulnar nerve
Volar carpal l.

Extensor pollicis longus tendon
Extensor carpi radialis brevis & longus t.
Abductor pollicis longus tendon
Extensor pollicis brevis tendon
Flexor pollicis longus t.
Flexor carpi radialis t.
Median nerve
Flexor retinaculum

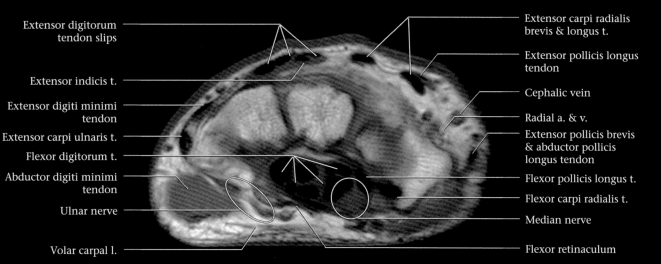

Extensor digitorum tendon slips
Extensor indicis t.
Extensor digiti minimi tendon
Extensor carpi ulnaris t.
Flexor digitorum t.
Abductor digiti minimi tendon
Ulnar nerve
Volar carpal l.

Extensor carpi radialis brevis & longus t.
Extensor pollicis longus tendon
Cephalic vein
Radial a. & v.
Extensor pollicis brevis & abductor pollicis longus tendon
Flexor pollicis longus t.
Flexor carpi radialis t.
Median nerve
Flexor retinaculum

(Top) Mid carpal tunnel. Median nerve is slightly flattened as it passes deep to flexor retinaculum & remains superficial to flexor pollicis longus. Ulnar nerve, artery & veins lie lateral to pisiform & may divide near pisiform into deep & superficial branches. **(Bottom)** Median nerve stippled apperance is evident as it becomes slightly more flattened in mid carpal tunnel. Ulnar nerve, superficial branch, continues distally over tip of hook of hamate while deep branch passes through pisohamate hiatus. Radial nerve is no longer evident.

NEUROVASCULAR STRUCTURES

CORONAL GRE & AXIAL T1 MR, CARPAL TUNNEL

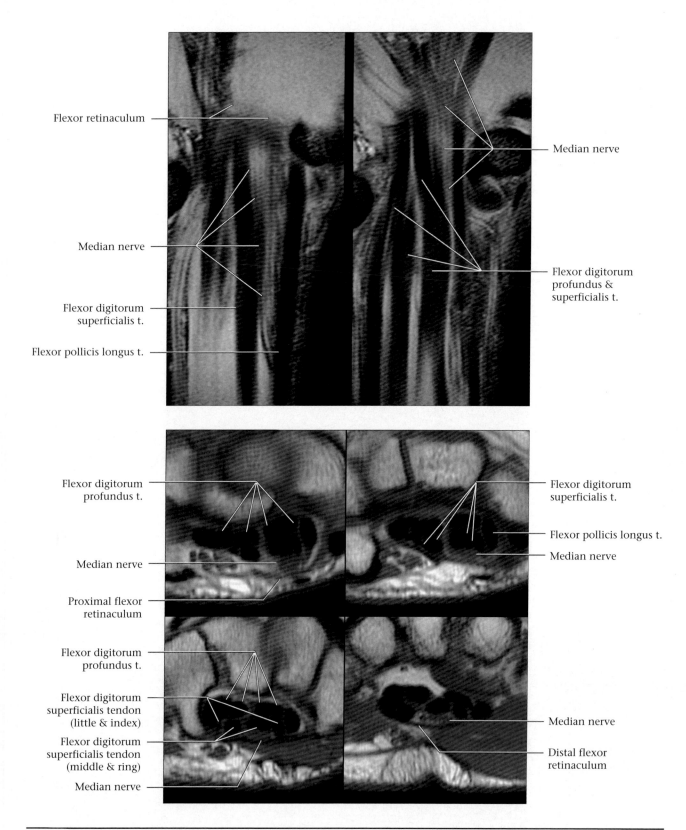

Flexor retinaculum

Median nerve

Median nerve

Flexor digitorum
superficialis t.

Flexor pollicis longus t.

Flexor digitorum
profundus &
superficialis t.

Flexor digitorum
profundus t.

Median nerve

Proximal flexor
retinaculum

Flexor digitorum
superficialis t.

Flexor pollicis longus t.

Median nerve

Flexor digitorum
profundus t.

Flexor digitorum
superficialis tendon
(little & index)

Flexor digitorum
superficialis tendon
(middle & ring)

Median nerve

Median nerve

Distal flexor
retinaculum

(Top) Selected coronal images (superficial to deep). Median nerve has a striated appearance as it travels from proximal to distal, accompanied by flexor digitorum & flexor pollicis longus tendons. **(Bottom)** Selected axial images (proximal to distal). Upper left: Proximal carpal tunnel with rounded median nerve, flexor digitorum & flexor pollicis longus tendons deep to nerve. Upper right: Mid carpal tunnel with median nerve volar & radial to tendons. Lower left: Mid carpal tunnel with tendons deep to median nerve & organized in layers with middle & ring superficialis tendons lying volar to little & index tendons. Profundus tendons lie across carpal tunnel base with little finger tendon most medial & index finger tendon most radial. Lower right: Median nerve is diminished in size & flattened as it branches to terminal branches.

Wrist

NEUROVASCULAR STRUCTURES

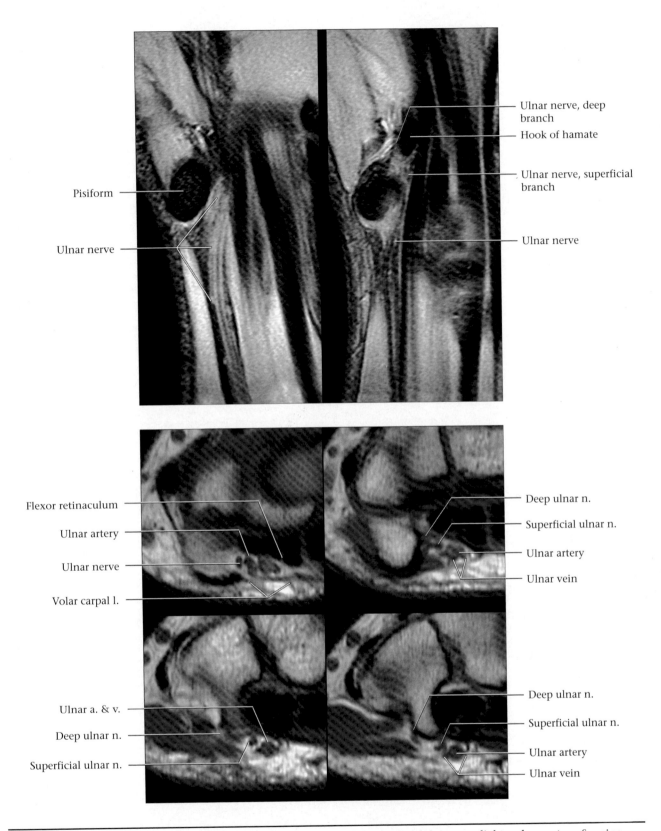

Ulnar nerve, deep branch

Hook of hamate

Ulnar nerve, superficial branch

Ulnar nerve

Pisiform

Ulnar nerve

Flexor retinaculum

Ulnar artery

Ulnar nerve

Volar carpal l.

Deep ulnar n.

Superficial ulnar n.

Ulnar artery

Ulnar vein

Ulnar a. & v.

Deep ulnar n.

Superficial ulnar n.

Deep ulnar n.

Superficial ulnar n.

Ulnar artery

Ulnar vein

(Top) Selected coronal images (superficial to deep). Ulnar nerve passes distal, lying medial to ulnar artery & veins, passing lateral to pisiform where it divides into superficial & deep branches with deep branch curving medially through pisohamate hiatus. **(Bottom)** Selected axial images (proximal to distal). Upper left: Proximal Guyon canal with volar carpal ligament forming roof & flexor retinaculum forming floor of canal. Upper right: Ulnar nerve divides, at mid pisiform, into superficial & deep branches. Lower left: Superficial ulnar nerve passes volar to tip of hamate hook & deep ulnar nerve courses medially through pisohamate hiatus. Lower right: Ulnar nerve branches continue distally supplying sensory (superficial) & motor (deep) to ulnar wrist & hand.

NEUROVASCULAR STRUCTURES

GRAPHICS, VOLAR & DORSAL ARTERIES & VEINS

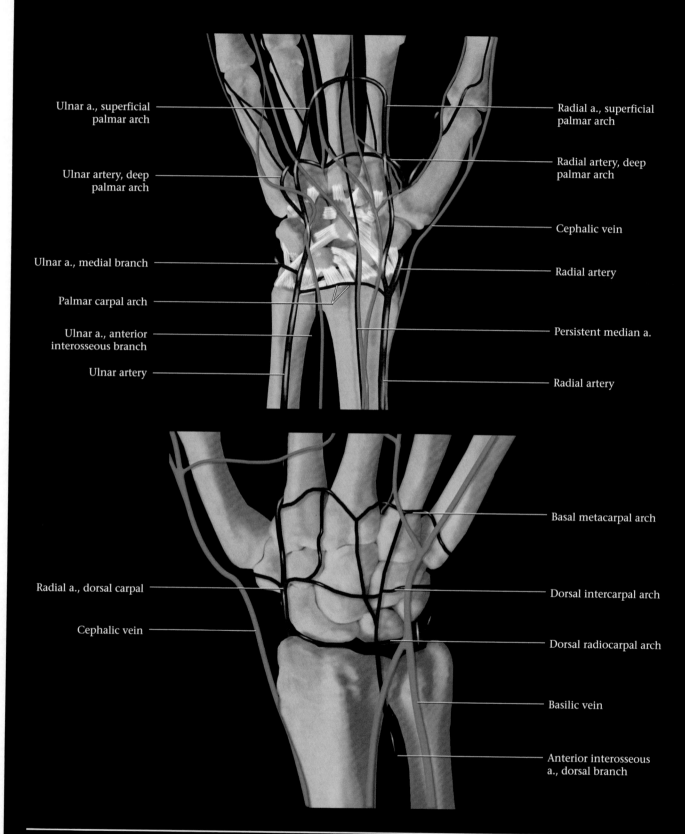

Ulnar a., superficial palmar arch

Ulnar artery, deep palmar arch

Ulnar a., medial branch

Palmar carpal arch

Ulnar a., anterior interosseous branch

Ulnar artery

Radial a., superficial palmar arch

Radial artery, deep palmar arch

Cephalic vein

Radial artery

Persistent median a.

Radial artery

Radial a., dorsal carpal

Cephalic vein

Basal metacarpal arch

Dorsal intercarpal arch

Dorsal radiocarpal arch

Basilic vein

Anterior interosseous a., dorsal branch

(Top) Volar arteries & veins. Each carpal arch has a variable contribution from ulnar, radial & anterior interosseous (a branch of ulnar artery) arteries. Venous plexus varies but flows into two main venous systems, basilic & cephalic. **(Bottom)** Three dorsal carpal arches are formed with variable contributions of radial, ulnar & anterior interosseous arteries. Basilic vein lies dorsal & ulnar while cephalic vein is radial.

NEUROVASCULAR STRUCTURES

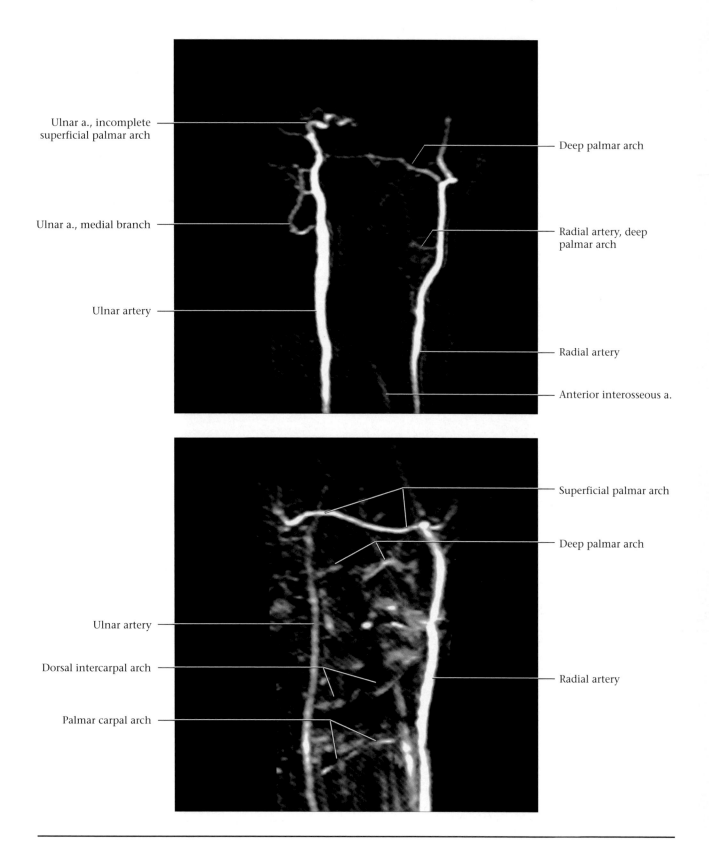

Ulnar a., incomplete superficial palmar arch

Deep palmar arch

Ulnar a., medial branch

Radial artery, deep palmar arch

Ulnar artery

Radial artery

Anterior interosseous a.

Superficial palmar arch

Deep palmar arch

Ulnar artery

Dorsal intercarpal arch

Palmar carpal arch

Radial artery

(Top) Contrast-enhanced angiography reveals major vessels but many smaller branches will not be seen. While deep palmar arch is identified, superficial palmar arch is incomplete. Note prominent ulnar arterial contribution to wrist & hand in this patient. (Bottom) Contrast-enhanced angiography (in different patient) shows radial artery to be dominant. Image was obtained later in scanning sequence. Superficial & deep palmar arches have contributions from both radial & ulnar arteries.

AXIAL T1 & T2 FS MR, ARTERIES & VEINS

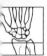

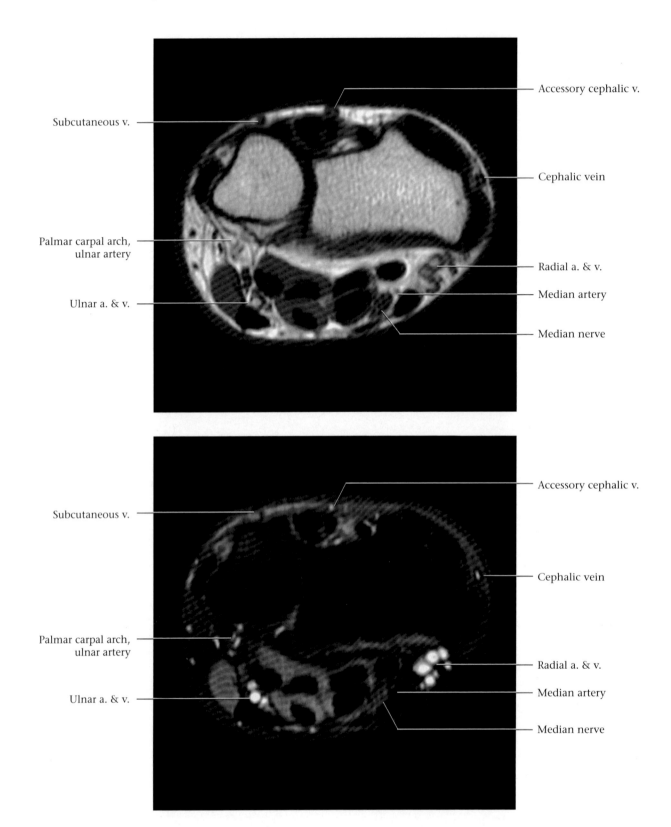

Subcutaneous v.

Accessory cephalic v.

Cephalic vein

Palmar carpal arch, ulnar artery

Radial a. & v.

Median artery

Ulnar a. & v.

Median nerve

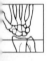

Subcutaneous v.

Accessory cephalic v.

Cephalic vein

Palmar carpal arch, ulnar artery

Radial a. & v.

Median artery

Ulnar a. & v.

Median nerve

(Top) Series of four selected axial T1 MR, paired with T2 FS MR at same level (proximal to distal). At distal radioulnar joint, radial & ulnar arteries are readily apparent with accompanying veins paralleling their course. **(Bottom)** Axial T2 MR at same level with fat-suppression shows multiple small veins strrounding radial & ulnar arteries.

Wrist

III

130

NEUROVASCULAR STRUCTURES

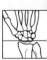

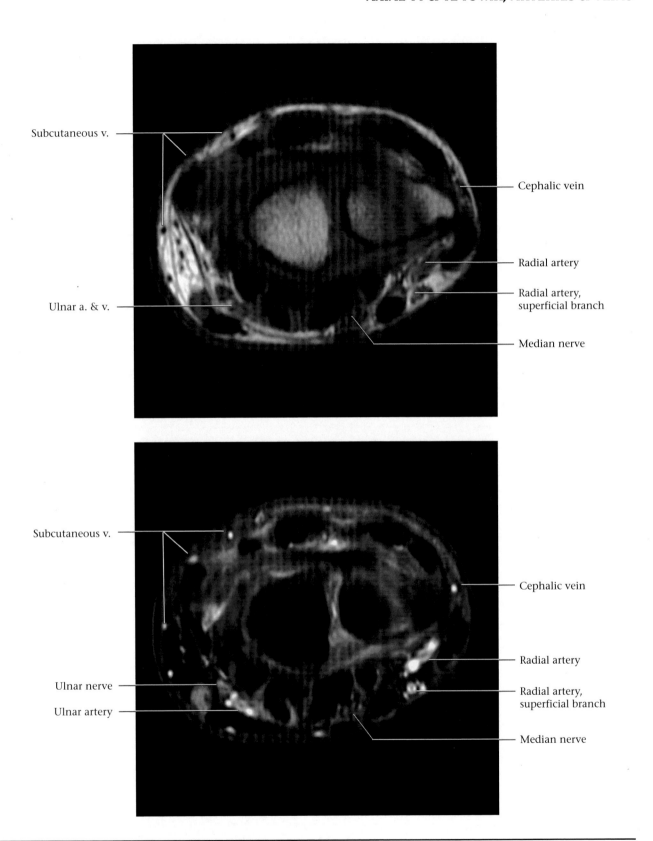

Subcutaneous v.

Cephalic vein

Radial artery

Radial artery, superficial branch

Ulnar a. & v.

Median nerve

Subcutaneous v.

Cephalic vein

Radial artery

Ulnar nerve

Radial artery, superficial branch

Ulnar artery

Median nerve

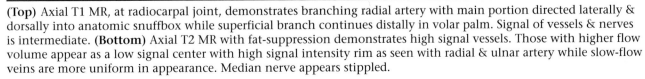

(Top) Axial T1 MR, at radiocarpal joint, demonstrates branching radial artery with main portion directed laterally & dorsally into anatomic snuffbox while superficial branch continues distally in volar palm. Signal of vessels & nerves is intermediate. **(Bottom)** Axial T2 MR with fat-suppression demonstrates high signal vessels. Those with higher flow volume appear as a low signal center with high signal intensity rim as seen with radial & ulnar artery while slow-flow veins are more uniform in appearance. Median nerve appears stippled.

AXIAL T1 & T2 FS MR, ARTERIES & VEINS

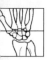

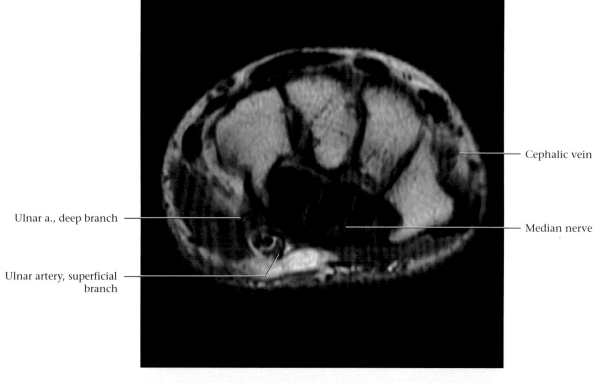

Cephalic vein

Ulnar a., deep branch

Median nerve

Ulnar artery, superficial branch

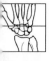

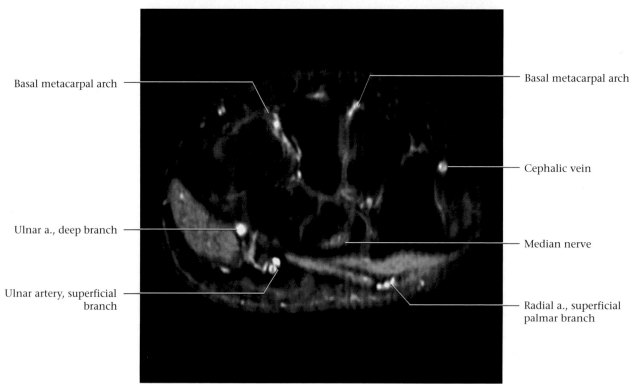

Basal metacarpal arch

Basal metacarpal arch

Cephalic vein

Ulnar a., deep branch

Median nerve

Ulnar artery, superficial branch

Radial a., superficial palmar branch

(Top) Axial T1 MR, at mid carpal tunnel (hook of hamate/trapezial ridge), demonstrates ulnar artery & veins within Guyon canal. Median nerve is deep to flexor retinaculum. (Bottom) Axial T2 MR with fat-suppression reveals ulnar artery has branched with deep branch traveling distally to form deep palmar arch while superficial branch will form superficial palmar arch.

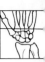

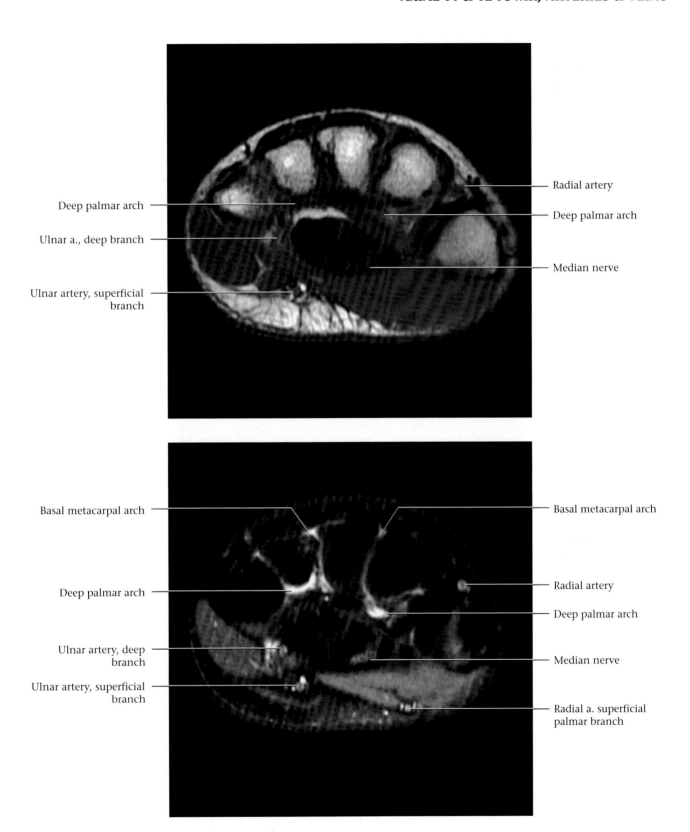

Deep palmar arch

Ulnar a., deep branch

Ulnar artery, superficial branch

Radial artery

Deep palmar arch

Median nerve

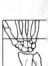

Basal metacarpal arch

Deep palmar arch

Ulnar artery, deep branch

Ulnar artery, superficial branch

Basal metacarpal arch

Radial artery

Deep palmar arch

Median nerve

Radial a. superficial palmar branch

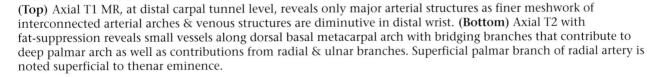

(Top) Axial T1 MR, at distal carpal tunnel level, reveals only major arterial structures as finer meshwork of interconnected arterial arches & venous structures are diminutive in distal wrist. (Bottom) Axial T2 with fat-suppression reveals small vessels along dorsal basal metacarpal arch with bridging branches that contribute to deep palmar arch as well as contributions from radial & ulnar branches. Superficial palmar branch of radial artery is noted superficial to thenar eminence.

Wrist

III

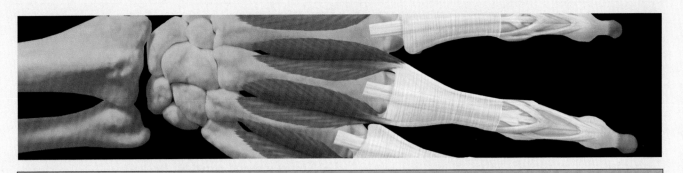

SECTION IV: Hand

HAND OVERVIEW

Terminology

Abbreviations
- Abductor digiti minimi (ADM)
- Abductor pollicis brevis (APB)
- Carpometacarpal (CMC)
- Distal interphalangeal (joint) (DIP)
- Dorsal palmar arch (DPA)
- Extensor digitorum communis (EDC)
- Extensor pollicis longus (EPL)
- Extension, extensor (ext.)
- Flexor digiti minimi (FDM)
- Flexor digitorum profundus (FDP)
- Flexor digitorum superficialis (FDS)
- Flexion, flexor (flex.)
- Flexor pollicis brevis (FPB)
- Flexor pollicis longus (FPL)
- Interosseus membrane (IOM)
- Interphalangeal (joint) (IP)
- Metacarpal (MC)
- Metacarpophalangeal (joint) (MCP)
- Opponens digiti minimi (ODM)
- Opponens pollicis (OP)
- Phalanx (phal.)
- Proximal interphalangeal (joint) (PIP)
- Retinaculum, retinacular (retinac)
- Signal-to-noise ratio (SNR)
- Superficial palmar arch (SPA)
- Volar plate (VP)

Definitions
- For this text, the hand will be defined as beginning at the carpometacarpal joint
- In anatomic position, the hand is in supination
- Radial: Toward radius and synonymous with lateral(ly)
- Ulnar: Toward ulna and synonymous with medial(ly)
- Mesial: Toward midline of structure
  - In the hand, for example, 3rd digit is more mesial than 2nd and 4th digits, which are more mesial than 1st and 5th digits

Osseus Anatomy

Metacarpals
- Comprised of a base, diaphysis, neck and head (from proximal to distal)
- Normal ossification center (epiphysis) is distal (head) for digits 2-5 and proximal (base) for 1st digit
- Bases are trapezoidal in shape (broader dorsally) with concave articular surface
- 1st metacarpal articulates with trapezium
- 2nd-5th metacarpals articulate with trapezoid, capitate, and hamate (both 4th and 5th) respectively, as well as with one another
- Diaphysis is roughly triangular in cross-section with apex volarly: Creating medial and lateral volar surfaces and dorsal surface
- Diaphysis is gently concave volarly (convex dorsally) throughout its proximal to distal course
- Head is relatively spherical with shallow groove volarly and short notches laterally and medially

- Volar groove of head transmits flexor tendons in extension and accommodates VP (especially in flexion)
- Lateral and medial notches are origin of collateral ligament complex

Phalanges
- 3 each (proximal, middle, and distal) for digits 2-5
- 2 (proximal and distal) for 1st digit
- Comprised of base, diaphysis, and head
- Ossification center (epiphysis) is proximal (base)
- Heads are bicondylar volarly with condyles separated by shallow groove
- Groove transmits flexor tendons in extension and accommodates VP (especially in flexion)
- Proximal articular surfaces of proximal phalanges are uniformly concave
- Proximal articular surfaces of middle and distal phalanges are biconcave with a median ridge running anteroposteriorly
- Median ridge tracks in groove between condyles: Helps prevent lateral translation

Muscles of Hand

See "Flexor Mechanism and Palmar Hand" Section for
- Flexor digitorum superficialis, flexor digitorum profundus, flexor pollicis longus, thenars, hypothenars, adductor pollicis, and palmar interossei

See "Extensor Mechanism and Joints" Section for
- Extensor digitorum communis, extensor indicis, extensor digiti minimi, lumbricals, dorsal interossei, extensor pollicis longus, and extensor pollicis brevis

Vessels of Hand
- Both superficial palmar arch and deep palmar arch run from radial artery to ulnar artery
  - Ulnar artery primarily supplies the superficial palmar arch
  - Radial artery primarily supplies the deep palmar arch

Radial Artery: Proximal to Distal
- 1) At radiocarpal joint level gives off contribution to SPA volarly which pierces APB before joining SPA
- 2) Travels superficially (superficial to EPL and ext. retinac.) around radial aspect of wrist to travel dorsally in anatomic snuffbox
- 3) Distal to snuffbox, gives off branch which splits into princeps pollicis and radialis indicis arteries
- 4) Dives deep in interspace between 1st and 2nd metacarpals
- 5) Travels between heads of 1st dorsal interosseus and adductor pollicis muscles before forming DPA
- 6) DPA runs between flexor tendons and metacarpals

Ulnar Artery: Proximal to Distal
- 1) Runs superficial to flexor retinaculum

- 2) Passes radial to pisiform
- 3) Gives off deep branch to DPA just proximal to hook of hamate which runs between ADM and FDM
- 4) Forms SPA which runs between palmar aponeurosis and flexor tendons
- 5) Arterial supply to lateral aspect 5th digit usually entirely from ulnar artery

Common Palmar Digital Arteries

- Between metacarpal necks and heads in 2nd, 3rd, and 4th interspaces
- Variably supplied by SPA and DPA

Proper Digital Arteries

- Arise at MCP joint level
- Run in subcutaneous fat along lateral aspects of digits

Nerves of Hand

Median Nerve

- Travels in carpal tunnel
- After exiting carpal tunnel, gives off recurrent branch (motor supply to thenars)
- In hand, motor to thenars (OP, APB, and FPB) as well as 1st and 2nd lumbricals
- Sensory
  ○ Palmar surface: Radial ½ of palm, digits 1-3 and radial ½ 4th digit
  ○ Dorsal surface: Just distal to PIP to fingertip digits 1-3 and radial ½ of 4th

Ulnar Nerve

- In hand, motor to hypothenars (ODM, ADM, and FDM), all interossei, 3rd and 4th lumbricals, and adductor pollicis
- Sensory
  ○ From radiocarpal joint to fingertips of 5th and ulnar ½ of 4th digits: Both volarly and dorsally

Radial Nerve

- **Not usually seen on routine imaging**
- No motor innervation in hand
- Sensory
  ○ Dorsal surface from radiocarpal joint to just distal to PIP joints for digits 1-3 and radial ½ of 4th digit

Imaging Modalities

Radiographs

- **Generally the first modality in all instances**
- Standard views
  ○ PA and lateral often sufficient
  ○ Obliques may help by decreasing superimposition of digits
  ○ Ball-catcher's view useful for evaluation of erosions (arthritis)

MR

- Most useful for evaluation of soft tissue injuries, masses, marrow abnormalities (including evaluation of occult fractures), synovitis, and infectious processes
- High SNR required when evaluating small structures within a small structure (the hand)

○ High field strength magnet
  ■ At least 1.5 Tesla generally recommended
  ■ Increasing magnet strength = improved SNR
○ Small field of view
○ Minimize motion by maximizing patient comfort and minimizing scan times
○ Centering hand within magnet bore improves SNR
  ■ Patient prone or supine with arm over head: This is often less comfortable than arm at side and may result in more motion
  ■ Can also be done with patient supine and hand over abdomen if hand is supported on platform separate from patient: Prevents respiratory motion
- Coils
  ○ Circumferential coils are generally preferred
    ■ Dedicated combined hand and wrist coils available
    ■ Dedicated wrist coils generally will not accommodate entire hand, but area of interest can be placed in center
    ■ Knee coils can be used if nothing else available: Place hand on folded towels to center in coil
    ■ Dedicated finger coils exist
  ○ Surface coils
    ■ Poorer fat-saturation than circumferential coils
    ■ Lose signal as distance from surface coil increases
    ■ Place area of interest on surface (i.e., do not put palm down to image extensor tendons)
- Best plane for imaging
  ○ Flexor tendons: Axial and sagittal
  ○ Extensor tendons: Axial and sagittal
  ○ Tendon sheaths: Axial > sagittal
  ○ Musculature: Axial > coronal and sagittal
  ○ Pulleys: Axial > sagittal
  ○ Collateral ligaments: Coronal and axial
  ○ Volar plate: Sagittal > axial

Ultrasound

- Highly operator dependent
  ○ For this reason (as well as lack of reader experience and comfort), not routinely used for MSK imaging in the United States
    ■ Most common exception would be imaging of suspected ganglion
    ■ Can be useful for evaluation of tendons in those with contraindication to MR
- Linear, high frequency (at least 8 MHz) transducer needed for MSK imaging
  ○ At least 12 MHz transducer should be used as depth of penetration needed is usually ≤ 1 cm

CT

- Not routinely used
  ○ Can be useful for evaluating complex fractures, evaluating neoplasms for evidence of subtle osseous or chondroid matrix, or evaluation of suspected osteoid osteoma

Angiography

- Generally done for evaluation of suspected embolization, arterial injury, vasculitis, and surgical planning

○ Conventional angiography gives best resolution, ability to tailor exam real-time, and possibility of intervention

○ MR angiography can be done when conventional angio is unavailable or contraindicated

Nuclear Medicine

- Rarely used for suspicion of osteomyelitis, reflex sympathetic dystrophy, occult fracture, surgical planning (e.g., viability evaluation in frostbite), and (very) rare osteoid osteoma of tubular bones of the hand

Imaging Pitfalls

- Magic angle phenomenon
  - Seen with short TE sequences (predominately T1, proton density, and some gradient echo sequences)
  - Occurs when structures composed of parallel fibers (almost exclusively tendons) are oriented at 55° to main magnetic vector
  - **Lack of increased signal in same location on long TE (usually T2 or STIR) sequences confirms magic angle**
  - Most likely to be seen in flexor tendons on sagittal views (when imaged in flexion) and in tendons of 1st digit in coronal plane
- When hand is imaged (with MR) with fingers in flexion, the lumbricals can be pulled into the carpal tunnel
  - Not to be mistaken for a mass or proximal origin of lumbricals (a normal variant)
- Inhomogeneous fat-saturation
  - Can be mistaken for pathologic high signal
  - More likely to be seen when
    - Coil not in center of magnet
    - Field of view is smaller
    - Coil not circumferential
- **A small amount of fluid is normal in tendon sheaths**
  - When fluid becomes circumferential about a tendon, it is usually pathologic
- Collateral ligament complex of MCP joints are often intermediate signal and heterogeneous on MR
  - Do not mistake for pathology: Compare to other collateral ligaments and evaluate continuity
- Anisotropy
  - Ultrasound artifact that occurs in structures composed of parallel fibers
    - Tendons > ligaments and muscles
  - When angle of incidence of ultrasound beam is not at or near 90° (with respect to parallel fibers), echogenicity may change
  - Hypoechoic defects are pathologic only if they persist without change regardless of changing orientation of transducer

Normal Variants

Osseous

- Accessory ossification center at base of MCs 2-5 or distal aspect of 1st MC

○ Normal ossification centers are reverse of above, i.e., distal aspects of MCs 2-5 and base of 1st MC

○ Occasionally mistaken for fracture

- Especially when small cleft remains at lateral aspects of physeal line 2° to incomplete fusion

- Small round or oval notches at lateral bases of proximal phalanges
  - May be mistaken for erosions; however, **erosions typically involve MC heads first**
- Sesamoids
  - Up to 2 sesamoids can be present at each MCP joint and at 3rd DIP joint
  - 1 sesamoid can be present at each DIP joint
  - Sesamoids are usually embedded in VP
  - No documentation of sesamoids occurring at PIP joints
- Accessory ossification centers of epiphyses at bases of phalanges
  - May be mistaken for fractures, especially when small and lateral
- Trapezium secundarium
  - Accessory ossification center at ulnar aspect of 1st CMC joint
  - May be mistaken for an avulsion fracture, especially when small
- Triphalangeal thumb
- Bifid distal phalanx

Muscular

- May be mistaken for neoplasm or other pathology
- **Follow muscle signal on all imaging sequences**
- Not uncommon: Prevalence in normal population given in parentheses where known
  - Accessory abductor digiti minimi (24%)
    - Muscle located palmar and lateral (radial) to pisiform is diagnostic
  - Proximal origin of lumbricals (22%)
    - Lumbricals in carpal tunnel **when fingers are extended** is diagnostic
    - Lumbricals may normally migrate proximally into carpal tunnel when fingers are flexed
  - Extensor digitorum manus brevis (1-3%)
    - Muscle belly associated with EDC tendons distal to CMC joint is diagnostic
  - Palmaris longus variants
    - Normal muscle belly should be only in the proximal half of the forearm, and the tendon inserts on/in the palmar aponeurosis
    - Variants may have a distal muscle belly, digastric muscle bellies, or muscle along almost entirety of the expected course of the tendon
    - Muscle tissue in the midline superficial to the flexor retinaculum at the level of the carpus is diagnostic
    - Not to be confused with the Palmaris brevis (normal structure) which is ulnar (not midline) and more distal (level of CMC joint)
  - Digastric flexor digitorum superficialis of 2nd digit
    - A second muscle belly is present in the mid-portion of the FDS tendon to the 2nd digit at mid-metacarpal level

3D CT RECONSTRUCTION, TENDON INJURY ZONES

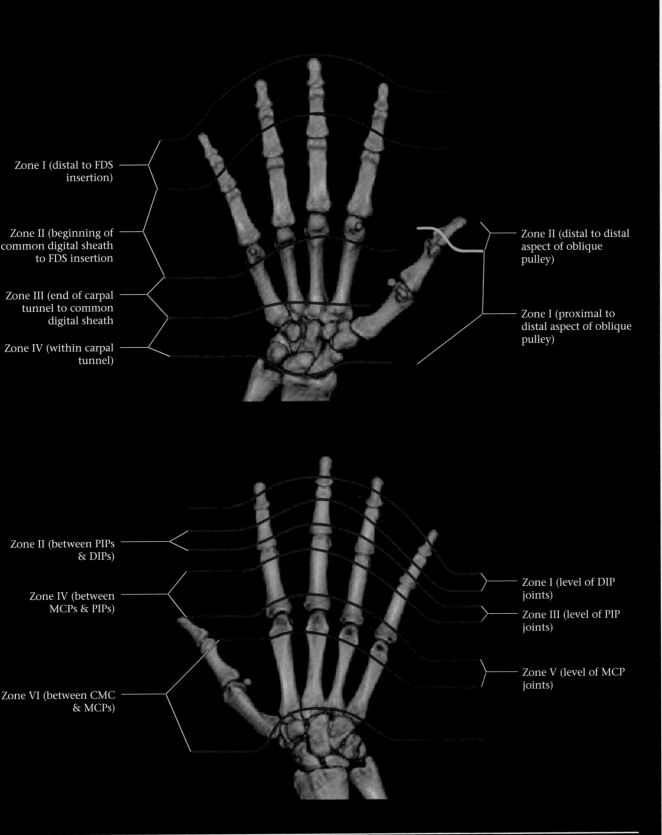

Zone I (distal to FDS insertion)

Zone II (beginning of common digital sheath to FDS insertion

Zone III (end of carpal tunnel to common digital sheath

Zone IV (within carpal tunnel)

Zone II (distal to distal aspect of oblique pulley)

Zone I (proximal to distal aspect of oblique pulley)

Zone II (between PIPs & DIPs)

Zone IV (between MCPs & PIPs)

Zone VI (between CMC & MCPs)

Zone I (level of DIP joints)

Zone III (level of PIP joints)

Zone V (level of MCP joints)

(Top) A modification of Verdan original tendon injury zones is now utilized for flexor tendon injuries. Establishing the zone of injury can be useful for the hand surgeon. Additional useful information includes: 1) Complete vs. incomplete disruption (when incomplete, the transverse width of the tendon disruption should be estimated). 2) When complete disruption is encountered, the level to which the tendon ends are retracted, and the distance between the tendon ends should be given. Injury zones for the thumb are not widely accepted. The most referenced zoning system for the thumb is illustrated. **(Bottom)** Verdan extensor injury zones. When extensor mechanism injury is encountered, information for the flexor injury zones should be given. No established zone classification for the thumb exists.

HAND OVERVIEW

3D CT RECONSTRUCTION, VOLAR ORIGINS AND INSERTIONS

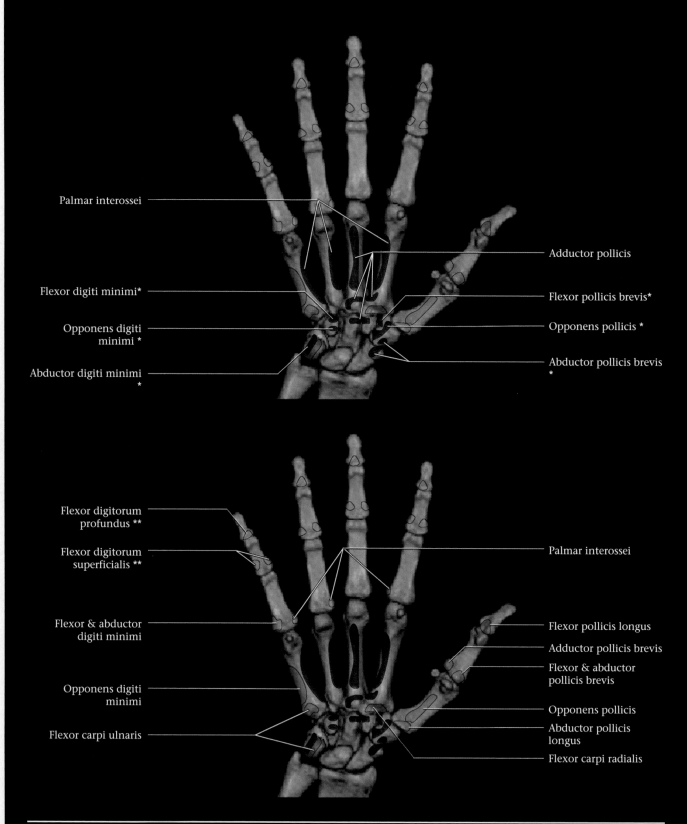

Palmar interossei

Flexor digiti minimi*

Opponens digiti minimi *

Abductor digiti minimi *

Adductor pollicis

Flexor pollicis brevis*

Opponens pollicis *

Abductor pollicis brevis *

Flexor digitorum profundus **

Flexor digitorum superficialis **

Flexor & abductor digiti minimi

Opponens digiti minimi

Flexor carpi ulnaris

Palmar interossei

Flexor pollicis longus

Adductor pollicis brevis

Flexor & abductor pollicis brevis

Opponens pollicis

Abductor pollicis longus

Flexor carpi radialis

(Top) Volar surface origins (red). * Indicates that in addition to bony origin as illustrated, muscle also arises from the flexor retinaculum. **(Bottom)** Volar surface insertions (blue). ** Indicates pattern is repeated on digits 2-5 despite lack of labels on image.

Hand

IV

6

3D CT RECONSTRUCTION, DORSAL ORIGINS AND INSERTIONS

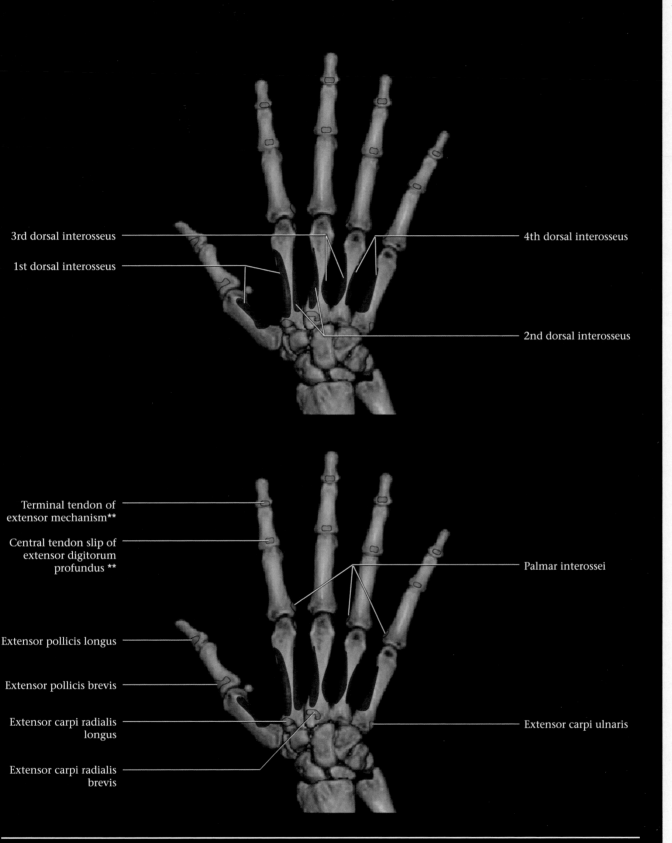

3rd dorsal interosseus

1st dorsal interosseus

4th dorsal interosseus

2nd dorsal interosseus

Terminal tendon of extensor mechanism**

Central tendon slip of extensor digitorum profundus **

Palmar interossei

Extensor pollicis longus

Extensor pollicis brevis

Extensor carpi radialis longus

Extensor carpi ulnaris

Extensor carpi radialis brevis

(Top) Dorsal surface origins (red). **(Bottom)** Dorsal surface insertions (blue). ** Indicates pattern is repeated on digits 2-5 despite lack of labels on image.

RADIOGRAPH, POSTEROANTERIOR

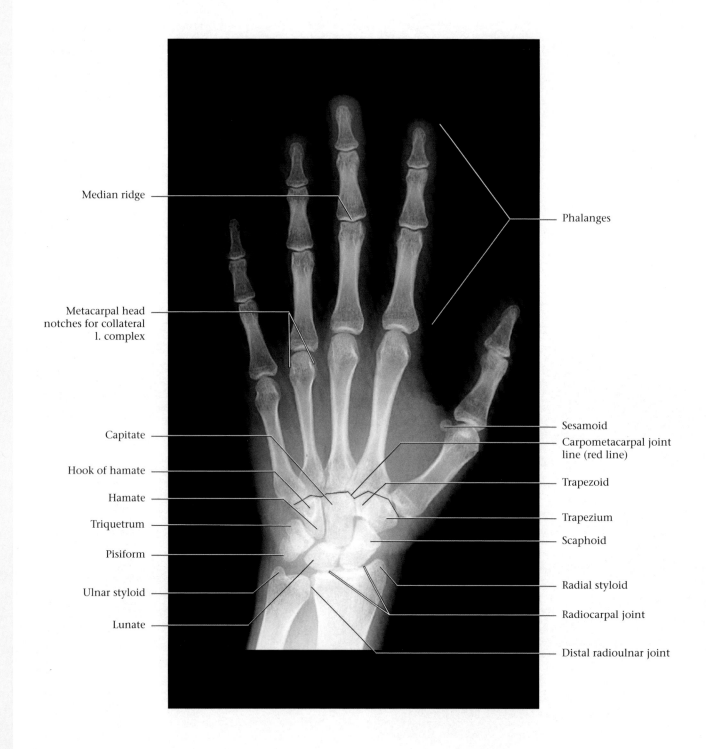

Median ridge

Metacarpal head notches for collateral l. complex

Capitate

Hook of hamate

Hamate

Triquetrum

Pisiform

Ulnar styloid

Lunate

Phalanges

Sesamoid

Carpometacarpal joint line (red line)

Trapezoid

Trapezium

Scaphoid

Radial styloid

Radiocarpal joint

Distal radioulnar joint

The dorsolateral grooves of the metacarpal heads (indicated on the fourth digit here) are the sites of origin for the collateral ligament complexes of the MCP joints. They are routinely seen on radiographs and should not be mistaken for pathology. On a PA radiograph of the hand, one should be able to trace the carpometacarpal joint (as indicated by the red line) as a continuous up and down "zig-zag". Inability to do so should raise the suspicion of a dislocation.

HAND OVERVIEW

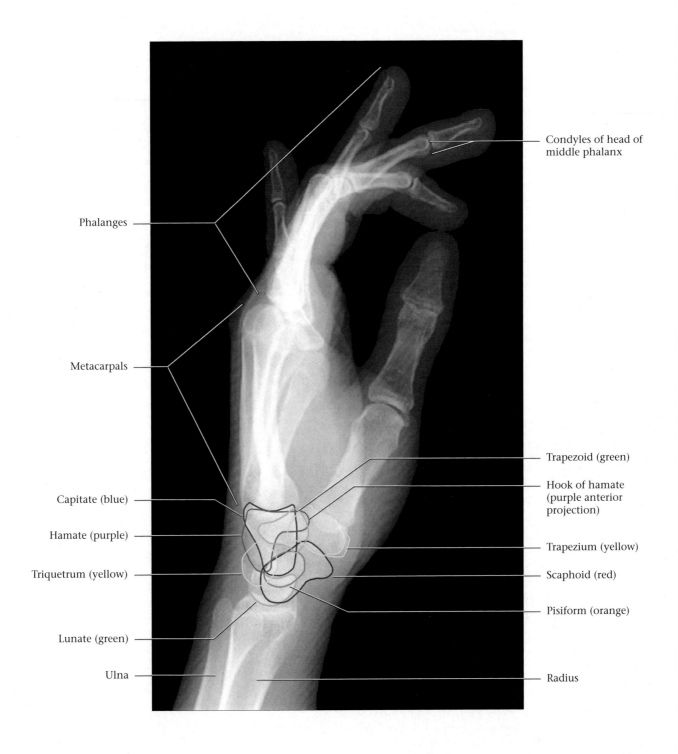

Phalanges

Metacarpals

Capitate (blue)

Hamate (purple)

Triquetrum (yellow)

Lunate (green)

Ulna

Condyles of head of middle phalanx

Trapezoid (green)

Hook of hamate (purple anterior projection)

Trapezium (yellow)

Scaphoid (red)

Pisiform (orange)

Radius

Lateral radiograph of the hand with carpal bones outlined. There should always be a coaxial (though not necessarily parallel) relationship between the radius, lunate, capitate, and 3rd metacarpal.

GRAPHIC, DORSAL INTEROSSEI

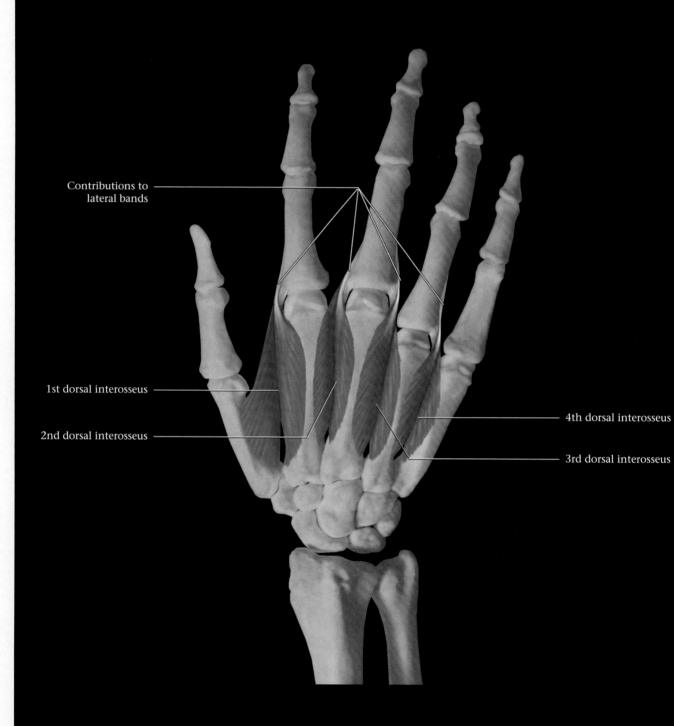

Contributions to
lateral bands

1st dorsal interosseus

2nd dorsal interosseus

4th dorsal interosseus

3rd dorsal interosseus

The tendons of the dorsal interossei (along with the tendons of the palmar interossei and tendons of the lumbricals) help form the lateral bands. Note how each interosseus only contributes fibers to the mesial-most adjacent lateral band. The dorsal interossei do not contribute any lateral band fibers to the 1st or 5th digits.

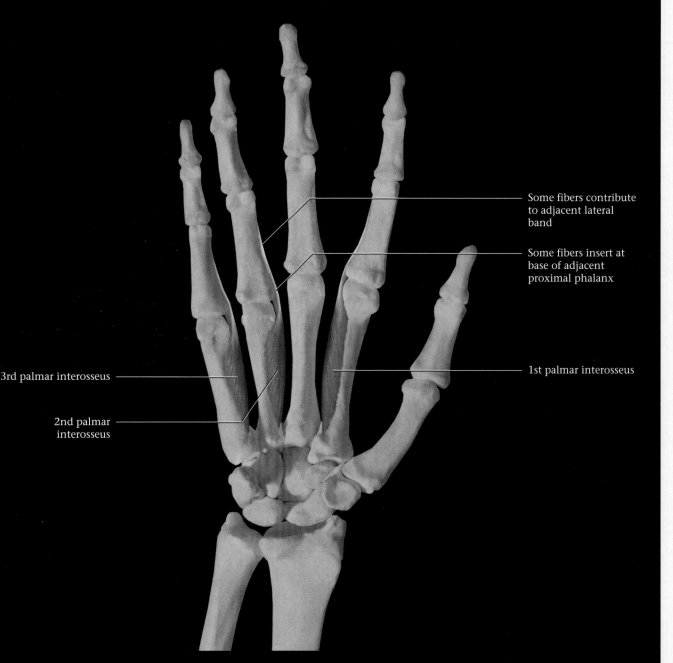

3rd palmar interosseus

2nd palmar interosseus

Some fibers contribute to adjacent lateral band

Some fibers insert at base of adjacent proximal phalanx

1st palmar interosseus

The palmar interossei insert at both the bases of the adjacent proximal phalanges as well as the adjacent lateral bands. The 2nd and 3rd palmar interossei contribute to the radial lateral bands of the 4th and 5th digits respectively, whereas the 1st palmar interosseus contributes to the ulnar lateral band of the 2nd digit.

HAND OVERVIEW

GRAPHICS, THENARS AND HYPOTHENARS: DEEP TO SUPERFICIAL

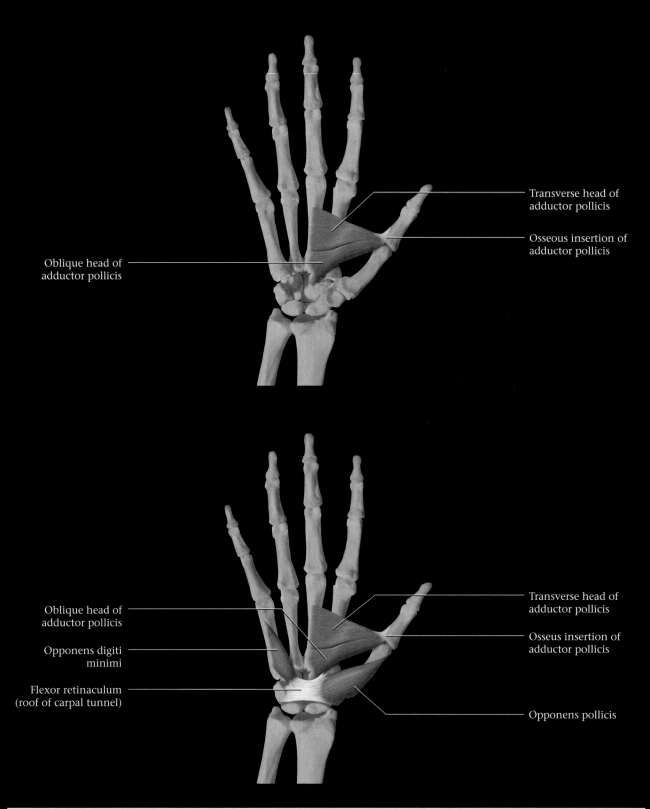

Transverse head of adductor pollicis

Osseous insertion of adductor pollicis

Oblique head of adductor pollicis

Oblique head of adductor pollicis

Opponens digiti minimi

Flexor retinaculum (roof of carpal tunnel)

Transverse head of adductor pollicis

Osseus insertion of adductor pollicis

Opponens pollicis

(Top) Although technically not one of the thenar muscles, the adductor pollicis is often grouped with them due to proximity. The osseus insertion is as shown in the graphic. The adductor pollicis also inserts on the volar plate and the extensor hood of the thumb. The contribution of the adductor pollicis to the extensor hood of the 1st digit cannot be seen here as it is dorsal and lateral to the MCP joint in this projection. The radial artery passes between the two heads of the adductor pollicis from dorsal to volar before forming the deep palmar arch. **(Bottom)** The two opponens (pollicis and digiti minimi) muscles have been added. Note that in addition to their osseous origins, these muscles also arise from the flexor retinaculum (which is the roof of the carpal tunnel).

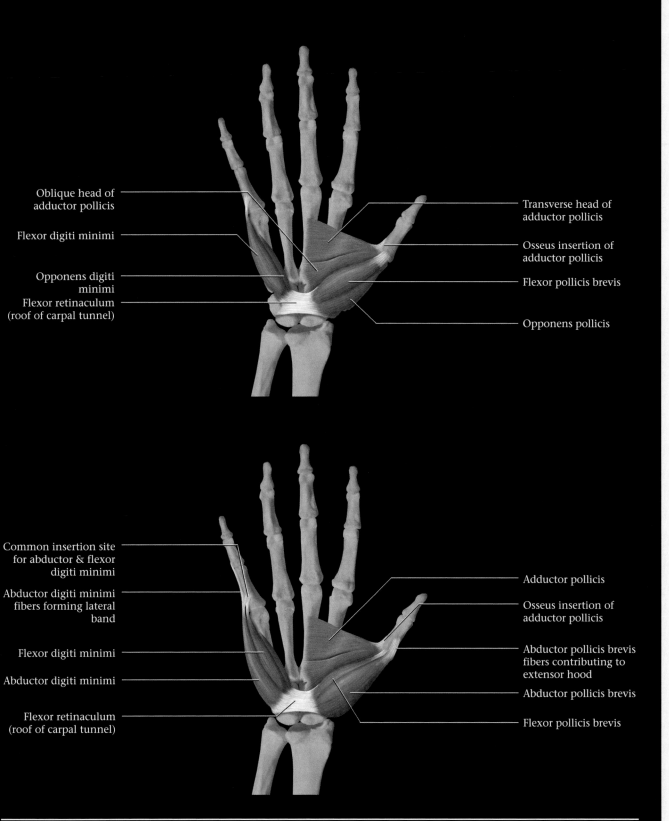

Oblique head of adductor pollicis

Flexor digiti minimi

Opponens digiti minimi

Flexor retinaculum (roof of carpal tunnel)

Transverse head of adductor pollicis

Osseus insertion of adductor pollicis

Flexor pollicis brevis

Opponens pollicis

Common insertion site for abductor & flexor digiti minimi

Abductor digiti minimi fibers forming lateral band

Flexor digiti minimi

Abductor digiti minimi

Flexor retinaculum (roof of carpal tunnel)

Adductor pollicis

Osseus insertion of adductor pollicis

Abductor pollicis brevis fibers contributing to extensor hood

Abductor pollicis brevis

Flexor pollicis brevis

(Top) In this graphic, the two flexor (pollicis brevis and digiti minimi) muscles have been added. As before, they originate from the flexor retinaculum as well as from their osseous origins. **(Bottom)** In this graphic, the abductor (pollicis brevis and digiti minimi) muscles have been added. Note that the abductor digiti minimi shares a combined osseus insertion at the base of the 5th proximal phalanx with the flexor digiti minimi. In addition, it gives off fibers to form the ulnar lateral band for the 5th digit. Similarly, the abductor pollicis brevis shares an osseus insertion with the flexor pollicis brevis as well as contributing fibers to the extensor hood of the 1st digit.

GRAPHICS, LUMBRICAL MUSCLES AND NERVES

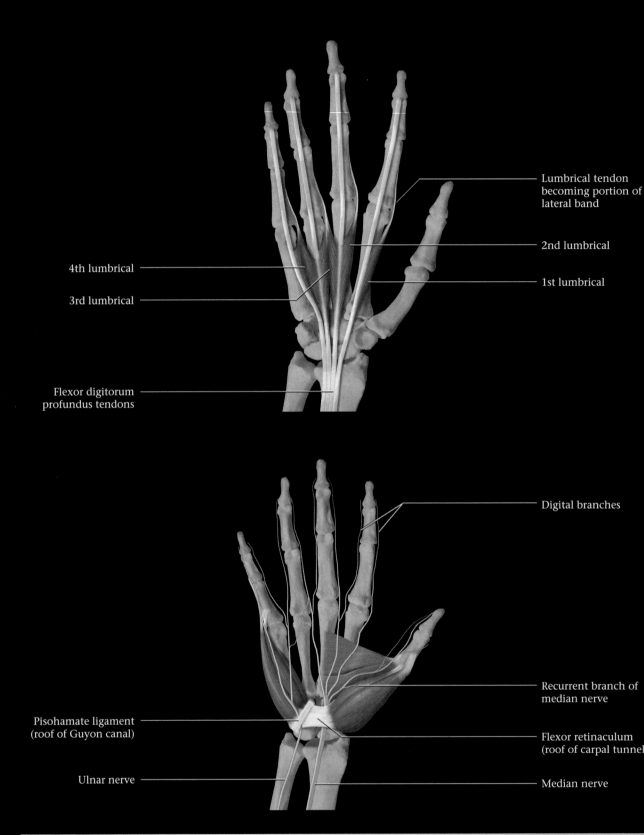

Lumbrical tendon becoming portion of lateral band

2nd lumbrical

1st lumbrical

4th lumbrical

3rd lumbrical

Flexor digitorum profundus tendons

Digital branches

Recurrent branch of median nerve

Pisohamate ligament (roof of Guyon canal)

Flexor retinaculum (roof of carpal tunnel

Ulnar nerve

Median nerve

(Top) The lumbricals originate from the flexor digitorum profundus tendons as shown. Note how the 1st and 2nd lumbricals arise only from the tendons to the 2nd and 3rd digits respectively (unipennate), whereas the 3rd and 4th lumbrical arise from the tendons to both the 3rd & 4th and the 4th & 5th digits respectively (bipennate). **(Bottom)** The median nerve travels deep to the flexor retinaculum (within the carpal tunnel). The ulnar nerve travels superficial to the flexor retinaculum and deep to the pisohamate ligament (within Guyon canal). Both are prone to compression syndromes within these fibroosseous tunnels. Motor supply of the median nerve is to the thenars (via the recurrent branch) and the 1st & 2nd lumbricals. Ulnar nerve motor supply is to all the intrinsic muscles of the hand not supplied by the median nerve. Muscle atrophy should prompt an evaluation of the supplying nerve.

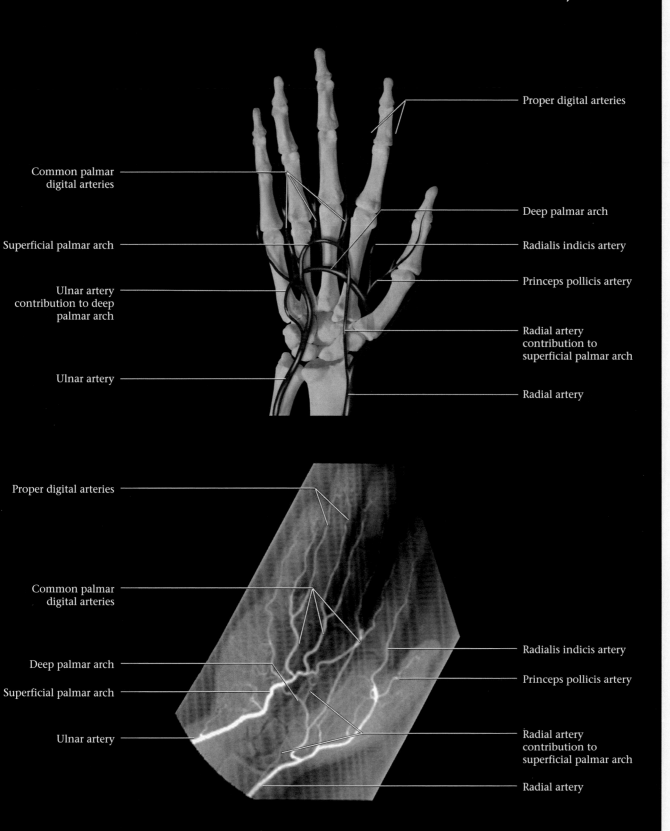

Proper digital arteries

Common palmar digital arteries

Deep palmar arch

Superficial palmar arch

Radialis indicis artery

Princeps pollicis artery

Ulnar artery contribution to deep palmar arch

Radial artery contribution to superficial palmar arch

Ulnar artery

Radial artery

Proper digital arteries

Common palmar digital arteries

Deep palmar arch

Superficial palmar arch

Radialis indicis artery

Princeps pollicis artery

Ulnar artery

Radial artery contribution to superficial palmar arch

Radial artery

(Top) After giving off its contribution to the superficial palmar arch, the radial artery travels around the radial aspect of the wrist to the dorsum of the hand where it travels in the anatomic snuffbox. It then dives into the 1st interspace between the heads of the 1st dorsal interosseus as well as ovetween the transverse and oblique heads of the adductor pollicis before forming the deep palmar arch. **(Bottom)** Conventional angiogram of the arteries of the hand. Digital subtraction was not utilized in this case so that the relationship of the arteries to the underlying bony architecture could be demonstrated.

AXIAL T1 MR, LEFT HAND

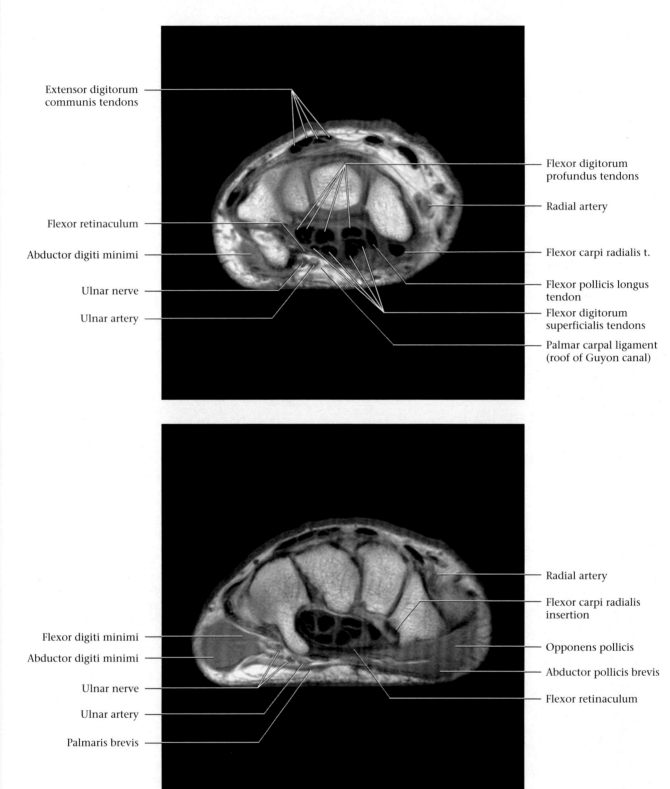

Extensor digitorum communis tendons

Flexor digitorum profundus tendons

Radial artery

Flexor retinaculum

Abductor digiti minimi

Flexor carpi radialis t.

Ulnar nerve

Flexor pollicis longus tendon

Ulnar artery

Flexor digitorum superficialis tendons

Palmar carpal ligament (roof of Guyon canal)

Flexor digiti minimi

Abductor digiti minimi

Radial artery

Flexor carpi radialis insertion

Opponens pollicis

Ulnar nerve

Abductor pollicis brevis

Ulnar artery

Flexor retinaculum

Palmaris brevis

(Top) First in series of axial T1 MR images of the left hand. Note the ulnar artery and nerve in Guyon canal. Also note the ghosting (pulsation) artifact from the radial artery at the radial aspect of the dorsal wrist. This artifact can occasionally help locate the normal vascular structures. **(Bottom)** Axial MR image of the left hand at the level of hook of hamate. Note the thenar muscles originating from the flexor retinaculum. At the level of the hook of the hamate, the ulnar artery generally passes anterior or anteromedial to the hook, whereas the ulnar nerve and its branches generally pass lateral to the hook.

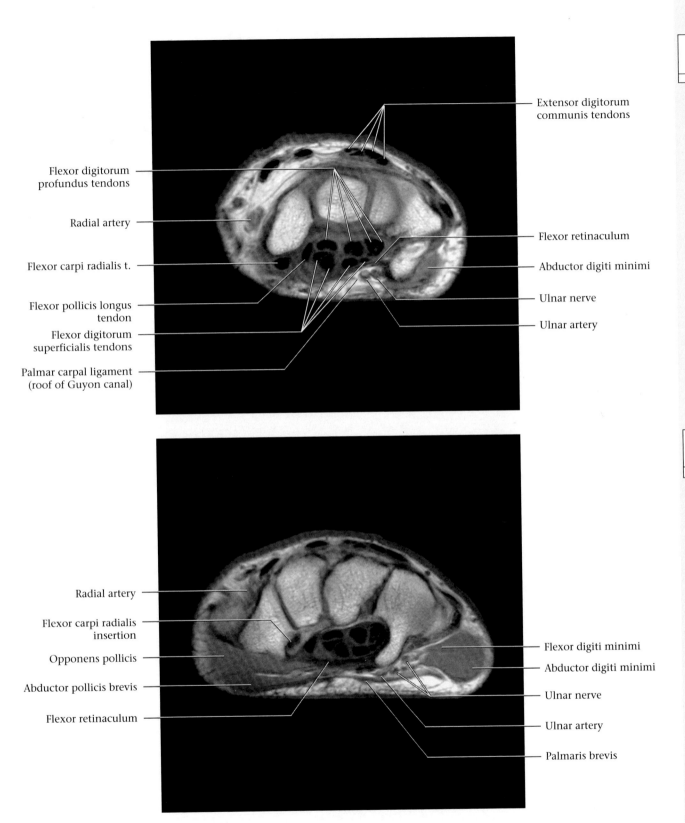

Extensor digitorum communis tendons

Flexor digitorum profundus tendons

Radial artery

Flexor carpi radialis t.

Flexor pollicis longus tendon

Flexor digitorum superficialis tendons

Palmar carpal ligament (roof of Guyon canal)

Flexor retinaculum

Abductor digiti minimi

Ulnar nerve

Ulnar artery

Radial artery

Flexor carpi radialis insertion

Opponens pollicis

Abductor pollicis brevis

Flexor retinaculum

Flexor digiti minimi

Abductor digiti minimi

Ulnar nerve

Ulnar artery

Palmaris brevis

(Top) First in series of axial T1 MR images of the right hand. Note the ulnar artery and nerve in Guyon canal. Also note the ghosting (pulsation) artifact from the radial artery at the radial aspect of the dorsal wrist. This artifact can occasionally help locate the normal vascular structures. **(Bottom)** Axial MR image of the right hand at the level of hook of hamate. Note the thenar muscles originating from the flexor retinaculum. At the level of the hook of the hamate, the ulnar artery generally passes anterior or anteromedial to the hook, whereas the ulnar nerve and its branches generally pass lateral to the hook.

AXIAL T1 MR, LEFT HAND

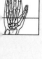

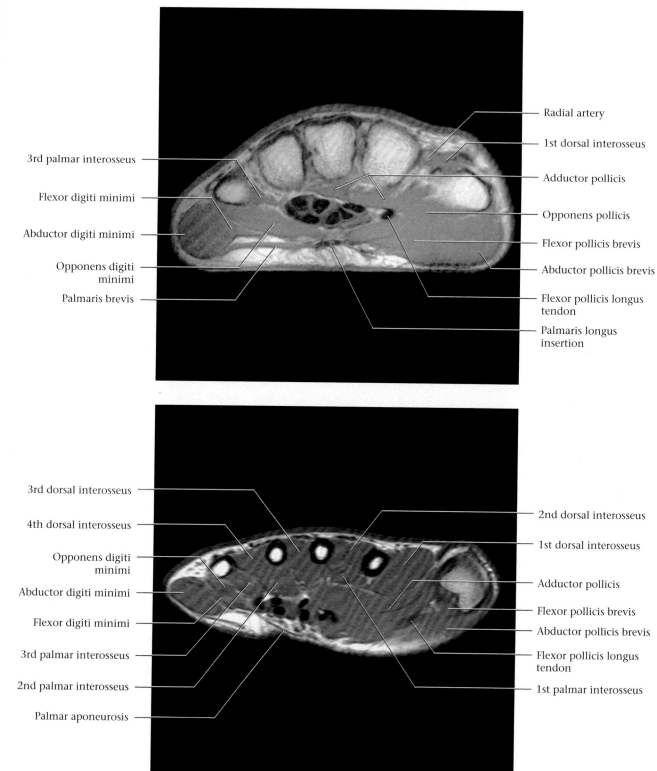

Top image labels:

3rd palmar interosseus

Flexor digiti minimi

Abductor digiti minimi

Opponens digiti minimi

Palmaris brevis

Radial artery

1st dorsal interosseus

Adductor pollicis

Opponens pollicis

Flexor pollicis brevis

Abductor pollicis brevis

Flexor pollicis longus tendon

Palmaris longus insertion

Bottom image labels:

3rd dorsal interosseus

4th dorsal interosseus

Opponens digiti minimi

Abductor digiti minimi

Flexor digiti minimi

3rd palmar interosseus

2nd palmar interosseus

Palmar aponeurosis

2nd dorsal interosseus

1st dorsal interosseus

Adductor pollicis

Flexor pollicis brevis

Abductor pollicis brevis

Flexor pollicis longus tendon

1st palmar interosseus

(Top) Axial T1 MR image of the left hand through the level of the metacarpal heads. The palmaris longus inserts onto the palmar aponeurosis (a fascial layer superficial to the flexor retinaculum) and can be identified as a midline thickening of the palmar aponeurosis. It is a relatively insignificant muscle, and as such, its long tendon is often sacrificed for tendon repairs at other sites. **(Bottom)** Axial T1 MR image of the left hand through the mid-metacarpals. At this level, we are beyond the carpal tunnel, and as such, the muscle intensity foci adjacent to the flexor tendons (although not labeled on this image) are the beginnings of the lumbrical muscles.

HAND OVERVIEW

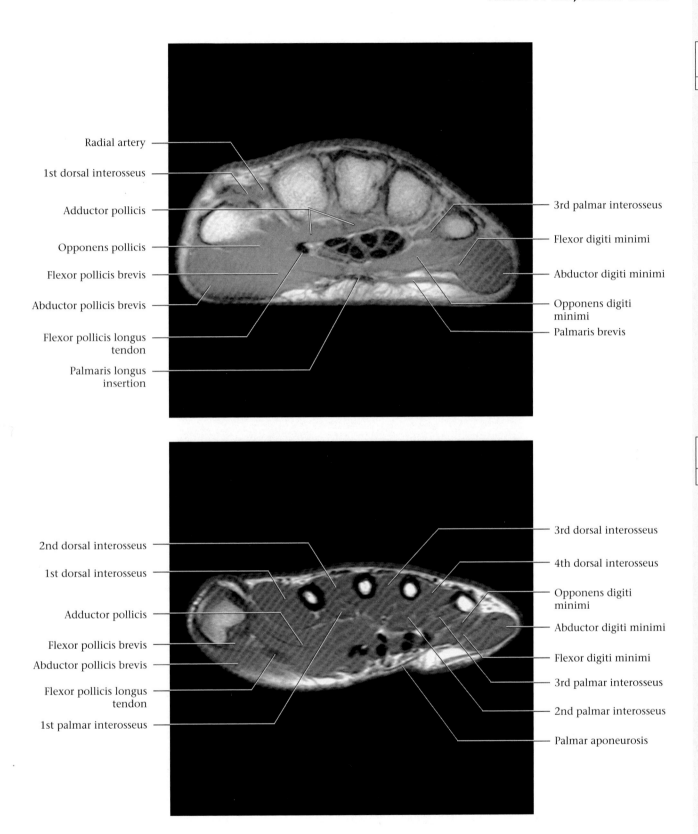

Radial artery

1st dorsal interosseus

Adductor pollicis

Opponens pollicis

Flexor pollicis brevis

Abductor pollicis brevis

Flexor pollicis longus tendon

Palmaris longus insertion

3rd palmar interosseus

Flexor digiti minimi

Abductor digiti minimi

Opponens digiti minimi

Palmaris brevis

2nd dorsal interosseus

1st dorsal interosseus

Adductor pollicis

Flexor pollicis brevis

Abductor pollicis brevis

Flexor pollicis longus tendon

1st palmar interosseus

3rd dorsal interosseus

4th dorsal interosseus

Opponens digiti minimi

Abductor digiti minimi

Flexor digiti minimi

3rd palmar interosseus

2nd palmar interosseus

Palmar aponeurosis

(Top) Axial T1 MR image of the right hand through the level of the metacarpal heads. The palmaris longus inserts onto the palmar aponeurosis (a fascial layer superficial to the flexor retinaculum) and can be identified as a midline thickening of the palmar aponeurosis. It is a relatively insignificant muscle, and as such, its long tendon is often sacrificed for tendon repairs at other sites. **(Bottom)** Axial T1 MR image of the right hand through the level of the mid-metacarpals. At this level, we are beyond the carpal tunnel, and as such, the muscle intensity foci adjacent to the flexor tendons (although not labeled on this image) are the beginnings of the lumbrical muscles.

Hand

IV

19

AXIAL T1 MR, LEFT HAND

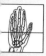

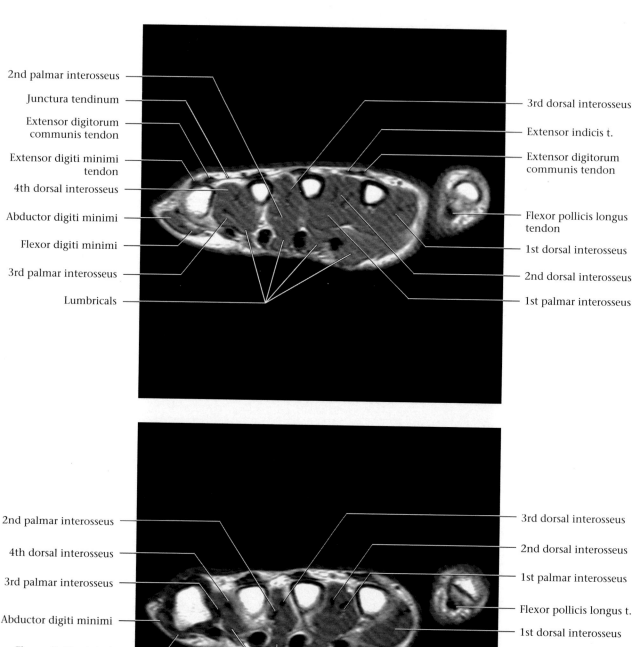

2nd palmar interosseus

Junctura tendinum

Extensor digitorum communis tendon

Extensor digiti minimi tendon

4th dorsal interosseus

Abductor digiti minimi

Flexor digiti minimi

3rd palmar interosseus

Lumbricals

3rd dorsal interosseus

Extensor indicis t.

Extensor digitorum communis tendon

Flexor pollicis longus tendon

1st dorsal interosseus

2nd dorsal interosseus

1st palmar interosseus

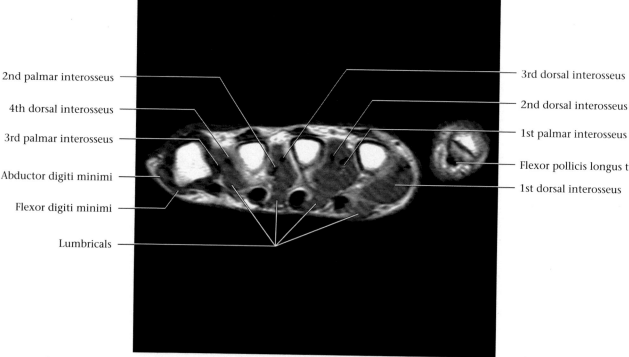

2nd palmar interosseus

4th dorsal interosseus

3rd palmar interosseus

Abductor digiti minimi

Flexor digiti minimi

Lumbricals

3rd dorsal interosseus

2nd dorsal interosseus

1st palmar interosseus

Flexor pollicis longus t.

1st dorsal interosseus

(Top) Axial T1 MR image of the left hand through the distal metacarpal diaphyses. The juncturae tendinum are fibrous bands which interconnect the extensor tendons of digits 2-5 just proximal to the MCP joints. These fibrous bands help prevent lateral translation of the extensor tendons over the metacarpals. Because of these interconnections, digital extension can be relatively preserved in the face of a complete transection of a single extensor digitorum communis tendon proximal to the juncturae, and such an injury may not be evident clinically. **(Bottom)** Axial T1 MR image of the left hand through the metacarpal heads.

HAND OVERVIEW

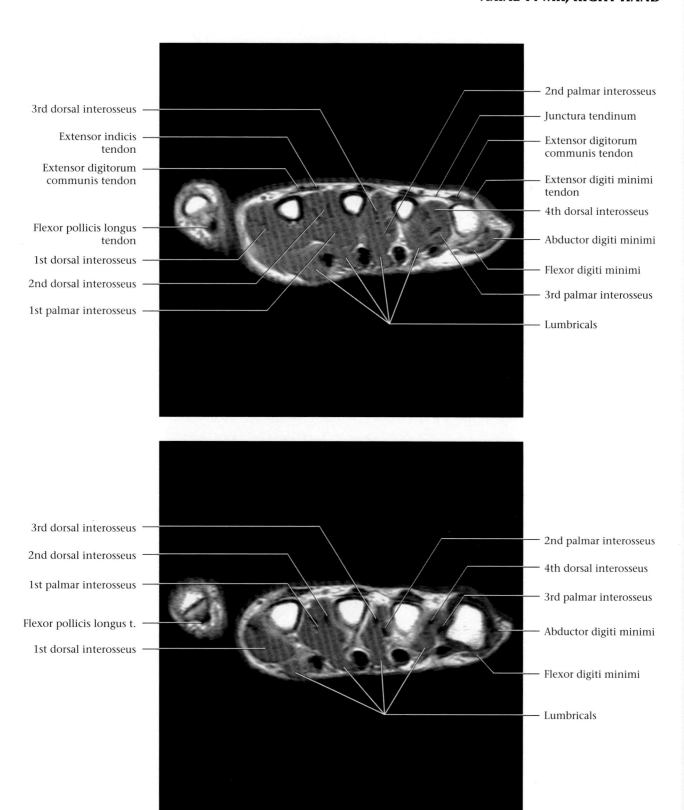

3rd dorsal interosseus

Extensor indicis tendon

Extensor digitorum communis tendon

Flexor pollicis longus tendon

1st dorsal interosseus

2nd dorsal interosseus

1st palmar interosseus

2nd palmar interosseus

Junctura tendinum

Extensor digitorum communis tendon

Extensor digiti minimi tendon

4th dorsal interosseus

Abductor digiti minimi

Flexor digiti minimi

3rd palmar interosseus

Lumbricals

3rd dorsal interosseus

2nd dorsal interosseus

1st palmar interosseus

Flexor pollicis longus t.

1st dorsal interosseus

2nd palmar interosseus

4th dorsal interosseus

3rd palmar interosseus

Abductor digiti minimi

Flexor digiti minimi

Lumbricals

(Top) Axial T1 MR image of the right hand through the distal metacarpal diaphyses. The juncturae tendinum are fibrous bands which interconnect the extensor tendons of digits 2-5 just proximal to the MCP joints. These fibrous bands help prevent lateral translation of the extensor tendons over the metacarpals. Because of these interconnections, digital extension can be relatively preserved in the face of a complete transection of a single extensor digitorum communis tendon proximal to the juncturae, and such an injury may not be evident clinically. **(Bottom)** Axial T1 MR images of the right hand through the metacarpal heads.

Hand

IV

HAND OVERVIEW

AXIAL T1 MR, LEFT HAND

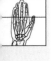

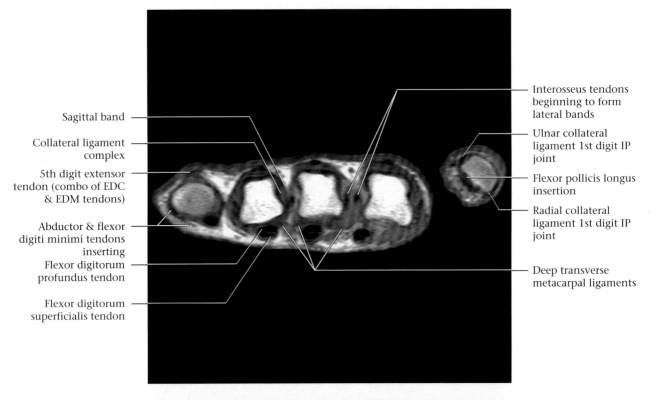

Sagittal band

Collateral ligament complex

5th digit extensor tendon (combo of EDC & EDM tendons)

Abductor & flexor digiti minimi tendons inserting

Flexor digitorum profundus tendon

Flexor digitorum superficialis tendon

Interosseus tendons beginning to form lateral bands

Ulnar collateral ligament 1st digit IP joint

Flexor pollicis longus insertion

Radial collateral ligament 1st digit IP joint

Deep transverse metacarpal ligaments

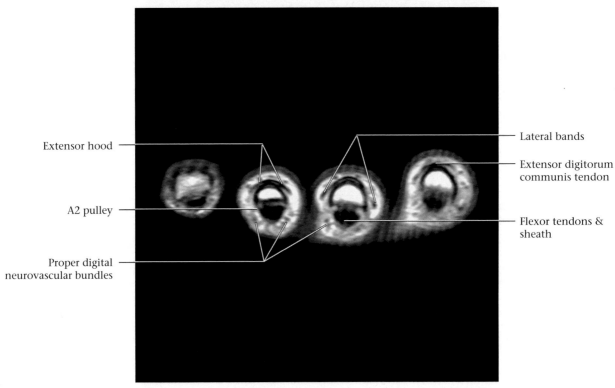

Extensor hood

A2 pulley

Proper digital neurovascular bundles

Lateral bands

Extensor digitorum communis tendon

Flexor tendons & sheath

(Top) Axial T1 MR image of the left hand slightly more distally through the metacarpal heads. The lateral notches of the MC heads are the sites of origin of the collateral ligaments which are the intermediate signal structures deep to the sagittal and lateral bands. The deep transverse metacarpal ligaments connect the volar plates of digits 2-5. **(Bottom)** Axial T1 MR image of the left hand through the proximal phalanges. The lateral bands can be defined as the lateral thickenings of the extensor hood, and the EDC tendon can be defined as the central thickening of the extensor hood. We know we are still in the lateral bands instead of the conjoined tendons as we are still proximal to the PIP joints.

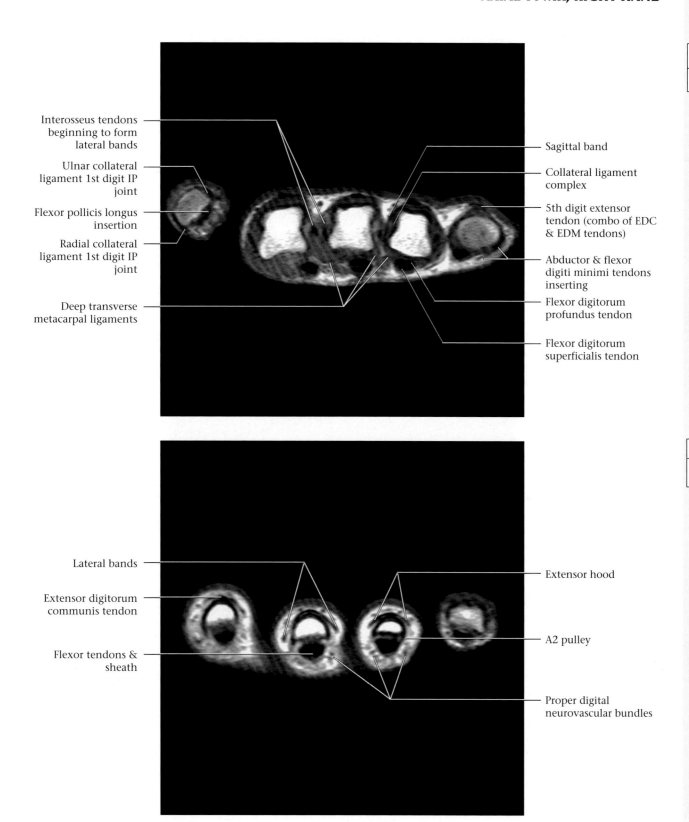

Interosseus tendons beginning to form lateral bands

Ulnar collateral ligament 1st digit IP joint

Flexor pollicis longus insertion

Radial collateral ligament 1st digit IP joint

Deep transverse metacarpal ligaments

Sagittal band

Collateral ligament complex

5th digit extensor tendon (combo of EDC & EDM tendons)

Abductor & flexor digiti minimi tendons inserting

Flexor digitorum profundus tendon

Flexor digitorum superficialis tendon

Lateral bands

Extensor digitorum communis tendon

Flexor tendons & sheath

Extensor hood

A2 pulley

Proper digital neurovascular bundles

(Top) Axial T1 MR image of the right hand slightly more distally through the metacarpal heads. The lateral notches of the MC heads are the sites of origin of the collateral ligaments which are the intermediate signal structures deep to the sagittal and lateral bands. The deep transverse metacarpal ligaments connect the volar plates of digits 2-5.
(Bottom) Axial T1 MR image of the right hand through the proximal phalanges. The lateral bands can be defined as the lateral thickenings of the extensor hood, and the EDC tendon can be defined as the central thickening of the extensor hood. We know we are still in the lateral bands instead of the conjoined tendons as we are still proximal to the PIP joints.

Hand

IV

CORONAL T1 MR, LEFT HAND

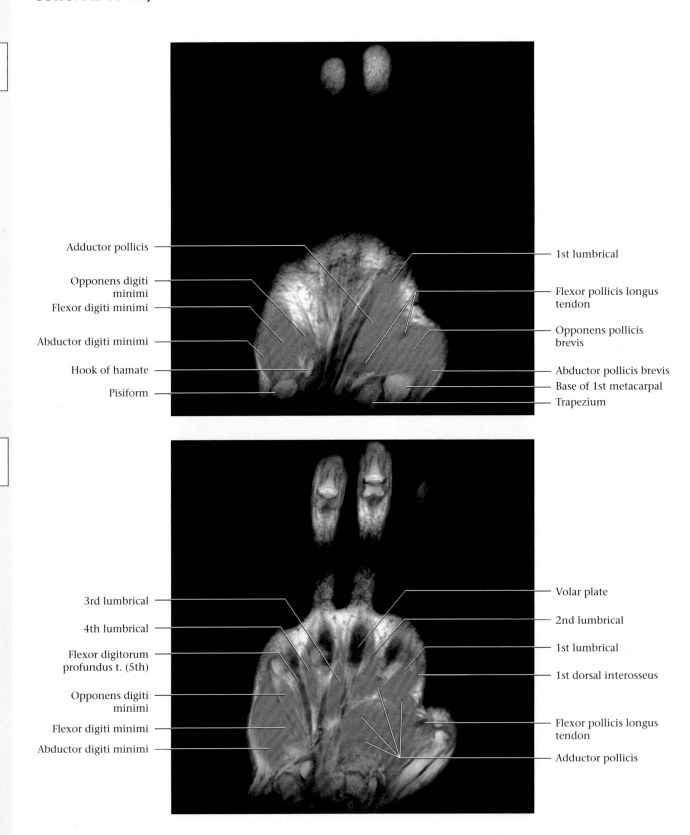

(Top) First in series of coronal T1 MR images of the left hand. This is located far volarly. **(Bottom)** Coronal T1 MR image of the left hand, through the deeper palmar structures. At this level, we happen to catch a portion of the MCP volar plates of digits 2-5 (only labeled on the third digit in this image). It can be determined that these are volar plates by their location and thickness. Note how much thicker they are compared to the flexor tendons.

HAND OVERVIEW

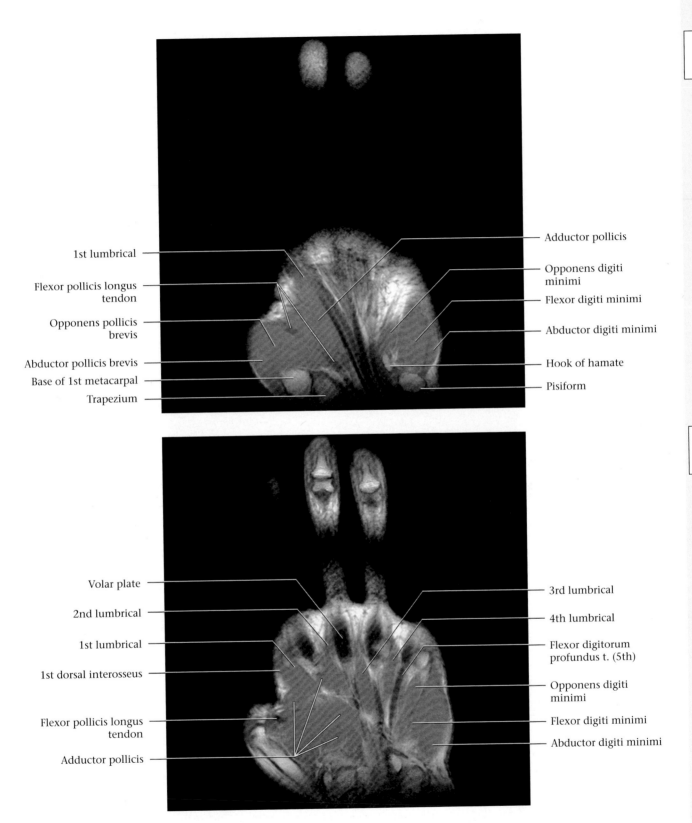

Top image labels:

- 1st lumbrical
- Flexor pollicis longus tendon
- Opponens pollicis brevis
- Abductor pollicis brevis
- Base of 1st metacarpal
- Trapezium
- Adductor pollicis
- Opponens digiti minimi
- Flexor digiti minimi
- Abductor digiti minimi
- Hook of hamate
- Pisiform

Bottom image labels:

- Volar plate
- 2nd lumbrical
- 1st lumbrical
- 1st dorsal interosseus
- Flexor pollicis longus tendon
- Adductor pollicis
- 3rd lumbrical
- 4th lumbrical
- Flexor digitorum profundus t. (5th)
- Opponens digiti minimi
- Flexor digiti minimi
- Abductor digiti minimi

(Top) First in series of coronal T1 MR images of the right hand. This is located far volarly. **(Bottom)** Coronal T1 MR image of the right hand through the deeper palmar structures. At this level, we happen to catch a portion of the MCP volar plates of digits 2-5 (only labeled on the third digit in this image). It can be determined that these are volar plates by their location and thickness. Note how much thicker they are compared to the flexor tendons.

CORONAL T1 MR, LEFT HAND

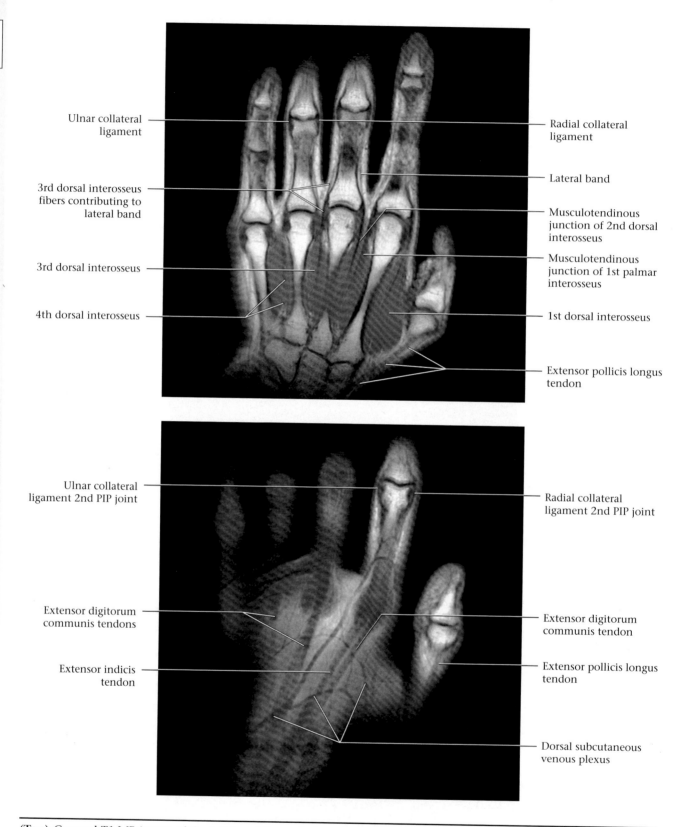

Ulnar collateral ligament

3rd dorsal interosseus fibers contributing to lateral band

3rd dorsal interosseus

4th dorsal interosseus

Radial collateral ligament

Lateral band

Musculotendinous junction of 2nd dorsal interosseus

Musculotendinous junction of 1st palmar interosseus

1st dorsal interosseus

Extensor pollicis longus tendon

Ulnar collateral ligament 2nd PIP joint

Extensor digitorum communis tendons

Extensor indicis tendon

Radial collateral ligament 2nd PIP joint

Extensor digitorum communis tendon

Extensor pollicis longus tendon

Dorsal subcutaneous venous plexus

(Top) Coronal T1 MR image of the left hand through the metacarpals. Although the dorsal interossei are predominately imaged in this plane, some of the 1st palmar interosseus is visible in the 2nd interspace. You can tell that this is palmar interosseus since it is contributing fibers from its musculotendinous junction to the ulnar lateral band of the 2nd digit instead of the radial lateral band of the 3rd digit (as the 2nd dorsal interosseus does). **(Bottom)** Coronal T1 MR image of the left hand (dorsal) demonstrates a few of the extensor digitorum communis tendons as well as the extensor indicis tendon. Note that the collateral ligaments of the PIP joints (and DIP joints as well, although not seen here) do not arise from the lateral notches of the heads of the phalanges as they do in their counterparts (the lateral notches of the metacarpal heads) at the MCP joints.

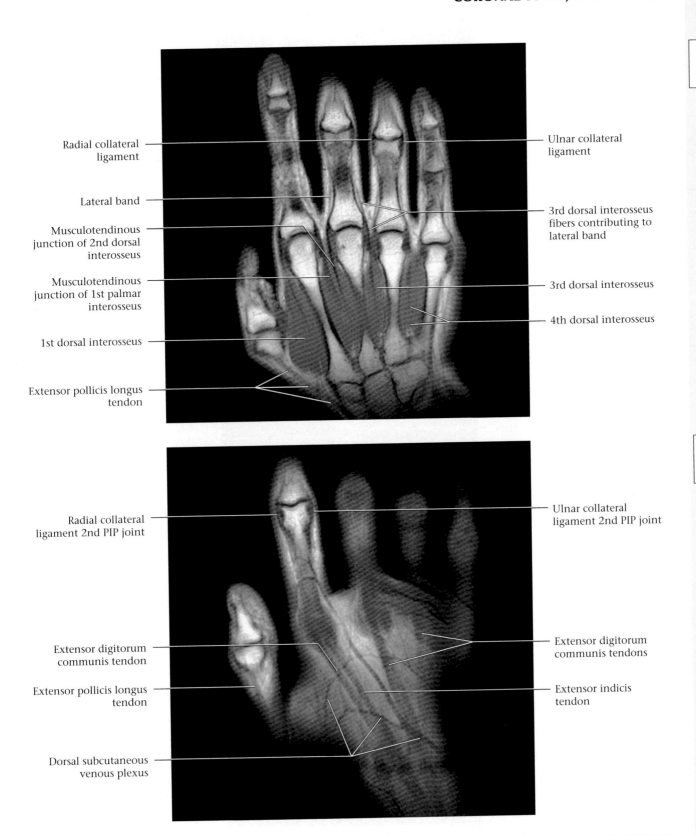

Radial collateral ligament

Lateral band

Musculotendinous junction of 2nd dorsal interosseus

Musculotendinous junction of 1st palmar interosseus

1st dorsal interosseus

Extensor pollicis longus tendon

Ulnar collateral ligament

3rd dorsal interosseus fibers contributing to lateral band

3rd dorsal interosseus

4th dorsal interosseus

Radial collateral ligament 2nd PIP joint

Extensor digitorum communis tendon

Extensor pollicis longus tendon

Dorsal subcutaneous venous plexus

Ulnar collateral ligament 2nd PIP joint

Extensor digitorum communis tendons

Extensor indicis tendon

(Top) Coronal T1 MR image of the right hand through the metacarpals. Although the dorsal interossei are predominately imaged in this plane, some of the 1st palmar interosseus is visible in the 2nd interspace. You can tell that this is palmar interosseus since it is contributing fibers from its musculotendinous junction to the ulnar lateral band of the 2nd digit instead of the radial lateral band of the 3rd digit (as the 2nd dorsal interosseus does). **(Bottom)** Coronal T1 MR image of the right hand (dorsal) demonstrates a few of the extensor digitorum communis tendons as well as the extensor indicis tendon. Note that the collateral ligaments of the PIP joints (and DIP joints as well, although not seen here) do not arise from the lateral notches of the heads of the phalanges as they do in their counterparts (the lateral notches of the metacarpal heads) at the MCP joints.

SAGITTAL T1 MR, RIGHT HAND

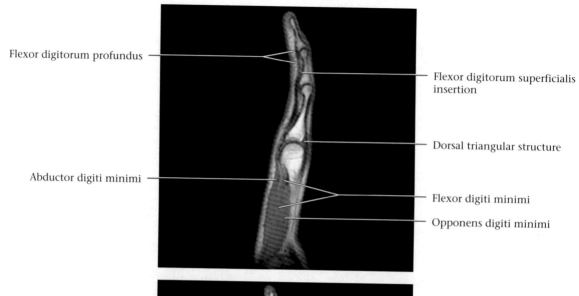

Flexor digitorum profundus — | — Flexor digitorum superficialis insertion

— Dorsal triangular structure

Abductor digiti minimi — | — Flexor digiti minimi

— Opponens digiti minimi

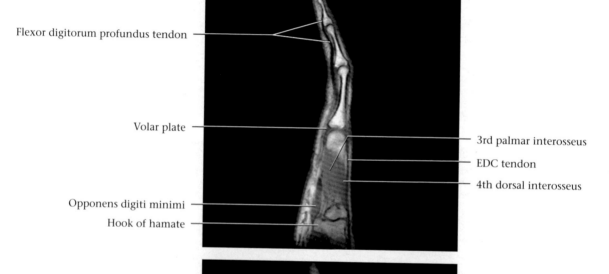

Flexor digitorum profundus tendon —

Volar plate — | — 3rd palmar interosseus

— EDC tendon

— 4th dorsal interosseus

Opponens digiti minimi —

Hook of hamate —

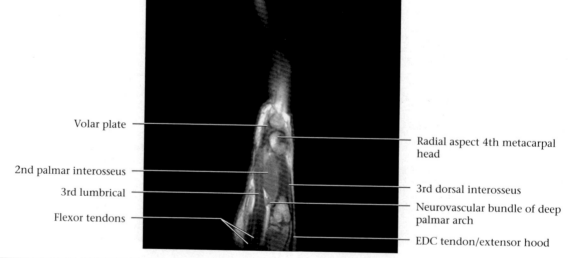

Volar plate — | — Radial aspect 4th metacarpal head

2nd palmar interosseus — | — 3rd dorsal interosseus

3rd lumbrical — | — Neurovascular bundle of deep palmar arch

Flexor tendons — | — EDC tendon/extensor hood

(Top) First of six sagittal T1 MR images of the right hand, at the level of the 5th digit. The dorsal triangular structure is a triangular-shaped vascularized fibrous structure of unknown significance which can be identified on MR and ultrasound imaging. **(Middle)** Sagittal T1 MR image of the right hand through the level of the 4th digit. **(Bottom)** Sagittal T1 MR image of the right hand obtained between the 3rd and 4th digits.

HAND OVERVIEW

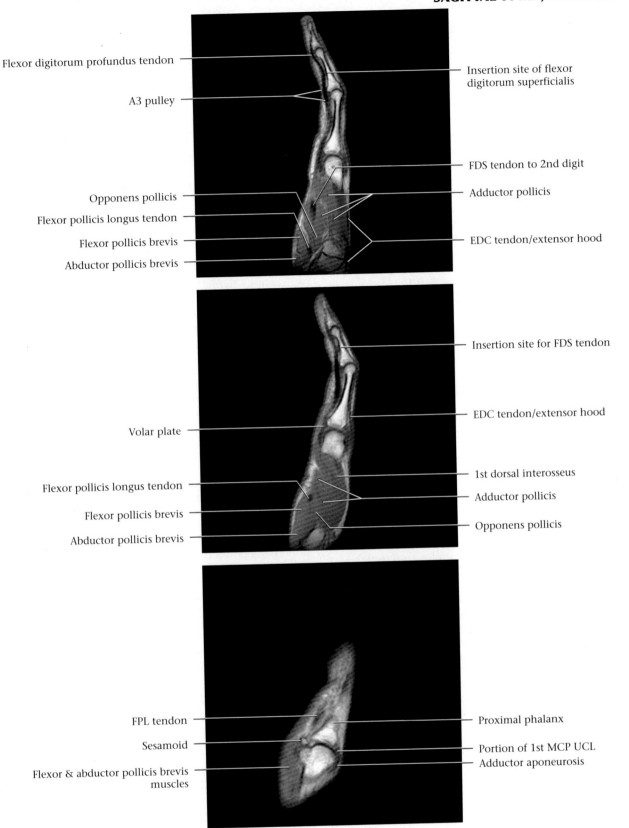

Flexor digitorum profundus tendon

A3 pulley

Insertion site of flexor digitorum superficialis

FDS tendon to 2nd digit

Opponens pollicis

Flexor pollicis longus tendon

Flexor pollicis brevis

Abductor pollicis brevis

Adductor pollicis

EDC tendon/extensor hood

Insertion site for FDS tendon

EDC tendon/extensor hood

Volar plate

Flexor pollicis longus tendon

Flexor pollicis brevis

Abductor pollicis brevis

1st dorsal interosseus

Adductor pollicis

Opponens pollicis

FPL tendon

Sesamoid

Flexor & abductor pollicis brevis muscles

Proximal phalanx

Portion of 1st MCP UCL

Adductor aponeurosis

(Top) Sagittal T1 MR image of the right hand through the 3rd digit. Although not routinely seen, the A3 pulley can be identified in this image as a slight, focal thickening of the flexor tendons just superficial to the PIP joint. (Middle) Sagittal T1 MR image of the right hand through the 2nd digit. Note the slight prominence of low signal on the volar surface of the middle phalanx. This is the insertion site of the flexor digitorum superficialis. (Bottom) Sagittal T1 MR image of the right hand obtained obliquely through the thumb metacarpal phalangeal joint. As this is a true sagittal image with respect to the hand, it is an oblique plane mid-way between sagittal and coronal with respect to the true axis of the thumb (1st digit). As such, the ulnar aspect of the MCP joint of the thumb is image right.

Hand

FLEXOR MECHANISM AND PALMAR HAND

Extrinsic Flexor Musculature: Digits 2 through 5

Flexor Digitorum Superficialis (FDS)
- Origin: Common flexor tendon (medial humeral epicondyle) of elbow and mid-radius
- Insertion: Volar plates of the proximal interphalangeal joints as well as the bases of the middle phalanges of digits 2 through 5
- Innervation: Median nerve
- Superficialis tendons split at level of the bases of proximal phalanges, forming two distinct tendon slips
  - Slips pass circumferentially around the lateral aspects of flexor digitorum profundus tendon before inserting deep to the FDP tendon
  - This forms a "tunnel" through which the Flexor digitorum profundus tendon passes
  - Just proximal to their insertion level, some fibers from each slip of FDS tendon decussate to the contralateral insertion site of the same digit
- Flexes both the metacarpophalangeal joints (aided by lumbricals and interossei) and proximal interphalangeal joints of digits 2 through 5

Flexor Digitorum Profundus (FDP)
- Origin: Proximal and mid radius, as well as the interosseus membrane
- Insertion: Volar plates of the distal interphalangeal joints as well as the bases of the distal phalanges of digits 2 through 5
- Innervation: Ulnar and median nerves
- Flexes the distal interphalangeal joints, and to lesser extent, the metacarpophalangeal (aided by lumbricals and interossei) and proximal interphalangeal joints of digits 2 through 5

Vinculum Breve and Longum
- Vinculum breve (short) and vinculum longum (long) are focal fibrovascular bands which course between the flexor tendons and volar surfaces of the phalanges
- Each of the flexor digitorum superficialis and flexor digitorum profundus tendons has one vinculum breve (distally) and one vinculum longum (proximally)
- Although not usually seen on routine imaging, these are important structures as they provide nutrients (via small vascular channels) to the flexor tendons

Extrinsic Flexor Musculature 1st Digit

Flexor Pollicis Longus (FPL)
- Origin: Mid-radius and interosseus membrane
- Insertion: Base of distal phalanx of 1st digit
- Innervation: Anterior interosseus nerve (branch of median nerve)
- Flexes 1st digit interphalangeal and metacarpophalangeal joints

Flexor Pulleys
- Focal thickenings of fibrous tissue of the common digital tendon sheaths
- Flexor pulleys serve to focally anchor tendon sheaths to volar surface of their respective digits at mechanically strategic points

Anular Pulleys Digits 2 through 5
- Denoted with **A for anular** and a number
  - Numbered 1 through 5 from proximal to distal
- **Odd** numbered pulleys are superficial to **oval** parts of digits (i.e., joints)
  - A1 pulley is located at level of metacarpophalangeal joint
  - A3 pulley is located at level of proximal interphalangeal joint
  - A5 pulley is located at level of distal interphalangeal joint
  - Odd numbered pulleys attach to underlying volar plates
- **Even** numbered pulleys are superficial to **elegant** waists (mid diaphyses) of phalanges
  - A2 pulley is located at level of mid-diaphysis of proximal phalanx
  - A4 pulley is located at level of mid-diaphysis of distal phalanx
  - Even numbered pulleys attach to underlying periosteum
- A2 and A4 pulleys are the **most important clinically** (for normal finger flexion), and are the only pulleys usually seen on **routine** imaging
- Evaluation for pulley rupture (with MR) should be performed with the fingers both in extension (as is routine) **and flexion**
- Pulley injury can be identified if discontinuity of a pulley is directly visualized (which is rare), but is more commonly inferred by "bowstringing" of flexor tendons
- "Bowstringing" of flexor tendons refers to an abnormal increase in distance between flexor tendons and underlying bones during flexion
- "Internal" comparison to the other fingers can give one an idea of the "normal" distance between the flexor tendons and the volar bony surface of the finger

Cruciform Pulleys Digits 2 through 5
- Not identified on routine imaging
  - Denoted with **C for cruciform** and a number
    - Numbered 1 through 3 from proximal to distal

Pulley System 1st Digit
- A1 pulley: Level of metacarpophalangeal joint
- Oblique pulley: Runs from ulnar aspect of proximal phalanx to radial aspect of distal phalanx
  - Crosses interphalangeal joint, so becomes lax in flexion
- A2 pulley: Level of interphalangeal joint
  - **Clinically, the most important pulley for flexion of thumb**
- **Av pulley: Variable in position** and may be anywhere over the proximal half of the proximal phalanx

Thenars and Hypothenars
- Thenars: Opponens pollicis, abductor pollicis brevis, and flexor pollicis brevis

FLEXOR MECHANISM AND PALMAR HAND

- o Origin: All originate from the flexor retinaculum and tubercle of the trapezium
  - Abductor pollicis brevis also originates from the tubercle of the scaphoid
- o Insertion: Abductor pollicis brevis and flexor pollicis brevis share a combined insertion at the lateral base of the proximal phalanx of the 1st digit
  - The Abductor pollicis brevis also contributes fibers to the extensor hood of the 1st digit (thumb)
- o Insertion: Opponens pollicis inserts on the proximal two-thirds of the volar diaphysis of the 1st metacarpal
- o Innervation: All by recurrent branch of median nerve
- o Actions
  - The Abductor pollicis brevis aids in extension of the joints of the 1st digit via its contributions to the extensor hood
  - Actions of the thenars are otherwise as their name implies
- Hypothenars: Opponens digiti minimi, abductor digiti minimi, and flexor digiti minimi
  - o Origin: Flexor digiti minimi and opponens digiti minimi originate from the flexor retinaculum and the hook of the Hamate
  - o Origin: Abductor digiti minimi originates from the pisiform
  - o Insertion: Flexor digiti minimi and abductor digiti minimi share a combined insertion on the ulnar base of the proximal phalanx of the 5th digit
    - Abductor digiti minimi also contributes fibers to the ulnar lateral band and extensor hood of the 5th digit
  - o Insertion: Opponens digiti minimi inserts on the proximal and mid diaphysis of the 5th metacarpal
  - o Innervation: All by ulnar nerve
  - o Actions
    - The Abductor digiti minimi aids flexion of the metacarpophalangeal joint and extension of the interphalangeal joint of the 5th digit via its contributions to the 5th digit ulnar lateral band and extensor hood
    - Actions of the hypothenars are otherwise as their name implies

Adductor Pollicis

- Comprised of oblique (proximal) and transverse (distal) heads
- Origin: Capitate, trapezoid, 2nd and 3rd metacarpals
- Insertion: Ulnar base of the proximal phalanx of the 1st digit, 1st digit interphalangeal joint volar plate, and it contributes fibers to the extensor hood of the 1st digit (which forms the adductor aponeurosis)
- Innervation: Ulnar nerve
- Actions: Adducts the thumb toward the 3rd digit and aids in extension of the thumb interphalangeal joint (via its contribution to extensor hood of 1st digit)

- Although often grouped with the thenar muscles (by virtue of proximity), the adductor pollicis is distinct from them, as it is separated from thenar muscles by a fascial plane, and innervated by ulnar nerve (as opposed to median nerve)

Palmar Interossei

- Denoted 1 through 3 from radial to ulnar
- Origin: Mesial palmar diaphyses of the 2nd, 4th, and 5th metacarpals
- Insertion: Mesial lateral bands and mesial aspect of the bases of proximal phalanges of the same digit from which they originate
- Innervation: Ulnar nerve
- Actions: Adduct digits and assists lumbricals with flexion of the metacarpophalangeal joints and extension of the interphalangeal joints of digits 2, 4, and 5

Tendon Sheaths

- Common flexor sheath (also known as the ulnar bursa)
  - o Contains the flexor digitorum superficialis and profundus tendons
  - o Begins just proximal to the carpal tunnel
  - o Extends to just beyond the level of the carpal tunnel over digits 2 through 4
  - o Encompasses the 5th digit flexor tendons over their entire course (to level of distal interphalangeal joint)
- Common digital sheaths (digits 2 through 4)
  - o Encompasses the flexor tendons from the level of the metacarpal necks to the bases of the distal phalanges
  - o Common digital sheaths may connect to the ulnar bursa (common flexor sheath) proximally in up to 10% of population
    - This possible connection is important as **it may provide a route for spread of infection** from digits 2 through 4 to common flexor sheath (and vice versa)
- Flexor pollicis longus tendon sheath (also known as radial bursa)
  - o Encompasses flexor pollicis longus tendon from just proximal to the beginning of the carpal tunnel to the level of its insertion (level of interphalangeal joint of thumb)
  - o It occasionally communicates with ulnar bursa (common flexor sheath) at level of carpal tunnel as a normal variant
    - This possible connection is important as **it can allow spread of infection**
- Tendon sheaths are lined by synovium
- Synovial fluid produced by the flexor sheath synovium bathes the flexor tendons with nutrients and decreases friction for smooth tendon motion during flexion

Hand

IV

31

GRAPHIC, FLEXOR MECHANISM COMPOSITE

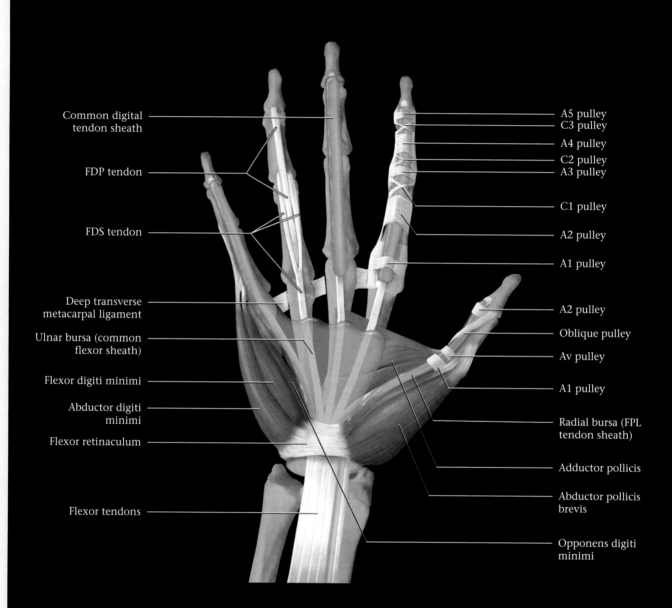

Common digital tendon sheath

FDP tendon

FDS tendon

Deep transverse metacarpal ligament

Ulnar bursa (common flexor sheath)

Flexor digiti minimi

Abductor digiti minimi

Flexor retinaculum

Flexor tendons

A5 pulley
C3 pulley
A4 pulley
C2 pulley
A3 pulley
C1 pulley
A2 pulley
A1 pulley
A2 pulley
Oblique pulley
Av pulley
A1 pulley
Radial bursa (FPL tendon sheath)
Adductor pollicis
Abductor pollicis brevis
Opponens digiti minimi

Pulley system for the 3rd-5th digits is identical to that demonstrated for the 2nd digit. Common digital sheath of the 4th digit is removed to show the relationship of the FDS and FDP tendons. The deep transverse metacarpal ligaments connect the volar plates (not shown) of digits 2-5. Although there is overlap of the radial and ulnar bursae in this image, these structures normally do not communicate. It is, however, important to know that the radial and ulnar bursae may communicate as a normal variation in a small percentage of the population. Similarly, any one or more of the common digital sheaths may communicate with the radial bursa in up to 10% of the normal population. These normal variant bursal communications are important as they can provide routes for more extensive spread of infection.

FLEXOR MECHANISM AND PALMAR HAND

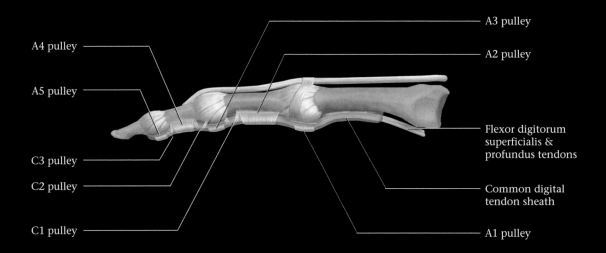

A3 pulley

A2 pulley

A4 pulley

A5 pulley

Flexor digitorum
superficialis &
profundus tendons

C3 pulley

C2 pulley

Common digital
tendon sheath

C1 pulley

A1 pulley

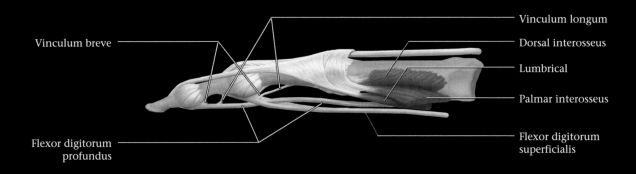

Vinculum longum

Vinculum breve

Dorsal interosseus

Lumbrical

Palmar interosseus

Flexor digitorum
profundus

Flexor digitorum
superficialis

(Top) Graphic of the lateral finger shows the flexor pulley system and common digital sheath. **(Bottom)** Graphic of the lateral finger shows the relationship of the two separate flexor tendons. Note how the FDP tendon passes through the "split" of the FDS tendon. Each FDS and FDP tendon has a vinculum longum and a vinculum breve. Although not normally seen on routine imaging, these structures are important as they provide vascular supply and a portion of the nutrients to the flexor tendons. Synovial fluid produced by the tendon sheaths also provides nutrients for the tendons.

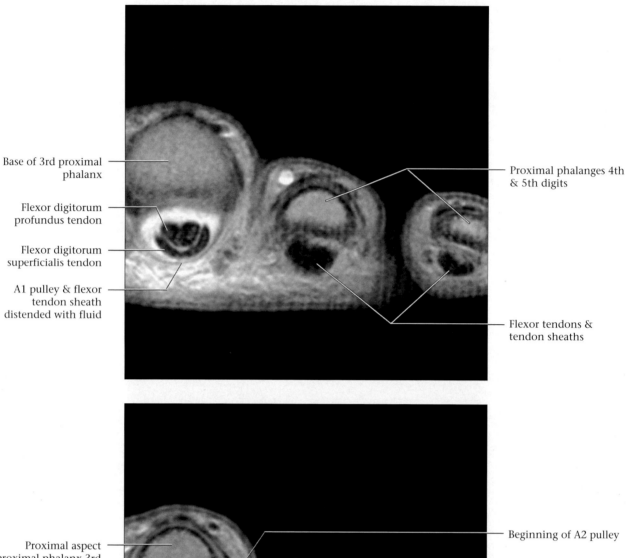

Base of 3rd proximal phalanx

Flexor digitorum profundus tendon

Flexor digitorum superficialis tendon

A1 pulley & flexor tendon sheath distended with fluid

Proximal phalanges 4th & 5th digits

Flexor tendons & tendon sheaths

Proximal aspect proximal phalanx 3rd digit

Flexor digitorum profundus tendon

Tendon sheath

Flexor digitorum superficialis tendon

Beginning of A2 pulley

Proximal phalanges 4th & 5th digits

A2 pulley

Flexor tendons

(Top) First of six axial PD FS MR images of the fingers. The flexor tendons and tendon sheaths are often inseparable from one another on routine imaging unless outlined by pathologic fluid (as in the third digit in this example). **(Bottom)** The FDS tendon splits at the proximal aspect of the proximal phalanx as demonstrated in the third digit. The same relationship exists in the 4th digit in this image, but delineation of the tendons as separate structures is difficult without the pathologic tendon sheath fluid present in the third digit.

FLEXOR MECHANISM AND PALMAR HAND

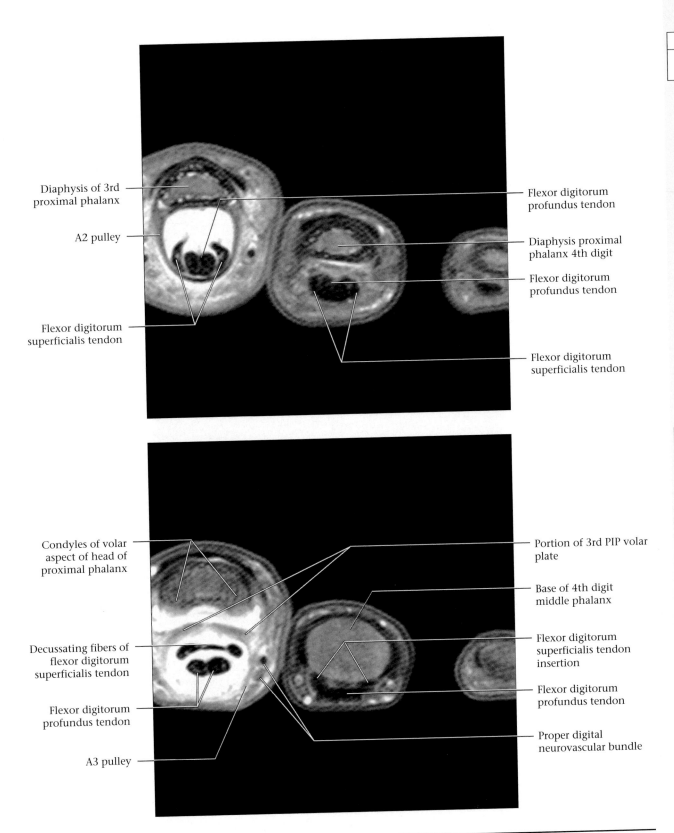

Diaphysis of 3rd proximal phalanx

A2 pulley

Flexor digitorum superficialis tendon

Flexor digitorum profundus tendon

Diaphysis proximal phalanx 4th digit

Flexor digitorum profundus tendon

Flexor digitorum superficialis tendon

Condyles of volar aspect of head of proximal phalanx

Decussating fibers of flexor digitorum superficialis tendon

Flexor digitorum profundus tendon

A3 pulley

Portion of 3rd PIP volar plate

Base of 4th digit middle phalanx

Flexor digitorum superficialis tendon insertion

Flexor digitorum profundus tendon

Proper digital neurovascular bundle

(Top) After the FDS tendon splits, it travels laterally around the FDP tendon from superficial to deep. In the 4th digit here, even without pathologic fluid for contrast, the flexor tendons can be seen as separate structures. The A2 Pulley can be identified by its location and thickness (compare to thickness of tendon sheath on the next image). **(Bottom)** In the 4th digit, the slips of the FDS tendon are beginning to insert on the volar aspect of the proximal portion of the middle phalanx. In the 3rd digit, the decussation of fibers from one slip of the FDS tendon to the other can be seen. Note the volar bicondylar shape of the head of the 3rd proximal phalanx vs. the oval shape of the base of 4th middle phalanx.

Hand

IV

3

AXIAL PD FS MR, RIGHT HAND

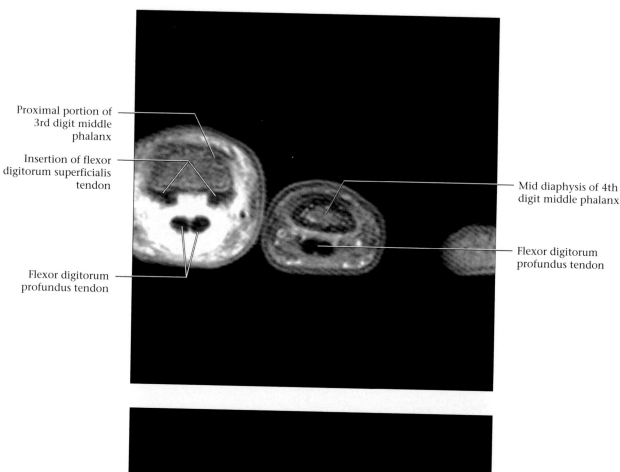

Proximal portion of 3rd digit middle phalanx

Insertion of flexor digitorum superficialis tendon

Flexor digitorum profundus tendon

Mid diaphysis of 4th digit middle phalanx

Flexor digitorum profundus tendon

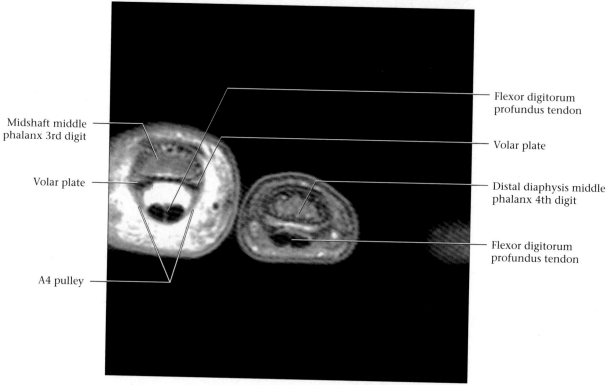

Midshaft middle phalanx 3rd digit

Volar plate

A4 pulley

Flexor digitorum profundus tendon

Volar plate

Distal diaphysis middle phalanx 4th digit

Flexor digitorum profundus tendon

(Top) In the 3rd digit, the FDS tendons insert on the volar aspect of the proximal portion of the middle phalanx. In the 4th digit, we are already beyond the insertion of the FDS tendon, and accordingly, only one tendon (the FDP tendon) is seen. **(Bottom)** Understanding the normal location of the pulleys allows identification of the A4 pulley at the midshaft of the middle phalanx 3rd digit. Additionally, note that the pulley is thicker than the normal tendon sheath: Compare to previous image where the normal tendon sheath is barely (if at all) discernible.

FLEXOR MECHANISM AND PALMAR HAND

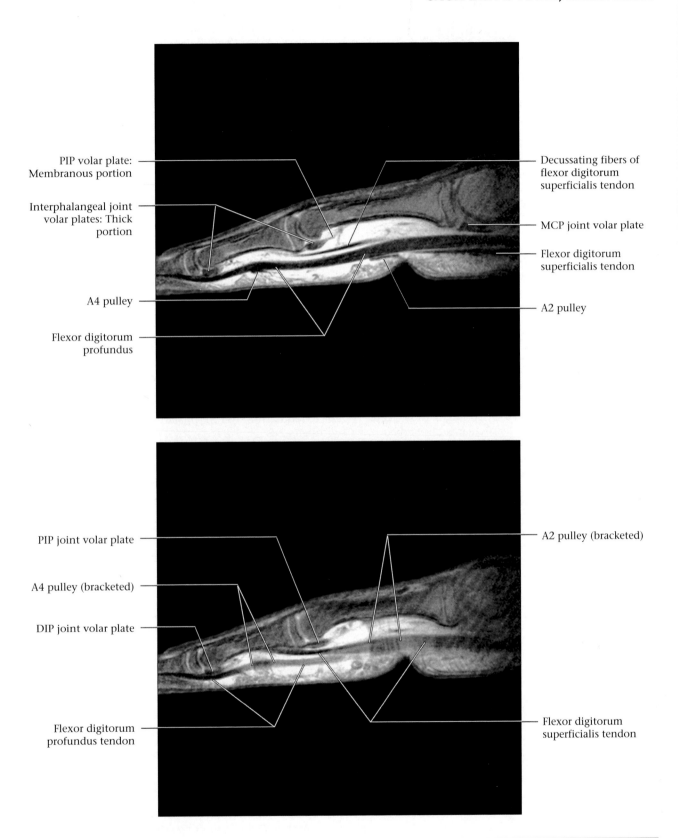

PIP volar plate: Membranous portion

Interphalangeal joint volar plates: Thick portion

A4 pulley

Flexor digitorum profundus

Decussating fibers of flexor digitorum superficialis tendon

MCP joint volar plate

Flexor digitorum superficialis tendon

A2 pulley

PIP joint volar plate

A4 pulley (bracketed)

DIP joint volar plate

Flexor digitorum profundus tendon

A2 pulley (bracketed)

Flexor digitorum superficialis tendon

(Top) First of two sagittal PD FS MR images of 3rd digit. This is the same digit from the previous axial series. As before, pathologic fluid is present within and about the common digital tendon sheath providing excellent contrast for delineation of normal structures. In this image, the FDS tendon appears discontinuous; however, remember that the FDS tendon splits and its slips pass lateral to the FDP tendon from just distal to the MCP joint until its decussation. Note the thin membranous portion of the volar plate of the PIP joint (not normally seen). In this plane, only the volar-most portions of the A2 and A4 pulleys can be seen. **(Bottom)** This image is slightly more lateral than the previous image. In this plane, we see that the FDS tendon is intact. We are also just lateral enough to catch some of the lateral portions of the A2 and A4 pulleys.

EXTENSOR MECHANISM AND JOINTS

Extensor Mechanism: Digits 2-5

Extensor Digitorum Communis (EDC)

- Origin: Common extensor tendon (lateral humeral epicondyle)
  - Distinct extensor digitorum communis tendon to 5th digit is present in only approximately 50% of population
  - When distinct 5th digit EDC tendon is absent, fiber contributions from 4th digit EDC tendon and junctura tendinum form a "makeshift" 5th digit EDC tendon
- Insertion: Inserts as central slip on dorsal bases of middle phalanges and proximal interphalangeal joint capsules
  - Just proximal to proximal interphalangeal joints, extensor digitorum communis tendons trifurcate into a central slip and two lateral slips
  - Lateral slips each fuse with their adjacent lateral band to form conjoined tendons
  - Disruption of central slip (via laceration or avulsion) can allow proximal interphalangeal joint to flex and herniate between EDC tendon lateral slips and lateral bands during extension resulting in a Boutonniere deformity
    - Easy to diagnose when associated with avulsion of osseus insertion
    - If articular portion of avulsed fragment is greater than one-third of total articular surface, open reduction with internal fixation is usually required
    - **When boutonniere deformity is present without an associated osseus fragment, and there is no history or associated findings to suggest inflammatory arthritis or connective tissue disease, central slip disruption should be suspected**
- Innervation: Posterior interosseus nerve (branch of radial nerve)

Extensor Indicis (EI)

- Origin: Posterior, distal ulna and interosseus membrane
- Insertion: Extensor indicis tendon blends with 2nd digit extensor digitorum communis tendon and extensor hood
- Innervation: Posterior interosseus nerve (branch of radial nerve)
- Extensor indicis tendon is generally located slightly ulnar and deep to 2nd digit extensor digitorum communis tendon at level of metacarpophalangeal joint

Extensor Digiti Minimi (EDM)

- Origin: Common extensor tendon (lateral humeral epicondyle)
  - In most cases, exists as two distinct tendons over wrist and 5th metacarpal
- Insertion
  - Two tendons of extensor digiti minimi fuse with one another and with 5th digit extensor digitorum communis tendon (if it exists), or, in its absence, with its "makeshift" counterpart
  - This combined extensor tendon inserts on dorsal base of proximal phalanx of 5th digit and also blends with joint capsule of 5th proximal interphalangeal joint
- Innervation: Posterior interosseus nerve (branch of radial nerve)
- Extensor digiti minimi tendons are generally located slightly ulnar and deep to 5th digit extensor digitorum communis tendon (or its equivalent) at level of metacarpophalangeal joint

Lumbricals

- Numbered 1-4 from radial to ulnar
- Origin: Flexor digitorum profundus tendons begin just distal to carpal tunnel
- Insertion: Radial lateral bands of digits 2-5
- Innervation
  - 1st and 2nd lumbricals: Median nerve
  - 3rd and 4th lumbricals: Ulnar nerve
- Extends interphalangeal joints and flexes metacarpophalangeal joints of digits 2-5

Dorsal Interossei

- Numbered 1-4 from radial to ulnar
- Origin: Dorsolateral metacarpal diaphyses
- Insertion: Mesial-most (in hand) adjacent lateral bands of digits 2-4
- Innervation: Ulnar nerve
- Extends 2nd-5th interphalangeal joints and abducts digits 2-5

Lateral Bands/Conjoined Tendons

- Lateral bands are formed by lumbrical and interosseus muscle tendons
  - Exception: Abductor digiti minimi forms ulnar lateral band of 5th digit
- At level of the distal aspect of proximal interphalangeal joints, lateral bands fuse with lateral slips of extensor digitorum communis tendons to form conjoined tendons
- At level of the distal interphalangeal joint, conjoined tendons fuse to form terminal tendons
- Terminal tendons insert on dorsal bases of distal phalanges and fuse with distal interphalangeal joint capsules of digits 2-5
- Just proximal to the level of distal interphalangeal joints, conjoined tendons are interconnected by a short band of transverse fibers called triangular ligament
  - Triangular ligament helps prevent lateral translation/volar subluxation of conjoined tendons
- Sudden forced flexion of an extended distal interphalangeal joint may cause terminal tendon to avulse its osseus insertion (a.k.a. mallet finger or baseball finger)
  - If articular surface involvement is greater than one-third of total articular surface, open reduction and internal fixation is generally required

Extensor Hood

- Begins just proximal to metacarpophalangeal joints and terminates just proximal to proximal interphalangeal joints

EXTENSOR MECHANISM AND JOINTS

- Dorsal hood of fibers oriented nearly perpendicular to long axis of extensor tendons
- Fibers of extensor hood interdigitate with extensor digitorum communis (and extensor indicis and digiti minimi) tendons to help prevent lateral translation
- Sagittal band
  - Proximal-most fibers of extensor hood
    - Located at metacarpophalangeal joint level
  - Attached to volar plate volarly
  - Prevents lateral translation of extensor digitorum communis tendons at metacarpophalangeal joint level
- Fibers of distal portion of extensor hood extend over dorsum of finger from one lateral band to opposite lateral band of same digit

Extensor Mechanism 1st Digit

Extensor Pollicis Longus (EPL)
- Origin: Mid-ulna and interosseus membrane
- Insertion: Dorsal base of 1st digit distal phalanx
  - Also interdigitates with fibers of extensor hood
- Innervation: Posterior interosseus nerve (branch of radial nerve)
- Extends both metacarpophalangeal and interphalangeal joints of 1st digit

Extensor Pollicis Brevis (EPB)
- Origin: Distal radius and interosseus membrane
- Insertion: Dorsal base of 1st digit proximal phalanx
  - Also interdigitates with fibers of extensor hood
- Innervation: Posterior interosseus nerve (branch of radial nerve)
- Extends 1st digit metacarpophalangeal joint

Extensor Hood
- Formed by fibers from adductor pollicis ulnarly and abductor pollicis brevis radially
- Aids extension of interphalangeal joint
- Adductor pollicis contribution to extensor hood is also known as adductor aponeurosis
  - Ulnar collateral ligament of 1st metacarpophalangeal joint is especially prone to tearing in forced abduction and extension
    - Such an injury is commonly referred to as gamekeeper's thumb or skier's thumb
  - **When ulnar collateral ligament is torn, the position of its proximal free end with respect to adductor aponeurosis is of utmost importance**
    - If proximal portion is displaced superficial to adductor aponeurosis,it is referred to as Stener lesion, and surgery is usually required as the displaced proximal stump will not spontaneously reduce
    - If proximal portion remains deep to adductor aponeurosis, conservative management may suffice as in situ fibrosis can provide adequate stability

Joints

Metacarpophalangeal Joints: Synovial Condylar Joints
- Allows flexion, as well as minimal extension, abduction, and adduction

Interphalangeal Joints: Synovial Hinge Joints
- Allows flexion and minimal extension

Volar Plate
- Constitutes majority of volar aspect of joint capsules of **all** metacarpophalangeal and interphalangeal joints
- Distally, volar plate is thick and firmly attached to volar base of adjacent phalanx
- In central aspect of the thick portion of volar plate (mid-sagittal plane) there is a normal, focal defect known as central recess
  - This should not be mistaken for pathology
- Proximally, volar plate is thin (membranous portion) and redundant in order to accommodate full range of motion
- With forced extension or posterior dislocation at a metacarpophalangeal or interphalangeal joint, volar plate may avulse
  - When volar plate avulses its osseus insertion, an intra-articular fracture results
  - If articular portion of avulsed fragment is greater than one-third of total articular surface, open reduction and internal fixation generally is required
- Volar plates of digits 2-5 are attached to one another at metacarpophalangeal joints by deep transverse metacarpal ligaments

Collateral Ligament Complex
- Constitutes majority of lateral aspects of joint capsules of **all** metacarpophalangeal and interphalangeal joints
- Comprised of main and accessory components
- Fibers of both main and accessory collateral ligaments course obliquely from dorsal (proximally) to volar (distally); albeit, at slightly different obliquities
- Main collateral ligament inserts on volar/lateral base of next distal-most adjacent phalanx
- Accessory collateral ligament inserts on mid to distal volar plate
- Collateral ligaments of metacarpophalangeal joints are normally heterogeneous in signal
  - Similar appearance of other collateral ligaments should help prevent one from mistaking this appearance for pathology

Bare Areas
- Intra-articular bone not covered by cartilage
- Location of initial erosions in inflammatory arthritis
- At metacarpophalangeal joint, metacarpal head is usually involved by erosions before adjacent proximal phalanx

GRAPHIC, EXTENSOR MECHANISM COMPOSITE

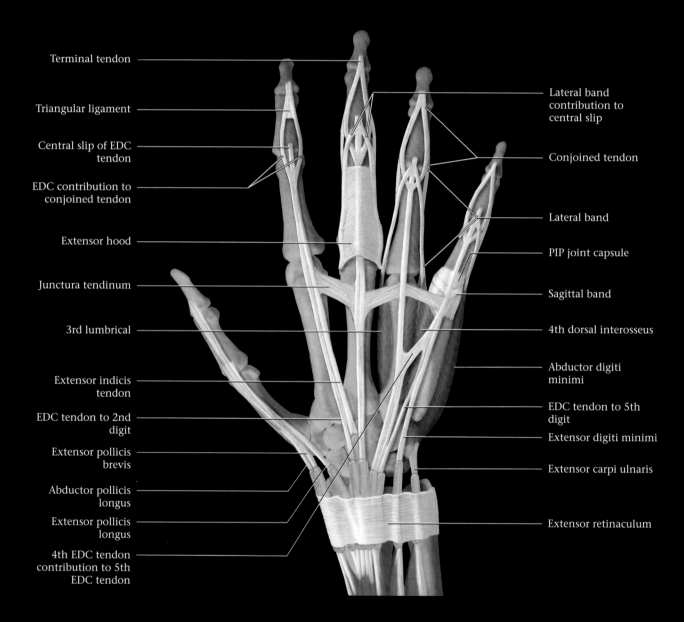

Terminal tendon

Triangular ligament

Central slip of EDC tendon

EDC contribution to conjoined tendon

Extensor hood

Junctura tendinum

3rd lumbrical

Extensor indicis tendon

EDC tendon to 2nd digit

Extensor pollicis brevis

Abductor pollicis longus

Extensor pollicis longus

4th EDC tendon contribution to 5th EDC tendon

Lateral band contribution to central slip

Conjoined tendon

Lateral band

PIP joint capsule

Sagittal band

4th dorsal interosseus

Abductor digiti minimi

EDC tendon to 5th digit

Extensor digiti minimi

Extensor carpi ulnaris

Extensor retinaculum

Extensor mechanism composite shows different components of extensor mechanism on different digits. With the exception of the extensor indicis, extensor digiti minimi, abductor digiti minimi, and 4th EDC tendon contribution to the 5th EDC tendon, any structure on any of the 2nd-5th digits can be extrapolated to any and all of the other 2nd-5th digits. Note that the 2nd extensor retinaculum compartment and its contents (the extensor carpi radialis longus and brevis tendons) are not included in this graphic. Although the abductor pollicis longus tendon travels in the 1st compartment of the extensor retinaculum, its insertion (not shown) is actually on the radial aspect of the volar surface of the base of the first metacarpal (refer to volar insertions graphic of the "Hand Overview" section).

EXTENSOR MECHANISM AND JOINTS

GRAPHIC, EXTENSOR MECHANISM DORSAL SURFACE, DIGITS 2-5

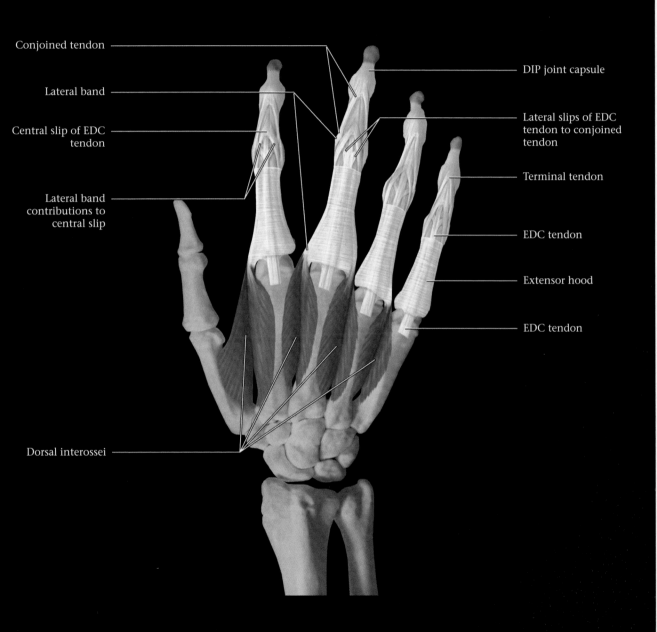

Conjoined tendon

Lateral band

Central slip of EDC tendon

Lateral band contributions to central slip

Dorsal interossei

DIP joint capsule

Lateral slips of EDC tendon to conjoined tendon

Terminal tendon

EDC tendon

Extensor hood

EDC tendon

This dorsal surface graphic of the extensor mechanism of digits 2-5 demonstrates the complex relationship of the various fiber bands. As in imaging, distinction of individual fiber bands is often difficult and must be inferred by knowledge of where the structure "should" be with respect to more easily identifiable structures (such as bones and joints).

GRAPHICS, EXTENSOR MECHANISM LATERAL FINGER & MCP JOINT

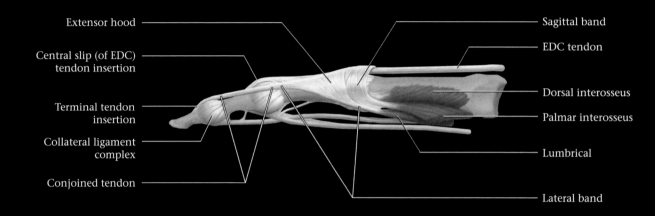

Extensor hood

Central slip (of EDC) tendon insertion

Terminal tendon insertion

Collateral ligament complex

Conjoined tendon

Sagittal band

EDC tendon

Dorsal interosseus

Palmar interosseus

Lumbrical

Lateral band

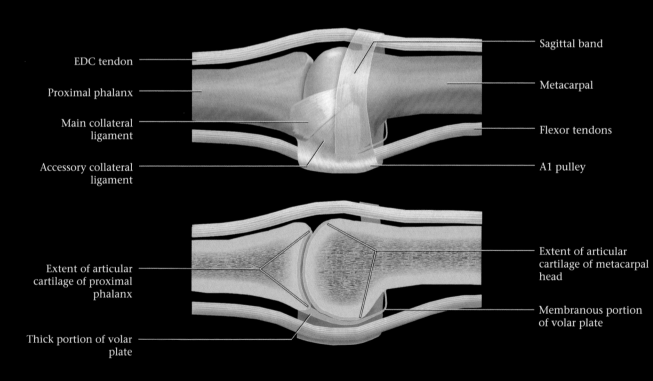

EDC tendon

Proximal phalanx

Main collateral ligament

Accessory collateral ligament

Sagittal band

Metacarpal

Flexor tendons

A1 pulley

Extent of articular cartilage of proximal phalanx

Thick portion of volar plate

Extent of articular cartilage of metacarpal head

Membranous portion of volar plate

(Top) Lateral view of the extensor components of the finger. The lateral band becomes the conjoined tendon after it receives the lateral slips of the EDC tendon (roughly at the level of the mid to distal PIP joint). The proximal-most fibers of the extensor hood known as the sagittal band run at a slightly different obliquity than those of the remainder of the extensor hood. **(Bottom)** Surface and cut-section graphics of the MCP joint. The collateral ligament complex is composed of two separate fiber bands. The main collateral ligament inserts on the base of the adjacent phalanx. The accessory collateral ligament inserts on the volar plate. The volar plate is thick distally; thin and redundant proximally. With the exception of the sagittal band (present only at the MCP joints), the anatomy in this graphic is duplicated in all MCP and IP joints in the hand.

EXTENSOR MECHANISM AND JOINTS

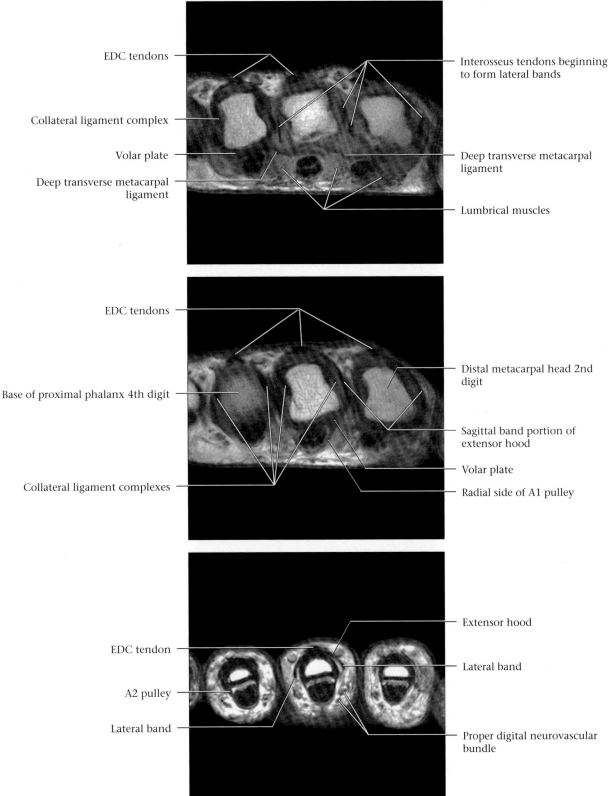

(Top) First of six axial PD MR images of the fingers. The deep transverse metacarpal ligaments interconnect the volar plates of digits 2-4. Note that the interossei pass dorsal and the lumbricals pass volar to the deep transverse metacarpal ligaments. The collateral ligament complexes are intermediate and somewhat heterogeneous in signal: This is normal. **(Middle)** Although a portion of the A1 pulley was captured on this image, it is not common to see this pulley on routine imaging. This was the only image in this series to visualize any of the A1 pulleys, and it only caught a portion of this structure. **(Bottom)** The A2 pulleys are visible on all digits in this image. The lateral bands of the 3rd digit are the lateral-most thickenings of the extensor hood. The EDC tendon is the central thickening of the extensor hood.

AXIAL PD MR, LEFT HAND

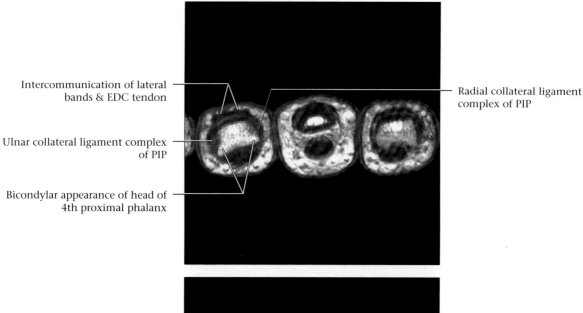

Intercommunication of lateral bands & EDC tendon

Ulnar collateral ligament complex of PIP

Bicondylar appearance of head of 4th proximal phalanx

Radial collateral ligament complex of PIP

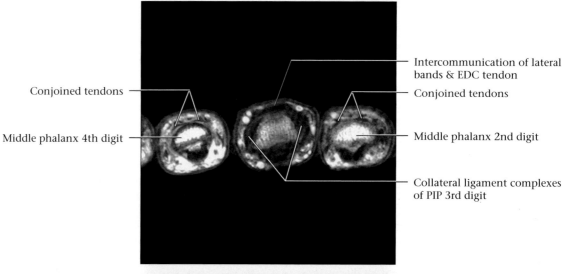

Conjoined tendons

Middle phalanx 4th digit

Intercommunication of lateral bands & EDC tendon

Conjoined tendons

Middle phalanx 2nd digit

Collateral ligament complexes of PIP 3rd digit

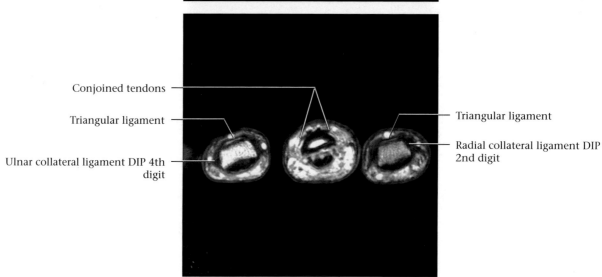

Conjoined tendons

Triangular ligament

Ulnar collateral ligament DIP 4th digit

Triangular ligament

Radial collateral ligament DIP 2nd digit

(Top) At the level of the distal diaphysis of the 3rd proximal phalanx, as this digit is longer than the others. In the 4th digit (image left), no distinct thickenings to define the lateral bands or EDC tendon can be discerned as these structures are sending fiber band contributions to one another. Note that the PIP collateral ligaments are relatively homogeneous and low signal, in contradistinction to the MCP collateral ligaments. **(Middle)** Distal to the 2nd and 4th PIP joints, the two distinct fiber bands over the dorsum of these digits are the conjoined tendons. **(Bottom)** The 3rd digit still shows two distinct conjoined tendons. The 2nd & 4th digits show a continuous dorsal fiber band which is the triangular ligament. As in the PIP Joints, the collateral ligaments of the DIP joints are relatively homogeneously low in signal.

EXTENSOR MECHANISM AND JOINTS

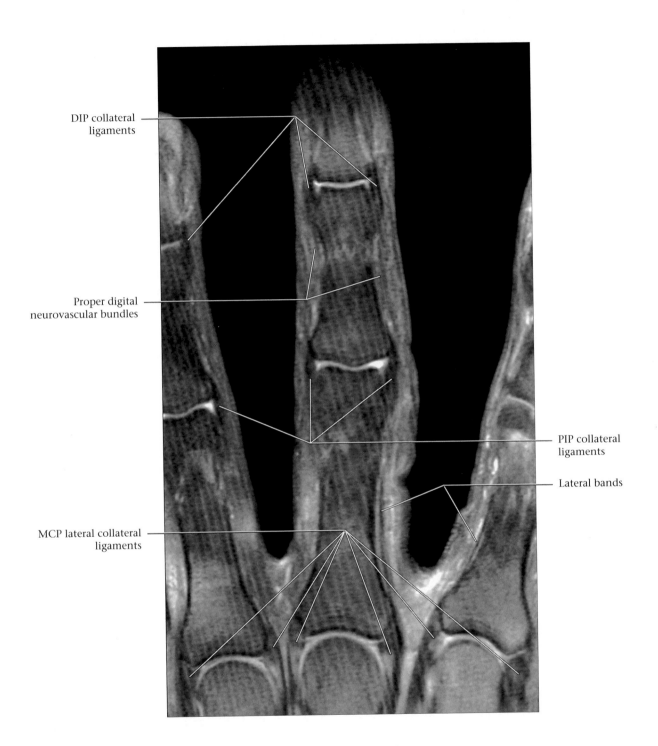

DIP collateral
ligaments

Proper digital
neurovascular bundles

PIP collateral
ligaments

Lateral bands

MCP lateral collateral
ligaments

Close-up coronal PD FS image centered on the 3rd digit which shows the differences in the collateral ligaments of the MCP joints compared to the interphalangeal joints. The collateral ligaments of the MCP joints are thicker and more heterogeneous and intermediate in signal than the collateral ligaments of the interphalangeal joints. Note the very small amount of normal fluid in the interphalangeal joints. A small amount of fluid can also be normally seen in the MCP joints despite not being demonstrated on this image.

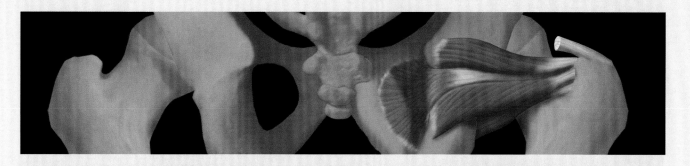

SECTION V: Hip and Pelvis

HIP AND PELVIS OVERVIEW

Terminology

Abbreviations
- Anterior superior iliac spine (ASIS)
- Avascular necrosis (AVN)
- Posterior superior iliac spine (PSIS)
- Structure supplied by nerve or artery (S)
- Slipped capital femoral epiphysis (SCFE)
- Sacroiliac joint (SI)

Gross Anatomy

Overview
- Pelvic ring composed of sacrum, coccyx, hip bone
  - Articulations: Lumbosacral, sacrococcygeal, sacroiliac, symphysis pubis
- Transmits body weight to lower extremities & absorbs forces from lower extremity
- Anteriorly tilted
  - Pelvic inlet 50° from horizontal
  - ASIS & anterosuperior pubis along same vertical axis
- Acetabulum faces inferomedially
  - Acetabular notch opens inferiorly
- Pattern of ossification
  - 3 primary centers: Ischium, ilium, pubis
    - Joined by triradiate cartilage; matures 15-16 y/o
  - 5 secondary centers: Iliac crest, anterior inferior iliac spine, ischial tuberosity, pubis, ASIS
    - Begin ossification puberty, mature 20-25 y/o
- Hip bone: Ischium, ilium, pubis
  - Articulation: Ball and socket hip joint (see "Hip Joint" section)
- Anatomic boundaries between pelvis & lower limb: External surfaces pelvic bones/sacrum/coccyx, iliac crest, inguinal ligament, symphysis pubis, ischiopubic rami, ischial tuberosity, sacrotuberous ligament

Bones
- **Coccyx**
  - Triangular shape
  - 3-5 rudimentary vertebra
  - Coccygeal cornua articulates with sacrum
- **Femur**
  - Femoral head is 2/3 sphere
    - Central cartilage void at fovea capitis
  - Neck connects shaft, head
    - Narrower near head, wider near trochanters
    - Allows shaft to clear acetabulum & pelvis during motion
    - **Subcapital** region: Head-neck junction
    - **Basicervical** region: Base of neck
  - Shaft: Circular cross section with thick ridge posteriorly (linea aspera)
  - Femoral neck/shaft angle (angle of inclination), (see "Measurements and Lines" section)
    - Smaller in women secondary to wider pelvis
  - Femoral anteversion/torsion angle/angle of declination: Anterior angulation neck relative to shaft (see "Measurements and Lines" section)
  - **Greater trochanter**: Lateral facing extension from superior femur

- **Lesser trochanter**: Conical projection arising posterior medial proximal diaphysis
    - Clinical note: En face visualization of lesser trochanter on radiographs indicates femoral external rotation
  - **Intertrochanteric line**: Anterior ridge connecting trochanters
    - Winds under lesser trochanter & continues posteriorly as spiral line
  - **Intertrochanteric ridge/crest**: Connects trochanters posteriorly
  - **Linea aspera**: Ridge along posterior femoral diaphysis
    - Divides proximally into medial & lateral lips
    - Medial lip blends with spiral line
    - Lateral lip blends with gluteal tuberosity
    - Distally divides into supracondylar lines
  - **Piriformis (trochanteric) fossa**: Deepening posteriorly between greater trochanter & femoral neck
    - Insertion site of hip external rotators
  - Condyles (see "Knee Overview" section)
- **Ilium**
  - Thin ala & 2 large columns
  - Concave internal **iliac fossa**
  - Convex external **auricular surface** (gluteal fossa)
  - **Arcuate line** marks inferior aspect iliac fossa
  - Superior **iliac crest** with overhanging external lip extends from ASIS to posterior superior iliac spine
    - **Tubercle** of iliac crest at anterosuperior margin
  - Anterior protuberances: **Anterior superior iliac spine, anterior inferior iliac spine**
    - Shallow notch between
  - Posterior protuberances: **Posterior superior iliac spine, posterior inferior iliac spine**
  - Forms 2/5 acetabulum
  - Clinical note: Use superior aspect iliac crest on physical examination or radiographs to identify the L4/5 level
- **Ischium**
  - V-shaped bone with body & ramus
  - Apex is **ischial tuberosity**
  - **Ischial spine**: Oriented posteromedially
    - Greater sciatic notch above (see "Posterior Pelvis" section)
    - Lesser sciatic notch below (see "Posterior Pelvis" section)
  - Ramus joins inferior pubic ramus forming ischiopubic ramus
  - Body forms 2/5 acetabulum
  - Clinical note: In seated position ischial tuberosities bear all body weight
- **Pubis**
  - Body & 2 rami
  - Bodies meet midline at symphysis pubis (see "Anterior Pelvis and Thigh" section)
  - **Iliopubic (iliopectineal) eminence** at junction with ilium
  - Inferior ramus part of **ischiopubic ramus**
  - **Pubic crest** along anterior superior border of symphysis & pubic bodies
  - **Pubic tubercle**: Lateral aspect pubic crest
    - Attachment inguinal ligament

- **Pecten**: Lateral ridge along superior ramus from pubic tubercle to arcuate line
- Body is 1/5 acetabulum
- Clinical note: Iliopubic eminence is common site of insufficiency fracture
- Clinical note: Iliopectineal thickening is often first site of Paget disease
- **Sacrum**
  - Triangular, concave anterior, convex posterior
  - Contains 5-6 fused rudimentary vertebra (variations of S1 segmentation are common)
  - 4 ridges & 4 anterior (ventral) neural foramina
    - Ridges remnants intervertebral discs
    - Clinical note: **Sacral arcs** are superior margin foramina; 2-3 should be visible, should be symmetric; absence indicates destructive process
  - **Sacral ala** (wings): Lateral aspect
  - Lamina fused posteriorly; cover spinal canal
  - **Median sacral crest**: Fusion spinous processes except S5 +/- S4
    - Incomplete fusion creates sacral hiatus
  - **Intermediate sacral crest**: Fusion articular processes
  - **Lateral sacral crest**: Tips fused transverse processes
  - **Sacral cornua**: Inferior articular facets S5
    - Articulate with coccyx (may be fibrous or fused)
  - Lateral surface: Articulate with ilium
    - Anterior auricular surface, synovial articulation
    - Posterior syndesmosis, insertion interosseous ligaments
  - **Sacral promontory**: Anterior superior projection S1
  - **Lumbosacral angle**: 130-160°

Muscles

- Anterior femoral muscles (see "Anterior Pelvis and Thigh" and "Thigh Overview" sections)
  - Knee extension & weak hip flexion
- Lateral femoral (gluteal) muscles (see "Lateral Hip" section)
  - Hip abduction & external rotation
- Medial femoral muscles (see "Thigh Overview" section)
  - Hip adduction & weak internal rotation, flexion
- Posterior femoral muscles (see "Thigh Overview" section)
  - Hip extension & knee flexion

Vessels

- **Femoral artery**: Continuation external iliac a. after passing beneath inguinal ligament
  - Bisects femoral triangle, enters adductor canal, traverses adductor hiatus, becomes popliteal a.
  - **Femoral vein**: Continuation popliteal v. in adductor hiatus
    - Becomes external iliac v. at inguinal ligament
    - Misnomer: Superficial femoral v.; part of deep venous system
  - See "Thigh Overview" section
- **Inferior gluteal artery**: Larger terminal branch anterior division internal iliac a.
  - Passes between S1 & S2 or S2 & S3
  - Exits pelvis through sciatic notch inferior to piriformis m.
  - Posteromedial to sciatic n.
  - S: Pelvic diaphragm, piriformis, quadratus femoris, upper hamstring & gluteus maximus m., sciatic n.

- **Inferior gluteal v.** travels with artery, drains into internal iliac v.
- **Obturator artery**: Branch anterior division internal iliac a.
  - Travels lateral pelvic wall; lateral to ureter, ductus deferens, peritoneum
  - Leaves pelvis via obturator canal, enters medial thigh
  - Acetabular branch via acetabular notch to ligamentum fovea capitis
  - 20% incidence aberrant artery from inferior epigastric a.
  - **Obturator v.** with a., drains into internal iliac v.
- **Superior gluteal artery**: Continuation posterior division internal iliac a.
  - Passes between lumbosacral trunk & S1 n.
  - Exits pelvis superior to piriformis m.
  - Divides
    - Superficial: S - gluteus maximus m.
    - Deep: S - gluteus medius & minimus m., tensor fascia lata
  - **Superior gluteal v.**: Travels with artery, drains into internal iliac v.

Nerves

- Pre-axial: Anterior to bone
- Post-axial: Posterior to bone
- **Lumbar plexus**: Ventral rami L1, L2, L3, portion of L4
  - Forms along anterior transverse processes within psoas major m.
  - Branches: Iliohypogastric: L1 ± T12; ilioinguinal: L1; genitofemoral: L1, L2 (pre-axial); lateral femoral cutaneous: L2, L3 (post-axial); obturator: L2, L3, L4 (pre-axial); accessory obturator: L3, L4 (pre-axial); femoral: L2, L3, L4 (post-axial)
    - Obturator & femoral ns. (see "Thigh Overview" section)
- **Sacral plexus**: **Lumbosacral trunk** (descending L4, anterior ramus L5), S1, S2, S3
  - Forms anterior surface piriformis & coccygeus ms.
  - Branches
    - Sciatic n. divides into tibial n.: L4, L5, S1, S2, S3 (pre-axial); common peroneal n.: L4, L5, S1, S2 (post-axial); (see "Posterior Pelvis" section)
    - Muscular branches: Piriformis: S1, S2; levator ani & coccygeus: S3, S4; quadratus femoris & inferior gemellus: L4, L5, S1; obturator internus & superior gemellus: L5, S1, S2
    - Superior gluteal n.: L4, L5, S1; inferior gluteal n.: L5, S1, S2; posterior femoral cutaneous n.: S1, S2, S3; perforating cutaneous n.: S2, S3; pudendal n.: S3, S4; pelvic splanchnic n.: S2, S3, S4; perineal branch S4
    - See "Posterior Pelvis" section
- **Coccygeal plexus**: S4, S5, coccygeal ns.
  - Supplies coccygeus & levator ani ms.
  - Branch: Anococcygeal n.

Other

- **Fascia lata**: Fascia encasing entire thigh
  - Superiorly attached to inguinal ligament
  - **Iliotibial tract** is lateral thickening
    - Attachments: Tubercle of iliac crest & lateral condyle tibia

HIP AND PELVIS OVERVIEW

- Insertion site portions of gluteus maximus & tensor fascia lata ms.
  - **Lateral intermuscular septum** separates vastus lateralis & biceps femoris ms.
  - **Medial intermuscular septum** separates adductor muscles & vastus medialis m.
  - **Saphenous opening** for saphenous v.
- **Gluteal fascia (aponeurosis)**: Between iliac crest & gluteus maximus m.
- **Greater (false) and lesser (true) pelvis**
  - Divided by pelvic inlet
  - Greater pelvis: Part of abdominal cavity
- **Obturator foramen**: Covered by obturator membrane
  - Boundaries: Pubis, ischium, superior pubic & ischiopubic rami
  - Reduces weight of pelvis
  - **Obturator canal**: Obturator a., v., n. thru membrane
- **Pelvic inlet**: Pelvic brim, sacral promontory, sacral ala, **linea terminalis** (arcuate line of ilium, pecten pubis, pubic crest)
- **Pelvic outlet**: Pubic arch, ischial tuberosities, sacrotuberous ligament, tip of coccyx
- **Teardrop**: Osseous margins ischium at anteroinferior fossa

Imaging Anatomy

Femur
- **Compressive & tensile** trabecular pattern upper femur
  - Principal compressive: Medial cortex neck to superior femoral head
  - Secondary compressive: Medial cortex shaft inferior to principle compressive trabecula
  - Principal tensile: Lateral cortex below greater trochanter to inferior femoral head
  - Secondary tensile: Lateral cortex below principle tensile, course adjacent to principal tensile, terminate after mid neck
  - Greater trochanteric: Lateral cortex to superior cortex greater trochanter; tensile
- **Ward triangle**: Bounded by principal compressive, secondary compressive, tensile trabeculae
- Clinical note: Trabecular pattern & Ward triangle examined to assess extent of osteoporosis

Acetabulum
- Conceptualize as inverted Y
  - Stem: Ilium
  - **Anterior column: Iliopubic column**
    - Anterior iliac crest to pubic symphysis
    - Radiographs: Iliopectineal line
  - **Posterior column: Ilioischial column**
    - Ilium from top sciatic notch to inferior ischium
    - Radiographs: Ilioischial line

Anatomy-Based Imaging Issues

Imaging Recommendations
- Radiographs: Pelvis (unless otherwise indicated cassette horizontal to floor, tube perpendicular to floor, patient supine, legs extended)
  - AP
  - Judet, obturator, or internal oblique: Patient 45° anterior oblique
    - Visualizes posterior acetabular rim, anterior acetabular column, obturator foramen, SI joint
  - Judet, iliac or external oblique: Patient 45° posterior oblique
    - Visualizes anterior acetabular rim, posterior acetabular column, iliac wing, ischial spine
  - Inlet: 40-50° caudad tube angulation
    - Visualizes rotational & anterior to posterior pelvic alignment
  - Outlet: 35-40° cranial tube angulation
    - Visualizes superior to inferior pelvic alignment
  - Sacrum: AP 35-40° cranial tube angulation
    - En face view sacrum & L5-S1 disc space
  - Coccyx: AP 15° caudad angulation
  - Sacrum and coccyx: Lateral
  - SI joints: AP, 30-35° cranial tube angulation
  - SI joints: Oblique; patient 25-30° posterior oblique
- Radiographs: Hip (unless otherwise indicated cassette horizontal to floor, tube perpendicular to floor, patient supine, legs extended)
  - AP
  - Frog lateral: Supine, knees & hips flexed, hip externally rotated, soles of feet together
    - Visualizes femoral head & upper femur
    - Used in pediatrics, evaluation AVN, SCFE
  - Axiolateral, shoot thru lateral, trauma lateral, groin lateral: Supine, opposite leg elevated/flexed, cassette vertical parallel femoral neck, tube parallels table & perpendicular to cassette
    - Keeps injured leg immobile
    - Evaluate suspected femoral neck fracture
  - Lauenstein lateral: Patient steep lateral affected side down, affected hip/knee flexed
    - Evaluate nontraumatic conditions femoral head, proximal femur, i.e., arthritis
  - False profile: Affected side 65° posterior oblique
    - Evaluate anterior femoral acetabular coverage (see "Measurements and Lines" section)
- CT
  - 5 mm thick reconstructed axial images entire pelvis
  - 2.5 mm thick reconstructed axial images through hip joint
    - Intra-articular fragments/bodies especially post-trauma
    - Contrast: Air for bodies, air + contrast for cartilage
  - 1-3 mm thick coronal and sagittal reconstructions
  - 3D imaging for fractures especially acetabulum
- MR
  - Fluid sensitive sequence to screen entire pelvis; coronal plane preferred
    - FOV: 32-44 cm; THK: 5-8 mm
  - T1 & fluid sensitive sequences painful side
    - Use surface coil
    - FOV: 14-26 cm, THK: 3-5 mm: Matrix 256 x 256
    - Sagittal, axial, coronal, oblique axial planes
- Arthrography, CT arthrography, MR arthrography, iliopsoas bursography (see "Hip Joint" section)

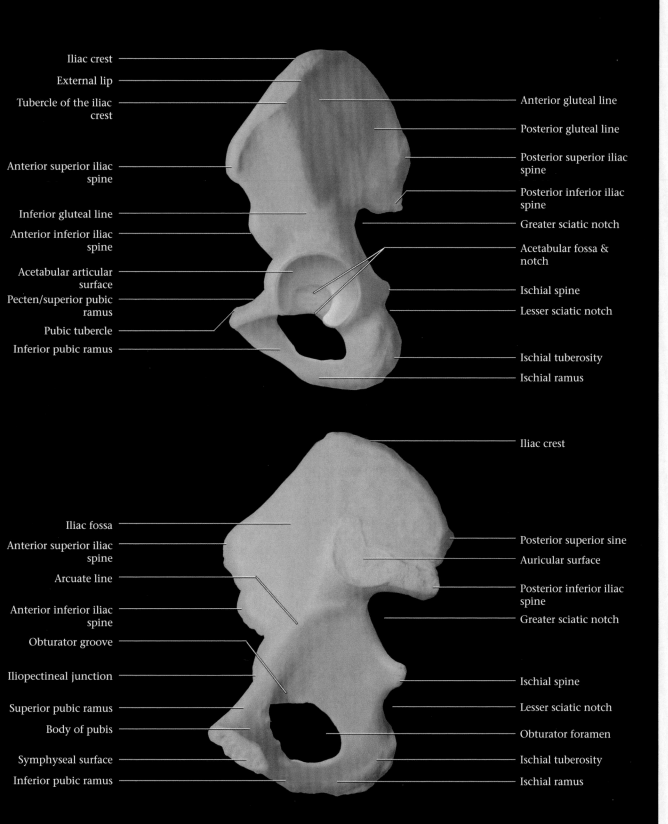

Iliac crest

External lip

Tubercle of the iliac crest

Anterior gluteal line

Posterior gluteal line

Anterior superior iliac spine

Posterior superior iliac spine

Posterior inferior iliac spine

Inferior gluteal line

Anterior inferior iliac spine

Greater sciatic notch

Acetabular fossa & notch

Acetabular articular surface

Pecten/superior pubic ramus

Ischial spine

Lesser sciatic notch

Pubic tubercle

Inferior pubic ramus

Ischial tuberosity

Ischial ramus

Iliac crest

Iliac fossa

Anterior superior iliac spine

Posterior superior sine

Arcuate line

Auricular surface

Anterior inferior iliac spine

Posterior inferior iliac spine

Obturator groove

Greater sciatic notch

Iliopectineal junction

Ischial spine

Superior pubic ramus

Lesser sciatic notch

Body of pubis

Obturator foramen

Symphyseal surface

Ischial tuberosity

Inferior pubic ramus

Ischial ramus

(Top) External surface of the pelvis. Note orientation with anterior superior iliac spine & symphysis pubis along the same vertical axis, acetabular notch inferior. **(Bottom)** Internal surface of the pelvis.

GRAPHICS, SACRUM

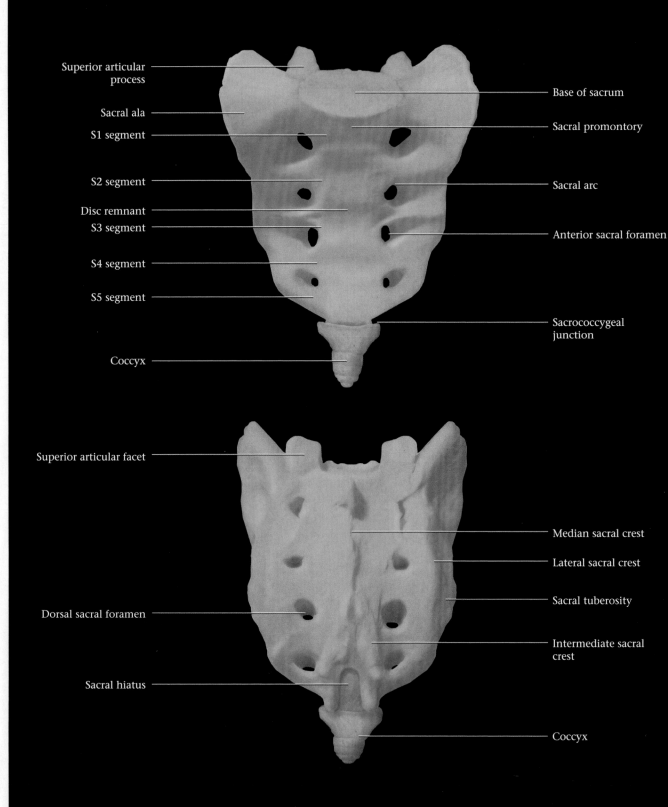

Superior articular process — Base of sacrum

Sacral ala — Sacral promontory

S1 segment

S2 segment — Sacral arc

Disc remnant
S3 segment — Anterior sacral foramen

S4 segment

S5 segment

Sacrococcygeal junction

Coccyx

Superior articular facet

Median sacral crest

Lateral sacral crest

Sacral tuberosity

Dorsal sacral foramen — Intermediate sacral crest

Sacral hiatus

Coccyx

(Top) Anterior view. The sacral promontory is the upper aspect of the S1 segment. The sacral ala are the lateral "wings" of the sacrum. Note the residual structures of the vertebral bodies including the disc remnants and neural foramina between each segment. (Bottom) Posterior view. The remnants of the vertebral body are not as readily appreciated as anteriorly. The medial sacral crest of the fused spinous processes, the intermediate sacral crest of the the fused articular processes and the lateral sacral crest of the fused transverse processes are all visible. The long and short dorsal sacroiliac ligaments attach to the lateral sacral crests. The incomplete fusion of the laminae in the lower sacrum creates the sacral hiatus. The hiatus is used as an access portal to the epidural space.

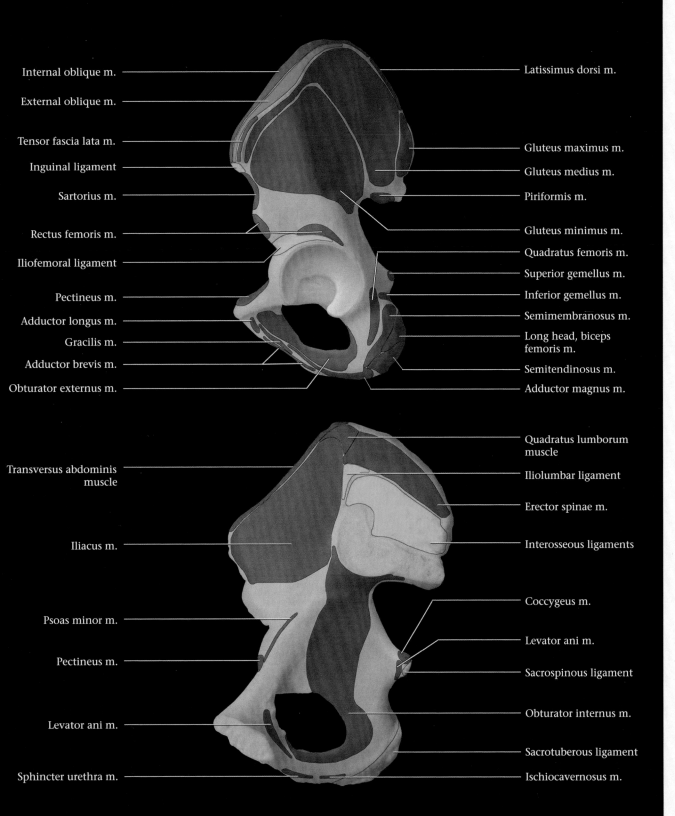

Internal oblique m.

External oblique m.

Tensor fascia lata m.

Inguinal ligament

Sartorius m.

Rectus femoris m.

Iliofemoral ligament

Pectineus m.

Adductor longus m.

Gracilis m.

Adductor brevis m.

Obturator externus m.

Latissimus dorsi m.

Gluteus maximus m.

Gluteus medius m.

Piriformis m.

Gluteus minimus m.

Quadratus femoris m.

Superior gemellus m.

Inferior gemellus m.

Semimembranosus m.

Long head, biceps femoris m.

Semitendinosus m.

Adductor magnus m.

Transversus abdominis muscle

Iliacus m.

Psoas minor m.

Pectineus m.

Levator ani m.

Sphincter urethra m.

Quadratus lumborum muscle

Iliolumbar ligament

Erector spinae m.

Interosseous ligaments

Coccygeus m.

Levator ani m.

Sacrospinous ligament

Obturator internus m.

Sacrotuberous ligament

Ischiocavernosus m.

(Top) Muscle and ligament attachments to the external surface of the pelvis. Note the relatively small origin of the tendon of the adductor longus muscle. The adductor brevis muscle is just deep to the longus muscle. The origin of the gracilis muscle is lateral to the adductor brevis muscle. The adductor magnus muscle has a broad origin with its posterior fibers in close proximity to the hamstring tendon origins. **(Bottom)** Muscle and ligament attachments to the internal surface of the pelvis. The muscles of the lower extremity include the iliacus, psoas, pectineus, and obturator internus muscles.

GRAPHICS, MUSCLES OF THIGH AT PELVIS

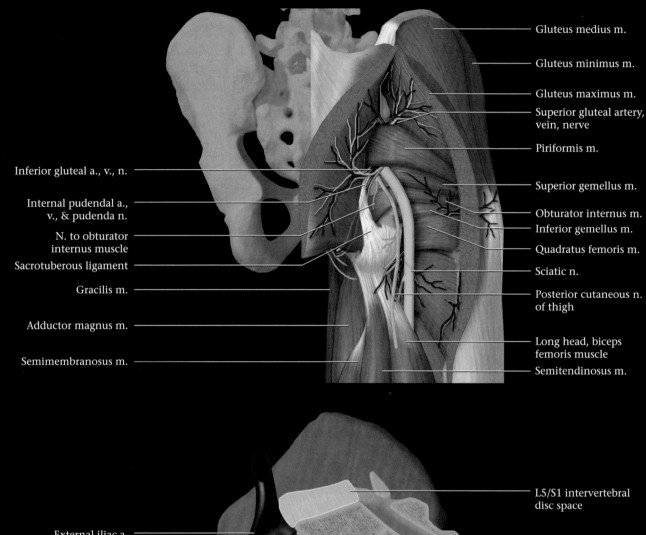

Gluteus medius m.

Gluteus minimus m.

Gluteus maximus m.

Superior gluteal artery, vein, nerve

Piriformis m.

Inferior gluteal a., v., n.

Internal pudendal a., v., & pudenda n.

N. to obturator internus muscle

Sacrotuberous ligament

Gracilis m.

Adductor magnus m.

Semimembranosus m.

Superior gemellus m.

Obturator internus m.

Inferior gemellus m.

Quadratus femoris m.

Sciatic n.

Posterior cutaneous n. of thigh

Long head, biceps femoris muscle

Semitendinosus m.

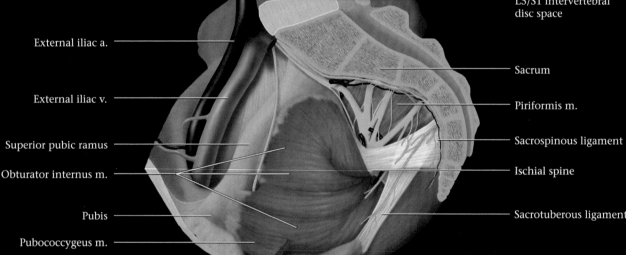

External iliac a.

External iliac v.

Superior pubic ramus

Obturator internus m.

Pubis

Pubococcygeus m.

Urogenital diaphragm

L5/S1 intervertebral disc space

Sacrum

Piriformis m.

Sacrospinous ligament

Ischial spine

Sacrotuberous ligament

Ischial tuberosity

(Top) The posterior structures of the proximal thigh at the level of the pelvis. The external rotators of the hip arise from the posterior surface of the pelvis. The adductor muscles of the thigh originate from the anterior structures of the pelvis. The sciatic nerve is the main innervation of the posterior muscles. Detailed descriptions of the external rotators, the greater sciatic notch and the adductor muscles are presented in the "Lateral Hip", "Posterior Pelvis", "Anterior Pelvis and Thigh" sections respectively. **(Bottom)** Medial view of the pelvic structures. The obturator internus muscle has an extensive origin from the inner aspect of the pelvis and funnels through the lesser sciatic notch before turning laterally to the piriformis fossa. The greater sciatic notch is filled with the piriformis muscle. The sacral plexus resides on the deep surface of the piriformis muscle.

HIP AND PELVIS OVERVIEW

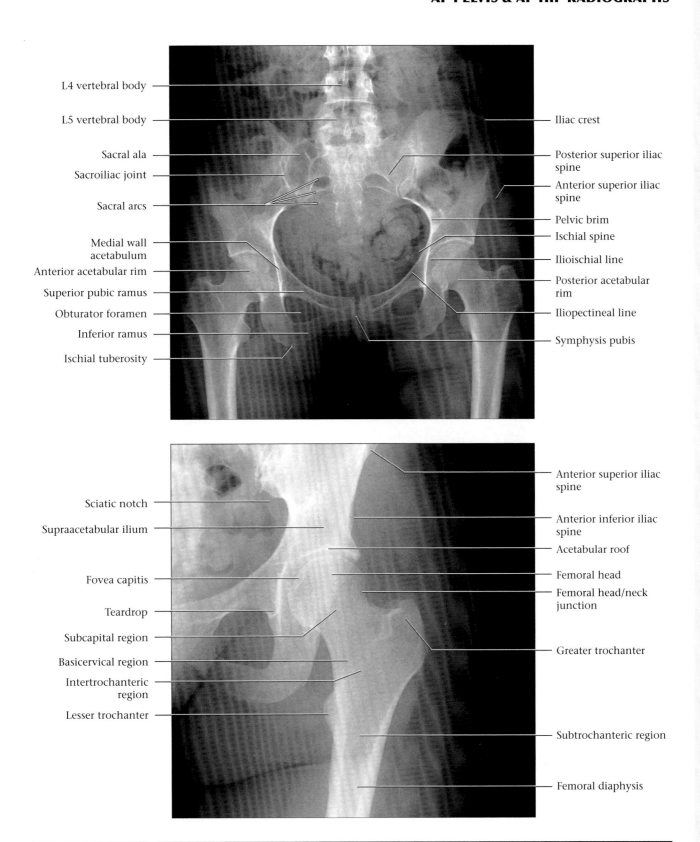

L4 vertebral body

L5 vertebral body

Sacral ala

Sacroiliac joint

Sacral arcs

Medial wall acetabulum

Anterior acetabular rim

Superior pubic ramus

Obturator foramen

Inferior ramus

Ischial tuberosity

Iliac crest

Posterior superior iliac spine

Anterior superior iliac spine

Pelvic brim

Ischial spine

Ilioischial line

Posterior acetabular rim

Iliopectineal line

Symphysis pubis

Sciatic notch

Supraacetabular ilium

Fovea capitis

Teardrop

Subcapital region

Basicervical region

Intertrochanteric region

Lesser trochanter

Anterior superior iliac spine

Anterior inferior iliac spine

Acetabular roof

Femoral head

Femoral head/neck junction

Greater trochanter

Subtrochanteric region

Femoral diaphysis

(Top) AP radiograph of the pelvis. Note continuity between the second sacral arc and the pelvic brim. Disruption of this continuity is a sign of malalignment. The symphysis pubis has a normal appearance. Multiple bony prominences are visible: Anterior superior & inferior iliac spines, posterior superior iliac spine, ischial spine, & pubic tubercle. The iliac crest extends from posterior to anterior superior iliac spines. The acetabular rims are visible. **(Bottom)** AP radiograph of the hip. The supra-acetabular ilium is above the acetabular roof. The thin medial acetabular wall overlaps the ilioischial line. The teardrop is present at the inferior aspect of the medial wall. The regions of the femoral neck are the subcapital region at the head-neck junction and the basicervical region adjacent to the intertrochanteric region.

LATERAL HIP RADIOGRAPHS

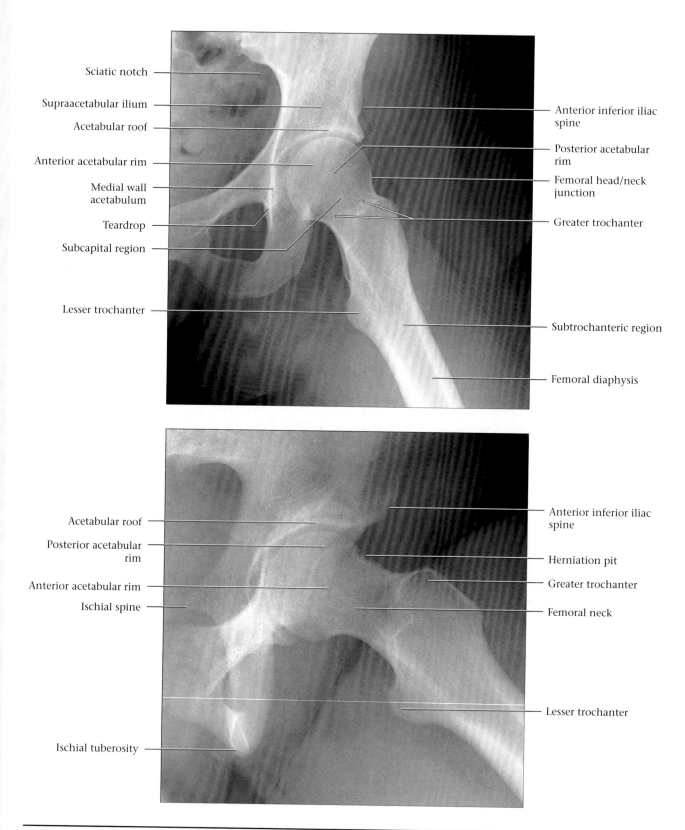

(Top) Frog lateral radiograph of the hip. The greater trochanter and femoral neck overlap. The femoral neck and shaft are in a straight line. As a result of the external rotation the anterior aspect of the femoral head is visible and the lesser trochanter is seen in profile. **(Bottom)** Lauenstein lateral of the hip. Similar to the frog lateral this view is obtained with posterior obliquity of the pelvis. Slightly different profiles of the greater trochanter and femoral neck are presented. The anterior aspect of the femoral head is well assessed. The relationship of the acetabular rims is reversed due to the obliquity. Note the herniation pit, located at the anterolateral aspect of the femoral neck. These may be seen normally, or be a part of the findings in femoral acetabular impingement. This view is frequently used in the workup of this syndrome.

HIP AND PELVIS OVERVIEW

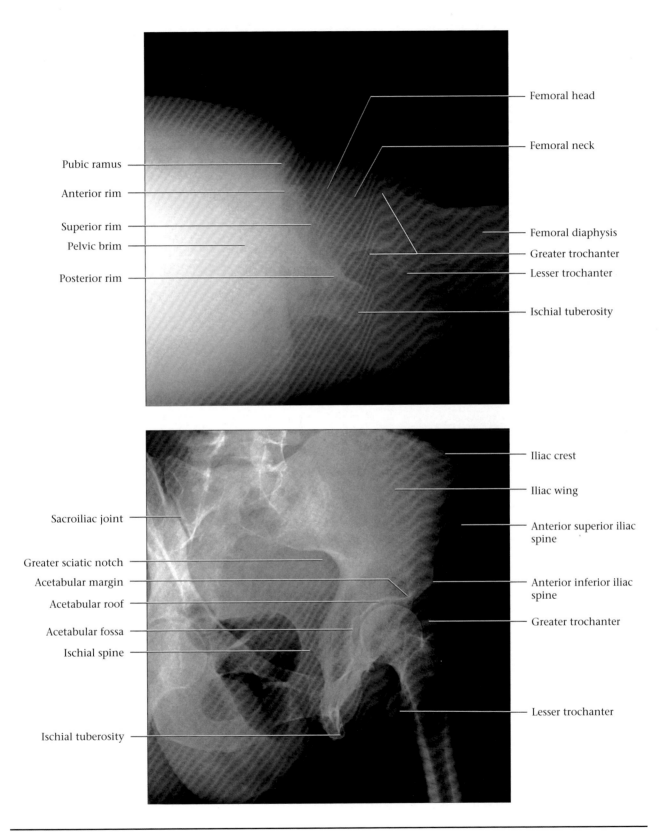

(Top) Axiolateral view of the hip most commonly used for suspected fracture or evaluation of acetabular version after total hip replacement. The prominence of the ischial tuberosity identifies the posterior aspect of the hip. Close inspection will reveal the triangular margins of the anterior and posterior acetabular rims. The superior rim is seen extending from anterior to posterior rim. The lesser trochanter is a posterior structure and the greater trochanter overlaps the femoral neck. **(Bottom)** False profile view of the left hip used to determine anterior acetabular coverage (see "Measurements and Lines" section). The anatomy is similar to the iliac oblique view although the obliquity is greater on this view (65 vs. 45 degrees). The anterior-most margin of the acetabular roof is seen and is a landmark for measurement.

RADIOGRAPHS, JUDET VIEWS

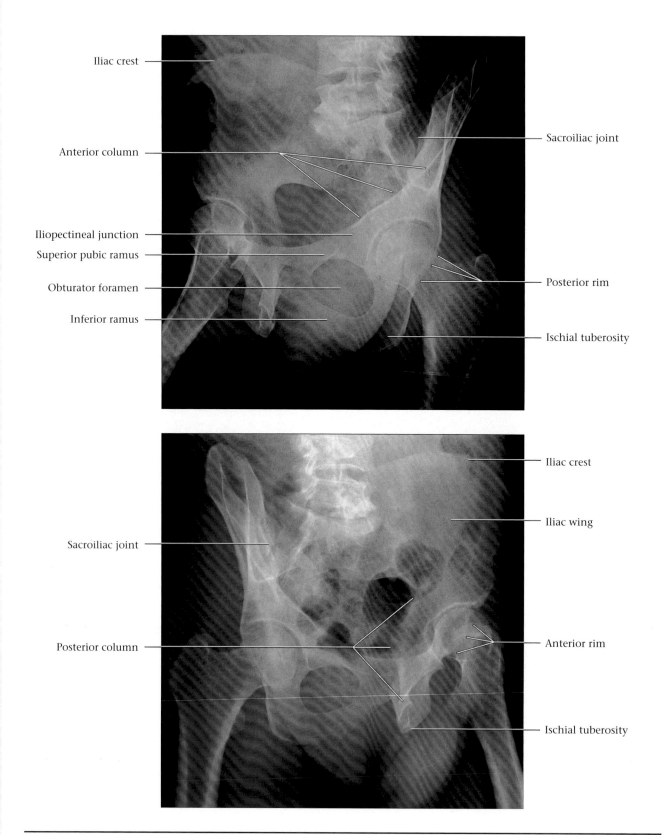

Iliac crest

Anterior column

Iliopectineal junction

Superior pubic ramus

Obturator foramen

Inferior ramus

Sacroiliac joint

Posterior rim

Ischial tuberosity

Sacroiliac joint

Posterior column

Iliac crest

Iliac wing

Anterior rim

Ischial tuberosity

(Top) Obturator (left anterior) oblique of the left hip (iliac oblique right hip). On this view the anterior or iliopectineal column of the acetabulum is seen in profile. The posterior acetabular rim is well visualized. **(Bottom)** Iliac (left posterior) oblique of the left hip (obturator oblique right hip). The posterior (ilioischial) column is profiled. The ischial spine protrudes from the posterior column (center limb of label). The anterior acetabular rim is well seen. Each oblique of the pelvis is an obturator oblique for one hip, iliac oblique for the other hip. For each hip one anterior and one posterior structure is profiled.

HIP AND PELVIS OVERVIEW

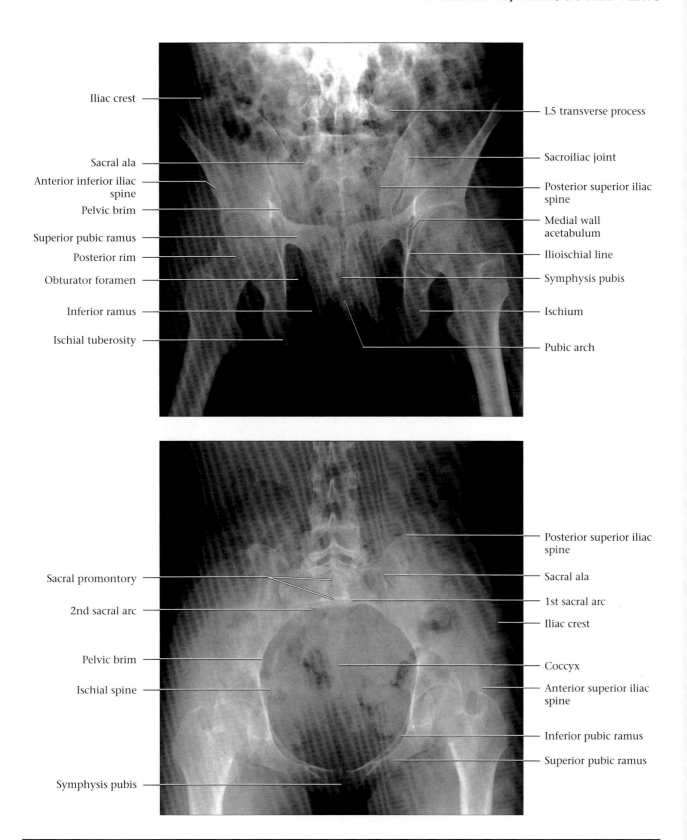

Iliac crest
Sacral ala
Anterior inferior iliac spine
Pelvic brim
Superior pubic ramus
Posterior rim
Obturator foramen
Inferior ramus
Ischial tuberosity

L5 transverse process
Sacroiliac joint
Posterior superior iliac spine
Medial wall acetabulum
Ilioischial line
Symphysis pubis
Ischium
Pubic arch

Sacral promontory
2nd sacral arc
Pelvic brim
Ischial spine
Symphysis pubis

Posterior superior iliac spine
Sacral ala
1st sacral arc
Iliac crest
Coccyx
Anterior superior iliac spine
Inferior pubic ramus
Superior pubic ramus

(Top) Outlet view of the pelvis used for determining superior to inferior displacements. On this radiograph note the relationship between the medial wall of the acetabulum and the ilioischial line. The pubic arch is well demonstrated in this projection. The arch is along the inferior margins of the inferior pubic rami. The pubic angle is the angle between the two inferior rami. **(Bottom)** Inlet view of the pelvis is used to assess anterior to posterior alignment within the pelvis. The pubic rami are nearly superimposed. The inferior ramus is slightly posterior to the superior ramus. The anterior and posterior iliac spines are well seen and the iliac crest between the two spines is laid out. Note continuity between the second sacral arc and the pelvic brim.

RADIOGRAPHS, SACRUM AND COCCYX

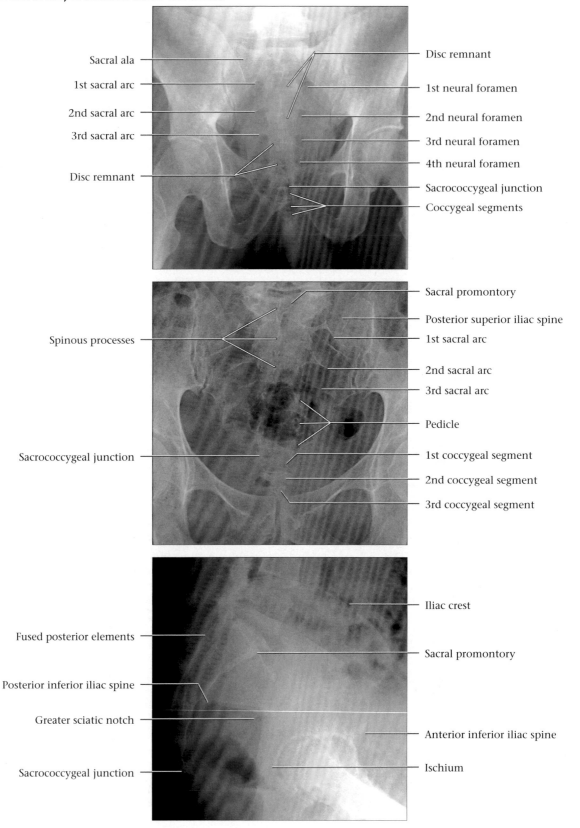

Sacral ala

1st sacral arc

2nd sacral arc

3rd sacral arc

Disc remnant

Disc remnant

1st neural foramen

2nd neural foramen

3rd neural foramen

4th neural foramen

Sacrococcygeal junction

Coccygeal segments

Spinous processes

Sacrococcygeal junction

Sacral promontory

Posterior superior iliac spine

1st sacral arc

2nd sacral arc

3rd sacral arc

Pedicle

1st coccygeal segment

2nd coccygeal segment

3rd coccygeal segment

Fused posterior elements

Posterior inferior iliac spine

Greater sciatic notch

Sacrococcygeal junction

Iliac crest

Sacral promontory

Anterior inferior iliac spine

Ischium

(Top) AP sacral radiograph. Each sacral segment is visualized with disc remnants between each segment. The nerve root exits below its respective segment just as in the lumbar spine. The neural foramina are easily appreciated. The sacral arcs are the superior margins of each neural foramina. **(Middle)** AP radiograph of the coccyx. The coccyx is projected above the anterior pelvic structures. Three coccygeal segments are visible. In this projection the pedicles and spinous processes of the sacral segments are visible. Looking past the sacrum the posterior superior iliac spine is present. The posterior inferior iliac spine is not easily identified on radiographs. **(Bottom)** Lateral view of the sacrum and coccyx. The entire pelvis is visible. The fused posterior elements can be appreciated. The greater sciatic notch is nicely demonstrated.

HIP AND PELVIS OVERVIEW

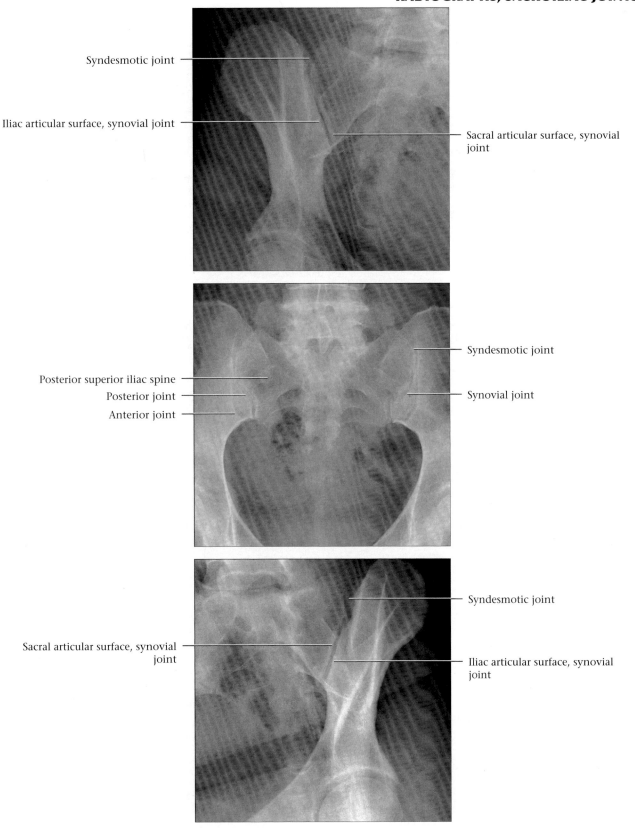

Syndesmotic joint

Iliac articular surface, synovial joint

Sacral articular surface, synovial joint

Posterior superior iliac spine

Posterior joint

Anterior joint

Syndesmotic joint

Synovial joint

Sacral articular surface, synovial joint

Syndesmotic joint

Iliac articular surface, synovial joint

(Top) In the left posterior oblique (right anterior oblique) the right sacroiliac joint is profiled and the articular surfaces delineated. The diagnostic usefulness of this view is limited. (Middle) AP radiograph of the sacroiliac joints. Two joints are visible. The lateral projecting joint is the anterior aspect of the joint, while the medial projecting joint is the posterior aspect of the joint. The superior 1/3 of the joint is syndesmotic. It appears as a widened "joint" and the articular surfaces are not congruent. Note the irregular but reciprocal contours of the articular surfaces of the synovial portion of the joint. This irregularity contributes to stability. This anatomy is discussed in the "Posterior Pelvis" section. (Bottom) In the right posterior oblique (left anterior oblique) position the articular surfaces of the left sacroiliac joint are profiled.

AXIAL T1 MR, UPPER PELVIS

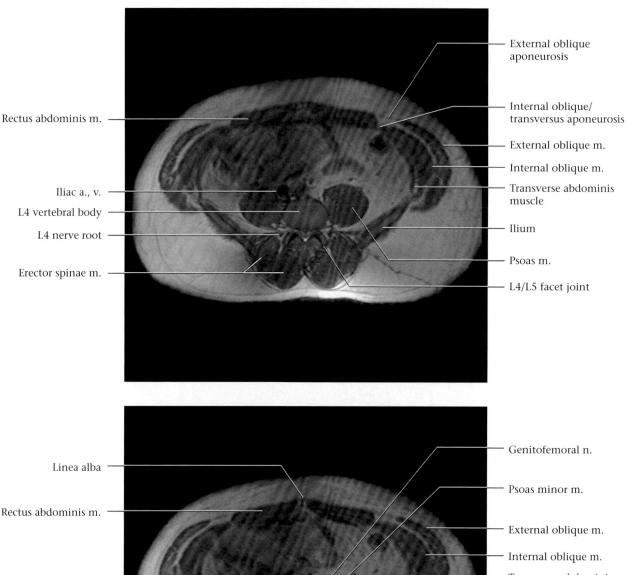

Rectus abdominis m.

Iliac a., v.

L4 vertebral body

L4 nerve root

Erector spinae m.

External oblique aponeurosis

Internal oblique/ transversus aponeurosis

External oblique m.

Internal oblique m.

Transverse abdominis muscle

Ilium

Psoas m.

L4/L5 facet joint

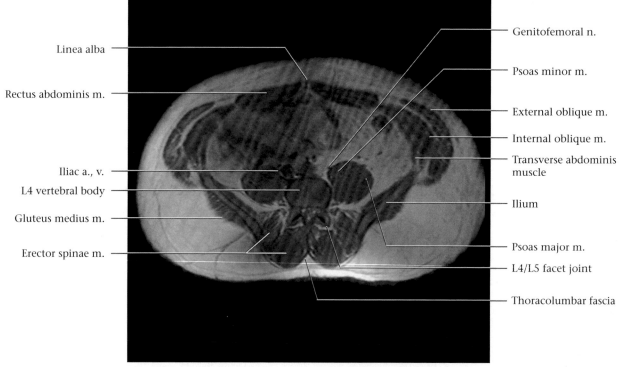

Linea alba

Rectus abdominis m.

Iliac a., v.

L4 vertebral body

Gluteus medius m.

Erector spinae m.

Genitofemoral n.

Psoas minor m.

External oblique m.

Internal oblique m.

Transverse abdominis muscle

Ilium

Psoas major m.

L4/L5 facet joint

Thoracolumbar fascia

(Top) First in series of thiry-four axial images of the pelvis, shown from superior to inferior. The three layers of the muscles of the lateral anterior abdominal wall are clearly visible. The psoas muscle courses inferiorly from its multifaceted spinal origin. The superior most aspect of the iliac crest corresponds to the L4/L5 intervertebral disc space. **(Bottom)** The aorta has just bifurcated. The paired rectus abdominis muscles in the center of the abdomen are visible.

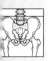

AXIAL T1 MR, UPPER PELVIS

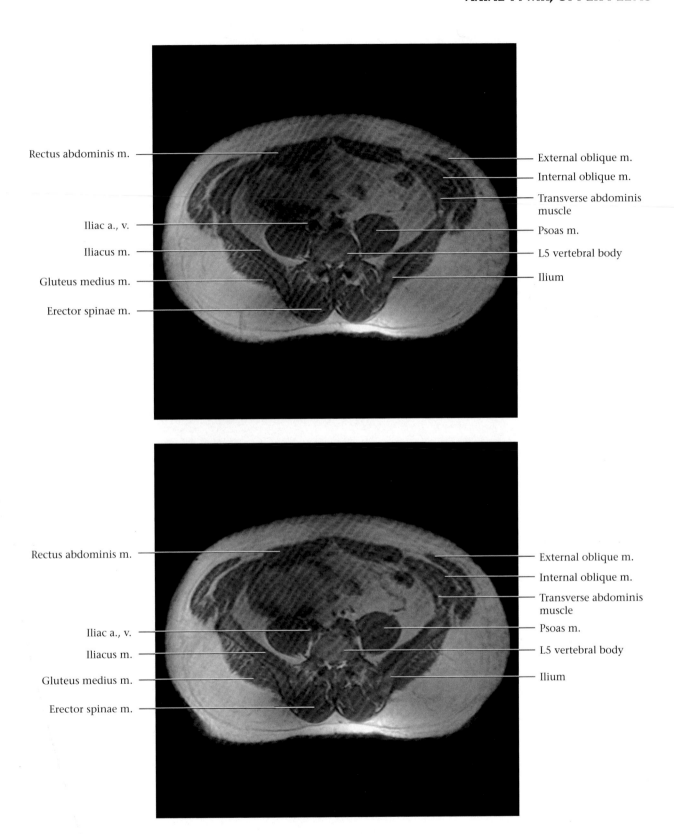

Rectus abdominis m. — External oblique m.

Internal oblique m.

Transverse abdominis muscle

Iliac a., v. — Psoas m.

Iliacus m. — L5 vertebral body

Gluteus medius m. — Ilium

Erector spinae m.

Rectus abdominis m. — External oblique m.

Internal oblique m.

Transverse abdominis muscle

Iliac a., v. — Psoas m.

Iliacus m. — L5 vertebral body

Gluteus medius m. — Ilium

Erector spinae m.

(Top) The gluteus medius muscle has the most superior origin of the gluteus muscles. The erector spinae muscles are a paired longitudinal muscle complex along the posterior aspect of the spine. **(Bottom)** The iliacus muscle has a broad origin from the deep surface of the ilium. Note the close association of the neurovascular bundle, coursing adjacent to the psoas. This association is maintained through the entire pelvis.

AXIAL T1 MR, UPPER PELVIS

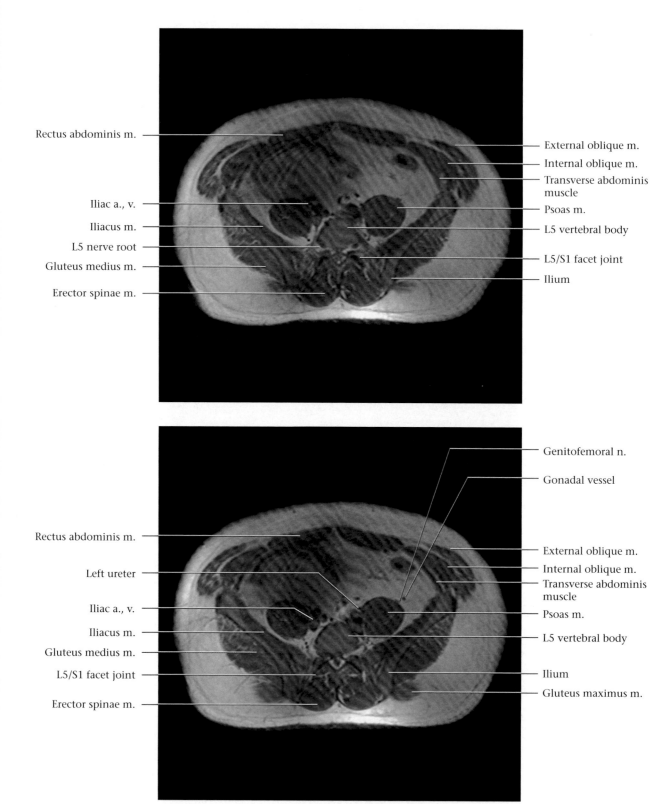

Rectus abdominis m.

External oblique m.

Internal oblique m.

Transverse abdominis muscle

Iliac a., v.

Psoas m.

Iliacus m.

L5 vertebral body

L5 nerve root

Gluteus medius m.

L5/S1 facet joint

Erector spinae m.

Ilium

Genitofemoral n.

Gonadal vessel

Rectus abdominis m.

External oblique m.

Left ureter

Internal oblique m.

Transverse abdominis muscle

Iliac a., v.

Psoas m.

Iliacus m.

L5 vertebral body

Gluteus medius m.

L5/S1 facet joint

Ilium

Erector spinae m.

Gluteus maximus m.

(Top) The L5 nerve root exits the neural foramina. The iliac vessels course along the medial aspect of the psoas muscle. Note that the iliacus & psoas remain separate through the majority of their pelvic course. **(Bottom)** The gluteus maximus muscle originates from the external surface of the ilium posterior to the gluteus medius muscle.

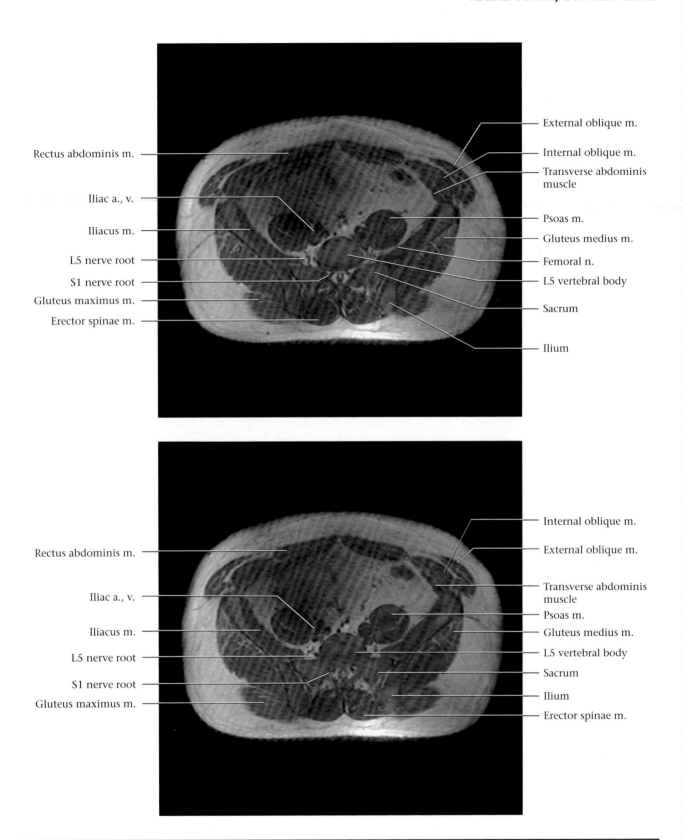

Rectus abdominis m.

Iliac a., v.

Iliacus m.

L5 nerve root

S1 nerve root

Gluteus maximus m.

Erector spinae m.

External oblique m.

Internal oblique m.

Transverse abdominis muscle

Psoas m.

Gluteus medius m.

Femoral n.

L5 vertebral body

Sacrum

Ilium

Rectus abdominis m.

Iliac a., v.

Iliacus m.

L5 nerve root

S1 nerve root

Gluteus maximus m.

Internal oblique m.

External oblique m.

Transverse abdominis muscle

Psoas m.

Gluteus medius m.

L5 vertebral body

Sacrum

Ilium

Erector spinae m.

(Top) The S1 nerve root has separated from the thecal sac. The transverse abdominis and internal oblique muscles are intimately related. They share a conjoined tendon/aponeurosis. The external oblique muscle is a more distinct muscle. **(Bottom)** Note the course of the L5 nerve root along the anterior aspect of the sacrum. The L5/S1 disc is partially visualized.

AXIAL T1 MR, UPPER PELVIS

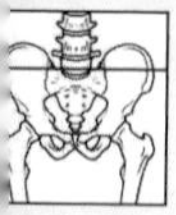

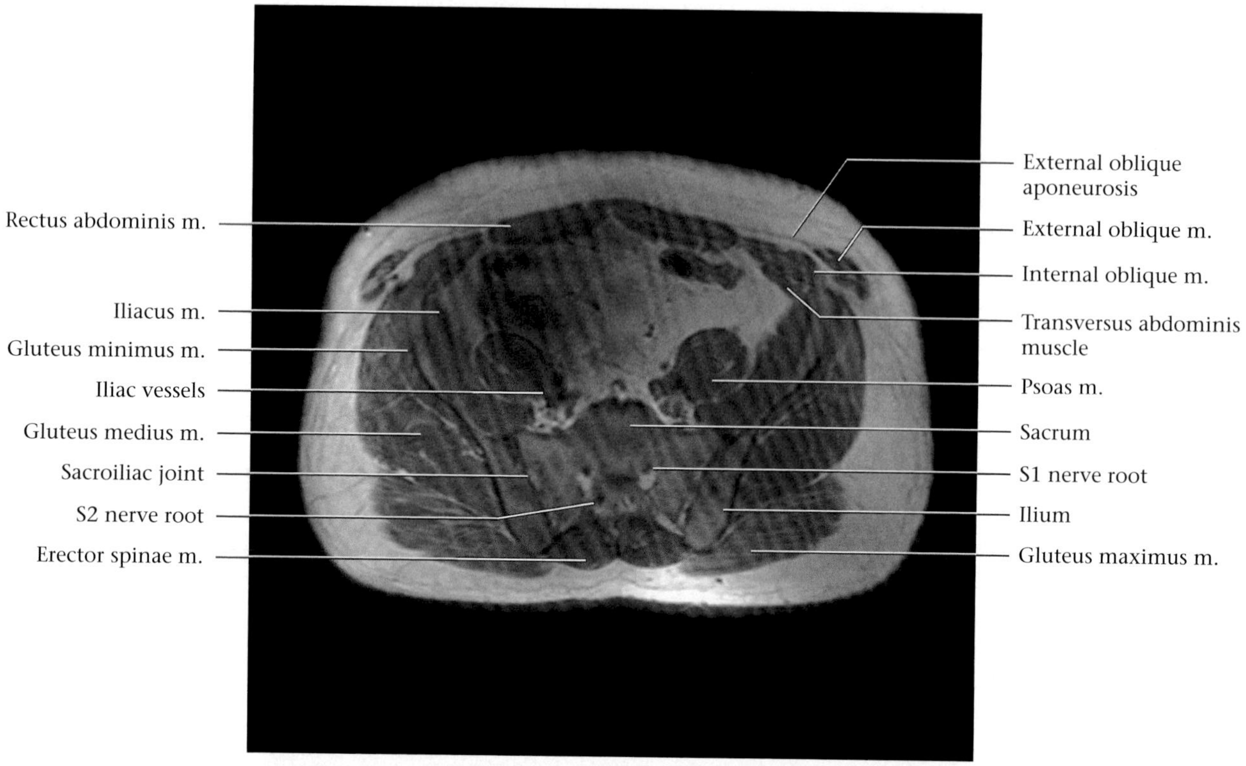
Rectus abdominis m.
Iliacus m.
Gluteus minimus m.
Iliac vessels
Gluteus medius m.
Sacroiliac joint
S2 nerve root
Erector spinae m.
External oblique aponeurosis
External oblique m.
Internal oblique m.
Transversus abdominis muscle
Psoas m.
Sacrum
S1 nerve root
Ilium
Gluteus maximus m.

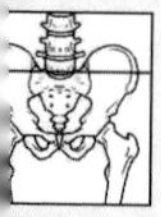

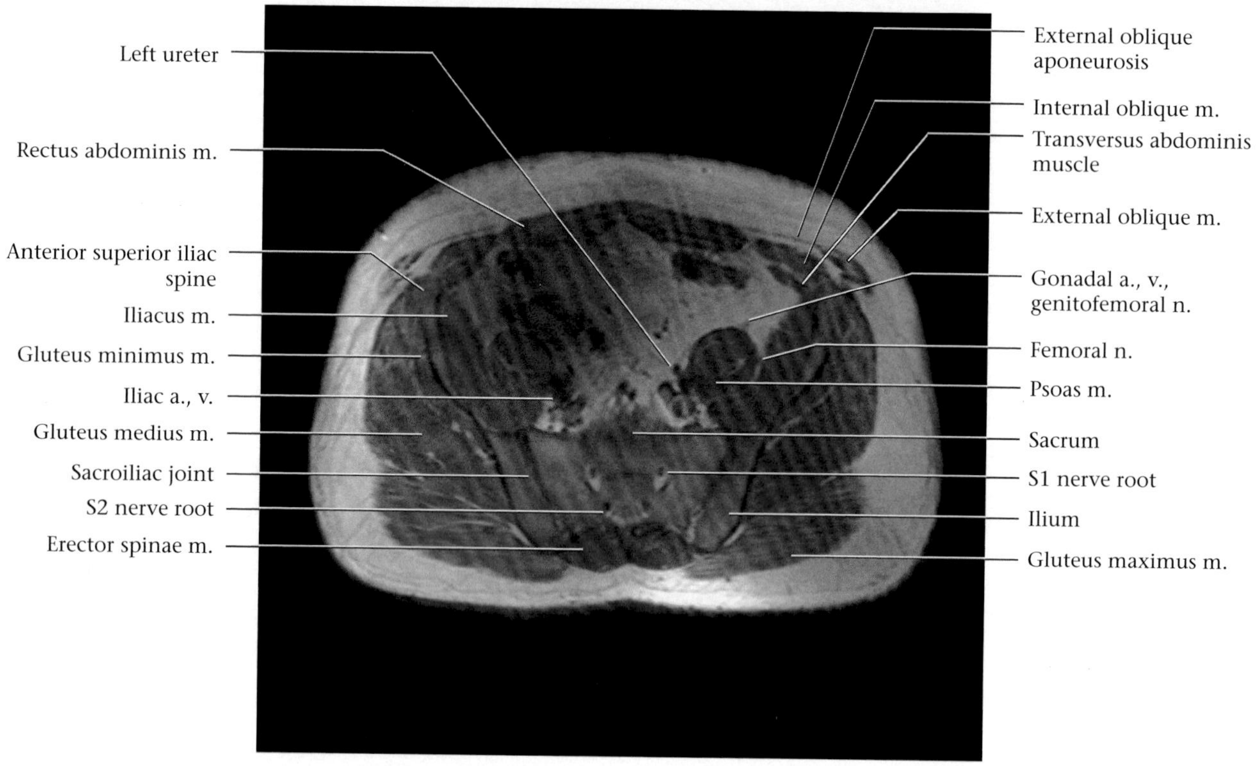
Left ureter
Rectus abdominis m.
Anterior superior iliac spine
Iliacus m.
Gluteus minimus m.
Iliac a., v.
Gluteus medius m.
Sacroiliac joint
S2 nerve root
Erector spinae m.
External oblique aponeurosis
Internal oblique m.
Transversus abdominis muscle
External oblique m.
Gonadal a., v., genitofemoral n.
Femoral n.
Psoas m.
Sacrum
S1 nerve root
Ilium
Gluteus maximus m.

(Top) The S2 nerve root is now apparent. The anterior synovial and posterior syndesmotic portions of the sacroiliac joint can be appreciated on this image. For more detail on this joint see "Posterior Pelvis". **(Bottom)** The origin of the gluteus minimus muscle is the most anterior of the gluteal muscles. The anterior superior iliac spine is seen as a bulbous enlargement from the anterior aspect of the ilium. It serves as the site of origin of the inguinal ligament. The ligament is the inferior edge of the external oblique aponeurosis.

HIP AND PELVIS OVERVIEW

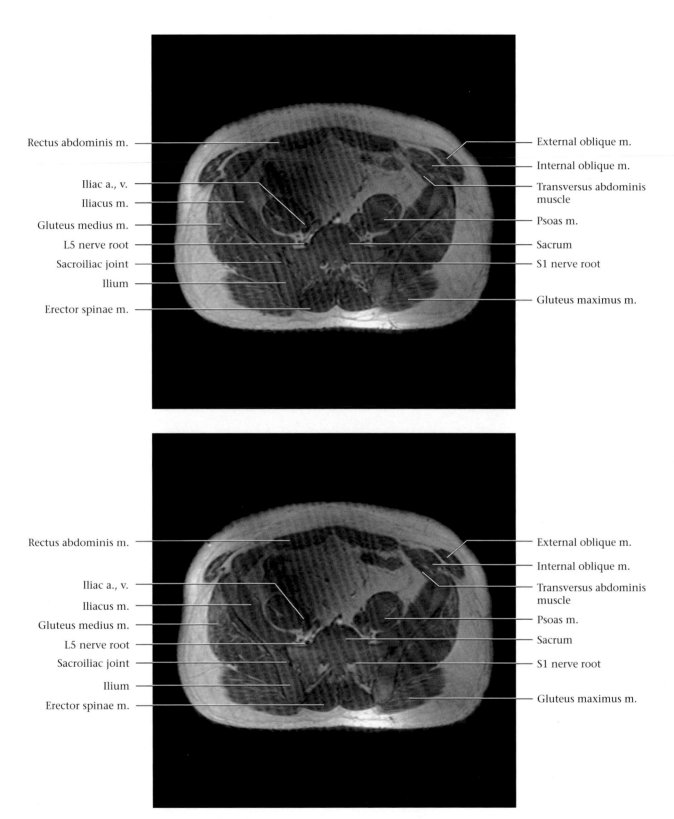

Rectus abdominis m. — External oblique m.

Internal oblique m.

Iliac a., v. — Transversus abdominis muscle

Iliacus m. —

Gluteus medius m. — Psoas m.

L5 nerve root — Sacrum

Sacroiliac joint — S1 nerve root

Ilium —

Erector spinae m. — Gluteus maximus m.

Rectus abdominis m. — External oblique m.

Internal oblique m.

Iliac a., v. — Transversus abdominis muscle

Iliacus m. —

Gluteus medius m. — Psoas m.

L5 nerve root — Sacrum

Sacroiliac joint — S1 nerve root

Ilium —

Erector spinae m. — Gluteus maximus m.

(Top) The gluteus maximus has an inferior and lateral course. At its superior aspect only a small portion of the muscle is visible. **(Bottom)** The erector spinae muscle complex diminishes in size as they near their inferior extent.

Hip and Pelvis

V

AXIAL T1 MR, MID PELVIS

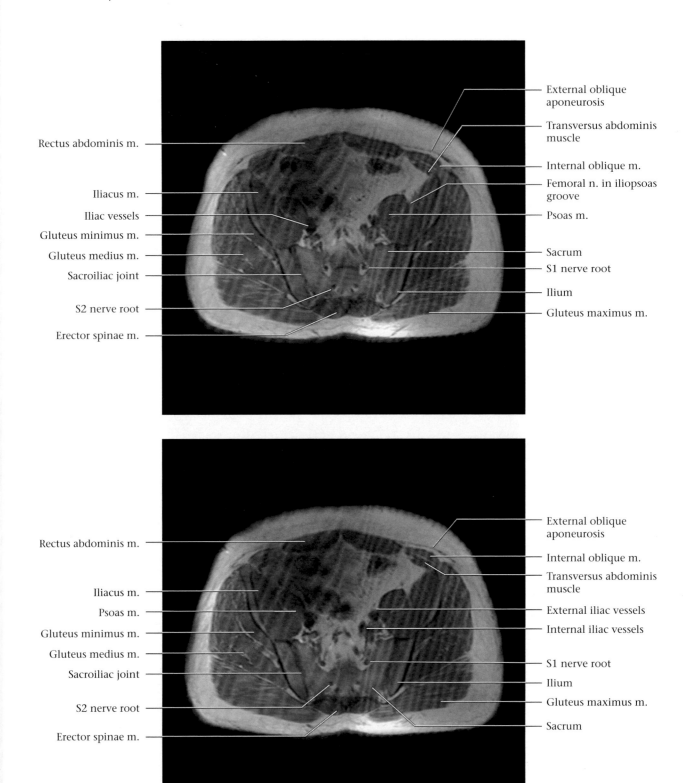

Top image labels (left): Rectus abdominis m., Iliacus m., Iliac vessels, Gluteus minimus m., Gluteus medius m., Sacroiliac joint, S2 nerve root, Erector spinae m.

Top image labels (right): External oblique aponeurosis, Transversus abdominis muscle, Internal oblique m., Femoral n. in iliopsoas groove, Psoas m., Sacrum, S1 nerve root, Ilium, Gluteus maximus m.

Bottom image labels (left): Rectus abdominis m., Iliacus m., Psoas m., Gluteus minimus m., Gluteus medius m., Sacroiliac joint, S2 nerve root, Erector spinae m.

Bottom image labels (right): External oblique aponeurosis, Internal oblique m., Transversus abdominis muscle, External iliac vessels, Internal iliac vessels, S1 nerve root, Ilium, Gluteus maximus m., Sacrum

(Top) Just below the anterior superior iliac spine the external oblique muscle belly is no longer visible. **(Bottom)** The iliac vessels have bifurcated. The internal iliac vessels will course posteriorly as they traverse the pelvis. At this more inferior level the sacroiliac joint is completely synovial.

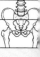

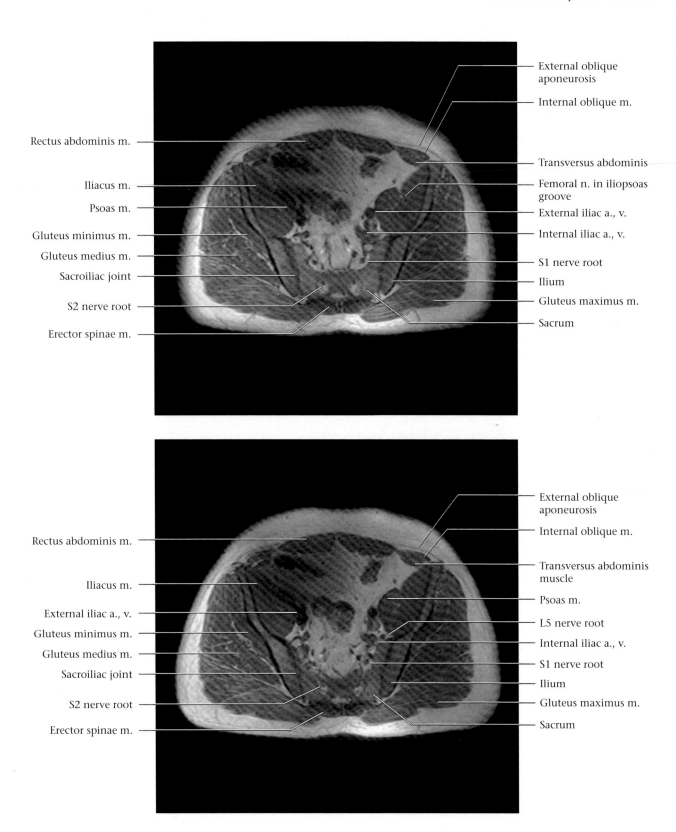

Rectus abdominis m.

Iliacus m.

Psoas m.

Gluteus minimus m.

Gluteus medius m.

Sacroiliac joint

S2 nerve root

Erector spinae m.

External oblique aponeurosis

Internal oblique m.

Transversus abdominis

Femoral n. in iliopsoas groove

External iliac a., v.

Internal iliac a., v.

S1 nerve root

Ilium

Gluteus maximus m.

Sacrum

Rectus abdominis m.

Iliacus m.

External iliac a., v.

Gluteus minimus m.

Gluteus medius m.

Sacroiliac joint

S2 nerve root

Erector spinae m.

External oblique aponeurosis

Internal oblique m.

Transversus abdominis muscle

Psoas m.

L5 nerve root

Internal iliac a., v.

S1 nerve root

Ilium

Gluteus maximus m.

Sacrum

(Top) Note the relative sizes of the gluteal muscles. **(Bottom)** The iliacus and psoas muscles are more difficult to identify as separate muscle bellies. Note how anterior the L5 nerve root is now located. The S1 nerve root is also moving anterior.

AXIAL T1 MR, MID PELVIS

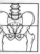

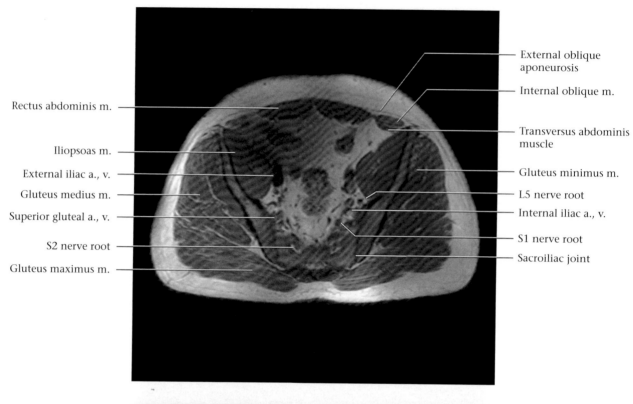

Rectus abdominis m.
Iliopsoas m.
External iliac a., v.
Gluteus medius m.
Superior gluteal a., v.
S2 nerve root
Gluteus maximus m.

External oblique aponeurosis
Internal oblique m.
Transversus abdominis muscle
Gluteus minimus m.
L5 nerve root
Internal iliac a., v.
S1 nerve root
Sacroiliac joint

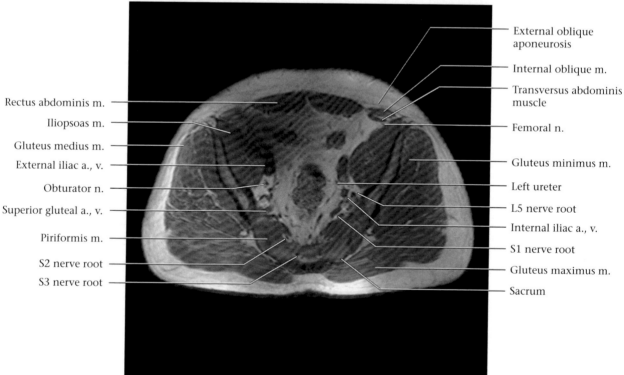

Rectus abdominis m.
Iliopsoas m.
Gluteus medius m.
External iliac a., v.
Obturator n.
Superior gluteal a., v.
Piriformis m.
S2 nerve root
S3 nerve root

External oblique aponeurosis
Internal oblique m.
Transversus abdominis muscle
Femoral n.
Gluteus minimus m.
Left ureter
L5 nerve root
Internal iliac a., v.
S1 nerve root
Gluteus maximus m.
Sacrum

(Top) Branches of the internal iliac vessels including the superior gluteal vessels are present within the pelvis. The external iliac vessels have maintained their position along the medial aspect of the psoas muscle. **(Bottom)** The obturator nerve is visible along the medial border of the psoas muscle posterior to the external iliac vessels. Its course is presented in greater detail in the "Posterior Pelvis" section.

AXIAL T1 MR, MID PELVIS

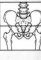

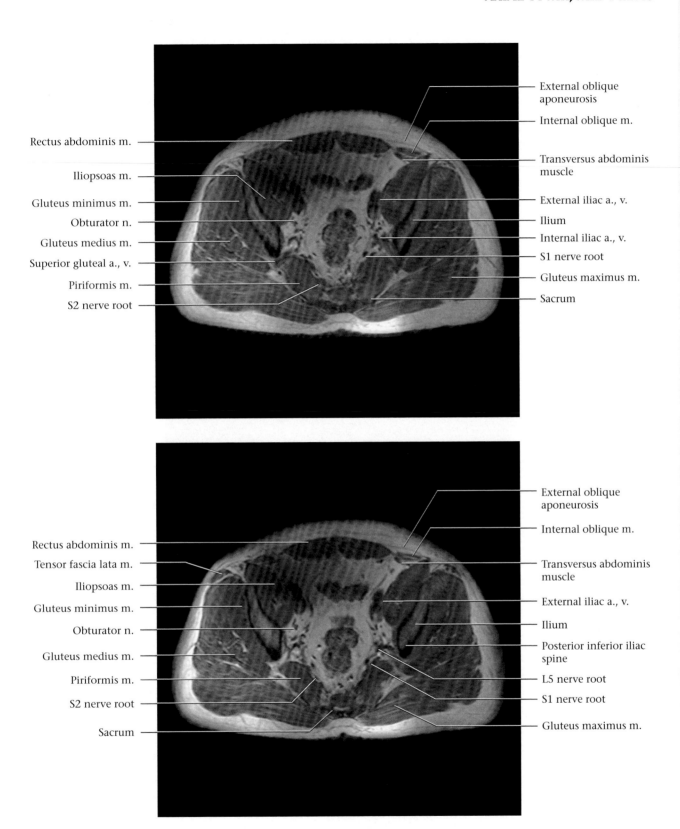

Rectus abdominis m.

Iliopsoas m.

Gluteus minimus m.

Obturator n.

Gluteus medius m.

Superior gluteal a., v.

Piriformis m.

S2 nerve root

External oblique aponeurosis

Internal oblique m.

Transversus abdominis muscle

External iliac a., v.

Ilium

Internal iliac a., v.

S1 nerve root

Gluteus maximus m.

Sacrum

Rectus abdominis m.

Tensor fascia lata m.

Iliopsoas m.

Gluteus minimus m.

Obturator n.

Gluteus medius m.

Piriformis m.

S2 nerve root

Sacrum

External oblique aponeurosis

Internal oblique m.

Transversus abdominis muscle

External iliac a., v.

Ilium

Posterior inferior iliac spine

L5 nerve root

S1 nerve root

Gluteus maximus m.

(Top) The superior gluteal vessels are exiting the pelvis along the superior border of the piriformis muscle. The internal oblique and transverse abdominis muscles are now more medially located than in more superior images. This position is consistent with their medial and inferior course. **(Bottom)** Muscle fibers of the tensor fascia lata are now visible. The posterior inferior iliac spine marks the superior posterior margin of the greater sciatic notch.

Hip and Pelvis

V

25

AXIAL T1 MR, MID PELVIS

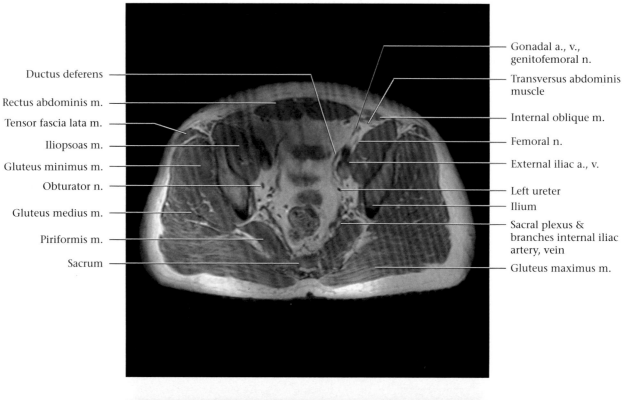

Ductus deferens

Rectus abdominis m.

Tensor fascia lata m.

Iliopsoas m.

Gluteus minimus m.

Obturator n.

Gluteus medius m.

Piriformis m.

Sacrum

Gonadal a., v., genitofemoral n.

Transversus abdominis muscle

Internal oblique m.

Femoral n.

External iliac a., v.

Left ureter

Ilium

Sacral plexus & branches internal iliac artery, vein

Gluteus maximus m.

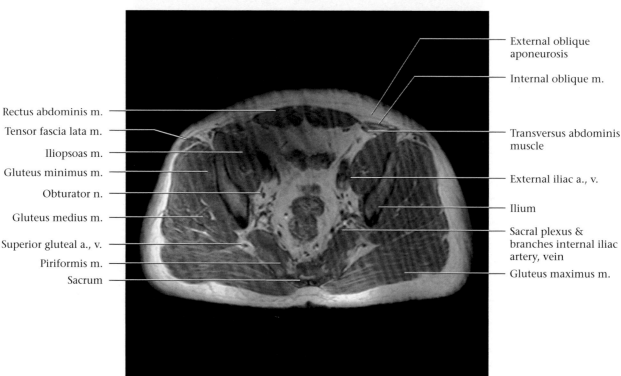

Rectus abdominis m.

Tensor fascia lata m.

Iliopsoas m.

Gluteus minimus m.

Obturator n.

Gluteus medius m.

Superior gluteal a., v.

Piriformis m.

Sacrum

External oblique aponeurosis

Internal oblique m.

Transversus abdominis muscle

External iliac a., v.

Ilium

Sacral plexus & branches internal iliac artery, vein

Gluteus maximus m.

(Top) A complex relationship exists between the branches of the internal iliac vessels and the nerve roots of the sacral plexus. These structures are identified along the deep surface of the piriformis muscle and are discussed in detail in the "Posterior Pelvis" section. **(Bottom)** Once they exists the pelvis the superior gluteal vessels travel in the fat plane deep to the gluteus maximus muscle.

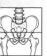
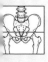

AXIAL T1 MR, MID PELVIS

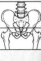

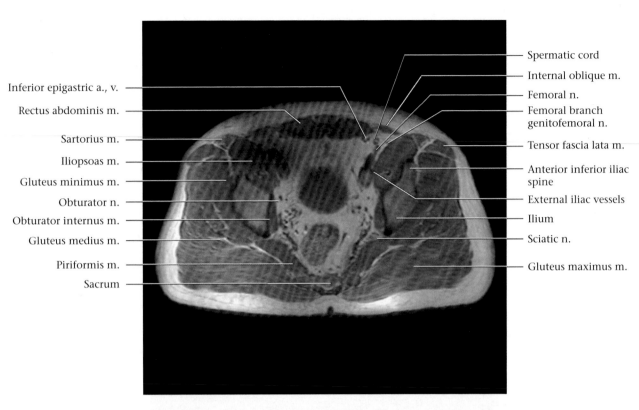

Top image labels (left): Inferior epigastric a., v. · Rectus abdominis m. · Sartorius m. · Iliopsoas m. · Gluteus minimus m. · Obturator n. · Obturator internus m. · Gluteus medius m. · Piriformis m. · Sacrum

Top image labels (right): Spermatic cord · Internal oblique m. · Femoral n. · Femoral branch genitofemoral n. · Tensor fascia lata m. · Anterior inferior iliac spine · External iliac vessels · Ilium · Sciatic n. · Gluteus maximus m.

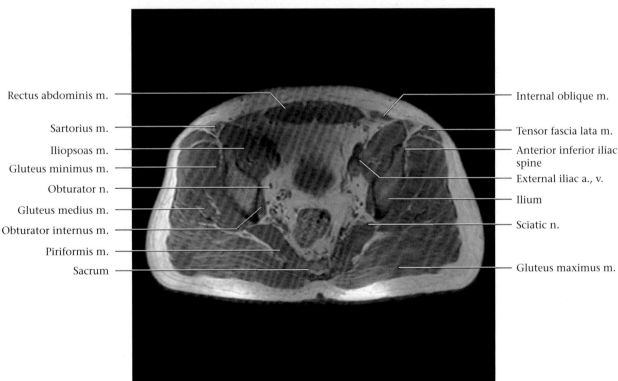

Bottom image labels (left): Rectus abdominis m. · Sartorius m. · Iliopsoas m. · Gluteus minimus m. · Obturator n. · Gluteus medius m. · Obturator internus m. · Piriformis m. · Sacrum

Bottom image labels (right): Internal oblique m. · Tensor fascia lata m. · Anterior inferior iliac spine · External iliac a., v. · Ilium · Sciatic n. · Gluteus maximus m.

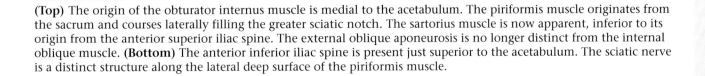

(Top) The origin of the obturator internus muscle is medial to the acetabulum. The piriformis muscle originates from the sacrum and courses laterally filling the greater sciatic notch. The sartorius muscle is now apparent, inferior to its origin from the anterior superior iliac spine. The external oblique aponeurosis is no longer distinct from the internal oblique muscle. **(Bottom)** The anterior inferior iliac spine is present just superior to the acetabulum. The sciatic nerve is a distinct structure along the lateral deep surface of the piriformis muscle.

AXIAL T1 MR, LOWER PELVIS

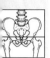

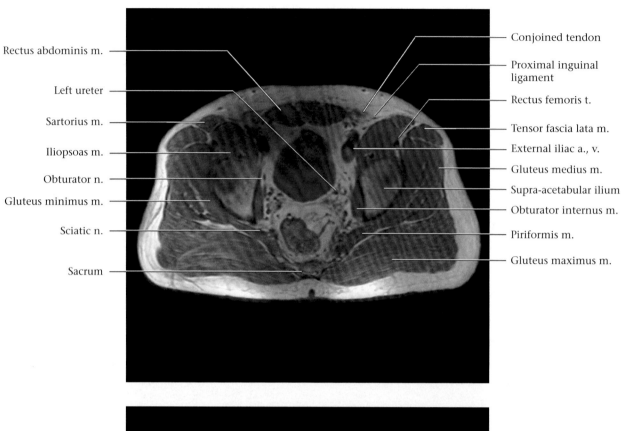

Rectus abdominis m.

Left ureter

Sartorius m.

Iliopsoas m.

Obturator n.

Gluteus minimus m.

Sciatic n.

Sacrum

Conjoined tendon

Proximal inguinal ligament

Rectus femoris t.

Tensor fascia lata m.

External iliac a., v.

Gluteus medius m.

Supra-acetabular ilium

Obturator internus m.

Piriformis m.

Gluteus maximus m.

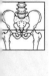

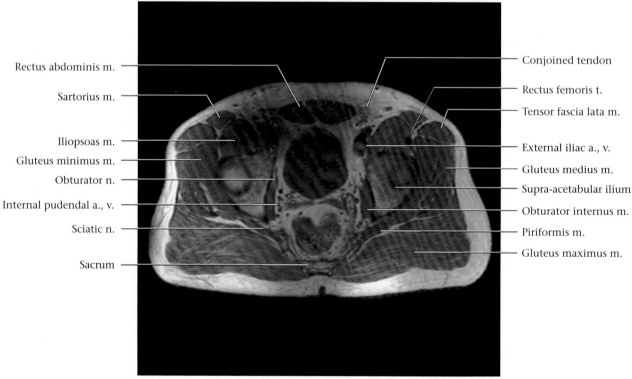

Rectus abdominis m.

Sartorius m.

Iliopsoas m.

Gluteus minimus m.

Obturator n.

Internal pudendal a., v.

Sciatic n.

Sacrum

Conjoined tendon

Rectus femoris t.

Tensor fascia lata m.

External iliac a., v.

Gluteus medius m.

Supra-acetabular ilium

Obturator internus m.

Piriformis m.

Gluteus maximus m.

(Top) The rectus femoris tendon is present between the iliopsoas muscle and gluteus minimus muscle after originating from the anterior inferior iliac spine. **(Bottom)** The inferior medial most aspect of the transverse abdominis and internal oblique muscles is evident as the conjoined tendon. Below this level the tendons are not distinct from the rectus abdominis muscle. The internal pudendal vessels are located posterior to the obturator nerve.

Hip and Pelvis

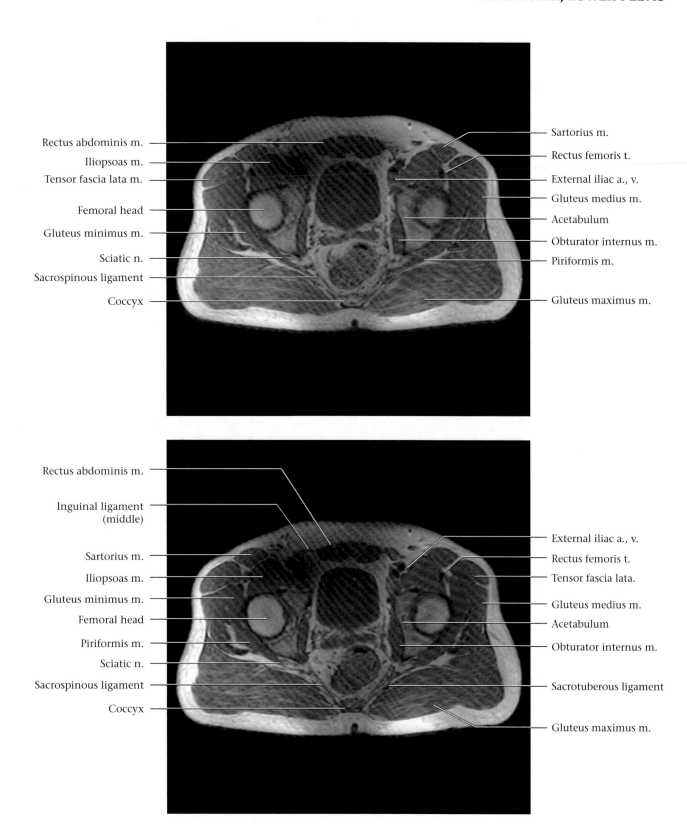
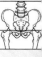

(Top) The sacrospinous ligament is visible. The iliopsoas muscle is intimately related to the anterior aspect of the hip joint. **(Bottom)** The sciatic nerve is present in its typical location just posterior to the acetabulum.

Hip and Pelvis

V

AXIAL T1 MR, LOWER PELVIS

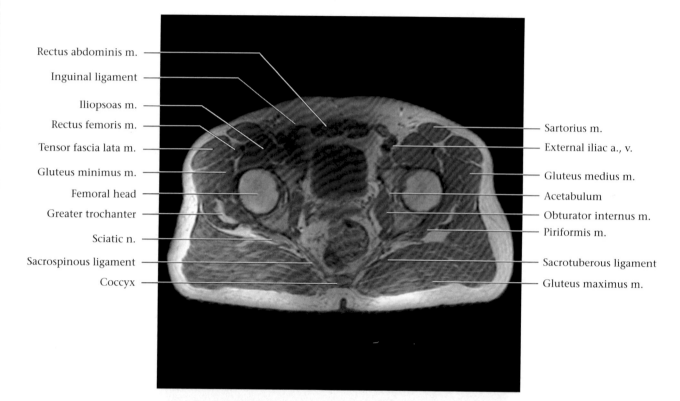

Rectus abdominis m.
Inguinal ligament
Iliopsoas m.
Rectus femoris m.
Tensor fascia lata m.
Gluteus minimus m.
Femoral head
Greater trochanter
Sciatic n.
Sacrospinous ligament
Coccyx

Sartorius m.
External iliac a., v.
Gluteus medius m.
Acetabulum
Obturator internus m.
Piriformis m.
Sacrotuberous ligament
Gluteus maximus m.

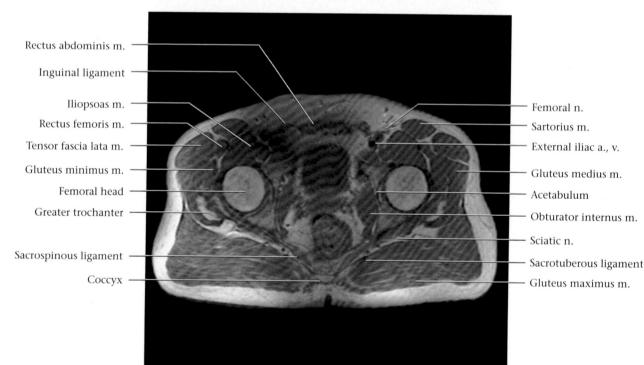

Rectus abdominis m.
Inguinal ligament
Iliopsoas m.
Rectus femoris m.
Tensor fascia lata m.
Gluteus minimus m.
Femoral head
Greater trochanter
Sacrospinous ligament
Coccyx

Femoral n.
Sartorius m.
External iliac a., v.
Gluteus medius m.
Acetabulum
Obturator internus m.
Sciatic n.
Sacrotuberous ligament
Gluteus maximus m.

(Top) The inguinal ligament is present just lateral to the rectus abdominis muscle. Like the muscles this structure also has an inferior medial course so that we only see segments and its most inferior extent will be medially located. **(Bottom)** Segments of the sacrotuberous ligament are present along the deep surface of the gluteus maximus muscle. The vertical orientation of this ligament means that only segments will be visible on axial images. For more detail on this structure see "Posterior Pelvis" section.

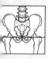
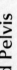

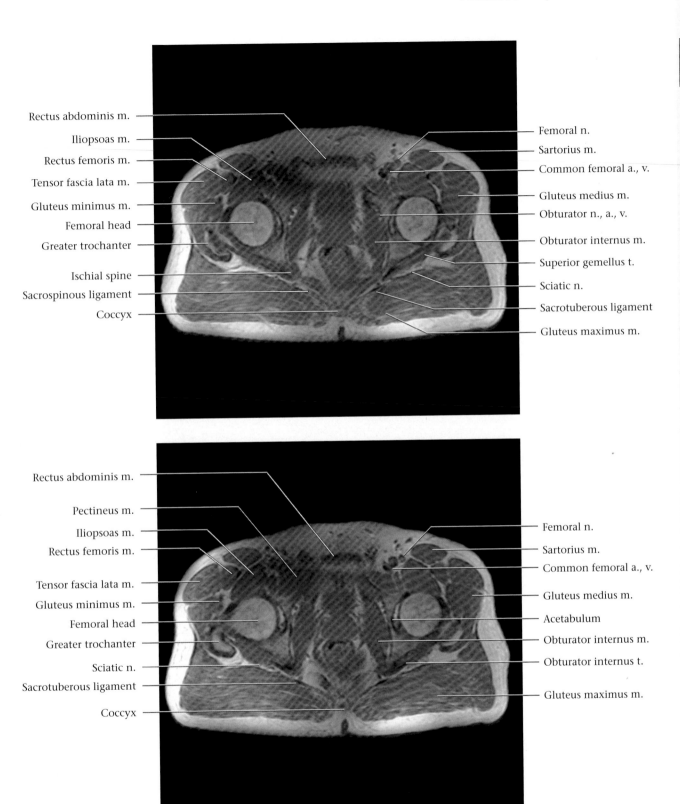

Rectus abdominis m.
Iliopsoas m.
Rectus femoris m.
Tensor fascia lata m.
Gluteus minimus m.
Femoral head
Greater trochanter
Ischial spine
Sacrospinous ligament
Coccyx

Femoral n.
Sartorius m.
Common femoral a., v.
Gluteus medius m.
Obturator n., a., v.
Obturator internus m.
Superior gemellus t.
Sciatic n.
Sacrotuberous ligament
Gluteus maximus m.

Rectus abdominis m.
Pectineus m.
Iliopsoas m.
Rectus femoris m.
Tensor fascia lata m.
Gluteus minimus m.
Femoral head
Greater trochanter
Sciatic n.
Sacrotuberous ligament
Coccyx

Femoral n.
Sartorius m.
Common femoral a., v.
Gluteus medius m.
Acetabulum
Obturator internus m.
Obturator internus t.
Gluteus maximus m.

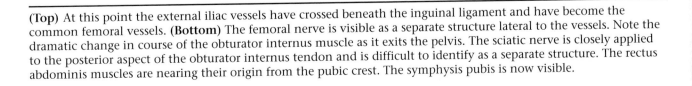

(Top) At this point the external iliac vessels have crossed beneath the inguinal ligament and have become the common femoral vessels. **(Bottom)** The femoral nerve is visible as a separate structure lateral to the vessels. Note the dramatic change in course of the obturator internus muscle as it exits the pelvis. The sciatic nerve is closely applied to the posterior aspect of the obturator internus tendon and is difficult to identify as a separate structure. The rectus abdominis muscles are nearing their origin from the pubic crest. The symphysis pubis is now visible.

AXIAL T1 MR, LOWER PELVIS

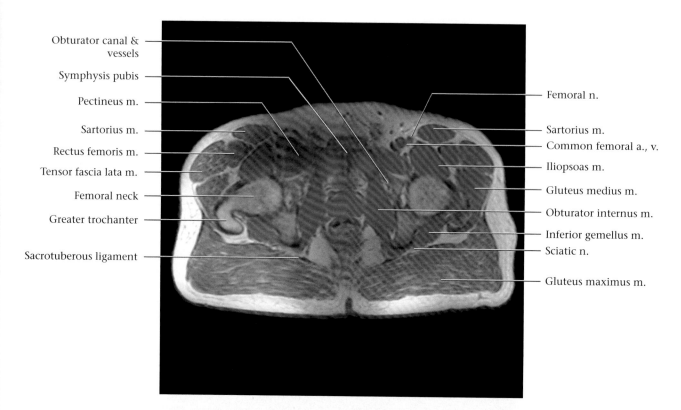

Obturator canal & vessels

Symphysis pubis

Pectineus m.

Sartorius m.

Rectus femoris m.

Tensor fascia lata m.

Femoral neck

Greater trochanter

Sacrotuberous ligament

Femoral n.

Sartorius m.

Common femoral a., v.

Iliopsoas m.

Gluteus medius m.

Obturator internus m.

Inferior gemellus m.

Sciatic n.

Gluteus maximus m.

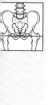

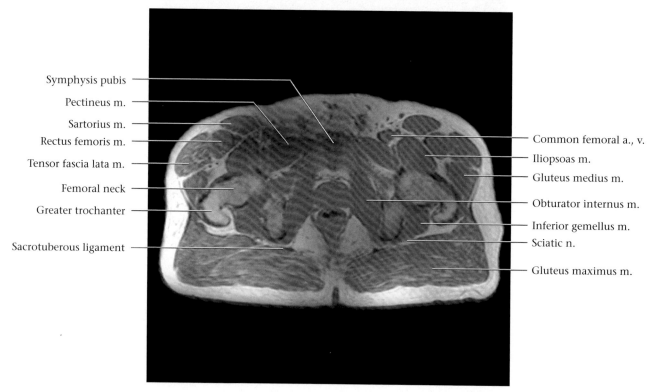

Symphysis pubis

Pectineus m.

Sartorius m.

Rectus femoris m.

Tensor fascia lata m.

Femoral neck

Greater trochanter

Sacrotuberous ligament

Common femoral a., v.

Iliopsoas m.

Gluteus medius m.

Obturator internus m.

Inferior gemellus m.

Sciatic n.

Gluteus maximus m.

(Top) Note the extension of tendon slips from the rectus abdominis along the anterior aspect of the symphysis pubis. These fibers serve to reinforce the joint. The adductor muscles of the thigh are now visible. The pectineus muscle is the most superior of these muscles. For a more thorough discussion of the adductor muscle origins see the "Anterior Pelvis and Thigh" section. **(Bottom)** At the opening of the obturator foramen the obturator internus covers the entire deep surface. The obturator externus muscle is not yet visible. To follow the structures of the thigh more inferiorly see the "Thigh Overview" section.

SAGITTAL T1 MR, MEDIAL PELVIS

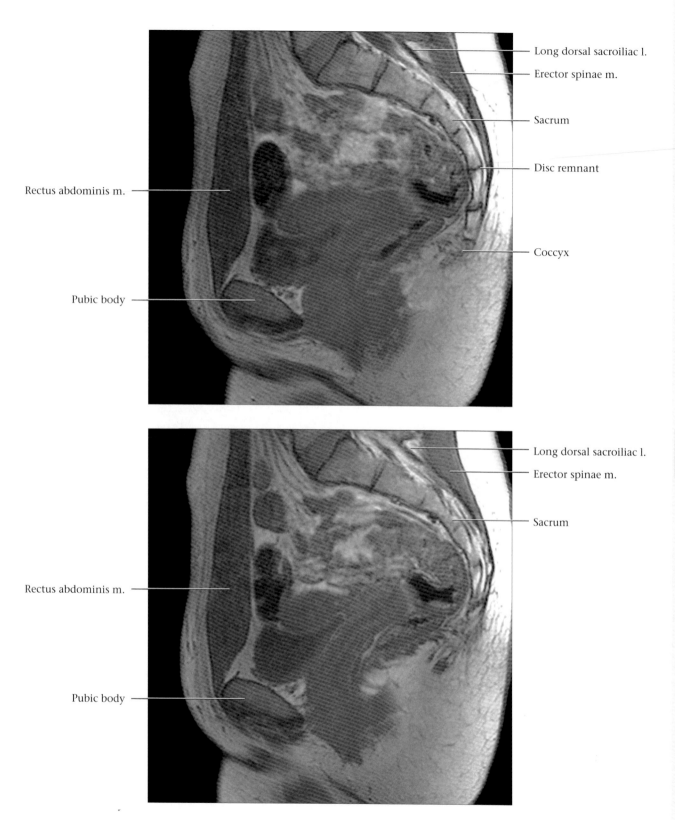

Long dorsal sacroiliac l.

Erector spinae m.

Sacrum

Disc remnant

Coccyx

Rectus abdominis m.

Pubic body

Long dorsal sacroiliac l.

Erector spinae m.

Sacrum

Rectus abdominis m.

Pubic body

(Top) First of thirty-eight sagittal images of the pelvis and upper thigh from medial to lateral. The sacrum and coccyx and their individual segments and disc remnants are easily appreciated. This image is off midline and the spinal canal is not present. **(Bottom)** The rectus abdominis muscle is a longitudinally oriented midline muscle that originates from the pubic crest and superior pubic ramus.

SAGITTAL T1 MR, MEDIAL PELVIS

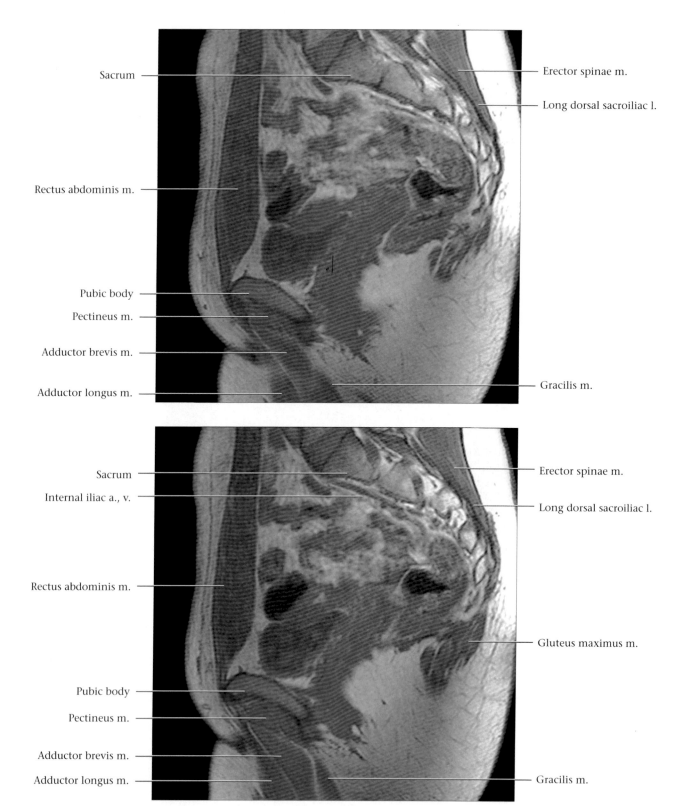

Sacrum — Erector spinae m.

Long dorsal sacroiliac l.

Rectus abdominis m.

Pubic body — Pectineus m. — Adductor brevis m. — Adductor longus m. — Gracilis m.

Sacrum — Erector spinae m.

Internal iliac a., v. — Long dorsal sacroiliac l.

Rectus abdominis m.

Gluteus maximus m.

Pubic body — Pectineus m. — Adductor brevis m. — Adductor longus m. — Gracilis m.

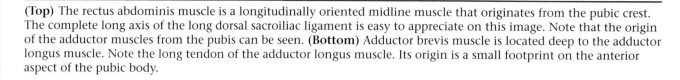

(Top) The rectus abdominis muscle is a longitudinally oriented midline muscle that originates from the pubic crest. The complete long axis of the long dorsal sacroiliac ligament is easy to appreciate on this image. Note that the origin of the adductor muscles from the pubis can be seen. **(Bottom)** Adductor brevis muscle is located deep to the adductor longus muscle. Note the long tendon of the adductor longus muscle. Its origin is a small footprint on the anterior aspect of the pubic body.

SAGITTAL T1 MR, MEDIAL PELVIS

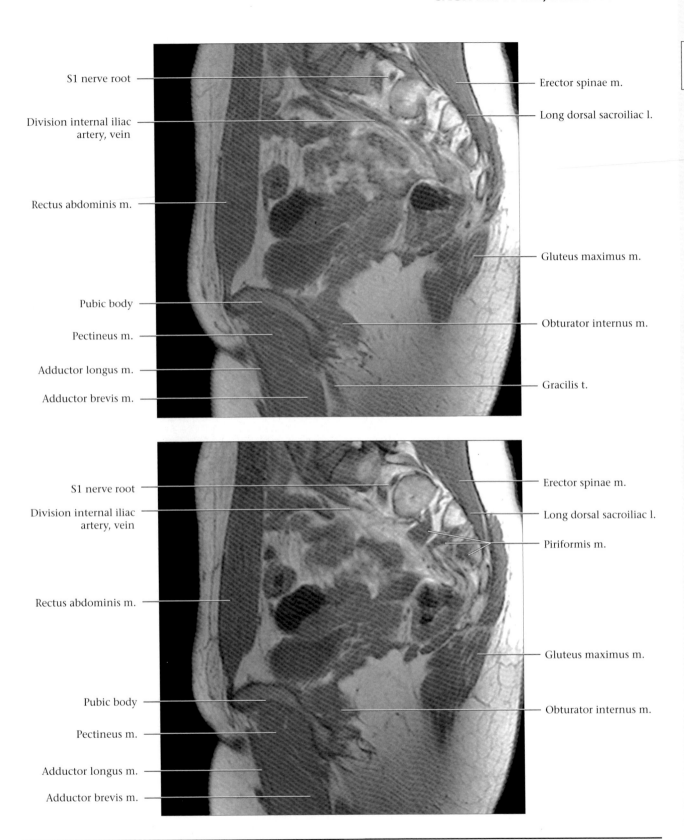

S1 nerve root — Erector spinae m.

Division internal iliac artery, vein — Long dorsal sacroiliac l.

Rectus abdominis m. — Gluteus maximus m.

Pubic body — Obturator internus m.

Pectineus m.

Adductor longus m. — Gracilis t.

Adductor brevis m.

S1 nerve root — Erector spinae m.

Division internal iliac artery, vein — Long dorsal sacroiliac l.

— Piriformis m.

Rectus abdominis m. — Gluteus maximus m.

Pubic body — Obturator internus m.

Pectineus m.

Adductor longus m.

Adductor brevis m.

(Top) The gracilis muscle is the most medial of the adductor muscles. It has a thin tendinous origin from the medial aspect of the inferior pubic ramus. **(Bottom)** The piriformis muscle takes origin from the anterior surface of the sacrum. The obturator internus muscles lines almost the entire deep surface of the pelvis.

Hip and Pelvis

V

35

SAGITTAL T1 MR, MEDIAL PELVIS

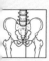

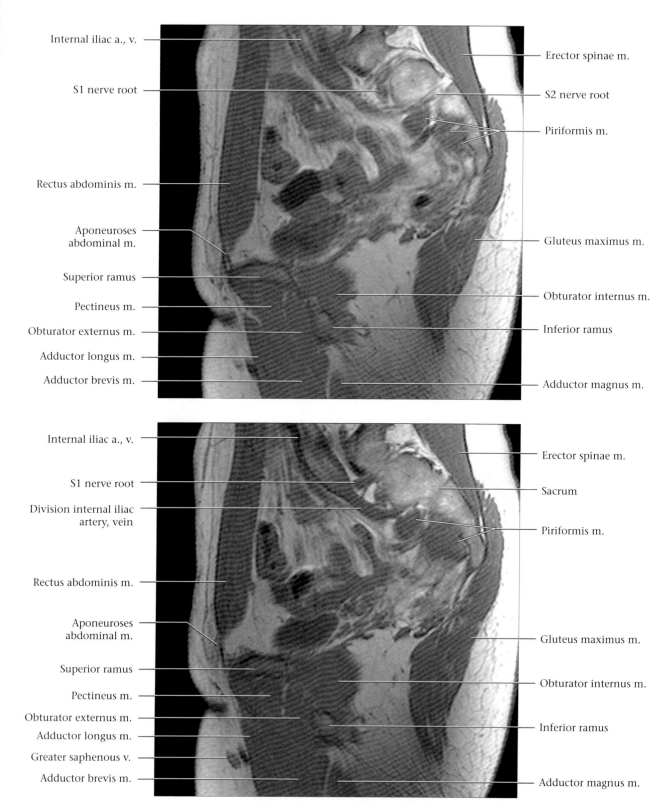

Internal iliac a., v.

S1 nerve root

Rectus abdominis m.

Aponeuroses abdominal m.

Superior ramus

Pectineus m.

Obturator externus m.

Adductor longus m.

Adductor brevis m.

Erector spinae m.

S2 nerve root

Piriformis m.

Gluteus maximus m.

Obturator internus m.

Inferior ramus

Adductor magnus m.

Internal iliac a., v.

S1 nerve root

Division internal iliac artery, vein

Rectus abdominis m.

Aponeuroses abdominal m.

Superior ramus

Pectineus m.

Obturator externus m.

Adductor longus m.

Greater saphenous v.

Adductor brevis m.

Erector spinae m.

Sacrum

Piriformis m.

Gluteus maximus m.

Obturator internus m.

Inferior ramus

Adductor magnus m.

(Top) The obturator foramen is between the superior and inferior pubic rami. The obturator internus and externus muscles arise from the respective surfaces of margins of the foramen and the membrane which covers the foramen. **(Bottom)** The adductor magnus muscle occupies the position assumed by the gracilis muscle on more medial images. The aponeuroses of the external and internal oblique and transversus abdominis muscles are present just lateral to the rectus abdominis muscle.

HIP AND PELVIS OVERVIEW

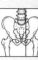

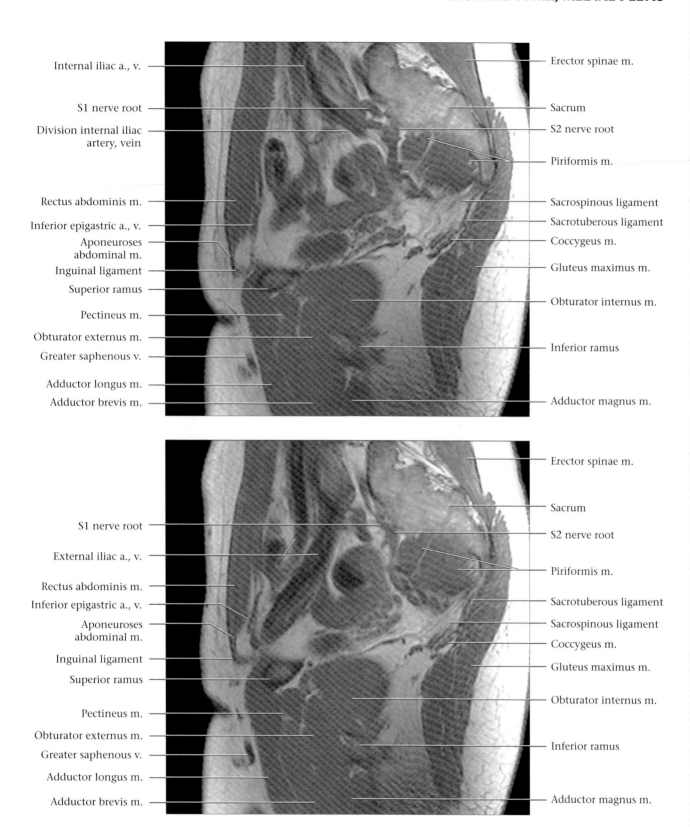

Internal iliac a., v. — Erector spinae m.

S1 nerve root — Sacrum

Division internal iliac artery, vein — S2 nerve root

— Piriformis m.

Rectus abdominis m. — Sacrospinous ligament

Inferior epigastric a., v. — Sacrotuberous ligament

Aponeuroses abdominal m. — Coccygeus m.

Inguinal ligament — Gluteus maximus m.

Superior ramus — Obturator internus m.

Pectineus m.

Obturator externus m.

Greater saphenous v. — Inferior ramus

Adductor longus m.

Adductor brevis m. — Adductor magnus m.

— Erector spinae m.

— Sacrum

S1 nerve root — S2 nerve root

External iliac a., v. — Piriformis m.

Rectus abdominis m.

Inferior epigastric a., v. — Sacrotuberous ligament

Aponeuroses abdominal m. — Sacrospinous ligament

— Coccygeus m.

Inguinal ligament — Gluteus maximus m.

Superior ramus — Obturator internus m.

Pectineus m.

Obturator externus m.

Greater saphenous v. — Inferior ramus

Adductor longus m.

Adductor brevis m. — Adductor magnus m.

(Top) The transverse abdominis and internal oblique tendons are present just lateral to the rectus abdominis muscle. The somewhat horizontal fibers of the sacrospinous ligament are deep to the more vertical fibers of the sacrotuberous ligament. **(Bottom)** This image bisects the long axis of the external iliac vessels. The inguinal ligament is the inferior edge of the aponeurosis of the external oblique muscle. The cross section of the pubic rami are presented.

SAGITTAL T1 MR, MEDIAL PELVIS

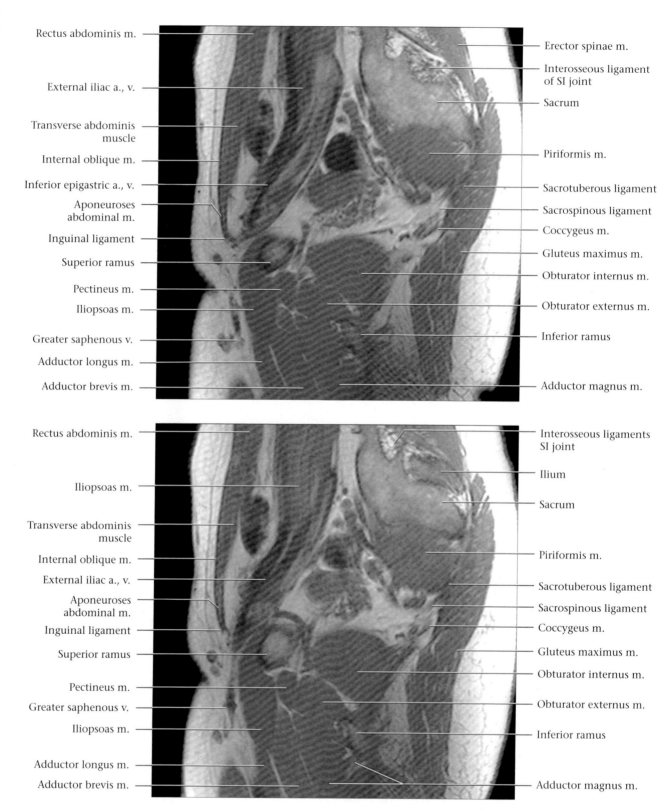

Rectus abdominis m.

External iliac a., v.

Transverse abdominis muscle

Internal oblique m.

Inferior epigastric a., v.

Aponeuroses abdominal m.

Inguinal ligament

Superior ramus

Pectineus m.

Iliopsoas m.

Greater saphenous v.

Adductor longus m.

Adductor brevis m.

Erector spinae m.

Interosseous ligament of SI joint

Sacrum

Piriformis m.

Sacrotuberous ligament

Sacrospinous ligament

Coccygeus m.

Gluteus maximus m.

Obturator internus m.

Obturator externus m.

Inferior ramus

Adductor magnus m.

Rectus abdominis m.

Iliopsoas m.

Transverse abdominis muscle

Internal oblique m.

External iliac a., v.

Aponeuroses abdominal m.

Inguinal ligament

Superior ramus

Pectineus m.

Greater saphenous v.

Iliopsoas m.

Adductor longus m.

Adductor brevis m.

Interosseous ligaments SI joint

Ilium

Sacrum

Piriformis m.

Sacrotuberous ligament

Sacrospinous ligament

Coccygeus m.

Gluteus maximus m.

Obturator internus m.

Obturator externus m.

Inferior ramus

Adductor magnus m.

(Top) The transition between the rectus abdominis muscle and the more lateral muscles is indistinct on sagittal images. The rectus abdominis muscle is wider superiorly than it is inferiorly; thus it extends onto more lateral images. The interosseous ligaments of the sacroiliac joint are seen in cross section. **(Bottom)** The adductor magnus muscle has two separate origins both of which are visible on this image. The ischiocondylar portion originates from the ischial tuberosity while the adductor portion originates from the inferior pubic ramus. This is the most lateral image on which the greater saphenous vein is present. It drains into the common femoral vein through the saphenous hiatus.

SAGITTAL T1 MR, LATERAL PELVIS

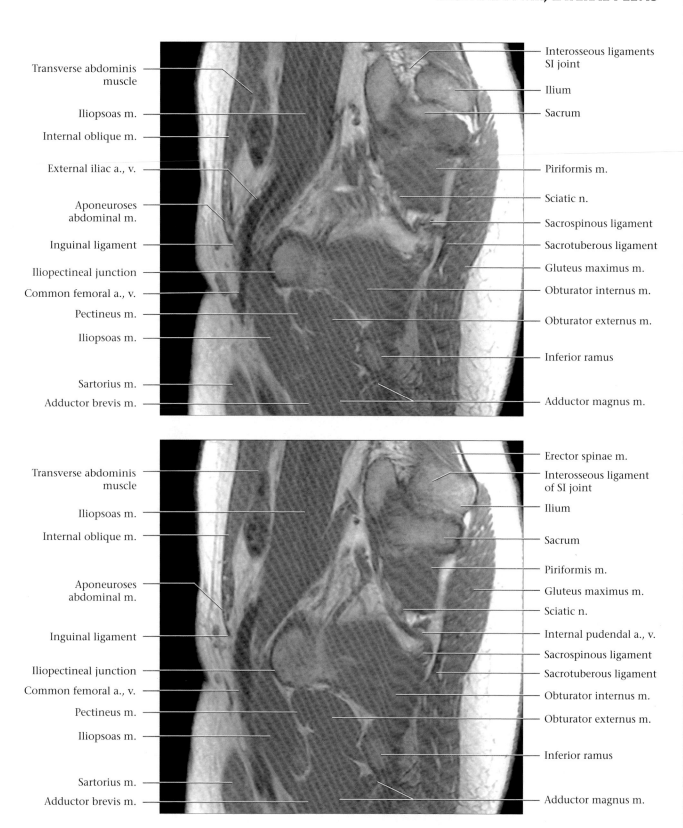

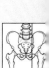

Transverse abdominis muscle

Iliopsoas m.

Internal oblique m.

External iliac a., v.

Aponeuroses abdominal m.

Inguinal ligament

Iliopectineal junction

Common femoral a., v.

Pectineus m.

Iliopsoas m.

Sartorius m.

Adductor brevis m.

Interosseous ligaments SI joint

Ilium

Sacrum

Piriformis m.

Sciatic n.

Sacrospinous ligament

Sacrotuberous ligament

Gluteus maximus m.

Obturator internus m.

Obturator externus m.

Inferior ramus

Adductor magnus m.

Transverse abdominis muscle

Iliopsoas m.

Internal oblique m.

Aponeuroses abdominal m.

Inguinal ligament

Iliopectineal junction

Common femoral a., v.

Pectineus m.

Iliopsoas m.

Sartorius m.

Adductor brevis m.

Erector spinae m.

Interosseous ligament of SI joint

Ilium

Sacrum

Piriformis m.

Gluteus maximus m.

Sciatic n.

Internal pudendal a., v.

Sacrospinous ligament

Sacrotuberous ligament

Obturator internus m.

Obturator externus m.

Inferior ramus

Adductor magnus m.

(Top) The external iliac vessels have crossed under the inguinal ligament to become the common femoral vessels. The sacroiliac joint is obliquely oriented and thus short segments will be seen on multiple images. The cross section of the iliopectineal junction is larger than the superior pubic ramus odicating transition from superior pubic ramus to acetabulum. **(Bottom)** The long axis of the iliopsoas muscle is present along the lateral aspect of the pelvis. The internal pudendal vessels exit the pelvis to wrap around the sacrospinous ligament and enter the perineum.

SAGITTAL T1 MR, LATERAL PELVIS

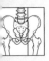

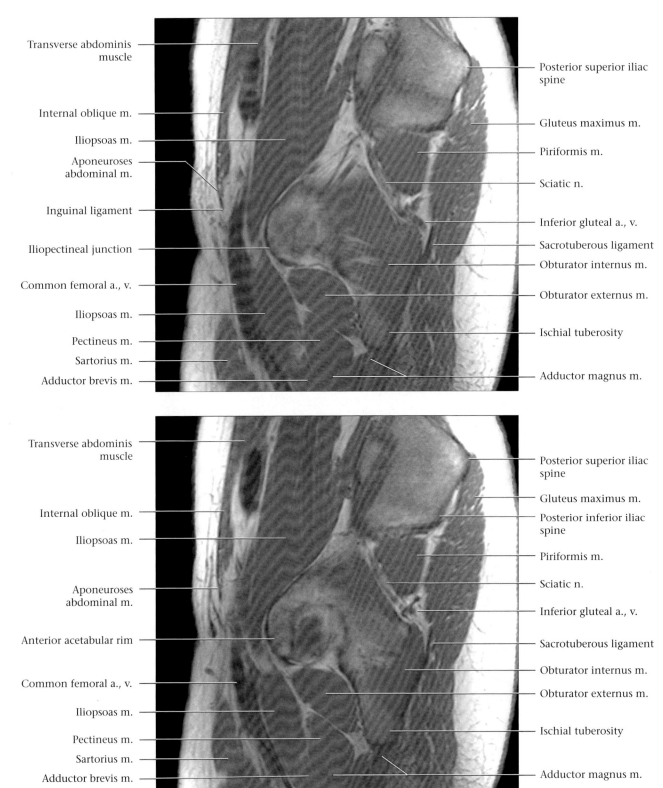

Transverse abdominis muscle

Internal oblique m.

Iliopsoas m.

Aponeuroses abdominal m.

Inguinal ligament

Iliopectineal junction

Common femoral a., v.

Iliopsoas m.

Pectineus m.

Sartorius m.

Adductor brevis m.

Posterior superior iliac spine

Gluteus maximus m.

Piriformis m.

Sciatic n.

Inferior gluteal a., v.

Sacrotuberous ligament

Obturator internus m.

Obturator externus m.

Ischial tuberosity

Adductor magnus m.

Transverse abdominis muscle

Internal oblique m.

Iliopsoas m.

Aponeuroses abdominal m.

Anterior acetabular rim

Common femoral a., v.

Iliopsoas m.

Pectineus m.

Sartorius m.

Adductor brevis m.

Posterior superior iliac spine

Gluteus maximus m.

Posterior inferior iliac spine

Piriformis m.

Sciatic n.

Inferior gluteal a., v.

Sacrotuberous ligament

Obturator internus m.

Obturator externus m.

Ischial tuberosity

Adductor magnus m.

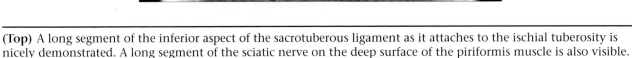

(Top) A long segment of the inferior aspect of the sacrotuberous ligament as it attaches to the ischial tuberosity is nicely demonstrated. A long segment of the sciatic nerve on the deep surface of the piriformis muscle is also visible. The inferior gluteal vessels are located just medial to the sciatic nerve. **(Bottom)** The posterior superior and inferior iliac spines are apparent. The inferior iliac spine marks the superior aspect of the greater sciatic notch.

SAGITTAL T1 MR, LATERAL PELVIS

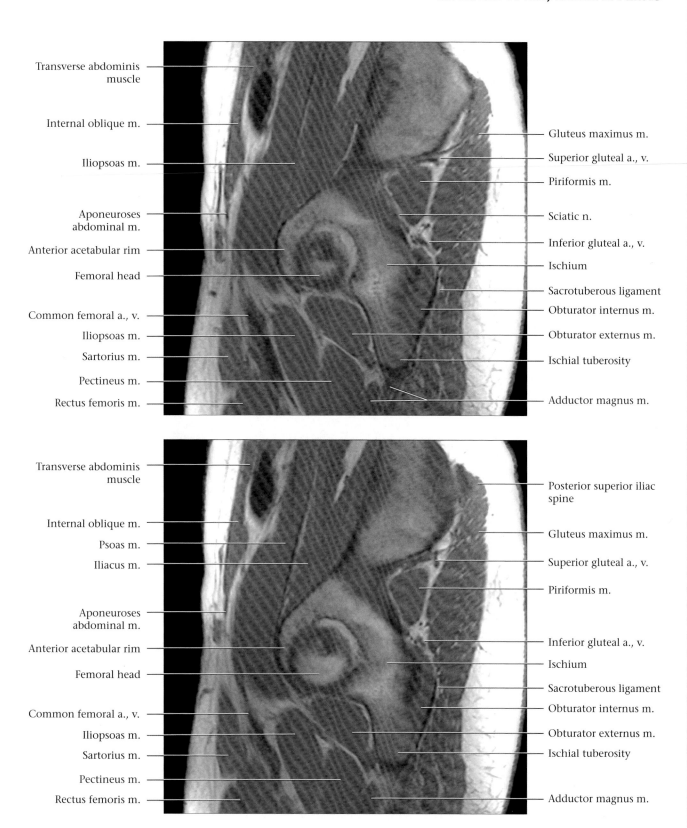

Transverse abdominis muscle

Internal oblique m.

Iliopsoas m.

Aponeuroses abdominal m.

Anterior acetabular rim

Femoral head

Common femoral a., v.

Iliopsoas m.

Sartorius m.

Pectineus m.

Rectus femoris m.

Gluteus maximus m.

Superior gluteal a., v.

Piriformis m.

Sciatic n.

Inferior gluteal a., v.

Ischium

Sacrotuberous ligament

Obturator internus m.

Obturator externus m.

Ischial tuberosity

Adductor magnus m.

Transverse abdominis muscle

Internal oblique m.

Psoas m.

Iliacus m.

Aponeuroses abdominal m.

Anterior acetabular rim

Femoral head

Common femoral a., v.

Iliopsoas m.

Sartorius m.

Pectineus m.

Rectus femoris m.

Posterior superior iliac spine

Gluteus maximus m.

Superior gluteal a., v.

Piriformis m.

Inferior gluteal a., v.

Ischium

Sacrotuberous ligament

Obturator internus m.

Obturator externus m.

Ischial tuberosity

Adductor magnus m.

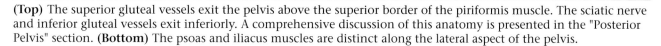

(Top) The superior gluteal vessels exit the pelvis above the superior border of the piriformis muscle. The sciatic nerve and inferior gluteal vessels exit inferiorly. A comprehensive discussion of this anatomy is presented in the "Posterior Pelvis" section. **(Bottom)** The psoas and iliacus muscles are distinct along the lateral aspect of the pelvis.

Hip and Pelvis

V

SAGITTAL T1 MR, LATERAL PELVIS

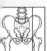
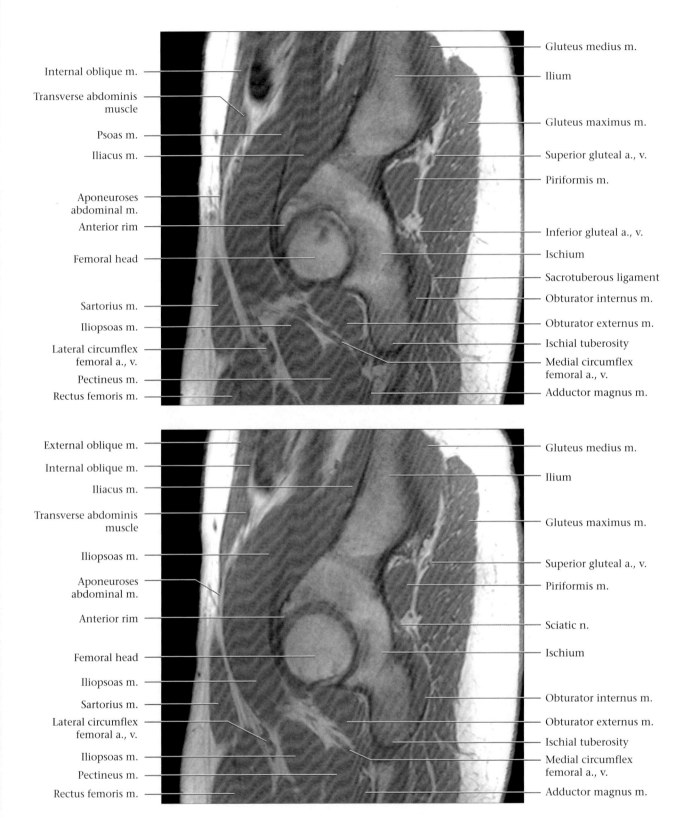

Internal oblique m.
Transverse abdominis muscle
Psoas m.
Iliacus m.
Aponeuroses abdominal m.
Anterior rim
Femoral head
Sartorius m.
Iliopsoas m.
Lateral circumflex femoral a., v.
Pectineus m.
Rectus femoris m.

Gluteus medius m.
Ilium
Gluteus maximus m.
Superior gluteal a., v.
Piriformis m.
Inferior gluteal a., v.
Ischium
Sacrotuberous ligament
Obturator internus m.
Obturator externus m.
Ischial tuberosity
Medial circumflex femoral a., v.
Adductor magnus m.

External oblique m.
Internal oblique m.
Iliacus m.
Transverse abdominis muscle
Iliopsoas m.
Aponeuroses abdominal m.
Anterior rim
Femoral head
Iliopsoas m.
Sartorius m.
Lateral circumflex femoral a., v.
Iliopsoas m.
Pectineus m.
Rectus femoris m.

Gluteus medius m.
Ilium
Gluteus maximus m.
Superior gluteal a., v.
Piriformis m.
Sciatic n.
Ischium
Obturator internus m.
Obturator externus m.
Ischial tuberosity
Medial circumflex femoral a., v.
Adductor magnus m.

(Top) The medial circumflex femoral vessels are found between the pectineus and iliopsoas muscles while the lateral circumflex femoral vessels are located deep to the sartorius and rectus femoris muscles. **(Bottom)** The rectus femoris muscle is now visible along the anterior aspect of the thigh. Note the inverted Y appearance of the ilium and acetabulum. The stem is the ilium and the anterior limb the anterior acetabulum and the posterior limb is the posterior column extending from the ilium through the ischium.

HIP AND PELVIS OVERVIEW

SAGITTAL T1 MR, LATERAL PELVIS

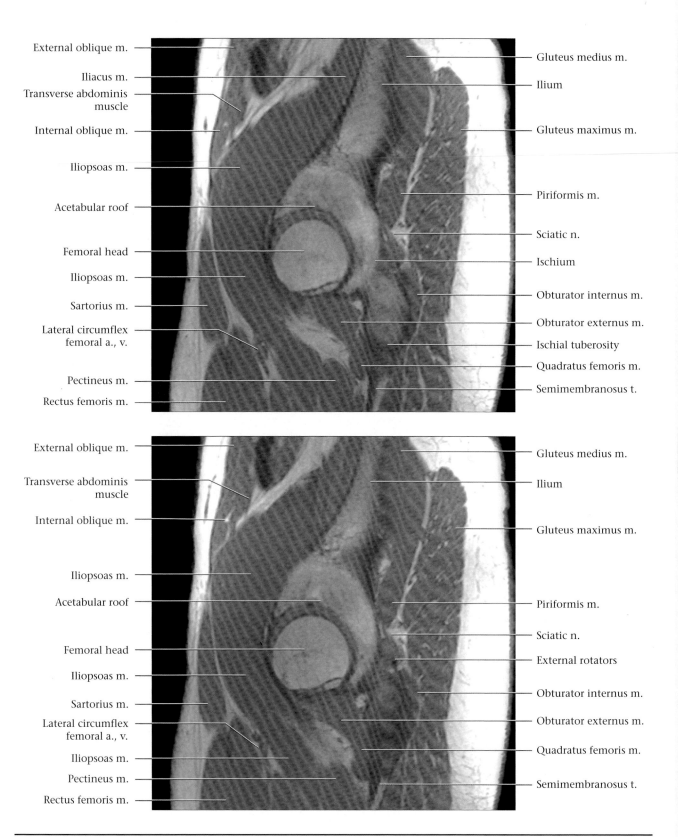

Top labels (left): External oblique m., Iliacus m., Transverse abdominis muscle, Internal oblique m., Iliopsoas m., Acetabular roof, Femoral head, Iliopsoas m., Sartorius m., Lateral circumflex femoral a., v., Pectineus m., Rectus femoris m.

Top labels (right): Gluteus medius m., Ilium, Gluteus maximus m., Piriformis m., Sciatic n., Ischium, Obturator internus m., Obturator externus m., Ischial tuberosity, Quadratus femoris m., Semimembranosus t.

Bottom labels (left): External oblique m., Transverse abdominis muscle, Internal oblique m., Iliopsoas m., Acetabular roof, Femoral head, Iliopsoas m., Sartorius m., Lateral circumflex femoral a., v., Iliopsoas m., Pectineus m., Rectus femoris m.

Bottom labels (right): Gluteus medius m., Ilium, Gluteus maximus m., Piriformis m., Sciatic n., External rotators, Obturator internus m., Obturator externus m., Quadratus femoris m., Semimembranosus t.

43

(Top) The three layers of the anterior lateral abdominal wall are now discernible. (Bottom) The external rotators of the hip are present along the posterior surface of the acetabulum. These muscles are well detailed in "Lateral Hip". Note also the origin of semimembranosus from the lateral portion of the ischial tuberosity.

Hip and Pelvis

V

SAGITTAL T1 MR, LATERAL PELVIS

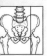

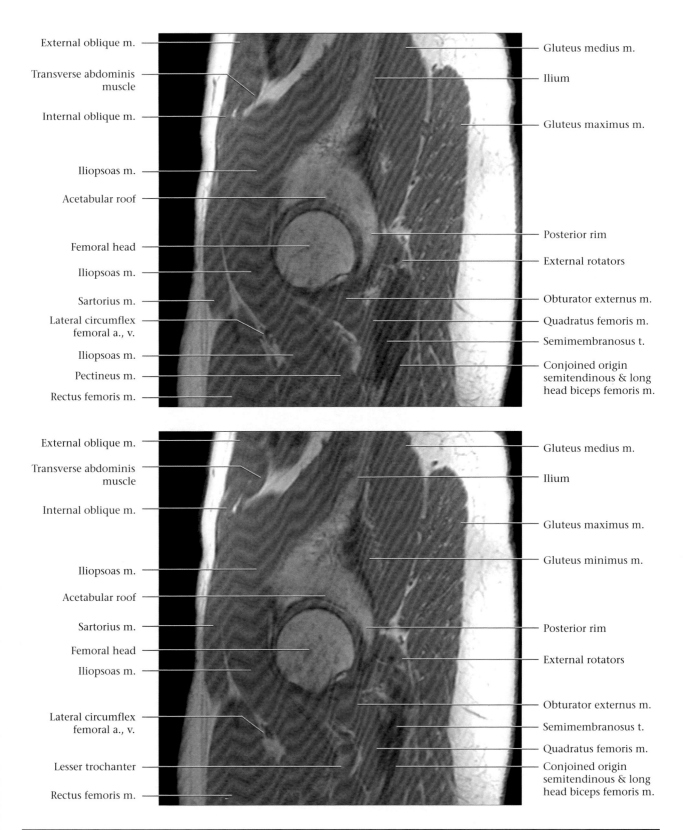

External oblique m.

Transverse abdominis muscle

Internal oblique m.

Iliopsoas m.

Acetabular roof

Femoral head

Iliopsoas m.

Sartorius m.

Lateral circumflex femoral a., v.

Iliopsoas m.

Pectineus m.

Rectus femoris m.

Gluteus medius m.

Ilium

Gluteus maximus m.

Posterior rim

External rotators

Obturator externus m.

Quadratus femoris m.

Semimembranosus t.

Conjoined origin semitendinous & long head biceps femoris m.

External oblique m.

Transverse abdominis muscle

Internal oblique m.

Iliopsoas m.

Acetabular roof

Sartorius m.

Femoral head

Iliopsoas m.

Lateral circumflex femoral a., v.

Lesser trochanter

Rectus femoris m.

Gluteus medius m.

Ilium

Gluteus maximus m.

Gluteus minimus m.

Posterior rim

External rotators

Obturator externus m.

Semimembranosus t.

Quadratus femoris m.

Conjoined origin semitendinous & long head biceps femoris m.

(Top) The sciatic nerve is not identifiable as a separate structure due to its close approximation to the external rotators of the hip. The conjoined origin of the semitendinosus and long head of the biceps femoris muscles takes origin from the ischial tuberosity posterior to the semimembranosus muscle origin. The quadratus femoris muscle also originates from the ischial tuberosity. The quadratus femoris muscle is deep to the hamstring tendons. **(Bottom)** The iliopsoas muscle inserts onto the lesser trochanter. The origin of the gluteus minimus muscle is visible on this image.

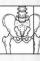

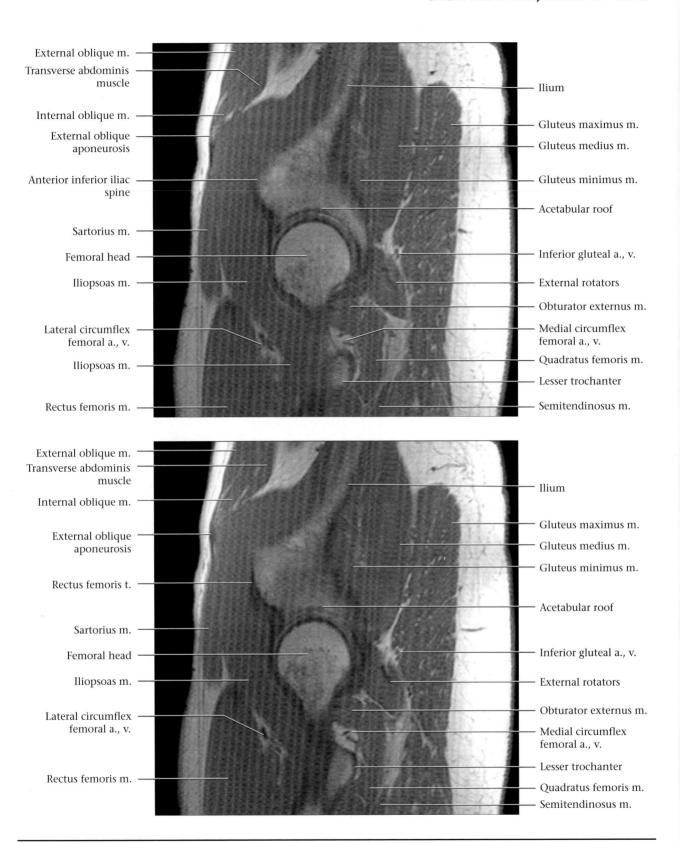

External oblique m.
Transverse abdominis muscle
Internal oblique m.
External oblique aponeurosis
Anterior inferior iliac spine
Sartorius m.
Femoral head
Iliopsoas m.
Lateral circumflex femoral a., v.
Iliopsoas m.
Rectus femoris m.

Ilium
Gluteus maximus m.
Gluteus medius m.
Gluteus minimus m.
Acetabular roof
Inferior gluteal a., v.
External rotators
Obturator externus m.
Medial circumflex femoral a., v.
Quadratus femoris m.
Lesser trochanter
Semitendinosus m.

External oblique m.
Transverse abdominis muscle
Internal oblique m.
External oblique aponeurosis
Rectus femoris t.
Sartorius m.
Femoral head
Iliopsoas m.
Lateral circumflex femoral a., v.
Rectus femoris m.

Ilium
Gluteus maximus m.
Gluteus medius m.
Gluteus minimus m.
Acetabular roof
Inferior gluteal a., v.
External rotators
Obturator externus m.
Medial circumflex femoral a., v.
Lesser trochanter
Quadratus femoris m.
Semitendinosus m.

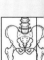

(Top) The anterior inferior iliac spine is an osseous protuberance just above the hip joint. **(Bottom)** The rectus femoris muscle originates from the anterior inferior iliac spine. The inferior gluteal vessels are still apparent along the deep surface of the gluteus maximus muscle. Although a discrete nerve is still not discernible the wisps of tissue adjacent to the inferior gluteal vessels are the sciatic nerve. The inguinal ligament is the most inferior edge of the external oblique aponeurosis.

SAGITTAL T1 MR, LATERAL PELVIS

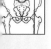

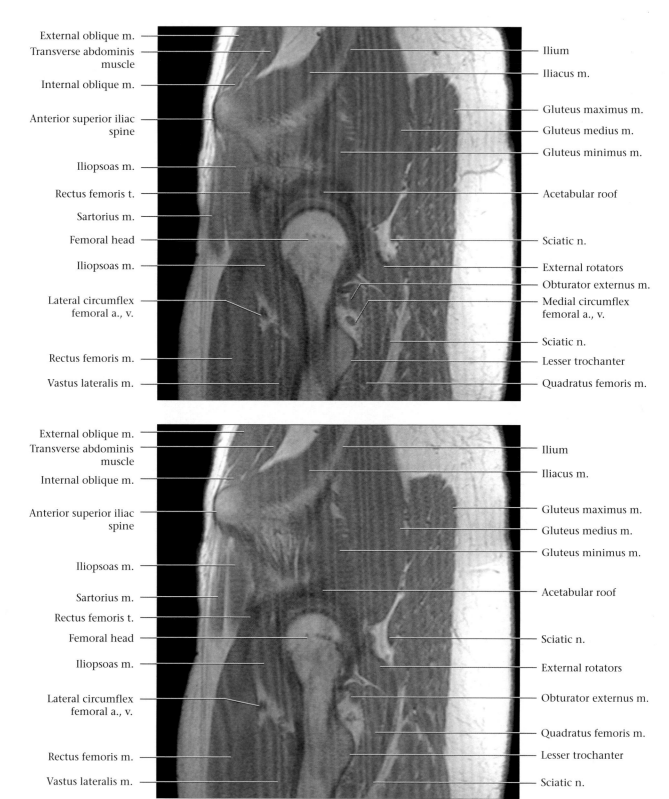

External oblique m.
Transverse abdominis muscle
Internal oblique m.
Anterior superior iliac spine
Iliopsoas m.
Rectus femoris t.
Sartorius m.
Femoral head
Iliopsoas m.
Lateral circumflex femoral a., v.
Rectus femoris m.
Vastus lateralis m.

Ilium
Iliacus m.
Gluteus maximus m.
Gluteus medius m.
Gluteus minimus m.
Acetabular roof
Sciatic n.
External rotators
Obturator externus m.
Medial circumflex femoral a., v.
Sciatic n.
Lesser trochanter
Quadratus femoris m.

External oblique m.
Transverse abdominis muscle
Internal oblique m.
Anterior superior iliac spine
Iliopsoas m.
Sartorius m.
Rectus femoris t.
Femoral head
Iliopsoas m.
Lateral circumflex femoral a., v.
Rectus femoris m.
Vastus lateralis m.

Ilium
Iliacus m.
Gluteus maximus m.
Gluteus medius m.
Gluteus minimus m.
Acetabular roof
Sciatic n.
External rotators
Obturator externus m.
Quadratus femoris m.
Lesser trochanter
Sciatic n.

(Top) The medial circumflex femoral vessels are now present posterior to the femur, having coursed around the medial aspect of the femoral neck. Note the posterior orientation of the lesser trochanter. The three layers of the anterior abdominal wall are all present and the separate muscles are easily discernible. Note also the origin of the sartorius muscle from the anterior superior iliac spine. **(Bottom)** A long segment of the sciatic nerve is seen closely applied to the posterior surface of the quadratus femoris tendon. It no longer has the fatty striations which were present within the nerve more superiorly.

HIP AND PELVIS OVERVIEW

SAGITTAL T1 MR, UPPER THIGH

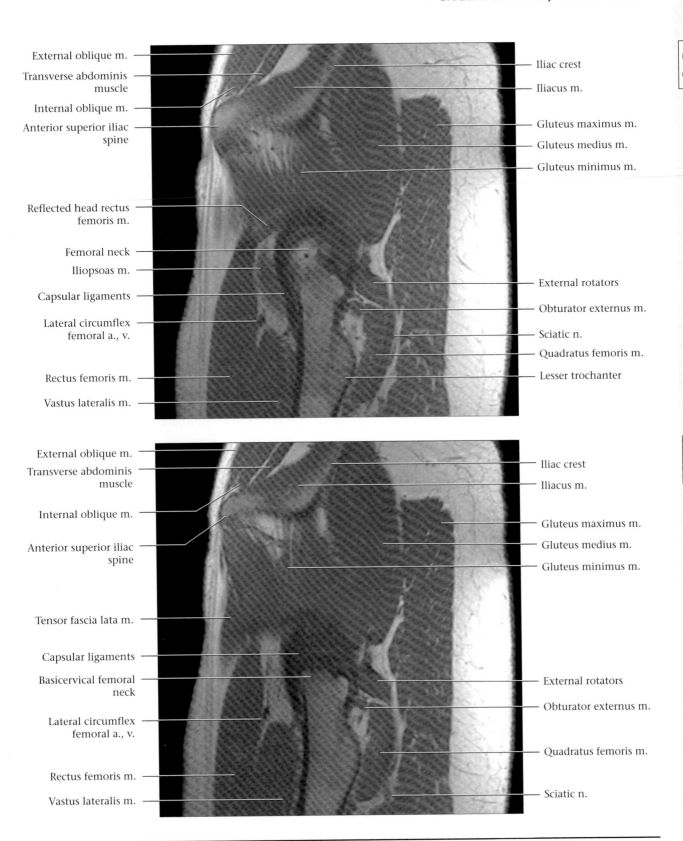

Top image labels (left): External oblique m.; Transverse abdominis muscle; Internal oblique m.; Anterior superior iliac spine; Reflected head rectus femoris m.; Femoral neck; Iliopsoas m.; Capsular ligaments; Lateral circumflex femoral a., v.; Rectus femoris m.; Vastus lateralis m.

Top image labels (right): Iliac crest; Iliacus m.; Gluteus maximus m.; Gluteus medius m.; Gluteus minimus m.; External rotators; Obturator externus m.; Sciatic n.; Quadratus femoris m.; Lesser trochanter

Bottom image labels (left): External oblique m.; Transverse abdominis muscle; Internal oblique m.; Anterior superior iliac spine; Tensor fascia lata m.; Capsular ligaments; Basicervical femoral neck; Lateral circumflex femoral a., v.; Rectus femoris m.; Vastus lateralis m.

Bottom image labels (right): Iliac crest; Iliacus m.; Gluteus maximus m.; Gluteus medius m.; Gluteus minimus m.; External rotators; Obturator externus m.; Quadratus femoris m.; Sciatic n.

(Top) The reflected head of the rectus femoris muscle is very nicely demonstrated on this image. It originates from a groove just above the acetabulum. The thick anterior joint capsule can be seen. Its anatomy is discussed in the "Hip Joint" section. **(Bottom)** Note the fibers of the gluteus minimus muscle arising from the auricular surface of the ilium.

Hip and Pelvis

V

47

SAGITTAL T1 MR, UPPER THIGH

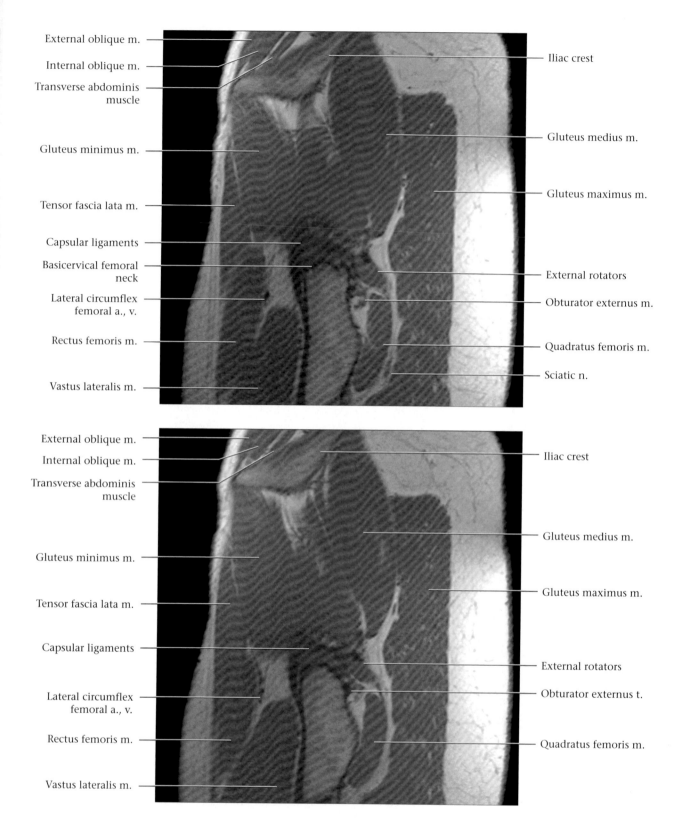

External oblique m.

Internal oblique m.

Transverse abdominis muscle

Gluteus minimus m.

Tensor fascia lata m.

Capsular ligaments

Basicervical femoral neck

Lateral circumflex femoral a., v.

Rectus femoris m.

Vastus lateralis m.

Iliac crest

Gluteus medius m.

Gluteus maximus m.

External rotators

Obturator externus m.

Quadratus femoris m.

Sciatic n.

External oblique m.

Internal oblique m.

Transverse abdominis muscle

Gluteus minimus m.

Tensor fascia lata m.

Capsular ligaments

Lateral circumflex femoral a., v.

Rectus femoris m.

Vastus lateralis m.

Iliac crest

Gluteus medius m.

Gluteus maximus m.

External rotators

Obturator externus t.

Quadratus femoris m.

(Top) The tensor fascia lata and rectus femoris muscles overlap each other, the rectus femoris muscle is more medial and on these lateral sagittal images more inferior. Note how far anteriorly the gluteus minimus is located. **(Bottom)** The external rotator muscles are closely related to the posterior and lateral aspect of the femoral neck as they approach their insertion site.

SAGITTAL T1 MR, UPPER THIGH

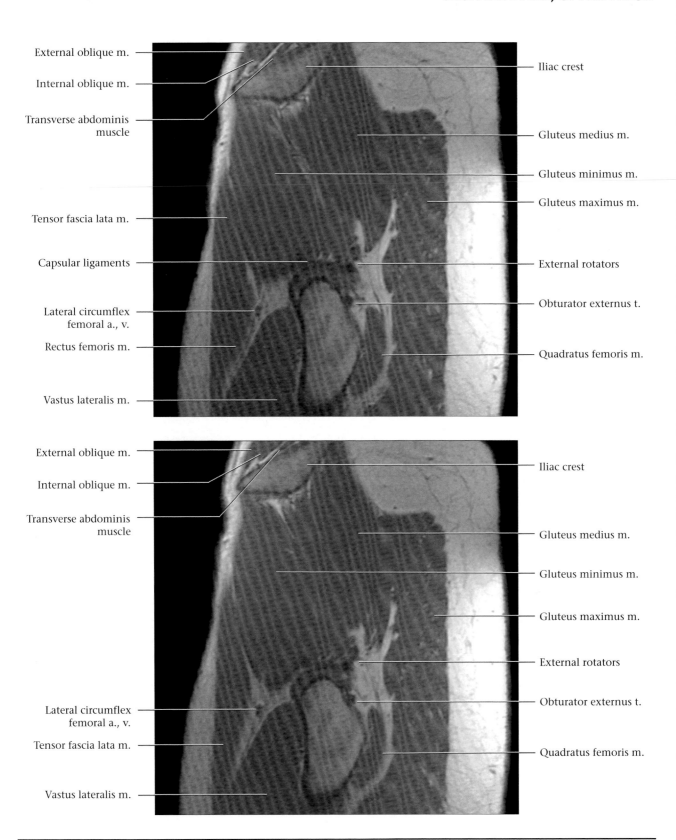

External oblique m.

Internal oblique m.

Transverse abdominis muscle

Tensor fascia lata m.

Capsular ligaments

Lateral circumflex femoral a., v.

Rectus femoris m.

Vastus lateralis m.

Iliac crest

Gluteus medius m.

Gluteus minimus m.

Gluteus maximus m.

External rotators

Obturator externus t.

Quadratus femoris m.

External oblique m.

Internal oblique m.

Transverse abdominis muscle

Lateral circumflex femoral a., v.

Tensor fascia lata m.

Vastus lateralis m.

Iliac crest

Gluteus medius m.

Gluteus minimus m.

Gluteus maximus m.

External rotators

Obturator externus t.

Quadratus femoris m.

(**Top**) The transverse abdominis muscle originates from the inner margin of the iliac crest. (**Bottom**) The vastus lateralis muscle has a relatively broad but not very long origin from the anterior aspect of the superior femoral diaphysis as seen on this image. Even though it is called the "lateralis" muscle in the upper thigh, this muscle wraps around the anterior aspect of the upper femur.

Hip and Pelvis

V

SAGITTAL T1 MR, UPPER THIGH

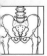

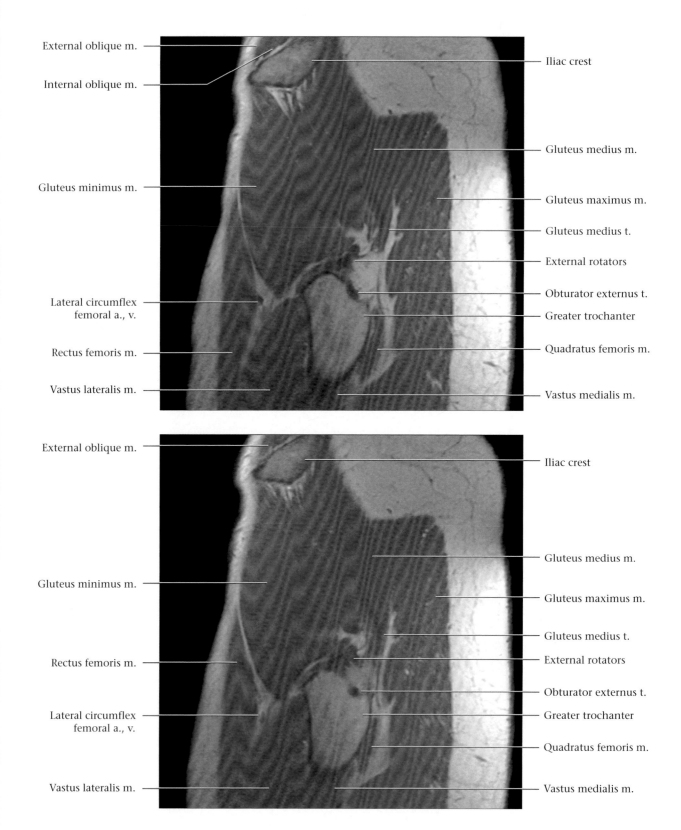

External oblique m. — — Iliac crest

Internal oblique m. —

— Gluteus medius m.

Gluteus minimus m. — — Gluteus maximus m.

— Gluteus medius t.

— External rotators

Lateral circumflex femoral a., v. — — Obturator externus t.

— Greater trochanter

Rectus femoris m. — — Quadratus femoris m.

Vastus lateralis m. — — Vastus medialis m.

External oblique m. — — Iliac crest

— Gluteus medius m.

Gluteus minimus m. — — Gluteus maximus m.

— Gluteus medius t.

Rectus femoris m. — — External rotators

— Obturator externus t.

Lateral circumflex femoral a., v. — — Greater trochanter

— Quadratus femoris m.

Vastus lateralis m. — — Vastus medialis m.

(Top) The internal oblique muscle originates from the superior aspect of the iliac crest. The gluteus medius tendon extends from the inferior border of that muscle. **(Bottom)** The gluteus medius tendon reaches towards the lateral facet of the greater trochanter. The obturator externus tendon is the most inferior tendon to insert onto the piriformis fossa located on the medial surface of the greater trochanter.

SAGITTAL T1 MR, UPPER THIGH

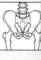

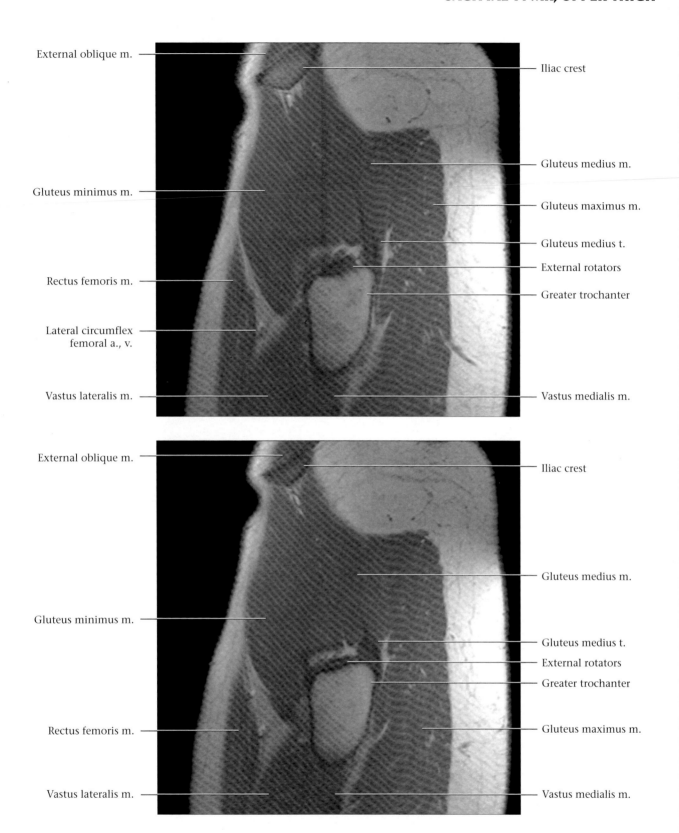

External oblique m. — — Iliac crest

— Gluteus medius m.

Gluteus minimus m. — — Gluteus maximus m.

— Gluteus medius t.
— External rotators

Rectus femoris m. — — Greater trochanter

Lateral circumflex femoral a., v. —

Vastus lateralis m. — — Vastus medialis m.

External oblique m. — — Iliac crest

— Gluteus medius m.

Gluteus minimus m. — — Gluteus medius t.
— External rotators
— Greater trochanter

Rectus femoris m. — — Gluteus maximus m.

Vastus lateralis m. — — Vastus medialis m.

(Top) The remaining external rotator tendons insert onto the piriformis fossa. The gluteus medius tendon inserts onto the greater trochanter. **(Bottom)** The vastus medialis tendon takes an origin from the upper anterior femoral diaphysis and the muscle belly lies deep to the vastus lateralis muscle in the upper thigh. For a discussion of anatomy lateral to this point see the "Lateral Hip" section.

CORONAL T1 MR, POSTERIOR PELVIS

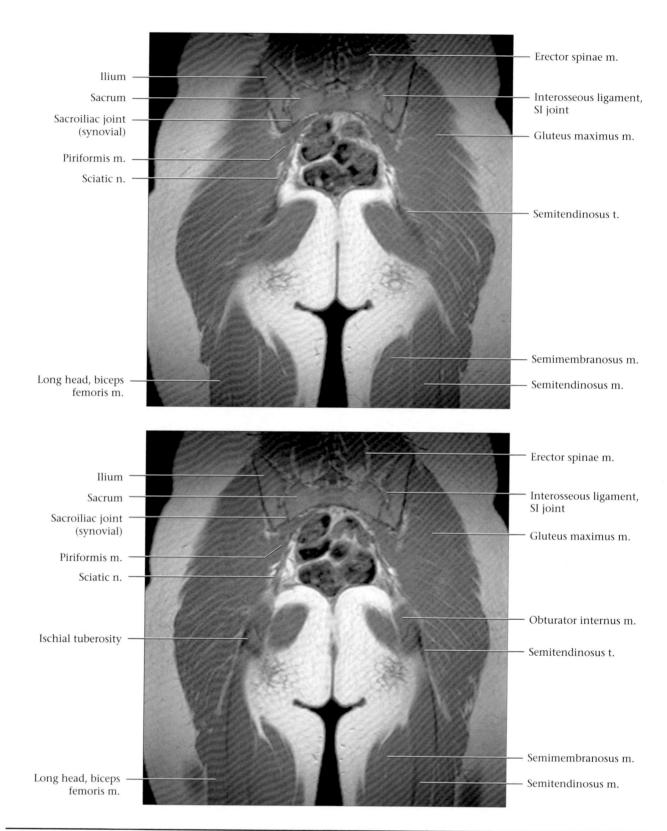

Ilium

Sacrum

Sacroiliac joint (synovial)

Piriformis m.

Sciatic n.

Long head, biceps femoris m.

Erector spinae m.

Interosseous ligament, SI joint

Gluteus maximus m.

Semitendinosus t.

Semimembranosus m.

Semitendinosus m.

Ilium

Sacrum

Sacroiliac joint (synovial)

Piriformis m.

Sciatic n.

Ischial tuberosity

Long head, biceps femoris m.

Erector spinae m.

Interosseous ligament, SI joint

Gluteus maximus m.

Obturator internus m.

Semitendinosus t.

Semimembranosus m.

Semitendinosus m.

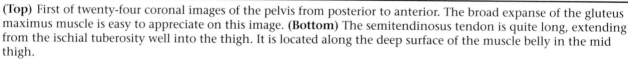

(Top) First of twenty-four coronal images of the pelvis from posterior to anterior. The broad expanse of the gluteus maximus muscle is easy to appreciate on this image. **(Bottom)** The semitendinosus tendon is quite long, extending from the ischial tuberosity well into the thigh. It is located along the deep surface of the muscle belly in the mid thigh.

CORONAL T1 MR, POSTERIOR PELVIS

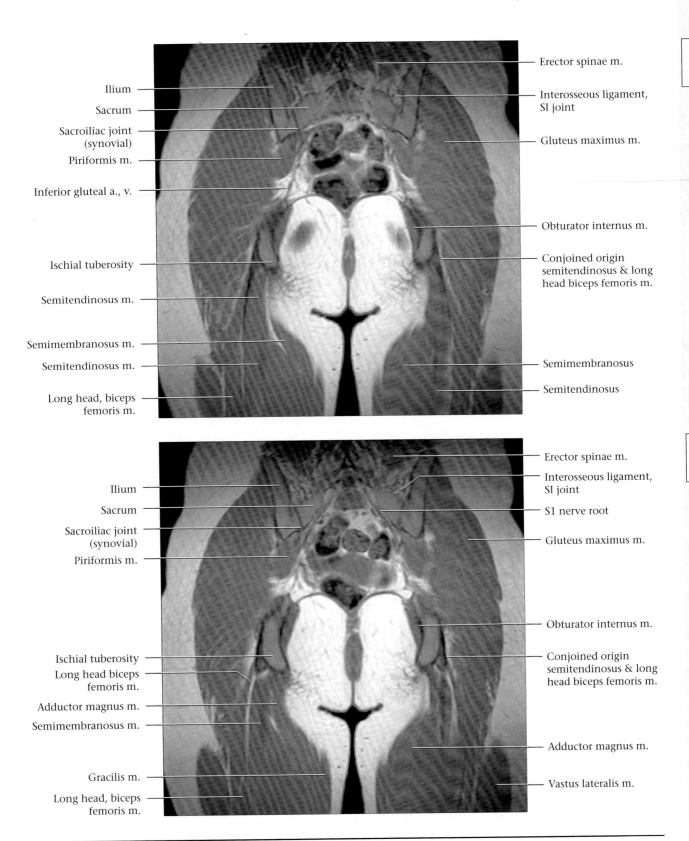

Erector spinae m.

Ilium

Interosseous ligament, SI joint

Sacrum

Sacroiliac joint (synovial)

Gluteus maximus m.

Piriformis m.

Inferior gluteal a., v.

Obturator internus m.

Conjoined origin semitendinosus & long head biceps femoris m.

Ischial tuberosity

Semitendinosus m.

Semimembranosus m.

Semitendinosus m.

Semimembranosus

Semitendinosus

Long head, biceps femoris m.

Erector spinae m.

Interosseous ligament, SI joint

Ilium

Sacrum

S1 nerve root

Sacroiliac joint (synovial)

Gluteus maximus m.

Piriformis m.

Obturator internus m.

Conjoined origin semitendinosus & long head biceps femoris m.

Ischial tuberosity

Long head biceps femoris m.

Adductor magnus m.

Semimembranosus m.

Adductor magnus m.

Gracilis m.

Vastus lateralis m.

Long head, biceps femoris m.

(Top) The inferior gluteal vessels follow the same course as the sciatic nerve. The vessels are located medial to the nerve. **(Bottom)** The proximal aspect of the hamstring tendons are visible. In the proximal thigh the semimembranosus muscle is purely membranous and is seen as a thin black slip. The ischiocondylar portion of the adductor magnus muscle is the most medial muscle, the long head of the biceps femoris is most lateral and the semitendinosus is in between. The membrane of the semimembranosus muscle is along the deep surface of the semitendinosus muscle. A long segment of the S1 nerve root is seen as it exits the neural foramina.

Hip and Pelvis

V

CORONAL T1 MR, POSTERIOR PELVIS

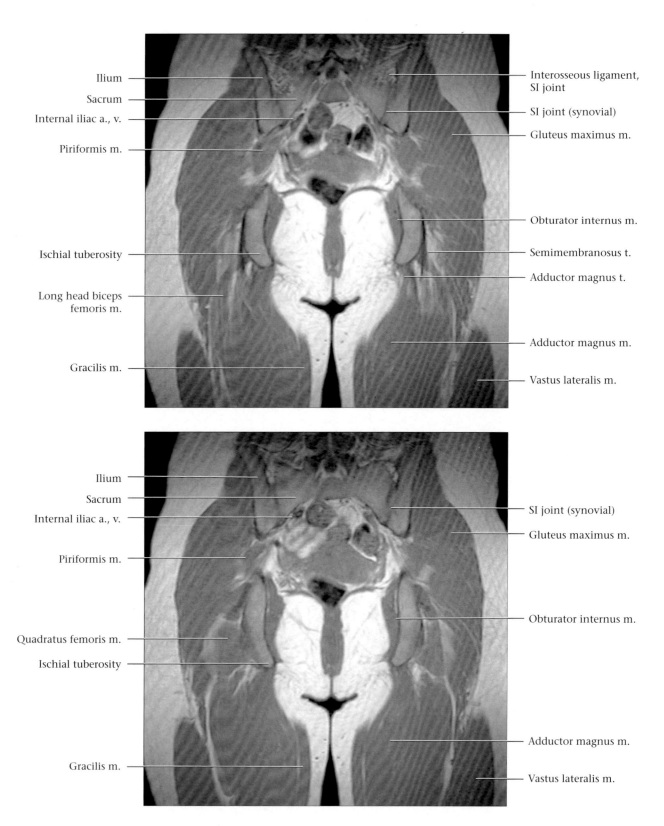

Ilium

Sacrum

Internal iliac a., v.

Piriformis m.

Ischial tuberosity

Long head biceps femoris m.

Gracilis m.

Interosseous ligament, SI joint

SI joint (synovial)

Gluteus maximus m.

Obturator internus m.

Semimembranosus t.

Adductor magnus t.

Adductor magnus m.

Vastus lateralis m.

Ilium

Sacrum

Internal iliac a., v.

Piriformis m.

Quadratus femoris m.

Ischial tuberosity

Gracilis m.

SI joint (synovial)

Gluteus maximus m.

Obturator internus m.

Adductor magnus m.

Vastus lateralis m.

(Top) The sacroiliac joint is composed of two different types of articulations, the thin anterior synovial portion of the joint, and the wider posterior syndesmotic portion of the joint. The strong interosseous ligaments connect to the two surfaces of the syndesmotic portion of the joint. (Bottom) The adductor magnus muscle dominates the posterior thigh. The gracilis muscle is the most medial muscle of the thigh. The vastus lateralis muscle occupies a large section of the lateral thigh.

HIP AND PELVIS OVERVIEW

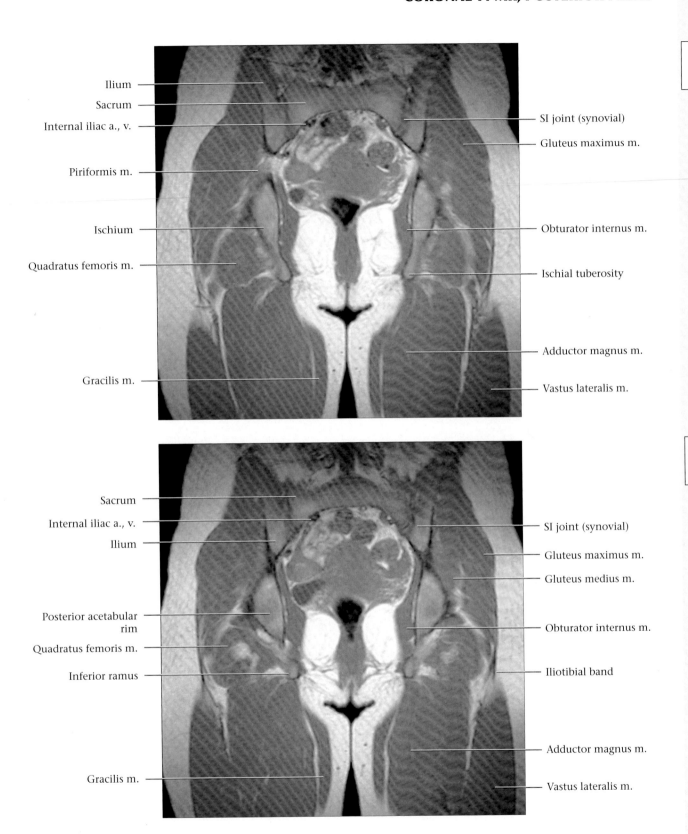

Top image labels:

- Ilium
- Sacrum
- Internal iliac a., v.
- Piriformis m.
- Ischium
- Quadratus femoris m.
- Gracilis m.
- SI joint (synovial)
- Gluteus maximus m.
- Obturator internus m.
- Ischial tuberosity
- Adductor magnus m.
- Vastus lateralis m.

Bottom image labels:

- Sacrum
- Internal iliac a., v.
- Ilium
- Posterior acetabular rim
- Quadratus femoris m.
- Inferior ramus
- Gracilis m.
- SI joint (synovial)
- Gluteus maximus m.
- Gluteus medius m.
- Obturator internus m.
- Iliotibial band
- Adductor magnus m.
- Vastus lateralis m.

(Top) The broad quadratus femoris muscle is seen coursing from the ischial tuberosity to the posterior aspect of the femur. **(Bottom)** The sacroiliac joint is now entirely synovial. The small inferior pubic ramus extends from the ischial tuberosity.

Hip and Pelvis

V

CORONAL T1 MR, POSTERIOR PELVIS

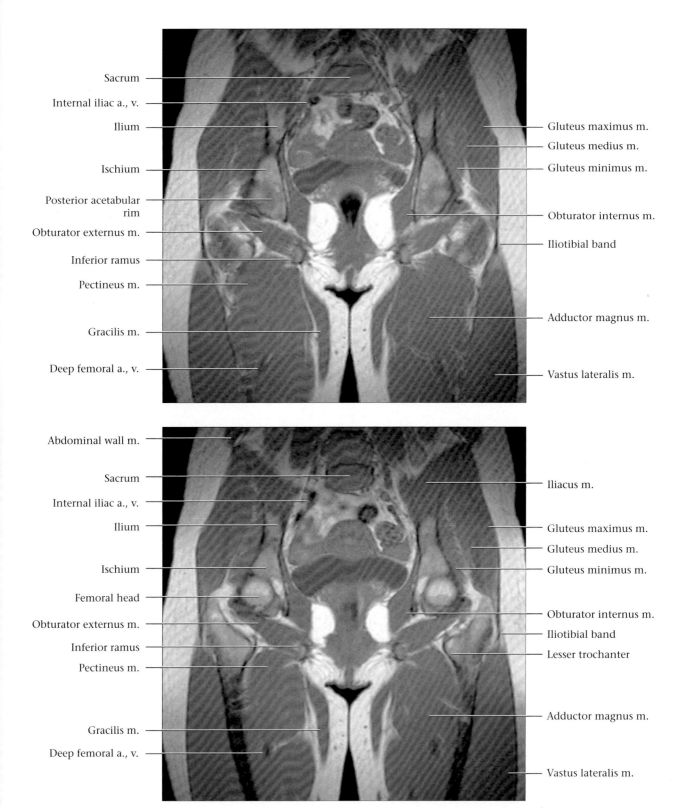

Sacrum

Internal iliac a., v.

Ilium

Ischium

Posterior acetabular rim

Obturator externus m.

Inferior ramus

Pectineus m.

Gracilis m.

Deep femoral a., v.

Gluteus maximus m.

Gluteus medius m.

Gluteus minimus m.

Obturator internus m.

Iliotibial band

Adductor magnus m.

Vastus lateralis m.

Abdominal wall m.

Sacrum

Internal iliac a., v.

Ilium

Ischium

Femoral head

Obturator externus m.

Inferior ramus

Pectineus m.

Gracilis m.

Deep femoral a., v.

Iliacus m.

Gluteus maximus m.

Gluteus medius m.

Gluteus minimus m.

Obturator internus m.

Iliotibial band

Lesser trochanter

Adductor magnus m.

Vastus lateralis m.

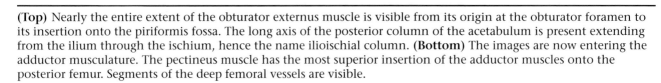

(Top) Nearly the entire extent of the obturator externus muscle is visible from its origin at the obturator foramen to its insertion onto the piriformis fossa. The long axis of the posterior column of the acetabulum is present extending from the ilium through the ischium, hence the name ilioischial column. **(Bottom)** The images are now entering the adductor musculature. The pectineus muscle has the most superior insertion of the adductor muscles onto the posterior femur. Segments of the deep femoral vessels are visible.

CORONAL T1 MR, MID PELVIS

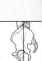
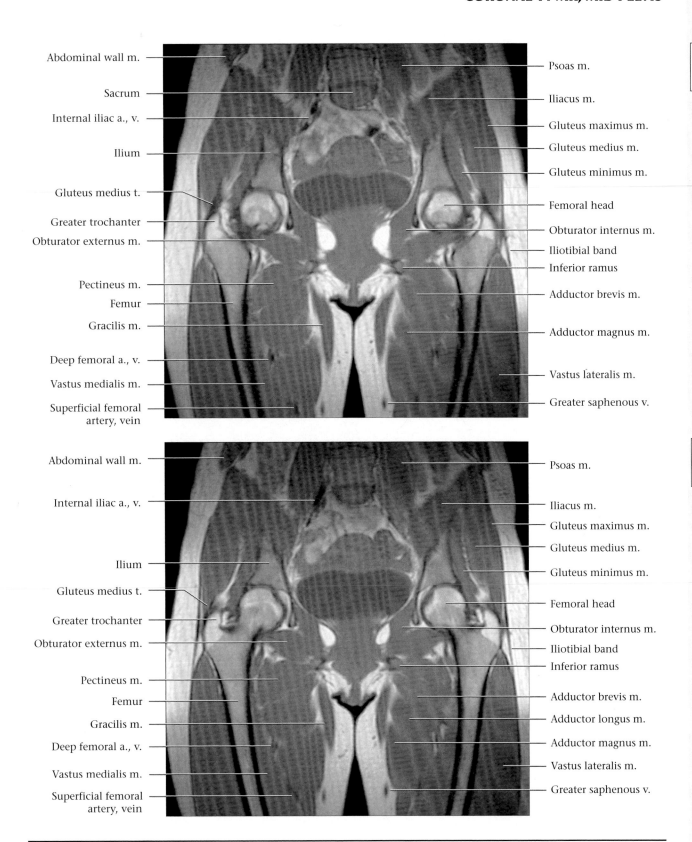

Abdominal wall m.

Sacrum

Internal iliac a., v.

Ilium

Gluteus medius t.

Greater trochanter

Obturator externus m.

Pectineus m.

Femur

Gracilis m.

Deep femoral a., v.

Vastus medialis m.

Superficial femoral artery, vein

Psoas m.

Iliacus m.

Gluteus maximus m.

Gluteus medius m.

Gluteus minimus m.

Femoral head

Obturator internus m.

Iliotibial band

Inferior ramus

Adductor brevis m.

Adductor magnus m.

Vastus lateralis m.

Greater saphenous v.

Abdominal wall m.

Internal iliac a., v.

Ilium

Gluteus medius t.

Greater trochanter

Obturator externus m.

Pectineus m.

Femur

Gracilis m.

Deep femoral a., v.

Vastus medialis m.

Superficial femoral artery, vein

Psoas m.

Iliacus m.

Gluteus maximus m.

Gluteus medius m.

Gluteus minimus m.

Femoral head

Obturator internus m.

Iliotibial band

Inferior ramus

Adductor brevis m.

Adductor longus m.

Adductor magnus m.

Vastus lateralis m.

Greater saphenous v.

(Top) The images are now entering the adductor musculature. The pectineus muscle has the most superior insertion of the adductor muscles onto the posterior femur. Segments of the deep femoral vessels are visible. **(Bottom)** Note the general relationship of the major vessels of the thigh. The greater saphenous vein is medial within the subcutaneous fat, the superficial femoral vessels are medial to the deep femoral vessels.

Hip and Pelvis

V

CORONAL T1 MR, MID PELVIS

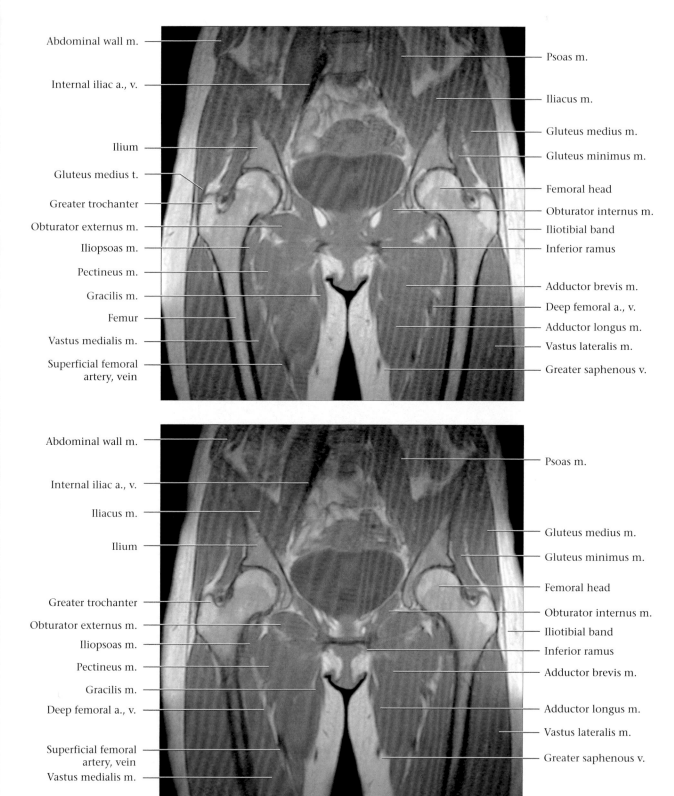

Abdominal wall m.

Internal iliac a., v.

Ilium

Gluteus medius t.

Greater trochanter

Obturator externus m.

Iliopsoas m.

Pectineus m.

Gracilis m.

Femur

Vastus medialis m.

Superficial femoral artery, vein

Psoas m.

Iliacus m.

Gluteus medius m.

Gluteus minimus m.

Femoral head

Obturator internus m.

Iliotibial band

Inferior ramus

Adductor brevis m.

Deep femoral a., v.

Adductor longus m.

Vastus lateralis m.

Greater saphenous v.

Abdominal wall m.

Internal iliac a., v.

Iliacus m.

Ilium

Greater trochanter

Obturator externus m.

Iliopsoas m.

Pectineus m.

Gracilis m.

Deep femoral a., v.

Superficial femoral artery, vein

Vastus medialis m.

Psoas m.

Gluteus medius m.

Gluteus minimus m.

Femoral head

Obturator internus m.

Iliotibial band

Inferior ramus

Adductor brevis m.

Adductor longus m.

Vastus lateralis m.

Greater saphenous v.

(Top) The gluteus medius tendon inserts onto the lateral facet of the greater trochanter. **(Bottom)** Note how difficult it is to identify the inferior pubic ramus. The external rotator tendons are seen just medial to the greater trochanter as they insert onto the piriformis fossa. The tendons are not labeled. This anatomy is presented in the "Lateral Hip" section.

CORONAL T1 MR, MID PELVIS

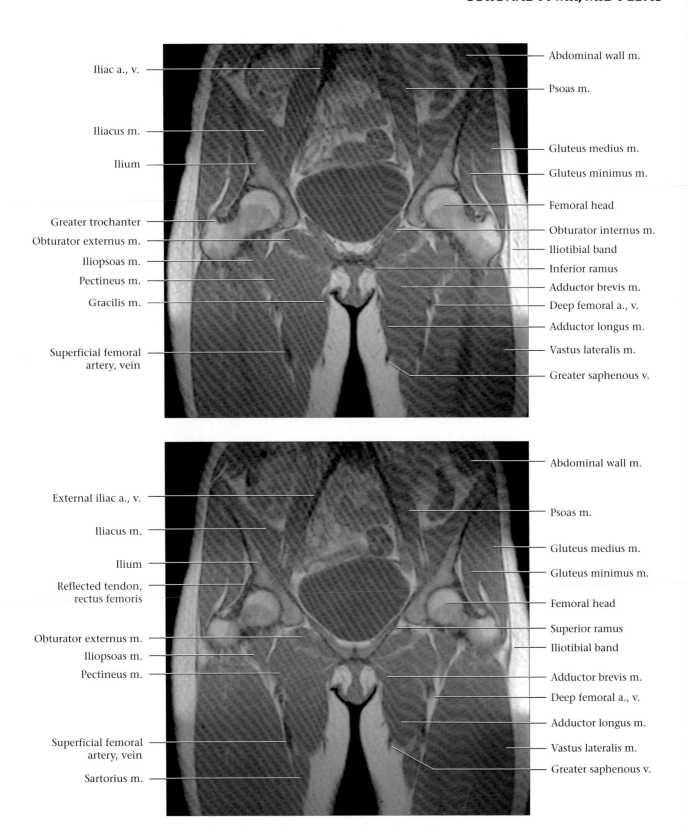

Top image labels:
- Iliac a., v.
- Iliacus m.
- Ilium
- Greater trochanter
- Obturator externus m.
- Iliopsoas m.
- Pectineus m.
- Gracilis m.
- Superficial femoral artery, vein
- Abdominal wall m.
- Psoas m.
- Gluteus medius m.
- Gluteus minimus m.
- Femoral head
- Obturator internus m.
- Iliotibial band
- Inferior ramus
- Adductor brevis m.
- Deep femoral a., v.
- Adductor longus m.
- Vastus lateralis m.
- Greater saphenous v.

Bottom image labels:
- External iliac a., v.
- Iliacus m.
- Ilium
- Reflected tendon, rectus femoris
- Obturator externus m.
- Iliopsoas m.
- Pectineus m.
- Superficial femoral artery, vein
- Sartorius m.
- Abdominal wall m.
- Psoas m.
- Gluteus medius m.
- Gluteus minimus m.
- Femoral head
- Superior ramus
- Iliotibial band
- Adductor brevis m.
- Deep femoral a., v.
- Adductor longus m.
- Vastus lateralis m.
- Greater saphenous v.

(Top) The iliopsoas muscle travels along the medial aspect of the joint as it courses posteriorly to its insertion onto the lesser trochanter. **(Bottom)** The gluteus minimus tendon inserts onto the anterior facet of the greater trochanter. The common femoral vessels have just bifurcated into deep femoral and superficial femoral vessels. The vastus lateralis muscle wraps the entire anterior aspect of the upper femur.

Hip and Pelvis

V

CORONAL T1 MR, MID PELVIS

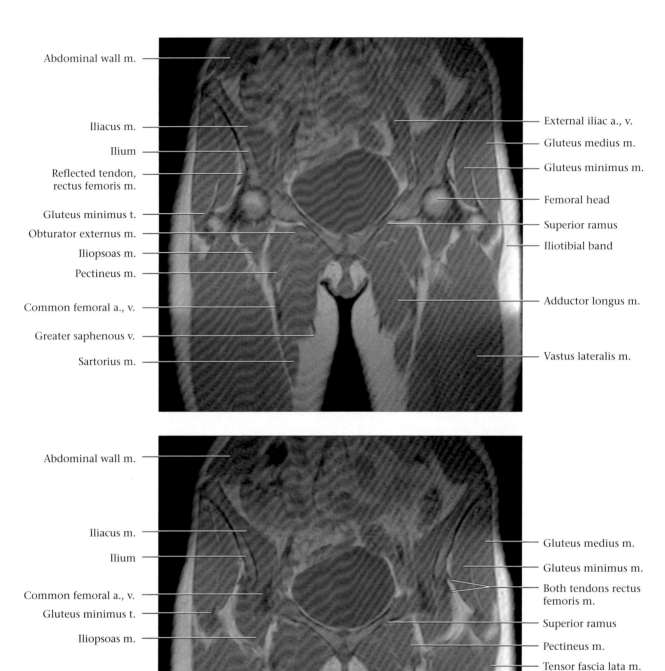

Abdominal wall m.

Iliacus m.

Ilium

Reflected tendon, rectus femoris m.

Gluteus minimus t.

Obturator externus m.

Iliopsoas m.

Pectineus m.

Common femoral a., v.

Greater saphenous v.

Sartorius m.

External iliac a., v.

Gluteus medius m.

Gluteus minimus m.

Femoral head

Superior ramus

Iliotibial band

Adductor longus m.

Vastus lateralis m.

Abdominal wall m.

Iliacus m.

Ilium

Common femoral a., v.

Gluteus minimus t.

Iliopsoas m.

Common femoral a., v.

Greater saphenous v.

Sartorius m.

Gluteus medius m.

Gluteus minimus m.

Both tendons rectus femoris m.

Superior ramus

Pectineus m.

Tensor fascia lata m.

Adductor longus m.

Vastus lateralis m.

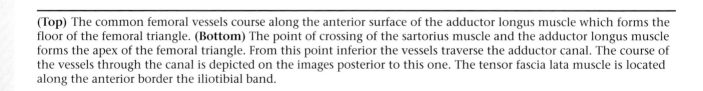

(Top) The common femoral vessels course along the anterior surface of the adductor longus muscle which forms the floor of the femoral triangle. **(Bottom)** The point of crossing of the sartorius muscle and the adductor longus muscle forms the apex of the femoral triangle. From this point inferior the vessels traverse the adductor canal. The course of the vessels through the canal is depicted on the images posterior to this one. The tensor fascia lata muscle is located along the anterior border the iliotibial band.

CORONAL T1 MR, ANTERIOR PELVIS

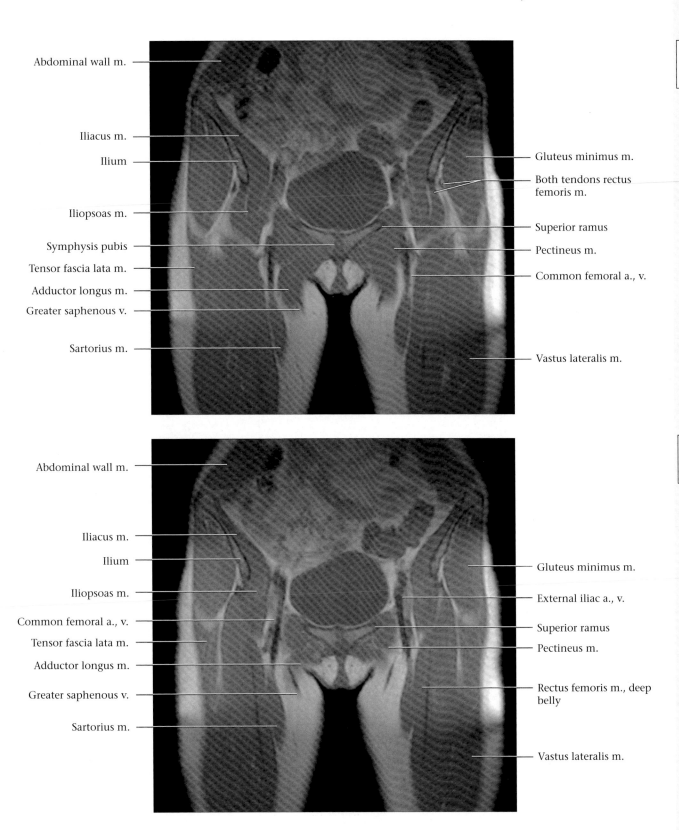

Abdominal wall m.

Iliacus m.

Ilium

Iliopsoas m.

Symphysis pubis

Tensor fascia lata m.

Adductor longus m.

Greater saphenous v.

Sartorius m.

Gluteus minimus m.

Both tendons rectus femoris m.

Superior ramus

Pectineus m.

Common femoral a., v.

Vastus lateralis m.

Abdominal wall m.

Iliacus m.

Ilium

Iliopsoas m.

Common femoral a., v.

Tensor fascia lata m.

Adductor longus m.

Greater saphenous v.

Sartorius m.

Gluteus minimus m.

External iliac a., v.

Superior ramus

Pectineus m.

Rectus femoris m., deep belly

Vastus lateralis m.

(Top) The symphysis pubis is the articulation of the anterior aspect of the pelvis. **(Bottom)** The external iliac vessels are medial to the iliopsoas muscle as those structures enter the thigh. As the vessels pass beneath the inguinal ligament; they become the common femoral vessels. The femoral nerve is the most lateral structure entering the femoral triangle. It is not identifiable on this examination.

CORONAL T1 MR, ANTERIOR PELVIS

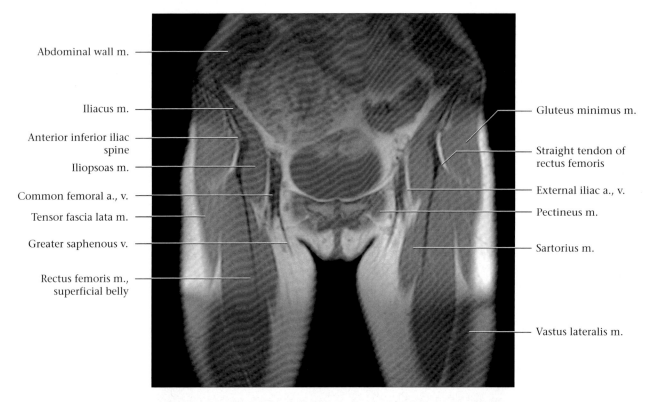

Abdominal wall m.

Iliacus m.

Anterior inferior iliac spine

Iliopsoas m.

Common femoral a., v.

Tensor fascia lata m.

Greater saphenous v.

Rectus femoris m., superficial belly

Gluteus minimus m.

Straight tendon of rectus femoris

External iliac a., v.

Pectineus m.

Sartorius m.

Vastus lateralis m.

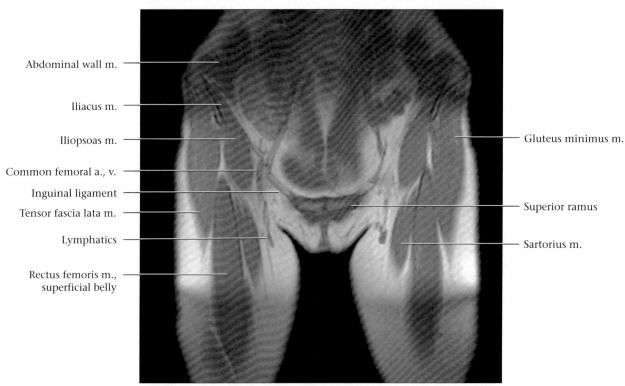

Abdominal wall m.

Iliacus m.

Iliopsoas m.

Common femoral a., v.

Inguinal ligament

Tensor fascia lata m.

Lymphatics

Rectus femoris m., superficial belly

Gluteus minimus m.

Superior ramus

Sartorius m.

(Top) The junction of the greater saphenous vein and common femoral vein is nicely seen on this image. The rectus femoris muscle originates from the anterior inferior iliac spine and supraacetabular ilium. The pectineus muscle has the most lateral origin of the muscles arising from the superior pubic ramus. **(Bottom)** A short segment of the inguinal ligament is visible near its attachment to the pubic tubercle. The lymphatics are the most lateral structures at the entrance to the femoral triangle.

CORONAL T1 MR, ANTERIOR PELVIS

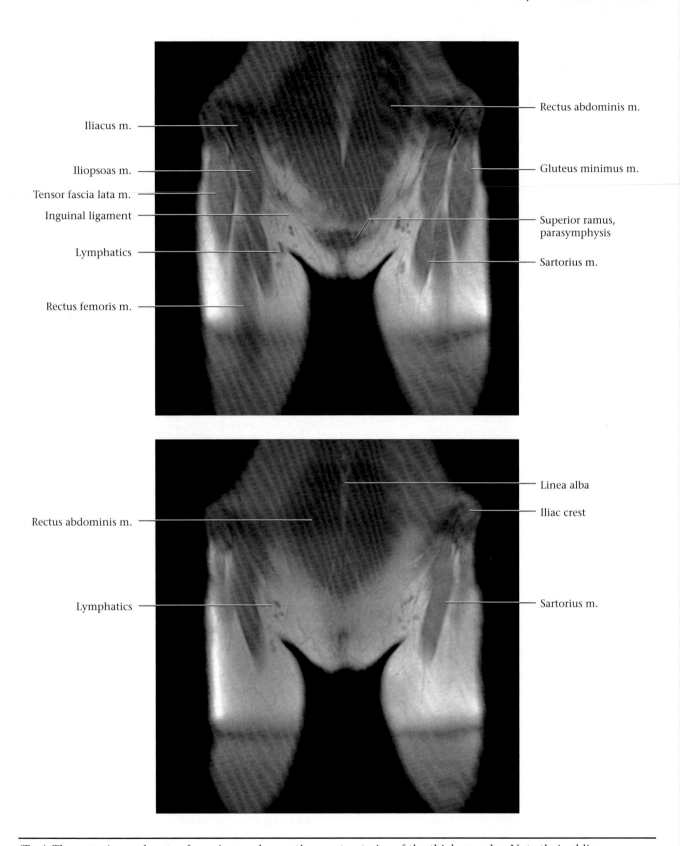

Iliacus m.

Iliopsoas m.

Tensor fascia lata m.

Inguinal ligament

Lymphatics

Rectus femoris m.

Rectus abdominis m.

Gluteus minimus m.

Superior ramus, parasymphysis

Sartorius m.

Rectus abdominis m.

Lymphatics

Linea alba

Iliac crest

Sartorius m.

(Top) The sartorius and rectus femoris muscles are the most anterior of the thigh muscles. Note their oblique orientation from superior lateral to inferior medial. A rich supply of lymphatics is present in the anterior thigh. (Bottom) The paired midline rectus abdominis muscles are visible. The muscles originate (not insert) from the superior pubic ramus and pubic crest. For more details see the "Anterior Pelvis and Thigh" section.

MEASUREMENTS AND LINES

Terminology

Abbreviations
- Purpose (P)
- Imaging examination on which measurement performed (E)
- Construction of measurement (C)
- Normal range (R)
- Abnormal range (A)

Anatomy-Based Imaging Issues

- **Acetabular protrusion**
  - P: Medial position of acetabulum relative to pelvis
  - E: AP radiograph pelvis or hip
  - C: Identify medial wall acetabulum, ilioischial line
  - Measure distance between ilioischial line & medial wall acetabulum
  - R: Medial wall acetabulum in close proximity to ilioischial line
  - A: Medial wall medial to ilioischial line
    - > 3 mm in men abnormal
    - > 6 mm in women abnormal
- **Acetabular angle/index**
  - P: Lateral acetabular coverage of femoral head
    - Developmental dysplasia
  - E: AP radiograph pelvis
  - Construction
    - Draw Hilgenreiner line (line H)
    - Draw line center femoral head to lateral margin acetabulum (line 2)
  - Measure angle between line H & line 2
  - R: Up to 30°
    - Age dependent
  - A: Greater than 30° suggests dysplasia
- **Acetabular version**: AP radiograph
  - P: Anterior to posterior acetabular angulation relative to pelvis
    - Abnormal may cause impingement by native or replaced hip
  - E: AP radiograph; extremely sensitive to positioning
  - Construction
    - Identify acetabular rims
    - Assess position of anterior rim to posterior rim
  - R: Anterior and posterior rims form an inverted "V", with anterior rim medial to posterior rim
  - A: Anterior rim lateral to posterior rim
    - May be focal especially superiorly
  - A: Alternative: Posterior rim medial to center femoral head
- **Acetabular version**: CT
  - P: Anterior to posterior acetabular angulation relative to pelvis
    - Abnormal may cause femoroacetabular impingement of native or replaced hip
  - E: Choose axial CT image at widest point femoral head
  - C: Construction
    - Draw pelvic horizontal axis line thru ischial tuberosities or posterior ischium
    - Draw line perpendicular to horizontal (line 1)
    - Draw line thru rims of acetabulum (line 2)
    - Measure angle between lines 1 & 2
  - R: Anteversion normal state
    - **Anteversion**: Anteriorly facing acetabular opening
    - (Line 2 ends medial to line 1)
  - A: Retroversion
    - **Retroversion**: Posteriorly facing acetabular opening
    - (Line 2 ends lateral to line 1)
    - Symptoms not likely until > 15°
- **Acetabular version**: Axiolateral hip radiograph
  - P: Determination of anterior to posterior acetabular angulation relative to pelvis
    - Abnormal may cause femoroacetabular impingement of native or replaced hip
  - E: Axiolateral or groin lateral radiograph
  - C: Construction
    - Draw horizontal line of pelvis; assume edge of film is representative (line 1)
    - Draw line through acetabular rims (line 2)
    - Measure angle between lines 1 and 2
  - R: Anteversion (angle open anteriorly)
  - A: Retroversion (angle open posteriorly)
- **Alpha (α) angle**
  - P: Determination of femoral head-neck offset
    - Lack of offset (or cutback) between femoral head and neck may cause femoroacetabular impingement
  - E: Oblique axial MR, CT, radiograph
  - C: Construction
    - Identify center of femoral head (point C)
    - Create best fit circle of femoral head (circle H)
    - Draw long axis femoral neck through point C (line 1)
    - Identify junction of femoral neck and circle 1 (point J)
    - Draw line through point C and point J (line 2)
    - Measure angle between lines 1 and 2
  - R: 50° or less is normal
  - A: Greater than 50° abnormal
- **Center-edge angle (of Wiberg)**
  - P: Determine lateral acetabular coverage of femoral head
    - Developmental dysplasia
    - Must be older than 5 years for measurement to be valid
  - E: AP radiograph pelvis
  - C: Construction
    - Identify center of femoral head
    - Draw Hilgenreiner line (line H)
    - Draw line perpendicular to line H through center of femoral head (line 1)
    - Draw line center of femoral head to lateral edge acetabular roof (line 2)
    - Measure angle between lines 1 and 3
  - R: Greater than 25°
  - A: Less than 20°
- **Center edge angle**: False profile view
  - Also known as **VCA (vertical center anterior margin) angle**
  - P: Determine anterior acetabular coverage of femoral head
    - Developmental dysplasia
    - Performed in adults

MEASUREMENTS AND LINES

- ○ E: False profile view hip
- ○ C: Construction
  - ■ Identify center of femoral head
  - ■ Draw long axis of pelvis (line 1); assume edge of film is representative
  - ■ Draw line from center of femoral head to anterior edge of acetabulum (line 2)
  - ■ Measure angle between lines 1 and 2
- ○ R: 20° or greater
- ○ A: Less than 20°
- **Femoral anteversion**
  - ○ P: Anterior rotation femoral neck relative to shaft
    - ■ In toeing/out toeing
    - ■ Femoroacetabular impingement
  - ○ E: Axial CT images hip & knee
  - ○ C: Construction
    - ■ Draw long axis femoral neck (line 1)
    - ■ Draw intercondylar line distal femur (line 2)
    - ■ Measure angle between lines 1 and 2
    - ■ Need to transpose line from one image to the other or superimpose images
  - ○ Alternative measure on workstation
    - ■ Measure angle line 1 relative to horizontal (angle 1)
    - ■ Measure angle line 2 relative to horizontal (angle 2)
    - ■ Subtract angle 2 from angle 1
  - ○ R: 30-40° at birth, 8-15° adult (men < women)
  - ○ A: Increased angle
    - ■ Excessive femoral anteversion: Medial femoral torsion
    - ■ Adult up to 25-30° not definitely abnormal
    - ■ Under 3 years old < 45° normal
  - ○ See "Knee Overview" section
- **Femoral angle of inclination (neck-shaft angle)**
  - ○ P: Determine angulation femoral neck relative to shaft
  - ○ E: AP radiograph hip, femur or pelvis
  - ○ C: Construction
    - ■ Long axis femoral neck (line 1)
    - ■ Long axis femoral diaphysis (line 2)
  - ○ Measure angle between line 1 & line 2
  - ○ R: 140-150° birth, 125° adult
  - ○ A: Decreased angle: **Coxa vara**
  - ○ A: Increased angle: **Coxa valga**
- **Hilgenreiner line**
  - ○ P: Establish horizontal axis of pelvis; used as landmark line for other measurements
  - ○ E: AP pelvis radiograph
  - ○ C: Drawn between inferior margins of teardrop or triradiate cartilage
- **Lateral migration femoral head**
  - ○ P: Relationship between femoral head & acetabulum
    - ■ Developmental dysplasia
  - ○ E: AP pelvis
  - ○ C: Hilgenreiner line & Perkin line (see below)
    - ■ Divides acetabulum into quadrants
  - ○ R: Normal head/metaphyseal beak in lower inner corner of quadrants
  - ○ A: Dislocated head upper outer quadrant
- **Leg length**
  - ○ P: Identify leg length discrepancy
  - ○ E: Examinations
    - ■ Radiographs with ruler between legs; spot images hip, knee, ankle
    - ■ CT scout image pelvis to ankle
    - ■ CT axial images hip, knee, ankle
  - ○ C1: Identify landmarks
    - ■ Superior iliac crest (I)
    - ■ Superior femoral head (F)
    - ■ Center medial femoral condyle (M)
    - ■ Center tibial plafond (T)
  - ○ C2: Identify landmark positions
    - ■ Radiograph: Draw horizontal line from anatomic point to ruler
    - ■ CT scout: On workstation identify slice position at each point of interest, record location
    - ■ CT axial images: Identify slice position for each point of interest, record location
  - ○ C3: Measurement: Subtract positions to determine length
    - ■ Femoral length: F - M
    - ■ Tibial length: M - T
    - ■ Overall length: F - T
    - ■ Overall length: I - T (accounts for acetabular/pelvic disease)
  - ○ R: Post-op correct to 1 cm difference
  - ○ A: Greater than 2 cm discrepancy is significant
- **Mechanical axis**
  - ○ P: Axis of weight transmission through lower extremity
    - ■ Abnormal leads to osteoarthritis
    - ■ Abnormal may result from arthritis
  - ○ E: Mechanical axis or long cassette view, weight-bearing
    - ■ Entire lower extremity hip to ankle
  - ○ C: Draw line from center of femoral head to center tibial plafond (line M)
  - ○ R: Line M passes through center of knee
  - ○ A: Medial or lateral deviation of line M at knee
- **Perkin line**
  - ○ Vertical line lateral acetabular roof perpendicular to Hilgenreiner line
- **Shenton line**
  - ○ P: Relationship femur to acetabulum
    - ■ Developmental dysplasia
  - ○ E: AP pelvis
  - ○ C: Line medial cortex femoral neck through superior obturator foramen
  - ○ R: Continuous line
  - ○ A: Interrupted line

Selected References

1. Notzli HP et al: The contour of the femoral head-neck junction as a predictor for the risk of anterior impingement. J Bone Joint Surg. 84:556-560, 2002
2. Reynolds D et al: Retroversion of the acetabulum. J Bone Joint Surg. 81-B:281-288, 1999
3. Tonnis D et al: Diminished femoral antetorsion syndrome: a cause of pain and osteoarthritis. J Ped Orthop. 11:419-431, 1991

MEASUREMENTS AND LINES

RADIOGRAPHS, ACETABULAR PROTRUSION; FEMORAL INCLINATION: MECHANICAL AXIS

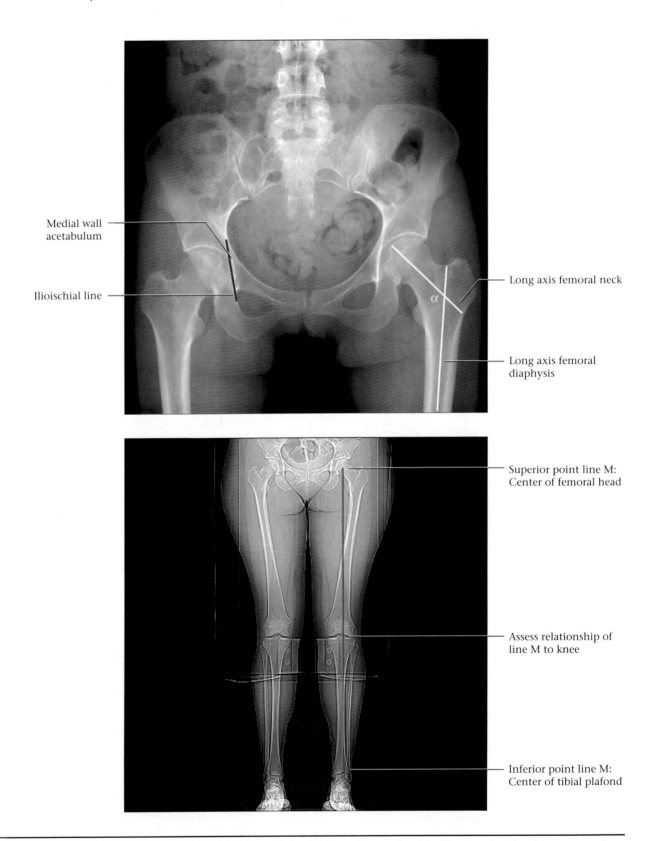

Medial wall acetabulum

Ilioischial line

Long axis femoral neck

Long axis femoral diaphysis

Superior point line M: Center of femoral head

Assess relationship of line M to knee

Inferior point line M: Center of tibial plafond

(Top) Determination of femoral angle of inclination of the left hip. The angle of inclination (angle α) is measured between the long axis of the femoral diaphysis and the long axis of the femoral neck. To assess for acetabular protrusio the relationship of the medial wall to the ilioischial line is determined. In this normal hip the medial wall of the acetabulum is within 6 mm of the ilioischial line. Thus no protrusio deformity is present. **(Bottom)** Determination of the mechanical axis (line M). With a normal mechanical axis the main force of weight is through the center of the knee.

MEASUREMENTS AND LINES

RADIOGRAPH & MR: ACETABULAR ANGLE, LATERAL MIGRATION HEAD, ALPHA ANGLE

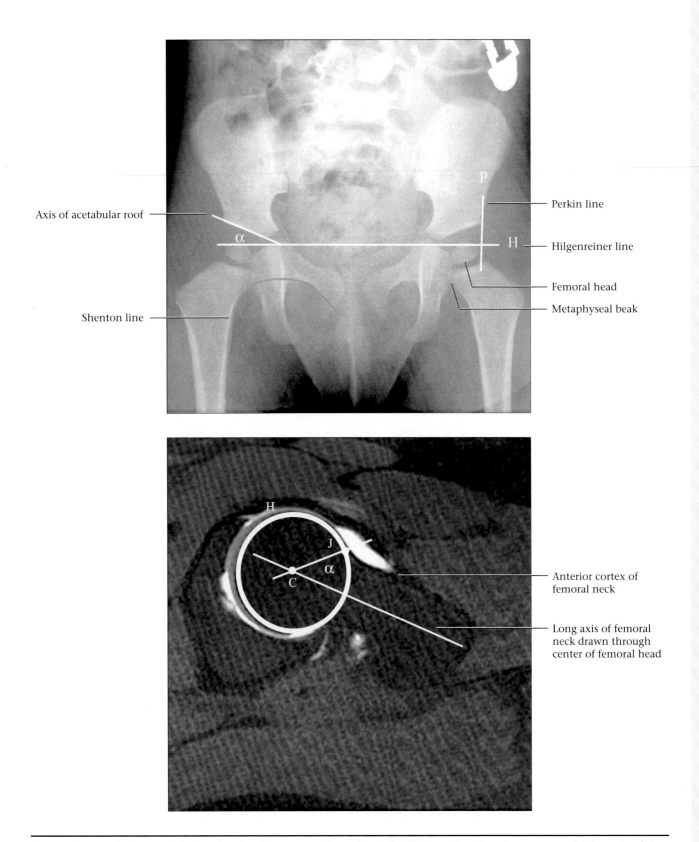

(Top) The acetabular angle/index (angle α) is measured on the right. Hilgenreiner line is constructed. The axis of the acetabular roof is drawn (see left hip for anatomic reference). The angle formed by these two lines is measured. Lateral migration of the femoral head is determined on the left. Hilgenreiner and Perkin lines are constructed. In this normal hip the head & metaphyseal beak are in the inferior medial quadrant formed by these lines. A normal Shenton line is present on the right, with continuous curvature extending from the obturator foramen to femoral metaphysis. (Bottom) The alpha (α) angle is constructed on oblique axial image. Critical points include: Circle H - best fit to perimeter of femoral head, point C - center of femoral head, point J - junction of circle H & anterior femoral neck, line CJ, long axis of femoral neck through point C.

AP & FALSE PROFILE RADIOGRAPHS, CENTER EDGE ANGLE

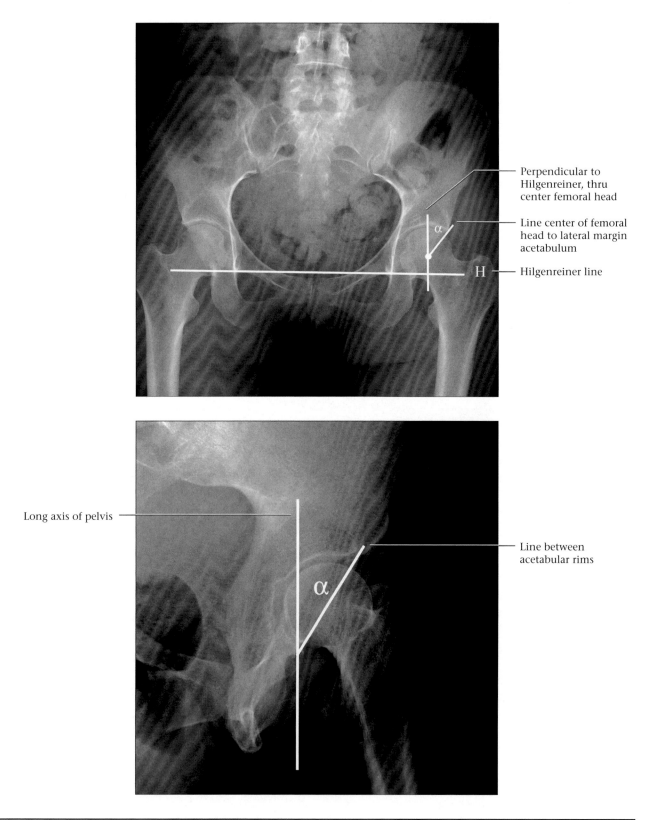

Perpendicular to Hilgenreiner, thru center femoral head

Line center of femoral head to lateral margin acetabulum

Hilgenreiner line

Long axis of pelvis

Line between acetabular rims

(Top) On an AP radiograph the center edge angle (angle α) of the acetabulum is constructed. This angle measures lateral acetabular coverage of the femoral head. **(Bottom)** The vertical center edge angle or VCA angle (angle α) is constructed on the false profile view of the hip. This angle measures anterior acetabular coverage of the femoral head. The long axis of the pelvis is a parallel to the edge of the film and is often depicted as going through the center of the femoral head, parallel to this line. The angled line extends from the acetabular rim through the center of the femoral head.

MEASUREMENTS AND LINES

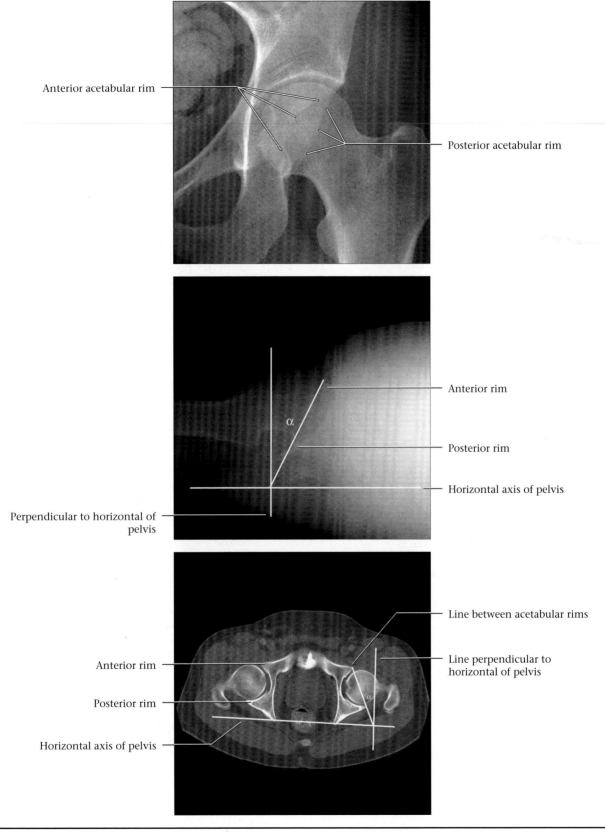

(Top) Acetabular version as determined by radiographic assessment. The relationship of the two acetabular rims is assessed. The anterior rim should be medial to the posterior rim. The posterior rim should be lateral to the center of the femoral head. (Middle) Acetabular version (angle α) measured on an axiolateral view of the hip. The horizontal axis of the pelvis is assumed to be parallel to the edge of the film. A perpendicular line to this axis is drawn. A line is then drawn through the two rims of the acetabulum. (Bottom) Acetabular version (angle α) as measured on axial CT image. The patient must be well positioned so that the hip joints are each imaged through the same point. The horizontal axis of the pelvis is drawn through the posterior aspects of the ischium. A perpendicular line to this line is constructed. A line is then drawn between the acetabular rims.

Hip and Pelvis

V

69

ANTERIOR PELVIS AND THIGH

Terminology

Abbreviations
- Anterior superior iliac spine (ASIS)
- Muscle insertion (I)
- Muscle function (F)
- Field of view (FOV)
- Nerve supply (N)
- Muscle origin (O)
- Section thickness (THK)

Imaging Anatomy

Anterior Pelvis: Osseous Anatomy
- **Bodies of pubis** articulate midline at symphysis pubis
- **Superior & inferior rami** extend from pubis
- **Pecten:** Ridge posterior aspect superior pubis
  - Origin pectineus m.
  - Insertion conjoined tendon
- **Pubic crest:** Superior surface anterior aspect pubic body
  - Insertion transversus abdominis & external oblique ms.
  - Origin rectus abdominis m.
- **Pubic tubercle:** Small protuberance lateral border pubic crest
  - Attachment inguinal ligament
- **Pubic arch:** Undersurface of ischiopubic (inferior) rami
  - Major differential feature between male & female pelvis
  - Wider (near 90°) in women
- **Pubic angle:** Between ischiopubic (inferior) rami

Symphysis Pubis
- Cartilaginous joint between pubic bodies
- Hyaline cartilage along articular surfaces
- Fibrocartilaginous intra-articular disc
  - Internal cleft with advancing age
  - Thicker in females
- **Superior pubic ligament:** Laterally extends to pubic tubercles
- **Inferior pubic ligament (arcuate pubic ligament)**
- Reinforced anteriorly by converging fibers rectus femoris, external abdominal oblique, adductor longus & brevis ms.
- Contributes little to pelvic stability
  - Diastasis up to 2.5 cm with intact posterior ligaments & maintenance pelvic stability
- Abnormal motion: 2 mm superior to inferior
  - Flamingo views, see following
- Normal width may be up to 7 mm

Adductor Musculature (see "Thigh Overview" section)
- Contributors to groin pain
  - Tenoperiosteal injuries adductor longus m.
  - Avulsion gracilis m.
- **Adductor longus m.:** Thin tendon arises from medial superior pubic ramus
  - Overlies origins gracilis, adductor brevis & magnus ms.

- **Gracilis m.:** Origin from anterior symphysis pubis & entire inferior pubic ramus
  - Origin medial to adductor brevis m., deep to adductor longus m.

Anterior Abdominal Wall
- Contributors to groin pain
  - Hernia
    - Sportsman hernia: Apparent only with straining, prehernia condition
  - Injuries rectus abdominis m. insertion
  - Abnormalities conjoined tendon
  - Posterior inguinal wall deficiency
  - Tear external oblique aponeurosis at exit iliohypogastric n.
  - Ilioinguinal n. irritation
- F: Trunk flexion, side to side bending, rotation; compress abdominal cavity, elevate diaphragm
- N: Intercostal 7-11, subcostal, iliohypogastric, ilioinguinal
  - **Iliohypogastric n.:** Traverses internal oblique m. anterior to ASIS, traverses external oblique m. above superficial inguinal ring
  - **Ilioinguinal n.:** Traverses internal oblique m. adjacent to deep inguinal ring, courses through inguinal canal
- Abdominal wall muscles
  - **Rectus abdominis:** Paired midline muscles
    - O: Superior pubic ramus, pubic crest
    - I: Xiphoid process, costal cartilages 5-7
  - **External oblique:** Most superficial
    - O: Ribs 5-12
    - I: Pubic crest, anterior iliac crest, linea alba
    - Inguinal ligament: Lower border of aponeurosis
  - **Internal oblique:** Between external oblique, transversus abdominis
    - O: Lateral inguinal ligament, iliac crest, thoracolumbar fascia
    - I: Pecten (conjoined tendon), pubic crest, inferior aspect ribs 10-12, linea alba
    - Origin anterior to deep inguinal ring
    - Insertion lateral to rectus abdominis m., posterior & medial to superficial inguinal ring
    - Arches over inguinal canal forming roof
  - **Transversus abdominis:** Deepest
    - O: Iliac crest, posterior aspect of lateral inguinal ligament, thoracolumbar fascia
    - I: Pubic crest, pecten (conjoined tendon), linea alba
    - Remains posterior to inguinal canal
    - **Transversalis fascia** along deep surface
  - **Conjoined tendon (inguinal falx):** Conjoined insertion internal oblique & transversus abdominis ms. onto pecten
    - Inconsistently present
  - **Linea alba:** Aponeurotic junction rectus femoris, transverse abdominis, internal & external oblique ms.
    - Between rectus abdominis muscle bellies
- **Rectus sheath:** Anatomy below umbilicus
  - Anterior: Aponeuroses internal oblique, external oblique, transversus abdominis ms.
  - Posterior: Peritoneum

ANTERIOR PELVIS AND THIGH

Inguinal Ligament

- Thickening inferior border external oblique aponeurosis
  - **Lacunar ligament:** Deep fibers of inguinal l., arched & posteriorly directed to insert lateral to pubic tubercle
    - Medial wall subinguinal space
    - **Pectineal ligament:** Lateral most fibers lacunar l., insert along pecten
  - **Reflected inguinal ligament:** Fibers of inguinal l. travel beyond pubic tubercle to interdigitate with contralateral external oblique aponeurosis
- Attachments: ASIS & pubic tubercle
- Separates lower extremity from pelvis
- Fascia lata attaches to inferior border
- **Subinguinal space:** Deep to inguinal ligament
  - Passageway for femoral vessels & nerve, iliopsoas m. into femoral triangle
  - External iliac vessels become femoral vessels once enter space
- **Iliopubic tract**
  - Thickening inferior border transversalis fascia
  - Deep & parallel to inguinal ligament

Inguinal Canal

- Anterior wall: External oblique aponeurosis & internal oblique m.
- Posterior wall: Transversalis fascia & conjoined tendon
- Roof: Lower border internal oblique m.
- Floor: Iliopubic tract lateral, inguinal ligament midportion, lacunar ligament medial
- Entrance: **Deep inguinal ring**
  - Located midinguinal ligament
  - Opening of evaginated transversalis fascia through which spermatic cord/round ligament pass
- Exit: Superficial inguinal ring
  - **Superficial inguinal ring:** Division of external oblique aponeurosis lateral to pubic tubercle
    - **Lateral crus:** Inserts pubic tubercle
    - **Medial crus:** Inserts pubic crest
    - **Intercrural fibers:** Superficial to canal; run medial crus to lateral crus
- Oblique orientation medial & inferior
  - Obliquity protections against hernia formation
  - Obliquity accounts for changing boundaries from lateral to medial
- Contents: Ilioinguinal nerve; male - spermatic cord, female - round ligament; associated vessels
  - Covered by evaginated transversalis fascia
- Clinical note: **Hernias**
  - Direct inguinal hernia from weak posterior inguinal wall
    - Medial to inferior epigastric a.
    - Lateral to spermatic cord
    - Not in deep inguinal ring
    - No preformed sac
    - Transversalis fascia covers
  - Indirect inguinal hernia through patent processus vaginalis into deep inguinal ring
    - **Processus vaginalis:** Peritoneal diverticulum that follows descending testes, usually closes off
    - Lateral to inferior epigastric a.
    - Within spermatic cord
    - More common overall
    - More common in men
    - May enter scrotum/labia
  - All hernias exit superficial inguinal ring
  - Inguinal hernias medial & superior to pubic tubercle
  - See "Thigh Overview" for femoral hernias

Clinical Notes

- Groin pain
  - Vague term attributable to multitude of causes including internal derangements hip, symphysis pubis, abdominal wall ms., adductor ms., stress fractures femur & pelvis
- Pubalgia
  - Groin pain, indeterminate physical examination

Anatomy-Based Imaging Issues

Imaging Recommendations

- Radiographs
  - AP pelvis: General assessment
  - Pelvic inlet: Anterior to posterior displacement
    - Usually post-trauma
  - Pelvic outlet: Superior to inferior displacement
    - Usually post-trauma
  - Flamingo views: Instability
    - AP pelvis, weightbearing on each lower extremity
    - Used occasionally for chronic injury, groin pain
- CT
  - Assess osseous integrity
  - 2.5 mm thick reconstructions
- MR
  - Coronal, axial images preferred
  - T1-weighted, fluid sensitive sequences, no contrast
  - FOV: 18-30 cm, THK: 3-5 mm, Matrix: 256 x 256
  - Surface coil
  - Prone position may eliminate motion artifacts
  - Screen entire pelvis: Fluid sensitive coronal
- Joint puncture
  - Uncommon
  - Indications: Infection, anesthetic & steroid injection
  - Arthrography: Diagnose adductor avulsions
- Herniography
  - Contrast injection abdominal cavity to identify outpouchings (hernias)

Imaging Pitfalls

- Osteitis pubis
  - Widening/narrowing, osteopenia/sclerosis, fragmentation, erosions/cysts, beaking/osteophytes, instability, bone marrow edema
  - Common with advancing age
  - Likely result of chronic repetitive stress
  - Reserve term for imaging findings with or without symptoms
    - Correlate with symptoms in athlete
    - When associated symptoms, traumatic osteitis pubis or pubic bone stress injury
- Hernias
  - Little successful imaging for early hernias
  - Herniography not in widespread use
  - Ultrasound may be useful for sportsman hernia

RADIOGRAPH & GRAPHIC, SYMPHYSIS PUBIS

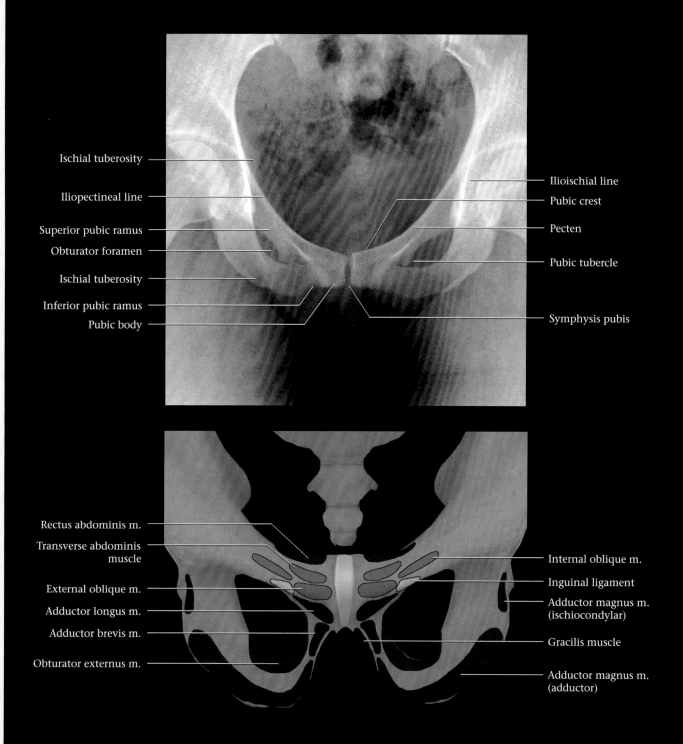

Ischial tuberosity

Iliopectineal line

Superior pubic ramus

Obturator foramen

Ischial tuberosity

Inferior pubic ramus

Pubic body

Ilioischial line

Pubic crest

Pecten

Pubic tubercle

Symphysis pubis

Rectus abdominis m.

Transverse abdominis muscle

External oblique m.

Adductor longus m.

Adductor brevis m.

Obturator externus m.

Internal oblique m.

Inguinal ligament

Adductor magnus m. (ischiocondylar)

Gracilis muscle

Adductor magnus m. (adductor)

(Top) AP radiograph coned down to the anterior pelvis. The symphysis pubis and the different regions of the pubic body and the pubic rami are evident. (Bottom) Anterior view of the anterior pelvis and the associated muscle attachments. A number of muscles take origin or insert onto the anterior aspect of the pelvis. These muscles aid in movement and stabilization of the trunk as well as movement and stabilization of the leg.

AXIAL T1 MR, SYMPHYSIS PUBIS & ADDUCTOR MUSCLES

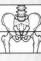

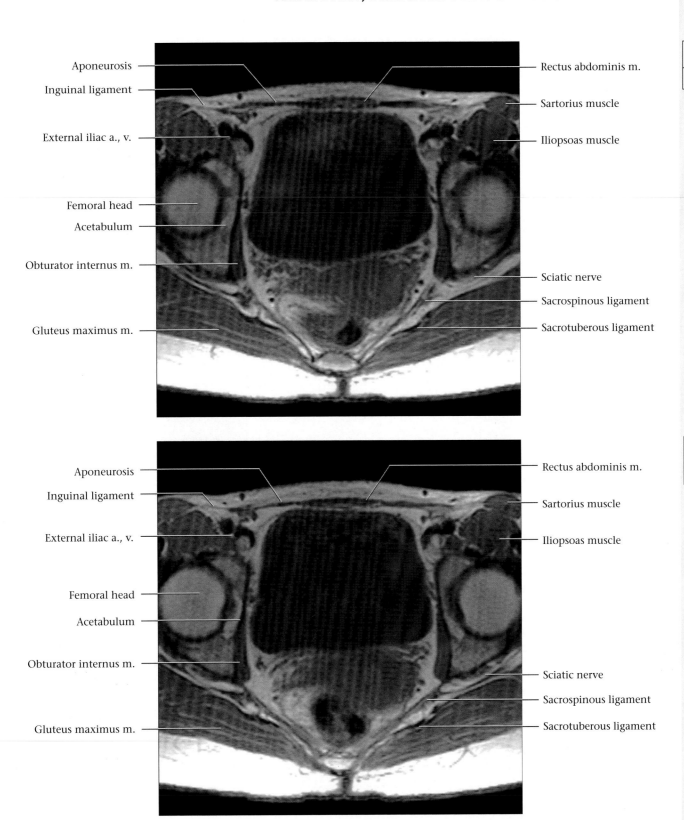

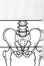

Aponeurosis
Inguinal ligament
External iliac a., v.
Femoral head
Acetabulum
Obturator internus m.
Gluteus maximus m.
Rectus abdominis m.
Sartorius muscle
Iliopsoas muscle
Sciatic nerve
Sacrospinous ligament
Sacrotuberous ligament

Aponeurosis
Inguinal ligament
External iliac a., v.
Femoral head
Acetabulum
Obturator internus m.
Gluteus maximus m.
Rectus abdominis m.
Sartorius muscle
Iliopsoas muscle
Sciatic nerve
Sacrospinous ligament
Sacrotuberous ligament

(Top) Axial images from superior to inferior. The rectus abdominis muscles are paired midline muscles. At this level the external and internal abdominal oblique and transversus muscle bellies are no longer visible. The aponeuroses of these muscles have joined together. **(Bottom)** The inguinal ligament is the inferior border of the external oblique aponeurosis. Its orientation is from superolateral to inferomedial. On axial images it is seen along the lateral edge of the fused aponeuroses.

Hip and Pelvis

∨

AXIAL T1 MR, SYMPHYSIS PUBIS & ADDUCTOR MUSCLES

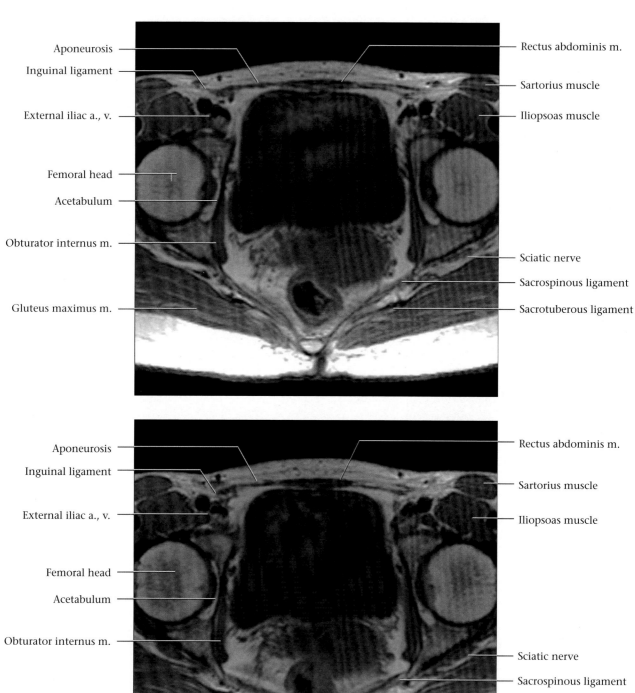

Aponeurosis — Rectus abdominis m.

Inguinal ligament — Sartorius muscle

External iliac a., v. — Iliopsoas muscle

Femoral head

Acetabulum

Obturator internus m. — Sciatic nerve

— Sacrospinous ligament

Gluteus maximus m. — Sacrotuberous ligament

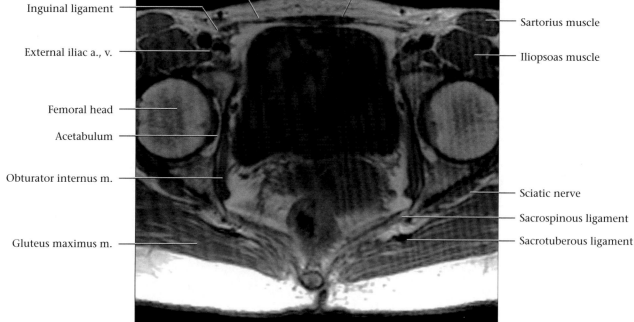

Aponeurosis — Rectus abdominis m.

Inguinal ligament — Sartorius muscle

External iliac a., v. — Iliopsoas muscle

Femoral head

Acetabulum

Obturator internus m. — Sciatic nerve

— Sacrospinous ligament

Gluteus maximus m. — Sacrotuberous ligament

(Top) The inguinal ligament is a landmark separating the pelvis from thigh. In the axial plane the structures lateral to the ligament are within the thigh. The structures medial and deep are within the pelvis. **(Bottom)** The external iliac vessels are deep to the inguinal ligament.

AXIAL T1 MR, SYMPHYSIS PUBIS & ADDUCTOR MUSCLES

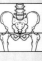

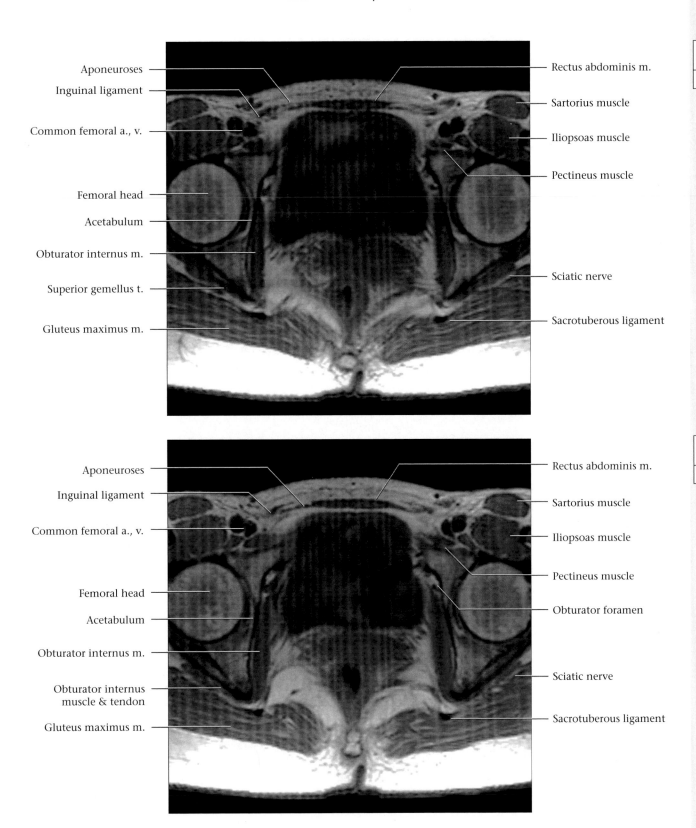

Aponeuroses

Inguinal ligament

Common femoral a., v.

Femoral head

Acetabulum

Obturator internus m.

Superior gemellus t.

Gluteus maximus m.

Rectus abdominis m.

Sartorius muscle

Iliopsoas muscle

Pectineus muscle

Sciatic nerve

Sacrotuberous ligament

Aponeuroses

Inguinal ligament

Common femoral a., v.

Femoral head

Acetabulum

Obturator internus m.

Obturator internus muscle & tendon

Gluteus maximus m.

Rectus abdominis m.

Sartorius muscle

Iliopsoas muscle

Pectineus muscle

Obturator foramen

Sciatic nerve

Sacrotuberous ligament

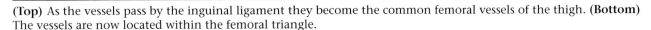

(Top) As the vessels pass by the inguinal ligament they become the common femoral vessels of the thigh. **(Bottom)** The vessels are now located within the femoral triangle.

Hip and Pelvis

V

AXIAL T1 MR, SYMPHYSIS PUBIS & ADDUCTOR MUSCLES

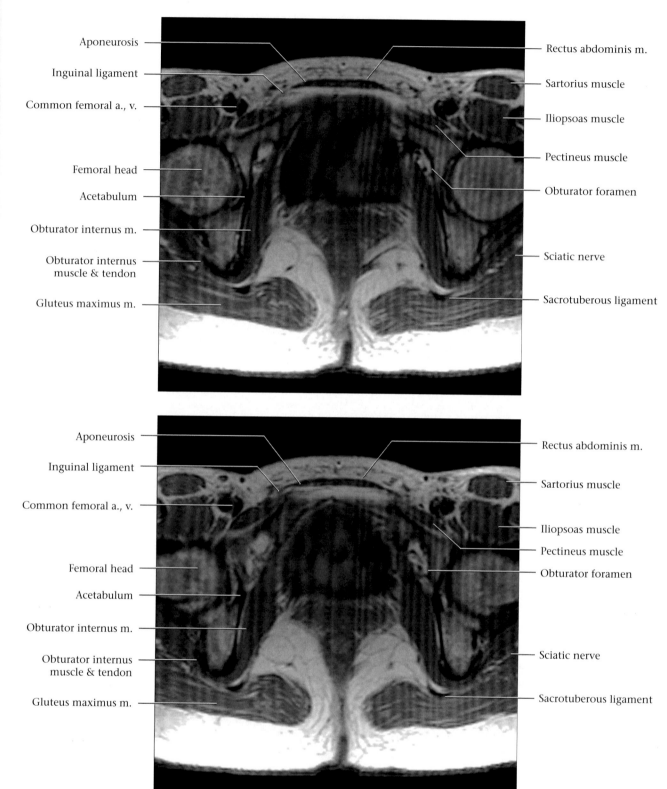

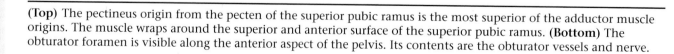

(Top) The pectineus origin from the pecten of the superior pubic ramus is the most superior of the adductor muscle origins. The muscle wraps around the superior and anterior surface of the superior pubic ramus. **(Bottom)** The obturator foramen is visible along the anterior aspect of the pelvis. Its contents are the obturator vessels and nerve.

AXIAL T1 MR, SYMPHYSIS PUBIS & ADDUCTOR MUSCLES

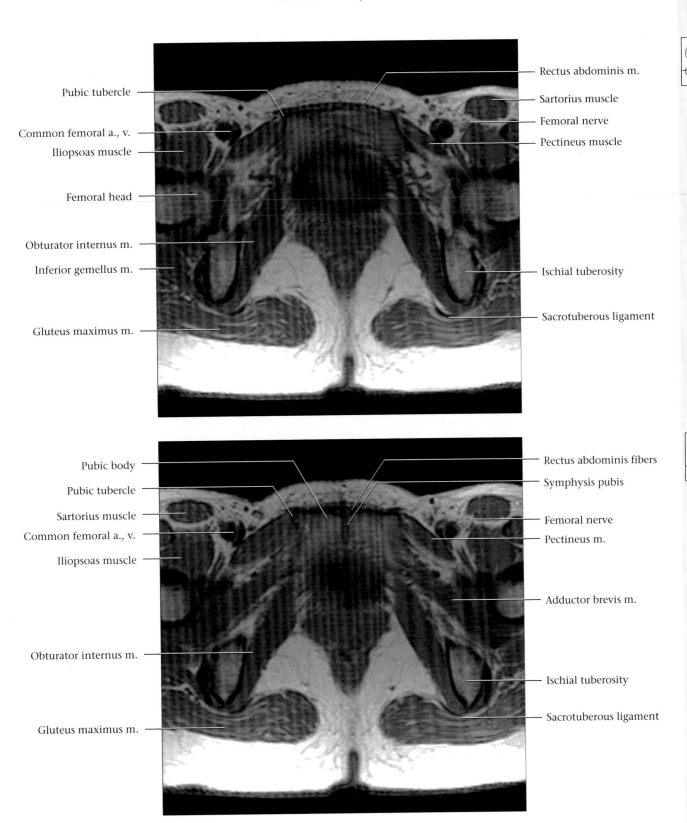

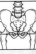

Top image labels:

Pubic tubercle

Common femoral a., v.

Iliopsoas muscle

Femoral head

Obturator internus m.

Inferior gemellus m.

Gluteus maximus m.

Rectus abdominis m.

Sartorius muscle

Femoral nerve

Pectineus muscle

Ischial tuberosity

Sacrotuberous ligament

Bottom image labels:

Pubic body

Pubic tubercle

Sartorius muscle

Common femoral a., v.

Iliopsoas muscle

Obturator internus m.

Gluteus maximus m.

Rectus abdominis fibers

Symphysis pubis

Femoral nerve

Pectineus m.

Adductor brevis m.

Ischial tuberosity

Sacrotuberous ligament

(Top) The femoral nerve has been traveling along the lateral aspect of the artery on all images superior to this one; however this is the first image on which it can be identified. It is the most lateral structure in the femoral triangle. **(Bottom)** The protrusion of the pubic tubercle from pelvis anterior surface of pubic body is apparent. This tubercle is the site of the medial attachment of the inguinal ligament. Fibers from the rectus abdominis muscle travel beyond the muscle to serve as reinforcements to the anterior aspect of the symphysis pubis.

AXIAL T1 MR, SYMPHYSIS PUBIS & ADDUCTOR MUSCLES

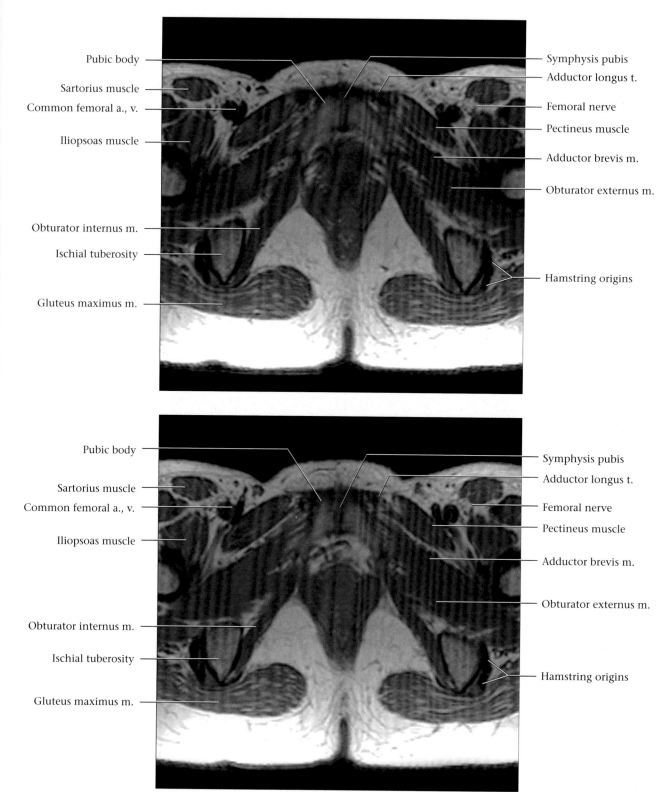

Left labels (top image):
Pubic body
Sartorius muscle
Common femoral a., v.
Iliopsoas muscle
Obturator internus m.
Ischial tuberosity
Gluteus maximus m.

Right labels (top image):
Symphysis pubis
Adductor longus t.
Femoral nerve
Pectineus muscle
Adductor brevis m.
Obturator externus m.
Hamstring origins

Left labels (bottom image):
Pubic body
Sartorius muscle
Common femoral a., v.
Iliopsoas muscle
Obturator internus m.
Ischial tuberosity
Gluteus maximus m.

Right labels (bottom image):
Symphysis pubis
Adductor longus t.
Femoral nerve
Pectineus muscle
Adductor brevis m.
Obturator externus m.
Hamstring origins

(Top) The origin of the obturator externus muscle includes the obturator membrane which is not visible on these images. Its origin from the pubic margin of the foramen is readily appreciated. **(Bottom)** The adductor longus muscle originates via a long tendon from a small region of the anterior pubic body inferior to the pubic crest.

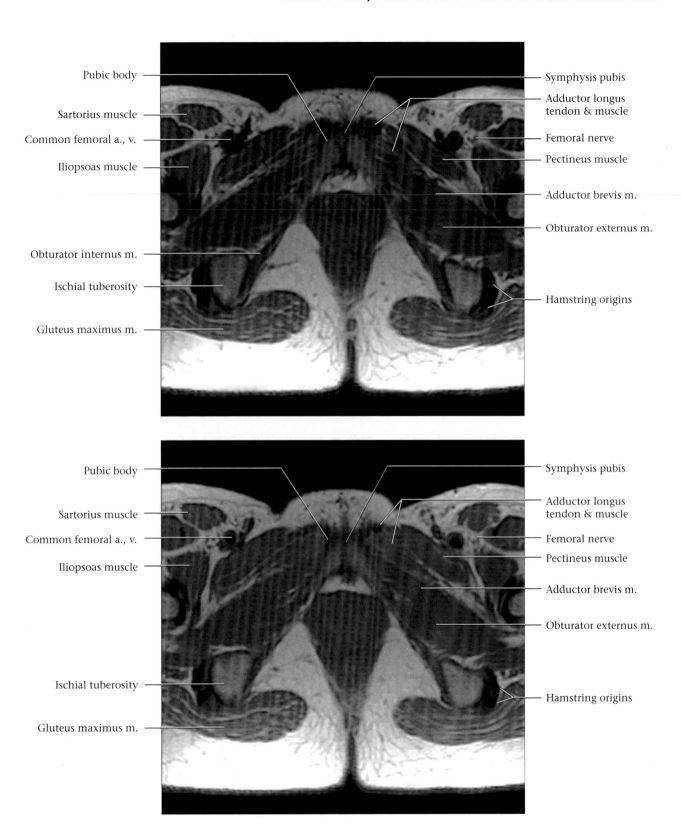

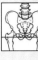

(Top) The origin of the adductor brevis muscle is from the anterior surface of the inferior pubic ramus just distal to the symphysis pubis. The adductor brevis muscle is located deep and lateral to the adductor longus muscle. **(Bottom)** The adductor brevis muscle is located anterior to the obturator externus muscle and on axial images may be difficult to separate from that muscle.

AXIAL T1 MR, SYMPHYSIS PUBIS & ADDUCTOR MUSCLES

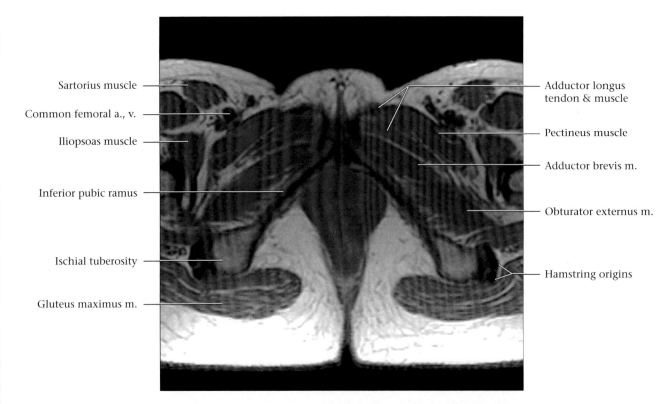

Sartorius muscle

Common femoral a., v.

Iliopsoas muscle

Inferior pubic ramus

Ischial tuberosity

Gluteus maximus m.

Adductor longus tendon & muscle

Pectineus muscle

Adductor brevis m.

Obturator externus m.

Hamstring origins

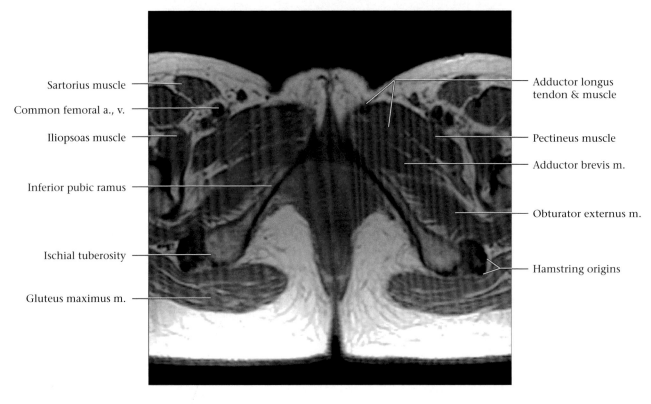

Sartorius muscle

Common femoral a., v.

Iliopsoas muscle

Inferior pubic ramus

Ischial tuberosity

Gluteus maximus m.

Adductor longus tendon & muscle

Pectineus muscle

Adductor brevis m.

Obturator externus m.

Hamstring origins

(Top) From anterior to posterior in the upper thigh the adductor muscles are pectineus, adductor longus and adductor brevis respectively. **(Bottom)** In the coronal plane the pectineus and adductor longus muscles lie in the same plane. The origin of the gracilis muscle is from the inferior pubic ramus and inferior surface of the symphysis pubis. For images of the origin of this tendon and anatomy inferior to this level see " Thigh Overview" section.

Hip and Pelvis

V

CORONAL T1 MR, SYMPHYSIS PUBIS & ADDUCTOR MUSCLES

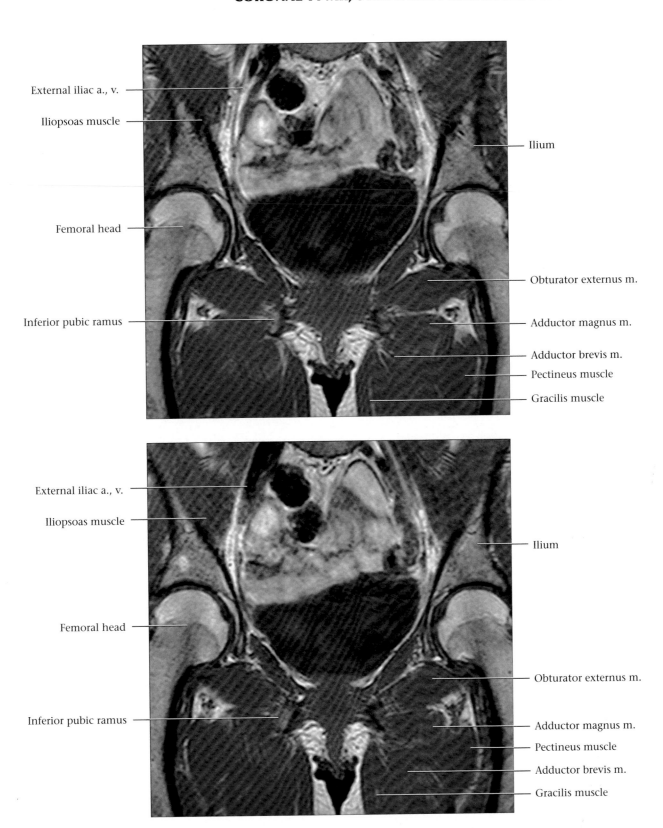

External iliac a., v.

Iliopsoas muscle

Ilium

Femoral head

Obturator externus m.

Inferior pubic ramus

Adductor magnus m.

Adductor brevis m.

Pectineus muscle

Gracilis muscle

External iliac a., v.

Iliopsoas muscle

Ilium

Femoral head

Obturator externus m.

Inferior pubic ramus

Adductor magnus m.

Pectineus muscle

Adductor brevis m.

Gracilis muscle

(Top) Coronal images of the anterior pelvis from posterior to anterior. The obturator externus and internus muscles are seen along the inner and outer margins of the foramen. The adductor muscles are difficult to distinguish from one another. The adductor magnus is the most posterior of these muscles. Its uppermost fibers are horizontally oriented. **(Bottom)** In the anterior to posterior direction the adductor brevis muscle is located between the adductor magnus and adductor longus muscle. Therefore these three muscles may not be seen in the same plane. The adductor brevis fibers travel lateral and inferior.

Hip and Pelvis

V

CORONAL T1 MR, SYMPHYSIS PUBIS & ADDUCTOR MUSCLES

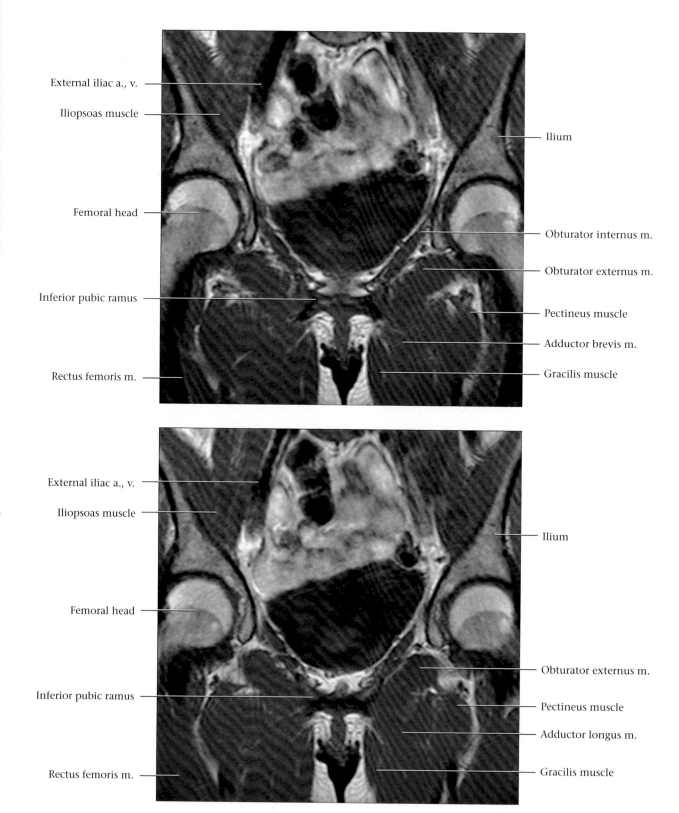

External iliac a., v.

Iliopsoas muscle

Femoral head

Inferior pubic ramus

Rectus femoris m.

Ilium

Obturator internus m.

Obturator externus m.

Pectineus muscle

Adductor brevis m.

Gracilis muscle

External iliac a., v.

Iliopsoas muscle

Femoral head

Inferior pubic ramus

Rectus femoris m.

Ilium

Obturator externus m.

Pectineus muscle

Adductor longus m.

Gracilis muscle

(Top) The gracilis muscle is the most medial of the adductor muscles. **(Bottom)** The pectineus muscle is located lateral to the adductor longus and brevis muscles. The pectineus muscle has the most medial insertion of these muscles onto the posterior aspect of the femur.

CORONAL T1 MR, SYMPHYSIS PUBIS & ADDUCTOR MUSCLES

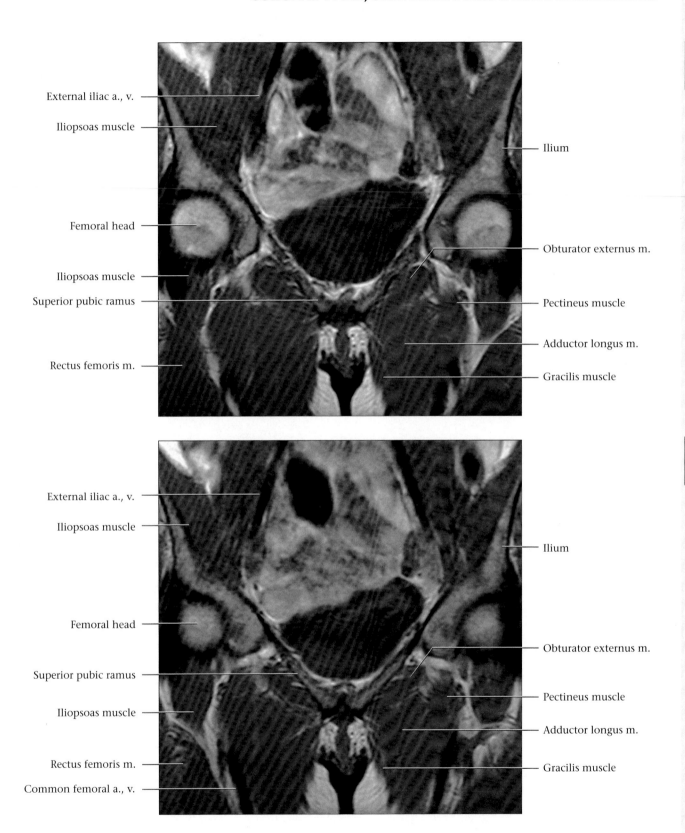

External iliac a., v.

Iliopsoas muscle

Femoral head

Iliopsoas muscle

Superior pubic ramus

Rectus femoris m.

Ilium

Obturator externus m.

Pectineus muscle

Adductor longus m.

Gracilis muscle

External iliac a., v.

Iliopsoas muscle

Femoral head

Superior pubic ramus

Iliopsoas muscle

Rectus femoris m.

Common femoral a., v.

Ilium

Obturator externus m.

Pectineus muscle

Adductor longus m.

Gracilis muscle

(Top) Recognition of the superior pubic ramus is one landmark that will help identify the adductor longus muscle and differentiate it from the adductor brevis muscle. **(Bottom)** The adductor longus muscle forms the medial border of the femoral triangle. Thus, the vessels may be used as landmarks for differentiation of the adductor longus and brevis muscles in the coronal plane.

CORONAL T1 MR, SYMPHYSIS PUBIS & ADDUCTOR MUSCLES

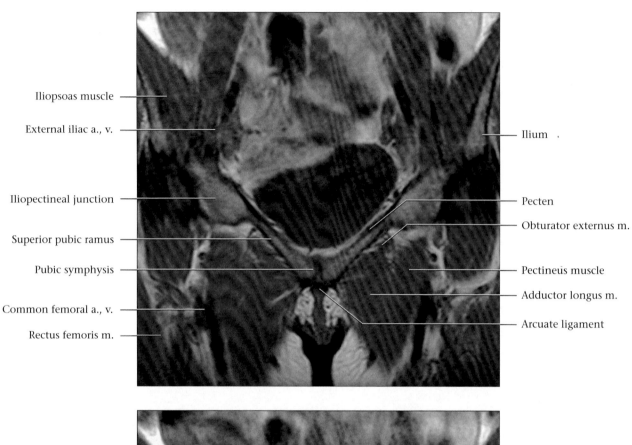

Iliopsoas muscle

External iliac a., v.

Iliopectineal junction

Superior pubic ramus

Pubic symphysis

Common femoral a., v.

Rectus femoris m.

Ilium

Pecten

Obturator externus m.

Pectineus muscle

Adductor longus m.

Arcuate ligament

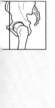

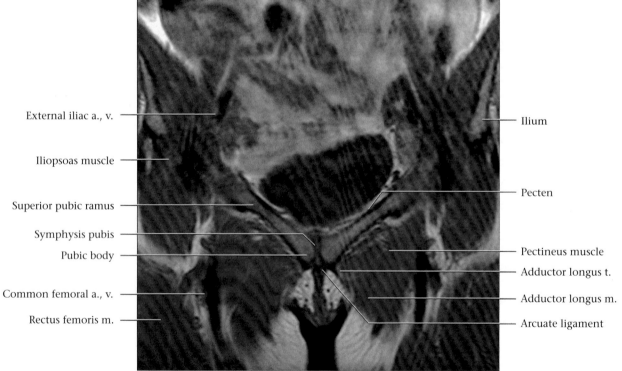

External iliac a., v.

Iliopsoas muscle

Superior pubic ramus

Symphysis pubis

Pubic body

Common femoral a., v.

Rectus femoris m.

Ilium

Pecten

Pectineus muscle

Adductor longus t.

Adductor longus m.

Arcuate ligament

(Top) The arcuate ligament is a relatively thick structure which helps to reinforce the inferior aspect of the symphysis pubis. The ridge along the superior pubic ramus is known as the pecten. **(Bottom)** Note the small area of origin of the adductor longus tendon.

ANTERIOR PELVIS AND THIGH

CORONAL T1 MR, SYMPHYSIS PUBIS & ADDUCTOR MUSCLES

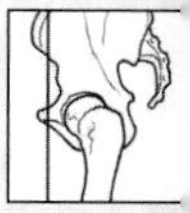

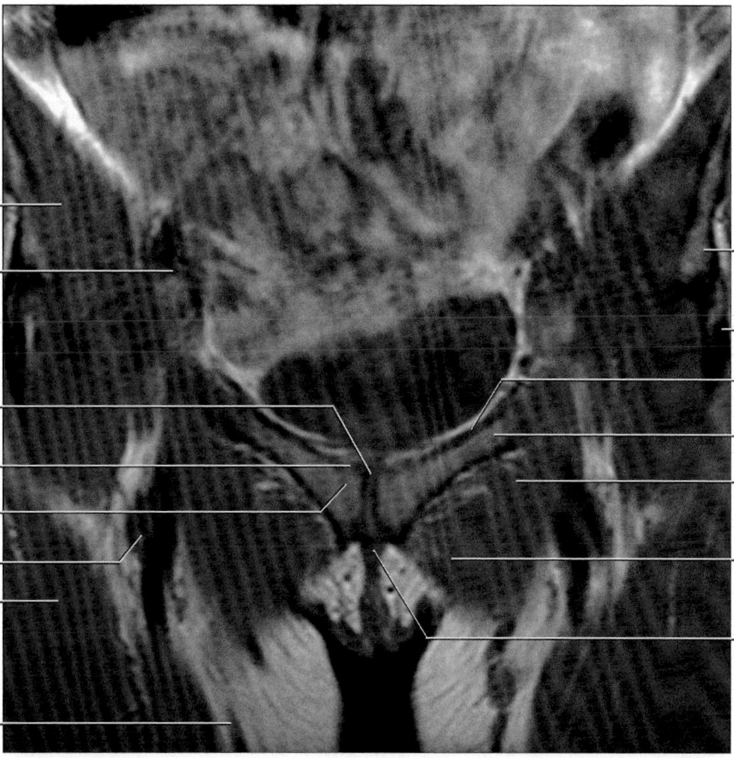

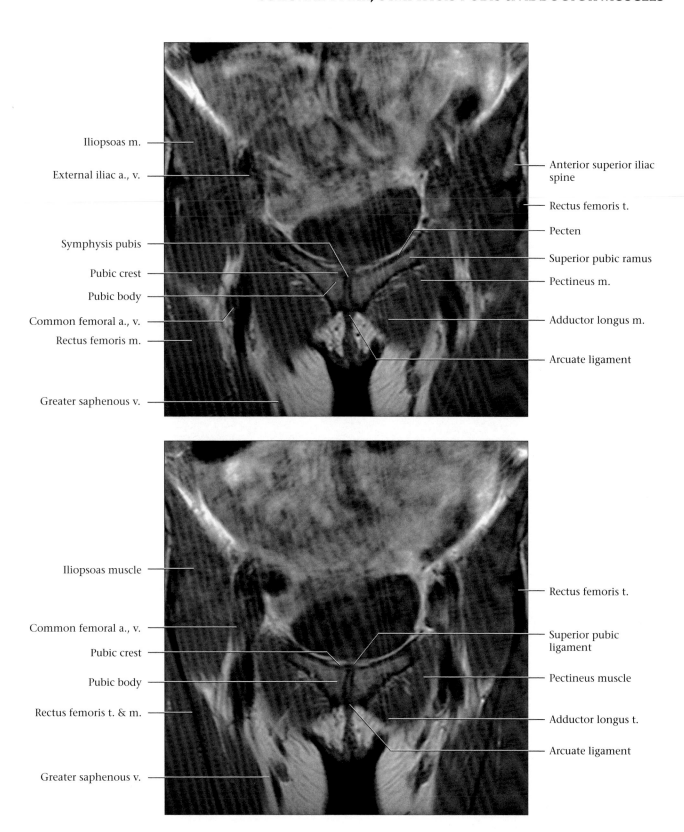

Iliopsoas m.
External iliac a., v.
Symphysis pubis
Pubic crest
Pubic body
Common femoral a., v.
Rectus femoris m.
Greater saphenous v.
Anterior superior iliac spine
Rectus femoris t.
Pecten
Superior pubic ramus
Pectineus m.
Adductor longus m.
Arcuate ligament

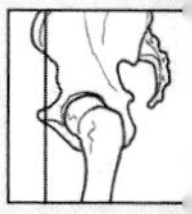

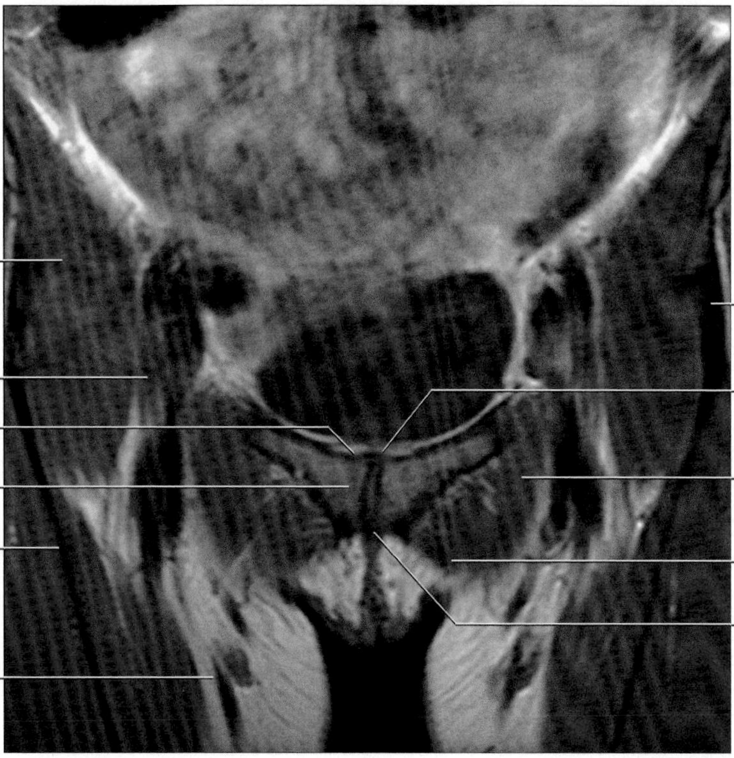

Iliopsoas muscle
Common femoral a., v.
Pubic crest
Pubic body
Rectus femoris t. & m.
Greater saphenous v.
Rectus femoris t.
Superior pubic ligament
Pectineus muscle
Adductor longus t.
Arcuate ligament

(Top) The adductor longus muscle is in close proximity to the symphysis pubis. Dysfunction or injury to the adductor longus muscle may contribute to instability of the symphysis. **(Bottom)** The relatively small superior pubic ligament is visible on this image.

CORONAL T1 MR, SYMPHYSIS PUBIS & ADDUCTOR MUSCLES

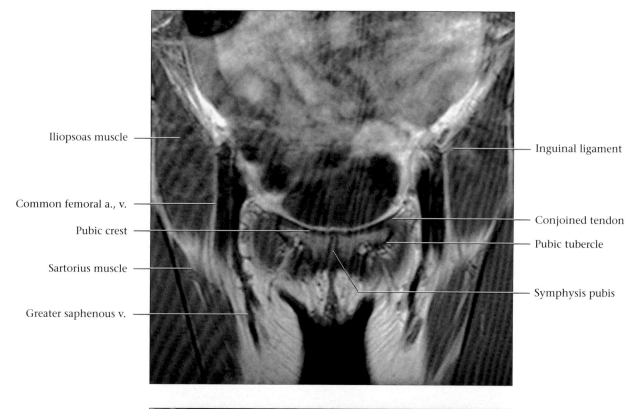

Iliopsoas muscle

Common femoral a., v.

Pubic crest

Sartorius muscle

Greater saphenous v.

Inguinal ligament

Conjoined tendon

Pubic tubercle

Symphysis pubis

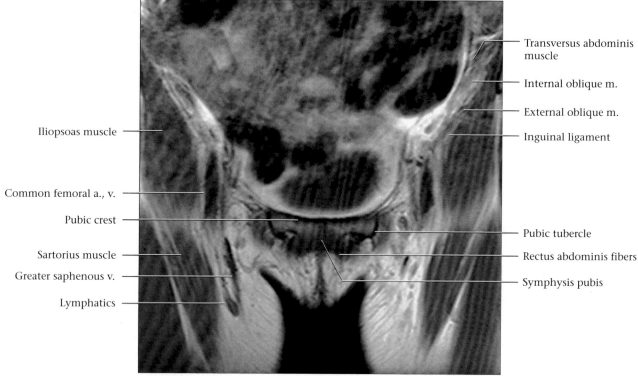

Iliopsoas muscle

Common femoral a., v.

Pubic crest

Sartorius muscle

Greater saphenous v.

Lymphatics

Transversus abdominis muscle

Internal oblique m.

External oblique m.

Inguinal ligament

Pubic tubercle

Rectus abdominis fibers

Symphysis pubis

(Top) The pubic tubercles are easy to visualize on this image. The pubic crest is the superior portion of the pubic body medial to the tubercle. The conjoined tendon of the obturator internus and transversus abdominis muscles inserts onto the pubic crest. (Bottom) The inguinal ligament orientation from superolateral to inferomedial is easy to appreciate on this image. Note the vessels as they cross beneath the ligament to enter the femoral triangle.

CORONAL T1 MR, SYMPHYSIS PUBIS & ADDUCTOR MUSCLES

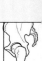

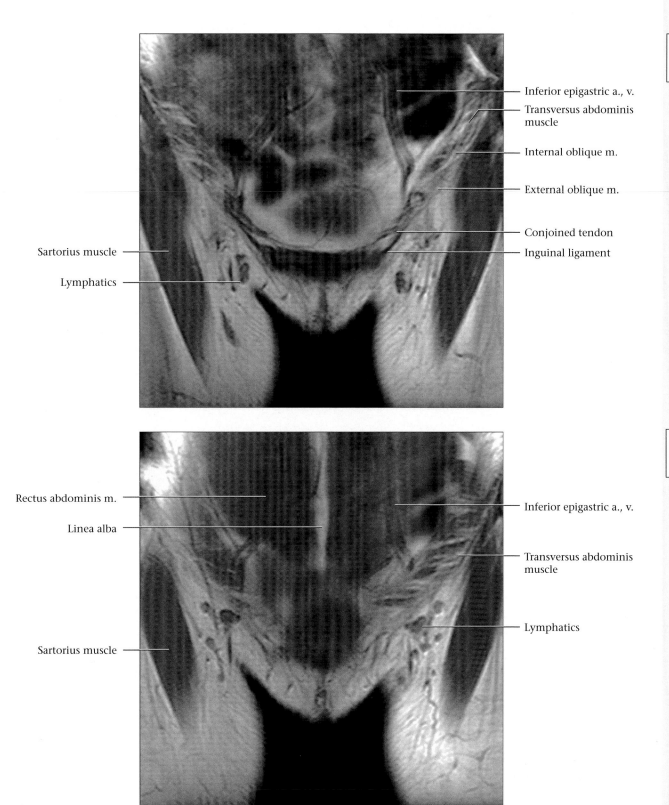

Inferior epigastric a., v.

Transversus abdominis muscle

Internal oblique m.

External oblique m.

Conjoined tendon

Inguinal ligament

Sartorius muscle

Lymphatics

Rectus abdominis m.

Linea alba

Inferior epigastric a., v.

Transversus abdominis muscle

Lymphatics

Sartorius muscle

(Top) The lateral aspect of the anterior abdominal wall consists of three layers. The transverse abdominis fibers are the deepest and are horizontally oriented. The middle layer, internal oblique muscle, is comprised of muscle fibers which are oriented from the iliac crest upward and medially. The external oblique fibers are oriented from superolateral to inferomedial. **(Bottom)** The anterior abdominal wall consists of the paired midline rectus abdominis muscle with longitudinally oriented muscle fibers. The inferior epigastric vessels are located along the lateral aspect of these muscle bellies.

Hip and Pelvis

V

SAGITTAL T1 MR, SYMPHYSIS PUBIS & ADDUCTOR MUSCLES

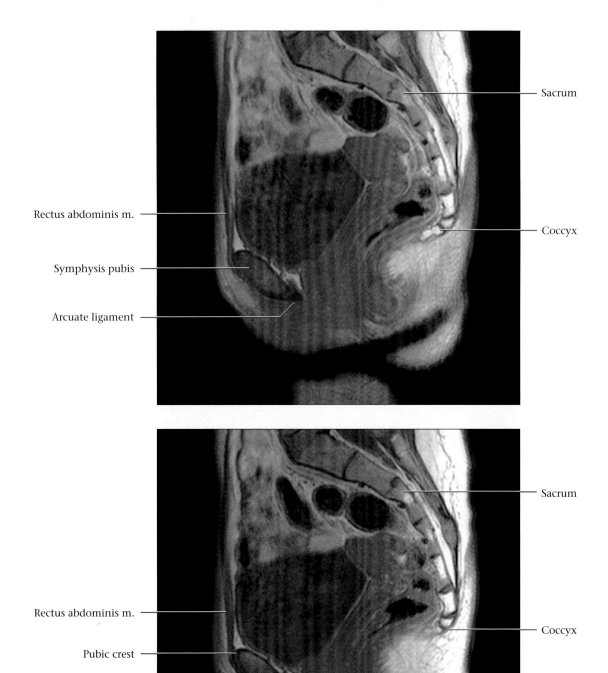

Rectus abdominis m.

Symphysis pubis

Arcuate ligament

Sacrum

Coccyx

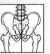

Rectus abdominis m.

Pubic crest

Symphysis pubis

Arcuate ligament

Sacrum

Coccyx

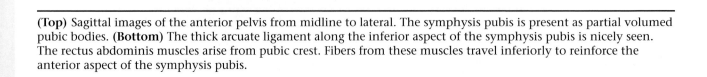

(Top) Sagittal images of the anterior pelvis from midline to lateral. The symphysis pubis is present as partial volumed pubic bodies. **(Bottom)** The thick arcuate ligament along the inferior aspect of the symphysis pubis is nicely seen. The rectus abdominis muscles arise from pubic crest. Fibers from these muscles travel inferiorly to reinforce the anterior aspect of the symphysis pubis.

ANTERIOR PELVIS AND THIGH

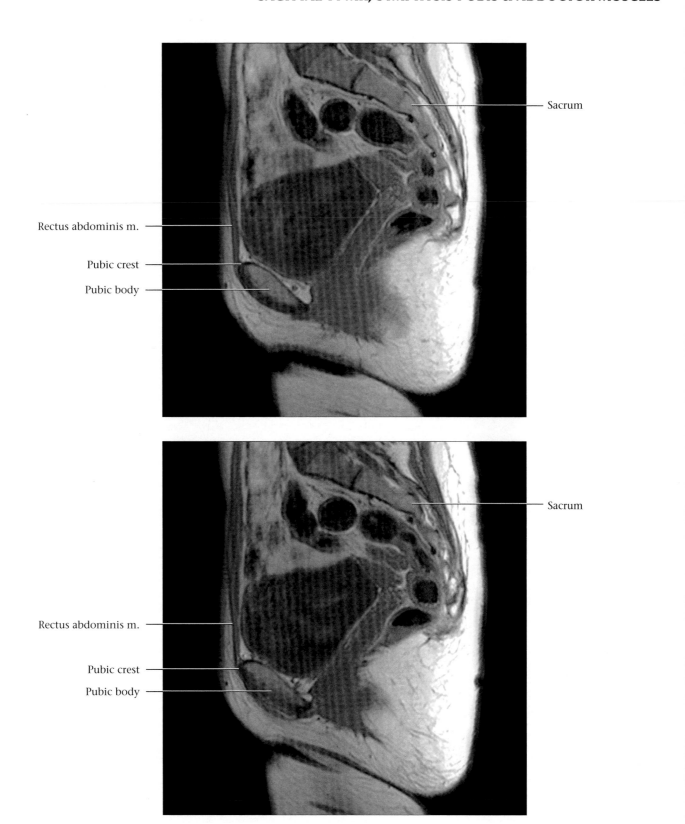

(Top) The elongated short axis of the pubic body is visible. (Bottom) Note how the rectus abdominis muscle thins from superior to inferior.

SAGITTAL T1 MR, SYMPHYSIS PUBIS & ADDUCTOR MUSCLES

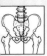

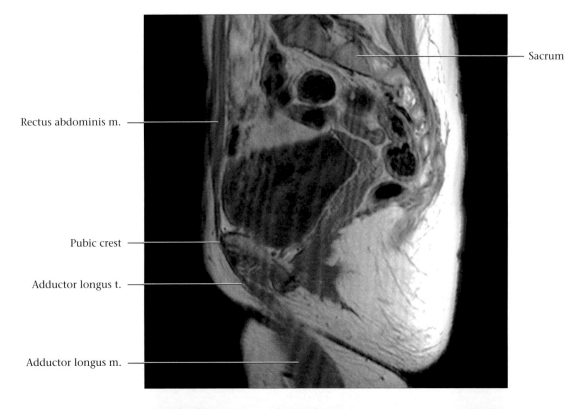

Rectus abdominis m.

Pubic crest

Adductor longus t.

Adductor longus m.

Sacrum

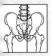

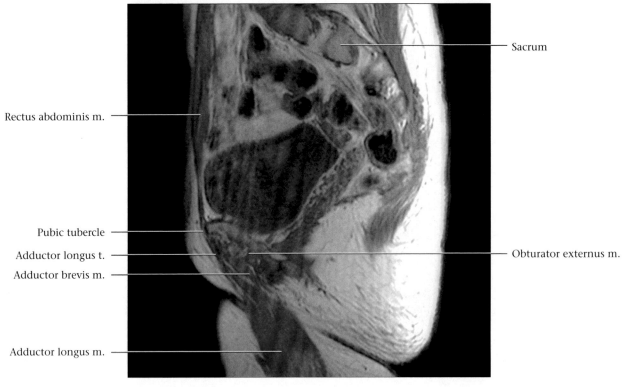

Rectus abdominis m.

Pubic tubercle

Adductor longus t.

Adductor brevis m.

Adductor longus m.

Sacrum

Obturator externus m.

(Top) The small site of origin of the adductor longus muscle is well depicted on this image. The pubic body thins along its lateral aspect prior to giving rise to the pubic rami. **(Bottom)** The anterior protrusion of the pubic tubercle is apparent. The adductor brevis muscle lies deep to the adductor longus muscle. The obturator externus muscle is deep to the adductor brevis muscle.

SAGITTAL T1 MR, SYMPHYSIS PUBIS & ADDUCTOR MUSCLES

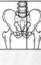

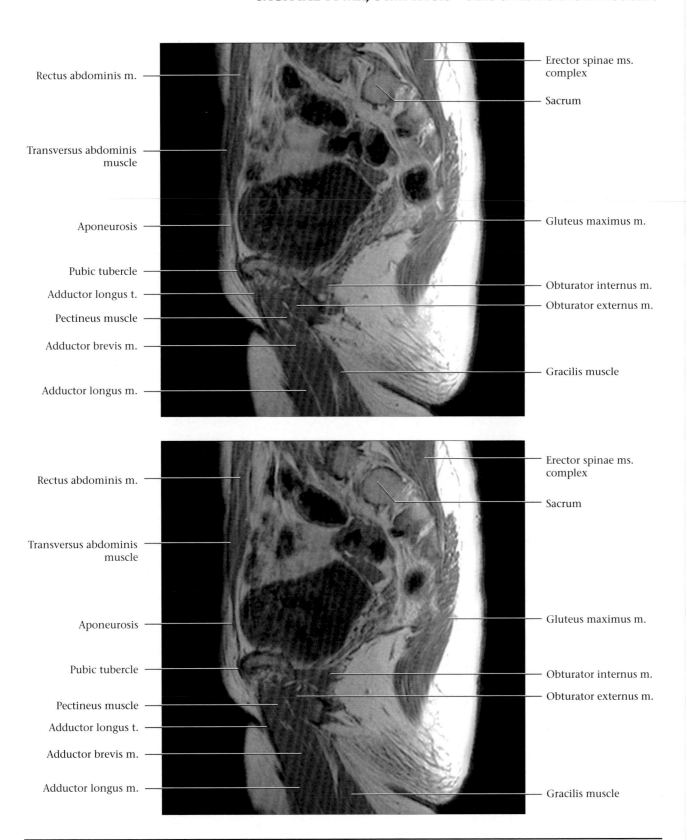

Rectus abdominis m.

Transversus abdominis muscle

Aponeurosis

Pubic tubercle

Adductor longus t.

Pectineus muscle

Adductor brevis m.

Adductor longus m.

Erector spinae ms. complex

Sacrum

Gluteus maximus m.

Obturator internus m.

Obturator externus m.

Gracilis muscle

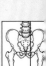

Rectus abdominis m.

Transversus abdominis muscle

Aponeurosis

Pubic tubercle

Pectineus muscle

Adductor longus t.

Adductor brevis m.

Adductor longus m.

Erector spinae ms. complex

Sacrum

Gluteus maximus m.

Obturator internus m.

Obturator externus m.

Gracilis muscle

(Top) The transition from the rectus abdominis muscle to the lateral abdominal muscles is not a distinct transition. The gracilis muscle takes origin from the inferior pubic ramus and that origin is nicely seen on this image. **(Bottom)** The thin fused aponeuroses of the lateral abdominal muscles is located along the inferior and lateral aspect of the abdominal wall. The inguinal ligament is formed by the lower border of the external oblique aponeurosis. The attachment of that structure to the pubic tubercle is visualized here.

Hip and Pelvis

V

SAGITTAL T1 MR, SYMPHYSIS PUBIS & ADDUCTOR MUSCLES

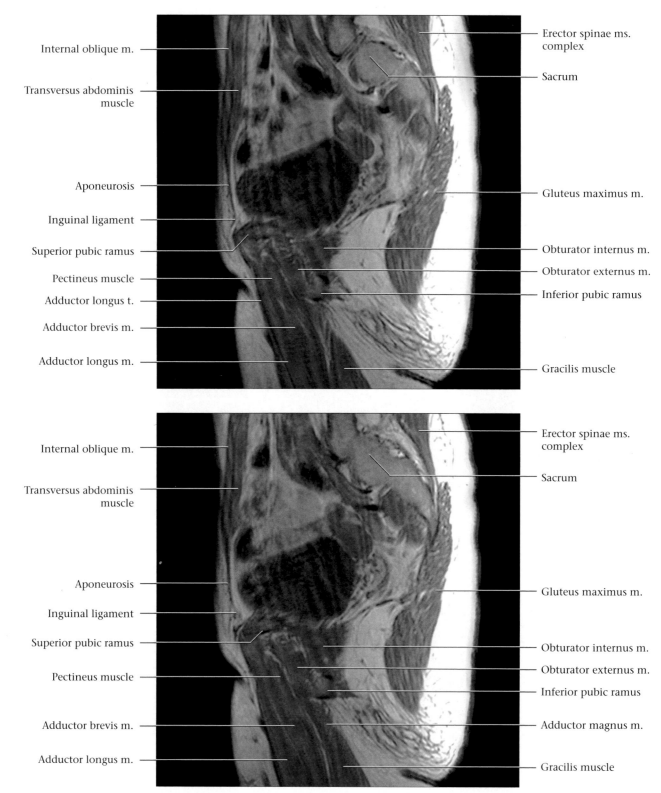

Internal oblique m.

Transversus abdominis muscle

Aponeurosis

Inguinal ligament

Superior pubic ramus

Pectineus muscle

Adductor longus t.

Adductor brevis m.

Adductor longus m.

Erector spinae ms. complex

Sacrum

Gluteus maximus m.

Obturator internus m.

Obturator externus m.

Inferior pubic ramus

Gracilis muscle

Internal oblique m.

Transversus abdominis muscle

Aponeurosis

Inguinal ligament

Superior pubic ramus

Pectineus muscle

Adductor brevis m.

Adductor longus m.

Erector spinae ms. complex

Sacrum

Gluteus maximus m.

Obturator internus m.

Obturator externus m.

Inferior pubic ramus

Adductor magnus m.

Gracilis muscle

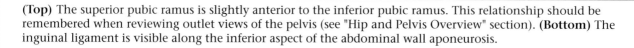

(Top) The superior pubic ramus is slightly anterior to the inferior pubic ramus. This relationship should be remembered when reviewing outlet views of the pelvis (see "Hip and Pelvis Overview" section). **(Bottom)** The inguinal ligament is visible along the inferior aspect of the abdominal wall aponeurosis.

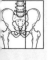
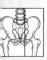

ANTERIOR PELVIS AND THIGH

SAGITTAL T1 MR, SYMPHYSIS PUBIS & ADDUCTOR MUSCLES

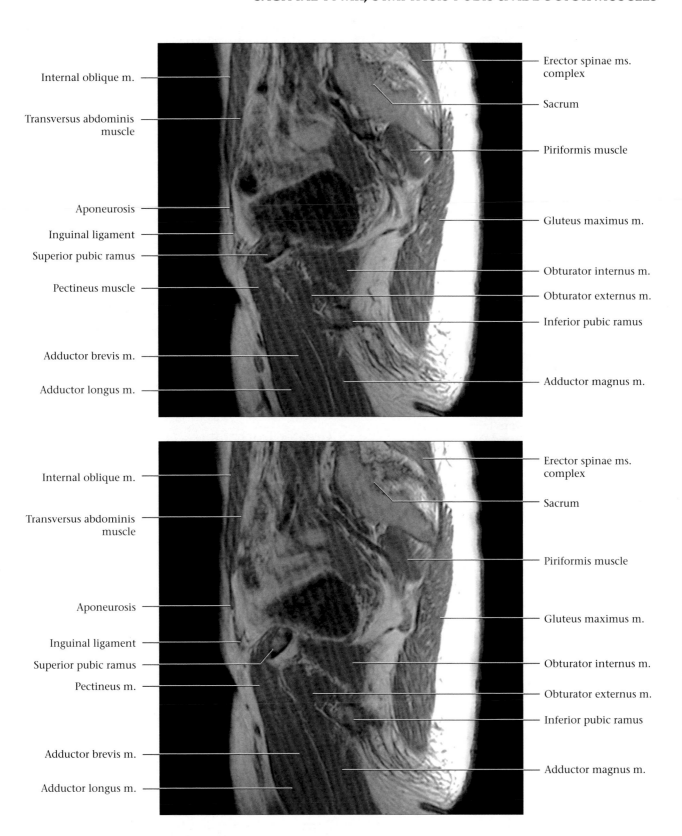

Internal oblique m.

Transversus abdominis muscle

Aponeurosis

Inguinal ligament

Superior pubic ramus

Pectineus muscle

Adductor brevis m.

Adductor longus m.

Erector spinae ms. complex

Sacrum

Piriformis muscle

Gluteus maximus m.

Obturator internus m.

Obturator externus m.

Inferior pubic ramus

Adductor magnus m.

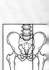

Internal oblique m.

Transversus abdominis muscle

Aponeurosis

Inguinal ligament

Superior pubic ramus

Pectineus m.

Adductor brevis m.

Adductor longus m.

Erector spinae ms. complex

Sacrum

Piriformis muscle

Gluteus maximus m.

Obturator internus m.

Obturator externus m.

Inferior pubic ramus

Adductor magnus m.

(Top) Note the transition from gracilis muscle to adductor magnus muscle as the images move from medial to lateral. The origin of the pectineus muscle from the pecten of the superior pubis ramus and its wrapping over the top of the ramus is well visualized on this image. **(Bottom)** Note how the pectineus muscle and adductor longus muscle lie in the same coronal plane. For anatomy lateral to this location refer to "Hip and Pelvis Overview" and "Thigh Overview" sections.

LATERAL HIP

Terminology

Abbreviations
- Anterior superior iliac spine (ASIS)
- Function (F)
- Greater (Gr)
- Muscle insertion (I)
- Nerve supply (N)
- Muscle origin (O)

Imaging Anatomy

Lateral Femoral (Gluteal) Muscles
- Post-axial: Gluteus maximus, gluteus medius, gluteus minimus, tensor fascia lata, piriformis
- Pre-axial: Obturator internus & externus, superior gemellus, inferior gemellus, quadratus femoris
- Common function: Hip abduction, external rotation
  - Variable, see individual functions
- **Gemellus inferior***
  - O: Ischial tuberosity
  - I: Piriformis fossa
  - N: N. to quadratus femoris m.
  - F: Hip external rotation & weak abduction
- **Gemellus superior***
  - O: Ischial spine
  - I: Piriformis fossa
  - N: N. to obturator internus m.
  - F: Hip external rotation, weak abduction
- **Gluteus maximus**
  - O: Posterior gluteal line (ilium), posterior sacrum & coccyx, sacrotuberous ligament
  - I: Iliotibial tract, gluteal tuberosity
  - N: Inferior gluteal
  - F: Hip extensor, hip abduction & external rotation
- **Gluteus medius**
  - O: Between anterior & posterior gluteal lines (ilium)
  - I: Lateral & superoposterior facets greater trochanter
  - N: Superior gluteal
  - F: Hip abduction & internal rotation
- **Gluteus minimus**
  - O: External ilium between ant. & inf. gluteal lines
  - I: Anterior facet greater trochanter
  - N: Superior gluteal
  - F: Hip abduction & internal rotation
- **Obturator externus**: Medial femoral muscle
  - See "Thigh Overview" section
- **Obturator internus***
  - O: Internal surface obturator foramen & membrane
  - I: Piriformis fossa (joins with gemelli tendons)
  - N: L5, S1, S2
  - F: Hip external rotation, weak abduction
- **Piriformis**
  - O: Anterior sacrum, sacrotuberous ligament
  - I: Greater trochanter (may fuse with obturator internus & gemellus ms.)
  - N: S1, S2
  - F: Hip external rotation, assists abduction
- **Tensor fascia lata**
  - O: External lip anterior iliac crest, external ASIS, notch below spine
  - I: Iliotibial tract
  - N: Superior gluteal
  - F: Hip flexion, abduction & weak internal rotation
- **Quadratus femoris**
  - O: Lateral ischial tuberosity
  - I: Quadrate line, intertrochanteric crest femur
  - N: L4, L5, S1
  - F: Strong hip external rotation
- ***Triceps coxae**: Obturator internus, superior & inferior gemelli function as one unit

Rotator Cuff of Hip
- Gluteus medius & minimus tendons, trochanteric bursa, subgluteus medius & minimus bursa
- Clinical note: Experiences same pathologic abnormalities as rotator cuff of shoulder
  - Typically elderly women
  - Athletes uncommonly affected

Bursa
- Trochanteric: Gr. trochanter & gluteus maximus m.
- Ischiogluteal: Ischial tuberosity & gluteus maximus m.
- Subgluteus medius: Gr. trochanter & gluteus medius
- Subgluteus minimus: Gr. trochanter & gluteus minimus m.
- Gluteofemoral: Iliotibial tract & vastus lateralis m.; also termed subcutaneus or superficial trochanteric
- Bursa of obturator internus: Muscle & ischium
- Obturator externus bursa: Synovial protrusion beneath inferior border

Greater Trochanter
- Anterior facet: Insertion gluteus minimus m.
- Lateral facet: Insertion gluteus medius m.
- Superoposterior: Insertion gluteus medius m.: Horizontal surface, most cranial portion trochanter
- Posterior: No tendon insertion, covered by trochanteric bursa

Other
- **Iliotibial tract**: Thickening lateral aspect fascia lata
  - O: Tubercle iliac crest
  - I: Anterolateral tibial condyle

Piriformis Fossa
- Between posterior femoral neck & posterior medial surface greater trochanter
- Site of insertion for piriformis, superior & inferior gemelli, obturator internus

Anatomy-Based Imaging Issues

Imaging Recommendations
- MR: Rotator cuff lesions
  - Sagittal & coronal images
  - Proton density & T2WI to characterize
  - FOV, 14-26 mm: THK, 3-5 mm: Matrix, 256 x 256

Selected References
1. Pfirrmann CW et al: Greater trochanter of the hip: attachment of the abductor mechanism and a complex of three bursae--MR imaging and MR bursography in cadavers and MR imaging in asymptomatic volunteers. Radiology. 221(2):469-77, 2001

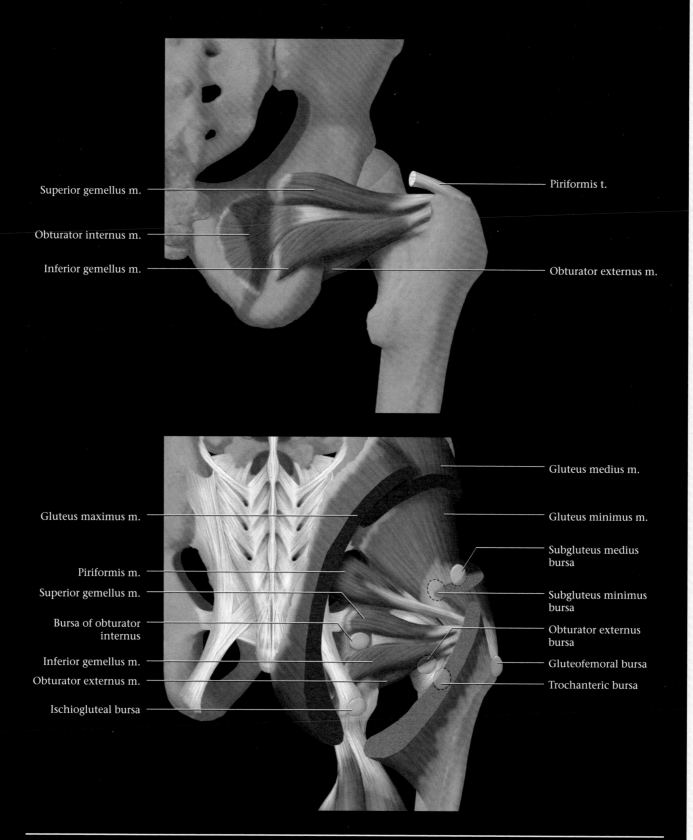

Superior gemellus m.

Obturator internus m.

Inferior gemellus m.

Piriformis t.

Obturator externus m.

Gluteus maximus m.

Piriformis m.

Superior gemellus m.

Bursa of obturator internus

Inferior gemellus m.

Obturator externus m.

Ischiogluteal bursa

Gluteus medius m.

Gluteus minimus m.

Subgluteus medius bursa

Subgluteus minimus bursa

Obturator externus bursa

Gluteofemoral bursa

Trochanteric bursa

(Top) Deep external rotators of the hip; the two gemelli and obturator internus insert together on the piriformis fossa and function together as the triceps coxae. **(Bottom)** Posterolateral structures of the hip, demonstrating the complex bursal system about the hip. Note that the gluteus maximus, gluteus minimus, and obturator internus have been cut away to demonstrate the underlying structures. Note also that the gluteofemoral bursa is also known as the subcutaneous or superficial trochanteric bursa.

AXIAL T1 MR, EXTERNAL ROTATORS & CUFF

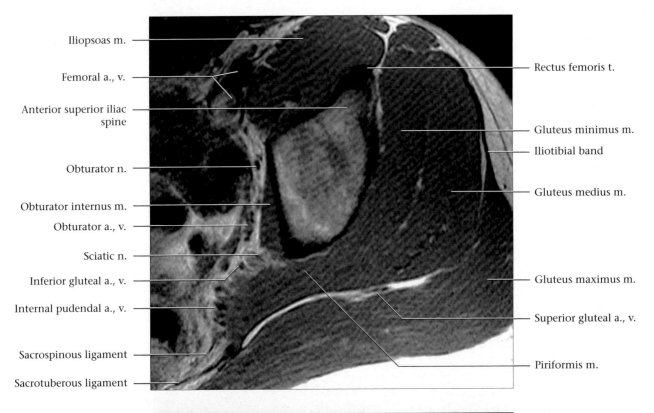

Iliopsoas m.

Femoral a., v.

Anterior superior iliac spine

Obturator n.

Obturator internus m.

Obturator a., v.

Sciatic n.

Inferior gluteal a., v.

Internal pudendal a., v.

Sacrospinous ligament

Sacrotuberous ligament

Rectus femoris t.

Gluteus minimus m.

Iliotibial band

Gluteus medius m.

Gluteus maximus m.

Superior gluteal a., v.

Piriformis m.

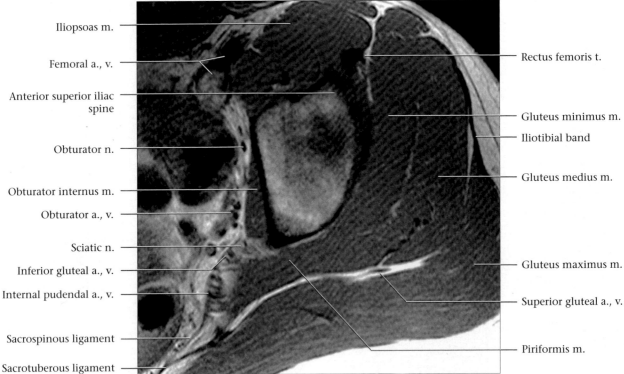

Iliopsoas m.

Femoral a., v.

Anterior superior iliac spine

Obturator n.

Obturator internus m.

Obturator a., v.

Sciatic n.

Inferior gluteal a., v.

Internal pudendal a., v.

Sacrospinous ligament

Sacrotuberous ligament

Rectus femoris t.

Gluteus minimus m.

Iliotibial band

Gluteus medius m.

Gluteus maximus m.

Superior gluteal a., v.

Piriformis m.

(Top) First of twenty axial images of the lateral aspect of the hip from superior to inferior. At this level of the buttocks the gluteal muscles have already arisen from the lateral surface of the ilium. From deep to superficial they are the gluteus minimus, medius and maximus muscles. **(Bottom)** The obturator internus muscle has the deepest origin of the external rotators. It originates within the pelvis along the obturator foramen. A portion of its origin extends superiorly to the inner margin of the ilium along the medial wall of the acetabulum. At this relatively superior level the obturator nerve and vessels are separated. The nerve has traveled from the posterior margin of the psoas muscle while the vessels are branches of the anterior division of the internal iliac vessels.

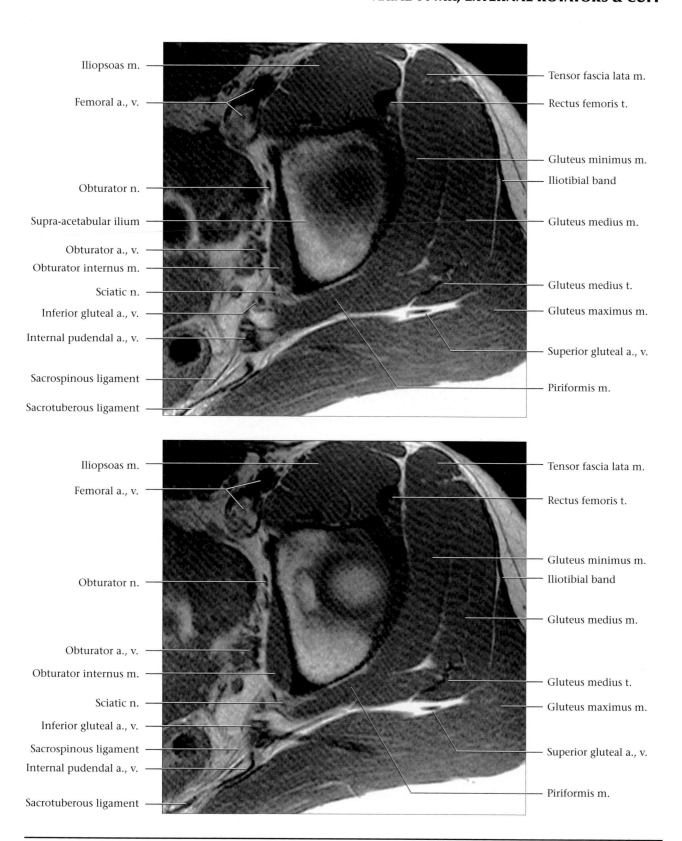

Iliopsoas m.

Femoral a., v.

Obturator n.

Supra-acetabular ilium

Obturator a., v.

Obturator internus m.

Sciatic n.

Inferior gluteal a., v.

Internal pudendal a., v.

Sacrospinous ligament

Sacrotuberous ligament

Tensor fascia lata m.

Rectus femoris t.

Gluteus minimus m.

Iliotibial band

Gluteus medius m.

Gluteus medius t.

Gluteus maximus m.

Superior gluteal a., v.

Piriformis m.

Iliopsoas m.

Femoral a., v.

Obturator n.

Obturator a., v.

Obturator internus m.

Sciatic n.

Inferior gluteal a., v.

Sacrospinous ligament

Internal pudendal a., v.

Sacrotuberous ligament

Tensor fascia lata m.

Rectus femoris t.

Gluteus minimus m.

Iliotibial band

Gluteus medius m.

Gluteus medius t.

Gluteus maximus m.

Superior gluteal a., v.

Piriformis m.

(Top) The gluteus medius tendon forms within the substance of the muscle along the posterior aspect of the muscle belly. **(Bottom)** As it exits the pelvis and courses towards the greater trochanter the piriformis muscle rapidly tapers in size.

AXIAL T1 MR, EXTERNAL ROTATORS & CUFF

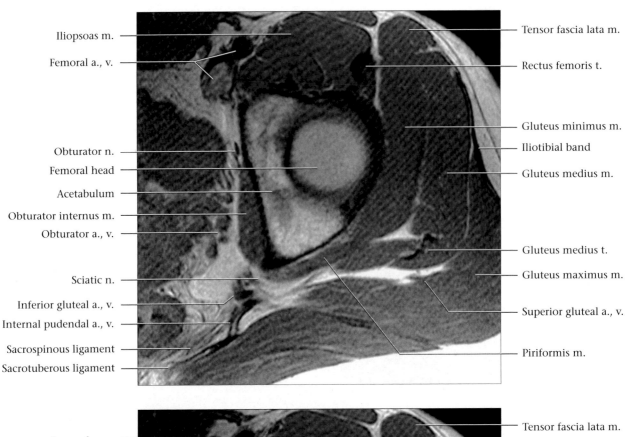

Iliopsoas m.
Femoral a., v.
Obturator n.
Femoral head
Acetabulum
Obturator internus m.
Obturator a., v.
Sciatic n.
Inferior gluteal a., v.
Internal pudendal a., v.
Sacrospinous ligament
Sacrotuberous ligament

Tensor fascia lata m.
Rectus femoris t.
Gluteus minimus m.
Iliotibial band
Gluteus medius m.
Gluteus medius t.
Gluteus maximus m.
Superior gluteal a., v.
Piriformis m.

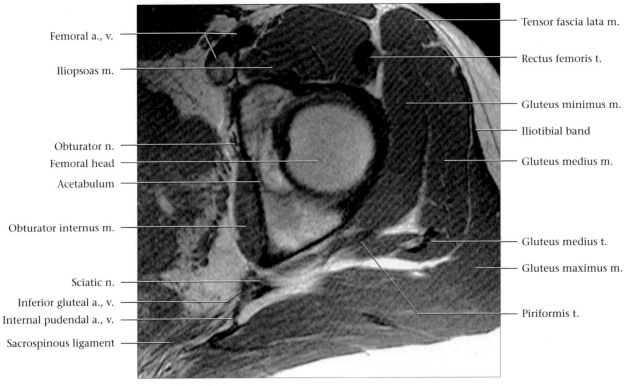

Femoral a., v.
Iliopsoas m.
Obturator n.
Femoral head
Acetabulum
Obturator internus m.
Sciatic n.
Inferior gluteal a., v.
Internal pudendal a., v.
Sacrospinous ligament

Tensor fascia lata m.
Rectus femoris t.
Gluteus minimus m.
Iliotibial band
Gluteus medius m.
Gluteus medius t.
Gluteus maximus m.
Piriformis t.

(Top) From superior to inferior along the posterior rim of the acetabulum the deeper external rotators are in close proximity to one another and often difficult to definitively identify. The piriformis muscle is the most superior of these muscles as seen here at the superior aspect of the hip joint. **(Bottom)** The piriformis tendon is seen on this image. Note the position of the sciatic nerve where it might be mistaken for a portion of the piriformis muscle belly.

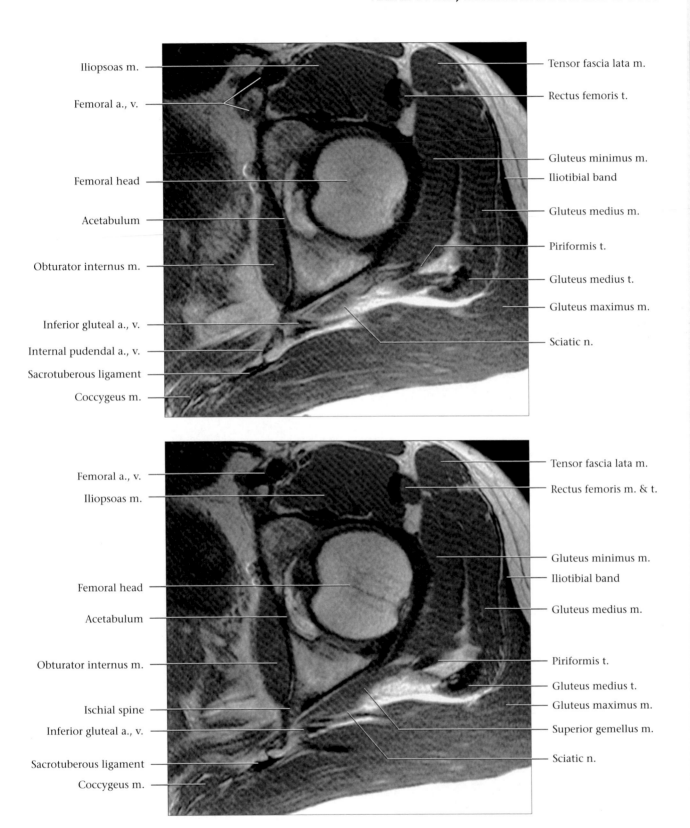

Iliopsoas m.

Femoral a., v.

Femoral head

Acetabulum

Obturator internus m.

Inferior gluteal a., v.

Internal pudendal a., v.

Sacrotuberous ligament

Coccygeus m.

Tensor fascia lata m.

Rectus femoris t.

Gluteus minimus m.

Iliotibial band

Gluteus medius m.

Piriformis t.

Gluteus medius t.

Gluteus maximus m.

Sciatic n.

Femoral a., v.

Iliopsoas m.

Femoral head

Acetabulum

Obturator internus m.

Ischial spine

Inferior gluteal a., v.

Sacrotuberous ligament

Coccygeus m.

Tensor fascia lata m.

Rectus femoris m. & t.

Gluteus minimus m.

Iliotibial band

Gluteus medius m.

Piriformis t.

Gluteus medius t.

Gluteus maximus m.

Superior gemellus m.

Sciatic n.

(Top) The gluteus medius tendon becomes better defined along the inferior aspect of the muscle. On this image taken between the piriformis muscle superiorly and the triceps coxae muscle inferiorly, the sciatic nerve is visible as a distinct structure. On the more inferior images it will be difficult to identify due to its close proximity to the gemelli muscles. **(Bottom)** The superior gemellus muscle arises from the superior aspect of the lateral surface of the ischial spine. The muscle is located just inferior to the piriformis muscle. Note how the sciatic nerve might be mistaken for a portion of the superior gemellus muscle belly.

Hip and Pelvis

V

AXIAL T1 MR, EXTERNAL ROTATORS & CUFF

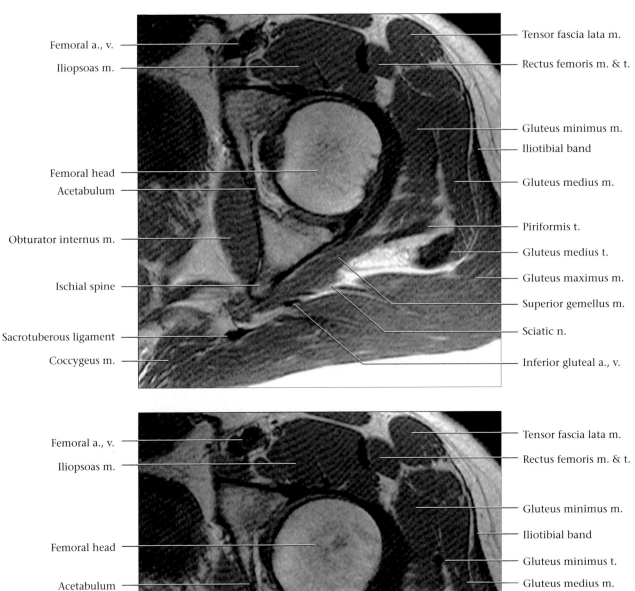

Femoral a., v. — Tensor fascia lata m.
Iliopsoas m. — Rectus femoris m. & t.
— Gluteus minimus m.
— Iliotibial band
Femoral head — Gluteus medius m.
Acetabulum —
Obturator internus m. — Piriformis t.
— Gluteus medius t.
— Gluteus maximus m.
Ischial spine — Superior gemellus m.
— Sciatic n.
Sacrotuberous ligament —
Coccygeus m. — Inferior gluteal a., v.

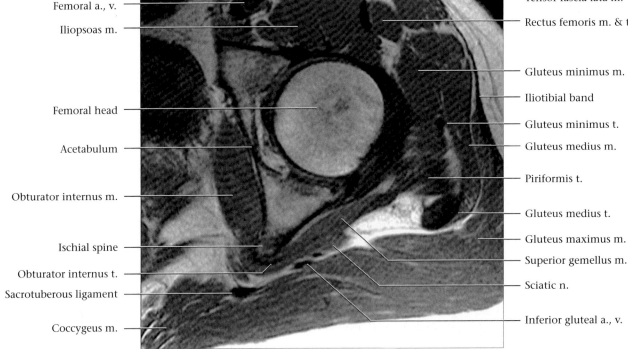

Femoral a., v. — Tensor fascia lata m.
Iliopsoas m. — Rectus femoris m. & t.
— Gluteus minimus m.
— Iliotibial band
Femoral head — Gluteus minimus t.
— Gluteus medius m.
Acetabulum — Piriformis t.
Obturator internus m. — Gluteus medius t.
— Gluteus maximus m.
Ischial spine — Superior gemellus m.
Obturator internus t. — Sciatic n.
Sacrotuberous ligament —
Coccygeus m. — Inferior gluteal a., v.

(Top) On this image the origin of the superior gemellus muscle is easy to appreciate. The piriformis tendon and gluteus medius tendon are in close proximity to one another. The gluteus medius tendon inserts onto the superior border of the greater trochanter while the piriformis tendon is the most superior tendon to insert into the piriformis fossa along the medial border of the greater trochanter. **(Bottom)** As the obturator internus muscle exits the pelvis it abruptly turns laterally, wrapping around the ischial spine just below the origin of the superior gemellus muscle.

Hip and Pelvis

LATERAL HIP

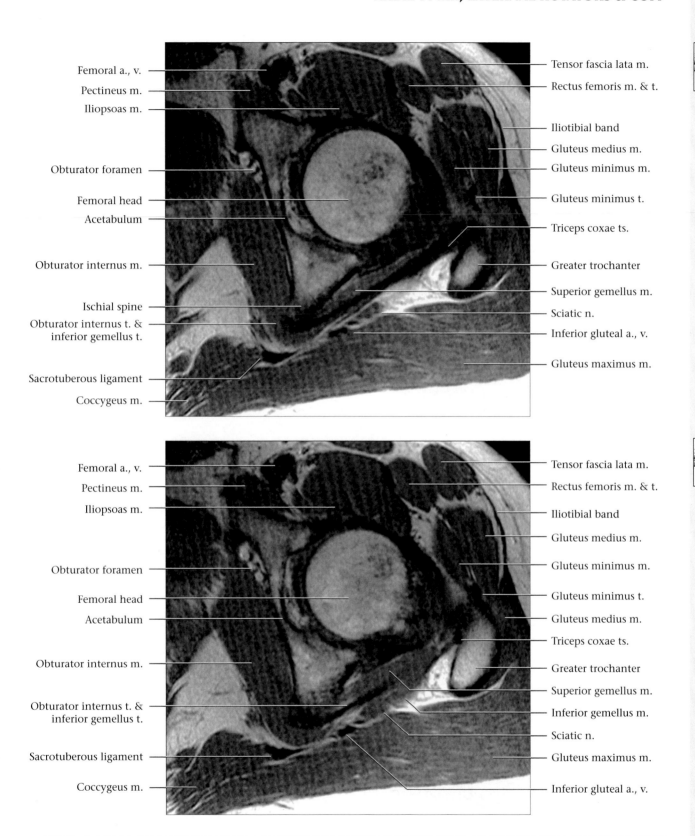

Top image labels (left):
- Femoral a., v.
- Pectineus m.
- Iliopsoas m.
- Obturator foramen
- Femoral head
- Acetabulum
- Obturator internus m.
- Ischial spine
- Obturator internus t. & inferior gemellus t.
- Sacrotuberous ligament
- Coccygeus m.

Top image labels (right):
- Tensor fascia lata m.
- Rectus femoris m. & t.
- Iliotibial band
- Gluteus medius m.
- Gluteus minimus m.
- Gluteus minimus t.
- Triceps coxae ts.
- Greater trochanter
- Superior gemellus m.
- Sciatic n.
- Inferior gluteal a., v.
- Gluteus maximus m.

Bottom image labels (left):
- Femoral a., v.
- Pectineus m.
- Iliopsoas m.
- Obturator foramen
- Femoral head
- Acetabulum
- Obturator internus m.
- Obturator internus t. & inferior gemellus t.
- Sacrotuberous ligament
- Coccygeus m.

Bottom image labels (right):
- Tensor fascia lata m.
- Rectus femoris m. & t.
- Iliotibial band
- Gluteus medius m.
- Gluteus minimus m.
- Gluteus minimus t.
- Gluteus medius m.
- Triceps coxae ts.
- Greater trochanter
- Superior gemellus m.
- Inferior gemellus m.
- Sciatic n.
- Gluteus maximus m.
- Inferior gluteal a., v.

(Top) The obturator internus tendon forms as the muscle wraps around the ischial spine. In this individual the tendon immediately fuses with the inferior gemellus tendon as the latter arises from the lateral border of the ischial spine. The entire course of this tendon can be appreciated on this image. Its insertion onto the medial border of the greater trochanter is well seen. **(Bottom)** The origin of the inferior gemellus tendon is nicely demonstrated on this image. The gluteus minimus tendon can now be identified. Like the gluteus medius tendon, the gluteus minimus tendon forms along the posterior aspect of the muscle. The obturator foramen is visible along the anterior aspect of the obturator internus muscle. The contents of the foramen are the obturator nerve, artery and vein.

Hip and Pelvis

V

LATERAL HIP

AXIAL T1 MR, EXTERNAL ROTATORS & CUFF

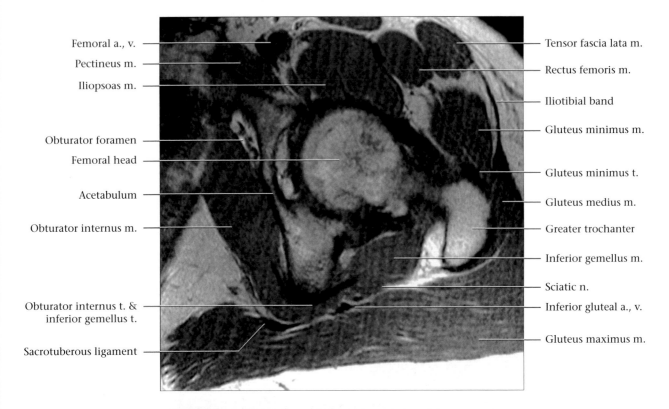

Femoral a., v.
Pectineus m.
Iliopsoas m.

Obturator foramen
Femoral head

Acetabulum

Obturator internus m.

Obturator internus t. &
inferior gemellus t.

Sacrotuberous ligament

Tensor fascia lata m.
Rectus femoris m.
Iliotibial band
Gluteus minimus m.

Gluteus minimus t.

Gluteus medius m.

Greater trochanter

Inferior gemellus m.

Sciatic n.

Inferior gluteal a., v.

Gluteus maximus m.

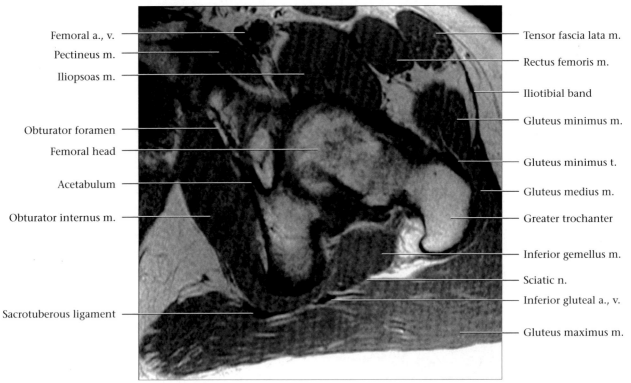

Femoral a., v.
Pectineus m.
Iliopsoas m.

Obturator foramen
Femoral head

Acetabulum

Obturator internus m.

Sacrotuberous ligament

Tensor fascia lata m.
Rectus femoris m.
Iliotibial band
Gluteus minimus m.

Gluteus minimus t.

Gluteus medius m.

Greater trochanter

Inferior gemellus m.

Sciatic n.

Inferior gluteal a., v.

Gluteus maximus m.

(Top) The muscle belly of the inferior gemellus muscle arises from the tendon several centimeters lateral to the origin of the tendon. In this individual the muscle belly wraps the inferior surface of the fused tendon of the obturator internus and superior gemellus muscles. Because the deeper layer of hip external rotators follows a course that is oriented from inferomedial to superomedial the muscle belly of the inferior gemellus muscle is seen inferior to its insertion. **(Bottom)** The gluteus minimus tendon inserts onto the anterior facet of the greater trochanter. This insertion is located inferior to the insertion of the gluteus medius muscle. Note how the sciatic nerve continues to be difficult to separate from the adjacent muscles.

AXIAL T1 MR, EXTERNAL ROTATORS & CUFF

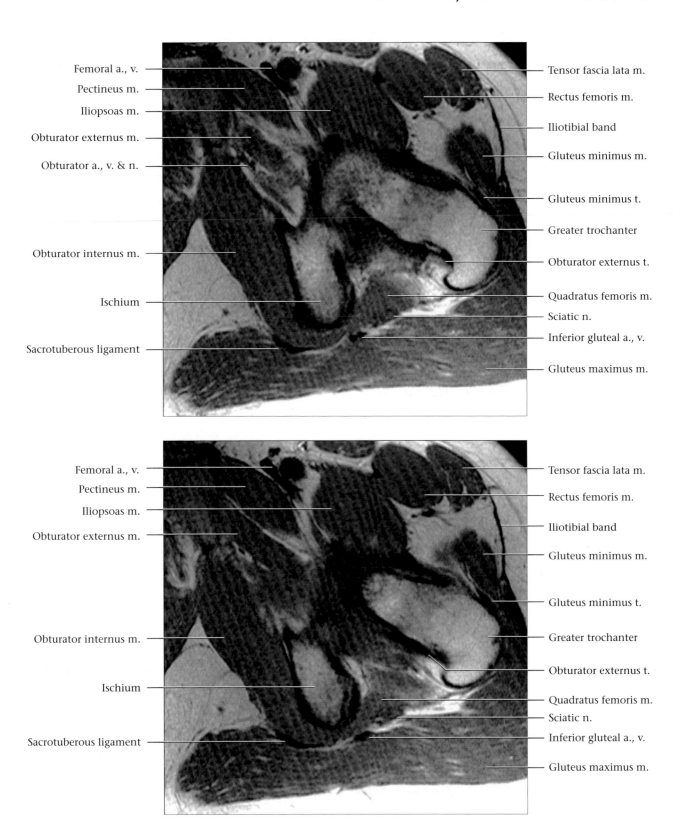

Femoral a., v.
Pectineus m.
Iliopsoas m.
Obturator externus m.
Obturator a., v. & n.

Obturator internus m.

Ischium

Sacrotuberous ligament

Tensor fascia lata m.
Rectus femoris m.
Iliotibial band
Gluteus minimus m.

Gluteus minimus t.

Greater trochanter

Obturator externus t.

Quadratus femoris m.
Sciatic n.
Inferior gluteal a., v.

Gluteus maximus m.

Femoral a., v.
Pectineus m.
Iliopsoas m.
Obturator externus m.

Obturator internus m.

Ischium

Sacrotuberous ligament

Tensor fascia lata m.
Rectus femoris m.
Iliotibial band
Gluteus minimus m.

Gluteus minimus t.

Greater trochanter

Obturator externus t.

Quadratus femoris m.
Sciatic n.
Inferior gluteal a., v.

Gluteus maximus m.

(Top) The obturator externus tendon is the most inferior tendon to insert into the piriformis fossa. This muscle also has a complex three dimensional orientation and on this image its origin is seen medially while its insertion is seen laterally. The intervening muscle, however, is only visible on more inferior images. **(Bottom)** The muscle belly of the gluteus minimus muscle remains visible as the tendon inserts onto the anterior facet of the greater trochanter. The muscle belly will continue inferiorly for several more images. The quadratus femoris muscle takes origin from the lateral surface of the ischial tuberosity superior to the hamstring muscles.

Hip and Pelvis

V

AXIAL T1 MR, EXTERNAL ROTATORS & CUFF

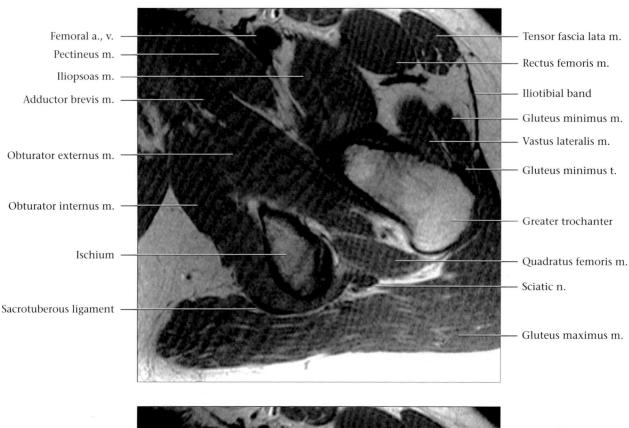

Femoral a., v.
Pectineus m.
Iliopsoas m.
Adductor brevis m.
Obturator externus m.
Obturator internus m.
Ischium
Sacrotuberous ligament

Tensor fascia lata m.
Rectus femoris m.
Iliotibial band
Gluteus minimus m.
Vastus lateralis m.
Gluteus minimus t.
Greater trochanter
Quadratus femoris m.
Sciatic n.
Gluteus maximus m.

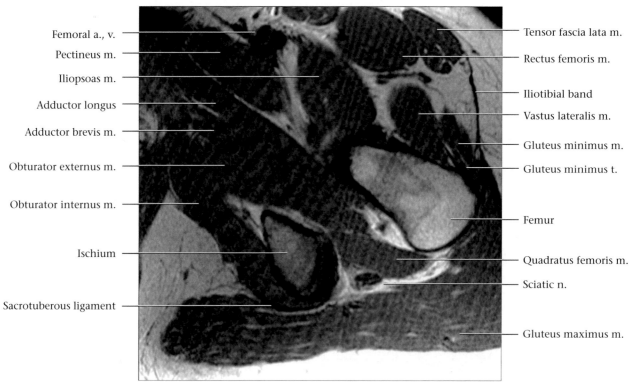

Femoral a., v.
Pectineus m.
Iliopsoas m.
Adductor longus
Adductor brevis m.
Obturator externus m.
Obturator internus m.
Ischium
Sacrotuberous ligament

Tensor fascia lata m.
Rectus femoris m.
Iliotibial band
Vastus lateralis m.
Gluteus minimus m.
Gluteus minimus t.
Femur
Quadratus femoris m.
Sciatic n.
Gluteus maximus m.

(Top) The full extent of the obturator externus muscle is easy to appreciate on this image extending from the external margins of the obturator foramen to the piriformis fossa. **(Bottom)** At its origin the vastus lateralis muscle is in close relationship to the inferior most extent of the gluteus minimus muscle along the anterior aspect of the femur.

LATERAL HIP

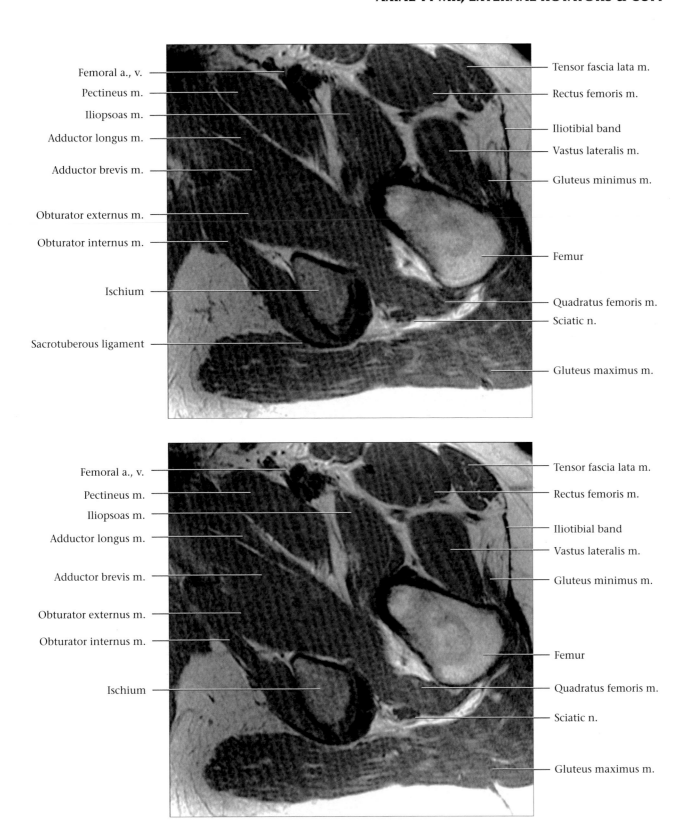

Femoral a., v.
Pectineus m.
Iliopsoas m.
Adductor longus m.
Adductor brevis m.
Obturator externus m.
Obturator internus m.
Ischium
Sacrotuberous ligament

Tensor fascia lata m.
Rectus femoris m.
Iliotibial band
Vastus lateralis m.
Gluteus minimus m.
Femur
Quadratus femoris m.
Sciatic n.
Gluteus maximus m.

Femoral a., v.
Pectineus m.
Iliopsoas m.
Adductor longus m.
Adductor brevis m.
Obturator externus m.
Obturator internus m.
Ischium

Tensor fascia lata m.
Rectus femoris m.
Iliotibial band
Vastus lateralis m.
Gluteus minimus m.
Femur
Quadratus femoris m.
Sciatic n.
Gluteus maximus m.

(Top) The insertion of the quadratus femoris muscle onto the posterior aspect of the femur is well seen here. It is superior to the insertion of the pectineus muscle and lateral to the insertion of the gluteus maximus muscle. **(Bottom)** The sciatic nerve travels along the posterior aspect of the quadratus femoris muscle. It finally becomes a distinct structure. The obturator internus muscle is still visible covering the entire inner aspect of the obturator foramen. As with many of the other external rotator muscles it has a complex three dimensional orientation. While the muscle belly is quite large it funnels to a very narrow structure that courses through the lesser sciatic notch and makes the abrupt lateral turn towards the greater trochanter. For anatomy more inferior to this level see "Thigh Overview" section.

SAGITTAL T1 MR, EXTERNAL ROTATORS & CUFF

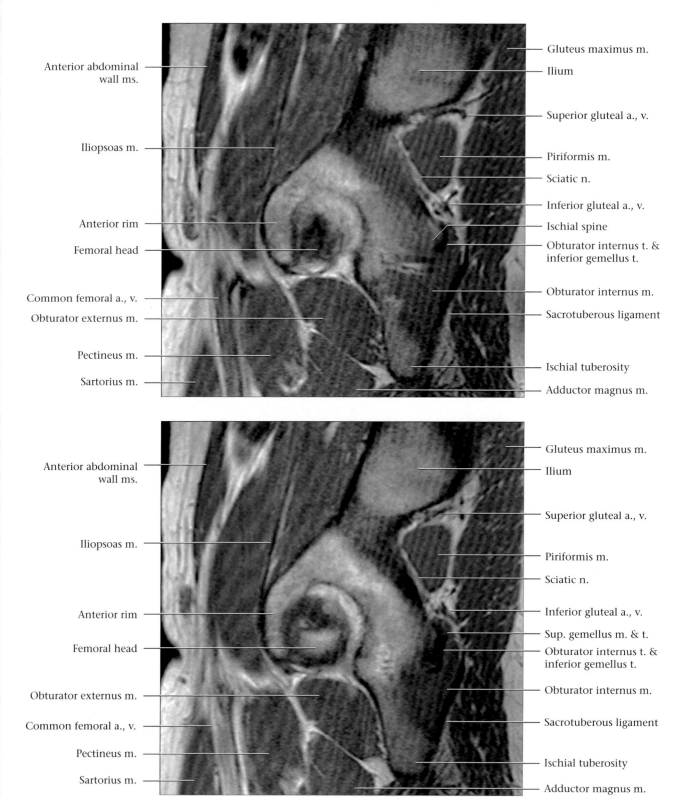

Anterior abdominal wall ms.

Iliopsoas m.

Anterior rim

Femoral head

Common femoral a., v.

Obturator externus m.

Pectineus m.

Sartorius m.

Gluteus maximus m.

Ilium

Superior gluteal a., v.

Piriformis m.

Sciatic n.

Inferior gluteal a., v.

Ischial spine

Obturator internus t. & inferior gemellus t.

Obturator internus m.

Sacrotuberous ligament

Ischial tuberosity

Adductor magnus m.

Anterior abdominal wall ms.

Iliopsoas m.

Anterior rim

Femoral head

Obturator externus m.

Common femoral a., v.

Pectineus m.

Sartorius m.

Gluteus maximus m.

Ilium

Superior gluteal a., v.

Piriformis m.

Sciatic n.

Inferior gluteal a., v.

Sup. gemellus m. & t.

Obturator internus t. & inferior gemellus t.

Obturator internus m.

Sacrotuberous ligament

Ischial tuberosity

Adductor magnus m.

(Top) First of twenty six sagittal images of the lateral hip from medial to lateral. For detail of the more medial anatomy see "Posterior Pelvis" section. The images are immediately lateral to the ischial spine. The gemelli muscles both originate from the outer aspect of the ischial spine. In this patient the tendons of the obturator internus and inferior gemellus muscle are fused. Fusion between the obturator internus tendons and the gemelli tendons is common. The piriformis tendon may also join the fused tendon. **(Bottom)** The muscle belly of the superior gemellus is visible. It is superior to the obturator internus tendon. The piriformis muscle is well above the other external rotators of the hip at this point. A few fibers of the ischiocondylar portion of the adductor magnus muscle (not labeled) are seen arising from the medial aspect of the ischial tuberosity.

SAGITTAL T1 MR, EXTERNAL ROTATORS & CUFF

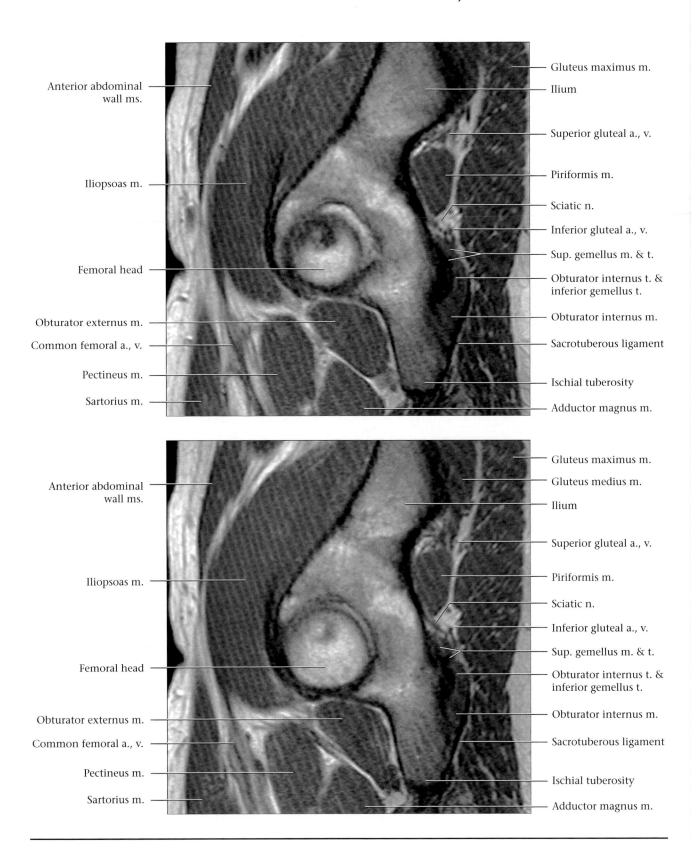

Anterior abdominal wall ms.

Iliopsoas m.

Femoral head

Obturator externus m.

Common femoral a., v.

Pectineus m.

Sartorius m.

Gluteus maximus m.

Ilium

Superior gluteal a., v.

Piriformis m.

Sciatic n.

Inferior gluteal a., v.

Sup. gemellus m. & t.

Obturator internus t. & inferior gemellus t.

Obturator internus m.

Sacrotuberous ligament

Ischial tuberosity

Adductor magnus m.

Anterior abdominal wall ms.

Iliopsoas m.

Femoral head

Obturator externus m.

Common femoral a., v.

Pectineus m.

Sartorius m.

Gluteus maximus m.

Gluteus medius m.

Ilium

Superior gluteal a., v.

Piriformis m.

Sciatic n.

Inferior gluteal a., v.

Sup. gemellus m. & t.

Obturator internus t. & inferior gemellus t.

Obturator internus m.

Sacrotuberous ligament

Ischial tuberosity

Adductor magnus m.

(Top) The tendon of the superior gemellus muscle is located along the inferior border of the muscle in close proximity to the fused tendons of the obturator internus and inferior gemellus muscles. The obturator externus muscle is anteriorly located relative to the ischium and the other external rotator tendons. (Bottom) The sciatic nerve is located along the inferior border of the piriformis muscle as it enters the lower extremity. The muscle belly of the obturator internus tapers as it courses along the posterior aspect of the hip joint.

Hip and Pelvis

V

SAGITTAL T1 MR, EXTERNAL ROTATORS & CUFF

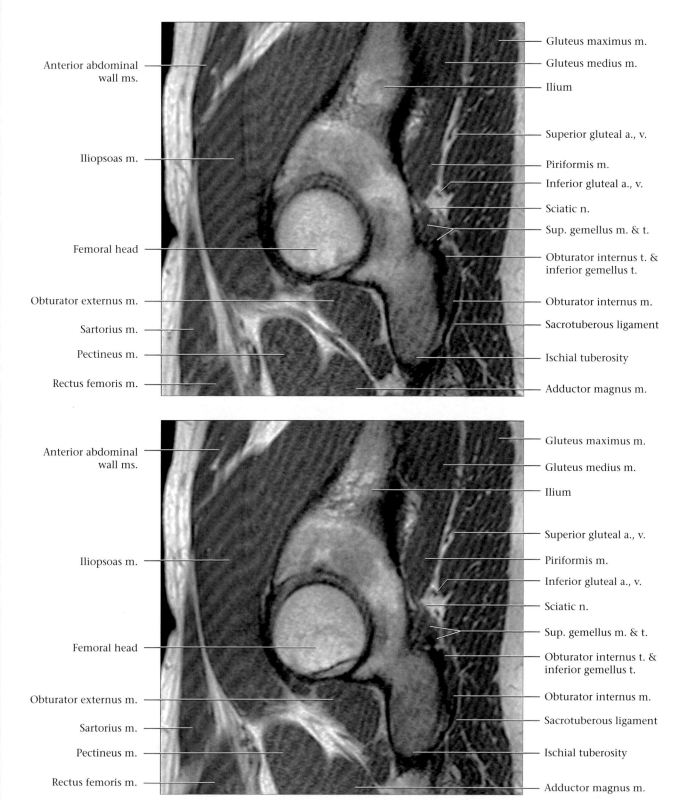

Top image labels (left):
- Anterior abdominal wall ms.
- Iliopsoas m.
- Femoral head
- Obturator externus m.
- Sartorius m.
- Pectineus m.
- Rectus femoris m.

Top image labels (right):
- Gluteus maximus m.
- Gluteus medius m.
- Ilium
- Superior gluteal a., v.
- Piriformis m.
- Inferior gluteal a., v.
- Sciatic n.
- Sup. gemellus m. & t.
- Obturator internus t. & inferior gemellus t.
- Obturator internus m.
- Sacrotuberous ligament
- Ischial tuberosity
- Adductor magnus m.

Bottom image labels (left):
- Anterior abdominal wall ms.
- Iliopsoas m.
- Femoral head
- Obturator externus m.
- Sartorius m.
- Pectineus m.
- Rectus femoris m.

Bottom image labels (right):
- Gluteus maximus m.
- Gluteus medius m.
- Ilium
- Superior gluteal a., v.
- Piriformis m.
- Inferior gluteal a., v.
- Sciatic n.
- Sup. gemellus m. & t.
- Obturator internus t. & inferior gemellus t.
- Obturator internus m.
- Sacrotuberous ligament
- Ischial tuberosity
- Adductor magnus m.

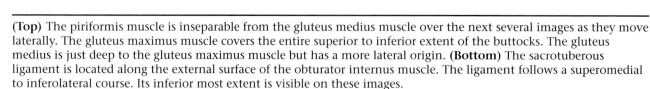

(Top) The piriformis muscle is inseparable from the gluteus medius muscle over the next several images as they move laterally. The gluteus maximus muscle covers the entire superior to inferior extent of the buttocks. The gluteus medius is just deep to the gluteus maximus muscle but has a more lateral origin. **(Bottom)** The sacrotuberous ligament is located along the external surface of the obturator internus muscle. The ligament follows a superomedial to inferolateral course. Its inferior most extent is visible on these images.

Hip and Pelvis

SAGITTAL T1 MR, EXTERNAL ROTATORS & CUFF

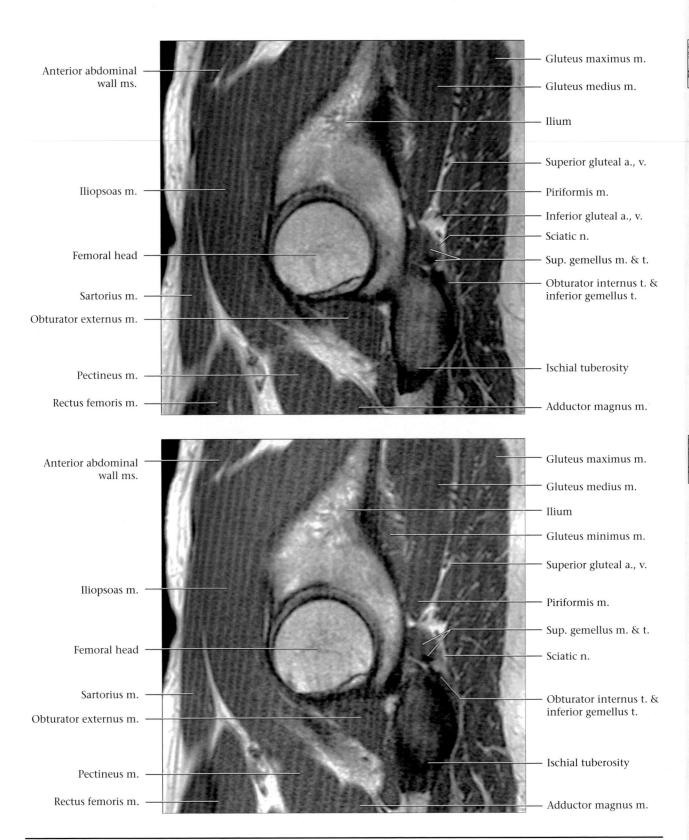

Top image labels:

Left side:
- Anterior abdominal wall ms.
- Iliopsoas m.
- Femoral head
- Sartorius m.
- Obturator externus m.
- Pectineus m.
- Rectus femoris m.

Right side:
- Gluteus maximus m.
- Gluteus medius m.
- Ilium
- Superior gluteal a., v.
- Piriformis m.
- Inferior gluteal a., v.
- Sciatic n.
- Sup. gemellus m. & t.
- Obturator internus t. & inferior gemellus t.
- Ischial tuberosity
- Adductor magnus m.

Bottom image labels:

Left side:
- Anterior abdominal wall ms.
- Iliopsoas m.
- Femoral head
- Sartorius m.
- Obturator externus m.
- Pectineus m.
- Rectus femoris m.

Right side:
- Gluteus maximus m.
- Gluteus medius m.
- Ilium
- Gluteus minimus m.
- Superior gluteal a., v.
- Piriformis m.
- Sup. gemellus m. & t.
- Sciatic n.
- Obturator internus t. & inferior gemellus t.
- Ischial tuberosity
- Adductor magnus m.

(Top) The sciatic nerve drapes along the posterior surfaces of the external rotator muscles and tendons and is difficult to identify as a separate structure. The inferior gluteal vessels are not discernible as discrete structures in the far lateral aspect of the buttocks. The superior gluteal vessels remain visible. **(Bottom)** Along the lateral most margin of the ischium the obturator externus muscle moves posteriorly gaining proximity to the other external rotator tendons.

Hip and Pelvis

V

SAGITTAL T1 MR, EXTERNAL ROTATORS & CUFF

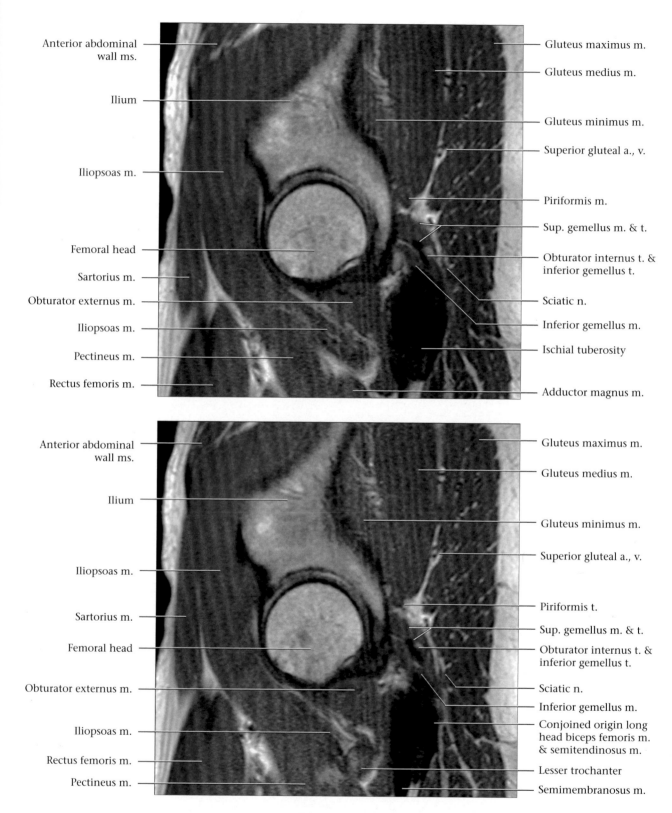

Top image labels (left): Anterior abdominal wall ms.; Ilium; Iliopsoas m.; Femoral head; Sartorius m.; Obturator externus m.; Iliopsoas m.; Pectineus m.; Rectus femoris m.

Top image labels (right): Gluteus maximus m.; Gluteus medius m.; Gluteus minimus m.; Superior gluteal a., v.; Piriformis m.; Sup. gemellus m. & t.; Obturator internus t. & inferior gemellus t.; Sciatic n.; Inferior gemellus m.; Ischial tuberosity; Adductor magnus m.

Bottom image labels (left): Anterior abdominal wall ms.; Ilium; Iliopsoas m.; Sartorius m.; Femoral head; Obturator externus m.; Iliopsoas m.; Rectus femoris m.; Pectineus m.

Bottom image labels (right): Gluteus maximus m.; Gluteus medius m.; Gluteus minimus m.; Superior gluteal a., v.; Piriformis t.; Sup. gemellus m. & t.; Obturator internus t. & inferior gemellus t.; Sciatic n.; Inferior gemellus m.; Conjoined origin long head biceps femoris m. & semitendinosus m.; Lesser trochanter; Semimembranosus m.

(Top) The gluteus minimus muscle origin is the deepest and most lateral of the gluteal muscles. The superior gluteal vessels are still visible as they travel in the fat plane deep to the gluteus maximus muscle. Lateral to the ischium the obturator externus muscle courses posteriorly to join the other external rotators of the hip. **(Bottom)** The inferior gemellus muscle belly appears in a relatively lateral position in this individual. It is located inferior to the obturator internus tendon. The piriformis tendon is now visible, located at the inferior most aspect of the gluteus medius muscle. The tendon of the semimembranosus muscle is located anterior to the conjoined tendon of the long head of the biceps femoris muscle and the semitendinosus muscle.

SAGITTAL T1 MR, EXTERNAL ROTATORS & CUFF

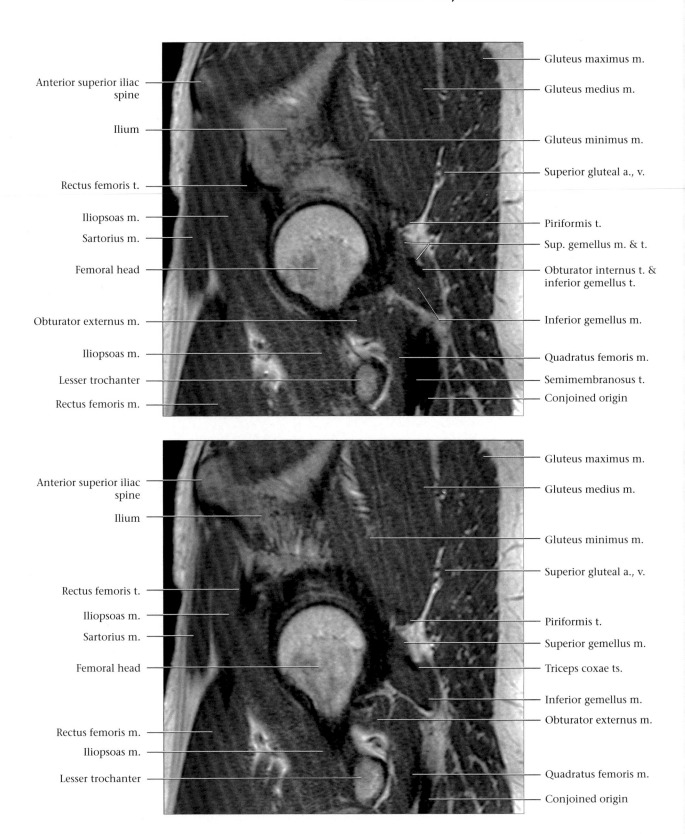

Anterior superior iliac spine

Ilium

Rectus femoris t.

Iliopsoas m.

Sartorius m.

Femoral head

Obturator externus m.

Iliopsoas m.

Lesser trochanter

Rectus femoris m.

Gluteus maximus m.

Gluteus medius m.

Gluteus minimus m.

Superior gluteal a., v.

Piriformis t.

Sup. gemellus m. & t.

Obturator internus t. & inferior gemellus t.

Inferior gemellus m.

Quadratus femoris m.

Semimembranosus t.

Conjoined origin

Anterior superior iliac spine

Ilium

Rectus femoris t.

Iliopsoas m.

Sartorius m.

Femoral head

Rectus femoris m.

Iliopsoas m.

Lesser trochanter

Gluteus maximus m.

Gluteus medius m.

Gluteus minimus m.

Superior gluteal a., v.

Piriformis t.

Superior gemellus m.

Triceps coxae ts.

Inferior gemellus m.

Obturator externus m.

Quadratus femoris m.

Conjoined origin

(Top) The superior gemellus tendon has now fused with the tendons of the obturator internus and inferior gemellus muscles. These three muscles act in concert and are also known as the triceps coxae. The quadratus femoris muscle takes origin from the lateral aspect of the ischial tuberosity deep to the hamstring tendons. **(Bottom)** The obturator externus muscle has now assumed a more posterior position and will travel with the other external rotators along the posterior aspect of the hip joint. The medial circumflex femoral vessels (not labeled) are just inferior to the obturator externus muscle (see "Hip and Pelvis Overview" section). The sciatic nerve is not identifiable on these images. The obturator internus muscle and the gemelli muscles function together and are known as the triceps coxae muscles. The tendons of the muscles often fuse as in this individual.

Hip and Pelvis

V

SAGITTAL T1 MR, EXTERNAL ROTATORS & CUFF

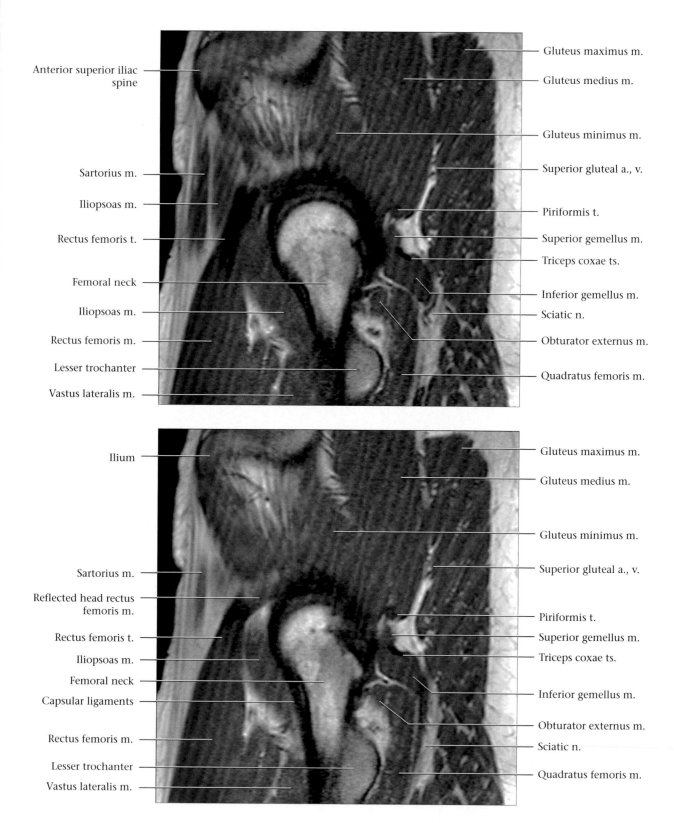

(Top) The sciatic nerve is now visible as it travels below the border of the inferior gemellus muscle. Once it assumes its position along the posterior hip the obturator externus muscle rapidly decreases in size. **(Bottom)** The relationships of the external rotators is apparent. Along the deep layer of muscles, the most superior tendon is the piriformis, followed by superior gemellus, obturator internus, inferior gemellus then obturator externus. These muscles all insert onto the piriformis fossa. The quadratus femoris muscle is deep to the gluteus maximus muscle and inserts medial to that muscle on the posterior aspect of the femur. The gluteus minimus and medius muscles both insert onto the greater trochanter.

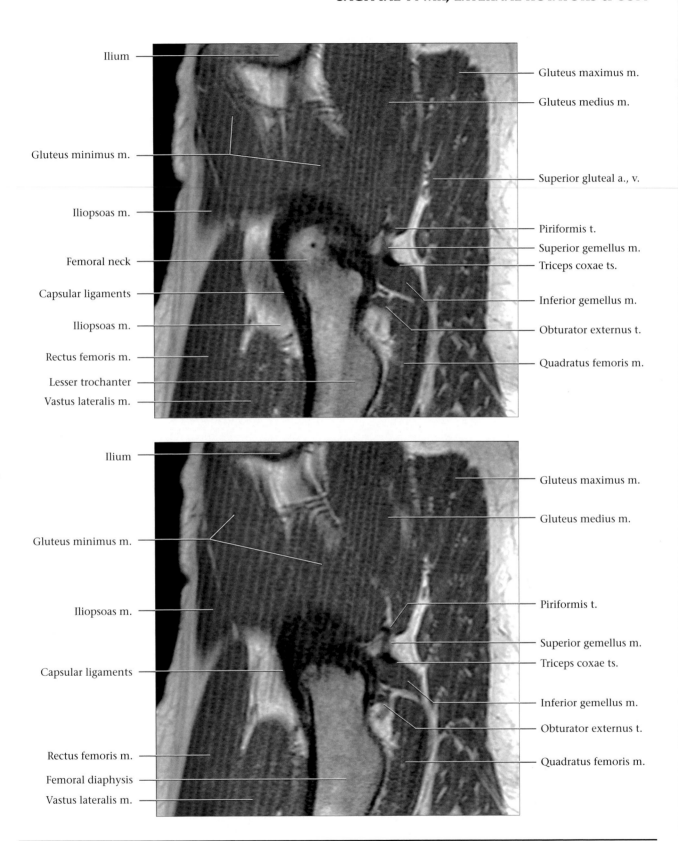

Top image labels (left): Ilium, Gluteus minimus m., Iliopsoas m., Femoral neck, Capsular ligaments, Iliopsoas m., Rectus femoris m., Lesser trochanter, Vastus lateralis m.

Top image labels (right): Gluteus maximus m., Gluteus medius m., Superior gluteal a., v., Piriformis t., Superior gemellus m., Triceps coxae ts., Inferior gemellus m., Obturator externus t., Quadratus femoris m.

Bottom image labels (left): Ilium, Gluteus minimus m., Iliopsoas m., Capsular ligaments, Rectus femoris m., Femoral diaphysis, Vastus lateralis m.

Bottom image labels (right): Gluteus maximus m., Gluteus medius m., Piriformis t., Superior gemellus m., Triceps coxae ts., Inferior gemellus m., Obturator externus t., Quadratus femoris m.

(Top) The broad origin of the gluteus minimus muscle from the anterior aspect of the auricular surface of the ilium can be easily appreciated on this image and the more lateral images. **(Bottom)** The gluteus medius muscle begins to taper inferiorly. This tapering will lead to formation of its tendon.

SAGITTAL T1 MR, EXTERNAL ROTATORS & CUFF

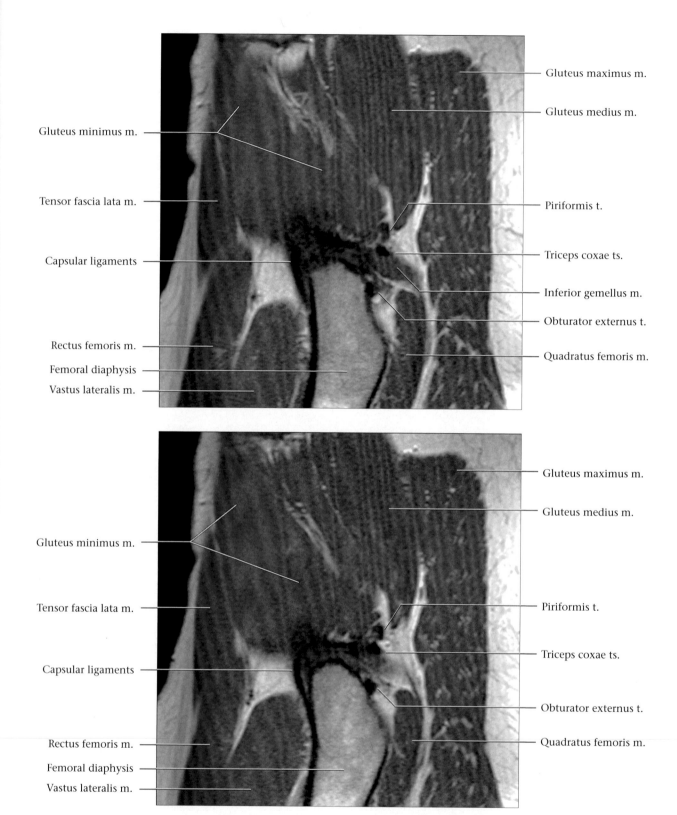

(Top) The broad expanse of the gluteus minimus muscle covers both anterior and superior surfaces of the joint. **(Bottom)** The inferior taper of the gluteus medius muscle is now well-defined. Note the orientation of the fibers within the muscle. Their long axis follows the taper of the muscle.

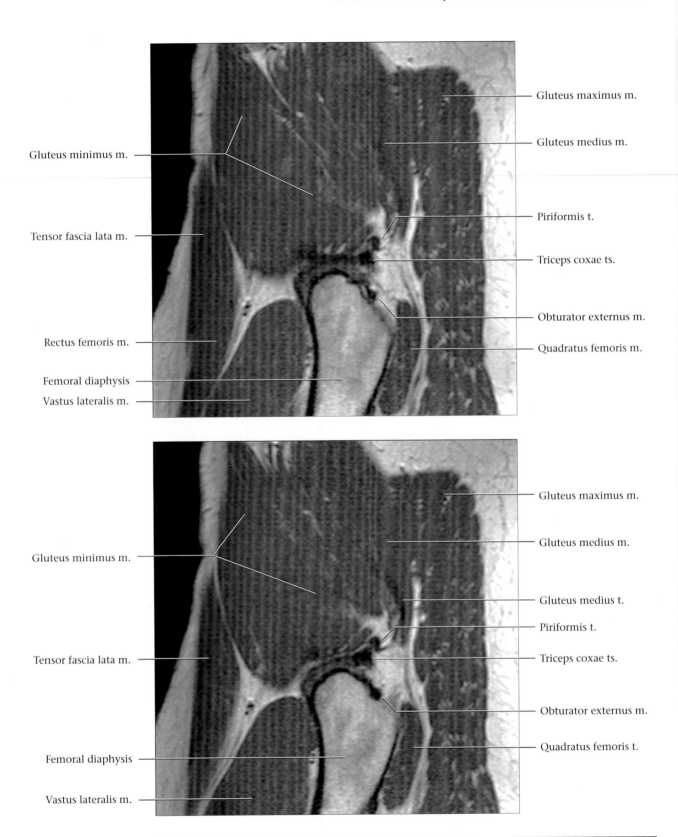

Gluteus minimus m.

Tensor fascia lata m.

Rectus femoris m.

Femoral diaphysis
Vastus lateralis m.

Gluteus maximus m.

Gluteus medius m.

Piriformis t.

Triceps coxae ts.

Obturator externus m.

Quadratus femoris m.

Gluteus minimus m.

Tensor fascia lata m.

Femoral diaphysis

Vastus lateralis m.

Gluteus maximus m.

Gluteus medius m.

Gluteus medius t.

Piriformis t.

Triceps coxae ts.

Obturator externus m.

Quadratus femoris t.

(Top) The piriformis tendon is deep to the gluteus medius muscle. It is closely related to the obturator internus and gemelli tendons. **(Bottom)** The gluteus medius tendon is now easily seen.

Hip and Pelvis

V

SAGITTAL T1 MR, EXTERNAL ROTATORS & CUFF

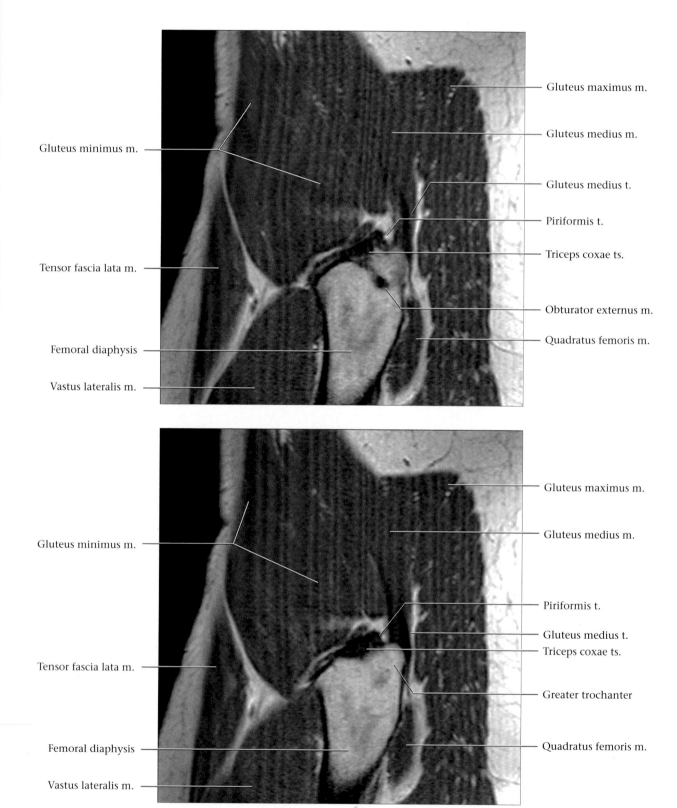

(Top) The obturator externus tendon inserts along the inferior-most aspect of the piriformis fossa. The fossa is located along the mesial surface of the greater trochanter. **(Bottom)** The piriformis tendon and the obturator internus and gemelli muscles insert at the piriformis fossa, superior to the obturator externus tendon. The gluteus medius tendon inserts onto the lateral facet of the greater trochanter. The gluteus medius tendon has two components, one which is coronally oriented and the other more sagittally oriented. The coronally oriented component is visible here.

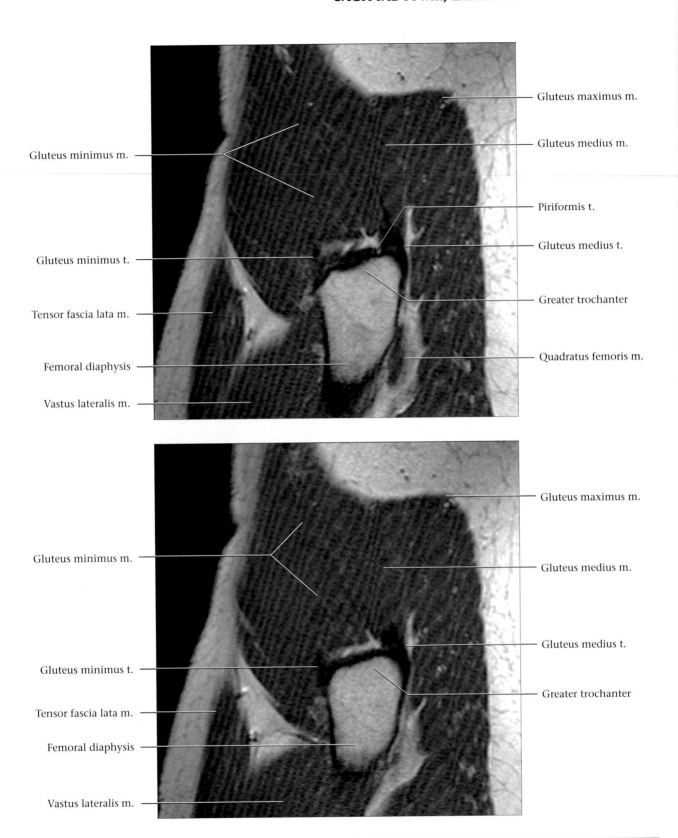

(Top) The tendon of the gluteus minimus muscle is not as well-defined as the tendon of the gluteus medius muscle. **(Bottom)** The gluteus minimus tendon inserts onto the anterior facet of the greater trochanter.

SAGITTAL T1 MR, EXTERNAL ROTATORS & CUFF

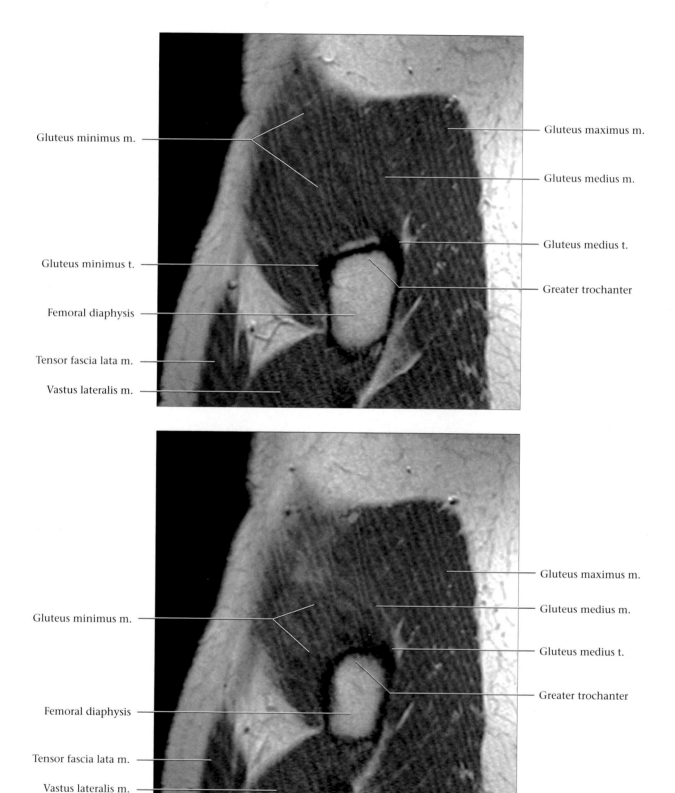

Gluteus minimus m.
Gluteus maximus m.
Gluteus medius m.
Gluteus minimus t.
Gluteus medius t.
Greater trochanter
Femoral diaphysis
Tensor fascia lata m.
Vastus lateralis m.

Gluteus minimus m.
Gluteus maximus m.
Gluteus medius m.
Gluteus medius t.
Greater trochanter
Femoral diaphysis
Tensor fascia lata m.
Vastus lateralis m.

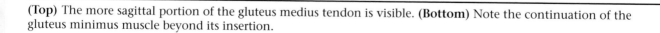

(Top) The more sagittal portion of the gluteus medius tendon is visible. (Bottom) Note the continuation of the gluteus minimus muscle beyond its insertion.

LATERAL HIP

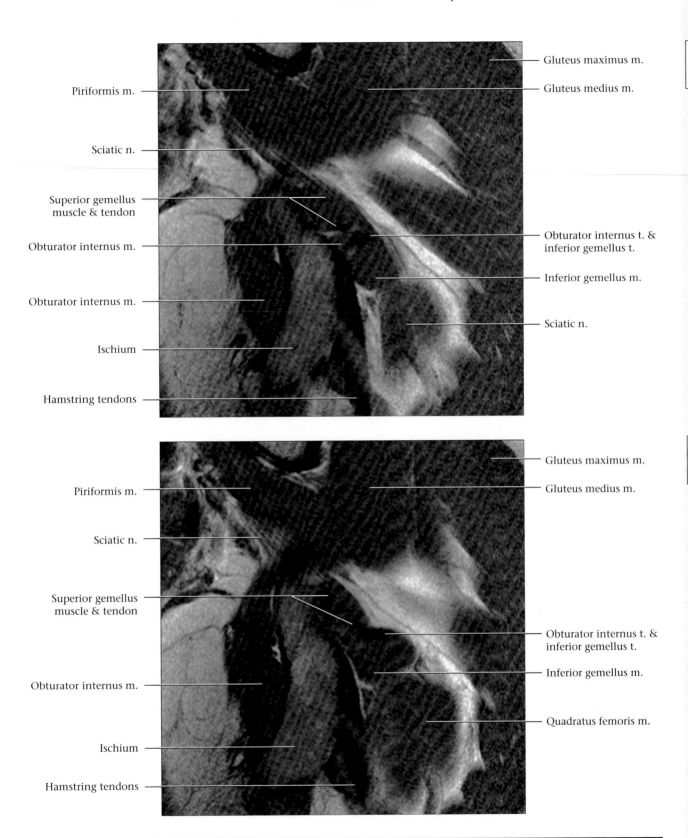

Top image labels:
- Piriformis m.
- Sciatic n.
- Superior gemellus muscle & tendon
- Obturator internus m.
- Obturator internus m.
- Ischium
- Hamstring tendons
- Gluteus maximus m.
- Gluteus medius m.
- Obturator internus t. & inferior gemellus t.
- Inferior gemellus m.
- Sciatic n.

Bottom image labels:
- Piriformis m.
- Sciatic n.
- Superior gemellus muscle & tendon
- Obturator internus m.
- Ischium
- Hamstring tendons
- Gluteus maximus m.
- Gluteus medius m.
- Obturator internus t. & inferior gemellus t.
- Inferior gemellus m.
- Quadratus femoris m.

(Top) First of fourteen coronal images of the lateral aspect of the left hip from posterior to anterior. This image is just anterior to the ischial spine. The superior to inferior relationships of the deeper layer of the external rotators is easily appreciated. The piriformis muscle is the most superior. Of the muscles intimately related to the ischial spine the superior gemellus muscle is most superior. Its tendon is along the inferior surface of the muscle belly. **(Bottom)** The obturator internus tendon is located between the superior and inferior gemellus muscles. The tendons of the obturator internus muscle and inferior gemellus muscles are fused in this individual.

Hip and Pelvis

V

CORONAL T1 MR, EXTERNAL ROTATORS & CUFF

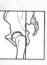

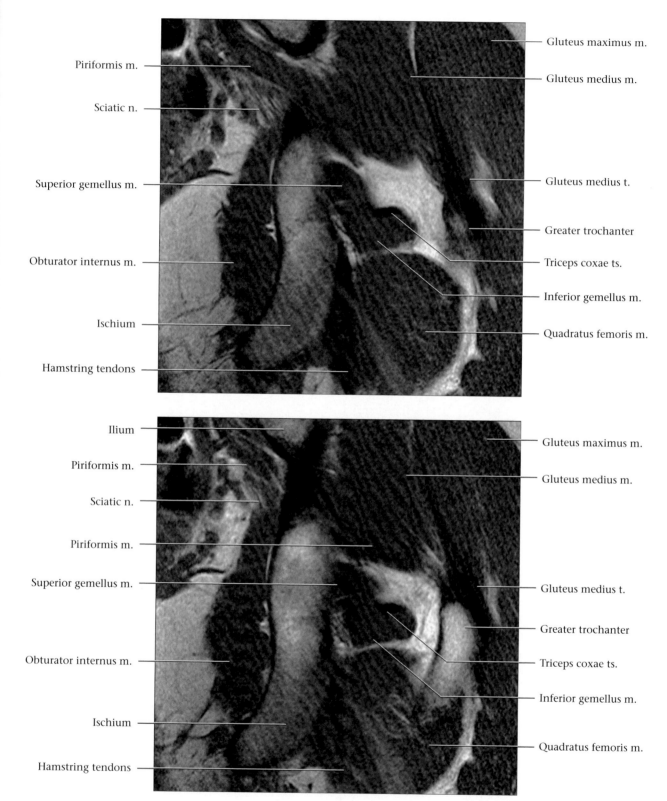

Piriformis m.

Sciatic n.

Superior gemellus m.

Obturator internus m.

Ischium

Hamstring tendons

Gluteus maximus m.

Gluteus medius m.

Gluteus medius t.

Greater trochanter

Triceps coxae ts.

Inferior gemellus m.

Quadratus femoris m.

Ilium

Piriformis m.

Sciatic n.

Piriformis m.

Superior gemellus m.

Obturator internus m.

Ischium

Hamstring tendons

Gluteus maximus m.

Gluteus medius m.

Gluteus medius t.

Greater trochanter

Triceps coxae ts.

Inferior gemellus m.

Quadratus femoris m.

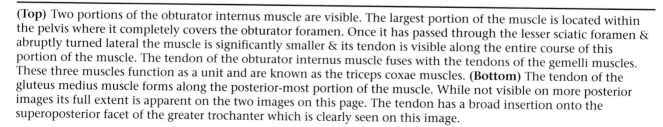

(Top) Two portions of the obturator internus muscle are visible. The largest portion of the muscle is located within the pelvis where it completely covers the obturator foramen. Once it has passed through the lesser sciatic foramen & abruptly turned lateral the muscle is significantly smaller & its tendon is visible along the entire course of this portion of the muscle. The tendon of the obturator internus muscle fuses with the tendons of the gemelli muscles. These three muscles function as a unit and are known as the triceps coxae muscles. **(Bottom)** The tendon of the gluteus medius muscle forms along the posterior-most portion of the muscle. While not visible on more posterior images its full extent is apparent on the two images on this page. The tendon has a broad insertion onto the superoposterior facet of the greater trochanter which is clearly seen on this image.

CORONAL T1 MR, EXTERNAL ROTATORS & CUFF

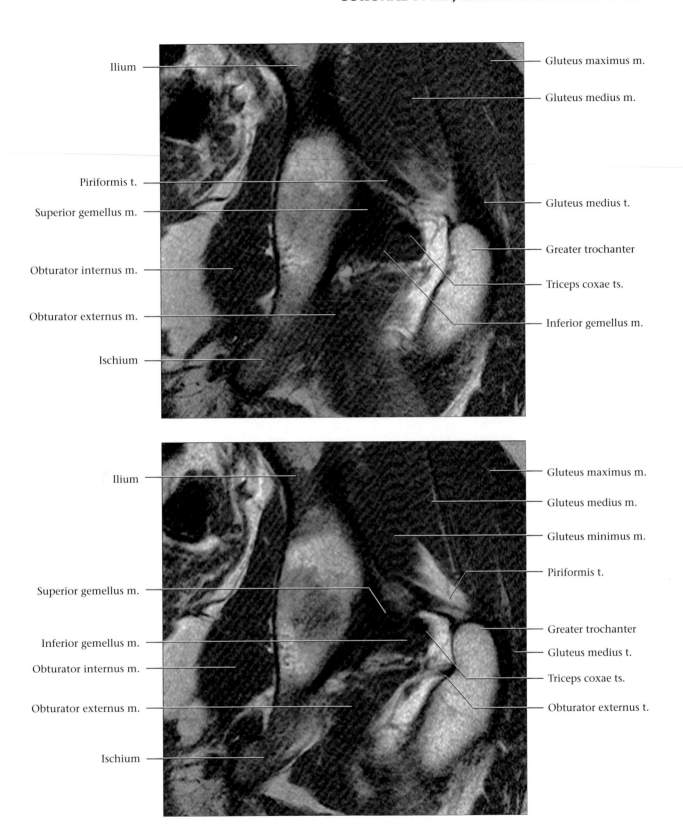

(Top image labels)

Ilium — Gluteus maximus m.

Gluteus medius m.

Piriformis t. — Gluteus medius t.

Superior gemellus m. — Greater trochanter

Obturator internus m. — Triceps coxae ts.

Obturator externus m. — Inferior gemellus m.

Ischium

(Bottom image labels)

Ilium — Gluteus maximus m.

Gluteus medius m.

Gluteus minimus m.

Piriformis t.

Superior gemellus m. — Greater trochanter

Inferior gemellus m. — Gluteus medius t.

Obturator internus m. — Triceps coxae ts.

Obturator externus m. — Obturator externus t.

Ischium

(Top) As it courses laterally the tendon of the piriformis muscle develops. This tendon is the most superior tendon to insert into the piriformis fossa. The second portion of the gluteus medius tendon inserts along the lateral facet of the greater trochanter. The transition between the two insertion sites is visible on this image. The insertion onto the lateral facet extends more inferiorly than the insertion onto the superoposterior facet. (Bottom) The piriformis tendon inserts onto the medial aspect of the greater trochanter, a region known as the piriformis fossa. Note the oblique superomedial to inferolateral course of the tendon. Compare this to the orientation of triceps coxae tendon on more anterior images. The obturator externus tendon is the most inferior tendon inserting into the piriformis fossa.

Hip and Pelvis

V

CORONAL T1 MR, EXTERNAL ROTATORS & CUFF

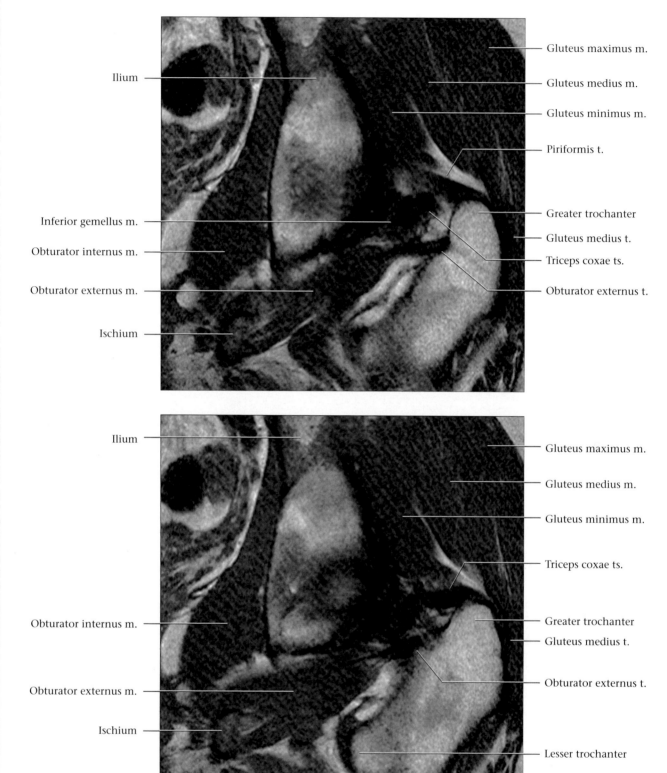

Top image labels:
- Ilium
- Inferior gemellus m.
- Obturator internus m.
- Obturator externus m.
- Ischium
- Gluteus maximus m.
- Gluteus medius m.
- Gluteus minimus m.
- Piriformis t.
- Greater trochanter
- Gluteus medius t.
- Triceps coxae ts.
- Obturator externus t.

Bottom image labels:
- Ilium
- Obturator internus m.
- Obturator externus m.
- Ischium
- Gluteus maximus m.
- Gluteus medius m.
- Gluteus minimus m.
- Triceps coxae ts.
- Greater trochanter
- Gluteus medius t.
- Obturator externus t.
- Lesser trochanter

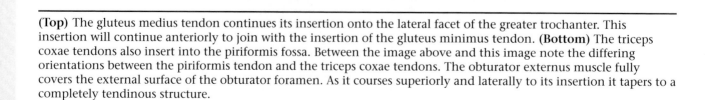

(Top) The gluteus medius tendon continues its insertion onto the lateral facet of the greater trochanter. This insertion will continue anteriorly to join with the insertion of the gluteus minimus tendon. **(Bottom)** The triceps coxae tendons also insert into the piriformis fossa. Between the image above and this image note the differing orientations between the piriformis tendon and the triceps coxae tendons. The obturator externus muscle fully covers the external surface of the obturator foramen. As it courses superiorly and laterally to its insertion it tapers to a completely tendinous structure.

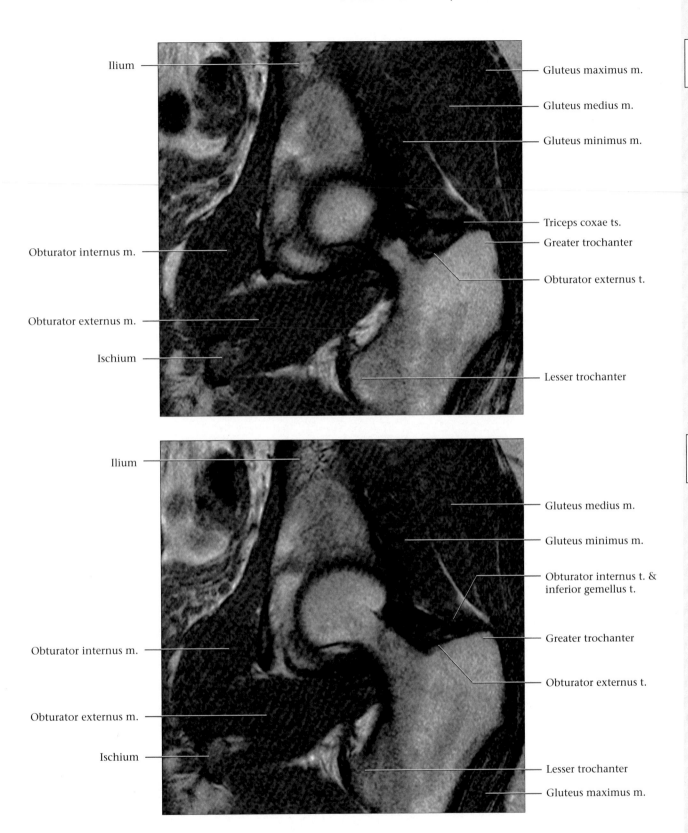

Labels (top image):
- Ilium
- Gluteus maximus m.
- Gluteus medius m.
- Gluteus minimus m.
- Triceps coxae ts.
- Greater trochanter
- Obturator internus m.
- Obturator externus t.
- Obturator externus m.
- Ischium
- Lesser trochanter

Labels (bottom image):
- Ilium
- Gluteus medius m.
- Gluteus minimus m.
- Obturator internus t. & inferior gemellus t.
- Greater trochanter
- Obturator internus m.
- Obturator externus t.
- Obturator externus m.
- Ischium
- Lesser trochanter
- Gluteus maximus m.

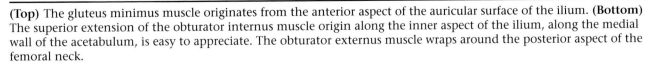

(Top) The gluteus minimus muscle originates from the anterior aspect of the auricular surface of the ilium. **(Bottom)** The superior extension of the obturator internus muscle origin along the inner aspect of the ilium, along the medial wall of the acetabulum, is easy to appreciate. The obturator externus muscle wraps around the posterior aspect of the femoral neck.

Hip and Pelvis

V

CORONAL T1 MR, EXTERNAL ROTATORS & CUFF

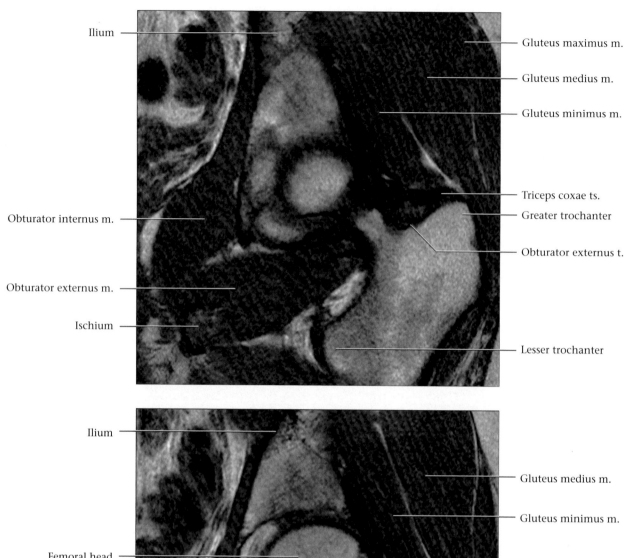

Ilium — Gluteus maximus m.

Gluteus medius m.

Gluteus minimus m.

Triceps coxae ts.

Obturator internus m. — Greater trochanter

Obturator externus t.

Obturator externus m. —

Ischium — Lesser trochanter

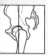

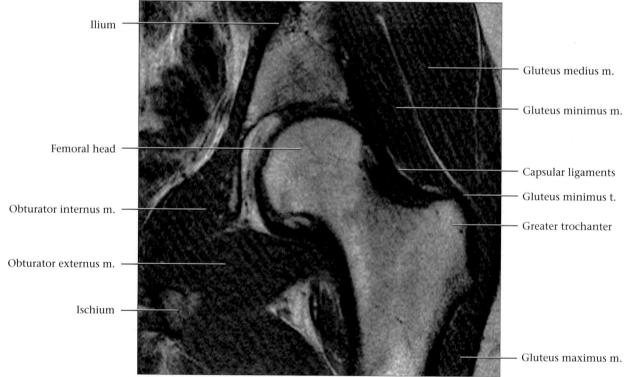

Ilium —

Gluteus medius m.

Gluteus minimus m.

Femoral head —

Capsular ligaments

Obturator internus m. — Gluteus minimus t.

Greater trochanter

Obturator externus m. —

Ischium —

Gluteus maximus m.

(Top) The gluteus minimus muscle originates from the anterior aspect of the auricular surface of the ilium. (Bottom) The gluteus minimus tendon is much shorter and thinner than the gluteus medius tendon.

CORONAL T1 MR, EXTERNAL ROTATORS & CUFF

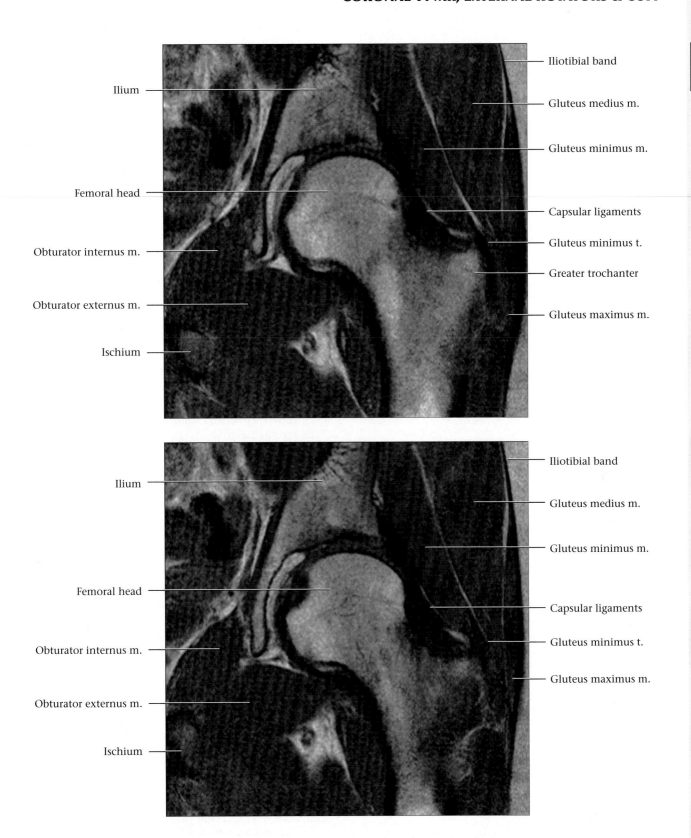

(Top) The gluteus minimus tendon inserts onto the anterior facet of the greater trochanter. Note how the gluteus medius muscle continues anteriorly to wrap around the anterior aspect of the gluteus minimus tendon. **(Bottom)** The gluteus medius and minimus muscle bellies continue anteriorly beyond their insertions onto the greater trochanter. For more anterior images see "Hip and Pelvis Overview" section.

POSTERIOR PELVIS

Terminology

Abbreviations
- Sacroiliac (SI) joint
- Structures (S): Supplied by a nerve or artery

Imaging Anatomy

Sacroiliac Joint
- Anterior synovial joint
  - Auricular surfaces sacrum & ilium
  - Distal 1/3 has synovial features
  - Upper 2/3 microscopically symphyseal, not synovial
- Posterior syndesmosis: Tuberosities sacrum & ilium
- Function: Primarily weight transfer axial to appendicular skeleton
  - Limited gliding & rotation
- Widening anteriorly can occur without instability
- Posterior widening indicates instability
- **Sacroiliac ligaments**
  - **Interosseous sacroiliac:** Within syndesmotic joint
    - Between tuberosities ilium & sacrum
    - Oriented superiorly & laterally
    - Weight transferred to sacrum, sacrum displaced inferiorly, force transmitted to ligaments, ligaments pull ilii inward, compress sacrum & interlocking surfaces SI joints
    - Extremely strong
  - **Anterior sacroiliac:** Weak ligaments
    - Mainly anterior joint capsule
  - **Posterior sacroiliac:** Posterior fibers interosseous ligament
    - **Short dorsal sacroiliac:** Horizontal; lateral sacral crest S1 & S2 to posterior iliac crest
    - **Long dorsal sacroiliac:** Vertical oblique; posterior superior iliac spine to lateral sacral crest S3, S4

Posterior Sacroiliac Ligaments of Pelvis
- Primary stabilizers of pelvis
  - Little contribution from anterior structures
- Resist rotational forces & vertical shear
- **Sacrotuberous:** Superior & inferior posterior iliac spines, sacrum & coccyx to ischial tuberosity
- **Sacrospinous:** Lateral sacrum & coccyx to ischial spine
- **Iliolumbar:** Tip L5 transverse process to iliac crest
- **Sacroiliac ligaments:** Interosseous, long & short dorsal
- Stages of **pelvic disruption**
  - Up to 2.5 cm disruption symphysis pubis with intact posterior ligaments
  - Symphysis > 8 cm likely posterior ligament disruption
  - Disrupt sacrospinous, anterior sacroiliac ligaments
    - Pelvis widens
    - Posterior superior iliac spines impinge on sacrum, limit widening
    - Rotation & shear stability preserved
    - CT: Anterior SI widened, posterior SI intact
  - Unilateral disruption sacrotuberous & posterior sacroiliac ligaments
    - Creates vertical & rotational instability
    - > 1 cm vertical or posterior displacement or rotation of ilium relative to sacrum
    - CT: Posterior SI widened
  - Bilateral disruption sacrotuberous & posterior sacroiliac ligaments
    - Completely disrupts ring
    - Separates spine from lower extremities

Greater Sciatic Foramen
- Greater sciatic notch converted to foramen by sacrospinous ligament
- Contents: 7 nerves, 3 sets of vessels, piriformis m.
- Passageway from pelvis to thigh
  - Structures identified as exiting pelvis above or below piriformis m.
    - Above: Superior gluteal a., v., n.
    - Below: Pudendal n., internal pudendal a., v., n. to obturator internus, sciatic n., inferior gluteal a., v., n., posterior cutaneous n. of thigh, n. to quadratus femoris m.
  - Relationship of structures
    - Most medial: Pudendal n.
    - Most lateral: Sciatic n.
    - N. to quadratus femoris m. deep to sciatic n.
- **Inferior gluteal artery**
  - Larger terminal branch anterior division internal iliac a.
  - Passes between S1 & S2 or S2 & S3
  - Exits pelvis inferior to piriformis m.
  - Posteromedial to sciatic n.
  - Prenatally continuous with popliteal a., remnant is artery to sciatic n.
  - S: Gluteus maximus, obturator internus, quadratus femoris, superior hamstrings ms.
  - **Inferior gluteal v.** travels with artery, drains into internal iliac v.
- **Inferior gluteal nerve**
  - Branch of sacral plexus
  - Exits pelvis inferior to piriformis m.
  - Posterior to sciatic n.
- **Superior gluteal artery**
  - Continuation posterior division internal iliac a.
  - Passes between lumbosacral trunk & S1
  - Exits pelvis superior to piriformis m.
  - Superficial branch: S - gluteus maximus m.
  - Deep branch: S - gluteus medius & minimus, tensor fascia lata ms.
  - **Superior gluteal v.** travels with artery, drains into internal iliac v.
- **Superior gluteal nerve**
  - Branch of sacral plexus
  - Exits pelvis superior to piriformis m.
- **Sciatic nerve**
  - Exits pelvis inferior to piriformis m.
  - Most lateral structure
  - See following page
- **Pudendal n. & internal pudendal vessels**
  - Exit inferior to piriformis m.
  - Nerve most medial structure
- **Nerve to obturator internus m.**
  - Exits pelvis inferior to piriformis m.

POSTERIOR PELVIS

Lesser Sciatic Foramen

- Lesser sciatic notch converted to foramen by intersection (crossing) sacrotuberous and sacrospinous ligaments
- **Pudendal n. & internal pudendal vessels**
  - Pass over sacrospinous ligament
  - Exit buttock, enter perineum
- **Obturator internus m.** (see "Lateral Hip" section)

Sacral Plexus

- Ventral rami L4, L5, S1, S2, S3, S4
  - L4, L5 enter as lumbosacral trunk
    - **Lumbosacral trunk:** Forms at pelvic brim; travels lateral anterior to SI joint, through psoas m. medial to obturator n.; joins sacral plexus
  - Superior gluteal a. passes between lumbosacral trunk & S1
  - S4 divided between sacral & coccygeal plexus
- Forms on anterior surface piriformis m. & coccygeus m.
- Branches
  - **Inferior gluteal n:** L5, S1, S2
    - Exits pelvis inferior to piriformis m. superficial to sciatic n.
    - S: Gluteus maximus m.
  - **N. to levator ani & coccygeus:** S3, S4
    - Exits plexus, enters muscle
  - **N. to obturator internus m. & superior gemellus m.:** L5, S1, S2
    - Exits pelvis inferior to piriformis m.
    - Lateral to internal pudendal a., v.
  - **N. to piriformis:** S1, S2
    - Exits plexus, enters muscle
  - **N. to quadratus femoris m. & inferior gemellus m.:** L4, L5, S1
    - Exits pelvis inferior to piriformis m., deep (anterior) to sciatic n.
    - Articular branch to hip
  - **Pelvic splanchnic:** S2, S3, S4
    - Travels anteriorly to join inferior hypogastric plexus
  - **Perineal branch S4**
    - Exits pelvis via coccygeus m.
  - **Perforating cutaneous n.:** S2, S3
    - Courses through sacrotuberous ligament
    - S: Skin medial buttock
  - **Posterior femoral cutaneous n. of thigh:** S1, S2, S3
    - Exits pelvis inferior to piriformis m.
    - S: Skin inferior buttock, posterior thigh, popliteal fossa, lateral perineum, upper medial thigh
  - **Pudendal:** S2, S3, S4
    - S: Perineum
  - **Sciatic n.:** L4, L5, S1, S2, S3
    - See below
  - **Superior gluteal n.:** L4, L5, S1
    - Exits pelvis superior to piriformis m.
    - Between gluteus medius & minimus ms.
    - S) gluteus medius & minimus, tensor fascia lata ms.

Sciatic Nerve

- 2 nerves in one sheath; typically divide at popliteal fossa
- Tibial n.: Pre-axial
- Common peroneal n.: Post-axial
- Largest nerve in body
- Exits pelvis inferior to piriformis m.
- Relationships
  - Deep to gluteus maximus m., biceps femoris m.
  - Midway between ischial tuberosity & greater trochanter
  - Posterior to obturator internus, quadratus femoris, adductor magnus ms.
- S: Posterior thigh, entire leg, entire foot
- Within thigh supplies
  - Tibial n.: Long head biceps femoris, semitendinosus, semimembranosus, ischiocondylar portion adductor magnus ms.
  - Common peroneal n.: Short head biceps femoris m.
- Anomalous relationship between sciatic n. & piriformis m. common
  - Undivided n. entirely below muscle 90%
  - Divided nerve one portion thru muscle, single one below 7.1%
  - Divided nerve above & below muscle 2.1%
  - Undivided nerve within muscle 0.8%
- Clinical note: Piriformis syndrome
  - Sciatic n. compression in greater sciatic notch
  - Causes: Nerve anomalies, fibrous bands, aberrant vessels, rare masses & hematoma
  - Clinically: Sciatica, no back pain
  - Diagnosis of exclusion

Anatomy-Based Imaging Issues

Imaging Recommendations

- MR: Soft tissue assessment
  - Diagnose masses, anatomic anomalies, other causes of nerve compression
  - Sequences
    - T1WI sagittal, axial, coronal provide anatomic assessment
    - STIR coronal
  - Parameters
    - FOV: 35-40 cm
    - THK: 5 mm, no gap
    - Matrix: 384 x 512
    - Limit coverage to sciatic notch
- MR: preferred modality for sacroiliitis
  - FOV: 30 cm
  - THK: 3 mm
  - Matrix 256 x 256
  - Oblique coronal & axial planes
    - Relative to sacral long axis
  - Intravenous contrast useful
    - Normal joint has no enhancement

Selected References

1. Puhakka KB et al: MR imaging of the normal sacroiliac joint with correlation to histology. Skeletal Radiol. 33(1):15-28, 2004
2. Beaton LE et al: The sciatic nerve and the piriformis muscle: their interrelation a possible cause of coccygodynia. J Bone Joint Surg. 20:686-8, 1938

POSTERIOR PELVIS

GRAPHICS, GREATER & LESSER SCIATIC NOTCH

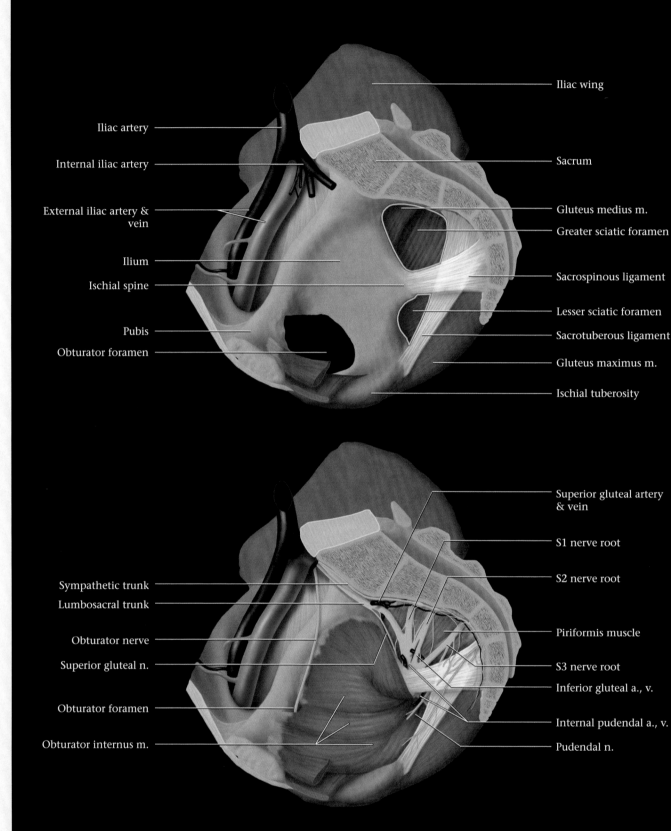

Iliac wing

Iliac artery

Internal iliac artery

Sacrum

External iliac artery & vein

Gluteus medius m.

Greater sciatic foramen

Ilium

Sacrospinous ligament

Ischial spine

Lesser sciatic foramen

Pubis

Sacrotuberous ligament

Obturator foramen

Gluteus maximus m.

Ischial tuberosity

Superior gluteal artery & vein

S1 nerve root

S2 nerve root

Sympathetic trunk

Lumbosacral trunk

Obturator nerve

Piriformis muscle

Superior gluteal n.

S3 nerve root

Inferior gluteal a., v.

Obturator foramen

Internal pudendal a., v.

Obturator internus m.

Pudendal n.

(Top) This view of the pelvis from the internal surface demonstrates the framework of the sciatic foramen. Each sciatic foramen is outlined in yellow. The greater sciatic notch is converted into a foramen by the vertically oriented sacrotuberous ligament. The intersection of the sacrotuberous and sacrospinous ligaments converts the lesser sciatic notch into a foramen. **(Bottom)** The obturator internus, piriformis muscles and sacral plexus now overlay the framework. The obturator internus muscles travel through the lesser sciatic notch as do the internal pudendal vessels and pudendal nerve.

POSTERIOR PELVIS

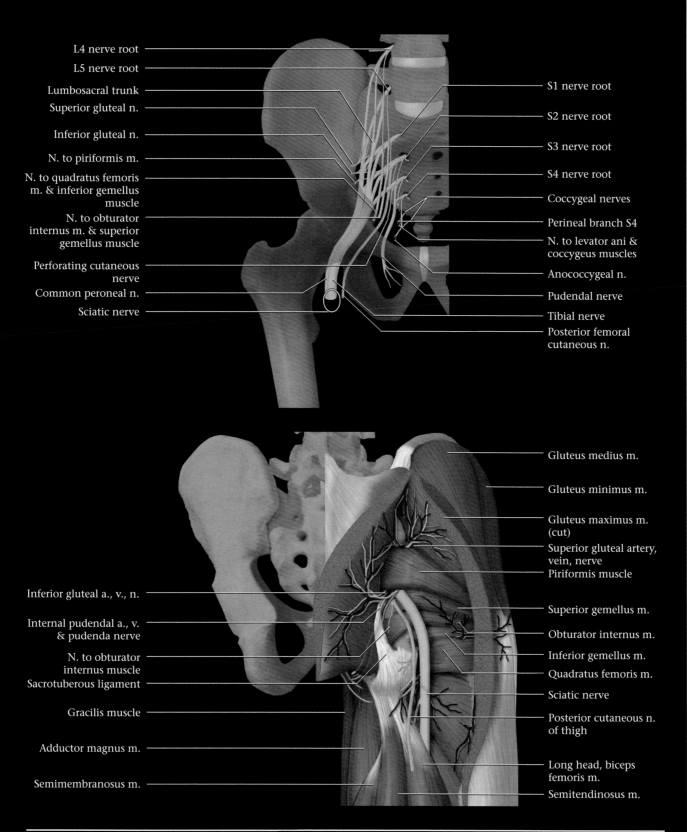

L4 nerve root
L5 nerve root
Lumbosacral trunk
Superior gluteal n.
Inferior gluteal n.
N. to piriformis m.
N. to quadratus femoris m. & inferior gemellus muscle
N. to obturator internus m. & superior gemellus muscle
Perforating cutaneous nerve
Common peroneal n.
Sciatic nerve

S1 nerve root
S2 nerve root
S3 nerve root
S4 nerve root
Coccygeal nerves
Perineal branch S4
N. to levator ani & coccygeus muscles
Anococcygeal n.
Pudendal nerve
Tibial nerve
Posterior femoral cutaneous n.

Inferior gluteal a., v., n.
Internal pudendal a., v. & pudenda nerve
N. to obturator internus muscle
Sacrotuberous ligament
Gracilis muscle
Adductor magnus m.
Semimembranosus m.

Gluteus medius m.
Gluteus minimus m.
Gluteus maximus m. (cut)
Superior gluteal artery, vein, nerve
Piriformis muscle
Superior gemellus m.
Obturator internus m.
Inferior gemellus m.
Quadratus femoris m.
Sciatic nerve
Posterior cutaneous n. of thigh
Long head, biceps femoris m.
Semitendinosus m.

(Top) The sacral plexus. The anterior (yellow) and posterior (green) divisions of the respective nerves are denoted. The common peroneal nerve is a post-axial nerve and the tibial nerve is a pre-axial nerve. **(Bottom)** This posterior view depicts the various structures that exit the pelvis through the greater sciatic notch. Note the superior gluteal vessels and nerve are the only structures above the piriformis muscle. All other structures exit inferior to the muscle.

Hip and Pelvis

V

GRAPHICS, SACROILIAC LIGAMENTS

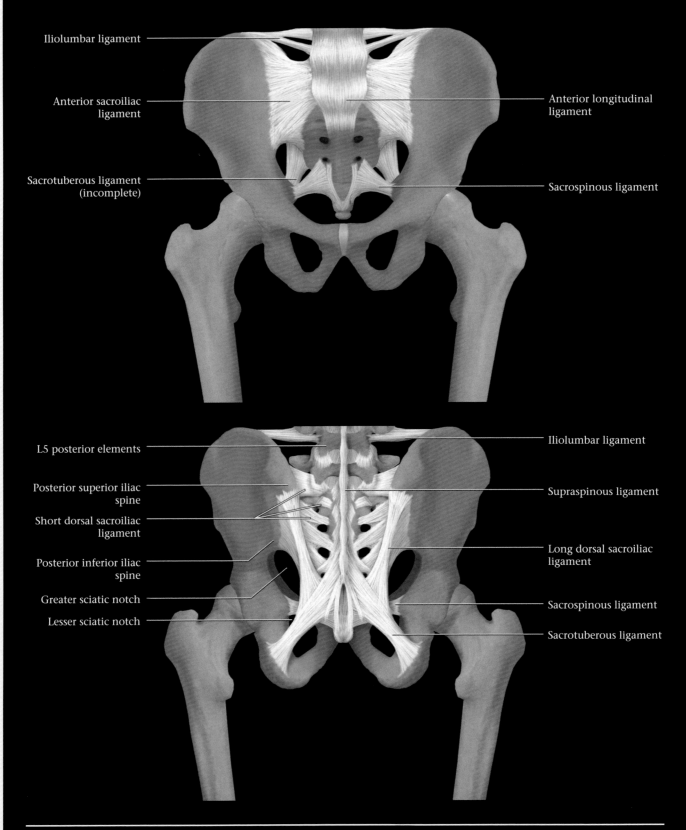

Iliolumbar ligament

Anterior sacroiliac ligament

Sacrotuberous ligament (incomplete)

Anterior longitudinal ligament

Sacrospinous ligament

L5 posterior elements

Posterior superior iliac spine

Short dorsal sacroiliac ligament

Posterior inferior iliac spine

Greater sciatic notch

Lesser sciatic notch

Iliolumbar ligament

Supraspinous ligament

Long dorsal sacroiliac ligament

Sacrospinous ligament

Sacrotuberous ligament

(Top) Anterior view of the ligaments of the sacroiliac joint and pelvis. The ventral ligaments of the sacroiliac joint are weak and composed primarily of joint capsule. **(Bottom)** Posterior view of the sacroiliac ligaments demonstrates the horizontal short dorsal sacroiliac ligaments and the vertically oriented long dorsal sacroiliac ligaments. The horizontally oriented iliolumbar ligaments are part of the posterior sacroiliac ligament complex.

POSTERIOR PELVIS

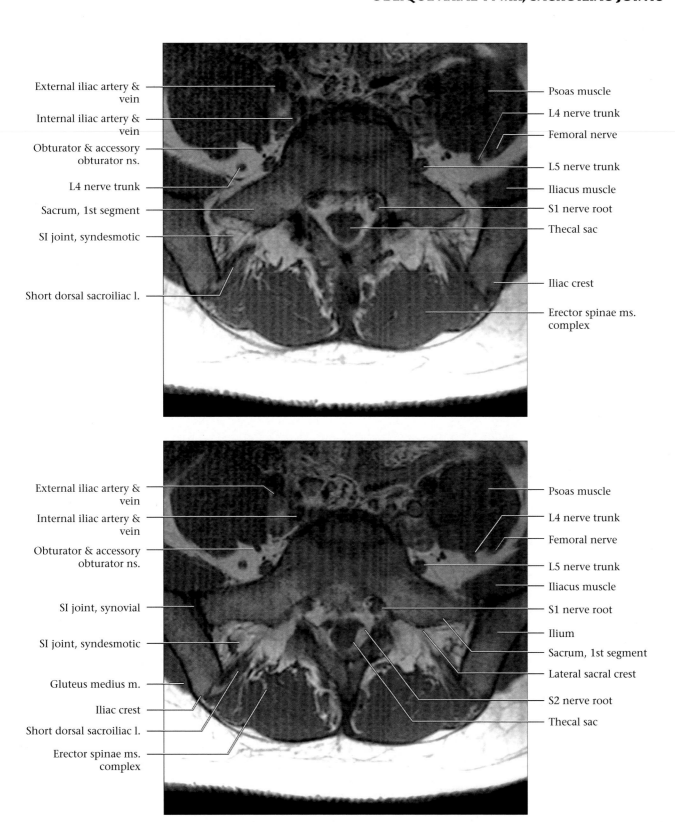

Top image labels (left):
- External iliac artery & vein
- Internal iliac artery & vein
- Obturator & accessory obturator ns.
- L4 nerve trunk
- Sacrum, 1st segment
- SI joint, syndesmotic
- Short dorsal sacroiliac l.

Top image labels (right):
- Psoas muscle
- L4 nerve trunk
- Femoral nerve
- L5 nerve trunk
- Iliacus muscle
- S1 nerve root
- Thecal sac
- Iliac crest
- Erector spinae ms. complex

Bottom image labels (left):
- External iliac artery & vein
- Internal iliac artery & vein
- Obturator & accessory obturator ns.
- SI joint, synovial
- SI joint, syndesmotic
- Gluteus medius m.
- Iliac crest
- Short dorsal sacroiliac l.
- Erector spinae ms. complex

Bottom image labels (right):
- Psoas muscle
- L4 nerve trunk
- Femoral nerve
- L5 nerve trunk
- Iliacus muscle
- S1 nerve root
- Ilium
- Sacrum, 1st segment
- Lateral sacral crest
- S2 nerve root
- Thecal sac

(Top) This series of axial images is obliquely oriented along the axial plane of the sacrum. The images cover from superior to inferior. By this level the L4 nerve trunk is still separate from L5 and has not yet formed the lumbosacral trunk. **(Bottom)** The synovial portion of the sacroiliac joint is now visible. Thin layers of articular cartilage are present within this portion of the joint and it is much narrower than the syndesmotic portion of the joint. The prominent lateral sacral crest is seen along the posterior sacral border. It is the site of origin of the short, and more inferiorly, long dorsal sacroiliac ligaments. The S2 nerve roots have separated from the thecal sac.

OBLIQUE AXIAL T1 MR, SACROILIAC JOINTS

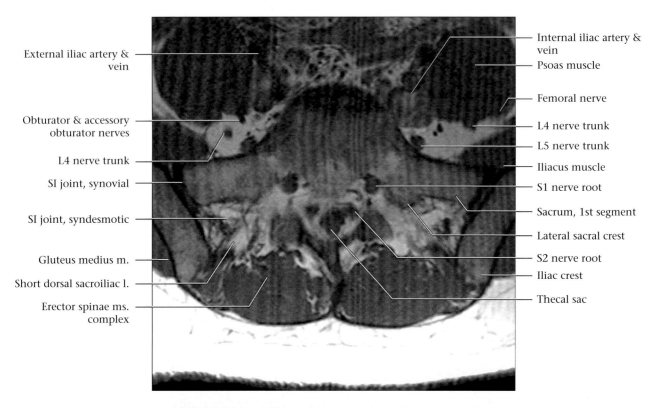

External iliac artery & vein

Obturator & accessory obturator nerves

L4 nerve trunk

SI joint, synovial

SI joint, syndesmotic

Gluteus medius m.

Short dorsal sacroiliac l.

Erector spinae ms. complex

Internal iliac artery & vein

Psoas muscle

Femoral nerve

L4 nerve trunk

L5 nerve trunk

Iliacus muscle

S1 nerve root

Sacrum, 1st segment

Lateral sacral crest

S2 nerve root

Iliac crest

Thecal sac

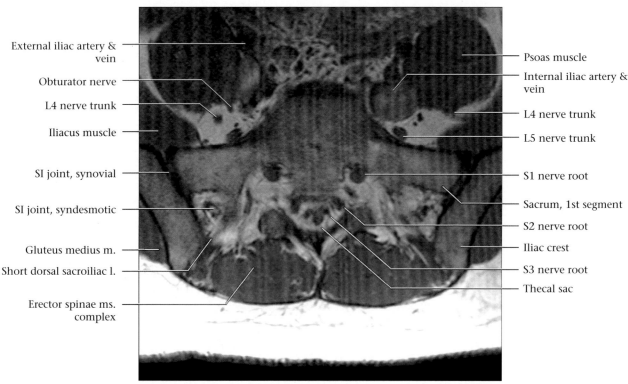

External iliac artery & vein

Obturator nerve

L4 nerve trunk

Iliacus muscle

SI joint, synovial

SI joint, syndesmotic

Gluteus medius m.

Short dorsal sacroiliac l.

Erector spinae ms. complex

Psoas muscle

Internal iliac artery & vein

L4 nerve trunk

L5 nerve trunk

S1 nerve root

Sacrum, 1st segment

S2 nerve root

Iliac crest

S3 nerve root

Thecal sac

(Top) Two articular surfaces of the ilium are present. The anterior articular surface is part of the synovial portion of the joint, & the posterior tuberosity is part of the syndesmosis of the sacroiliac joint. The femoral nerves are located posterior to the psoas muscle & are not separable on these images. The L4 nerve trunks are also posterior to the psoas; their relationships are different from side to side in this image. On the right the nerve is separated from the muscle while on the left it is more closely approximated to the muscle. The obturator nerve is located more medially along the posterior border of the psoas muscle. **(Bottom)** The S1 nerve roots are seen traveling anteriorly to exit the ventral neural foramina and the S3 nerve roots have now separated from the thecal sac.

Hip and Pelvis

V

POSTERIOR PELVIS

OBLIQUE AXIAL T1 MR, SACROILIAC JOINTS

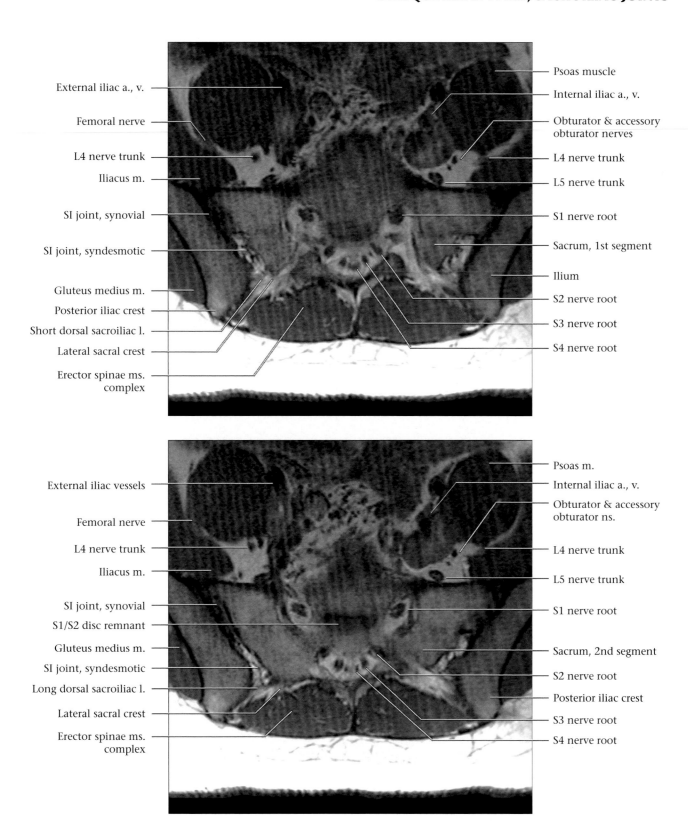

Top image labels (left):
- External iliac a., v.
- Femoral nerve
- L4 nerve trunk
- Iliacus m.
- SI joint, synovial
- SI joint, syndesmotic
- Gluteus medius m.
- Posterior iliac crest
- Short dorsal sacroiliac l.
- Lateral sacral crest
- Erector spinae ms. complex

Top image labels (right):
- Psoas muscle
- Internal iliac a., v.
- Obturator & accessory obturator nerves
- L4 nerve trunk
- L5 nerve trunk
- S1 nerve root
- Sacrum, 1st segment
- Ilium
- S2 nerve root
- S3 nerve root
- S4 nerve root

Bottom image labels (left):
- External iliac vessels
- Femoral nerve
- L4 nerve trunk
- Iliacus m.
- SI joint, synovial
- S1/S2 disc remnant
- Gluteus medius m.
- SI joint, syndesmotic
- Long dorsal sacroiliac l.
- Lateral sacral crest
- Erector spinae ms. complex

Bottom image labels (right):
- Psoas m.
- Internal iliac a., v.
- Obturator & accessory obturator ns.
- L4 nerve trunk
- L5 nerve trunk
- S1 nerve root
- Sacrum, 2nd segment
- S2 nerve root
- Posterior iliac crest
- S3 nerve root
- S4 nerve root

(Top) The obturator and accessory obturator nerves are seen traveling medially and posteriorly. They are located along the lateral aspect of the internal iliac vessels. The femoral nerves are tucked behind the psoas muscle and exit within the iliopsoas fat plane. The posterior most aspect of the ilium at this level is the iliac crest. The crest continues anteriorly to the anterior superior iliac spine and extends inferiorly to the posterior superior iliac spine. **(Bottom)** A remnant of the S1/S2 intervertebral disc is present and identifies the transition from the S1 to S2 sacral segments. Irregular but congruent articular surfaces of the sacroiliac joint are evident especially on the right. The irregularity contributes to stability.

Hip and Pelvis

V

133

OBLIQUE AXIAL T1 MR, SACROILIAC JOINTS

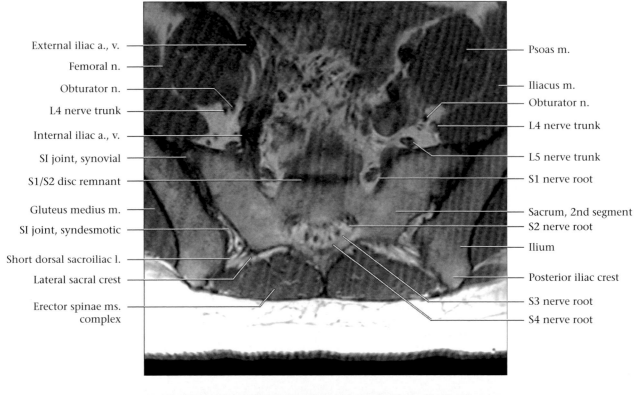

External iliac a., v.
Femoral n.
Obturator n.
L4 nerve trunk
Internal iliac a., v.
SI joint, synovial
S1/S2 disc remnant
Gluteus medius m.
SI joint, syndesmotic
Short dorsal sacroiliac l.
Lateral sacral crest
Erector spinae ms. complex

Psoas m.
Iliacus m.
Obturator n.
L4 nerve trunk
L5 nerve trunk
S1 nerve root
Sacrum, 2nd segment
S2 nerve root
Ilium
Posterior iliac crest
S3 nerve root
S4 nerve root

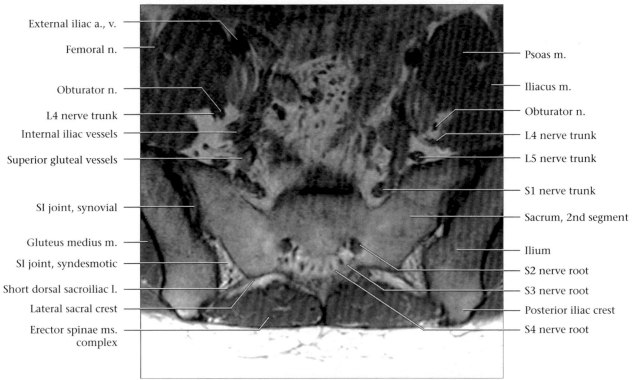

External iliac a., v.
Femoral n.
Obturator n.
L4 nerve trunk
Internal iliac vessels
Superior gluteal vessels
SI joint, synovial
Gluteus medius m.
SI joint, syndesmotic
Short dorsal sacroiliac l.
Lateral sacral crest
Erector spinae ms. complex

Psoas m.
Iliacus m.
Obturator n.
L4 nerve trunk
L5 nerve trunk
S1 nerve trunk
Sacrum, 2nd segment
Ilium
S2 nerve root
S3 nerve root
Posterior iliac crest
S4 nerve root

(Top) The S1 nerve roots have exited the ventral neural foramina. The synovial portion of the SI joint now occupies 1/2 of the anterior to posterior dimension of the entire joint. The synovial and syndesmotic portions of the SI joint are in the same orientation. The synovial portion is located more laterally, the syndesmotic portion more medially. This orientation explains the relationship of these portions of the joint as seen on AP radiographs. The iliac vessels have now branched into internal and external vessels. **(Bottom)** The short dorsal iliac ligaments are well depicted. Their horizontal orientation is easily appreciated and their attachments to the lateral crest of the sacrum and to the posterior iliac crest are well seen.

POSTERIOR PELVIS

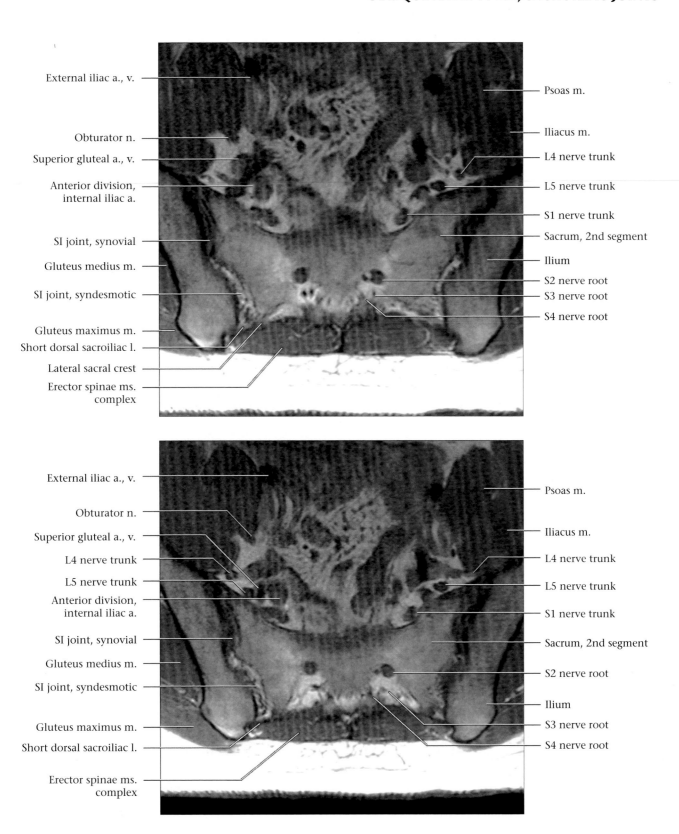

External iliac a., v. — Psoas m.

Obturator n. — Iliacus m.

Superior gluteal a., v. — L4 nerve trunk

Anterior division, internal iliac a. — L5 nerve trunk

— S1 nerve trunk

SI joint, synovial — Sacrum, 2nd segment

Gluteus medius m. — Ilium

SI joint, syndesmotic — S2 nerve root

— S3 nerve root

Gluteus maximus m. — S4 nerve root

Short dorsal sacroiliac l.

Lateral sacral crest

Erector spinae ms. complex

External iliac a., v. — Psoas m.

Obturator n. — Iliacus m.

Superior gluteal a., v. — L4 nerve trunk

L4 nerve trunk — L5 nerve trunk

L5 nerve trunk — S1 nerve trunk

Anterior division, internal iliac a.

SI joint, synovial — Sacrum, 2nd segment

Gluteus medius m. — S2 nerve root

SI joint, syndesmotic — Ilium

Gluteus maximus m. — S3 nerve root

Short dorsal sacroiliac l. — S4 nerve root

Erector spinae ms. complex

(Top) The L4 & L5 nerve trunks are converging to become the lumbosacral trunk, and that is converging with the S1 nerve trunk as they travel inferior and lateral to form the sacral plexus. The internal iliac artery has branched into anterior and posterior divisions. The femoral nerve is no longer visible since it is within the groove between the iliacus and psoas muscles. **(Bottom)** The irregularity of the articular surfaces of the sacroiliac joints is even greater at this level and is well appreciated on the left. While the joint surfaces are congruent, their undulating course prohibits any significant motion through the joint. The superior gluteal artery is the continuation of the posterior division of the internal iliac artery. It passes between the lumbosacral trunk (or in this case L5 since the lumbosacral nerve trunk has not yet converged) and S1 nerve root.

OBLIQUE AXIAL T1 MR, SACROILIAC JOINTS

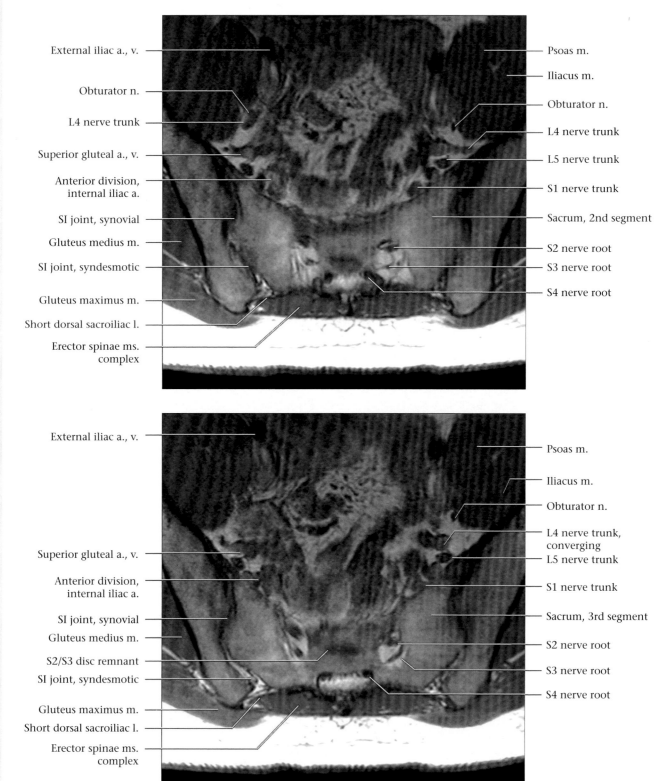

External iliac a., v.

Obturator n.

L4 nerve trunk

Superior gluteal a., v.

Anterior division,
internal iliac a.

SI joint, synovial

Gluteus medius m.

SI joint, syndesmotic

Gluteus maximus m.

Short dorsal sacroiliac l.

Erector spinae ms.
complex

Psoas m.

Iliacus m.

Obturator n.

L4 nerve trunk

L5 nerve trunk

S1 nerve trunk

Sacrum, 2nd segment

S2 nerve root

S3 nerve root

S4 nerve root

External iliac a., v.

Superior gluteal a., v.

Anterior division,
internal iliac a.

SI joint, synovial

Gluteus medius m.

S2/S3 disc remnant

SI joint, syndesmotic

Gluteus maximus m.

Short dorsal sacroiliac l.

Erector spinae ms.
complex

Psoas m.

Iliacus m.

Obturator n.

L4 nerve trunk,
converging

L5 nerve trunk

S1 nerve trunk

Sacrum, 3rd segment

S2 nerve root

S3 nerve root

S4 nerve root

(Top) A consistent relationship between the nerve roots of the sacral plexus and the adjacent vessels exists. The inferior gluteal vessels will pass from anterior to posterior between the S1 & S2 nerve roots or between the S2 & S3 nerve roots. The superior gluteal artery previously passed between the lumbosacral trunk (or L5 trunk) and S1. Note the "wandering" course of the right L4 nerve trunk; it kinks anteriorly and then posteriorly, while the left follows a straight course. Such alterations in course can be confusing. (Bottom) The S3 nerve root on the right has exited the ventral neural foramen. The orientation of the syndesmotic portion of the sacroiliac joint has changed from a more direct posterior orientation to an oblique orientation angle medially. A remnant of the S2/S3 intervertebral disc space helps identify the different sacral segments.

OBLIQUE AXIAL T1 MR, SACROILIAC JOINTS

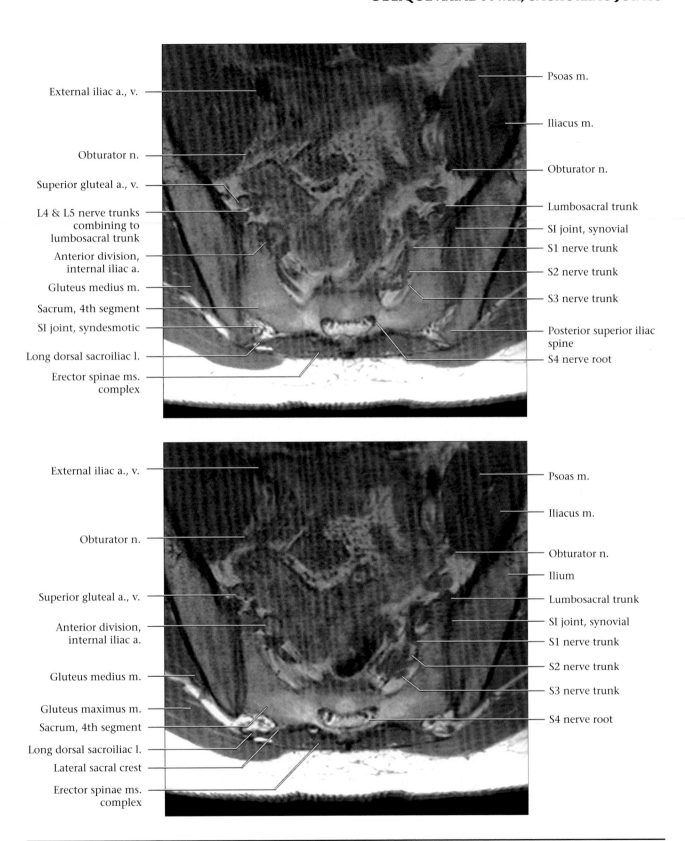

External iliac a., v.

Obturator n.

Superior gluteal a., v.

L4 & L5 nerve trunks
combining to
lumbosacral trunk

Anterior division,
internal iliac a.

Gluteus medius m.

Sacrum, 4th segment

SI joint, syndesmotic

Long dorsal sacroiliac l.

Erector spinae ms.
complex

Psoas m.

Iliacus m.

Obturator n.

Lumbosacral trunk

SI joint, synovial

S1 nerve trunk

S2 nerve trunk

S3 nerve trunk

Posterior superior iliac
spine

S4 nerve root

External iliac a., v.

Obturator n.

Superior gluteal a., v.

Anterior division,
internal iliac a.

Gluteus medius m.

Gluteus maximus m.

Sacrum, 4th segment

Long dorsal sacroiliac l.

Lateral sacral crest

Erector spinae ms.
complex

Psoas m.

Iliacus m.

Obturator n.

Ilium

Lumbosacral trunk

SI joint, synovial

S1 nerve trunk

S2 nerve trunk

S3 nerve trunk

S4 nerve root

(Top) The posterior superior iliac spine is evident. It marks the posterior extent of the iliac crest. The long dorsal sacroiliac ligaments attach superiorly at this site. Note the close proximity of the S2 and S3 nerve roots at this level. The transition from the third to the fourth sacral segments is marked by the S3 neural foramina. Note that L4 & L5 nerve trunks are combining to form the lumbosacral trunk on both sides. **(Bottom)** The S2 and S3 nerve trunks course anteriorly and laterally and will eventually join the lumbosacral trunk and S1 nerve trunk in formation of the sacral plexus. In this imaging plane the synovial portion of the sacroiliac joint continues more inferiorly than the syndesmotic portion.

OBLIQUE AXIAL T1 MR, SACROILIAC JOINTS

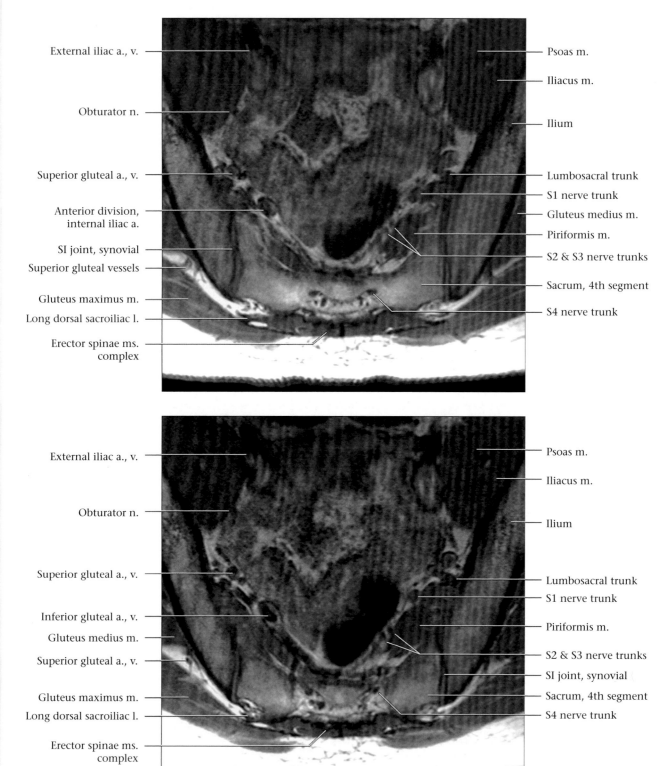

External iliac a., v. —
Obturator n. —
Superior gluteal a., v. —
Anterior division, internal iliac a. —
SI joint, synovial —
Superior gluteal vessels —
Gluteus maximus m. —
Long dorsal sacroiliac l. —
Erector spinae ms. complex —

— Psoas m.
— Iliacus m.
— Ilium
— Lumbosacral trunk
— S1 nerve trunk
— Gluteus medius m.
— Piriformis m.
— S2 & S3 nerve trunks
— Sacrum, 4th segment
— S4 nerve trunk

External iliac a., v. —
Obturator n. —
Superior gluteal a., v. —
Inferior gluteal a., v. —
Gluteus medius m. —
Superior gluteal a., v. —
Gluteus maximus m. —
Long dorsal sacroiliac l. —
Erector spinae ms. complex —

— Psoas m.
— Iliacus m.
— Ilium
— Lumbosacral trunk
— S1 nerve trunk
— Piriformis m.
— S2 & S3 nerve trunks
— SI joint, synovial
— Sacrum, 4th segment
— S4 nerve trunk

(Top) The sacroiliac joint is now completely synovial. Injections into the joint should be directed at this level to avoid injection of the syndesmosis. The superior most fibers of the piriformis muscle can be seen originating from the sacrum. **(Bottom)** The transition from the fourth to the fifth sacral segment is marked by the S4 neural foramina. The vertical fibers of the long dorsal sacroiliac ligaments are visible as is their origin from the lateral sacral crests. The structures of the sacral plexus and the associated vessels continue to move laterally along the deep surface of the piriformis muscle.

OBLIQUE AXIAL T1 MR, SACROILIAC JOINTS

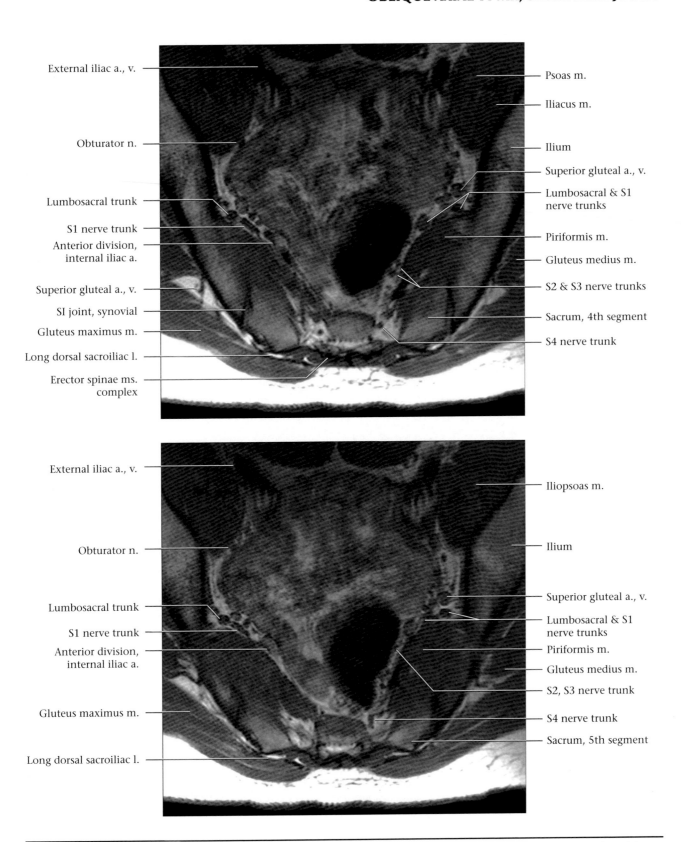

(Top) At this more inferior level the obturator nerve is beginning to course more posteriorly to its eventual position along the medial aspect of the obturator internus muscle. The S4 neural foramina marks the transition between the fourth and fifth sacral segments. **(Bottom)** The inferior most aspect of the sacroiliac joint is visible. Below this is the greater sciatic notch, which is primarily filled with the piriformis muscle.

Hip and Pelvis

V

OBLIQUE AXIAL T1 MR, SACROILIAC JOINTS

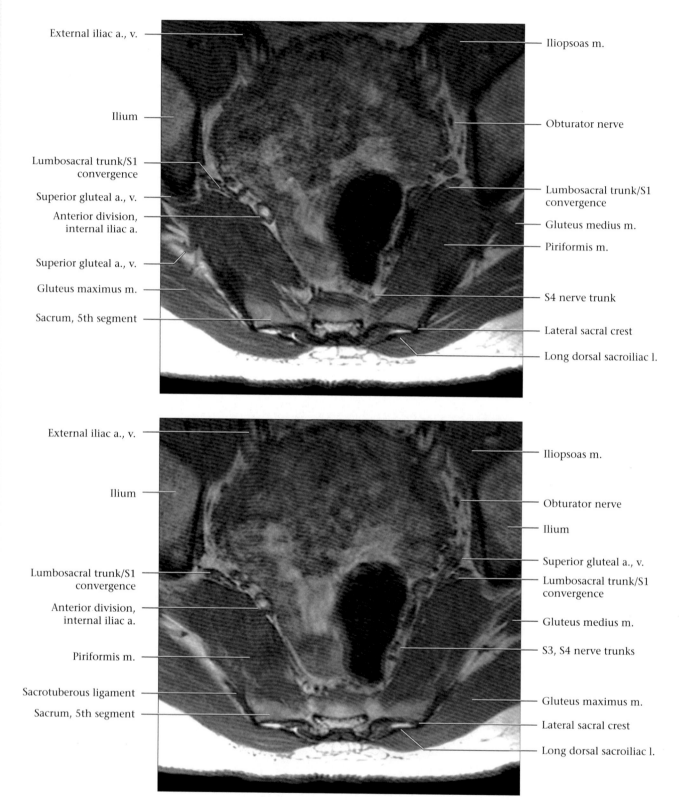

External iliac a., v.

Ilium

Lumbosacral trunk/S1 convergence

Superior gluteal a., v.

Anterior division, internal iliac a.

Superior gluteal a., v.

Gluteus maximus m.

Sacrum, 5th segment

Iliopsoas m.

Obturator nerve

Lumbosacral trunk/S1 convergence

Gluteus medius m.

Piriformis m.

S4 nerve trunk

Lateral sacral crest

Long dorsal sacroiliac l.

External iliac a., v.

Ilium

Lumbosacral trunk/S1 convergence

Anterior division, internal iliac a.

Piriformis m.

Sacrotuberous ligament

Sacrum, 5th segment

Iliopsoas m.

Obturator nerve

Ilium

Superior gluteal a., v.

Lumbosacral trunk/S1 convergence

Gluteus medius m.

S3, S4 nerve trunks

Gluteus maximus m.

Lateral sacral crest

Long dorsal sacroiliac l.

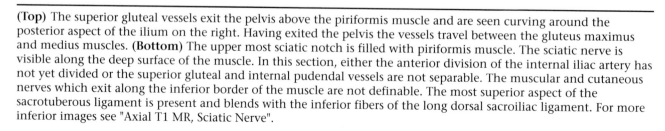

(Top) The superior gluteal vessels exit the pelvis above the piriformis muscle and are seen curving around the posterior aspect of the ilium on the right. Having exited the pelvis the vessels travel between the gluteus maximus and medius muscles. **(Bottom)** The upper most sciatic notch is filled with piriformis muscle. The sciatic nerve is visible along the deep surface of the muscle. In this section, either the anterior division of the internal iliac artery has not yet divided or the superior gluteal and internal pudendal vessels are not separable. The muscular and cutaneous nerves which exit along the inferior border of the muscle are not definable. The most superior aspect of the sacrotuberous ligament is present and blends with the inferior fibers of the long dorsal sacroiliac ligament. For more inferior images see "Axial T1 MR, Sciatic Nerve".

OBLIQUE CORONAL T1 MR, SI JOINTS & GREATER SCIATIC NOTCH

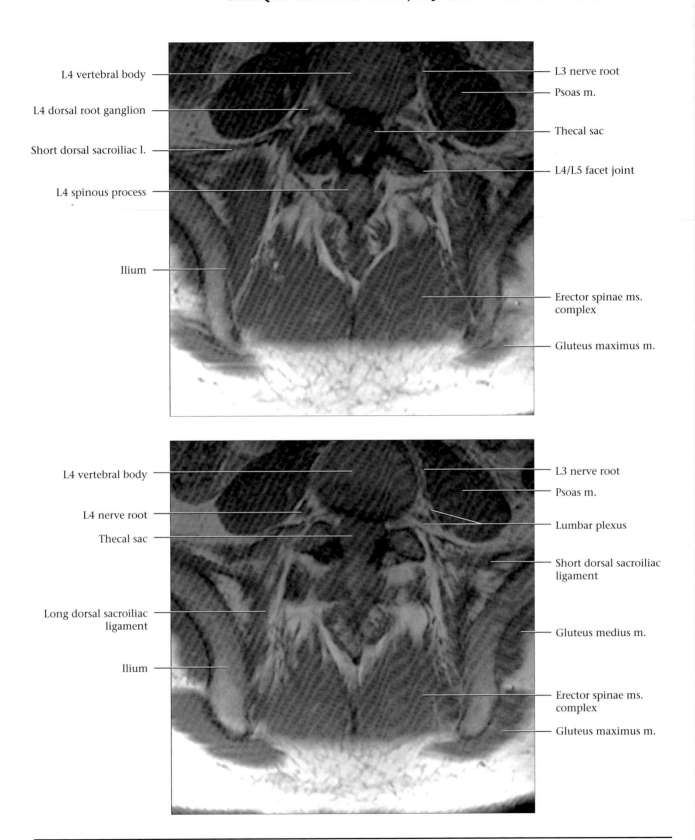

L4 vertebral body

L4 dorsal root ganglion

Short dorsal sacroiliac l.

L4 spinous process

Ilium

L3 nerve root

Psoas m.

Thecal sac

L4/L5 facet joint

Erector spinae ms. complex

Gluteus maximus m.

L4 vertebral body

L4 nerve root

Thecal sac

Long dorsal sacroiliac ligament

Ilium

L3 nerve root

Psoas m.

Lumbar plexus

Short dorsal sacroiliac ligament

Gluteus medius m.

Erector spinae ms. complex

Gluteus maximus m.

(Top) This series of coronal images is oriented along the long axis of the sacrum and begins posteriorly. The oblique coronal orientation presents the posterior elements in an unusual fashion, as seen here with visibility of the L4/5 facet joints and the L3 nerve root. **(Bottom)** The posterior ligaments of the sacroiliac joint are well depicted. The vertically oriented long dorsal sacroiliac ligaments and the horizontally oriented short dorsal sacroiliac ligament are visible. Portions of the lumbar plexus are seen.

OBLIQUE CORONAL T1 MR, SI JOINTS & GREATER SCIATIC NOTCH

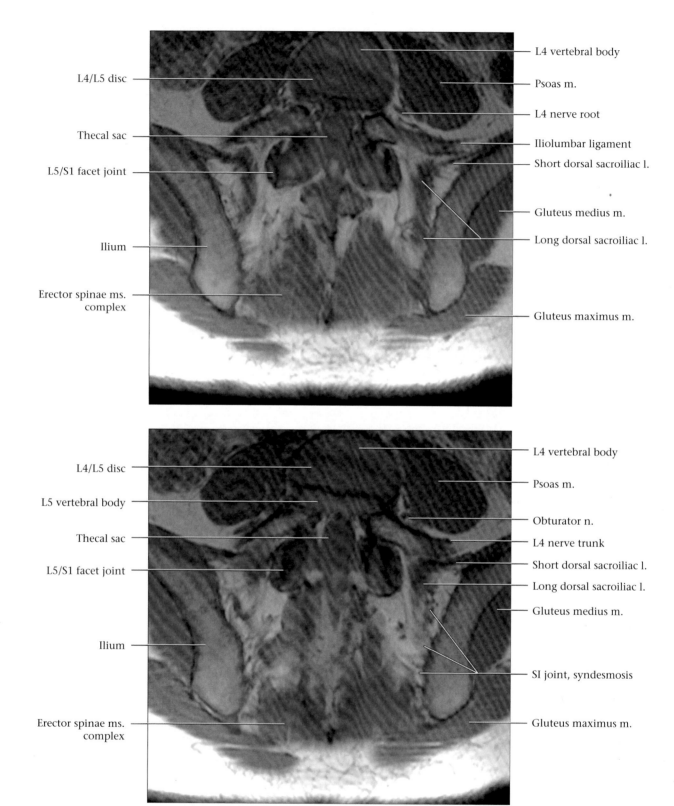

Top image labels:
- L4/L5 disc
- Thecal sac
- L5/S1 facet joint
- Ilium
- Erector spinae ms. complex
- L4 vertebral body
- Psoas m.
- L4 nerve root
- Iliolumbar ligament
- Short dorsal sacroiliac l.
- Gluteus medius m.
- Long dorsal sacroiliac l.
- Gluteus maximus m.

Bottom image labels:
- L4/L5 disc
- L5 vertebral body
- Thecal sac
- L5/S1 facet joint
- Ilium
- Erector spinae ms. complex
- L4 vertebral body
- Psoas m.
- Obturator n.
- L4 nerve trunk
- Short dorsal sacroiliac l.
- Long dorsal sacroiliac l.
- Gluteus medius m.
- SI joint, syndesmosis
- Gluteus maximus m.

(Top) The iliolumbar ligament extends from the tip of the L5 transverse process to the inner margin of the iliac crest. **(Bottom)** The dorsal sacroiliac ligaments are contiguous with the most posterior fibers of the interosseous ligaments and the transition is visible on this and the next image. The obturator nerve is present along the medial border of the psoas muscle.

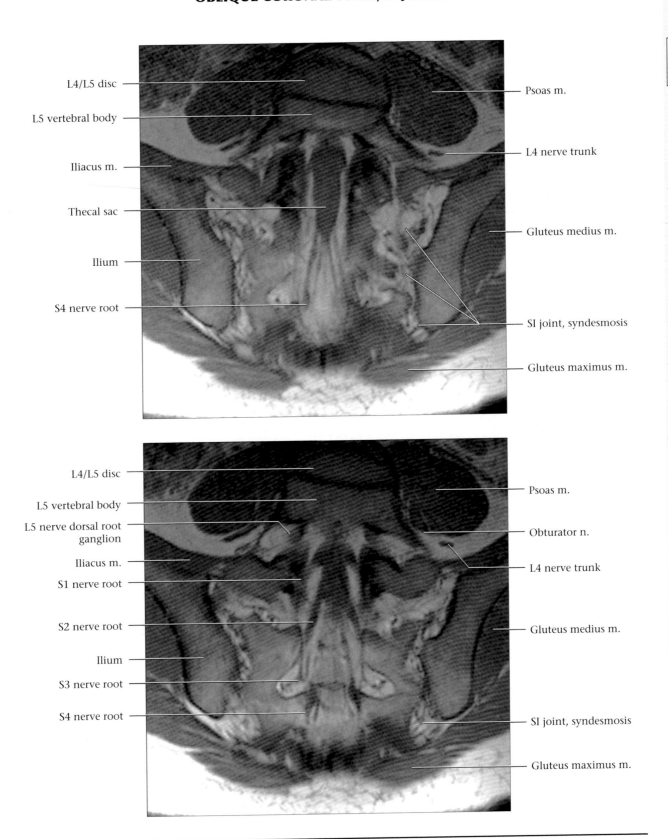

Top image labels (left): L4/L5 disc · L5 vertebral body · Iliacus m. · Thecal sac · Ilium · S4 nerve root

Top image labels (right): Psoas m. · L4 nerve trunk · Gluteus medius m. · SI joint, syndesmosis · Gluteus maximus m.

Bottom image labels (left): L4/L5 disc · L5 vertebral body · L5 nerve dorsal root ganglion · Iliacus m. · S1 nerve root · S2 nerve root · Ilium · S3 nerve root · S4 nerve root

Bottom image labels (right): Psoas m. · Obturator n. · L4 nerve trunk · Gluteus medius m. · SI joint, syndesmosis · Gluteus maximus m.

(Top) This imaging plane is through a long axis of the terminal aspect of the thecal sac. Multiple interosseous ligaments of the syndesmotic portion of the sacroiliac joint are still visible. Note their superior and lateral orientation. **(Bottom)** The L5, S1, S2, S3, S4 nerve roots arise from the thecal sac and course laterally and inferiorly and are directed anteriorly. The L5 nerve roots are within the neural foramina on this image.

OBLIQUE CORONAL T1 MR, SI JOINTS & GREATER SCIATIC NOTCH

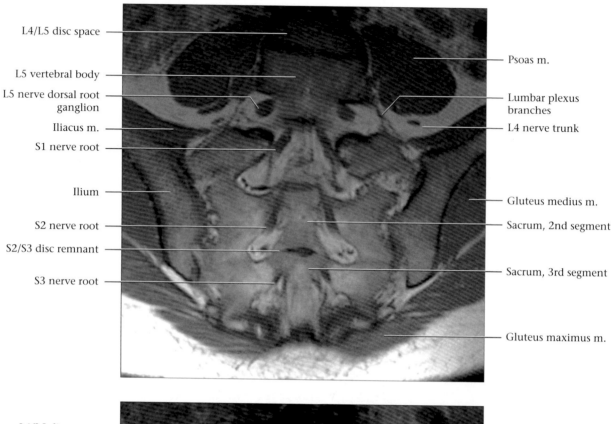

L4/L5 disc space

L5 vertebral body

L5 nerve dorsal root
ganglion

Iliacus m.

S1 nerve root

Ilium

S2 nerve root

S2/S3 disc remnant

S3 nerve root

Psoas m.

Lumbar plexus
branches

L4 nerve trunk

Gluteus medius m.

Sacrum, 2nd segment

Sacrum, 3rd segment

Gluteus maximus m.

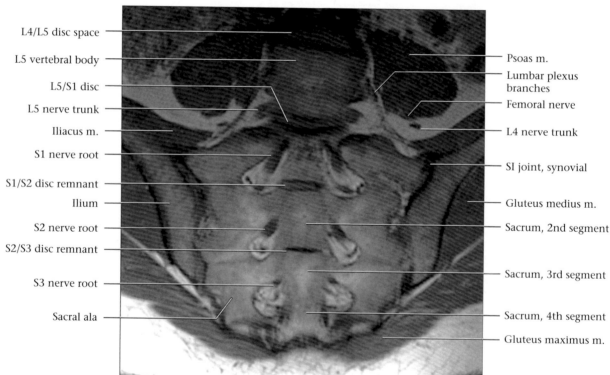

L4/L5 disc space

L5 vertebral body

L5/S1 disc

L5 nerve trunk

Iliacus m.

S1 nerve root

S1/S2 disc remnant

Ilium

S2 nerve root

S2/S3 disc remnant

S3 nerve root

Sacral ala

Psoas m.

Lumbar plexus
branches

Femoral nerve

L4 nerve trunk

SI joint, synovial

Gluteus medius m.

Sacrum, 2nd segment

Sacrum, 3rd segment

Sacrum, 4th segment

Gluteus maximus m.

(Top) The sacroiliac joint is transitioning from syndesmotic posteriorly to synovial more anteriorly. The sacral nerve roots are seen entering the neural foramina. **(Bottom)** A comparison of the intervertebral discs reveals a healthy thick L4/L5 disc and the normal slightly narrower L5/S1 disc. Remnants of the S1/S2 and S2/S3 intervertebral discs are visible within the sacrum. The anterior synovial portion of the sacroiliac joint is seen. This portion of the joint is thinner and articular cartilage is present within. This image through the long axis of the mid sacral body displays the full extent of the sacral ala.

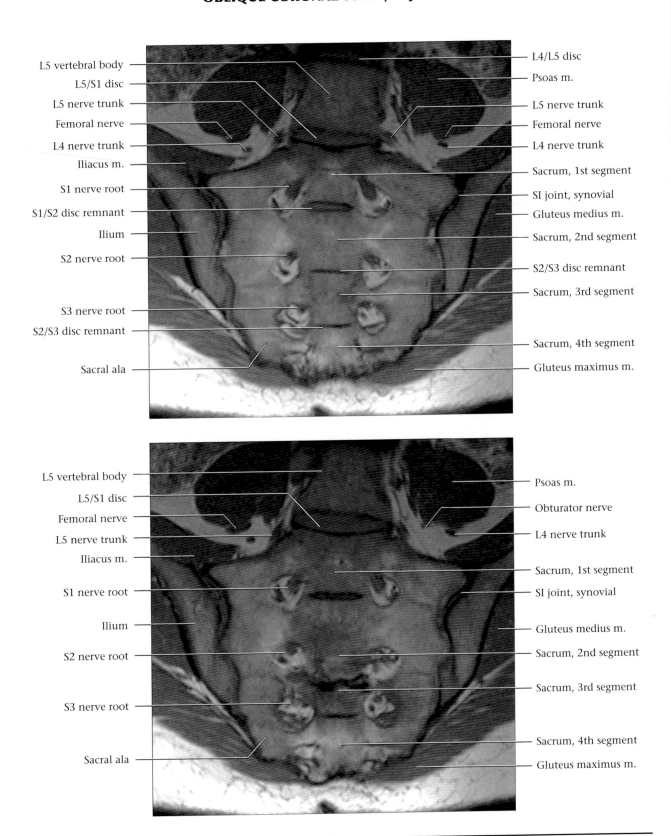

Top image labels (left):
- L5 vertebral body
- L5/S1 disc
- L5 nerve trunk
- Femoral nerve
- L4 nerve trunk
- Iliacus m.
- S1 nerve root
- S1/S2 disc remnant
- Ilium
- S2 nerve root
- S3 nerve root
- S2/S3 disc remnant
- Sacral ala

Top image labels (right):
- L4/L5 disc
- Psoas m.
- L5 nerve trunk
- Femoral nerve
- L4 nerve trunk
- Sacrum, 1st segment
- SI joint, synovial
- Gluteus medius m.
- Sacrum, 2nd segment
- S2/S3 disc remnant
- Sacrum, 3rd segment
- Sacrum, 4th segment
- Gluteus maximus m.

Bottom image labels (left):
- L5 vertebral body
- L5/S1 disc
- Femoral nerve
- L5 nerve trunk
- Iliacus m.
- S1 nerve root
- Ilium
- S2 nerve root
- S3 nerve root
- Sacral ala

Bottom image labels (right):
- Psoas m.
- Obturator nerve
- L4 nerve trunk
- Sacrum, 1st segment
- SI joint, synovial
- Gluteus medius m.
- Sacrum, 2nd segment
- Sacrum, 3rd segment
- Sacrum, 4th segment
- Gluteus maximus m.

(Top) The sacral ala continue to be well seen, as are the sacroiliac joints. The irregular interlocking articular surfaces of the sacroiliac joints are easy to appreciate. This irregularity significantly limits mobility and improves stability of the sacroiliac joint. **(Bottom)** The sacral nerve roots course forward within the neural foramina.

OBLIQUE CORONAL T1 MR, SI JOINTS & GREATER SCIATIC NOTCH

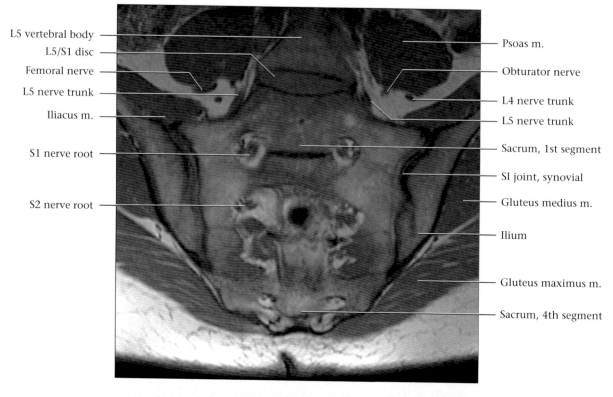

L5 vertebral body — Psoas m.
L5/S1 disc — Obturator nerve
Femoral nerve — L4 nerve trunk
L5 nerve trunk — L5 nerve trunk
Iliacus m. — Sacrum, 1st segment
S1 nerve root — SI joint, synovial
— Gluteus medius m.
S2 nerve root — Ilium
— Gluteus maximus m.
— Sacrum, 4th segment

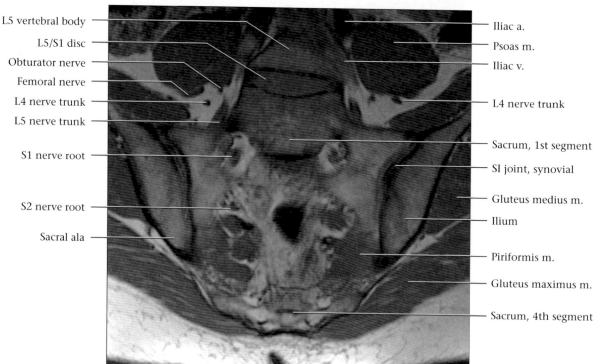

L5 vertebral body — Iliac a.
L5/S1 disc — Psoas m.
Obturator nerve — Iliac v.
Femoral nerve — L4 nerve trunk
L4 nerve trunk — L5 nerve trunk
— Sacrum, 1st segment
S1 nerve root — SI joint, synovial
— Gluteus medius m.
S2 nerve root — Ilium
Sacral ala — Piriformis m.
— Gluteus maximus m.
— Sacrum, 4th segment

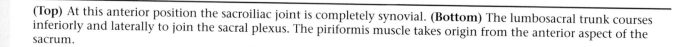

(Top) At this anterior position the sacroiliac joint is completely synovial. (Bottom) The lumbosacral trunk courses inferiorly and laterally to join the sacral plexus. The piriformis muscle takes origin from the anterior aspect of the sacrum.

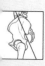

OBLIQUE CORONAL T1 MR, SI JOINTS & GREATER SCIATIC NOTCH

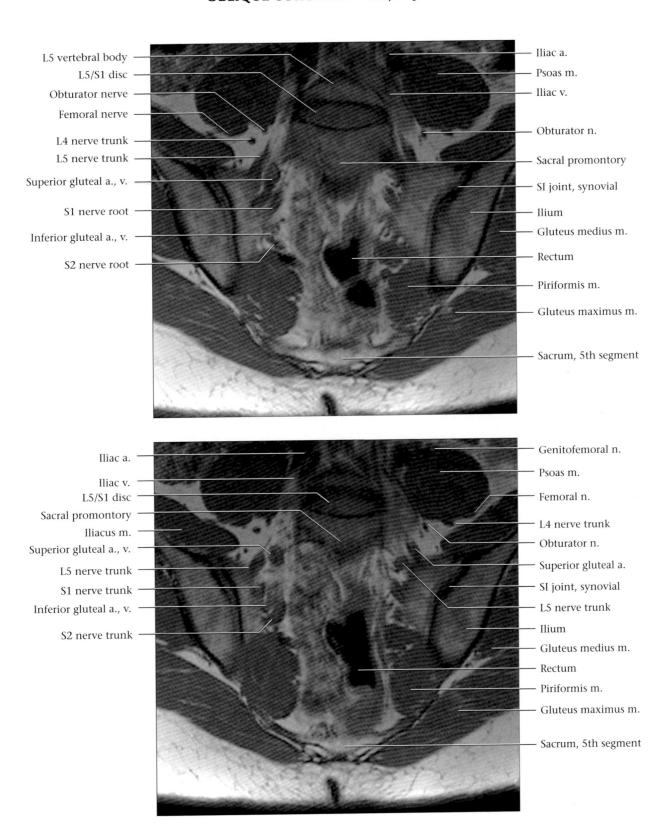

Top image labels (left): L5 vertebral body, L5/S1 disc, Obturator nerve, Femoral nerve, L4 nerve trunk, L5 nerve trunk, Superior gluteal a., v., S1 nerve root, Inferior gluteal a., v., S2 nerve root

Top image labels (right): Iliac a., Psoas m., Iliac v., Obturator n., Sacral promontory, SI joint, synovial, Ilium, Gluteus medius m., Rectum, Piriformis m., Gluteus maximus m., Sacrum, 5th segment

Bottom image labels (left): Iliac a., Iliac v., L5/S1 disc, Sacral promontory, Iliacus m., Superior gluteal a., v., L5 nerve trunk, S1 nerve trunk, Inferior gluteal a., v., S2 nerve trunk

Bottom image labels (right): Genitofemoral n., Psoas m., Femoral n., L4 nerve trunk, Obturator n., Superior gluteal a., SI joint, synovial, L5 nerve trunk, Ilium, Gluteus medius m., Rectum, Piriformis m., Gluteus maximus m., Sacrum, 5th segment

(Top) Along the anterior aspect of the sacrum the piriformis muscle is identified and its fibers are oriented laterally and inferiorly. The superior gluteal artery is seen passing between the lumbosacral trunk (or L5) and S1 nerve trunk as the artery courses posteriorly. The genitofemoral nerve is now apparent along the anterior aspect of the psoas muscle. **(Bottom)** The anterior division of the internal iliac artery has divided and the inferior gluteal vessels are now distinguishable. The vessels are located between the S1 and S2 nerve roots. The sacral promontory, the anterosuperior projection of S1, is well seen.

OBLIQUE CORONAL T1 MR, SI JOINTS & GREATER SCIATIC NOTCH

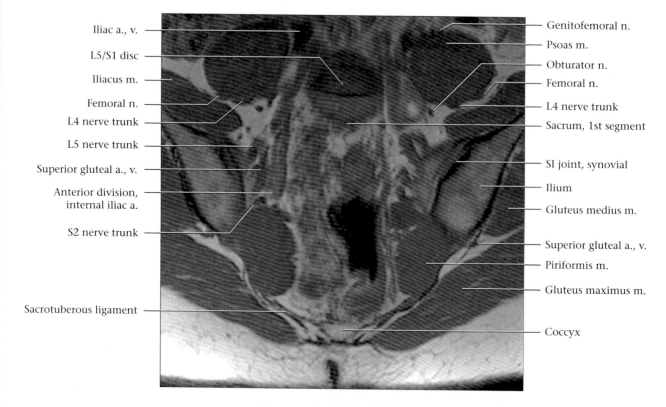

Iliac a., v. — L5/S1 disc — Iliacus m. — Femoral n. — L4 nerve trunk — L5 nerve trunk — Superior gluteal a., v. — Anterior division, internal iliac a. — S2 nerve trunk — Sacrotuberous ligament

Genitofemoral n. — Psoas m. — Obturator n. — Femoral n. — L4 nerve trunk — Sacrum, 1st segment — SI joint, synovial — Ilium — Gluteus medius m. — Superior gluteal a., v. — Piriformis m. — Gluteus maximus m. — Coccyx

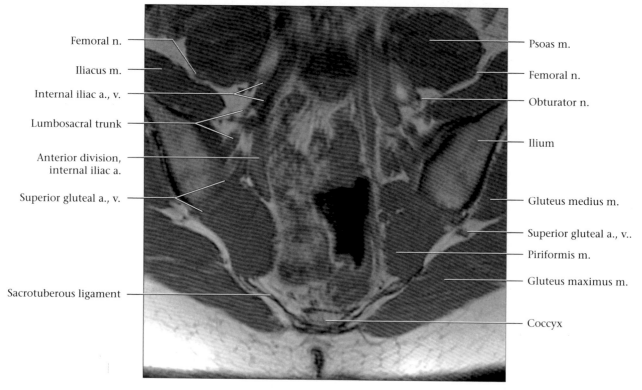

Femoral n. — Iliacus m. — Internal iliac a., v. — Lumbosacral trunk — Anterior division, internal iliac a. — Superior gluteal a., v. — Sacrotuberous ligament

Psoas m. — Femoral n. — Obturator n. — Ilium — Gluteus medius m. — Superior gluteal a., v.. — Piriformis m. — Gluteus maximus m. — Coccyx

(Top) The sacrotuberous ligament converts the greater sciatic notch into a foramen which is primarily filled with the piriformis muscle. The ligament is located inferiorly to the muscle. The internal iliac vessels have divided and the superior gluteal artery is the continuation of the posterior division. **(Bottom)** The superior gluteal vessels exit the pelvis above the superior border of the piriformis muscle on the right. The vessels are partial volumed with the adjacent piriformis muscle. On the left the vessels are seen deep to the gluteus maximus muscle after exiting the pelvis. Note that asymmetry can occur; the lumbosacral nerve trunk has formed on the right side, but L4 and L5 nerve trunks are still separate structures on the left.

POSTERIOR PELVIS

OBLIQUE CORONAL T1 MR, SI JOINTS & GREATER SCIATIC NOTCH

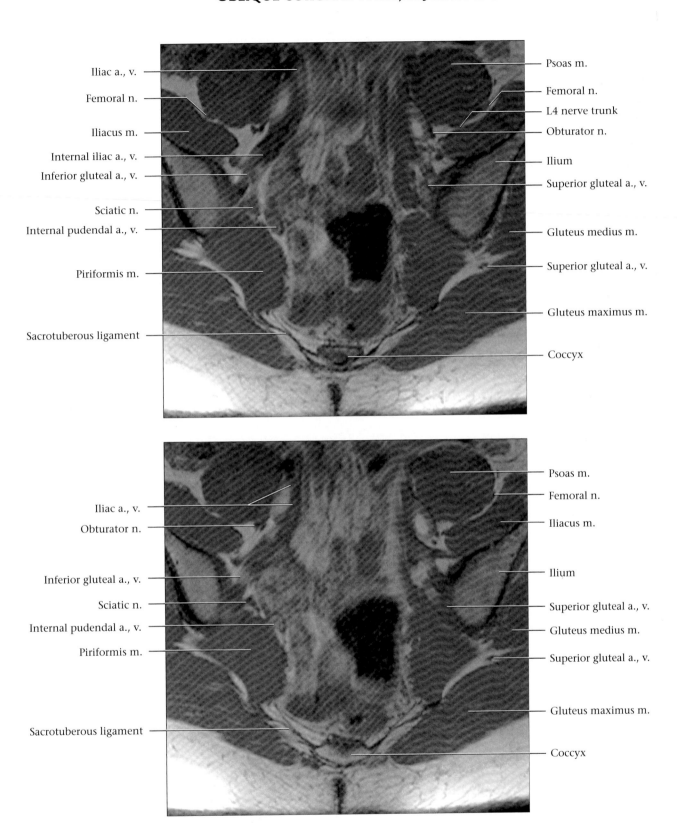

Labels (Top image):
- Iliac a., v.
- Femoral n.
- Iliacus m.
- Internal iliac a., v.
- Inferior gluteal a., v.
- Sciatic n.
- Internal pudendal a., v.
- Piriformis m.
- Sacrotuberous ligament
- Psoas m.
- Femoral n.
- L4 nerve trunk
- Obturator n.
- Ilium
- Superior gluteal a., v.
- Gluteus medius m.
- Superior gluteal a., v.
- Gluteus maximus m.
- Coccyx

Labels (Bottom image):
- Iliac a., v.
- Obturator n.
- Inferior gluteal a., v.
- Sciatic n.
- Internal pudendal a., v.
- Piriformis m.
- Sacrotuberous ligament
- Psoas m.
- Femoral n.
- Iliacus m.
- Ilium
- Superior gluteal a., v.
- Gluteus medius m.
- Superior gluteal a., v.
- Gluteus maximus m.
- Coccyx

(Top) The internal pudendal and inferior gluteal vessels are visible; they are the terminal branches of the anterior division of the internal iliac artery. The sciatic nerve, the largest branch of the sacral plexus is visible as a discrete structure. The obturator nerve is seen along the lateral aspect of the internal iliac vessels. It reaches this location by passing posterior to the common iliac vessels, a relationship not well depicted on these images. **(Bottom)** The superior gluteal vessels on the left are exiting the pelvis. The piriformis muscle fills the greater sciatic foramen which is bounded by the ilium superiorly and the sacrotuberous ligament inferiorly.

OBLIQUE CORONAL T1 MR, SI JOINTS & GREATER SCIATIC NOTCH

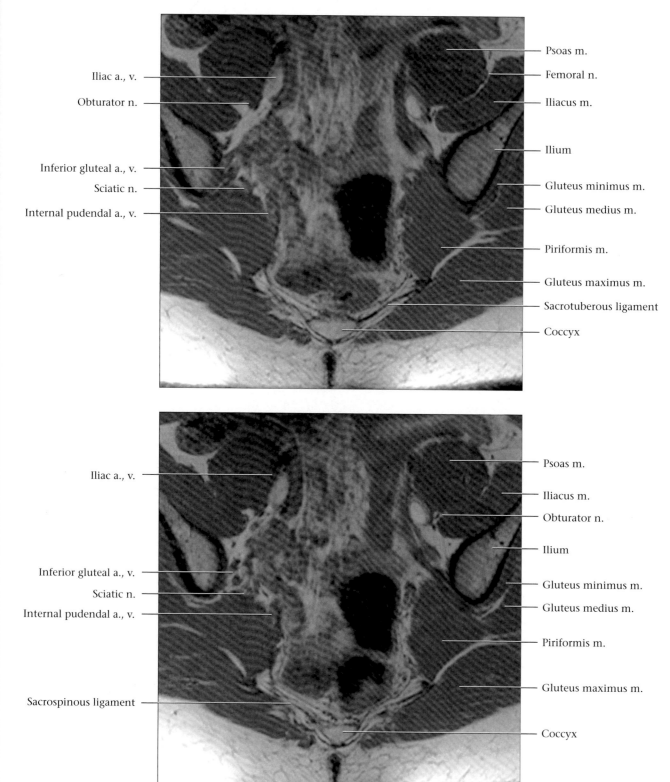

Iliac a., v.
Obturator n.

Inferior gluteal a., v.
Sciatic n.
Internal pudendal a., v.

Psoas m.
Femoral n.
Iliacus m.

Ilium

Gluteus minimus m.
Gluteus medius m.

Piriformis m.

Gluteus maximus m.
Sacrotuberous ligament
Coccyx

Iliac a., v.

Inferior gluteal a., v.
Sciatic n.
Internal pudendal a., v.

Sacrospinous ligament

Psoas m.

Iliacus m.
Obturator n.

Ilium

Gluteus minimus m.
Gluteus medius m.

Piriformis m.

Gluteus maximus m.

Coccyx

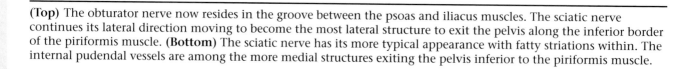

(Top) The obturator nerve now resides in the groove between the psoas and iliacus muscles. The sciatic nerve continues its lateral direction moving to become the most lateral structure to exit the pelvis along the inferior border of the piriformis muscle. (Bottom) The sciatic nerve has its more typical appearance with fatty striations within. The internal pudendal vessels are among the more medial structures exiting the pelvis inferior to the piriformis muscle.

POSTERIOR PELVIS

OBLIQUE CORONAL T1 MR, SI JOINTS & GREATER SCIATIC NOTCH

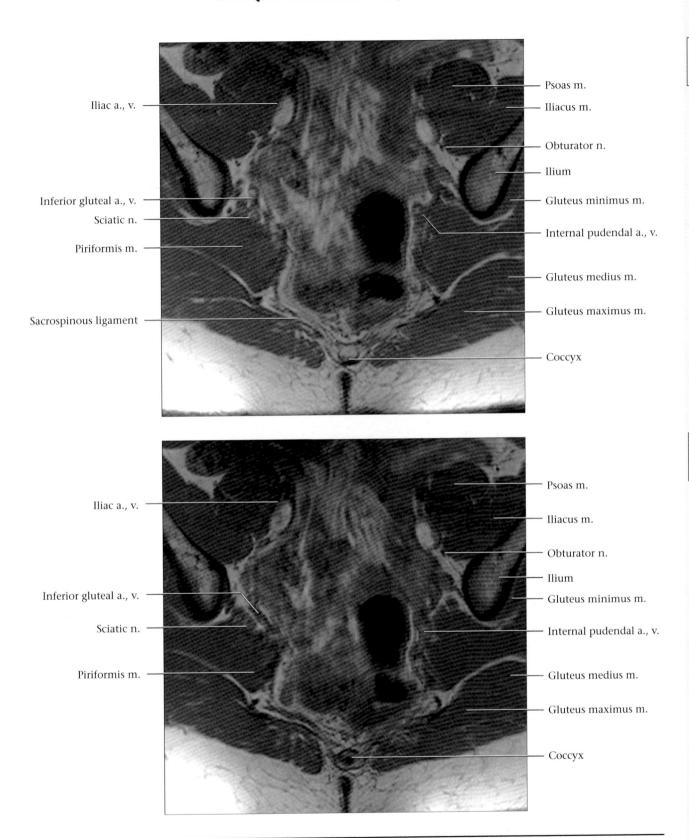

Iliac a., v. — Psoas m. — Iliacus m. — Obturator n. — Ilium — Gluteus minimus m. — Inferior gluteal a., v. — Sciatic n. — Internal pudendal a., v. — Piriformis m. — Gluteus medius m. — Gluteus maximus m. — Sacrospinous ligament — Coccyx

Iliac a., v. — Psoas m. — Iliacus m. — Obturator n. — Ilium — Inferior gluteal a., v. — Gluteus minimus m. — Sciatic n. — Internal pudendal a., v. — Piriformis m. — Gluteus medius m. — Gluteus maximus m. — Coccyx

(Top) The course of the piriformis muscle through the greater sciatic foramen is visible. This imaging plane erroneously creates the impression that the piriformis muscle is located between the gluteus minimus and medius muscles. See "Axial T1 MR, Sciatic Nerve" to understand its relationship to these muscles. Note the inferior gluteal vessels coursing from lateral to medial, posterior to the sciatic nerve. **(Bottom)** The sciatic nerve is more clearly seen on this image.

OBLIQUE CORONAL T1 MR, SI JOINTS & GREATER SCIATIC NOTCH

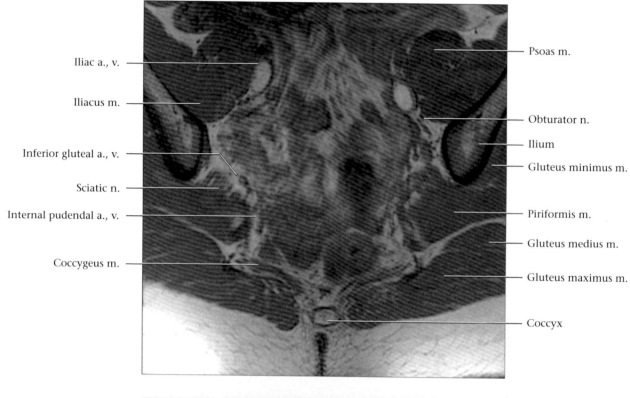

Iliac a., v. — Psoas m.

Iliacus m. — Obturator n.

Inferior gluteal a., v. — Ilium

Sciatic n. — Gluteus minimus m.

Internal pudendal a., v. — Piriformis m.

— Gluteus medius m.

Coccygeus m. — Gluteus maximus m.

— Coccyx

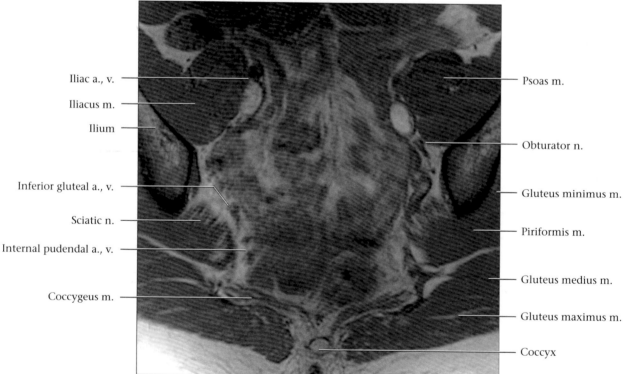

Iliac a., v. — Psoas m.

Iliacus m.

Ilium

Inferior gluteal a., v. — Obturator n.

Sciatic n. — Gluteus minimus m.

Internal pudendal a., v. — Piriformis m.

— Gluteus medius m.

Coccygeus m. — Gluteus maximus m.

— Coccyx

(Top) The inferior gluteal vessels are seen coursing to a more medial position. They exit the pelvis along the inferior border of the piriformis muscle in close proximity to the internal pudendal vessels. The pudendal nerve, which is the most medial structure along the inferior piriformis border, is not discernible. **(Bottom)** At this anterior position the inferior-most portion of the piriformis muscle is present. The sciatic nerve is the most lateral structure to exit the pelvis along the inferior border of the piriformis muscle.

POSTERIOR PELVIS

OBLIQUE CORONAL T1 MR, SI JOINTS & GREATER SCIATIC NOTCH

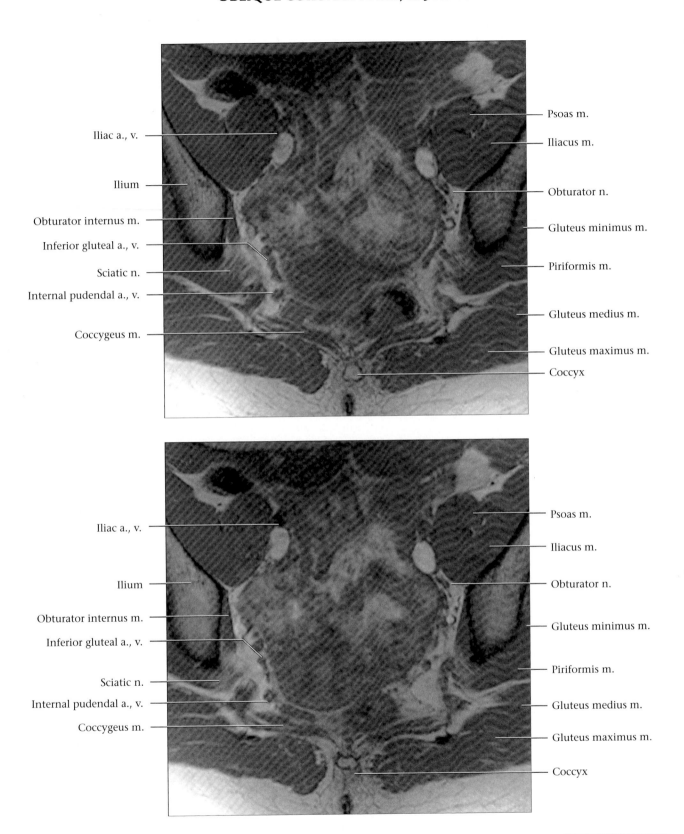

Top image labels:

Iliac a., v. · Ilium · Obturator internus m. · Inferior gluteal a., v. · Sciatic n. · Internal pudendal a., v. · Coccygeus m.

Psoas m. · Iliacus m. · Obturator n. · Gluteus minimus m. · Piriformis m. · Gluteus medius m. · Gluteus maximus m. · Coccyx

Bottom image labels:

Iliac a., v. · Ilium · Obturator internus m. · Inferior gluteal a., v. · Sciatic n. · Internal pudendal a., v. · Coccygeus m.

Psoas m. · Iliacus m. · Obturator n. · Gluteus minimus m. · Piriformis m. · Gluteus medius m. · Gluteus maximus m. · Coccyx

(Top) The sciatic nerve has exited the pelvis. Its longitudinal orientation is visible by the direction of the fatty striations within. The nerve is quite wide but relatively flat (see "Axial T1 MR, Sciatic Nerve"). The obturator nerve is seen coursing inferiorly to its eventual position along the inner border of the obturator internus muscle. **(Bottom)** The piriformis muscle is now a lateral structure, having passed through the notch. It is now traveling laterally to its insertion into the piriformis fossa of the hip. The sciatic nerve will continue its course, running inferiorly through the posterior thigh (see "Thigh Overview" section).

Hip and Pelvis

V

153

SAGITTAL T1 MR, GREATER SCIATIC NOTCH

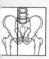

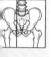

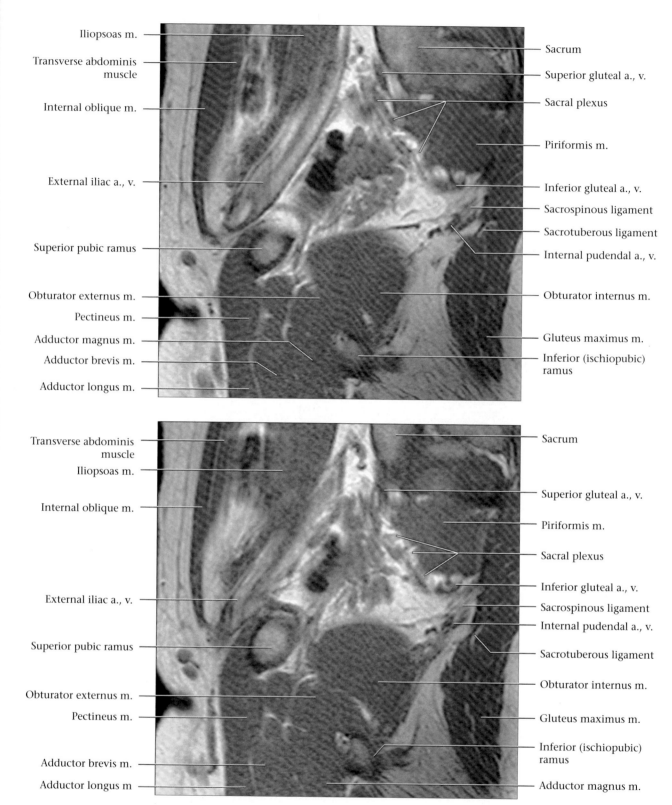

Iliopsoas m.

Transverse abdominis muscle

Internal oblique m.

External iliac a., v.

Superior pubic ramus

Obturator externus m.

Pectineus m.

Adductor magnus m.

Adductor brevis m.

Adductor longus m.

Sacrum

Superior gluteal a., v.

Sacral plexus

Piriformis m.

Inferior gluteal a., v.

Sacrospinous ligament

Sacrotuberous ligament

Internal pudendal a., v.

Obturator internus m.

Gluteus maximus m.

Inferior (ischiopubic) ramus

Transverse abdominis muscle

Iliopsoas m.

Internal oblique m.

External iliac a., v.

Superior pubic ramus

Obturator externus m.

Pectineus m.

Adductor brevis m.

Adductor longus m

Sacrum

Superior gluteal a., v.

Piriformis m.

Sacral plexus

Inferior gluteal a., v.

Sacrospinous ligament

Internal pudendal a., v.

Sacrotuberous ligament

Obturator internus m.

Gluteus maximus m.

Inferior (ischiopubic) ramus

Adductor magnus m.

(Top) This series of sagittal images from medial to lateral begins just lateral to midline. The sacral nerve roots are seen converging to form the sacral plexus on the deep surface of the piriformis muscle. The inferior gluteal and internal pudendal vessels are visible. **(Bottom)** The sacrospinous ligament is nicely seen. On this image the internal pudendal vessels are seen coursing around the ligament to travel from the buttocks to the perineum. The fibers of the sacrotuberous ligament are vertically oriented. They are seen as a thick band along the deep surface of the gluteus maximus muscle and they serve as a site of origin for that muscle.

SAGITTAL T1 MR, GREATER SCIATIC NOTCH

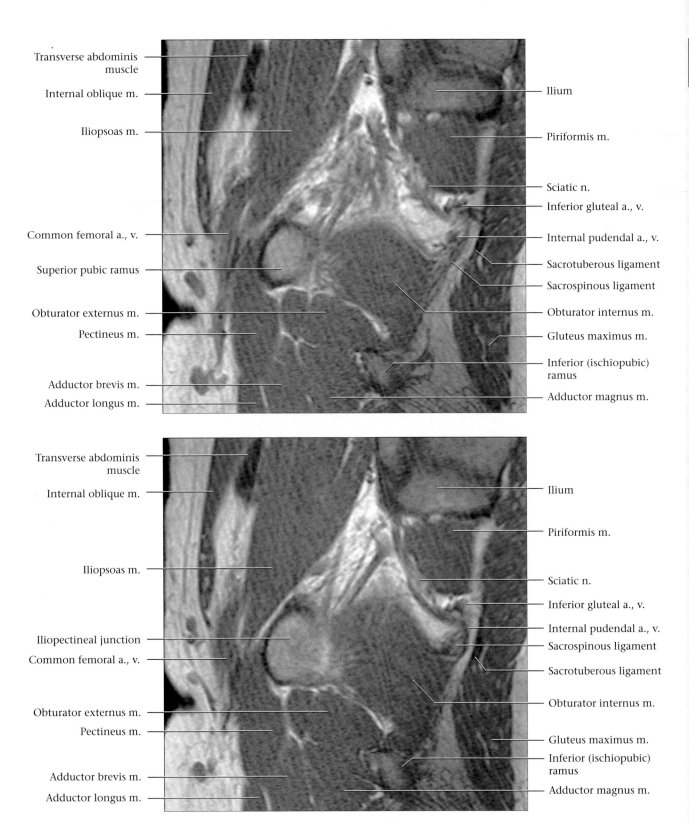

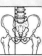

Top image labels:

Left side:
- Transverse abdominis muscle
- Internal oblique m.
- Iliopsoas m.
- Common femoral a., v.
- Superior pubic ramus
- Obturator externus m.
- Pectineus m.
- Adductor brevis m.
- Adductor longus m.

Right side:
- Ilium
- Piriformis m.
- Sciatic n.
- Inferior gluteal a., v.
- Internal pudendal a., v.
- Sacrotuberous ligament
- Sacrospinous ligament
- Obturator internus m.
- Gluteus maximus m.
- Inferior (ischiopubic) ramus
- Adductor magnus m.

Bottom image labels:

Left side:
- Transverse abdominis muscle
- Internal oblique m.
- Iliopsoas m.
- Iliopectineal junction
- Common femoral a., v.
- Obturator externus m.
- Pectineus m.
- Adductor brevis m.
- Adductor longus m.

Right side:
- Ilium
- Piriformis m.
- Sciatic n.
- Inferior gluteal a., v.
- Internal pudendal a., v.
- Sacrospinous ligament
- Sacrotuberous ligament
- Obturator internus m.
- Gluteus maximus m.
- Inferior (ischiopubic) ramus
- Adductor magnus m.

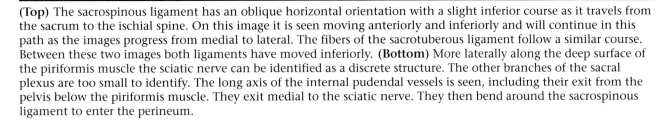

(Top) The sacrospinous ligament has an oblique horizontal orientation with a slight inferior course as it travels from the sacrum to the ischial spine. On this image it is seen moving anteriorly and inferiorly and will continue in this path as the images progress from medial to lateral. The fibers of the sacrotuberous ligament follow a similar course. Between these two images both ligaments have moved inferiorly. **(Bottom)** More laterally along the deep surface of the piriformis muscle the sciatic nerve can be identified as a discrete structure. The other branches of the sacral plexus are too small to identify. The long axis of the internal pudendal vessels is seen, including their exit from the pelvis below the piriformis muscle. They exit medial to the sciatic nerve. They then bend around the sacrospinous ligament to enter the perineum.

Hip and Pelvis

V

SAGITTAL T1 MR, GREATER SCIATIC NOTCH

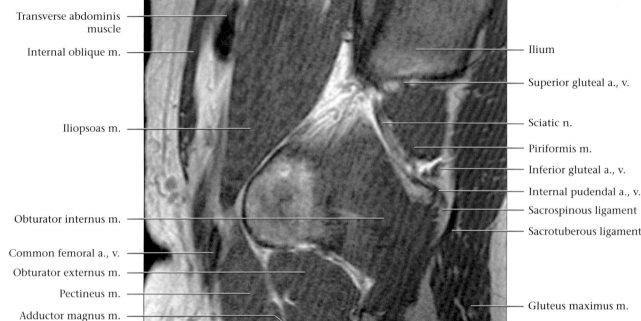

Transverse abdominis muscle

Internal oblique m.

Iliopsoas m.

Obturator internus m.

Common femoral a., v.

Obturator externus m.

Pectineus m.

Adductor magnus m.

Adductor brevis m.

Adductor longus m.

Ilium

Superior gluteal a., v.

Sciatic n.

Piriformis m.

Inferior gluteal a., v.

Internal pudendal a., v.

Sacrospinous ligament

Sacrotuberous ligament

Gluteus maximus m.

Inferior (ischiopubic) ramus

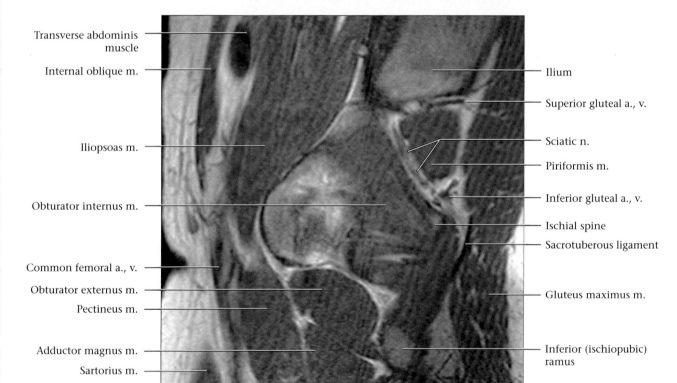

Transverse abdominis muscle

Internal oblique m.

Iliopsoas m.

Obturator internus m.

Common femoral a., v.

Obturator externus m.

Pectineus m.

Adductor magnus m.

Sartorius m.

Ilium

Superior gluteal a., v.

Sciatic n.

Piriformis m.

Inferior gluteal a., v.

Ischial spine

Sacrotuberous ligament

Gluteus maximus m.

Inferior (ischiopubic) ramus

(Top) The exit of the inferior gluteal vessels from the pelvis is seen by following the vessels from medial to lateral. Here they are just below the piriformis muscle and are in close proximity to the internal pudendal vessels. The distal attachment of the sacrospinous ligament onto the ischial spine is seen between this image as well as the next one. **(Bottom)** On this more lateral image the sacrotuberous ligament is seen only over a short segment and is more inferiorly positioned than on the more medial images. The sciatic nerve is beginning its exit from the pelvis. The superior gluteal vessels are well seen as they course along the superior border of the piriformis muscle to enter the buttocks.

SAGITTAL T1 MR, GREATER SCIATIC NOTCH

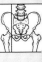

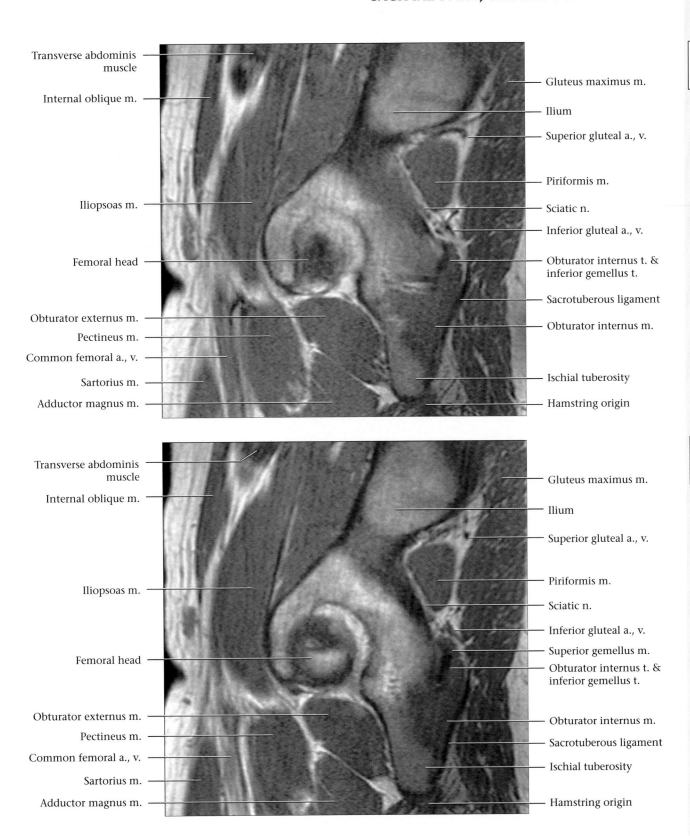

Top image labels (left): Transverse abdominis muscle, Internal oblique m., Iliopsoas m., Femoral head, Obturator externus m., Pectineus m., Common femoral a., v., Sartorius m., Adductor magnus m.

Top image labels (right): Gluteus maximus m., Ilium, Superior gluteal a., v., Piriformis m., Sciatic n., Inferior gluteal a., v., Obturator internus t. & inferior gemellus t., Sacrotuberous ligament, Obturator internus m., Ischial tuberosity, Hamstring origin

Bottom image labels (left): Transverse abdominis muscle, Internal oblique m., Iliopsoas m., Femoral head, Obturator externus m., Pectineus m., Common femoral a., v., Sartorius m., Adductor magnus m.

Bottom image labels (right): Gluteus maximus m., Ilium, Superior gluteal a., v., Piriformis m., Sciatic n., Inferior gluteal a., v., Superior gemellus m., Obturator internus t. & inferior gemellus t., Obturator internus m., Sacrotuberous ligament, Ischial tuberosity, Hamstring origin

(Top) Along the lateral aspect of the piriformis muscle the superior and inferior gluteal vessels are seen above and below the piriformis muscle respectively. The vessels are deep to the gluteal maximus muscle and will branch within this fat plane. **(Bottom)** The attachment of the sacrotuberous ligament onto the ischial tuberosity is seen. From medial to lateral the ligament has followed an inferior course. The external rotators of the hip are just now visible.

Hip and Pelvis

V

SAGITTAL T1 MR, GREATER SCIATIC NOTCH

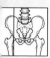

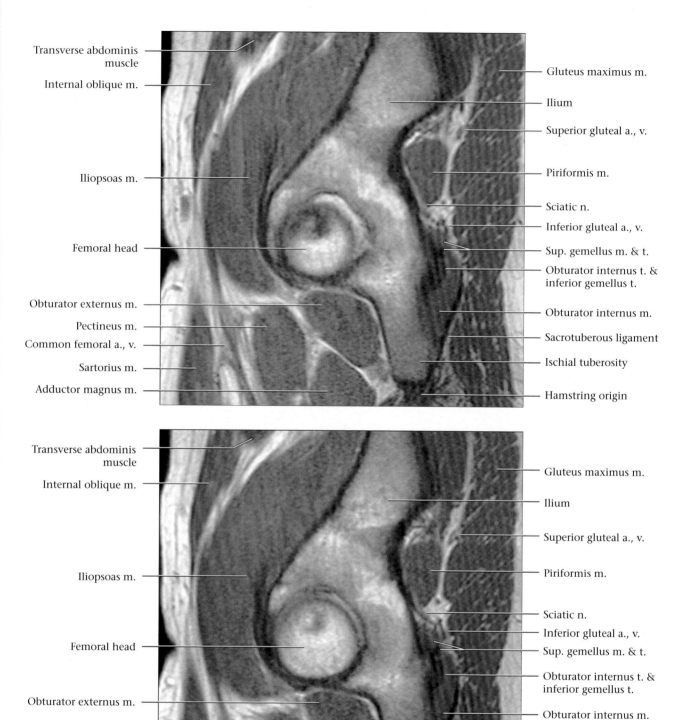

Transverse abdominis muscle — Gluteus maximus m.

Internal oblique m. — Ilium

— Superior gluteal a., v.

Iliopsoas m. — Piriformis m.

— Sciatic n.

— Inferior gluteal a., v.

Femoral head — Sup. gemellus m. & t.

— Obturator internus t. & inferior gemellus t.

Obturator externus m. — Obturator internus m.

Pectineus m. — Sacrotuberous ligament

Common femoral a., v. — Ischial tuberosity

Sartorius m. — Hamstring origin

Adductor magnus m.

Transverse abdominis muscle

Internal oblique m. — Gluteus maximus m.

— Ilium

— Superior gluteal a., v.

Iliopsoas m. — Piriformis m.

— Sciatic n.

— Inferior gluteal a., v.

Femoral head — Sup. gemellus m. & t.

— Obturator internus t. & inferior gemellus t.

Obturator externus m. — Obturator internus m.

Pectineus m. — Sacrotuberous ligament

Common femoral a., v. — Ischial tuberosity

Sartorius m. — Hamstring origin

Adductor magnus m.

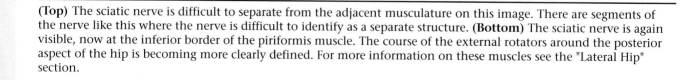

(Top) The sciatic nerve is difficult to separate from the adjacent musculature on this image. There are segments of the nerve like this where the nerve is difficult to identify as a separate structure. **(Bottom)** The sciatic nerve is again visible, now at the inferior border of the piriformis muscle. The course of the external rotators around the posterior aspect of the hip is becoming more clearly defined. For more information on these muscles see the "Lateral Hip" section.

Hip and Pelvis

V

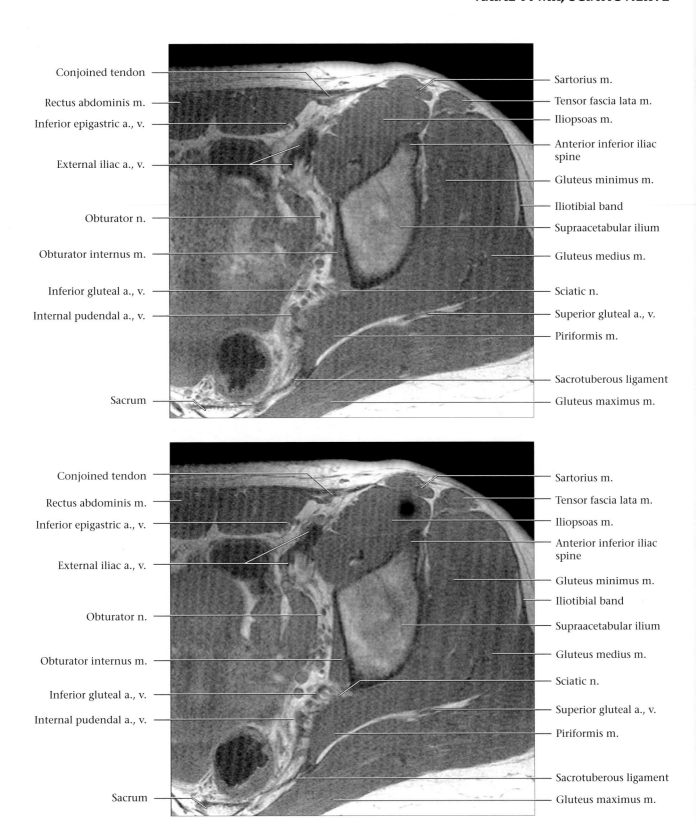

Top image labels (left):
- Conjoined tendon
- Rectus abdominis m.
- Inferior epigastric a., v.
- External iliac a., v.
- Obturator n.
- Obturator internus m.
- Inferior gluteal a., v.
- Internal pudendal a., v.
- Sacrum

Top image labels (right):
- Sartorius m.
- Tensor fascia lata m.
- Iliopsoas m.
- Anterior inferior iliac spine
- Gluteus minimus m.
- Iliotibial band
- Supraacetabular ilium
- Gluteus medius m.
- Sciatic n.
- Superior gluteal a., v.
- Piriformis m.
- Sacrotuberous ligament
- Gluteus maximus m.

Bottom image labels (left):
- Conjoined tendon
- Rectus abdominis m.
- Inferior epigastric a., v.
- External iliac a., v.
- Obturator n.
- Obturator internus m.
- Inferior gluteal a., v.
- Internal pudendal a., v.
- Sacrum

Bottom image labels (right):
- Sartorius m.
- Tensor fascia lata m.
- Iliopsoas m.
- Anterior inferior iliac spine
- Gluteus minimus m.
- Iliotibial band
- Supraacetabular ilium
- Gluteus medius m.
- Sciatic n.
- Superior gluteal a., v.
- Piriformis m.
- Sacrotuberous ligament
- Gluteus maximus m.

(Top) Axial MR series following the sciatic nerve. The midportion of the greater sciatic notch is at the level of the superior aspect of the hip joint. The superior gluteal vessels have already exited above the piriformis muscle (see "Oblique Axial T1 MR, Sacroiliac Joints"). The vessels are identified in the plane between the gluteus maximus and medius muscles. The sciatic nerve is assuming its position along the lateral aspect of the notch. The inferior gluteal vessels are just medial to the nerve and the internal pudendal vessels are the most medial of the visible structures. **(Bottom)** Like the piriformis muscle the sacrotuberous ligament has a lateral and inferior course. At this more superior position its lateral fibers are visible. It follows along the inferior aspect of the piriformis muscle, converting the greater sciatic notch into a foramen.

Hip and Pelvis

V

AXIAL T1 MR, SCIATIC NERVE

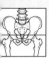

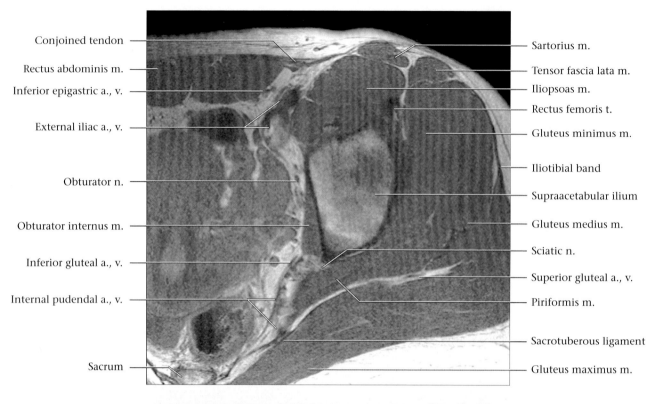

Conjoined tendon

Rectus abdominis m.

Inferior epigastric a., v.

External iliac a., v.

Obturator n.

Obturator internus m.

Inferior gluteal a., v.

Internal pudendal a., v.

Sacrum

Sartorius m.

Tensor fascia lata m.

Iliopsoas m.

Rectus femoris t.

Gluteus minimus m.

Iliotibial band

Supraacetabular ilium

Gluteus medius m.

Sciatic n.

Superior gluteal a., v.

Piriformis m.

Sacrotuberous ligament

Gluteus maximus m.

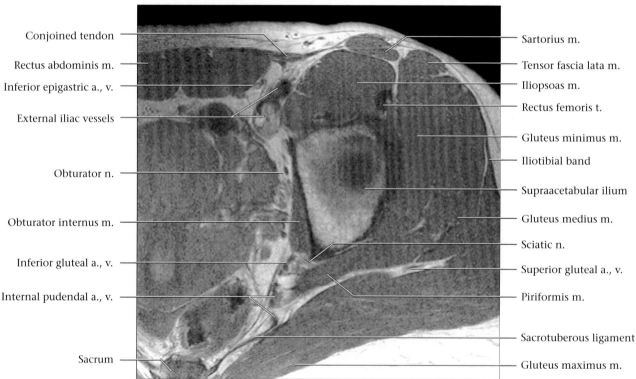

Conjoined tendon

Rectus abdominis m.

Inferior epigastric a., v.

External iliac vessels

Obturator n.

Obturator internus m.

Inferior gluteal a., v.

Internal pudendal a., v.

Sacrum

Sartorius m.

Tensor fascia lata m.

Iliopsoas m.

Rectus femoris t.

Gluteus minimus m.

Iliotibial band

Supraacetabular ilium

Gluteus medius m.

Sciatic n.

Superior gluteal a., v.

Piriformis m.

Sacrotuberous ligament

Gluteus maximus m.

(Top) The medial margin of the piriformis muscle moves lateral as the muscle extends inferiorly and there is a larger gap between the muscle and the sacrum than on the more superior images. The internal pudendal vessels are seen both within the pelvis and in the buttocks. As it exits the pelvis the sciatic nerve is identified by the fatty striations within. **(Bottom)** The sacral attachment of the sacrotuberous ligament is well visualized. More laterally it serves as a site of origin for the gluteus maximus muscle.

POSTERIOR PELVIS

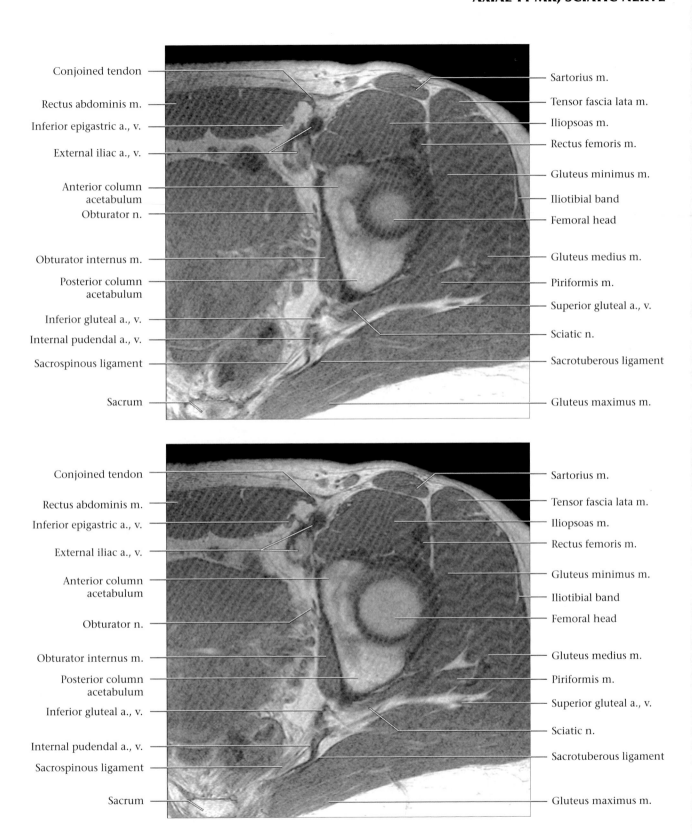

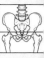

Top image labels (left): Conjoined tendon, Rectus abdominis m., Inferior epigastric a., v., External iliac a., v., Anterior column acetabulum, Obturator n., Obturator internus m., Posterior column acetabulum, Inferior gluteal a., v., Internal pudendal a., v., Sacrospinous ligament, Sacrum

Top image labels (right): Sartorius m., Tensor fascia lata m., Iliopsoas m., Rectus femoris m., Gluteus minimus m., Iliotibial band, Femoral head, Gluteus medius m., Piriformis m., Superior gluteal a., v., Sciatic n., Sacrotuberous ligament, Gluteus maximus m.

Bottom image labels (left): Conjoined tendon, Rectus abdominis m., Inferior epigastric a., v., External iliac a., v., Anterior column acetabulum, Obturator n., Obturator internus m., Posterior column acetabulum, Inferior gluteal a., v., Internal pudendal a., v., Sacrospinous ligament, Sacrum

Bottom image labels (right): Sartorius m., Tensor fascia lata m., Iliopsoas m., Rectus femoris m., Gluteus minimus m., Iliotibial band, Femoral head, Gluteus medius m., Piriformis m., Superior gluteal a., v., Sciatic n., Sacrotuberous ligament, Gluteus maximus m.

(Top) As it exits the pelvis the sciatic nerve is closely applied to the posterior column of the acetabulum. This osseous landmark can be used on other examinations such as CT where the soft tissue discrimination is not as great as MR. **(Bottom)** During its exit from the pelvis the sciatic nerve can be difficult to identify. Knowledge of its expected location can aid the search. Little variability in its position exits. At its most inferior extent the piriformis muscle is identified as a far lateral structure approaching its insertion into the piriformis fossa. The sacrospinous ligament is now visible. It is relatively horizontal in its orientation. It lies deep to the sacrotuberous ligament; the internal pudendal vessels upon leaving the pelvis immediately pass around this structure to enter the perineum.

Hip and Pelvis

V

AXIAL T1 MR, SCIATIC NERVE

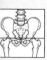

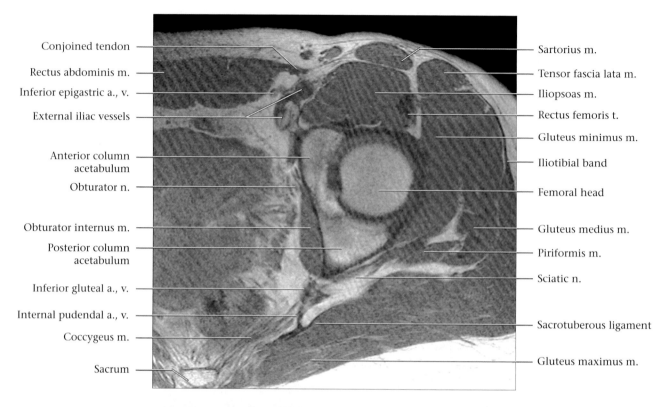

Conjoined tendon — — Sartorius m.
Rectus abdominis m. — — Tensor fascia lata m.
Inferior epigastric a., v. — — Iliopsoas m.
External iliac vessels — — Rectus femoris t.
Anterior column acetabulum — — Gluteus minimus m.
Obturator n. — — Iliotibial band
— Femoral head
Obturator internus m. — — Gluteus medius m.
Posterior column acetabulum — — Piriformis m.
Inferior gluteal a., v. — — Sciatic n.
Internal pudendal a., v. —
Coccygeus m. — — Sacrotuberous ligament
Sacrum — — Gluteus maximus m.

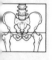

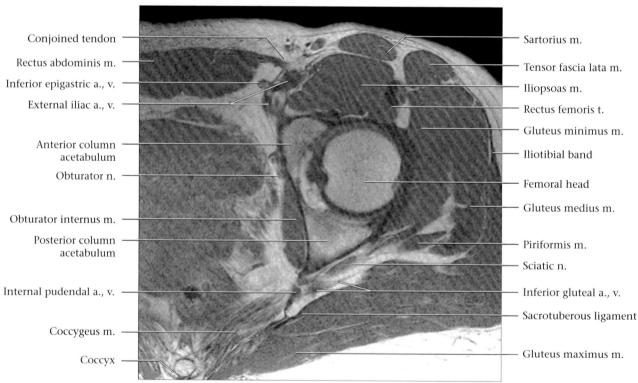

Conjoined tendon — — Sartorius m.
Rectus abdominis m. — — Tensor fascia lata m.
Inferior epigastric a., v. — — Iliopsoas m.
External iliac a., v. — — Rectus femoris t.
— Gluteus minimus m.
Anterior column acetabulum — — Iliotibial band
Obturator n. — — Femoral head
— Gluteus medius m.
Obturator internus m. —
Posterior column acetabulum — — Piriformis m.
— Sciatic n.
Internal pudendal a., v. — — Inferior gluteal a., v.
— Sacrotuberous ligament
Coccygeus m. —
Coccyx — — Gluteus maximus m.

(Top) The sciatic nerve continues to be difficult to identify as a discrete structure. This is a common appearance of the nerve at this point. **(Bottom)** The sciatic nerve is now visible as a discrete structure. It has its typical flattened ovoid shape. Upon exiting the pelvis the inferior gluteal artery branches. One of the branches is visible here coursing along the posterior aspect of the sciatic nerve. This vascular morphology may contribute to compression of the nerve and the development of piriformis syndrome.

CORONAL T1 MR, SCIATIC NERVE

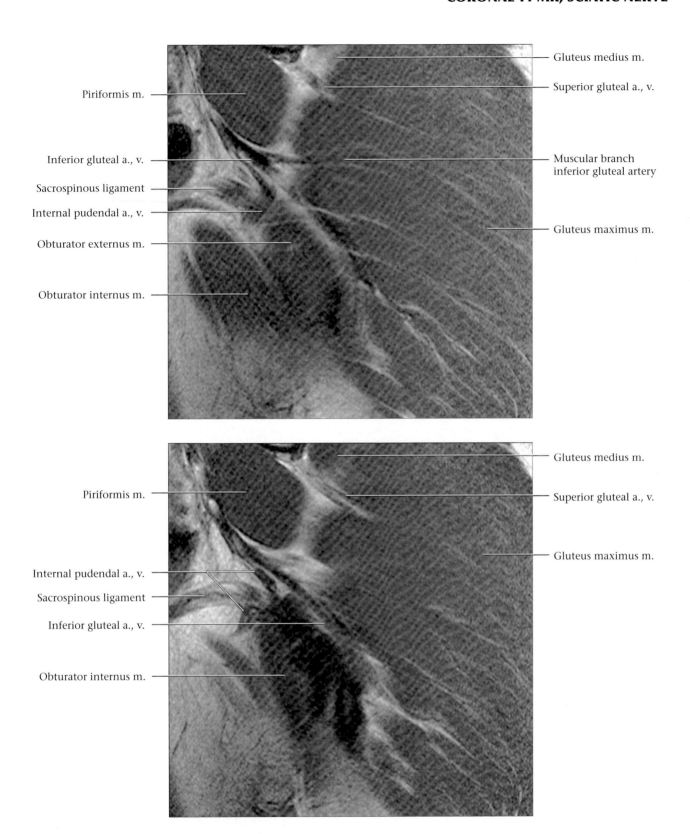

Piriformis m.

Inferior gluteal a., v.

Sacrospinous ligament

Internal pudendal a., v.

Obturator externus m.

Obturator internus m.

Gluteus medius m.

Superior gluteal a., v.

Muscular branch inferior gluteal artery

Gluteus maximus m.

Piriformis m.

Internal pudendal a., v.

Sacrospinous ligament

Inferior gluteal a., v.

Obturator internus m.

Gluteus medius m.

Superior gluteal a., v.

Gluteus maximus m.

(Top) This series of coronal images depicts the relationship of the structures exiting the pelvis via the greater sciatic notch. Those structures include the superior gluteal artery, which exits along the superior border of the piriformis muscle. The visible structures exiting along inferior border of the pelvis include the sciatic nerve, the inferior gluteal and internal pudendal vessels. Here, after the inferior gluteal artery exits the pelvis it has many branches (such as the large muscular branch which is visible on this image). The internal pudendal vessels immediately leave the buttocks by passing around the sacrospinous ligament to enter the lesser sciatic notch. **(Bottom)** The horizontally oriented fibers of the sacrospinous ligament are identified. The course of the internal pudendal vessels before and after piercing the ligament is seen.

CORONAL T1 MR, SCIATIC NERVE

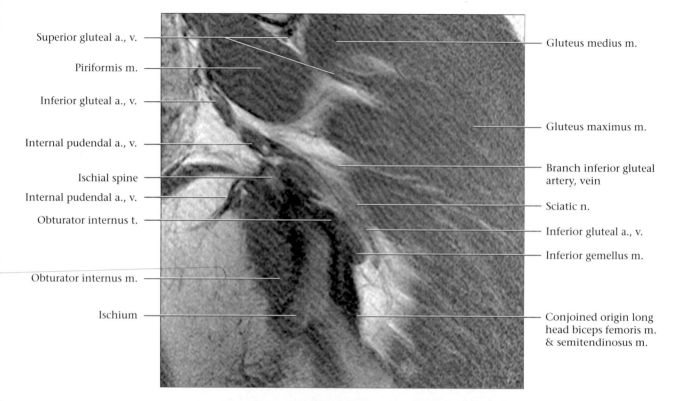

Superior gluteal a., v.

Piriformis m.

Inferior gluteal a., v.

Internal pudendal a., v.

Ischial spine

Internal pudendal a., v.

Obturator internus t.

Obturator internus m.

Ischium

Gluteus medius m.

Gluteus maximus m.

Branch inferior gluteal artery, vein

Sciatic n.

Inferior gluteal a., v.

Inferior gemellus m.

Conjoined origin long head biceps femoris m. & semitendinosus m.

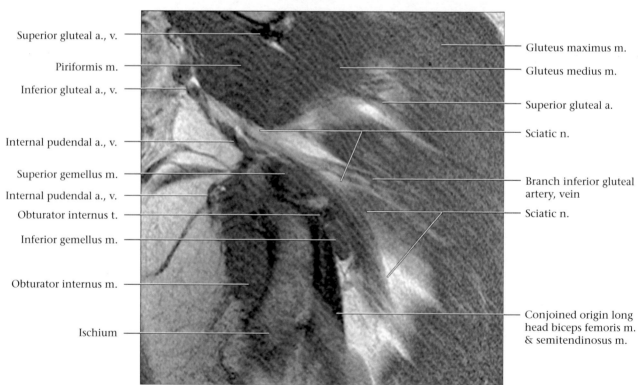

Superior gluteal a., v.

Piriformis m.

Inferior gluteal a., v.

Internal pudendal a., v.

Superior gemellus m.

Internal pudendal a., v.

Obturator internus t.

Inferior gemellus m.

Obturator internus m.

Ischium

Gluteus maximus m.

Gluteus medius m.

Superior gluteal a.

Sciatic n.

Branch inferior gluteal artery, vein

Sciatic n.

Conjoined origin long head biceps femoris m. & semitendinosus m.

(Top) Once exiting the pelvis the superior gluteal artery travels between the gluteus medius and maximus muscles. The inferior gluteal vessels and sciatic nerve are partial volumed together on this image. The inferior gluteal vessels and sciatic nerve travel in close proximity; the vessels travel along the medial aspect of the nerve. **(Bottom)** The sciatic nerve is the most lateral structure to exit along the inferior border of the piriformis muscle. The long axis of the sciatic nerve is nicely demonstrated. Its course posterior to the external rotators of the hip is easily appreciated.

POSTERIOR PELVIS

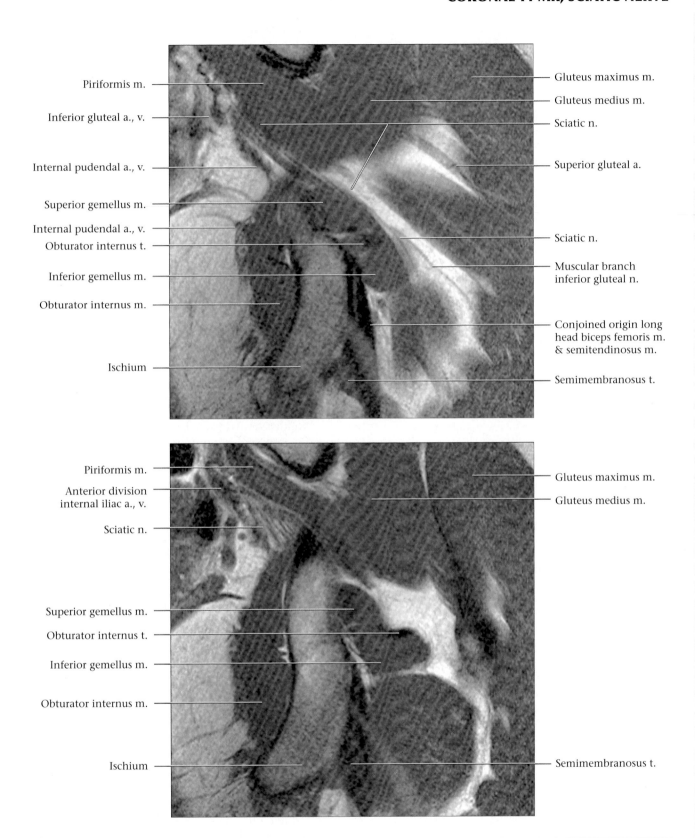

Piriformis m.

Inferior gluteal a., v.

Internal pudendal a., v.

Superior gemellus m.

Internal pudendal a., v.
Obturator internus t.

Inferior gemellus m.

Obturator internus m.

Ischium

Gluteus maximus m.

Gluteus medius m.

Sciatic n.

Superior gluteal a.

Sciatic n.

Muscular branch
inferior gluteal n.

Conjoined origin long
head biceps femoris m.
& semitendinosus m.

Semimembranosus t.

Piriformis m.

Anterior division
internal iliac a., v.

Sciatic n.

Superior gemellus m.

Obturator internus t.

Inferior gemellus m.

Obturator internus m.

Ischium

Gluteus maximus m.

Gluteus medius m.

Semimembranosus t.

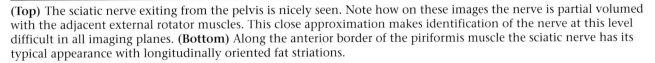

(Top) The sciatic nerve exiting from the pelvis is nicely seen. Note how on these images the nerve is partial volumed with the adjacent external rotator muscles. This close approximation makes identification of the nerve at this level difficult in all imaging planes. **(Bottom)** Along the anterior border of the piriformis muscle the sciatic nerve has its typical appearance with longitudinally oriented fat striations.

Hip and Pelvis

V

HIP JOINT

Imaging Anatomy

Overview

- Most stable articulation in body
- Greatest range of motion after glenohumeral joint
- Motion
  - Flexion with knee flexed limited by abdomen
  - Flexion with knee extended limited by hamstrings
  - Extension limited to 30° past vertical
  - Abduction without limitation
  - Adduction limited by opposite extremity
  - External rotation > internal
  - Internal rotation weakest motion
- Muscle/ligament balance
  - Anterior ligaments stronger than internal rotators
  - External rotators stronger than posterior ligaments
- Maximum stability in extension
  - Function of capsular ligaments

Acetabulum

- Formed by pubis, ilium, ischium
- Oriented anterior, inferior, lateral
- Covers > 50% femoral head
- Lunate surface along outer margin
  - Covered by horseshoe shaped articular cartilage
- Acetabular fossa: Central cartilage devoid region
  - Mainly ilium
- Acetabular notch: Osseous opening inferior margin
- Pulvinar: Fibrofatty tissue fills acetabular fossa
  - Covered by synovium: Extra-articular
- Consider as inverted Y: Transfers weight axial to appendicular skeleton
  - Anterior iliopubic (iliopectineal) column
  - Posterior ilioischial column
  - Stem: Ilium
- Anterior & posterior rims: Osseous margins of acetabulum
- Medial wall: Quadrilateral plate ilium
  - Radiographic acetabular line
- Teardrop: Radiographic conglomerate shadow
  - Lateral: Wall acetabular fossa
  - Medial: Anterior, inferior quadrilateral plate

Femoral Head

- 2/3 of sphere
- Covered by articular cartilage
  - Except central fovea capitis
  - Cartilage thickest superiorly
  - Cartilage thins at head/neck junction
- Fovea capitis: Central cartilage devoid depression on head
  - Attachment site ligamentum teres

Labrum

- Fibrocartilage
- Resides on acetabular rim
- May overlie articular cartilage
  - Labrocartilaginous cleft
    - Between articular cartilage & labrum
    - Anterosuperior, posteroinferior
    - Likely normal variant
- Joins transverse ligament at margins acetabular notch

- Labroligamentous sulci: Junction ligament & labrum
- Thickest posterior & superior
- Widest anterior & superior
- Vascular supply: Branches obturator, superior & inferior gluteal arteries
  - Mainly capsular surface
  - Articular surface avascular
    - Limited ability to repair
- Shape
  - Triangular 66-94%
    - Decreasing incidence with increasing age
  - Variants: Rounded, blunted, absent
  - Absent labra: Constellation absent anterior labrum & small remnant superiorly
    - 10-14% asymptomatic individuals
- MR signal
  - Typically low signal all sequences
  - Signal variations
    - Men > women
    - Increase incidence with increasing age
    - Most common anterior & superior
    - Intermediate T1 & proton density: 58%
    - Intermediate T2 signal: 37%
    - Bright T2 signal: 15%
    - Globular, linear, curvilinear
    - May extend to labral margins
    - Etiologies: Degeneration, fibrocartilaginous bundles (especially at base), osseous metaplasia (extension of rim into base)
- Function
  - Protect cartilage: Distributes forces by maintaining synovial fluid layer between articular surface
  - Prevents lateral translation femoral head

Joint Capsule

- 2 layers: Internal synovial; external fibrous
  - External forms capsular ligaments
- Attachments
  - Acetabulum
    - Base of labrum anteriorly & posteriorly
    - Several millimeters above labrum superiorly
    - Transverse ligament inferiorly
  - Femur
    - Anterior: Intertrochanteric line
    - Posterior: Proximal to intertrochanteric crest
    - Anterior attachment more lateral than posterior attachment
  - Perilabral recess: Between labrum & capsule
    - Smaller anterior & posterior
    - Larger superior
- External layer: Ligaments of joint capsule
  - Iliofemoral (Bigelow ligament)
    - Anterior, superior longitudinal spiral
    - Inverted Y-shape
    - Prevents hyperextension
    - Strongest ligament in body
    - Medial attachment anterior inferior iliac spine
  - Pubofemoral: Anterior, inferior, longitudinal spiral
    - Prevents hyperabduction
    - Medial attachment obturator crest pubis
  - Ischiofemoral: Posterior, longitudinal spiral
    - Weakest

- o **Zona orbicularis:** Deep, circular
- Synovial layer
  - o Longitudinally oriented folds/retinacula
  - o Retinacular arteries within folds

Bursa

- **Iliopsoas bursa**: Lateral and/or medial to tendon
  - o Communicates with hip joint between pubofemoral & iliofemoral ligaments: 10-14%
- **Obturator externus bursa:** Outpouching between zona orbicularis & ischiofemoral ligaments

Ligamentum Teres

- Attachments: Fovea capitis & transverse ligament
- Lined by synovium: Intracapsular, extra-articular
- Artery of ligamentum teres within
  - o Negligible supply femoral head
- Narrow superior, wider inferior
- Function unknown
- Tension in flexion, adduction, external rotation
- May be pain generator

Transverse Ligament

- Spans acetabular notch
  - o Completes socket of acetabulum
- Blends with labra at margins of notch
  - o Labroligamentous sulci at junction

Vascular Supply

- Branches of medial & lateral circumflex femoral, deep division superior gluteal, inferior gluteal arteries, a. of ligamentum teres (branch of obturator a.)

Innervation

- Branches from n. to rectus femoris, n. to quadratus femoris, anterior division obturator n., accessory obturator n., superior gluteal n.

Anatomy-Based Imaging Issues

Imaging Recommendations

- MR-arthrography preferred to assess intra-articular structures
- Arthrography/joint puncture
  - o Conventional arthrography primarily for joint replacement loosening
  - o Diagnostic & therapeutic injection with lidocaine, bupivacaine, steroids common
  - o Joint aspiration for infection common
  - o Patient position: Flexion & internal rotation maximizes joint volume
    - Bolster under knees
    - Knees & toes point inward (tape feet if needed)
  - o Needle direction: Straight down over center or lateral femoral head, or angle top greater trochanter to lateral femoral head
    - Avoid medial femoral head to avoid iliopsoas bursa
  - o Joint volume: 8-20 cc
  - o Hip communicates with iliopsoas bursa 10-14%
- MR arthrography
  - o Indications: Labral tears, loose bodies, cartilage defects

- o Inject 0.2 mmol gadopentetate dimeglumine
- o Image within 20-30 minutes
- o Fat suppressed T1-weighted or gradient echo images; one sequence without fat suppression
- o Screen entire pelvis with fluid sensitive sequence; coronal plane best
- o Imaging planes
  - Minimum 3 planes to fully visualize labrum
  - Axial, coronal, sagittal, oblique axial
  - Oblique axial: May replace axial, needed for alpha angle
  - Radial imaging may be useful
- CT arthrography
  - o Alternative if unable to undergo MR
  - o Acquire as thin as possible to maximize multiplanar reconstructions
  - o Consider interleaved acquisition
  - o Double contrast best: Small volume contrast 3-5 cc, air 5-7 cc
- Iliopsoas bursography
  - o Diagnostic: Snapping hip
  - o Therapeutic: Bursitis any cause
  - o Injection: Target superomedial femoral head/acetabular rim, hit bone, retract needle 3-5 mm
    - If hip replacement aim at tip lesser trochanter
  - o Diagnostic: Inject contrast first & evaluate tendon motion
    - Overdistention may diminish sensitivity
    - Volume for diagnostic: 3-5 cc
    - Repuncture for therapeutic
    - Abnormal motion: Sudden snap from flexion, abduction, external rotation to extension, adduction, internal rotation

Imaging Pitfalls

- Anterior labrocartilaginous cleft
  - o No definitive literature
  - o Controversy normal variant or pathologic
    - Likely normal variant
  - o Differential diagnosis: Labral detachment
    - Differential features: Smooth labral margins, smooth cartilage margins, intact attachment labrum & rim, absence other pathology

Selected References

1. Seldes RM et al: Anatomy, histologic features, and vascularity of the adult acetabular labrum. Clin Orthop Relat Res. (382):232-40, 2001
2. Tan V et al: Contribution of acetabular labrum to articulating surface area and femoral head coverage in adult hip joints: an anatomic study in cadavera. Am J Orthop. 30(11):809-12, 2001
3. Abe I et al: Acetabular labrum: abnormal findings at MR imaging in asymptomatic hips. Radiology. 216(2):576-81, 2000
4. Cotten A et al: Acetabular labrum: MRI in asymptomatic volunteers. J Comput Assist Tomogr. 22(1):1-7, 1998
5. Lecouvet FE et al: MR imaging of the acetabular labrum: variations in 200 asymptomatic hips. AJR Am J Roentgenol. 167(4):1025-8, 1996

GRAPHICS, JOINT CAPSULE AND LIGAMENTS

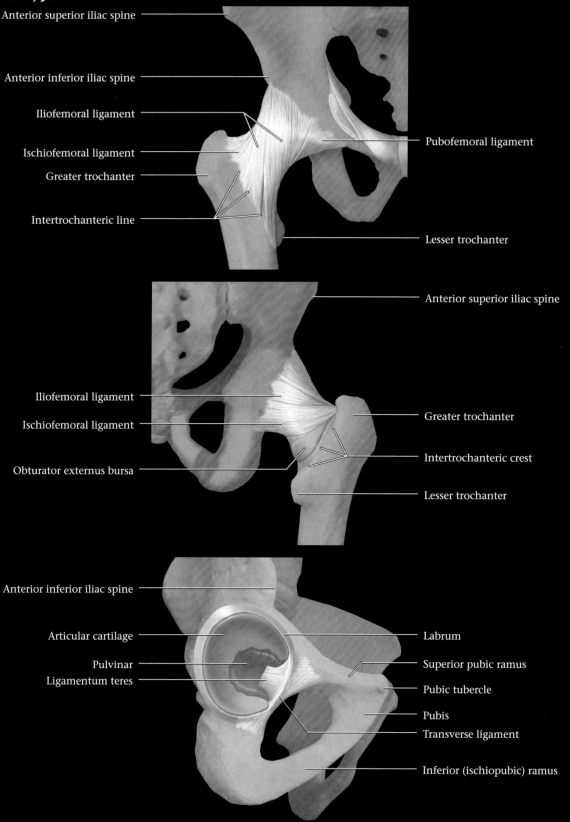

Anterior superior iliac spine

Anterior inferior iliac spine

Iliofemoral ligament

Ischiofemoral ligament

Greater trochanter

Intertrochanteric line

Pubofemoral ligament

Lesser trochanter

Anterior superior iliac spine

Iliofemoral ligament

Ischiofemoral ligament

Obturator externus bursa

Greater trochanter

Intertrochanteric crest

Lesser trochanter

Anterior inferior iliac spine

Articular cartilage

Pulvinar

Ligamentum teres

Labrum

Superior pubic ramus

Pubic tubercle

Pubis

Transverse ligament

Inferior (ischiopubic) ramus

(Top) Anterior ligaments. The longitudinal spiral of the iliofemoral and pubofemoral ligaments is well seen. Their attachments to the anterior inferior iliac spine and pubic aspect of the obturator foramen respectively are visible. The ischiofemoral ligament wraps over the superior aspect of the femoral neck to attach to the anterior femoral neck. **(Middle)** Posterior perspective. The longitudinal spiral of the ischiofemoral ligament is nicely seen. The obturator externus bursa protrudes from the joint along the inferior margin of the ischiofemoral ligament. **(Bottom)** External view of the acetabulum demonstrates the horseshoe shaped articular cartilage with the pulvinar within. The labrum resides on acetabular rim and blends with the transverse ligament. The ligamentum teres attaches to the transverse ligament.

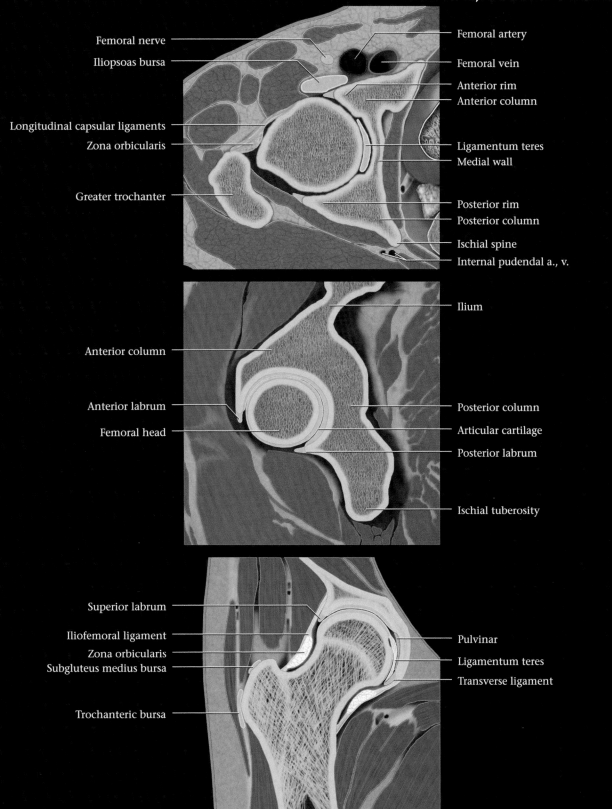

Femoral nerve

Iliopsoas bursa

Longitudinal capsular ligaments

Zona orbicularis

Greater trochanter

Femoral artery

Femoral vein

Anterior rim

Anterior column

Ligamentum teres

Medial wall

Posterior rim

Posterior column

Ischial spine

Internal pudendal a., v.

Ilium

Anterior column

Anterior labrum

Femoral head

Posterior column

Articular cartilage

Posterior labrum

Ischial tuberosity

Superior labrum

Iliofemoral ligament

Zona orbicularis

Subgluteus medius bursa

Trochanteric bursa

Pulvinar

Ligamentum teres

Transverse ligament

(Top) Axial representation of the hip joint. The iliopsoas bursa is closely approximated to the joint anteriorly. The ligamentum teres is seen in profile as a flattened structure. The two layers of the external capsule are visible, the more superficial longitudinal fibers and deep circular fibers. **(Middle)** Sagittal representation of the hip joint nicely demonstrates the inverted Y of the acetabulum. The ilium is the stem and the limbs are the anterior and posterior acetabular columns. **(Bottom)** This coronal image demonstrates many of the important structures of the hip joint. The longitudinally oriented fibers of the ligaments of the external joint capsule and the deeper circularly oriented fibers of the zona orbicularis are visible. Note the long axis of the ligamentum teres and its insertion onto the transverse ligament. The pulvinar fills the acetabular fossa.

HIP JOINT

RADIOGRAPHS, HIP & BURSAL INJECTIONS

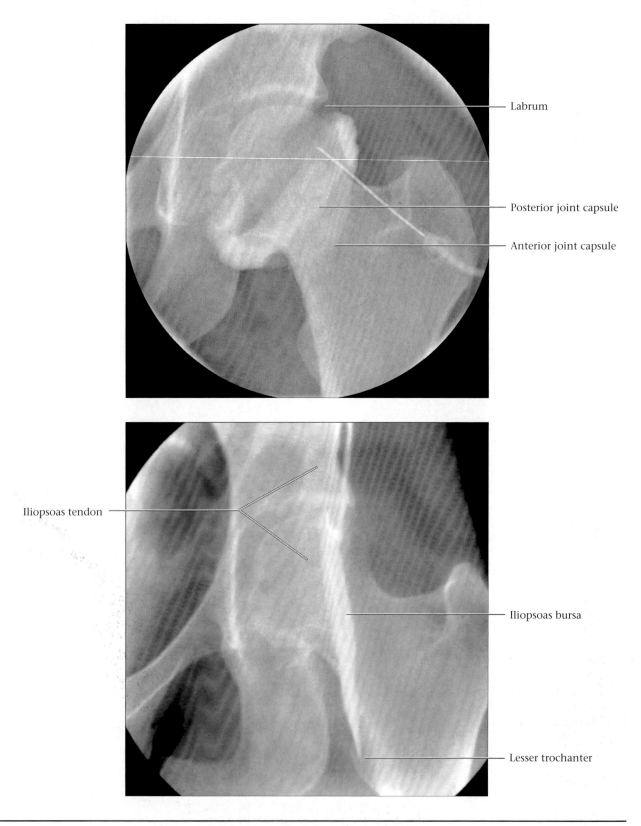

Labrum

Posterior joint capsule

Anterior joint capsule

Iliopsoas tendon

Iliopsoas bursa

Lesser trochanter

(Top) AP radiograph during injection of the hip joint. An oblique approach to the joint was used. Note that the posterior-most extension of contrast is medial to the most lateral extension of contrast anteriorly. The inferior margin of the labrum is outlined by contrast. **(Bottom)** Iliopsoas bursal injection. A direct approach is used. The needle is directed to hit the anterior rim, then withdrawn 5 mm. The contrast flows along the bursa inferiorly to the lesser trochanter. Variable superior extension of contrast may be seen. In this patient the superior extent is limited. The tendon is faintly outlined by contrast.

AXIAL GRE MR ARTHROGRAM

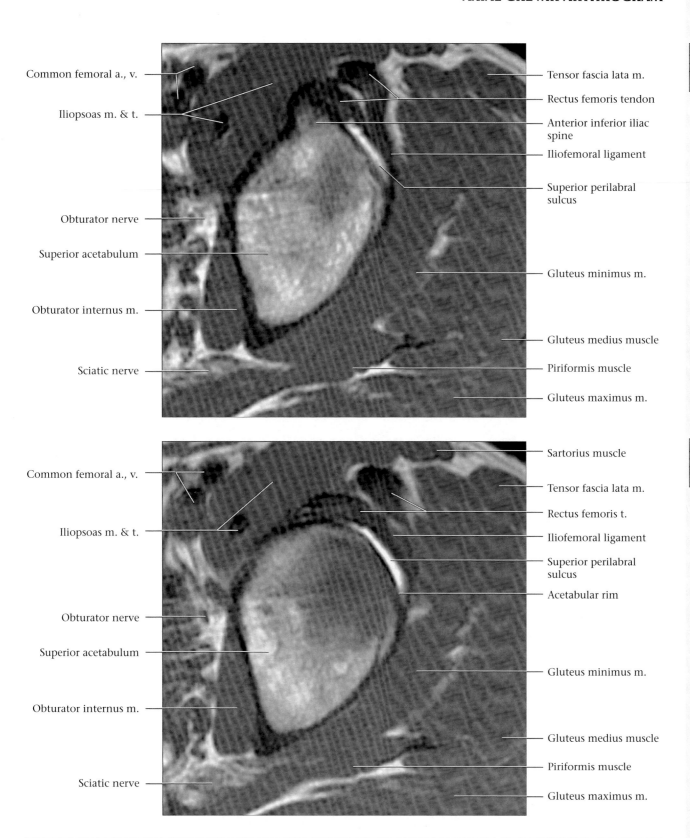

Common femoral a., v. — Tensor fascia lata m.

Iliopsoas m. & t. — Rectus femoris tendon

— Anterior inferior iliac spine

— Iliofemoral ligament

— Superior perilabral sulcus

Obturator nerve —

Superior acetabulum —

— Gluteus minimus m.

Obturator internus m. —

— Gluteus medius muscle

— Piriformis muscle

Sciatic nerve — — Gluteus maximus m.

— Sartorius muscle

Common femoral a., v. — — Tensor fascia lata m.

— Rectus femoris t.

Iliopsoas m. & t. — — Iliofemoral ligament

— Superior perilabral sulcus

— Acetabular rim

Obturator nerve —

Superior acetabulum —

— Gluteus minimus m.

Obturator internus m. —

— Gluteus medius muscle

— Piriformis muscle

Sciatic nerve — — Gluteus maximus m.

(Top) First of ten T1-weighted gradient echo axial images with intra-articular contrast from superior to inferior. The two heads of the rectus femoris muscle are visible. The direct head arises from the anterior inferior iliac spine, the indirect head has arisen from a groove above the acetabulum. **(Bottom)** At the superior aspect of the joint the contrast is within the superior perilabral sulcus between the joint capsule (iliofemoral ligament) and the acetabular rim.

Hip and Pelvis

∨

HIP JOINT

AXIAL GRE MR ARTHROGRAM

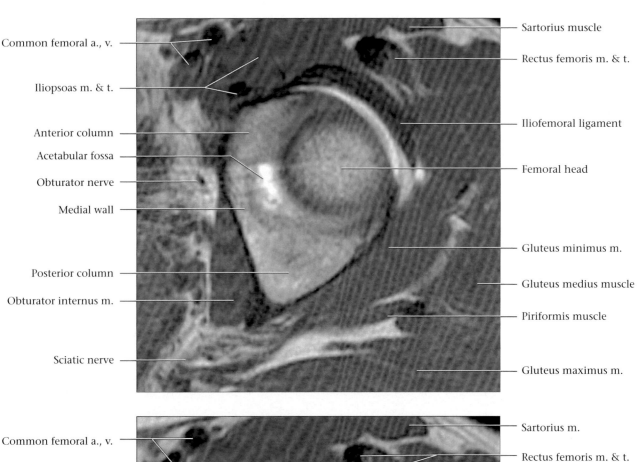

Common femoral a., v.

Iliopsoas m. & t.

Anterior column

Acetabular fossa

Obturator nerve

Medial wall

Posterior column

Obturator internus m.

Sciatic nerve

Sartorius muscle

Rectus femoris m. & t.

Iliofemoral ligament

Femoral head

Gluteus minimus m.

Gluteus medius muscle

Piriformis muscle

Gluteus maximus m.

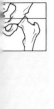

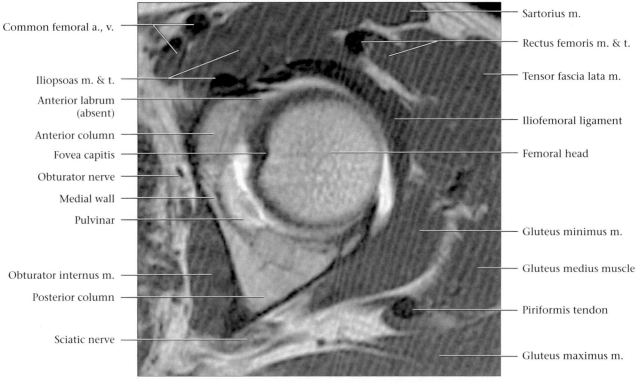

Common femoral a., v.

Iliopsoas m. & t.

Anterior labrum (absent)

Anterior column

Fovea capitis

Obturator nerve

Medial wall

Pulvinar

Obturator internus m.

Posterior column

Sciatic nerve

Sartorius m.

Rectus femoris m. & t.

Tensor fascia lata m.

Iliofemoral ligament

Femoral head

Gluteus minimus m.

Gluteus medius muscle

Piriformis tendon

Gluteus maximus m.

(Top) The acetabular notch (fossa) is visible as a contrast filled defect within the acetabulum. The thin medial wall is its osseous boundary. The iliofemoral ligament wraps over the anterior and superior aspect of the joint. **(Bottom)** A small defect is seen in the joint capsule just lateral to the iliopsoas muscle. This defect is the site of communication between the joint and the bursa. Contrast material fills the space between the joint capsule anterior rim in this patient with an absent labra. A small depression is seen on the femoral head. This is the fovea capitis which is devoid of cartilage.

HIP JOINT

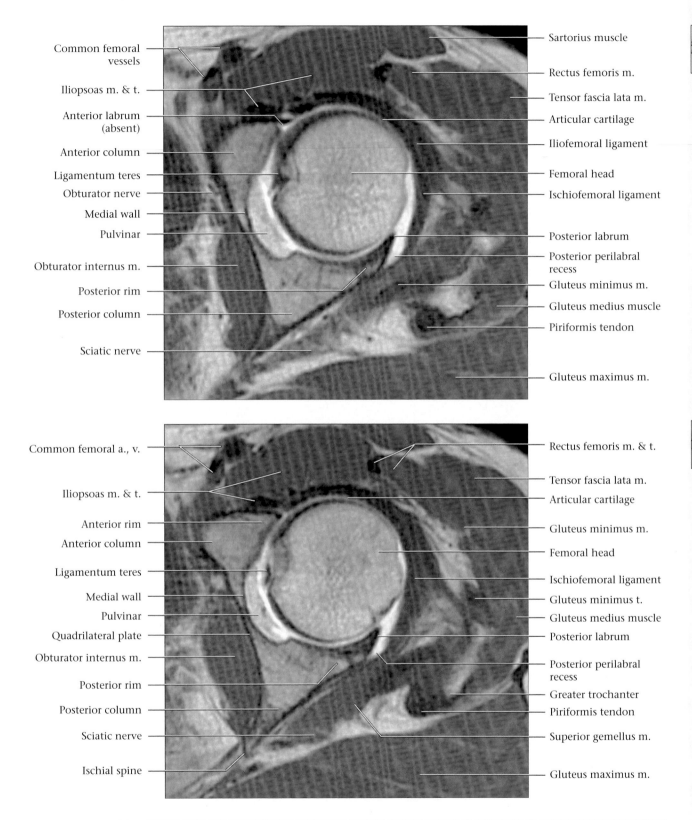

Top image labels (left):
- Common femoral vessels
- Iliopsoas m. & t.
- Anterior labrum (absent)
- Anterior column
- Ligamentum teres
- Obturator nerve
- Medial wall
- Pulvinar
- Obturator internus m.
- Posterior rim
- Posterior column
- Sciatic nerve

Top image labels (right):
- Sartorius muscle
- Rectus femoris m.
- Tensor fascia lata m.
- Articular cartilage
- Iliofemoral ligament
- Femoral head
- Ischiofemoral ligament
- Posterior labrum
- Posterior perilabral recess
- Gluteus minimus m.
- Gluteus medius muscle
- Piriformis tendon
- Gluteus maximus m.

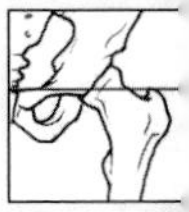

Bottom image labels (left):
- Common femoral a., v.
- Iliopsoas m. & t.
- Anterior rim
- Anterior column
- Ligamentum teres
- Medial wall
- Pulvinar
- Quadrilateral plate
- Obturator internus m.
- Posterior rim
- Posterior column
- Sciatic nerve
- Ischial spine

Bottom image labels (right):
- Rectus femoris m. & t.
- Tensor fascia lata m.
- Articular cartilage
- Gluteus minimus m.
- Femoral head
- Ischiofemoral ligament
- Gluteus minimus t.
- Gluteus medius muscle
- Posterior labrum
- Posterior perilabral recess
- Greater trochanter
- Piriformis tendon
- Superior gemellus m.
- Gluteus maximus m.

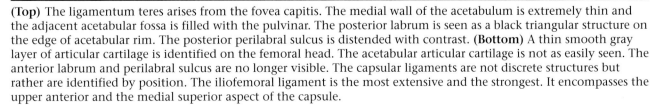

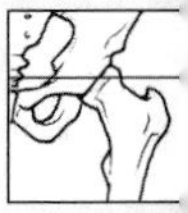

(Top) The ligamentum teres arises from the fovea capitis. The medial wall of the acetabulum is extremely thin and the adjacent acetabular fossa is filled with the pulvinar. The posterior labrum is seen as a black triangular structure on the edge of acetabular rim. The posterior perilabral sulcus is distended with contrast. **(Bottom)** A thin smooth gray layer of articular cartilage is identified on the femoral head. The acetabular articular cartilage is not as easily seen. The anterior labrum and perilabral sulcus are no longer visible. The capsular ligaments are not discrete structures but rather are identified by position. The iliofemoral ligament is the most extensive and the strongest. It encompasses the upper anterior and the medial superior aspect of the capsule.

Hip and Pelvis

V

HIP JOINT

AXIAL GRE MR ARTHROGRAM

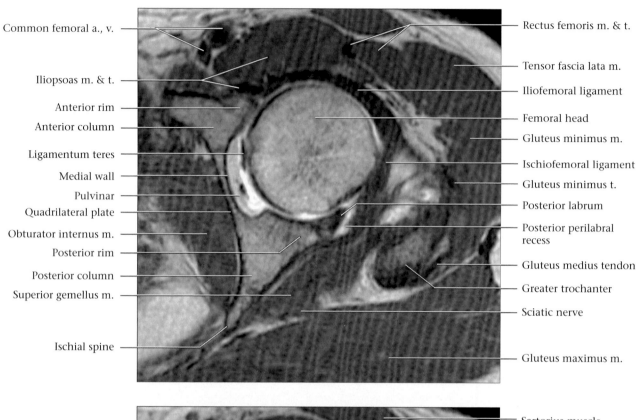

Common femoral a., v.

Iliopsoas m. & t.

Anterior rim

Anterior column

Ligamentum teres

Medial wall

Pulvinar

Quadrilateral plate

Obturator internus m.

Posterior rim

Posterior column

Superior gemellus m.

Ischial spine

Rectus femoris m. & t.

Tensor fascia lata m.

Iliofemoral ligament

Femoral head

Gluteus minimus m.

Ischiofemoral ligament

Gluteus minimus t.

Posterior labrum

Posterior perilabral recess

Gluteus medius tendon

Greater trochanter

Sciatic nerve

Gluteus maximus m.

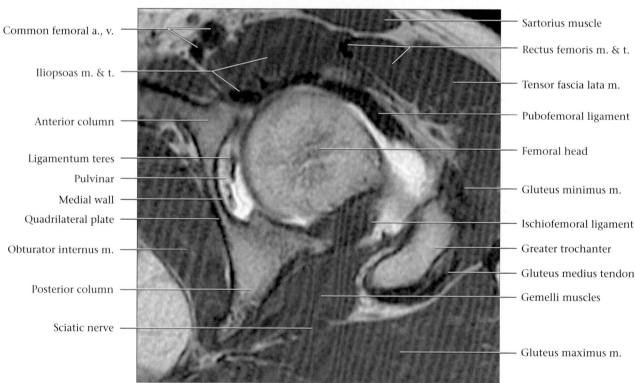

Common femoral a., v.

Iliopsoas m. & t.

Anterior column

Ligamentum teres

Pulvinar

Medial wall

Quadrilateral plate

Obturator internus m.

Posterior column

Sciatic nerve

Sartorius muscle

Rectus femoris m. & t.

Tensor fascia lata m.

Pubofemoral ligament

Femoral head

Gluteus minimus m.

Ischiofemoral ligament

Greater trochanter

Gluteus medius tendon

Gemelli muscles

Gluteus maximus m.

(Top) The ischiofemoral ligament courses from posterior to anterior over the lateral aspect of the femoral neck. Its origin from the ischium is well seen on this image. The flattened cross section of the ligamentum teres is present medial to the femoral head. **(Bottom)** The pubofemoral ligament covers the anterior inferior aspect of the joint. The thin medial wall of the acetabulum and the quadrilateral plate of the ilium are visible. These structures form the boundaries of the teardrop on radiographs.

Hip and Pelvis

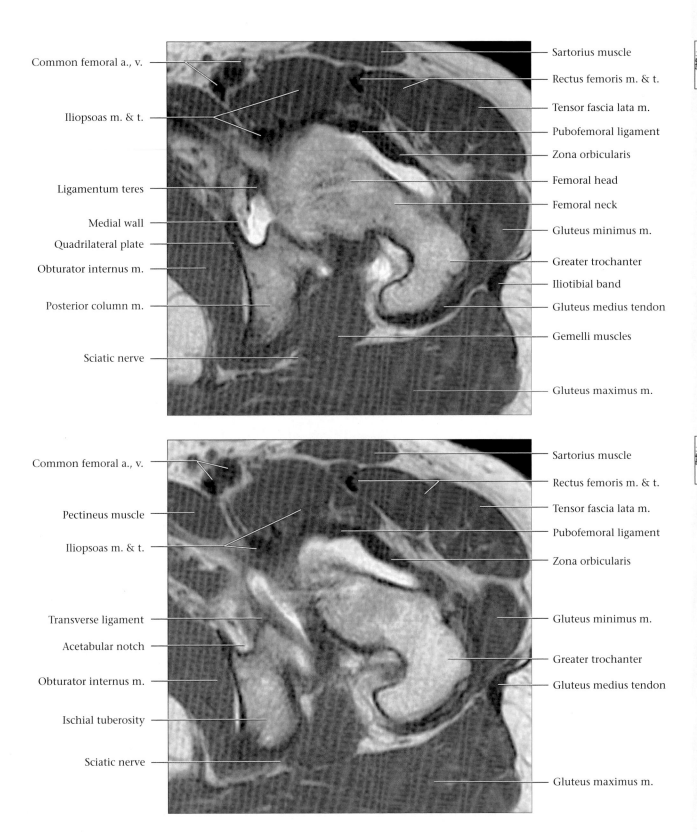

Common femoral a., v.

Iliopsoas m. & t.

Ligamentum teres

Medial wall

Quadrilateral plate

Obturator internus m.

Posterior column m.

Sciatic nerve

Sartorius muscle

Rectus femoris m. & t.

Tensor fascia lata m.

Pubofemoral ligament

Zona orbicularis

Femoral head

Femoral neck

Gluteus minimus m.

Greater trochanter

Iliotibial band

Gluteus medius tendon

Gemelli muscles

Gluteus maximus m.

Common femoral a., v.

Pectineus muscle

Iliopsoas m. & t.

Transverse ligament

Acetabular notch

Obturator internus m.

Ischial tuberosity

Sciatic nerve

Sartorius muscle

Rectus femoris m. & t.

Tensor fascia lata m.

Pubofemoral ligament

Zona orbicularis

Gluteus minimus m.

Greater trochanter

Gluteus medius tendon

Gluteus maximus m.

(Top) A focal area of thickening is seen in the lateral joint capsule at the site of the fibers of the zona orbicularis. The attachment of the ligamentum teres to the transverse ligament occurs in the inferior aspect of the joint. **(Bottom)** A short segment of the transverse ligament is seen at the posterior margin of the acetabular notch marking the inferior extent of the acetabulum and hip joint. Along the femoral neck note the more lateral extension of the anterior joint capsule compared to the posterior joint capsule.

Hip and Pelvis

V

OBLIQUE AXIAL T1 FS MR ARTHROGRAM

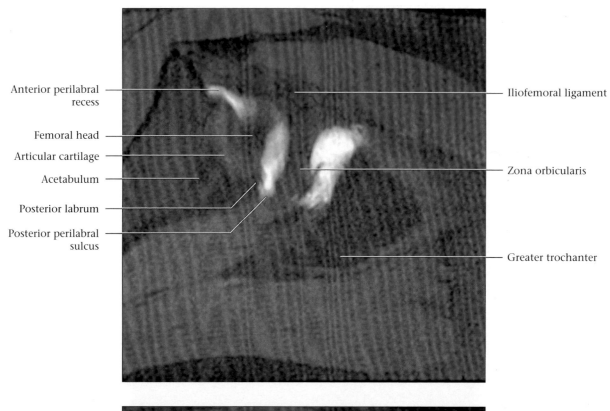

Anterior perilabral recess — Iliofemoral ligament

Femoral head

Articular cartilage

Acetabulum — Zona orbicularis

Posterior labrum

Posterior perilabral sulcus — Greater trochanter

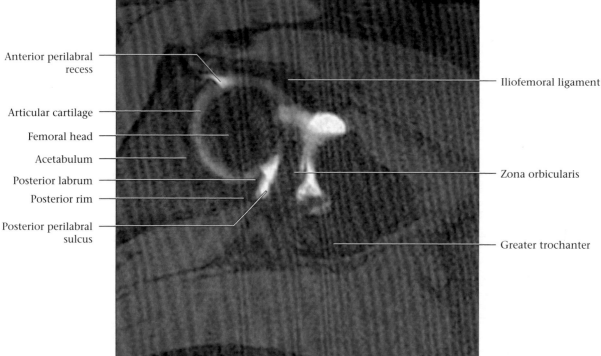

Anterior perilabral recess — Iliofemoral ligament

Articular cartilage

Femoral head

Acetabulum

Posterior labrum — Zona orbicularis

Posterior rim

Posterior perilabral sulcus — Greater trochanter

(Top) First of ten fat suppressed T1 weighted oblique axial images along the long axis of the femoral neck with intra-articular contrast. Images are from superior to inferior. At the superior aspect of the joint the anterior perilabral sulcus is seen. This individual has an absent anterosuperior labrum. The iliofemoral ligament is an anterior longitudinally oriented black structure. The circular orientation of the fibers of the zona orbicularis is also well seen. **(Bottom)** The articular cartilage is easily appreciated between the acetabulum and femoral head, although femoral and acetabular cartilage are not easily discernible as separate structures. The posterior labrum is the triangular structure at the tip of the posterior acetabular rim. Note the continuity of the fibers of the zona orbicularis with the focal area of thickening anteriorly described on the axial images.

HIP JOINT

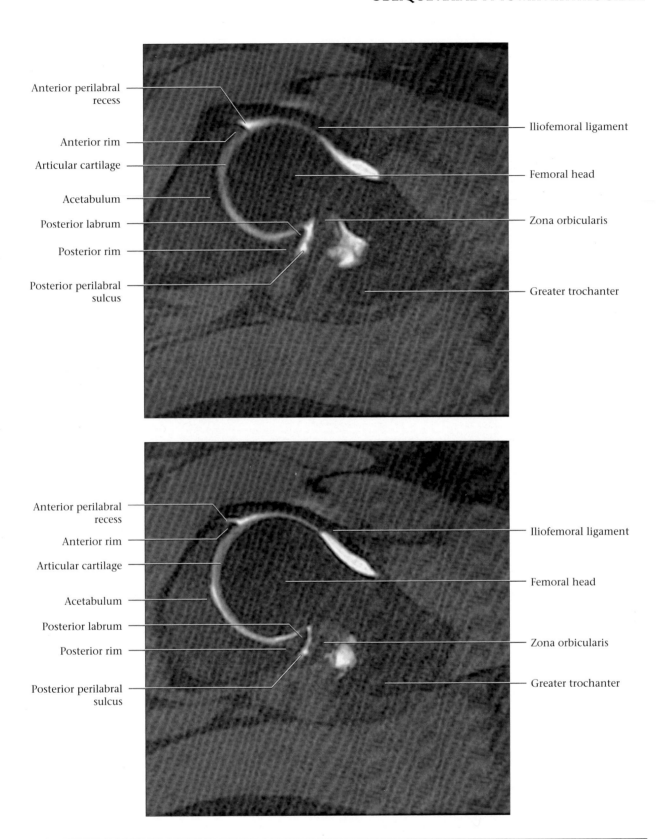

Anterior perilabral recess — Iliofemoral ligament

Anterior rim

Articular cartilage — Femoral head

Acetabulum

Posterior labrum — Zona orbicularis

Posterior rim

Posterior perilabral sulcus — Greater trochanter

Anterior perilabral recess — Iliofemoral ligament

Anterior rim

Articular cartilage — Femoral head

Acetabulum

Posterior labrum — Zona orbicularis

Posterior rim

Posterior perilabral sulcus — Greater trochanter

(Top) The posterior perilabral sulcus is prominent in part due to the laxity of the posterior joint secondary to slight external rotation. The anterior capsular structures are taut. **(Bottom)** At this level the articular cartilage of the femoral head is distinctly seen. The acetabular cartilage is normally extremely thin.

Hip and Pelvis

V

HIP JOINT

OBLIQUE AXIAL T1 FS MR ARTHROGRAM

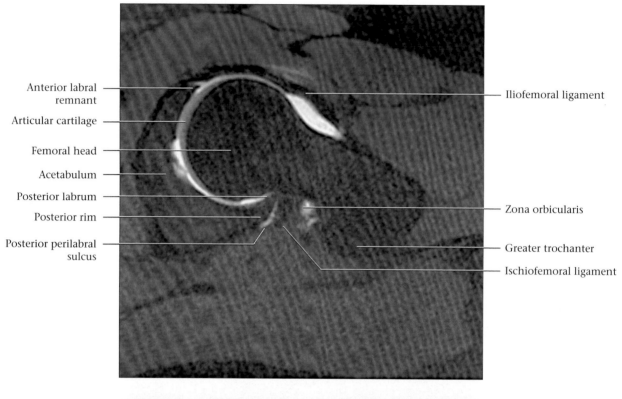

Anterior labral remnant

Articular cartilage

Femoral head

Acetabulum

Posterior labrum

Posterior rim

Posterior perilabral sulcus

Iliofemoral ligament

Zona orbicularis

Greater trochanter

Ischiofemoral ligament

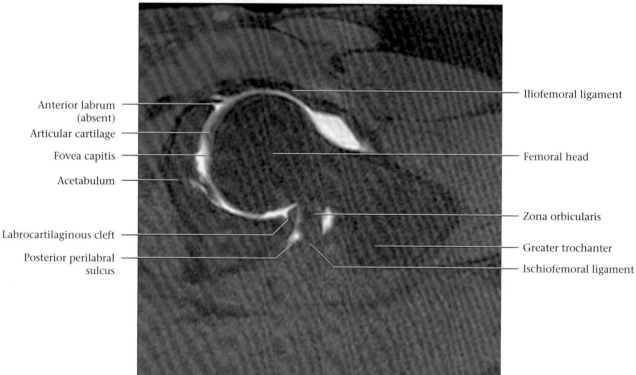

Anterior labrum (absent)

Articular cartilage

Fovea capitis

Acetabulum

Labrocartilaginous cleft

Posterior perilabral sulcus

Iliofemoral ligament

Femoral head

Zona orbicularis

Greater trochanter

Ischiofemoral ligament

(Top) At the anterior aspect of the joint a small triangular anterior labrum is present. Continuity between the fibers of the ischiofemoral ligament and the fibers of the zona orbicularis posteriorly can be appreciated on this image. (Bottom) A thin collection of contrast is identified posteriorly between the articular cartilage and the posterior labrum. This labrocartilaginous cleft is a normal variant. The cartilage of the femoral head thins at the margins of the fovea capitis.

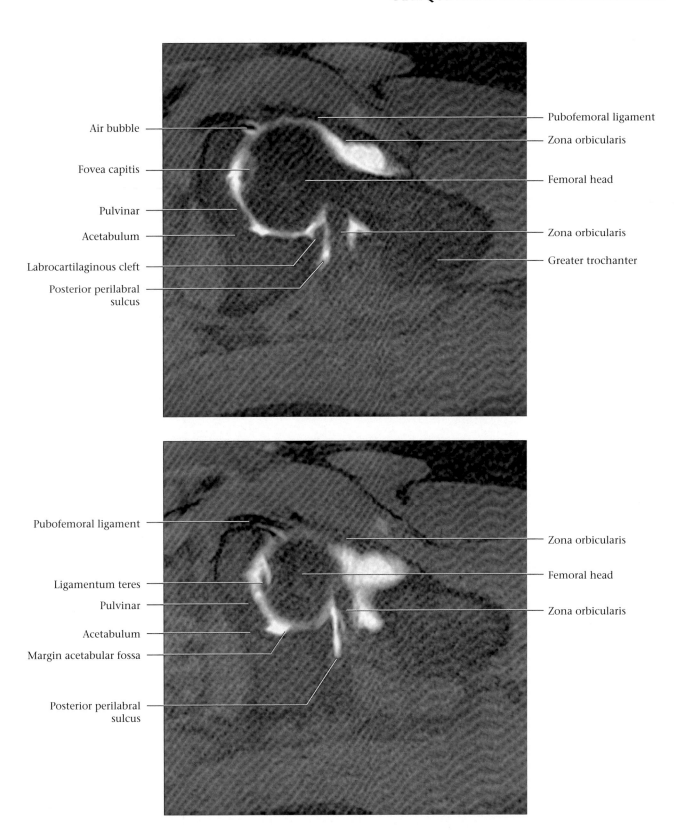

Air bubble — Pubofemoral ligament

Fovea capitis — Zona orbicularis

Pulvinar — Femoral head

Acetabulum —

Labrocartilaginous cleft — Zona orbicularis

Posterior perilabral sulcus — Greater trochanter

Pubofemoral ligament — Zona orbicularis

Ligamentum teres — Femoral head

Pulvinar — Zona orbicularis

Acetabulum —

Margin acetabular fossa —

Posterior perilabral sulcus —

(Top) The fovea capitis is an impression on the central portion of the femoral head. A small air bubble collects in the anterior perilabral recess. The pulvinar is difficult to appreciate as a distinct structure on fat suppressed images. It blends with the adjacent acetabulum. **(Bottom)** The attachment of the ligamentum teres to the fovea capitis is visible. At this inferior aspect of the joint the pubofemoral ligament forms the external layer of the joint capsule. Note the abrupt loss of acetabular articular cartilage at the posterior margin of the acetabular fossa.

HIP JOINT

OBLIQUE AXIAL T1 FS MR ARTHROGRAM

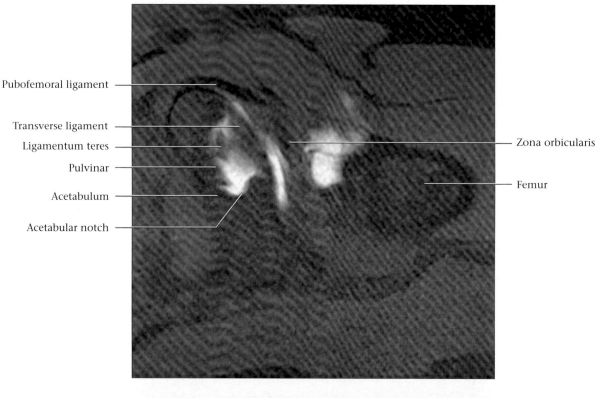

Pubofemoral ligament

Transverse ligament

Ligamentum teres

Pulvinar

Acetabulum

Acetabular notch

Zona orbicularis

Femur

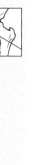

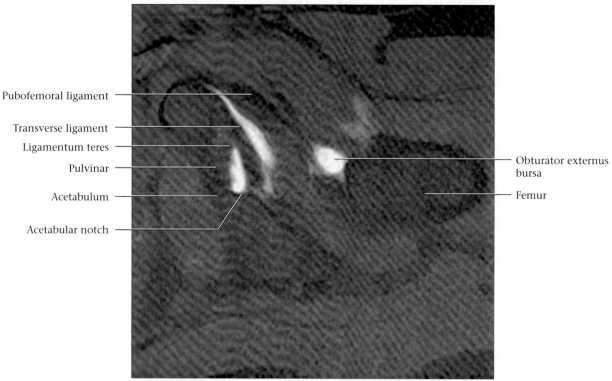

Pubofemoral ligament

Transverse ligament

Ligamentum teres

Pulvinar

Acetabulum

Acetabular notch

Obturator externus bursa

Femur

(Top) The posterior margin of the acetabular notch is easily appreciated. The fibers of the transverse ligament span the notch from anterior to posterior. The labra have blended with the transverse ligament by the level. **(Bottom)** The ligamentum teres attaches to the transverse ligament at the inferior aspect of the joint. The obturator externus bursa is an outpouching of the synovium from beneath the inferior margin of the obturator externus muscle along the posterior aspect of the joint.

HIP JOINT

CORONAL T1 FS MR ARTHROGRAM

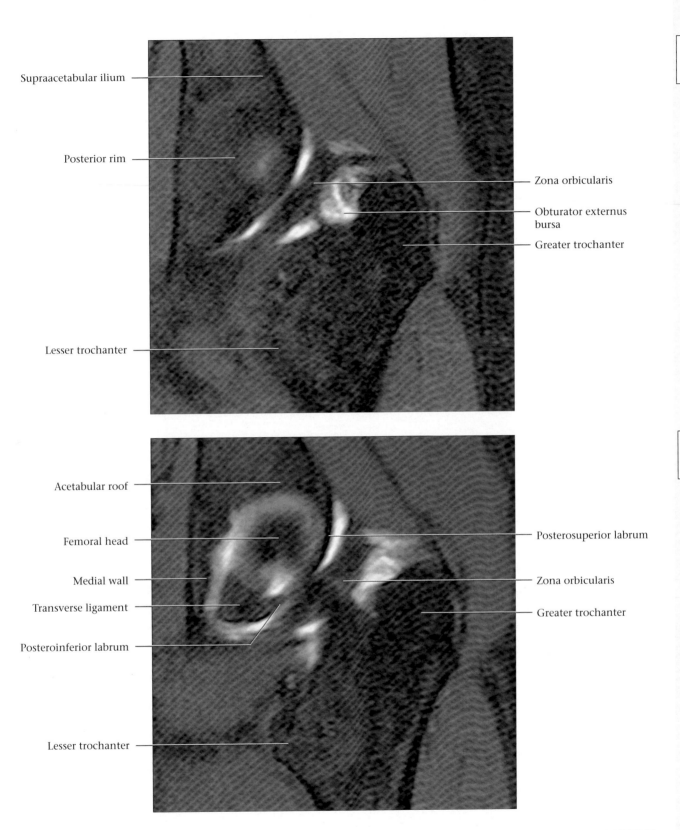

Supraacetabular ilium

Posterior rim

Lesser trochanter

Zona orbicularis

Obturator externus bursa

Greater trochanter

Acetabular roof

Femoral head

Medial wall

Transverse ligament

Posteroinferior labrum

Lesser trochanter

Posterosuperior labrum

Zona orbicularis

Greater trochanter

(Top) First of eight T1-weighted fat suppressed coronal images with intra-articular contrast from posterior to anterior. Images begin at the posterior acetabular rim. The fibers of the zona orbicularis are visible as a circular band of fibers. The obturator externus bursa is present as a posterior outpouching of the joint from beneath the inferior border of the obturator externus muscle (see "Lateral Hip" section). (Bottom) The entire course of the posterior labrum is seen. At the posterior margin of the acetabular notch the labrum blends with the transverse ligament.

Hip and Pelvis

V

181

CORONAL T1 FS MR ARTHROGRAM

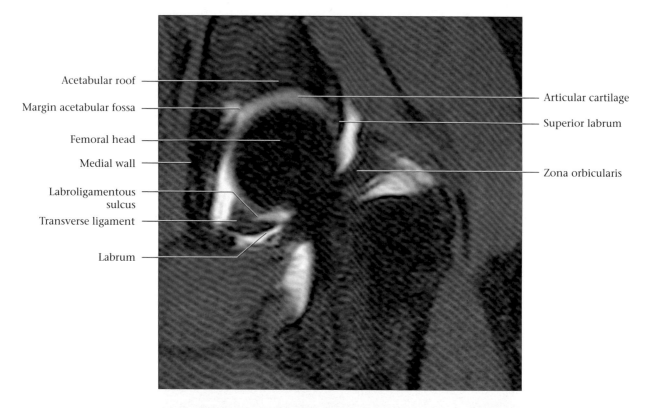

Acetabular roof

Margin acetabular fossa

Femoral head

Medial wall

Labroligamentous sulcus

Transverse ligament

Labrum

Articular cartilage

Superior labrum

Zona orbicularis

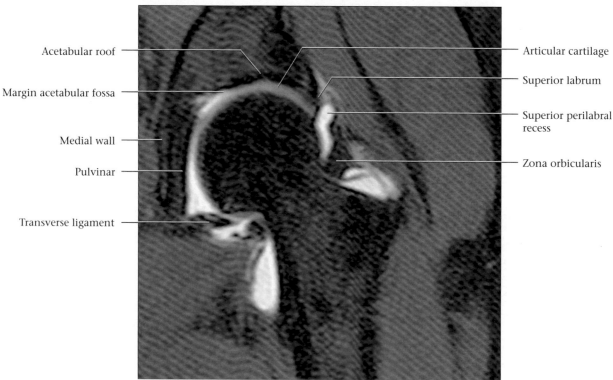

Acetabular roof

Margin acetabular fossa

Medial wall

Pulvinar

Transverse ligament

Articular cartilage

Superior labrum

Superior perilabral recess

Zona orbicularis

(Top) The labroligamentous sulcus is created at the junction of the posterior labrum and the transverse ligament. This sulcus should not be misinterpreted as labral pathology. The articular surfaces of the acetabulum and femoral head are discernible as two separate structures on this image. **(Bottom)** An abrupt loss of acetabular articular cartilage occurs at the medial margin of the acetabular fossa. The cross section of the transverse ligament is seen along the acetabular notch. It is triangular in shape similar to the labrum. The superior labrum is present as a small black triangular structure along the lateral margin of the acetabular roof.

HIP JOINT

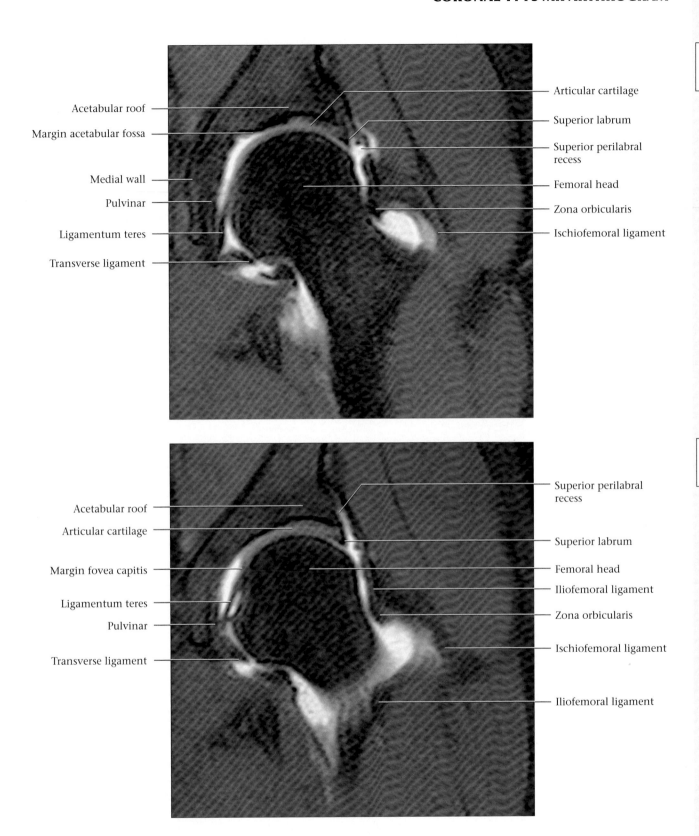

(Top) The superior labrum is nicely visualized. In this patient it overlaps the articular cartilage. A small air bubble is noted in the superior perilabral recess. The long axis of the ligamentum teres is seen extending from the fovea capitis to the transverse ligament. The ischiofemoral ligament is the most lateral of the capsular ligaments. With fat suppression it is difficult to visualize the pulvinar and adjacent medial wall of the acetabulum as separate structures. **(Bottom)** Superiorly the joint capsule inserts several millimeters above the acetabular rim creating a larger perilabral recess. The fovea capitis is the central depression on the femoral head. It is devoid of cartilage and an abrupt drop off of cartilage is seen at its edge.

CORONAL T1 FS MR ARTHROGRAM

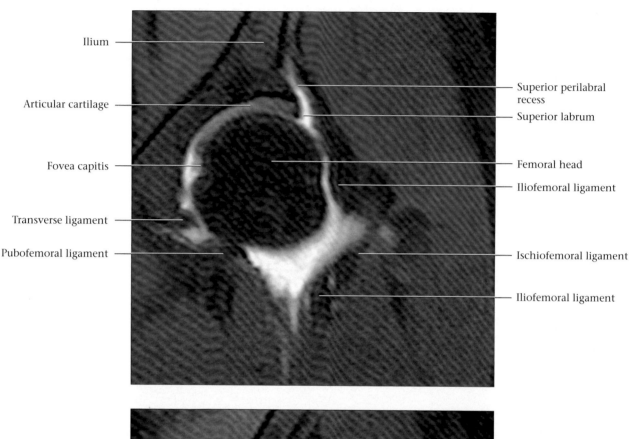

Ilium

Articular cartilage

Fovea capitis

Transverse ligament

Pubofemoral ligament

Superior perilabral recess

Superior labrum

Femoral head

Iliofemoral ligament

Ischiofemoral ligament

Iliofemoral ligament

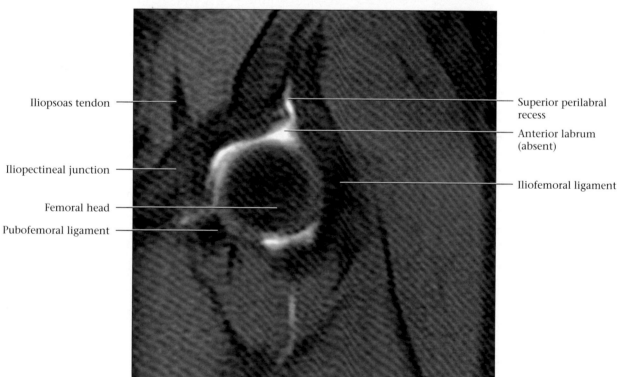

Iliopsoas tendon

Iliopectineal junction

Femoral head

Pubofemoral ligament

Superior perilabral recess

Anterior labrum (absent)

Iliofemoral ligament

(Top) Visualization of the articular cartilage is excellent in this portion of the joint. The superior labrum is also nicely demonstrated as a triangular structure along the acetabular rim. (Bottom) The pubofemoral ligament is the most inferior of the anterior external capsular ligaments. At this transition from superior to anterior labrum a contrast filled defect is seen at the expected location of the anterior labrum. This anatomic variant is not uncommon. The iliopsoas tendon is crossing the iliopectineal junction and its intimate relationship with the joint is easily appreciated.

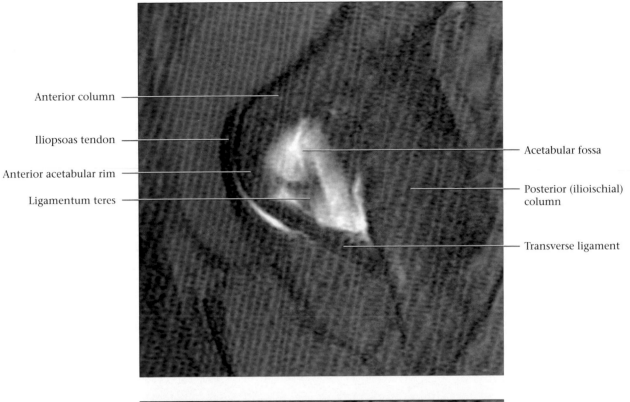

Anterior column

Iliopsoas tendon

Anterior acetabular rim

Ligamentum teres

Acetabular fossa

Posterior (ilioischial) column

Transverse ligament

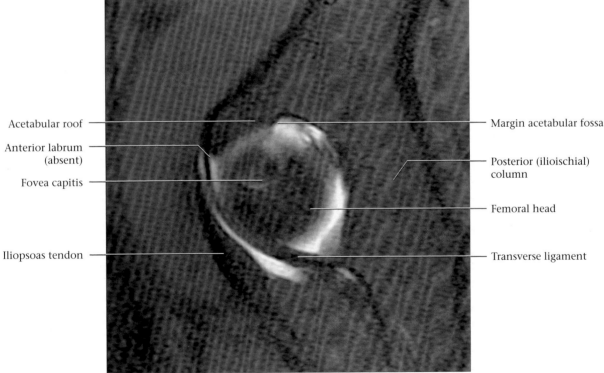

Acetabular roof

Anterior labrum (absent)

Fovea capitis

Iliopsoas tendon

Margin acetabular fossa

Posterior (ilioischial) column

Femoral head

Transverse ligament

(Top) First of ten fat suppressed T1-weighted sagittal images from medial to lateral with intra-articular contrast. This medial most image is through the acetabular notch. A segment of the long axis of the ligamentum teres is seen nearing its attachment to the transverse ligament. The horizontal fibers of the transverse ligament span the acetabular notch from anterior to posterior. The close relationship between the iliopsoas tendon and the anterior aspect of the joint is easily appreciated. **(Bottom)** More laterally the cross section of the "hip socket" is seen completed by the transverse ligament inferiorly. A small anterior perilabral recess is present and the anterior labrum is absent. The depression of the fovea capitis can be appreciated on the femoral head.

Hip and Pelvis

V

SAGITTAL T1 FS MR ARTHROGRAM

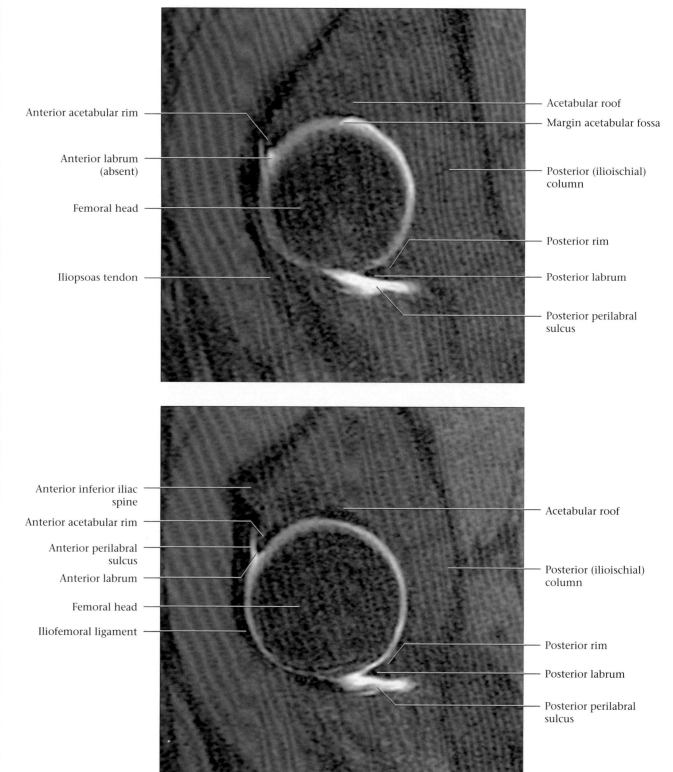

Anterior acetabular rim

Anterior labrum (absent)

Femoral head

Iliopsoas tendon

Acetabular roof

Margin acetabular fossa

Posterior (ilioischial) column

Posterior rim

Posterior labrum

Posterior perilabral sulcus

Anterior inferior iliac spine

Anterior acetabular rim

Anterior perilabral sulcus

Anterior labrum

Femoral head

Iliofemoral ligament

Acetabular roof

Posterior (ilioischial) column

Posterior rim

Posterior labrum

Posterior perilabral sulcus

(**Top**) The sharp margin of the articular cartilage at the edge of the acetabular fossa should not be confused with an articular cartilage defect. Anterior to the margin of the fossa the femoral and acetabular cartilage blend together imperceptibly. The posterior perilabral sulcus is quite prominent. (**Bottom**) On this image a small anterior labrum is seen on the anterior acetabular rim. The posterior labrum is well seen on the tip of the posterior acetabular rim and a prominent posterior perilabral sulcus is present. The attachment of the iliofemoral ligament to the anterior inferior iliac spine is well seen.

SAGITTAL T1 FS MR ARTHROGRAM

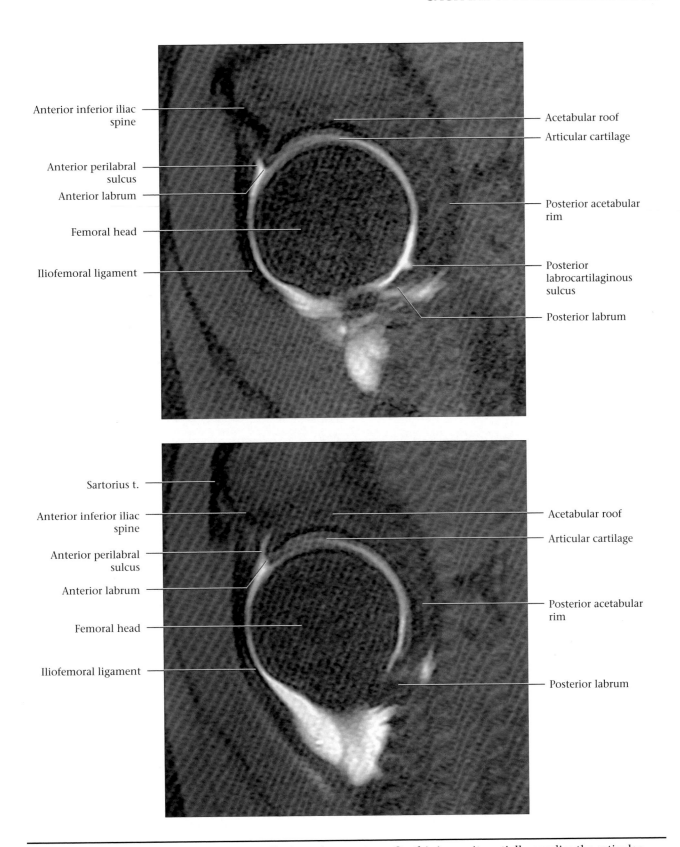

Anterior inferior iliac spine

Anterior perilabral sulcus

Anterior labrum

Femoral head

Iliofemoral ligament

Acetabular roof

Articular cartilage

Posterior acetabular rim

Posterior labrocartilaginous sulcus

Posterior labrum

Sartorius t.

Anterior inferior iliac spine

Anterior perilabral sulcus

Anterior labrum

Femoral head

Iliofemoral ligament

Acetabular roof

Articular cartilage

Posterior acetabular rim

Posterior labrum

(Top) The anterior labrum is visible as a small triangular structure. On this image it partially overlies the articular cartilage. A small perilabral recess is present. The articular cartilage of the femoral head and acetabulum are visible as separate structures. A small posterior labrocartilaginous sulcus is present. (Bottom) The anterior inferior iliac spine is visible. The attachment of the iliofemoral ligament to the spine is nicely demonstrated. A small anterior perilabral sulcus is present.

Hip and Pelvis

V

SAGITTAL T1 FS MR ARTHROGRAM

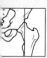

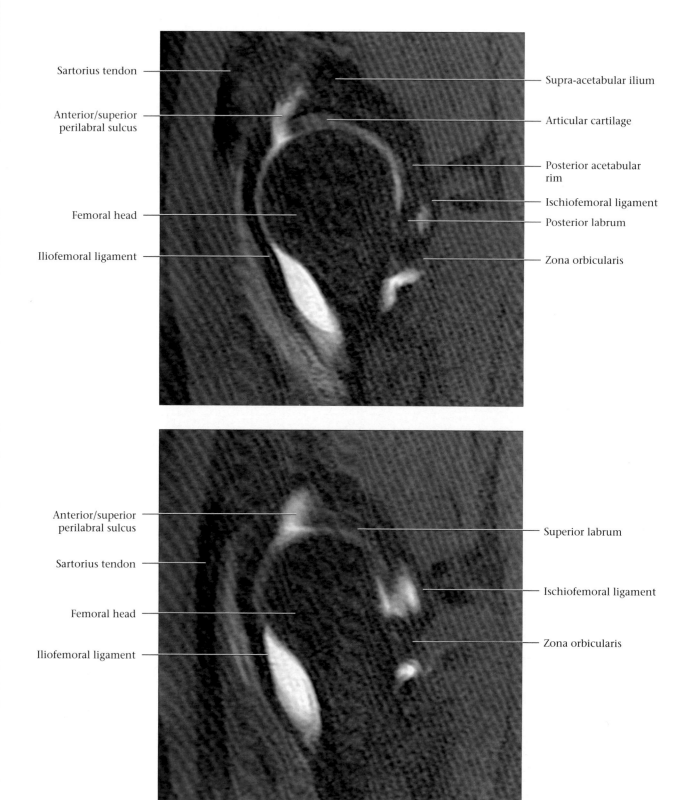

Sartorius tendon — Supra-acetabular ilium

Anterior/superior perilabral sulcus — Articular cartilage

Posterior acetabular rim

Ischiofemoral ligament

Femoral head — Posterior labrum

Iliofemoral ligament — Zona orbicularis

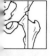

Anterior/superior perilabral sulcus — Superior labrum

Sartorius tendon

Ischiofemoral ligament

Femoral head

Iliofemoral ligament — Zona orbicularis

(Top) Note the thick iliofemoral ligament. This ligament must be pierced for successful joint puncture. On this image slight infiltration of the ligament with contrast is visible. **(Bottom)** The course of the superior labrum over the top of the femoral head is well appreciated on this image. Recognition of the labrum on sagittal images is crucial for determining the full anterior to posterior extent of labral tears. Cross referencing between images will aid in identification of the labrum in this plane. The circular fibers of the zona orbicularis can be well seen.

Hip and Pelvis

HIP JOINT

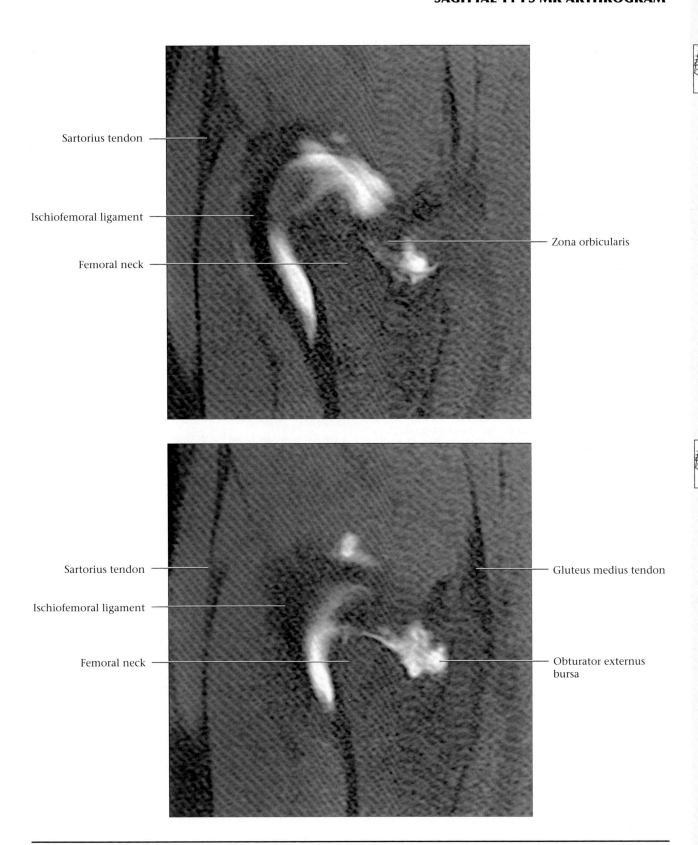

(Top) The ischiofemoral ligament is the most lateral of the external capsular ligaments. It passes from posterior to anterior at the lateral margin of the joint. **(Bottom)** The obturator externus bursa is an outpouching of the synovium beneath the inferior border of the obturator externus muscle (see "Lateral Hip" section). The anterior capsular insertion extends more laterally than the posterior capsular insertion.

Hip and Pelvis

V

THIGH OVERVIEW

Terminology

Abbreviations
- Anterior superior iliac spine (ASIS)
- Function (F)
- Muscle insertion (I)
- Nerve supply (N)
- Muscle origin (O)
- Structure supplied by a nerve or vessel (S)
- Sacroiliac joint (SI)

Imaging Anatomy

Compartment Anatomy
- **Compartmental anatomy is different from functional groupings below**
- Thigh divided into anterior, medial, and posterior compartments
  - **Anterior compartment**: Iliotibial tract, tensor fascia lata m., quadriceps ms., sartorius m.
  - **Medial compartment**: Gracilis m., adductor ms.
  - **Posterior compartment**: Hamstring ms., short head of biceps femoris m., sciatic n.
- Muscles at junction pelvis/thigh: Each considered separate compartment
  - Pectineus, iliopsoas, obturator externus, lateral femoral ms.
- Extensions from fascia lata divide compartments
  - Medial intermuscular septum: Anterior/medial
  - Lateral intermuscular septum: Anterior/lateral
  - Thin fascia separates medial, posterior compartments
- Clinical note: Compartment anatomy critical to tumor staging & biopsy planning
  - Cross compartment extension of tumor, contamination by biopsy requires change from limb salvage to amputation

Medial Femoral Muscles
- Common nerve: Obturator n., except pectineus m.
  - Anterior division: Adductor brevis & longus, gracilis muscles
  - Posterior division: Adductor portion adductor magnus m.
- Common function: Hip adduction; assist hip flexion, internal rotation
  - Except obturator externus m.
- Pre-axial muscles
- **Adductor brevis**
  - O: Inferior pubic ramus
  - I: Inferior 2/3 pectineal line, superior 1/2 medial lip linea aspera
- **Adductor longus**
  - O: Pubic body inferior to crest
  - I: Medial lip linea aspera
- **Adductor magnus**: Two separate muscles with different innervations & functions
  - Adductor portion
    - O: Ischiopubic ramus
    - I: Gluteal tuberosity, medial lip linea aspera, medial supracondylar line
  - Ischiocondylar portion: See "Posterior Femoral Muscles"
  - Adductor hiatus between 2 divisions of muscle in distal thigh
- **Gracilis**
  - O: Inferior pubic ramus, symphysis pubis
  - I: Medial proximal tibia (pes anserine)
  - F: Also assists knee flexion
- **Obturator externus**
  - O: External margins obturator foramen & membrane
  - I: Piriformis fossa
  - F: Hip external rotation only
- **Pectineus**
  - O: Superior pubic ramus, pecten
  - I: Pectineal line femur
  - Femoral n. ± accessory obturator n.
  - Unclear pre- or post-axial muscle
- See "Anterior Pelvis and Thigh" section

Anterior Femoral Muscles
- Common innervation: Femoral nerve
- Common function: Knee extension
  - Except sartorius m.
- Post-axial muscles
- **Articularis genu**
  - O: Anterior lower femur
  - I: Synovial membrane knee
  - N. to vastus intermedius
- **Rectus femoris**
  - O: Straight head - anterior inferior iliac spine, reflected head - groove above acetabulum
  - I: Superior patella, tibial tuberosity
  - F: Also hip flexion
  - Crosses 2 joints
- **Sartorius**: (Tailor's m.)
  - O: ASIS, notch below
  - I: Proximal medial tibia (pes anserine)
  - F: Hip flexion, abduction, external rotation; knee flexion
  - Crosses 2 joints
  - Longest muscle in body
  - Separate fascial covering
- **Vastus lateralis**
  - O: Superior intertrochanteric line femur, anterior & inferior greater trochanter, gluteal tuberosity, lateral lip linea aspera, lateral intermuscular septum
  - I: Lateral tibial condyle (lateral patellar retinaculum) superolateral patella (quadriceps tendon)
    - See "Extensor Mechanism and Retinacula" section
  - Largest quadriceps muscle
- **Vastus medialis**
  - O: Entire medial lip linea aspera, inferior intertrochanteric line, medial intermuscular septum
  - I: Tendon rectus femoris m., superomedial patella (quadriceps tendon), medial condyle tibia (medial patellar retinaculum)
    - See "Extensor Mechanism and Retinacula" section
- **Vastus intermedius**
  - O: Anterior & lateral femoral shaft, inferior lateral lip linea aspera, lateral intermuscular septum
  - I: Blends along deep aspect rectus femoris, vastus medialis, vastus lateralis ms.

THIGH OVERVIEW

- **Quadriceps femoris**: Rectus femoris, vastus lateralis, vastus medialis, vastus intermedius ms.
  - Common tendon of insertion onto superior, lateral, medial patella

Posterior Femoral Muscles

- Common nerve: Sciatic n.
  - Tibial division: Long head biceps femoris, semitendinosus, semimembranosus, ischiocondylar portion adductor magnus ms.
  - Common peroneal division: Short head biceps femoris m.
- Common functions: Hip extension, knee flexion
- Pre-axial muscles except short head biceps femoris m.
- **Biceps femoris**
  - Long head: O - ischial tuberosity (inferior, medial)
    - Common tendon with semitendinosus m.
  - Short head: O - lateral lip linea aspera femur, lateral supracondylar line, lateral intermuscular septum
    - Post-axial muscle
    - Not part of hamstring ms.
  - I: Fibular head, lateral condyle tibia
  - F: Also external rotation flexed knee
- **Semimembranosus**
  - O: Ischial tuberosity (superior, lateral)
  - I: Posterior medial condyle tibia, popliteal fascia
    - Some fibers extend to form oblique popliteal l. (see "Medial Support Systems" section)
  - F: Also internal rotation flexed knee
  - Membranous in upper thigh
- **Semitendinosus**
  - O: Ischial tuberosity (inferior, medial)
    - Common tendon long head biceps femoris m.
  - I: Medial proximal tibia (pes anserine)
  - F: Also internal rotation flexed knee
  - Entirely tendinous in distal thigh
- **Ischiocondylar portion of adductor magnus**
  - O: Ischial tuberosity
  - I: Adductor tubercle
  - Medial-most aspect adductor magnus m.
- **Hamstrings**: Long head biceps femoris, semimembranous, semitendinosus, ischiocondylar portion adductor magnus ms.
  - Does not include short head biceps femoris m.

Lateral Femoral (Gluteal) Muscles

- (See "Lateral Hip" section)

Other

- **Pes anserine** (see "Knee Overview" section)
  - Common aponeurosis for insertion gracilis, semitendinosus, sartorius tendons
  - Pes anserine bursa between tendons & tibia
- **Iliotibial tract/band:** Lateral thickening fascia lata
  - O: Tubercle iliac crest
  - I: Lateral condyle tibia
  - Insertion site tensor fascia lata m., portion of gluteus maximus m.

Hip Flexors

- Sartorius: Anterior femoral muscle
- Pectineus: Medial femoral muscle
- **Iliopsoas**: I - lesser trochanter
  - Iliacus

  - O: Iliac crest, iliac fossa, sacral ala, SI joint capsule
  - Femoral n.
- Psoas major
  - O: lateral vertebral body & intervertebral discs T12-L5, all lumbar transverse processes
  - L1, L2, L3
- Psoas minor
  - O: lateral vertebral body T12, L1 & T12-L1 intervertebral disc
  - L1, L2

Femoral Triangle

- Anterior wall: Inguinal ligament
- Posterior wall: Adductor longus & pectineus ms. (medial), iliopsoas m. (lateral)
- Medial border: Adductor longus m.
- Lateral border: Sartorius m.
- Apex: Crossing adductor longus & sartorius ms.
- Contents: Femoral n. & branches, femoral vessels, lymph node (Cloquet node), femoral sheath
  - Structures lateral to medial at entrance: NAVeL
    - Nerve, Artery, Vein, Lymphatics
- Femoral artery/vein relationships
  - Entrance: Artery lateral
  - Apex: Artery anterior
- Femoral n. branches within triangle
  - Saphenous n., & n. to vastus medialis only branches to exit triangle
- **Femoral sheath**: Transversalis fascia covers vessels proximally
  - 3 compartments
    - Lateral: Artery
    - Middle: Vein
    - Medial: Lymph node (femoral canal)
- **Femoral canal**: Medial compartment femoral sheath
  - Anterior border: Inguinal ligament
  - Posterior border: Pubic bone
  - Medial border: Lacunar ligament
  - Lateral border: Femoral v.
  - Entrance: **Femoral ring**
    - Anterior border: Medial inguinal ligament
    - Posterior border: Superior pubic ramus
    - Medial border: Lacunar ligament
    - Lateral border: Septum between femoral canal & femoral v.
    - Open to peritoneal cavity
  - Contents: Lymphatic vessels & nodes (**Cloquet node**), fat, connective tissue
  - Clinical note: **Femoral hernia**
    - Lateral & inferior to pubic tubercle
    - Travels femoral ring to femoral canal to saphenous opening to subcutaneous tissue
    - More common in women
    - Strangulation at femoral ring
    - Inguinal hernias: See "Anterior Pelvis and Thigh"

Adductor (Subsartorial or Hunter) Canal

- Fascial passageway for vessels midthigh
  - Boundaries are fascial surfaces of adjacent muscles
- Anteromedial border: Sartorius m.
- Anterolateral border: Vastus medialis m.
- Posterior border: Adductor longus & magnus ms.
- Entrance: Apex femoral triangle
- Exit: Adductor hiatus

- **Adductor hiatus**: Gap adductor magnus m. between adductor portion & ischiocondylar portion distal thigh
- Vessel passageway from thigh to popliteal fossa
- Vessels travel caudad & posterior within hiatus
- Contents: Femoral a. & v., saphenous n.
  - Nerve initially anterior to artery then medial
  - Artery anterior to vein
  - Descending geniculate a. arises in canal

Femoral Vessels
- Enter thigh deep to inguinal ligament, midpoint between ASIS & symphysis pubis
  - Change from external iliac vessels to common femoral vessels
- Upper thigh: Vessels within femoral triangle
  - Enter: Artery lateral to vein
  - Exit: Artery anterior
- Mid thigh: Vessels within adductor canal
  - Entrance: Artery anterior
  - Exit: Artery anterior
- Distal thigh: Exit adductor canal via adductor hiatus, enter popliteal fossa
- **Common femoral artery branches**
  - **Superficial epigastric, superficial circumflex iliac, superficial external pudendal** arise anteriorly
  - **Deep external pudendal** arises medially
    - May branch from medial circumflex femoral
  - Divides into superficial & deep branches
  - **Superficial femoral artery**
    - Branch: **Descending genicular**
  - **Deep femoral (profunda femoris)**
    - Arises laterally in femoral triangle
    - Dives between pectineus & adductor longus ms.
    - Medial to femur, deep to adductor longus m.
    - Branches in femoral triangle: **Medial circumflex femoral** (main supply femoral head & neck), lateral circumflex femoral, muscular branches
    - Branches in adductor canal: 3 perforating branches, descending genicular
    - Terminal branch: 4th perforating artery
- **Femoral vein:** Travels with artery
  - Tributaries: Deep femoral, descending genicular, lateral circumflex femoral, medial circumflex femoral, deep external pudendal, greater saphenous vs.
  - **Greater saphenous vein**
    - Longest vein in body
    - Toes to saphenous opening (fascia lata)
    - Tributaries: Accessory saphenous, superficial epigastric, superficial circumflex femoral, superficial external pudendal veins

Femoral Nerve
- L2, L3, L4, L5; post-axial
- Largest branch lumbar plexus
- Exits plexus lower psoas m.
- Travels in groove between psoas & iliacus ms.
- Exits pelvis beneath inguinal ligament, lateral to femoral vessels, enters femoral triangle
- Multiple branches in femoral triangle
  - Muscular branches: To pectineus, sartorius, rectus femoris, vastus lateralis, vastus medialis, vastus intermedius ms.

- Cutaneous nerves: Anterior femoral cutaneous, saphenous
  - Saphenous n. exits triangle, enters adductor canal
- Articular branches hip & knee

Obturator Nerve
- L2, L3, L4; pre-axial
- Branch lumbar plexus
- Relationships
  - Posterior to iliac vessels
  - Medial to psoas m.
  - Lateral to internal iliac vessels
- Via obturator foramen to thigh
- S: Adductor ms., hip & knee joints, skin medial distal thigh
- Accessory obturator n: L3, L4
  - Present in 9%

Sciatic Nerve
- L4, L5, S1, S2, S3
- Largest branch sacral plexus
- Two nerves in one sheath
  - Tibial n. (medial) & common peroneal n. (lateral)
  - Separate in lower thigh
- Exits pelvis inferior to piriformis m.
  - Anomalous relationship in 10%
  - See "Posterior Pelvis" section
- Crosses over superior gemellus, obturator internus, inferior gemellus, quadratus femoris, adductor magnus muscles
- Deep to long head biceps femoris m.
- Branches arising in thigh: Articular to hip, nerves to hamstring ms.
- **Tibial nerve:** Larger division of sciatic n.
  - S: Posterior femoral ms. except short head biceps femoris m.
- **Common peroneal nerve**
  - Oblique lateral course with biceps femoris m.
  - S: Short head biceps femoris m.
- See "Knee Overview" section

Anatomy-Based Imaging Issues

Imaging Recommendations
- Radiographs
  - Femur: AP & lateral views
    - Use film diagonal to cover greatest length
    - Likely need separate upper & lower coverage
- CT
  - Best for evaluation of known osseous abnormality
  - Acquire 0.625-1.25 mm to improve reconstructions
    - Consider interleaved acquisition
    - Reconstructions: 2-3 mm
- MR
  - Sequences
    - T1 & STIR ideal long axis
    - Fat suppressed T2 for axial plane
  - Parameters
    - Long axis thigh(s): FOV 35-40 mm; THK 5 mm
    - Single extremity axial: FOV 20 mm; THK 5-8 mm
    - Matrix: 256 x 256

THIGH OVERVIEW

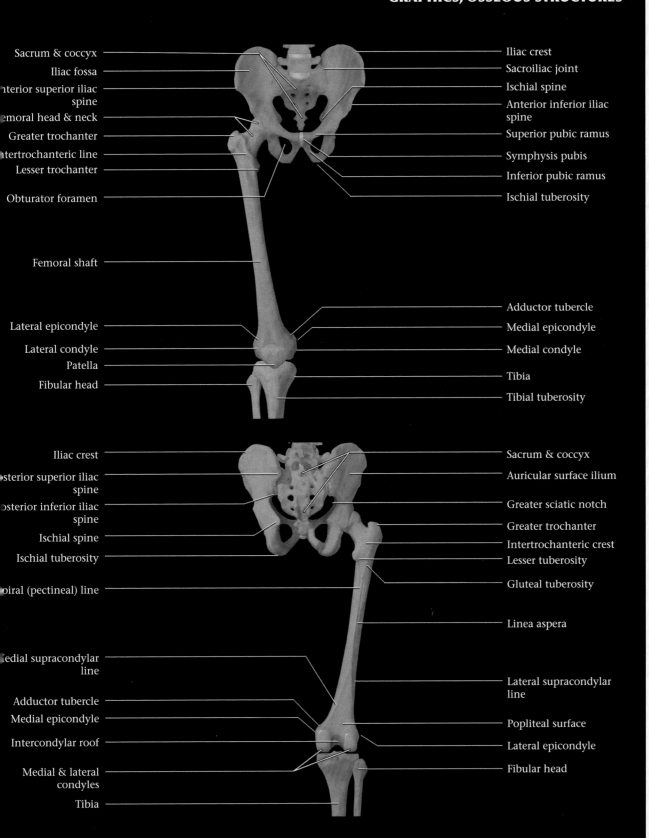

Sacrum & coccyx

Iliac fossa

Anterior superior iliac spine

Femoral head & neck

Greater trochanter

Intertrochanteric line

Lesser trochanter

Obturator foramen

Femoral shaft

Lateral epicondyle

Lateral condyle

Patella

Fibular head

Iliac crest

Sacroiliac joint

Ischial spine

Anterior inferior iliac spine

Superior pubic ramus

Symphysis pubis

Inferior pubic ramus

Ischial tuberosity

Adductor tubercle

Medial epicondyle

Medial condyle

Tibia

Tibial tuberosity

Iliac crest

Posterior superior iliac spine

Posterior inferior iliac spine

Ischial spine

Ischial tuberosity

Spiral (pectineal) line

Medial supracondylar line

Adductor tubercle

Medial epicondyle

Intercondylar roof

Medial & lateral condyles

Tibia

Sacrum & coccyx

Auricular surface ilium

Greater sciatic notch

Greater trochanter

Intertrochanteric crest

Lesser tuberosity

Gluteal tuberosity

Linea aspera

Lateral supracondylar line

Popliteal surface

Lateral epicondyle

Fibular head

(Top) Anterior view of the osseous structures of the pelvis and lower extremity. Note the downward tilt of the pelvis exposing the pelvic inlet. The obturator foramina reduce the bulk of the pelvis yet provide surface area for muscular origins. The ischial tuberosities are the weight bearing structures in the seated position. For more details of the structures surrounding the symphysis pubis see "Anterior Pelvis and Thigh" section. **(Bottom)** Posterior view of the osseous structures of the pelvis and lower extremity. A multitude of ridges are present along the posterior femur and serve as the sites of muscular origins and insertions. Note the posterior orientation of the lesser trochanter. The deep recess on the medial surface of the greater trochanter is the piriformis fossa, site of insertion of the external rotators of the hip.

GRAPHICS, MUSCLE ATTACHMENTS

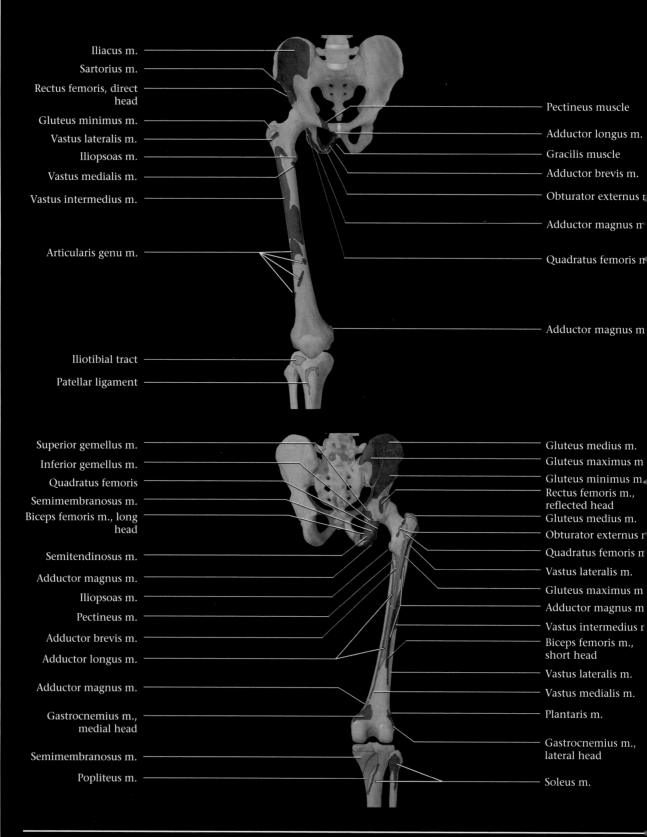

Iliacus m.

Sartorius m.

Rectus femoris, direct head

Gluteus minimus m.

Vastus lateralis m.

Iliopsoas m.

Vastus medialis m.

Vastus intermedius m.

Articularis genu m.

Iliotibial tract

Patellar ligament

Pectineus muscle

Adductor longus m.

Gracilis muscle

Adductor brevis m.

Obturator externus ι

Adductor magnus n

Quadratus femoris n

Adductor magnus m

Superior gemellus m.

Inferior gemellus m.

Quadratus femoris

Semimembranosus m.

Biceps femoris m., long head

Semitendinosus m.

Adductor magnus m.

Iliopsoas m.

Pectineus m.

Adductor brevis m.

Adductor longus m.

Adductor magnus m.

Gastrocnemius m., medial head

Semimembranosus m.

Popliteus m.

Gluteus medius m.

Gluteus maximus m

Gluteus minimus m.

Rectus femoris m., reflected head

Gluteus medius m.

Obturator externus ι

Quadratus femoris n

Vastus lateralis m.

Gluteus maximus m

Adductor magnus m

Vastus intermedius ι

Biceps femoris m., short head

Vastus lateralis m.

Vastus medialis m.

Plantaris m.

Gastrocnemius m., lateral head

Soleus m.

(Top) Muscle and ligament attachments of the anterior pelvis and femur. The vastus muscles are the primary musc arising from the anterior femur. The complex relationship of the adductor muscle origins at the symphysis pubis is presented in greater detail in the "Anterior Pelvis and Thigh" section. **(Bottom)** Muscle and ligament attachments o the posterior pelvis and femur. At the ischial tuberosity the semimembranosus muscle origin is superior and lateral the semitendinosus and long head of the biceps muscle origins. The gemelli muscles arise from the ischial spine. T sacrospinous ligament attaches to the medial aspect of the spine (not labeled). The adductor brevis muscle insertio is superior to the adductor longus muscle. The adductor magnus muscle insertion is lateral to the adductor longus muscle insertion. The gluteus maximus muscle has the most lateral insertion.

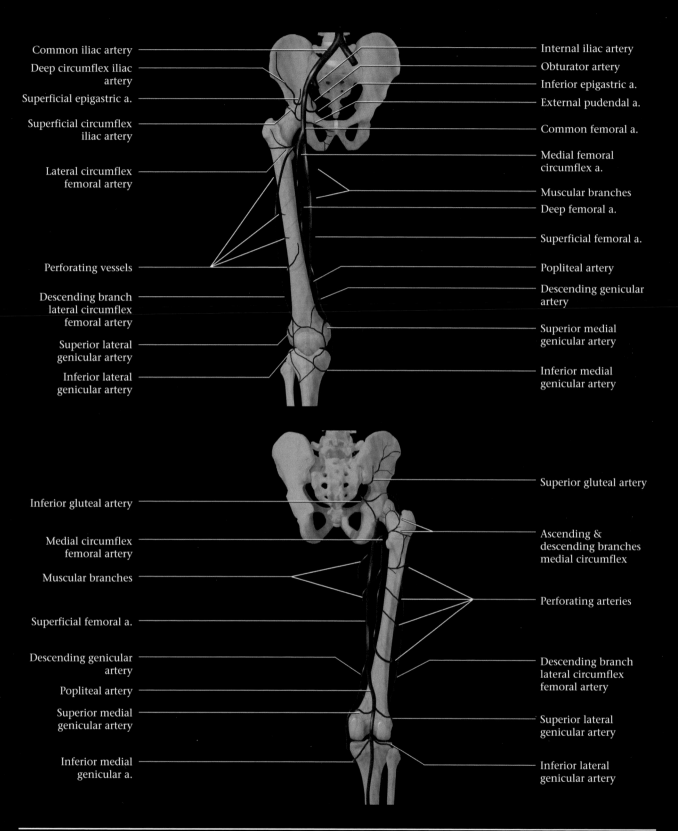

Common iliac artery

Deep circumflex iliac artery

Superficial epigastric a.

Superficial circumflex iliac artery

Lateral circumflex femoral artery

Perforating vessels

Descending branch lateral circumflex femoral artery

Superior lateral genicular artery

Inferior lateral genicular artery

Internal iliac artery

Obturator artery

Inferior epigastric a.

External pudendal a.

Common femoral a.

Medial femoral circumflex a.

Muscular branches

Deep femoral a.

Superficial femoral a.

Popliteal artery

Descending genicular artery

Superior medial genicular artery

Inferior medial genicular artery

Inferior gluteal artery

Medial circumflex femoral artery

Muscular branches

Superficial femoral a.

Descending genicular artery

Popliteal artery

Superior medial genicular artery

Inferior medial genicular a.

Superior gluteal artery

Ascending & descending branches medial circumflex

Perforating arteries

Descending branch lateral circumflex femoral artery

Superior lateral genicular artery

Inferior lateral genicular artery

(Top) Anterior view of the external iliac, femoral and popliteal arteries and their branches. **(Bottom)** Posterior view of the femoral and popliteal arteries and the superior and inferior gluteal arteries of the greater sciatic notch.

THIGH OVERVIEW

GRAPHICS, VEINS OF THIGH

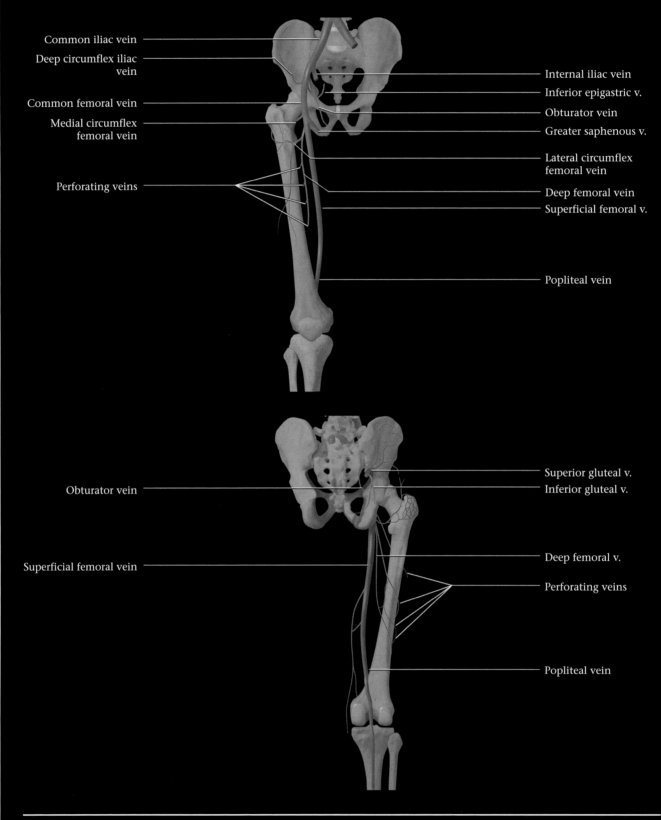

Common iliac vein

Deep circumflex iliac vein

Common femoral vein

Medial circumflex femoral vein

Perforating veins

Internal iliac vein

Inferior epigastric v.

Obturator vein

Greater saphenous v.

Lateral circumflex femoral vein

Deep femoral vein

Superficial femoral v.

Popliteal vein

Obturator vein

Superficial femoral vein

Superior gluteal v.

Inferior gluteal v.

Deep femoral v.

Perforating veins

Popliteal vein

(Top) Anterior view of the veins of the thigh. The veins typically follow the arterial tree. The main venous drainage is the superficial femoral vein which is actually a deep venous structure. Note the entrance of the greater saphenous vein into the femoral vein; it has no associated artery. **(Bottom)** Posterior view of the veins of the thigh and buttocks. The veins generally follow the arterial tree although more variability is seen within the venous system.

THIGH OVERVIEW

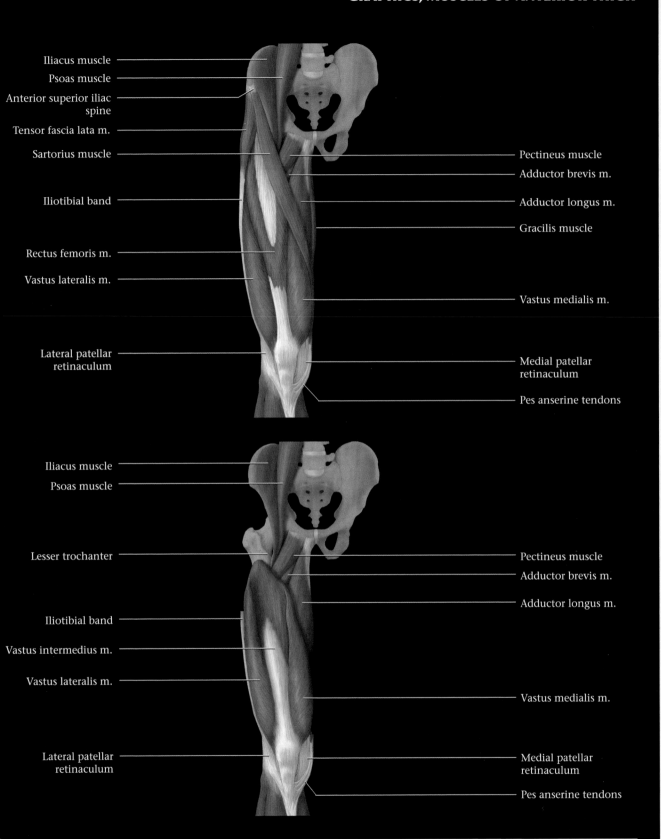

Iliacus muscle
Psoas muscle
Anterior superior iliac spine
Tensor fascia lata m.
Sartorius muscle
Iliotibial band
Rectus femoris m.
Vastus lateralis m.
Lateral patellar retinaculum

Pectineus muscle
Adductor brevis m.
Adductor longus m.
Gracilis muscle
Vastus medialis m.
Medial patellar retinaculum
Pes anserine tendons

Iliacus muscle
Psoas muscle
Lesser trochanter
Iliotibial band
Vastus intermedius m.
Vastus lateralis m.
Lateral patellar retinaculum

Pectineus muscle
Adductor brevis m.
Adductor longus m.
Vastus medialis m.
Medial patellar retinaculum
Pes anserine tendons

Top) Superficial muscles of the anterior thigh. The oblique course of the sartorius muscle is easily appreciated. The adductor brevis muscle is deep to the adductor longus and pectineus muscles. The most medial muscle is the gracilis. The vastus lateralis and medialis muscles continue to their insertions as the lateral and medial patellar retinacula respectively. **(Bottom)** Deep muscles of the anterior thigh. The vastus intermedius muscle is deep to the rectus femoris muscle. The vastus intermedius tendon muscle blends with the rectus femoris tendon along its deep surface. The iliopsoas muscle dives deep after crossing over the pelvic brim. With removal of the sartorius muscle a little more of the adductor brevis muscle is visible. The pes anserine tendons, the gracilis, sartorius and semitendinosus, have a conjoined insertion onto the proximal medial tibia.

THIGH OVERVIEW

GRAPHICS, MUSCLES OF POSTERIOR THIGH

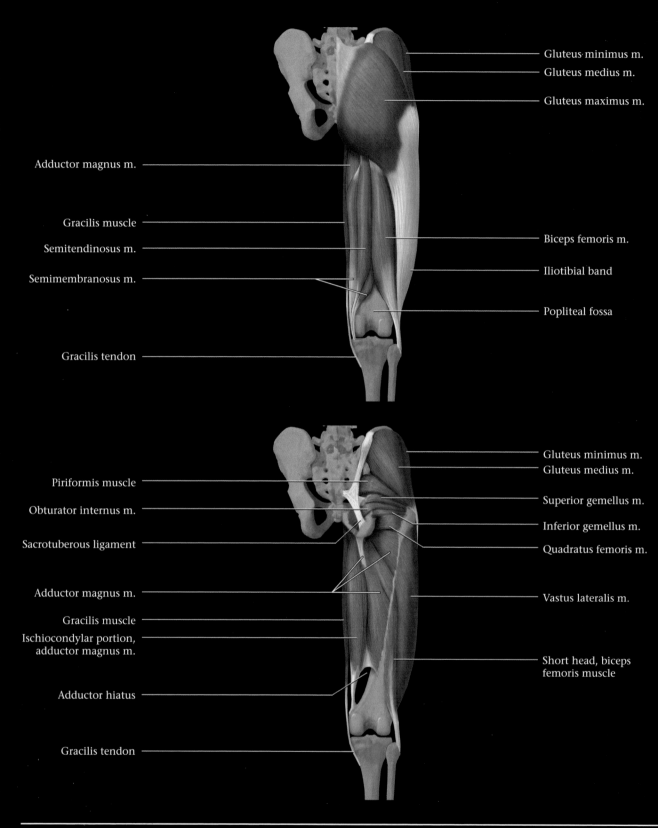

Gluteus minimus m.

Gluteus medius m.

Gluteus maximus m.

Adductor magnus m.

Gracilis muscle

Semitendinosus m.

Semimembranosus m.

Biceps femoris m.

Iliotibial band

Popliteal fossa

Gracilis tendon

Piriformis muscle

Obturator internus m.

Sacrotuberous ligament

Adductor magnus m.

Gracilis muscle

Ischiocondylar portion, adductor magnus m.

Adductor hiatus

Gracilis tendon

Gluteus minimus m.

Gluteus medius m.

Superior gemellus m.

Inferior gemellus m.

Quadratus femoris m.

Vastus lateralis m.

Short head, biceps femoris muscle

(Top) Superficial muscles of the posterior thigh. The gluteus muscles from anterior to posterior and deep to superficial are gluteus minimus, medius and maximus. The semitendinosus muscle is superficial to the semimembranosus muscle. At their origins the semimembranous muscle is more lateral as seen under the inferior edge of the gluteus maximus muscle. **(Bottom)** Deep muscles of the posterior thigh. With removal of the hamstring muscles the expansive adductor magnus muscle is visible. The separation of its two heads in the distal thigh forms the adductor hiatus. The external rotators of the hip arise from the posterior pelvis and insert in the piriformis fossa. The muscles are discussed in the "Lateral Hip" section. Note the piriformis muscle which fills the greater sciatic foramen and the obturator internus muscle within the lesser sciatic foramen.

THIGH OVERVIEW

GRAPHICS, MEDIAL PELVIS & THIGH

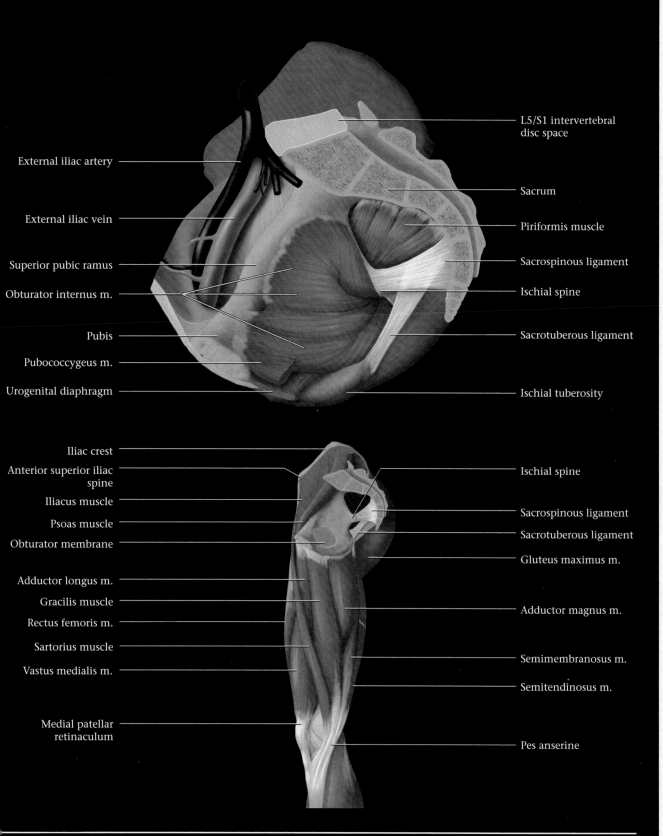

External iliac artery

External iliac vein

Superior pubic ramus

Obturator internus m.

Pubis

Pubococcygeus m.

Urogenital diaphragm

L5/S1 intervertebral disc space

Sacrum

Piriformis muscle

Sacrospinous ligament

Ischial spine

Sacrotuberous ligament

Ischial tuberosity

Iliac crest

Anterior superior iliac spine

Iliacus muscle

Psoas muscle

Obturator membrane

Adductor longus m.

Gracilis muscle

Rectus femoris m.

Sartorius muscle

Vastus medialis m.

Medial patellar retinaculum

Ischial spine

Sacrospinous ligament

Sacrotuberous ligament

Gluteus maximus m.

Adductor magnus m.

Semimembranosus m.

Semitendinosus m.

Pes anserine

(Top) Medial view of the pelvis muscles. The obturator internus muscle has an extensive origin from the inner aspect of the pelvis and then funnels through the lesser sciatic notch before turning laterally to the piriformis fossa. The greater sciatic notch is filled with the piriformis muscle. (Bottom) Medial muscles of the thigh. The gracilis muscle has a thin profile when viewed from the front, however when viewed from the side it is quite broad. The semimembranosus muscle runs along the deep surface of the semitendinous muscle and inserts onto the tibia posterior to the pes anserine tendons. Its insertion is hidden on this image. The iliopsoas muscle courses over the pelvic brim on its course to the lesser trochanter.

THIGH OVERVIEW

GRAPHICS, NERVES OF THIGH

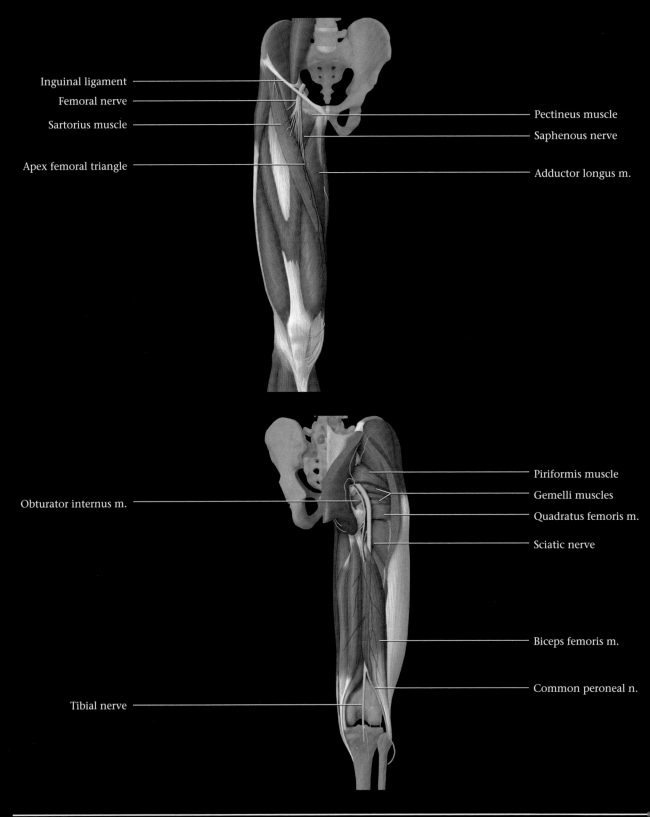

Inguinal ligament

Femoral nerve

Sartorius muscle

Apex femoral triangle

Pectineus muscle

Saphenous nerve

Adductor longus m.

Obturator internus m.

Piriformis muscle

Gemelli muscles

Quadratus femoris m.

Sciatic nerve

Biceps femoris m.

Common peroneal n.

Tibial nerve

(Top) Femoral nerve. After emerging from the groove between the psoas and iliacus muscles the nerve passes under the inguinal ligament to enter the femoral triangle. It immediately branches into muscular, cutaneous, & articular nerves. The only nerve to pass through the femoral triangle into the adductor canal is the saphenous nerve.
(Bottom) Sciatic nerve. The sciatic nerve enters the lower extremity by passing under the inferior border of the piriformis muscle. That anatomy is presented in greater detail in the "Posterior Pelvis" section. The sciatic nerve passes posterior to the external rotator tendons and then courses deep to the biceps femoris muscle. It separates into the tibial and common peroneal nerves in the distal thigh. The tibial nerve bisects the popliteal fossa. The common peroneal nerve follows the biceps femoris muscle around the fibular head.

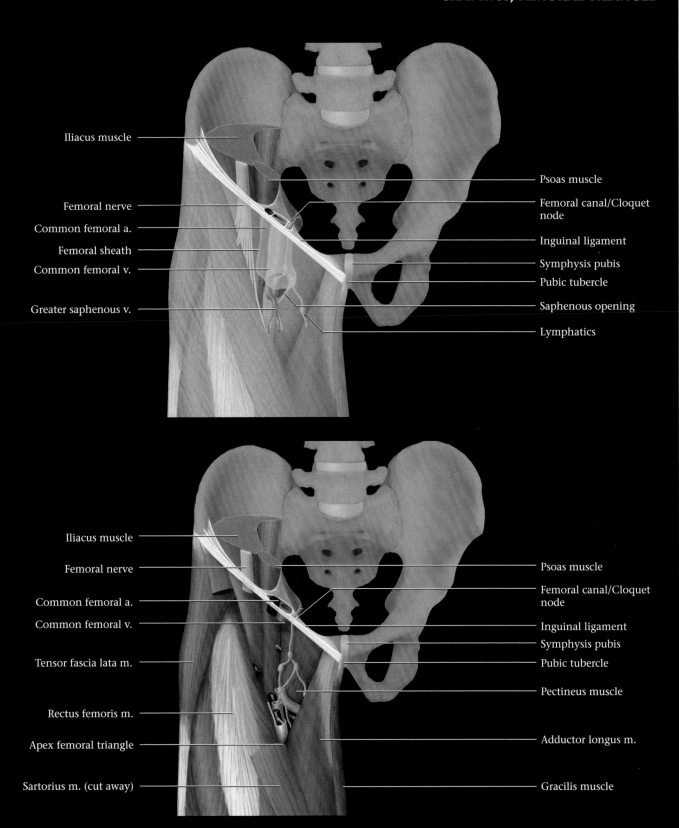

Iliacus muscle

Femoral nerve

Common femoral a.

Femoral sheath

Common femoral v.

Greater saphenous v.

Psoas muscle

Femoral canal/Cloquet node

Inguinal ligament

Symphysis pubis

Pubic tubercle

Saphenous opening

Lymphatics

Iliacus muscle

Femoral nerve

Common femoral a.

Common femoral v.

Tensor fascia lata m.

Rectus femoris m.

Apex femoral triangle

Sartorius m. (cut away)

Psoas muscle

Femoral canal/Cloquet node

Inguinal ligament

Symphysis pubis

Pubic tubercle

Pectineus muscle

Adductor longus m.

Gracilis muscle

(Top) The contents of the femoral triangle from lateral to medial (NAVeL) are femoral nerve, femoral artery & vein, lymphatics. The nerve lies superficial to the iliopsoas muscle. The lateral border of the triangle is the sartorius muscle. The anterior wall is the inguinal ligament. The fascia lata encases the structures of the thigh. The femoral sheath is the fascial covering over the proximal vessels. At the cut away proximal boundary note the septa dividing the sheath into compartments. The femoral canal is the medial compartment. **(Bottom)** Femoral triangle after removal of the fascia lata, sartorius muscle and the vessels. The apex of the triangle is at the crossing of sartorius and adductor longus muscles. The pectineus, adductor longus and iliopsoas muscles form the floor of the triangle.

THIGH OVERVIEW

RADIOGRAPHS, UPPER FEMUR

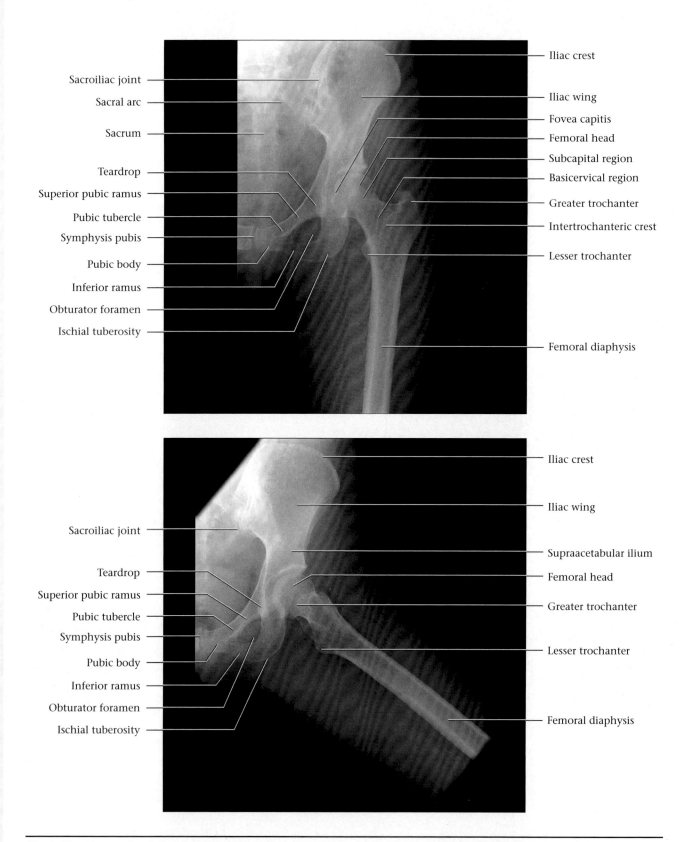

Sacroiliac joint

Sacral arc

Sacrum

Teardrop

Superior pubic ramus

Pubic tubercle

Symphysis pubis

Pubic body

Inferior ramus

Obturator foramen

Ischial tuberosity

Iliac crest

Iliac wing

Fovea capitis

Femoral head

Subcapital region

Basicervical region

Greater trochanter

Intertrochanteric crest

Lesser trochanter

Femoral diaphysis

Sacroiliac joint

Teardrop

Superior pubic ramus

Pubic tubercle

Symphysis pubis

Pubic body

Inferior ramus

Obturator foramen

Ischial tuberosity

Iliac crest

Iliac wing

Supraacetabular ilium

Femoral head

Greater trochanter

Lesser trochanter

Femoral diaphysis

(Top) AP radiograph of the proximal femur. Note the regions of the proximal femur: The subcapital region at the junction of the femoral head and neck, the basicervical region at the base of the femoral neck. For descriptive purposes fractures between the basicervical and subcapital oregions are referred to as transcervical (not labeled). In a well positioned AP femur the lesser trochanter points medial and posterior. The intertrochanteric crest, a posterior prominence connecting the two trochanters, is visible. The fovea capitis appears as a central depression on the femoral head. **(Bottom)** Lateral view of the proximal femur. With external rotation the lesser trochanter is now seen in profile, its inferior cortex blending with the cortex of the adjacent femoral neck. The femoral head, neck and greater trochanter are all overlapping.

THIGH OVERVIEW

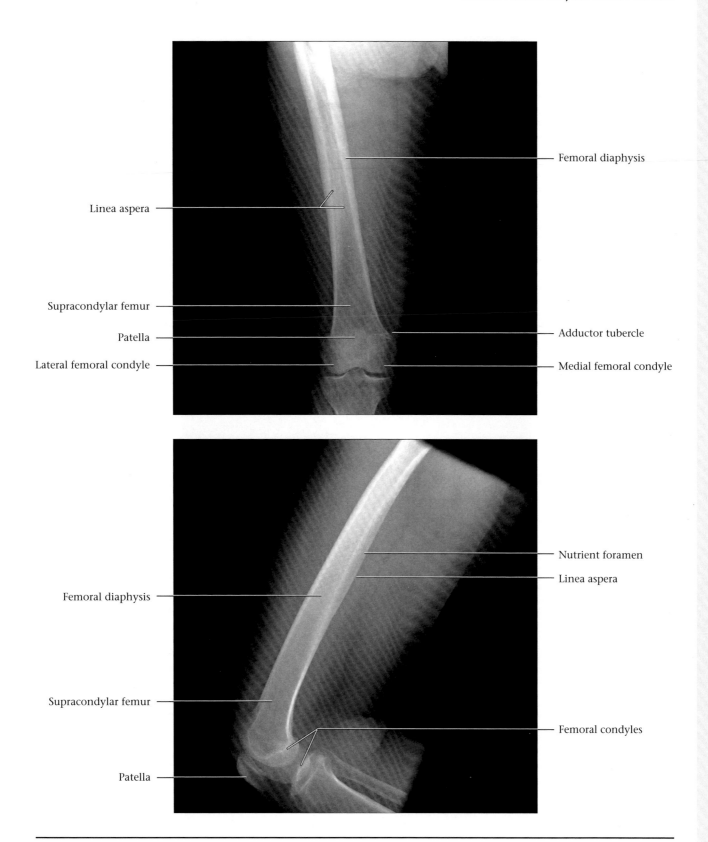

Femoral diaphysis

Linea aspera

Supracondylar femur

Patella

Lateral femoral condyle

Adductor tubercle

Medial femoral condyle

Nutrient foramen

Linea aspera

Femoral diaphysis

Supracondylar femur

Femoral condyles

Patella

(Top) AP radiograph of the distal femur. The anatomy is less complex than the proximal femur. The lips of the linea aspera are well visualized in this patient. The adductor tubercle is located just above the medial femoral condyle. The supracondylar region is a frequent site of fracture. **(Bottom)** Lateral radiograph of the distal femur. The thickened cortex of the linea aspera is apparent. A nutrient foramen (vascular channel) is also visible. The blood will enter the cortex and flow proximally. "To the elbow I go and from the knee I flee" will help one to remember the orientation of a vascular channel. The femoral condyles can be identified if the patella femoral groove can be seen on the lateral femoral condyle. In general the medial condyle is more rounded than the lateral. A more detailed description of the knee can be found in the "Knee Overview" section.

Hip and Pelvis

V

THIGH OVERVIEW

COMPARTMENTS OF THIGH

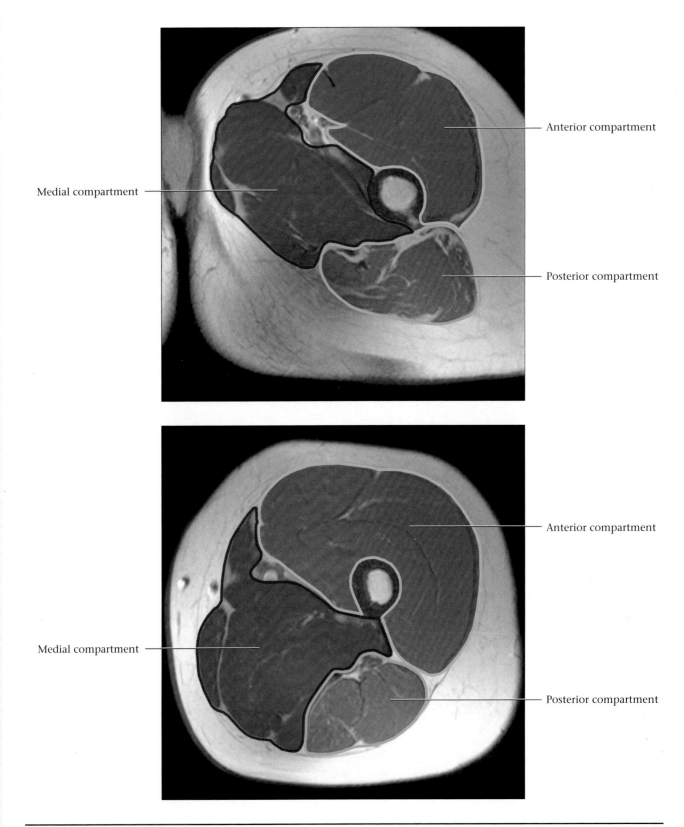

Anterior compartment

Medial compartment

Posterior compartment

Anterior compartment

Medial compartment

Posterior compartment

(Top) Compartment anatomy of the upper thigh. The femoral vessels and the femur are extracompartmental.
(Bottom) Compartment anatomy upper mid thigh. The sciatic nerve is located within the posterior compartment.

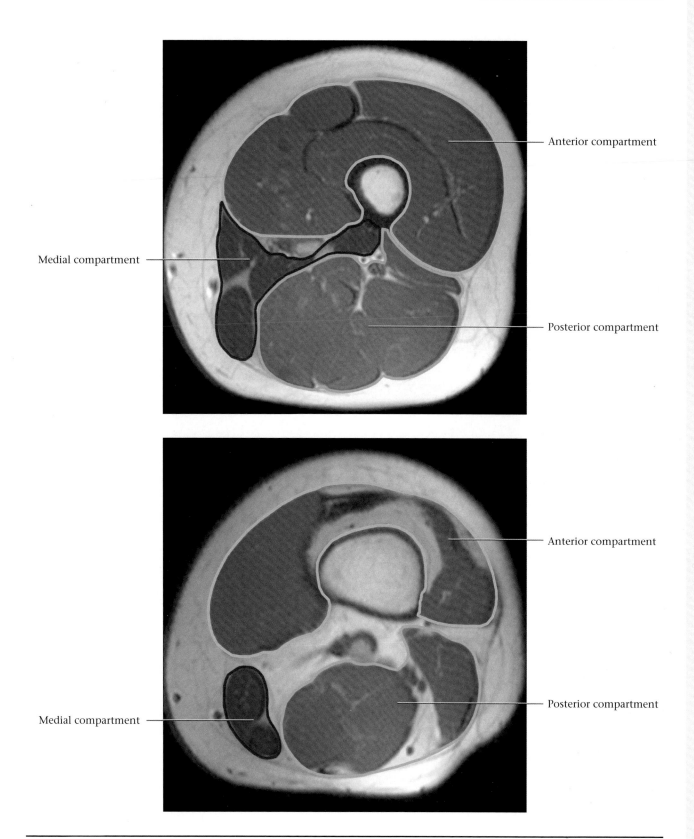

Anterior compartment

Medial compartment

Posterior compartment

Anterior compartment

Posterior compartment

Medial compartment

(Top) Compartmental anatomy lower mid thigh. At this level the medial compartment is quite small. The anterior and posterior compartments remain similar in size. **(Bottom)** Compartmental anatomy distal thigh. Most of the muscles of the medial compartment have already inserted onto the femur. Significant extracompartmental fat exists and extracompartmental extension of tumor is likely at this level.

THIGH OVERVIEW

AXIAL T1 MR, UPPER RIGHT THIGH

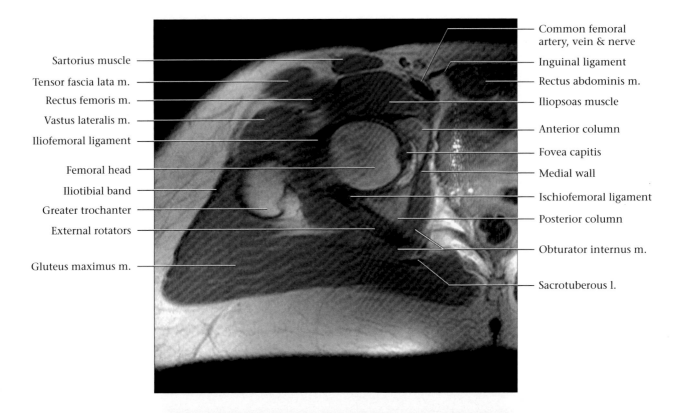

Sartorius muscle — Common femoral artery, vein & nerve
Tensor fascia lata m. — Inguinal ligament
Rectus femoris m. — Rectus abdominis m.
Vastus lateralis m. — Iliopsoas muscle
Iliofemoral ligament — Anterior column
Femoral head — Fovea capitis
Iliotibial band — Medial wall
Greater trochanter — Ischiofemoral ligament
External rotators — Posterior column
Gluteus maximus m. — Obturator internus m.
Sacrotuberous l.

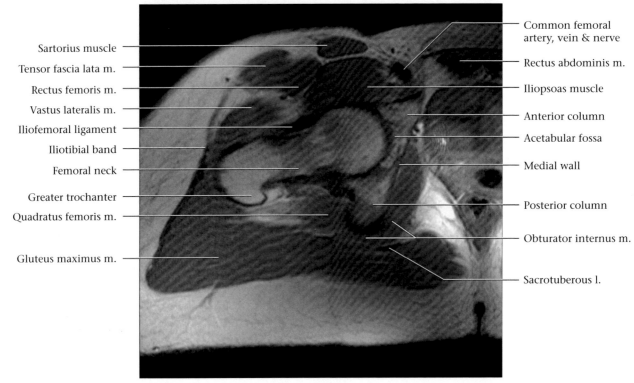

Sartorius muscle — Common femoral artery, vein & nerve
Tensor fascia lata m. — Rectus abdominis m.
Rectus femoris m. — Iliopsoas muscle
Vastus lateralis m. — Anterior column
Iliofemoral ligament — Acetabular fossa
Iliotibial band — Medial wall
Femoral neck — Posterior column
Greater trochanter — Obturator internus m.
Quadratus femoris m. — Sacrotuberous l.
Gluteus maximus m.

(Top) Axial images of the thigh from superior to inferior. The thigh begins at the inguinal ligament and the external surfaces of the pelvis. The superior-most aspect of the lower extremity is detailed in the "Hip Overview" section. This series of images begins at the inferior medial aspect of the inguinal ligament. The external iliac vessels have just entered the femoral triangle and become the common femoral vessels. The iliotibial band is present between the tensor fascia lata and gluteus maximus muscles. The obturator internus muscle has traveled through the lesser sciatic foramen and changed direction in the buttocks as it courses to the piriformis fossa. (Bottom) The sacrotuberous ligament is visible along the deep surface of the gluteus maximus muscle. The vastus lateralis muscle has the most proximal origin of the vastus muscles.

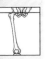

THIGH OVERVIEW

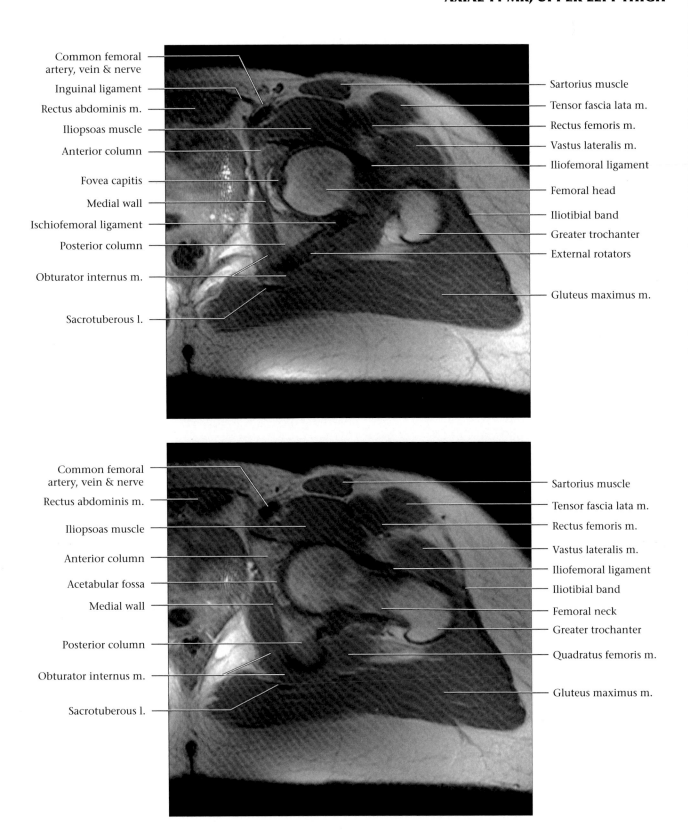

Top image labels (left):
- Common femoral artery, vein & nerve
- Inguinal ligament
- Rectus abdominis m.
- Iliopsoas muscle
- Anterior column
- Fovea capitis
- Medial wall
- Ischiofemoral ligament
- Posterior column
- Obturator internus m.
- Sacrotuberous l.

Top image labels (right):
- Sartorius muscle
- Tensor fascia lata m.
- Rectus femoris m.
- Vastus lateralis m.
- Iliofemoral ligament
- Femoral head
- Iliotibial band
- Greater trochanter
- External rotators
- Gluteus maximus m.

Bottom image labels (left):
- Common femoral artery, vein & nerve
- Rectus abdominis m.
- Iliopsoas muscle
- Anterior column
- Acetabular fossa
- Medial wall
- Posterior column
- Obturator internus m.
- Sacrotuberous l.

Bottom image labels (right):
- Sartorius muscle
- Tensor fascia lata m.
- Rectus femoris m.
- Vastus lateralis m.
- Iliofemoral ligament
- Iliotibial band
- Femoral neck
- Greater trochanter
- Quadratus femoris m.
- Gluteus maximus m.

(Top) Axial images of the thigh from superior to inferior. The thigh begins at the inguinal ligament and the external surfaces of the pelvis. The superior-most aspect of the lower extremity is detailed in the "Hip Overview" section. This series of images begins at the inferior medial aspect of the inguinal ligament. The external iliac vessels have just entered the femoral triangle and become the common femoral vessels. The iliotibial band is present between the tensor fascia lata and gluteus maximus muscles. The obturator internus muscle has traveled through the lesser sciatic foramen and changed direction in the buttocks as it courses to the piriformis fossa. **(Bottom)** The sacrotuberous ligament is visible along the deep surface of the gluteus maximus muscle. The vastus lateralis muscle has the most proximal origin of the vastus muscles.

Hip and Pelvis

V

THIGH OVERVIEW

AXIAL T1 MR, UPPER RIGHT THIGH

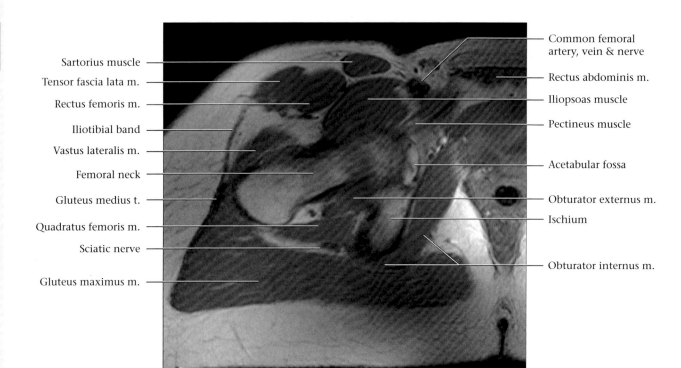

Sartorius muscle

Tensor fascia lata m.

Rectus femoris m.

Iliotibial band

Vastus lateralis m.

Femoral neck

Gluteus medius t.

Quadratus femoris m.

Sciatic nerve

Gluteus maximus m.

Common femoral artery, vein & nerve

Rectus abdominis m.

Iliopsoas muscle

Pectineus muscle

Acetabular fossa

Obturator externus m.

Ischium

Obturator internus m.

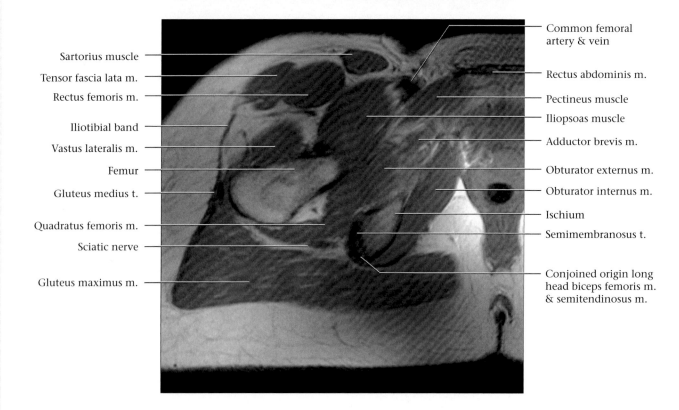

Sartorius muscle

Tensor fascia lata m.

Rectus femoris m.

Iliotibial band

Vastus lateralis m.

Femur

Gluteus medius t.

Quadratus femoris m.

Sciatic nerve

Gluteus maximus m.

Common femoral artery & vein

Rectus abdominis m.

Pectineus muscle

Iliopsoas muscle

Adductor brevis m.

Obturator externus m.

Obturator internus m.

Ischium

Semimembranosus t.

Conjoined origin long head biceps femoris m. & semitendinosus m.

(Top) On the more previous images the sciatic nerve was not distinguishable from the adjacent musculature. On this image it is now seen as a discrete structure. The tensor fascia lata and sartorius muscles are on a divergent course heading laterally and medially respectively. **(Bottom)** The obturator internus and externus muscles are seen on the respective surfaces of the obturator foramen. The obturator membrane separates the muscles. The iliopsoas muscle is tapering towards its insertion onto the lesser trochanter. The gluteus maximus muscle continues its significant coverage of the inferior aspect of the buttocks.

AXIAL T1 MR, UPPER LEFT THIGH

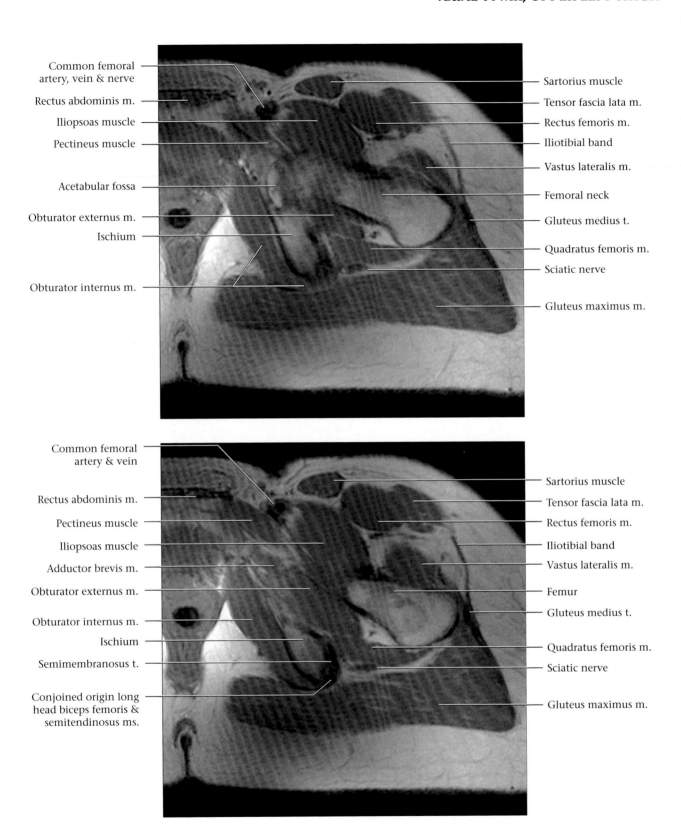

Common femoral artery, vein & nerve — Sartorius muscle

Rectus abdominis m. — Tensor fascia lata m.

Iliopsoas muscle — Rectus femoris m.

Pectineus muscle — Iliotibial band

— Vastus lateralis m.

Acetabular fossa — Femoral neck

Obturator externus m. — Gluteus medius t.

Ischium — Quadratus femoris m.

— Sciatic nerve

Obturator internus m. — Gluteus maximus m.

Common femoral artery & vein — Sartorius muscle

Rectus abdominis m. — Tensor fascia lata m.

Pectineus muscle — Rectus femoris m.

Iliopsoas muscle — Iliotibial band

Adductor brevis m. — Vastus lateralis m.

Obturator externus m. — Femur

Obturator internus m. — Gluteus medius t.

Ischium — Quadratus femoris m.

Semimembranosus t. — Sciatic nerve

Conjoined origin long head biceps femoris & semitendinosus ms. — Gluteus maximus m.

(Top) On the more previous images the sciatic nerve was not distinguishable from the adjacent musculature. On this image it is now seen as a discrete structure. The tensor fascia lata and sartorius muscles are on a divergent course heading laterally and medially respectively. **(Bottom)** The obturator internus and externus muscles are seen on the respective surfaces of the obturator foramen. The obturator membrane separates the muscles. The iliopsoas muscle is tapering towards its insertion onto the lesser trochanter. The gluteus maximus muscle continues its significant coverage of the inferior aspect of the buttocks.

Hip and Pelvis

V

THIGH OVERVIEW

AXIAL T1 MR, UPPER RIGHT THIGH

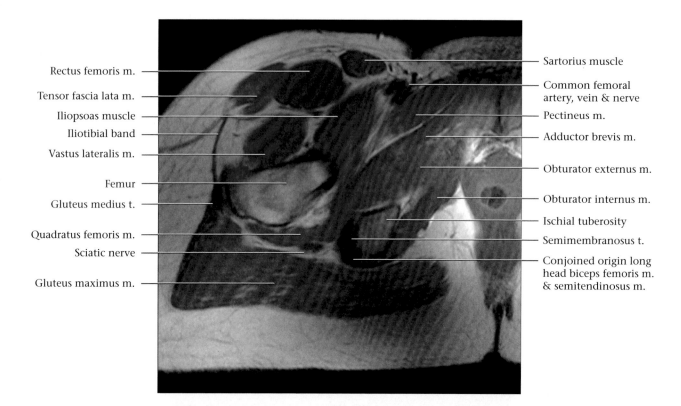

Rectus femoris m.
Tensor fascia lata m.
Iliopsoas muscle
Iliotibial band
Vastus lateralis m.
Femur
Gluteus medius t.
Quadratus femoris m.
Sciatic nerve
Gluteus maximus m.

Sartorius muscle
Common femoral artery, vein & nerve
Pectineus m.
Adductor brevis m.
Obturator externus m.
Obturator internus m.
Ischial tuberosity
Semimembranosus t.
Conjoined origin long head biceps femoris m. & semitendinosus m.

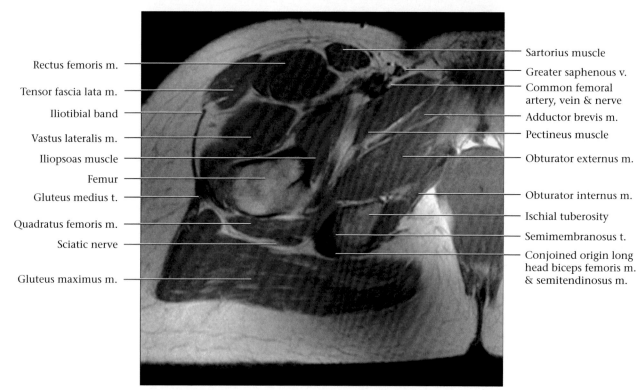

Rectus femoris m.
Tensor fascia lata m.
Iliotibial band
Vastus lateralis m.
Iliopsoas muscle
Femur
Gluteus medius t.
Quadratus femoris m.
Sciatic nerve
Gluteus maximus m.

Sartorius muscle
Greater saphenous v.
Common femoral artery, vein & nerve
Adductor brevis m.
Pectineus muscle
Obturator externus m.
Obturator internus m.
Ischial tuberosity
Semimembranosus t.
Conjoined origin long head biceps femoris m. & semitendinosus m.

(Top) The more superior and lateral origin of the semimembranosus muscle from the external surface of the ischial tuberosity and the more inferior and medial conjoined origin of the semitendinous and long head of the biceps femoris muscles are visible. The adductor brevis muscles lies deep to the pectineus muscle. **(Bottom)** The greater saphenous vein is feeding into the common femoral vein. The gluteus medius tendon has its insertion along the lateral facet of the greater trochanter. Except for the gluteus maximus muscle the quadratus femoris muscle is the most inferior of the external rotators of the hip and is recognized by its horizontal orientation deep to the gluteus maximus muscle.

THIGH OVERVIEW

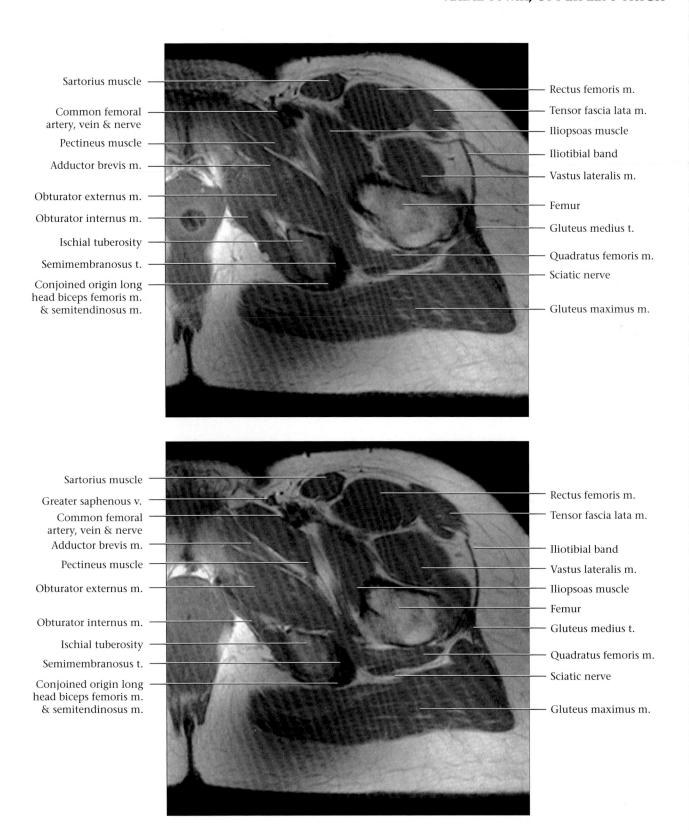

Top image labels (left):
- Sartorius muscle
- Common femoral artery, vein & nerve
- Pectineus muscle
- Adductor brevis m.
- Obturator externus m.
- Obturator internus m.
- Ischial tuberosity
- Semimembranosus t.
- Conjoined origin long head biceps femoris m. & semitendinosus m.

Top image labels (right):
- Rectus femoris m.
- Tensor fascia lata m.
- Iliopsoas muscle
- Iliotibial band
- Vastus lateralis m.
- Femur
- Gluteus medius t.
- Quadratus femoris m.
- Sciatic nerve
- Gluteus maximus m.

Bottom image labels (left):
- Sartorius muscle
- Greater saphenous v.
- Common femoral artery, vein & nerve
- Adductor brevis m.
- Pectineus muscle
- Obturator externus m.
- Obturator internus m.
- Ischial tuberosity
- Semimembranosus t.
- Conjoined origin long head biceps femoris m. & semitendinosus m.

Bottom image labels (right):
- Rectus femoris m.
- Tensor fascia lata m.
- Iliotibial band
- Vastus lateralis m.
- Iliopsoas muscle
- Femur
- Gluteus medius t.
- Quadratus femoris m.
- Sciatic nerve
- Gluteus maximus m.

(Top) The more superior and lateral origin of the semimembranosus muscle from the external surface of the ischial tuberosity and the more inferior and medial conjoined origin of the semitendinous and long head of the biceps femoris muscles are visible. The adductor brevis muscles lies deep to the pectineus muscle. **(Bottom)** The greater saphenous vein is feeding into the common femoral vein. The gluteus medius tendon has its insertion along the lateral facet of the greater trochanter. Except for the gluteus maximus muscle the quadratus femoris muscle is the most inferior of the external rotators of the hip and is recognized by its horizontal orientation deep to the gluteus maximus muscle.

THIGH OVERVIEW

AXIAL T1 MR, UPPER RIGHT THIGH

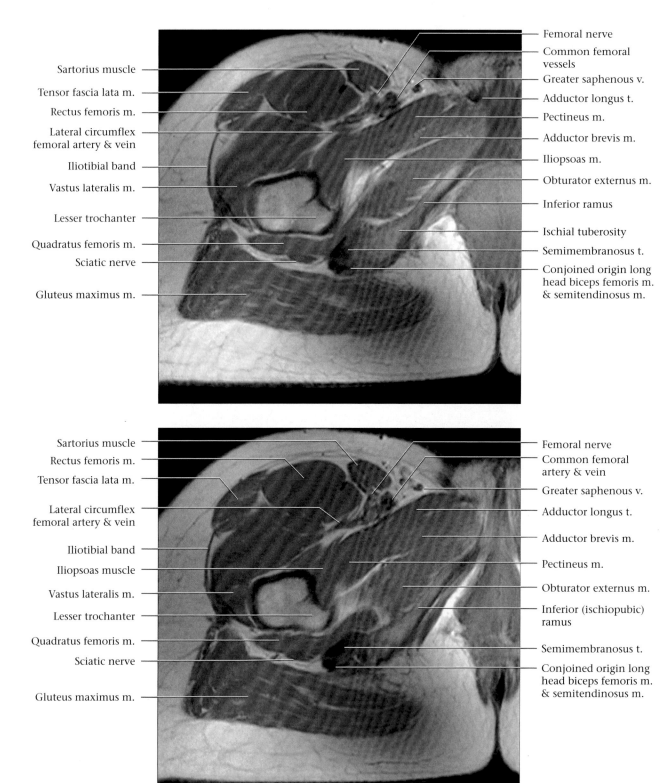

Sartorius muscle — Femoral nerve
Tensor fascia lata m. — Common femoral vessels
Rectus femoris m. — Greater saphenous v.
Lateral circumflex femoral artery & vein — Adductor longus t.
Iliotibial band — Pectineus m.
Vastus lateralis m. — Adductor brevis m.
Lesser trochanter — Iliopsoas m.
Quadratus femoris m. — Obturator externus m.
Sciatic nerve — Inferior ramus
Gluteus maximus m. — Ischial tuberosity
— Semimembranosus t.
— Conjoined origin long head biceps femoris m. & semitendinosus m.

Sartorius muscle — Femoral nerve
Rectus femoris m. — Common femoral artery & vein
Tensor fascia lata m. — Greater saphenous v.
Lateral circumflex femoral artery & vein — Adductor longus t.
Iliotibial band — Adductor brevis m.
Iliopsoas muscle — Pectineus m.
Vastus lateralis m. — Obturator externus m.
Lesser trochanter — Inferior (ischiopubic) ramus
Quadratus femoris m. — Semimembranosus t.
Sciatic nerve — Conjoined origin long head biceps femoris m. & semitendinosus m.
Gluteus maximus m.

(Top) The origin of the adductor longus muscle is via a small tendon from the pubic body. The adductor longus and pectineus muscle lie in the same plane and thus occupy the same position as images move from superior to inferior. This transition is demonstrated on these two images. **(Bottom)** The iliopsoas muscle inserts onto the lesser trochanter. The lateral circumflex femoral artery courses deep to the sartorius and rectus femoris muscles. Note the movement of the semimembranosus tendon from a more lateral to an anterior position relative to the semitendinosus and long head biceps femoris tendons.

THIGH OVERVIEW

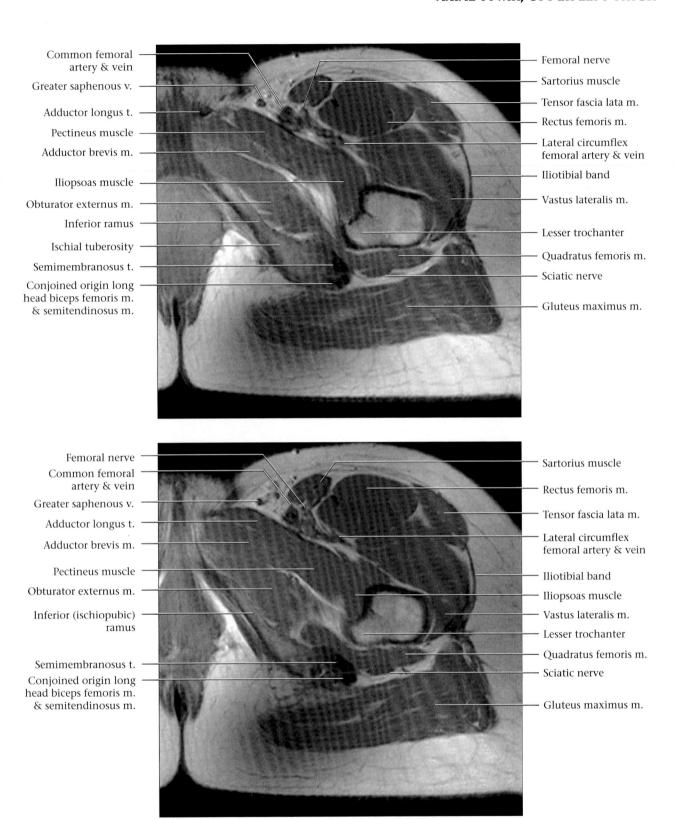

Top image labels (left):
- Common femoral artery & vein
- Greater saphenous v.
- Adductor longus t.
- Pectineus muscle
- Adductor brevis m.
- Iliopsoas muscle
- Obturator externus m.
- Inferior ramus
- Ischial tuberosity
- Semimembranosus t.
- Conjoined origin long head biceps femoris m. & semitendinosus m.

Top image labels (right):
- Femoral nerve
- Sartorius muscle
- Tensor fascia lata m.
- Rectus femoris m.
- Lateral circumflex femoral artery & vein
- Iliotibial band
- Vastus lateralis m.
- Lesser trochanter
- Quadratus femoris m.
- Sciatic nerve
- Gluteus maximus m.

Bottom image labels (left):
- Femoral nerve
- Common femoral artery & vein
- Greater saphenous v.
- Adductor longus t.
- Adductor brevis m.
- Pectineus muscle
- Obturator externus m.
- Inferior (ischiopubic) ramus
- Semimembranosus t.
- Conjoined origin long head biceps femoris m. & semitendinosus m.

Bottom image labels (right):
- Sartorius muscle
- Rectus femoris m.
- Tensor fascia lata m.
- Lateral circumflex femoral artery & vein
- Iliotibial band
- Iliopsoas muscle
- Vastus lateralis m.
- Lesser trochanter
- Quadratus femoris m.
- Sciatic nerve
- Gluteus maximus m.

(Top) The origin of the adductor longus muscle is via a small tendon from the pubic body. The adductor longus and pectineus muscle lie in the same plane and thus occupy the same position as images move from superior to inferior. This transition is demonstrated on these two images. **(Bottom)** The iliopsoas muscle inserts onto the lesser trochanter. The lateral circumflex femoral artery courses deep to the sartorius and rectus femoris muscles. Note the movement of the semimembranosus tendon from a more lateral to an anterior position relative to the semitendinosus and long head biceps femoris tendons.

Hip and Pelvis

V

THIGH OVERVIEW

AXIAL T1 MR, UPPER RIGHT THIGH

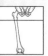

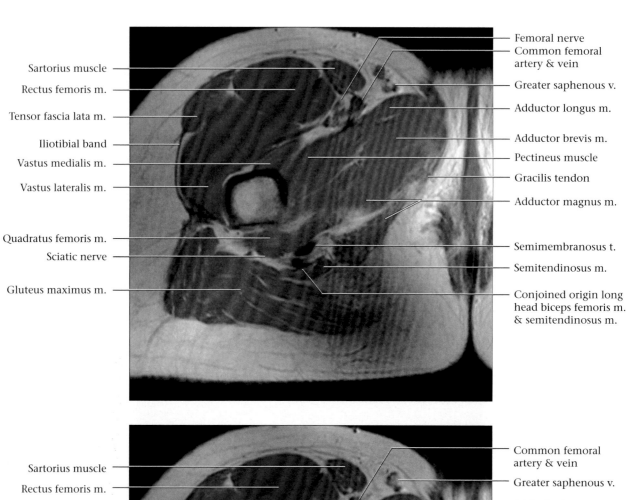

Sartorius muscle
Rectus femoris m.
Tensor fascia lata m.
Iliotibial band
Vastus medialis m.
Vastus lateralis m.
Quadratus femoris m.
Sciatic nerve
Gluteus maximus m.

Femoral nerve
Common femoral artery & vein
Greater saphenous v.
Adductor longus m.
Adductor brevis m.
Pectineus muscle
Gracilis tendon
Adductor magnus m.
Semimembranosus t.
Semitendinosus m.
Conjoined origin long head biceps femoris m. & semitendinosus m.

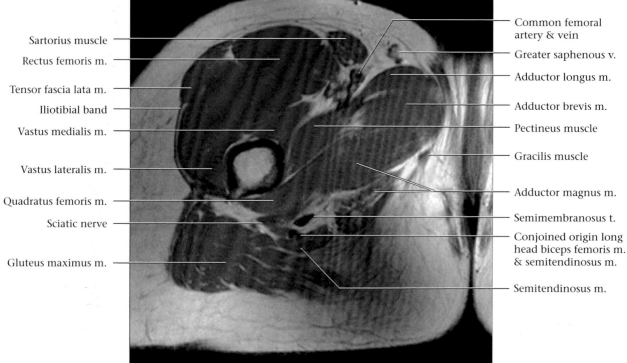

Sartorius muscle
Rectus femoris m.
Tensor fascia lata m.
Iliotibial band
Vastus medialis m.
Vastus lateralis m.
Quadratus femoris m.
Sciatic nerve
Gluteus maximus m.

Common femoral artery & vein
Greater saphenous v.
Adductor longus m.
Adductor brevis m.
Pectineus muscle
Gracilis muscle
Adductor magnus m.
Semimembranosus t.
Conjoined origin long head biceps femoris m. & semitendinosus m.
Semitendinosus m.

(Top) As images move more inferiorly the greater saphenous vein assumes a more superficial position. The vastus medialis origin from the proximal femoral diaphysis is seen and is deep to the vastus lateralis at this level. This is the most inferior image on which the femoral nerve can be identified. It branches entirely within the femoral triangle. The two origins of the adductor magnus muscle are visible. The more anterior adductor portion originates from the inferior pubic ramus, the more posterior portion of the muscle originates from the ischial tuberosity. **(Bottom)** The changing orientation between the semimembranosus and the other hamstring tendons continues. The semimembranosus tendon is now more medially positioned. These are the first images on which the thin gracilis tendon is visible. It is partial volumed with other structures above this level.

THIGH OVERVIEW

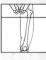

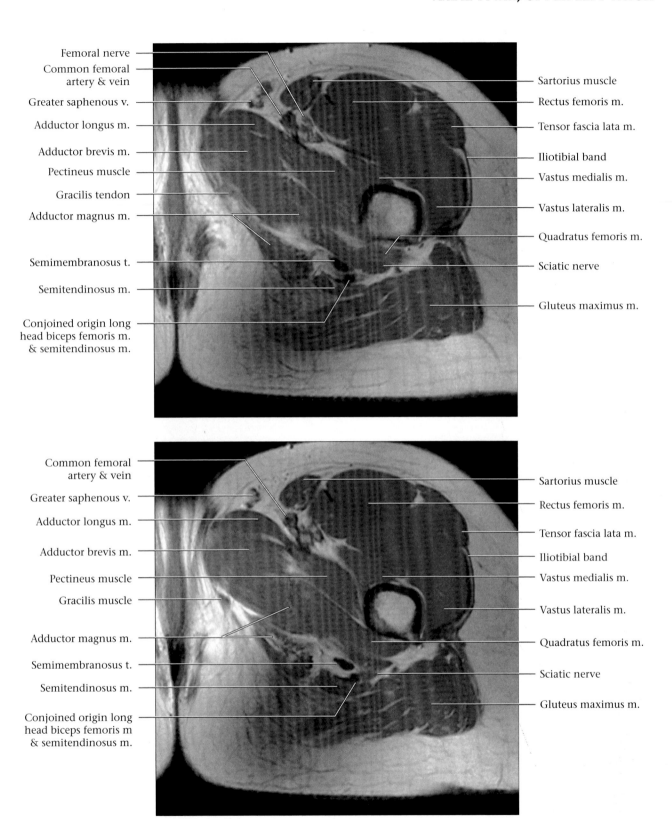

Femoral nerve
Common femoral artery & vein
Greater saphenous v.
Adductor longus m.
Adductor brevis m.
Pectineus muscle
Gracilis tendon
Adductor magnus m.
Semimembranosus t.
Semitendinosus m.
Conjoined origin long head biceps femoris m. & semitendinosus m.

Sartorius muscle
Rectus femoris m.
Tensor fascia lata m.
Iliotibial band
Vastus medialis m.
Vastus lateralis m.
Quadratus femoris m.
Sciatic nerve
Gluteus maximus m.

Common femoral artery & vein
Greater saphenous v.
Adductor longus m.
Adductor brevis m.
Pectineus muscle
Gracilis muscle
Adductor magnus m.
Semimembranosus t.
Semitendinosus m.
Conjoined origin long head biceps femoris m & semitendinosus m.

Sartorius muscle
Rectus femoris m.
Tensor fascia lata m.
Iliotibial band
Vastus medialis m.
Vastus lateralis m.
Quadratus femoris m.
Sciatic nerve
Gluteus maximus m.

(Top) As images move more inferiorly the greater saphenous vein assumes a more superficial position. The vastus medialis origin from the proximal femoral diaphysis is seen and is deep to the vastus lateralis at this level. This is the most inferior image on which the femoral nerve can be identified. It branches entirely within the femoral triangle. The two origins of the adductor magnus muscle are visible. The more anterior adductor portion originates from the inferior pubic ramus, the more posterior portion of the muscle originates from the ischial tuberosity. **(Bottom)** The changing orientation between the semimembranosus and the other hamstring tendons continues. The semimembranosus tendon is now more medially positioned. These are the first images on which the thin gracilis tendon is visible. It is partial volumed with other structures above this level.

Hip and Pelvis ∨

215

THIGH OVERVIEW

AXIAL T1 MR, UPPER RIGHT THIGH

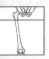

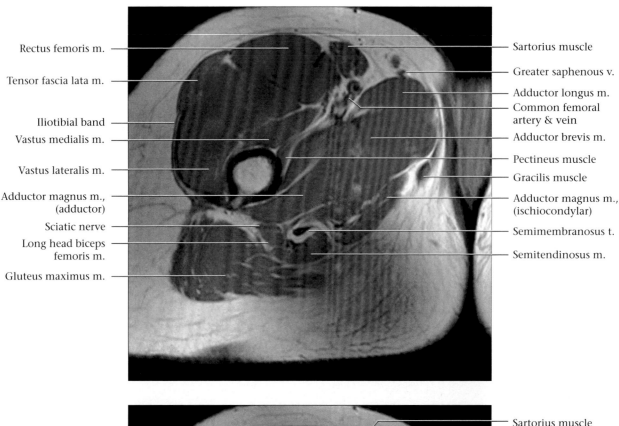

Rectus femoris m.

Tensor fascia lata m.

Iliotibial band

Vastus medialis m.

Vastus lateralis m.

Adductor magnus m., (adductor)

Sciatic nerve

Long head biceps femoris m.

Gluteus maximus m.

Sartorius muscle

Greater saphenous v.

Adductor longus m.

Common femoral artery & vein

Adductor brevis m.

Pectineus muscle

Gracilis muscle

Adductor magnus m., (ischiocondylar)

Semimembranosus t.

Semitendinosus m.

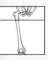

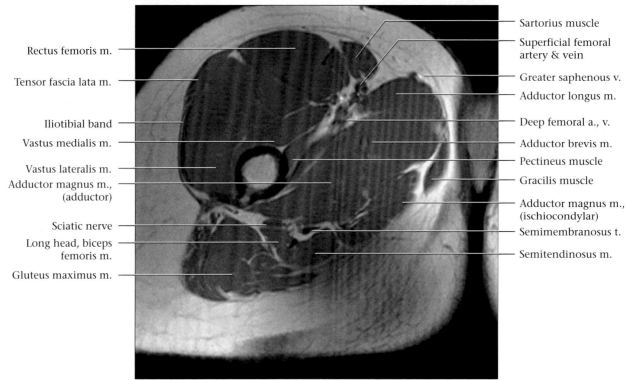

Rectus femoris m.

Tensor fascia lata m.

Iliotibial band

Vastus medialis m.

Vastus lateralis m.

Adductor magnus m., (adductor)

Sciatic nerve

Long head, biceps femoris m.

Gluteus maximus m.

Sartorius muscle

Superficial femoral artery & vein

Greater saphenous v.

Adductor longus m.

Deep femoral a., v.

Adductor brevis m.

Pectineus muscle

Gracilis muscle

Adductor magnus m., (ischiocondylar)

Semimembranosus t.

Semitendinosus m.

(Top) In the upper thigh the rectus femoris tendon is present along the anterior aspect of the muscle. The muscle bellies of the semitendinosus and long head of the biceps femoris muscles are now present. **(Bottom)** The common femoral vessels have divided into superficial and deep femoral vessels. The gracilis muscle is now visible. The tensor fascia lata muscle has assumed a more flattened profile. Thin slips of the pectineus and adductor brevis muscles are present as they insert along the posterior femur.

THIGH OVERVIEW

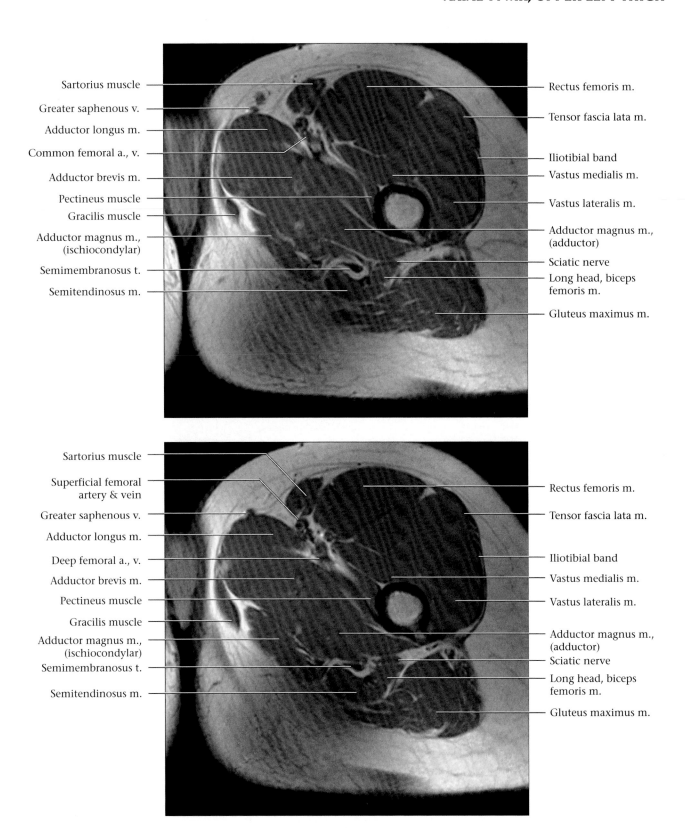

Sartorius muscle — Rectus femoris m.

Greater saphenous v. — Tensor fascia lata m.

Adductor longus m.

Common femoral a., v. — Iliotibial band
— Vastus medialis m.

Adductor brevis m.

Pectineus muscle — Vastus lateralis m.

Gracilis muscle

Adductor magnus m., — Adductor magnus m.,
(ischiocondylar) (adductor)

Semimembranosus t. — Sciatic nerve
— Long head, biceps
Semitendinosus m. femoris m.

— Gluteus maximus m.

Sartorius muscle

Superficial femoral
artery & vein — Rectus femoris m.

Greater saphenous v. — Tensor fascia lata m.

Adductor longus m.

Deep femoral a., v. — Iliotibial band

Adductor brevis m. — Vastus medialis m.

Pectineus muscle — Vastus lateralis m.

Gracilis muscle

Adductor magnus m., — Adductor magnus m.,
(ischiocondylar) (adductor)
— Sciatic nerve
Semimembranosus t. — Long head, biceps
femoris m.
Semitendinosus m.
— Gluteus maximus m.

(Top) In the upper thigh the rectus femoris tendon is present along the anterior aspect of the muscle. The muscle bellies of the semitendinosus and long head of the biceps femoris muscles are now present. **(Bottom)** The common femoral vessels have divided into superficial and deep femoral vessels. The gracilis muscle is now visible. The tensor fascia lata muscle has assumed a more flattened profile. Thin slips of the pectineus and adductor brevis muscles are present as they insert along the posterior femur.

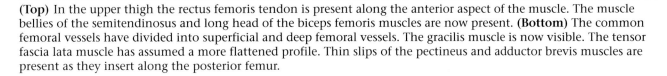

Hip and Pelvis

∨

AXIAL T1 MR, UPPER RIGHT THIGH

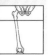

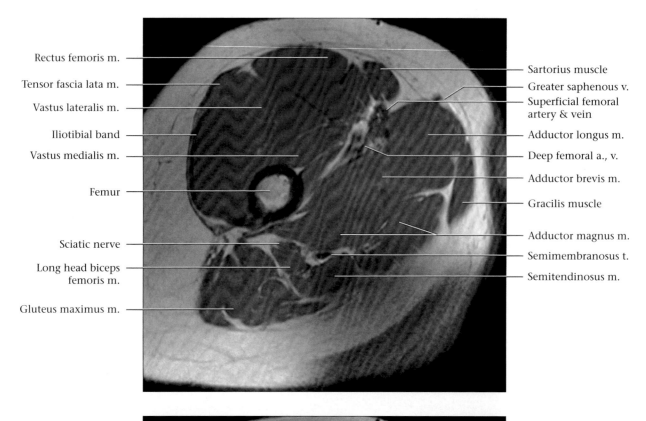

Rectus femoris m.
Tensor fascia lata m.
Vastus lateralis m.
Iliotibial band
Vastus medialis m.
Femur
Sciatic nerve
Long head biceps femoris m.
Gluteus maximus m.

Sartorius muscle
Greater saphenous v.
Superficial femoral artery & vein
Adductor longus m.
Deep femoral a., v.
Adductor brevis m.
Gracilis muscle
Adductor magnus m.
Semimembranosus t.
Semitendinosus m.

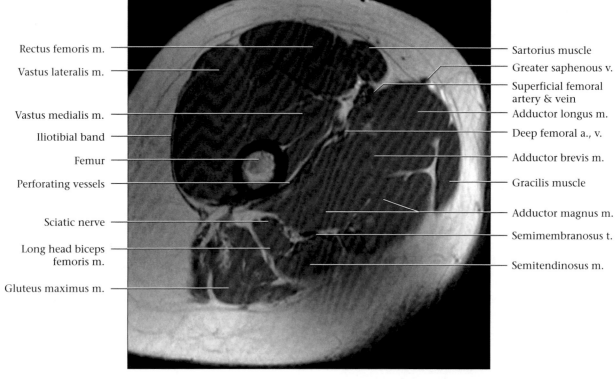

Rectus femoris m.
Vastus lateralis m.
Vastus medialis m.
Iliotibial band
Femur
Perforating vessels
Sciatic nerve
Long head biceps femoris m.
Gluteus maximus m.

Sartorius muscle
Greater saphenous v.
Superficial femoral artery & vein
Adductor longus m.
Deep femoral a., v.
Adductor brevis m.
Gracilis muscle
Adductor magnus m.
Semimembranosus t.
Semitendinosus m.

(Top) The two portions of the adductor magnus muscle are now in close proximity. The semimembranosus continues as a thin membranous slip through the proximal and mid thigh along the deep surface of the semitendinosus muscle. **(Bottom)** A large perforating artery is visible. It is a branch of the deep femoral artery. The tensor fascia lata muscle has completely inserted onto the iliotibial band. Throughout the thigh the sciatic nerve resides deep to the biceps femoris muscle.

THIGH OVERVIEW

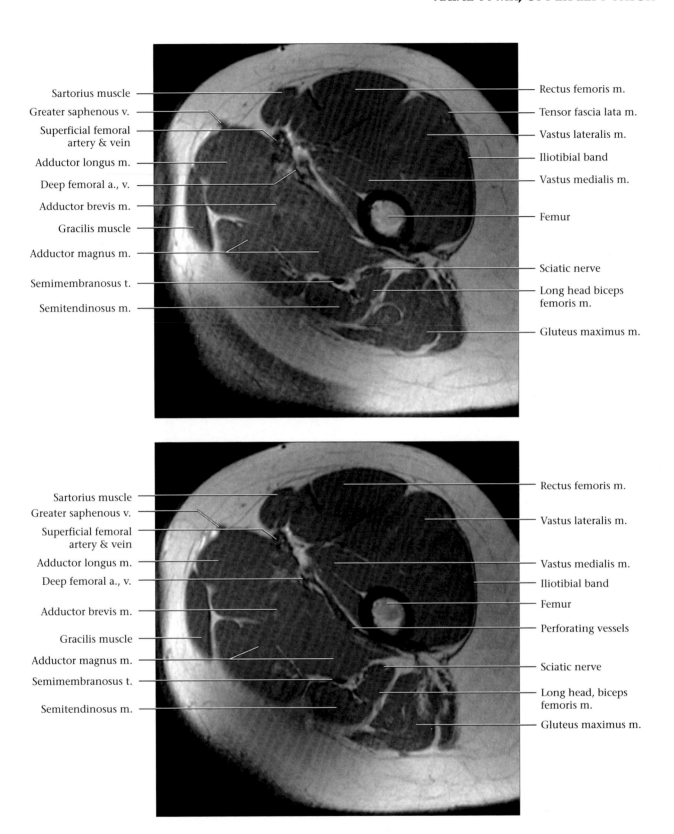

Sartorius muscle
Greater saphenous v.
Superficial femoral artery & vein
Adductor longus m.
Deep femoral a., v.
Adductor brevis m.
Gracilis muscle
Adductor magnus m.
Semimembranosus t.
Semitendinosus m.

Rectus femoris m.
Tensor fascia lata m.
Vastus lateralis m.
Iliotibial band
Vastus medialis m.
Femur
Sciatic nerve
Long head biceps femoris m.
Gluteus maximus m.

Sartorius muscle
Greater saphenous v.
Superficial femoral artery & vein
Adductor longus m.
Deep femoral a., v.
Adductor brevis m.
Gracilis muscle
Adductor magnus m.
Semimembranosus t.
Semitendinosus m.

Rectus femoris m.
Vastus lateralis m.
Vastus medialis m.
Iliotibial band
Femur
Perforating vessels
Sciatic nerve
Long head, biceps femoris m.
Gluteus maximus m.

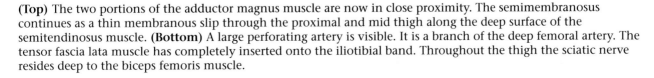

(Top) The two portions of the adductor magnus muscle are now in close proximity. The semimembranosus continues as a thin membranous slip through the proximal and mid thigh along the deep surface of the semitendinosus muscle. **(Bottom)** A large perforating artery is visible. It is a branch of the deep femoral artery. The tensor fascia lata muscle has completely inserted onto the iliotibial band. Throughout the thigh the sciatic nerve resides deep to the biceps femoris muscle.

Hip and Pelvis

V

THIGH OVERVIEW

AXIAL T1 MR, MID RIGHT THIGH

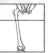

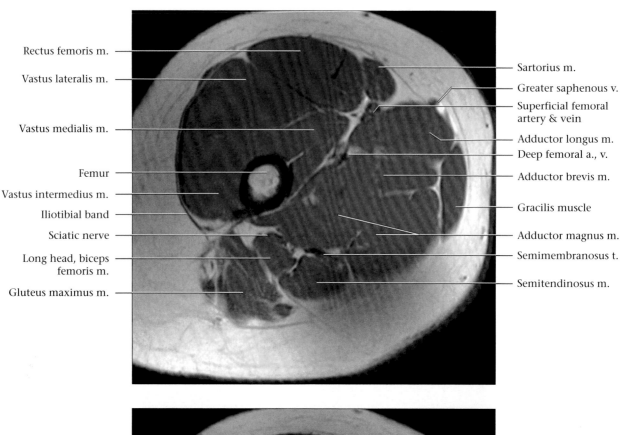

Rectus femoris m. — Sartorius m.
Vastus lateralis m. — Greater saphenous v.
— Superficial femoral artery & vein
Vastus medialis m. — Adductor longus m.
— Deep femoral a., v.
Femur — Adductor brevis m.
Vastus intermedius m. — Gracilis muscle
Iliotibial band —
Sciatic nerve — Adductor magnus m.
Long head, biceps femoris m. — Semimembranosus t.
Gluteus maximus m. — Semitendinosus m.

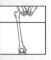

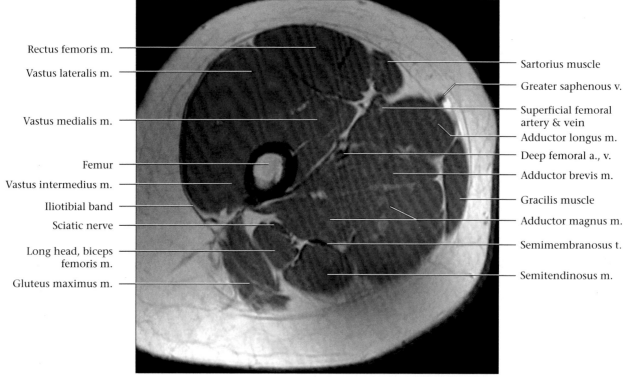

Rectus femoris m. — Sartorius muscle
Vastus lateralis m. — Greater saphenous v.
— Superficial femoral artery & vein
Vastus medialis m. — Adductor longus m.
— Deep femoral a., v.
Femur — Adductor brevis m.
Vastus intermedius m. — Gracilis muscle
Iliotibial band — Adductor magnus m.
Sciatic nerve —
Long head, biceps femoris m. — Semimembranosus t.
Gluteus maximus m. — Semitendinosus m.

(Top) Differentiation of the vastus muscles is difficult in the midthigh. Incomplete fat planes partially separate the muscles. The adductor muscles are slightly more distinct but often blend together in sections. **(Bottom)** The sartorius muscle continues its course across the thigh from anterior to medial. It is now located medial to the rectus femoris muscle. The inferior most aspect of the gluteus maximus muscle is visible. Its inferior most insertion is onto the distal upper 1/3 of the femur via the linea aspera. As the vessels course through the femoral triangle the artery assumes a more anterior position as seen on these images.

THIGH OVERVIEW

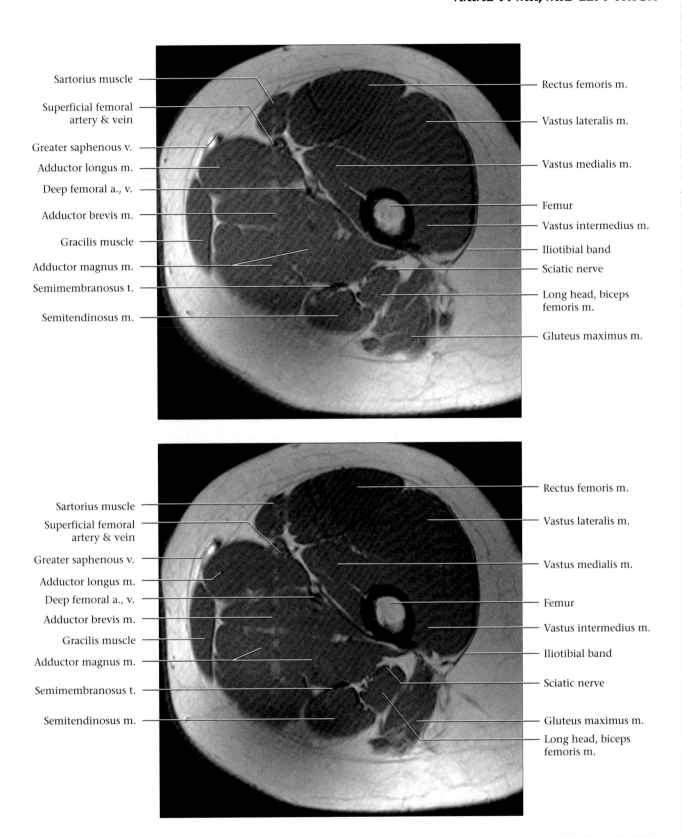

Top image labels (left): Sartorius muscle; Superficial femoral artery & vein; Greater saphenous v.; Adductor longus m.; Deep femoral a., v.; Adductor brevis m.; Gracilis muscle; Adductor magnus m.; Semimembranosus t.; Semitendinosus m.

Top image labels (right): Rectus femoris m.; Vastus lateralis m.; Vastus medialis m.; Femur; Vastus intermedius m.; Iliotibial band; Sciatic nerve; Long head, biceps femoris m.; Gluteus maximus m.

Bottom image labels (left): Sartorius muscle; Superficial femoral artery & vein; Greater saphenous v.; Adductor longus m.; Deep femoral a., v.; Adductor brevis m.; Gracilis muscle; Adductor magnus m.; Semimembranosus t.; Semitendinosus m.

Bottom image labels (right): Rectus femoris m.; Vastus lateralis m.; Vastus medialis m.; Femur; Vastus intermedius m.; Iliotibial band; Sciatic nerve; Gluteus maximus m.; Long head, biceps femoris m.

(Top) Differentiation of the vastus muscles is difficult in the midthigh. Incomplete fat planes partially separate the muscles. The adductor muscles are slightly more distinct but often blend together in sections. **(Bottom)** The sartorius muscle continues its course across the thigh from anterior to medial. It is now located medial to the rectus femoris muscle. The inferior most aspect of the gluteus maximus muscle is visible. Its inferior most insertion is onto the distal upper 1/3 of the femur via the linea aspera. As the vessels course through the femoral triangle the artery assumes a more anterior position as seen on these images.

Hip and Pelvis

V

AXIAL T1 MR, MID RIGHT THIGH

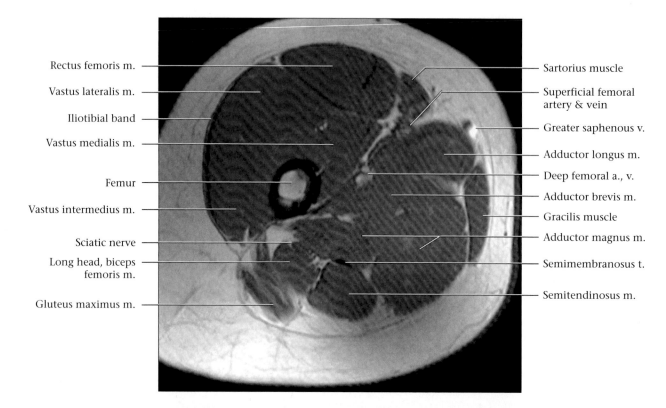

Rectus femoris m.

Vastus lateralis m.

Iliotibial band

Vastus medialis m.

Femur

Vastus intermedius m.

Sciatic nerve

Long head, biceps femoris m.

Gluteus maximus m.

Sartorius muscle

Superficial femoral artery & vein

Greater saphenous v.

Adductor longus m.

Deep femoral a., v.

Adductor brevis m.

Gracilis muscle

Adductor magnus m.

Semimembranosus t.

Semitendinosus m.

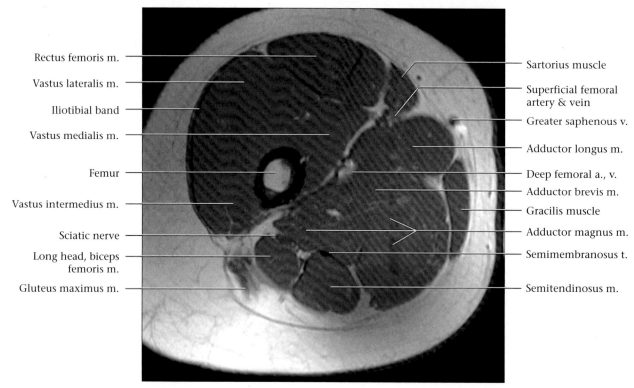

Rectus femoris m.

Vastus lateralis m.

Iliotibial band

Vastus medialis m.

Femur

Vastus intermedius m.

Sciatic nerve

Long head, biceps femoris m.

Gluteus maximus m.

Sartorius muscle

Superficial femoral artery & vein

Greater saphenous v.

Adductor longus m.

Deep femoral a., v.

Adductor brevis m.

Gracilis muscle

Adductor magnus m.

Semimembranosus t.

Semitendinosus m.

(Top) The semitendinosus muscle belly enlarges through the mid thigh. The muscle bellies of the semimembranosus and semitendinosus muscle share a reciprocal relationship. As the semitendinosus muscle becomes smaller along its inferior extent the semimembranosus muscle becomes larger. **(Bottom)** The vastus intermedius muscle origin is now visible. At this level the vastus lateralis muscle is anterior to the intermedius muscle and anterolateral to the vastus medialis muscle.

THIGH OVERVIEW

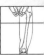

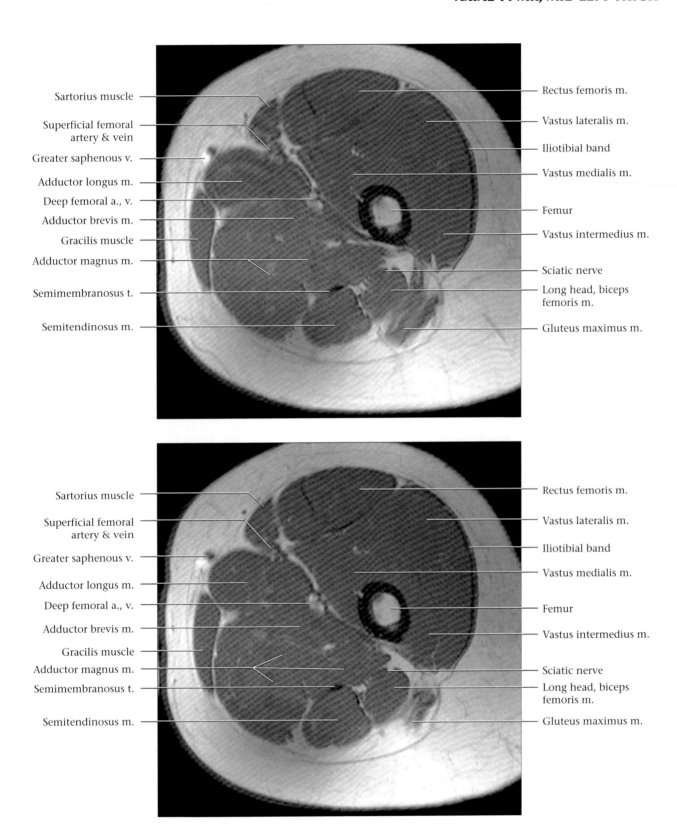

Sartorius muscle — Rectus femoris m.

Superficial femoral artery & vein — Vastus lateralis m.

Greater saphenous v. — Iliotibial band

Adductor longus m. — Vastus medialis m.

Deep femoral a., v. —

Adductor brevis m. — Femur

Gracilis muscle — Vastus intermedius m.

Adductor magnus m. —

Semimembranosus t. — Sciatic nerve

Semitendinosus m. — Long head, biceps femoris m.

— Gluteus maximus m.

Sartorius muscle — Rectus femoris m.

Superficial femoral artery & vein — Vastus lateralis m.

Greater saphenous v. — Iliotibial band

Adductor longus m. — Vastus medialis m.

Deep femoral a., v. —

Adductor brevis m. — Femur

Gracilis muscle — Vastus intermedius m.

Adductor magnus m. — Sciatic nerve

Semimembranosus t. — Long head, biceps femoris m.

Semitendinosus m. — Gluteus maximus m.

(Top) The semitendinosus muscle belly enlarges through the mid thigh. The muscle bellies of the semimembranosus and semitendinosus muscle share a reciprocal relationship. As the semitendinosus muscle becomes smaller along its inferior extent the semimembranosus muscle becomes larger. **(Bottom)** The vastus intermedius muscle origin is now visible. At this level the vastus lateralis muscle is anterior to the intermedius muscle and anterolateral to the vastus medialis muscle.

Hip and Pelvis

V

THIGH OVERVIEW

AXIAL T1 MR, MID RIGHT THIGH

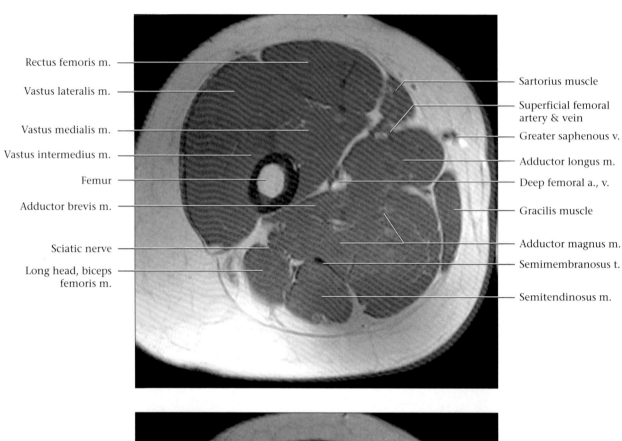

Rectus femoris m.

Vastus lateralis m.

Vastus medialis m.

Vastus intermedius m.

Femur

Adductor brevis m.

Sciatic nerve

Long head, biceps femoris m.

Sartorius muscle

Superficial femoral artery & vein

Greater saphenous v.

Adductor longus m.

Deep femoral a., v.

Gracilis muscle

Adductor magnus m.

Semimembranosus t.

Semitendinosus m.

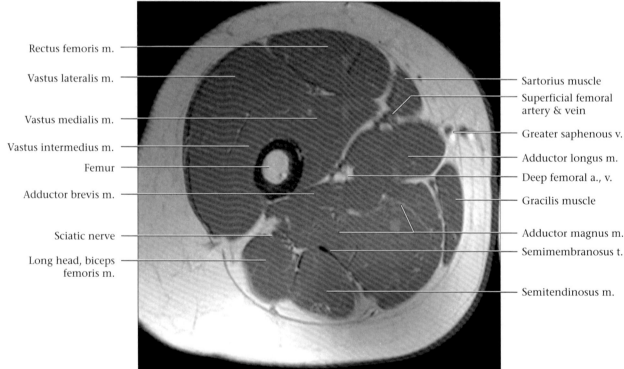

Rectus femoris m.

Vastus lateralis m.

Vastus medialis m.

Vastus intermedius m.

Femur

Adductor brevis m.

Sciatic nerve

Long head, biceps femoris m.

Sartorius muscle

Superficial femoral artery & vein

Greater saphenous v.

Adductor longus m.

Deep femoral a., v.

Gracilis muscle

Adductor magnus m.

Semimembranosus t.

Semitendinosus m.

(Top) Note the continuation of the superior tendon of the semitendinosus muscle along its deep lateral surface. The gracilis muscle follows a subtle posterior course from superior to inferior thigh. **(Bottom)** The vastus intermedius muscle wraps the anterior aspect of the femoral diaphysis. The adductor magnus is the largest mid-thigh muscle.

THIGH OVERVIEW

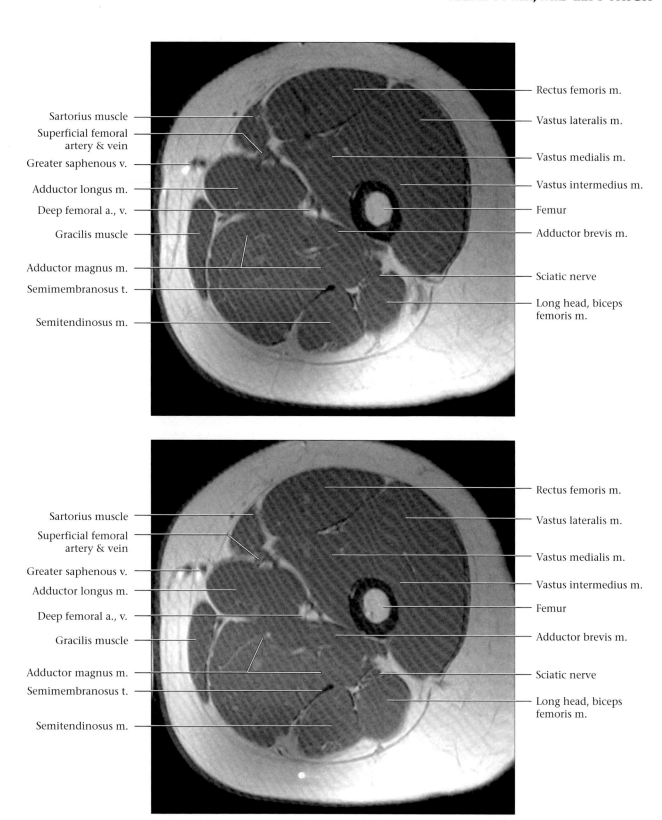

Sartorius muscle

Superficial femoral artery & vein

Greater saphenous v.

Adductor longus m.

Deep femoral a., v.

Gracilis muscle

Adductor magnus m.

Semimembranosus t.

Semitendinosus m.

Rectus femoris m.

Vastus lateralis m.

Vastus medialis m.

Vastus intermedius m.

Femur

Adductor brevis m.

Sciatic nerve

Long head, biceps femoris m.

Sartorius muscle

Superficial femoral artery & vein

Greater saphenous v.

Adductor longus m.

Deep femoral a., v.

Gracilis muscle

Adductor magnus m.

Semimembranosus t.

Semitendinosus m.

Rectus femoris m.

Vastus lateralis m.

Vastus medialis m.

Vastus intermedius m.

Femur

Adductor brevis m.

Sciatic nerve

Long head, biceps femoris m.

(Top) Note the continuation of the superior tendon of the semitendinosus muscle along its deep lateral surface. The gracilis muscle follows a subtle posterior course from superior to inferior thigh. **(Bottom)** The vastus intermedius muscle wraps the anterior aspect of the femoral diaphysis. The adductor magnus is the largest mid-thigh muscle.

Hip and Pelvis

V

AXIAL T1 MR, MID RIGHT THIGH

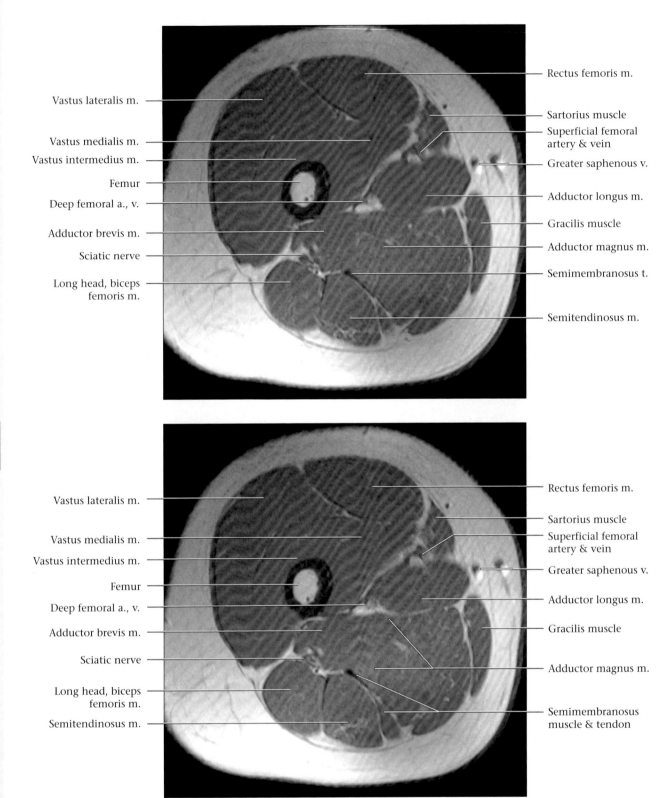

Labels (top image):
- Vastus lateralis m.
- Vastus medialis m.
- Vastus intermedius m.
- Femur
- Deep femoral a., v.
- Adductor brevis m.
- Sciatic nerve
- Long head, biceps femoris m.
- Rectus femoris m.
- Sartorius muscle
- Superficial femoral artery & vein
- Greater saphenous v.
- Adductor longus m.
- Gracilis muscle
- Adductor magnus m.
- Semimembranosus t.
- Semitendinosus m.

Labels (bottom image):
- Vastus lateralis m.
- Vastus medialis m.
- Vastus intermedius m.
- Femur
- Deep femoral a., v.
- Adductor brevis m.
- Sciatic nerve
- Long head, biceps femoris m.
- Semitendinosus m.
- Rectus femoris m.
- Sartorius muscle
- Superficial femoral artery & vein
- Greater saphenous v.
- Adductor longus m.
- Gracilis muscle
- Adductor magnus m.
- Semimembranosus muscle & tendon

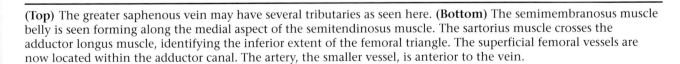

(Top) The greater saphenous vein may have several tributaries as seen here. (Bottom) The semimembranosus muscle belly is seen forming along the medial aspect of the semitendinosus muscle. The sartorius muscle crosses the adductor longus muscle, identifying the inferior extent of the femoral triangle. The superficial femoral vessels are now located within the adductor canal. The artery, the smaller vessel, is anterior to the vein.

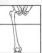

Hip and Pelvis

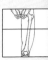

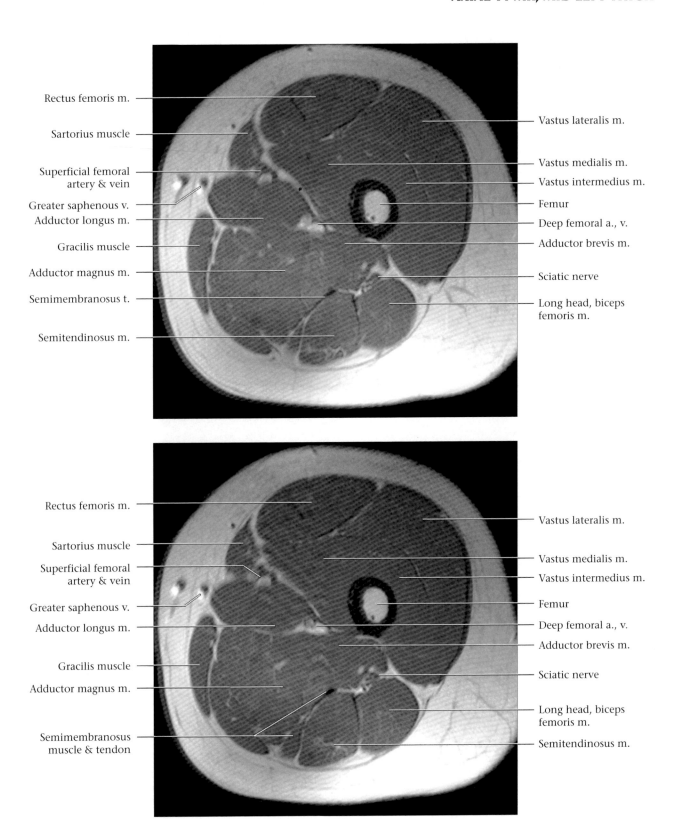

Rectus femoris m.

Sartorius muscle

Superficial femoral artery & vein

Greater saphenous v.
Adductor longus m.

Gracilis muscle

Adductor magnus m.

Semimembranosus t.

Semitendinosus m.

Vastus lateralis m.

Vastus medialis m.
Vastus intermedius m.

Femur

Deep femoral a., v.

Adductor brevis m.

Sciatic nerve

Long head, biceps femoris m.

Rectus femoris m.

Sartorius muscle

Superficial femoral artery & vein

Greater saphenous v.

Adductor longus m.

Gracilis muscle

Adductor magnus m.

Semimembranosus muscle & tendon

Vastus lateralis m.

Vastus medialis m.
Vastus intermedius m.

Femur

Deep femoral a., v.

Adductor brevis m.

Sciatic nerve

Long head, biceps femoris m.

Semitendinosus m.

(Top) The greater saphenous vein may have several tributaries as seen here. **(Bottom)** The semimembranosus muscle belly is seen forming along the medial aspect of the semitendinosus muscle. The sartorius muscle crosses the adductor longus muscle, identifying the inferior extent of the femoral triangle. The superficial femoral vessels are now located within the adductor canal. The artery, the smaller vessel, is anterior to the vein.

Hip and Pelvis

V

THIGH OVERVIEW

AXIAL T1 MR, MID RIGHT THIGH

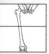

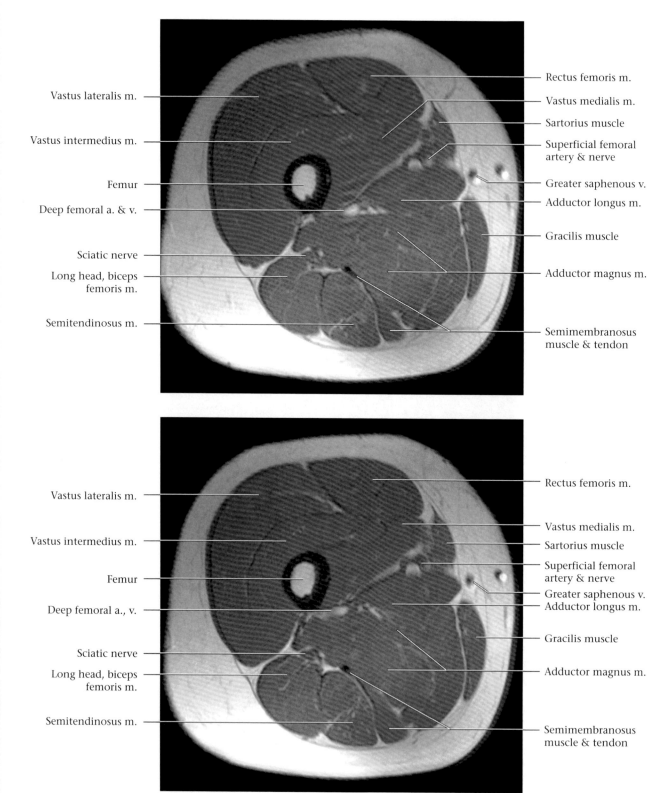

Vastus lateralis m.

Vastus intermedius m.

Femur

Deep femoral a. & v.

Sciatic nerve

Long head, biceps femoris m.

Semitendinosus m.

Rectus femoris m.

Vastus medialis m.

Sartorius muscle

Superficial femoral artery & nerve

Greater saphenous v.

Adductor longus m.

Gracilis muscle

Adductor magnus m.

Semimembranosus muscle & tendon

Vastus lateralis m.

Vastus intermedius m.

Femur

Deep femoral a., v.

Sciatic nerve

Long head, biceps femoris m.

Semitendinosus m.

Rectus femoris m.

Vastus medialis m.

Sartorius muscle

Superficial femoral artery & nerve

Greater saphenous v.

Adductor longus m.

Gracilis muscle

Adductor magnus m.

Semimembranosus muscle & tendon

(Top) The sartorius muscle continues its medial and now posterior course. It will eventually reside immediately anterior to the gracilis muscle. The adductor brevis muscle is no longer visible. It does not continue into the lower thigh. **(Bottom)** The semimembranosus muscle continues to enlarge. The long head of the biceps femoris muscle is at its largest mid thigh.

THIGH OVERVIEW

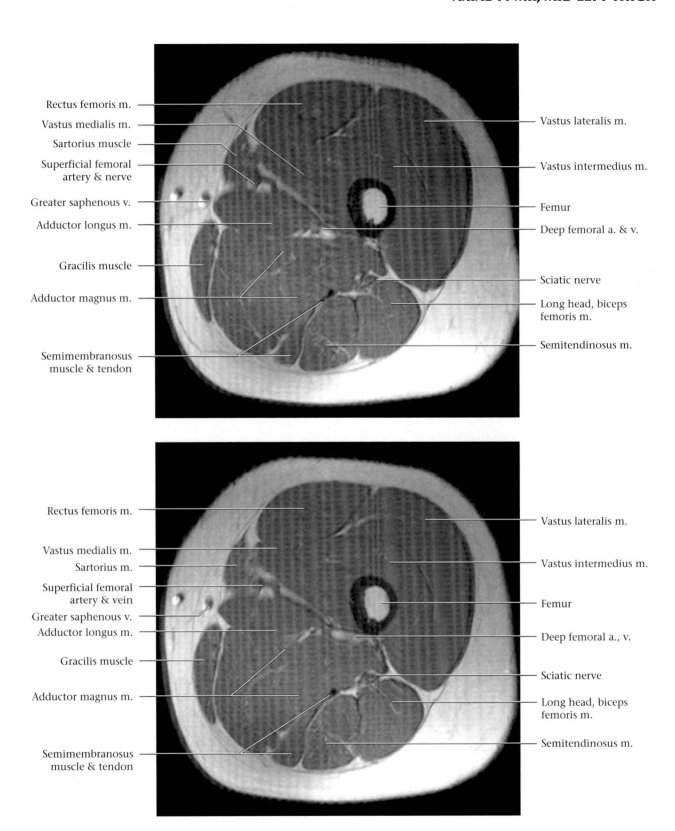

Rectus femoris m.

Vastus medialis m.

Sartorius muscle

Superficial femoral
artery & nerve

Greater saphenous v.

Adductor longus m.

Gracilis muscle

Adductor magnus m.

Semimembranosus
muscle & tendon

Vastus lateralis m.

Vastus intermedius m.

Femur

Deep femoral a. & v.

Sciatic nerve

Long head, biceps
femoris m.

Semitendinosus m.

Rectus femoris m.

Vastus medialis m.

Sartorius m.

Superficial femoral
artery & vein

Greater saphenous v.

Adductor longus m.

Gracilis muscle

Adductor magnus m.

Semimembranosus
muscle & tendon

Vastus lateralis m.

Vastus intermedius m.

Femur

Deep femoral a., v.

Sciatic nerve

Long head, biceps
femoris m.

Semitendinosus m.

(Top) The sartorius muscle continues its medial and now posterior course. It will eventually reside immediately anterior to the gracilis muscle. The adductor brevis muscle is no longer visible. It does not continue into the lower thigh. **(Bottom)** The semimembranosus muscle continues to enlarge. The long head of the biceps femoris muscle is at its largest mid thigh.

Hip and Pelvis

V

THIGH OVERVIEW

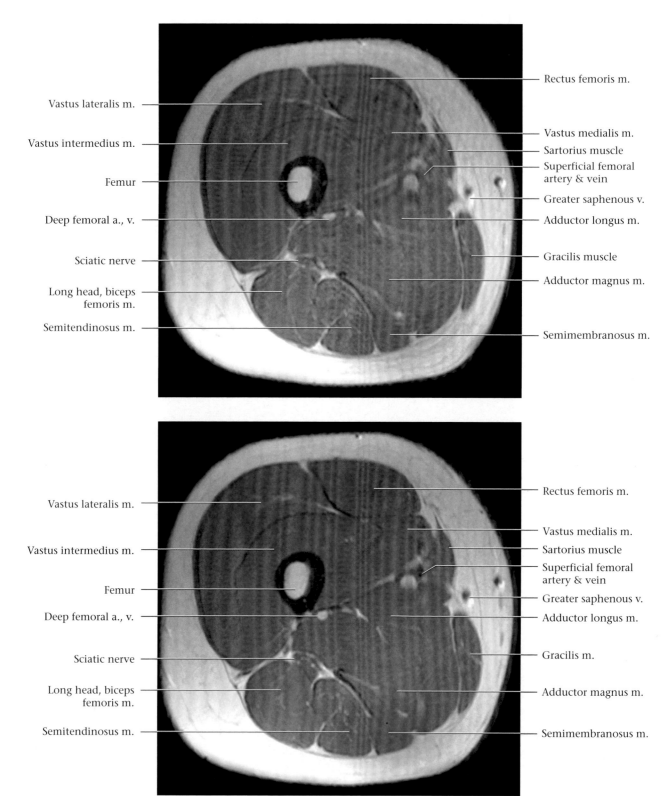

Vastus lateralis m.

Vastus intermedius m.

Femur

Deep femoral a., v.

Sciatic nerve

Long head, biceps femoris m.

Semitendinosus m.

Rectus femoris m.

Vastus medialis m.
Sartorius muscle
Superficial femoral artery & vein
Greater saphenous v.
Adductor longus m.

Gracilis muscle
Adductor magnus m.

Semimembranosus m.

Vastus lateralis m.

Vastus intermedius m.

Femur

Deep femoral a., v.

Sciatic nerve

Long head, biceps femoris m.

Semitendinosus m.

Rectus femoris m.

Vastus medialis m.
Sartorius muscle
Superficial femoral artery & vein
Greater saphenous v.
Adductor longus m.

Gracilis m.

Adductor magnus m.

Semimembranosus m.

(Top) The gracilis muscle continues its posterior course. The sartorius muscle moves closer to the gracilis muscle. **(Bottom)** The semimembranosus muscle belly increases in size as the semitendinosus muscle belly decreases in size. The adductor longus muscle lies anterior to the adductor magnus muscle throughout the thigh.

THIGH OVERVIEW

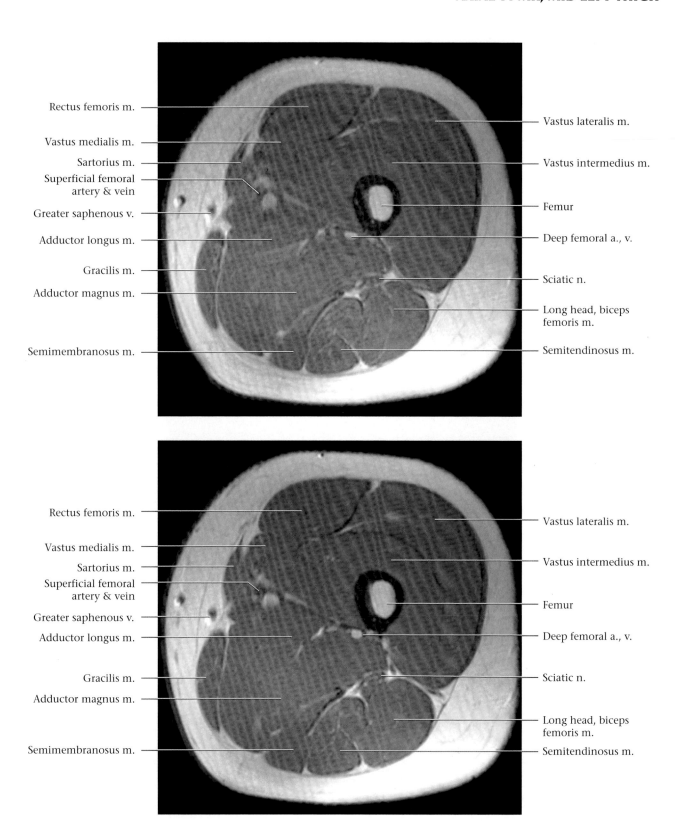

Rectus femoris m.

Vastus medialis m.

Sartorius m.

Superficial femoral artery & vein

Greater saphenous v.

Adductor longus m.

Gracilis m.

Adductor magnus m.

Semimembranosus m.

Vastus lateralis m.

Vastus intermedius m.

Femur

Deep femoral a., v.

Sciatic n.

Long head, biceps femoris m.

Semitendinosus m.

Rectus femoris m.

Vastus medialis m.

Sartorius m.

Superficial femoral artery & vein

Greater saphenous v.

Adductor longus m.

Gracilis m.

Adductor magnus m.

Semimembranosus m.

Vastus lateralis m.

Vastus intermedius m.

Femur

Deep femoral a., v.

Sciatic n.

Long head, biceps femoris m.

Semitendinosus m.

(Top) The gracilis muscle continues its posterior course. The sartorius muscle moves closer to the gracilis muscle.
(Bottom) The semimembranosus muscle belly increases in size as the semitendinosus muscle belly decreases in size. The adductor longus muscle lies anterior to the adductor magnus muscle throughout the thigh.

Hip and Pelvis

V

AXIAL T1 MR, MID RIGHT THIGH

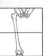

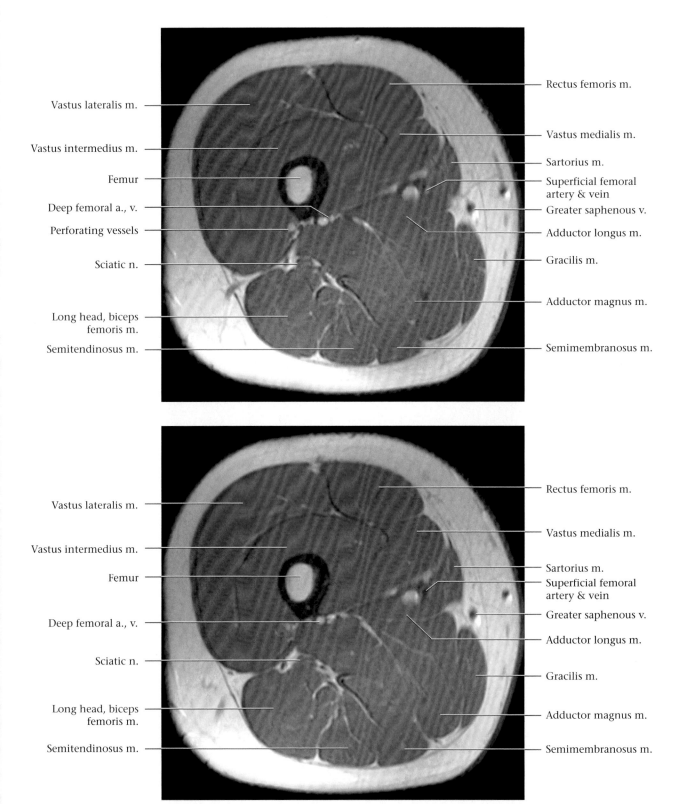

Vastus lateralis m. — — Rectus femoris m.

Vastus intermedius m. — — Vastus medialis m.

Femur — — Sartorius m.

Deep femoral a., v. — — Superficial femoral artery & vein

Perforating vessels — — Greater saphenous v.

— Adductor longus m.

Sciatic n. — — Gracilis m.

— Adductor magnus m.

Long head, biceps femoris m. —

Semitendinosus m. — — Semimembranosus m.

Vastus lateralis m. — — Rectus femoris m.

Vastus intermedius m. — — Vastus medialis m.

Femur — — Sartorius m.
— Superficial femoral artery & vein

Deep femoral a., v. — — Greater saphenous v.

— Adductor longus m.

Sciatic n. — — Gracilis m.

Long head, biceps femoris m. — — Adductor magnus m.

Semitendinosus m. — — Semimembranosus m.

(Top) Because of its oblique course and its own separate fascial covering, the sartorius muscle is often considered a separate compartment although it is commonly included within the medial compartment (see "Compartments of Thigh" pages). Superior to this level the muscle is not in direct continuity with the other muscles of the anterior compartment. **(Bottom)** The boundaries of the adductor canal are apparent: The sartorius, vastus medialis, adductor longus and adductor magnus muscles. The semimembranosus and semitendinosus muscle are of similar size. In the mid thigh the tendon of the rectus femoris muscle is located within the muscle belly.

AXIAL T1 MR, MID LEFT THIGH

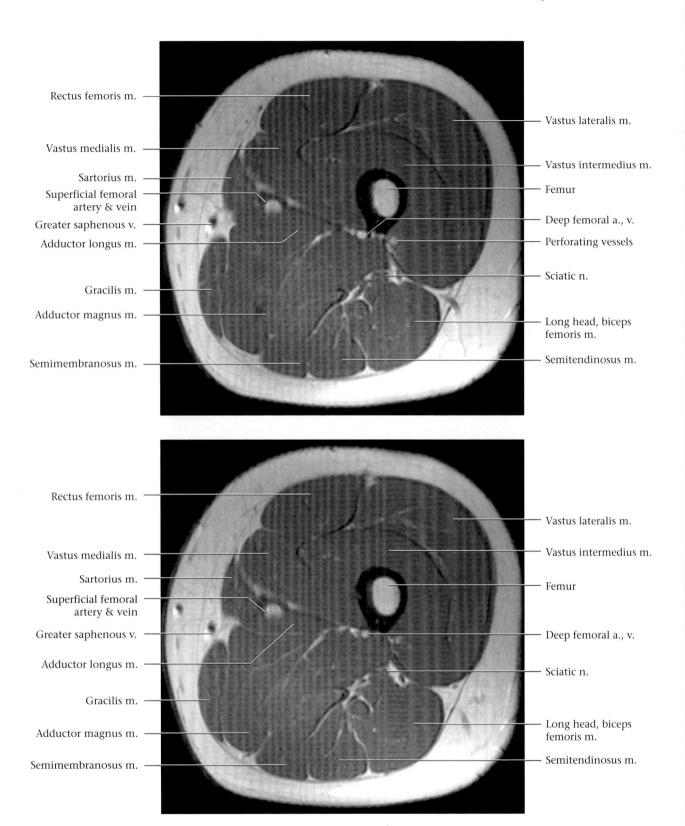

Rectus femoris m.

Vastus medialis m.

Sartorius m.

Superficial femoral artery & vein

Greater saphenous v.

Adductor longus m.

Gracilis m.

Adductor magnus m.

Semimembranosus m.

Vastus lateralis m.

Vastus intermedius m.

Femur

Deep femoral a., v.

Perforating vessels

Sciatic n.

Long head, biceps femoris m.

Semitendinosus m.

Rectus femoris m.

Vastus medialis m.

Sartorius m.

Superficial femoral artery & vein

Greater saphenous v.

Adductor longus m.

Gracilis m.

Adductor magnus m.

Semimembranosus m.

Vastus lateralis m.

Vastus intermedius m.

Femur

Deep femoral a., v.

Sciatic n.

Long head, biceps femoris m.

Semitendinosus m.

(Top) Because of its oblique course and its own separate fascial covering, the sartorius muscle is often considered a separate compartment although it is commonly included within the medial compartment (see "Compartments of Thigh" pages). Superior to this level the muscle is not in direct continuity with the other muscles of the anterior compartment. **(Bottom)** The boundaries of the adductor canal are apparent: The sartorius, vastus medialis, adductor longus and adductor magnus muscles. The semimembranosus and semitendinosus muscle are of similar size. In the mid thigh the tendon of the rectus femoris muscle is located within the muscle belly.

Hip and Pelvis

V

AXIAL T1 MR, MID RIGHT THIGH

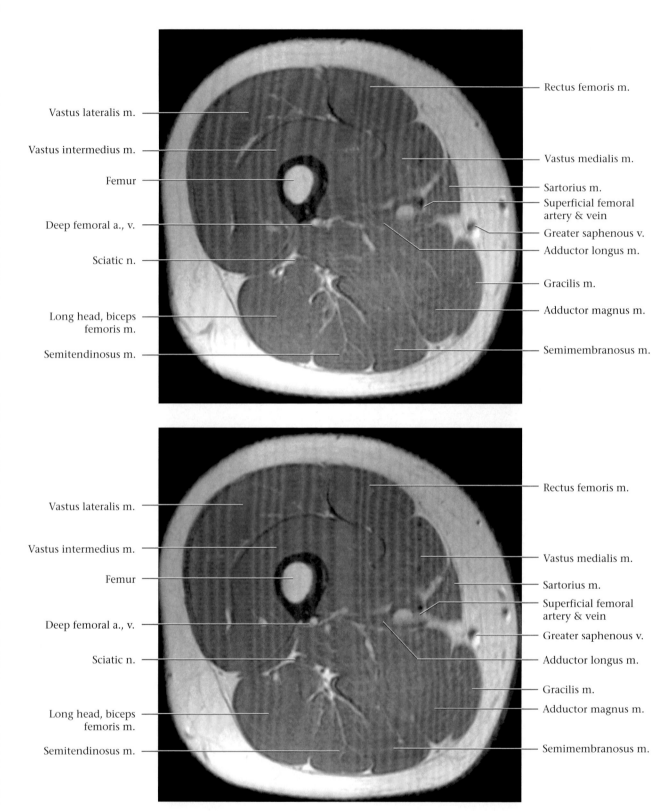

Labels (top image):
- Vastus lateralis m.
- Vastus intermedius m.
- Femur
- Deep femoral a., v.
- Sciatic n.
- Long head, biceps femoris m.
- Semitendinosus m.
- Rectus femoris m.
- Vastus medialis m.
- Sartorius m.
- Superficial femoral artery & vein
- Greater saphenous v.
- Adductor longus m.
- Gracilis m.
- Adductor magnus m.
- Semimembranosus m.

Labels (bottom image):
- Vastus lateralis m.
- Vastus intermedius m.
- Femur
- Deep femoral a., v.
- Sciatic n.
- Long head, biceps femoris m.
- Semitendinosus m.
- Rectus femoris m.
- Vastus medialis m.
- Sartorius m.
- Superficial femoral artery & vein
- Greater saphenous v.
- Adductor longus m.
- Gracilis m.
- Adductor magnus m.
- Semimembranosus m.

(Top) The deep femoral vessels have followed an inferior and lateral course from their point of branching in the upper thigh. They now course posterior to the femur. The inferior-most aspect of the adductor longus muscle is visible. The adductor magnus, gracilis and sartorius muscles are the only medial compartment muscles to continue into the distal thigh. **(Bottom)** The rectus femoris muscle is now nestled between the vastus medialis and lateralis muscles.

AXIAL T1 MR, MID LEFT THIGH

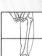

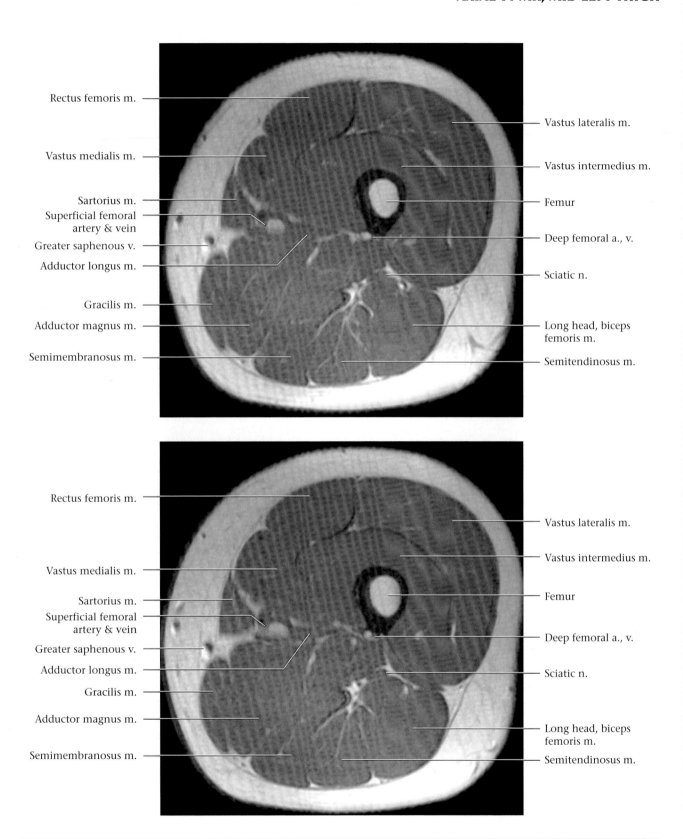

Rectus femoris m.

Vastus medialis m.

Sartorius m.

Superficial femoral artery & vein

Greater saphenous v.

Adductor longus m.

Gracilis m.

Adductor magnus m.

Semimembranosus m.

Vastus lateralis m.

Vastus intermedius m.

Femur

Deep femoral a., v.

Sciatic n.

Long head, biceps femoris m.

Semitendinosus m.

Rectus femoris m.

Vastus medialis m.

Sartorius m.

Superficial femoral artery & vein

Greater saphenous v.

Adductor longus m.

Gracilis m.

Adductor magnus m.

Semimembranosus m.

Vastus lateralis m.

Vastus intermedius m.

Femur

Deep femoral a., v.

Sciatic n.

Long head, biceps femoris m.

Semitendinosus m.

(Top) The deep femoral vessels have followed an inferior and lateral course from their point of branching in the upper thigh. They now course posterior to the femur. The inferior-most aspect of the adductor longus muscle is visible. The adductor magnus, gracilis and sartorius muscles are the only medial compartment muscles to continue into the distal thigh. **(Bottom)** The rectus femoris muscle is now nestled between the vastus medialis and lateralis muscles.

Hip and Pelvis

V

AXIAL T1 MR, MID RIGHT THIGH

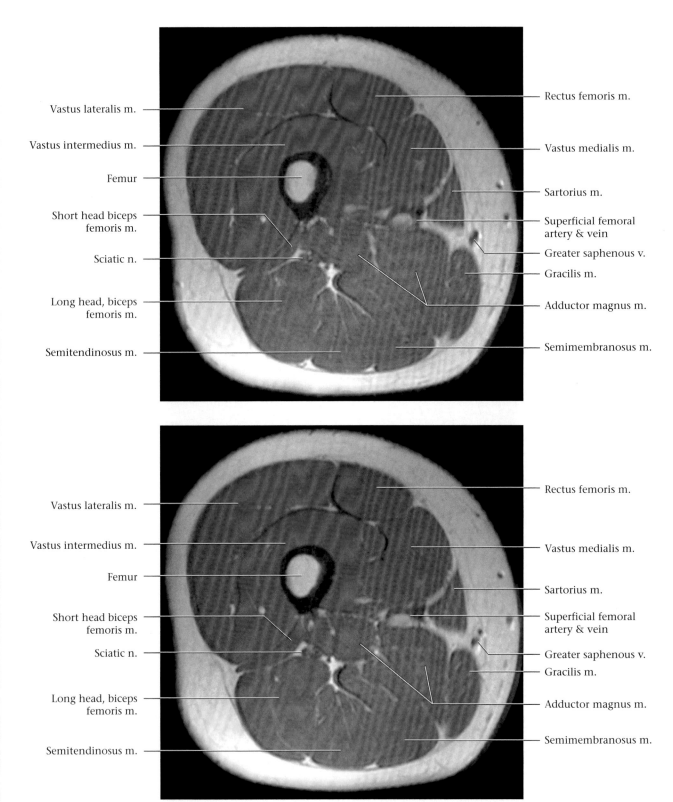

Vastus lateralis m. — Rectus femoris m.

Vastus intermedius m. — Vastus medialis m.

Femur — Sartorius m.

Short head biceps femoris m. — Superficial femoral artery & vein

Sciatic n. — Greater saphenous v.

Gracilis m.

Long head, biceps femoris m. — Adductor magnus m.

Semitendinosus m. — Semimembranosus m.

Vastus lateralis m. — Rectus femoris m.

Vastus intermedius m. — Vastus medialis m.

Femur — Sartorius m.

Short head biceps femoris m. — Superficial femoral artery & vein

Sciatic n. — Greater saphenous v.

Gracilis m.

Long head, biceps femoris m. — Adductor magnus m.

Semitendinosus m. — Semimembranosus m.

(Top) The origin of the short head of the biceps femoris muscle is in the midthigh. The terminal portion of the deep femoral vessels also occurs mid thigh. **(Bottom)** The vastus muscles are easily separated at this level. The sartorius and gracilis muscles are now in close proximity. The semimembranosus muscle is located medial to the semitendinous. At the ischial tuberosity it originated lateral to the semitendinosus, then crossed the deep surface of the semitendinosus tendon; its membranous portion resides on the deep surface of the muscle belly in the upper thigh.

THIGH OVERVIEW

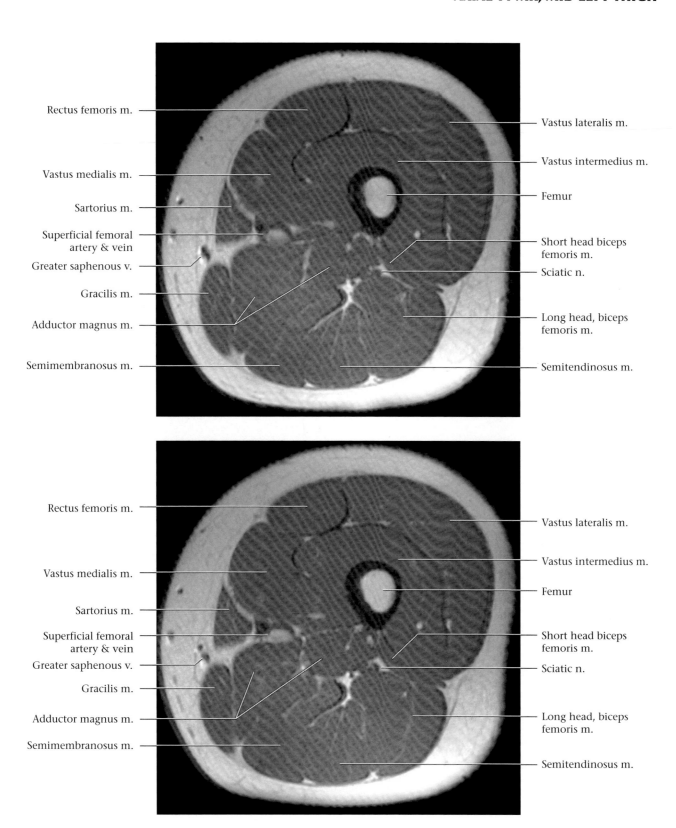

Rectus femoris m.

Vastus medialis m.

Sartorius m.

Superficial femoral
artery & vein

Greater saphenous v.

Gracilis m.

Adductor magnus m.

Semimembranosus m.

Vastus lateralis m.

Vastus intermedius m.

Femur

Short head biceps
femoris m.

Sciatic n.

Long head, biceps
femoris m.

Semitendinosus m.

Rectus femoris m.

Vastus medialis m.

Sartorius m.

Superficial femoral
artery & vein

Greater saphenous v.

Gracilis m.

Adductor magnus m.

Semimembranosus m.

Vastus lateralis m.

Vastus intermedius m.

Femur

Short head biceps
femoris m.

Sciatic n.

Long head, biceps
femoris m.

Semitendinosus m.

(Top) The origin of the short head of the biceps femoris muscle is in the midthigh. The terminal portion of the deep femoral vessels also occurs mid thigh. **(Bottom)** The vastus muscles are easily separated at this level. The sartorius and gracilis muscles are now in close proximity. The semimembranosus muscle is located medial to the semitendinous. At the ischial tuberosity it originated lateral to the semitendinosus, then crossed the deep surface of the semitendinosus tendon; its membranous portion resides on the deep surface of the muscle belly in the upper thigh.

Hip and Pelvis

V

237

THIGH OVERVIEW

AXIAL T1 MR, MID RIGHT THIGH

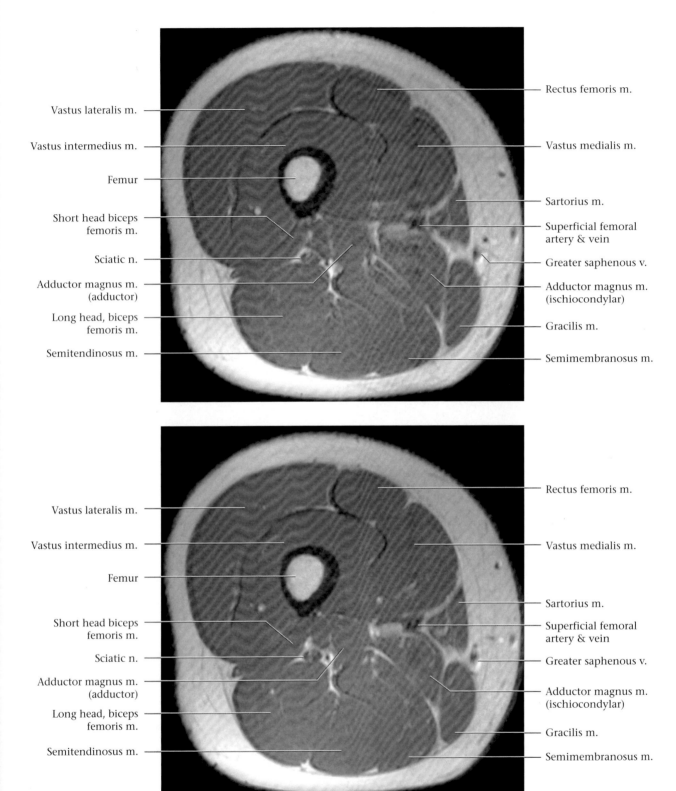

Vastus lateralis m.

Vastus intermedius m.

Femur

Short head biceps femoris m.

Sciatic n.

Adductor magnus m. (adductor)

Long head, biceps femoris m.

Semitendinosus m.

Rectus femoris m.

Vastus medialis m.

Sartorius m.

Superficial femoral artery & vein

Greater saphenous v.

Adductor magnus m. (ischiocondylar)

Gracilis m.

Semimembranosus m.

(Top) The ischiocondylar and adductor portions of the adductor magnus muscle are again separable as the adductor portion inserts onto the posterior femur. **(Bottom)** The tendon of the rectus femoris muscle is now located along the deep surface of the muscle. The muscle belly of the long head of the biceps femoris muscle continues to enlarge. The ischiocondylar portion of the adductor magnus muscle is now medial to the adductor portion of the muscle.

AXIAL T1 MR, MID LEFT THIGH

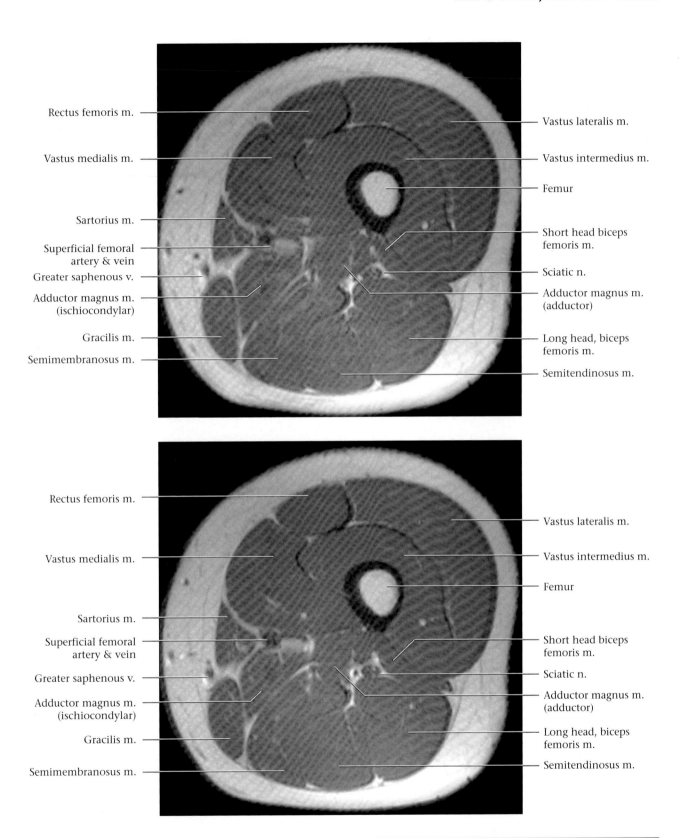

Rectus femoris m.

Vastus medialis m.

Sartorius m.

Superficial femoral artery & vein

Greater saphenous v.

Adductor magnus m. (ischiocondylar)

Gracilis m.

Semimembranosus m.

Vastus lateralis m.

Vastus intermedius m.

Femur

Short head biceps femoris m.

Sciatic n.

Adductor magnus m. (adductor)

Long head, biceps femoris m.

Semitendinosus m.

Rectus femoris m.

Vastus medialis m.

Sartorius m.

Superficial femoral artery & vein

Greater saphenous v.

Adductor magnus m. (ischiocondylar)

Gracilis m.

Semimembranosus m.

Vastus lateralis m.

Vastus intermedius m.

Femur

Short head biceps femoris m.

Sciatic n.

Adductor magnus m. (adductor)

Long head, biceps femoris m.

Semitendinosus m.

(Top) The ischiocondylar and adductor portions of the adductor magnus muscle are again separable as the adductor portion inserts onto the posterior femur. **(Bottom)** The tendon of the rectus femoris muscle is now located along the deep surface of the muscle. The muscle belly of the long head of the biceps femoris muscle continues to enlarge. The ischiocondylar portion of the adductor magnus muscle is now medial to the adductor portion of the muscle.

Hip and Pelvis

V

AXIAL T1 MR, MID RIGHT THIGH

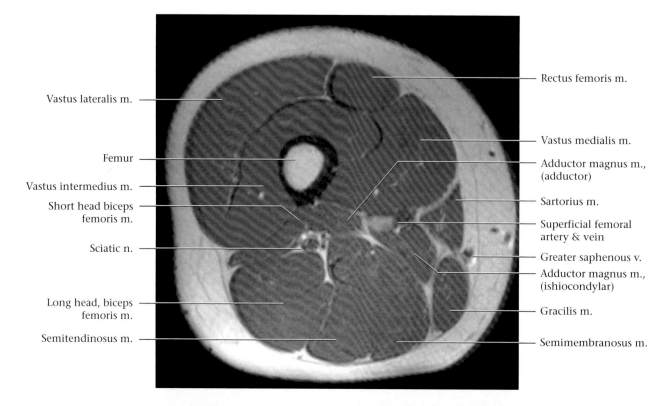

Vastus lateralis m.

Femur

Vastus intermedius m.

Short head biceps femoris m.

Sciatic n.

Long head, biceps femoris m.

Semitendinosus m.

Rectus femoris m.

Vastus medialis m.

Adductor magnus m., (adductor)

Sartorius m.

Superficial femoral artery & vein

Greater saphenous v.

Adductor magnus m., (ishiocondylar)

Gracilis m.

Semimembranosus m.

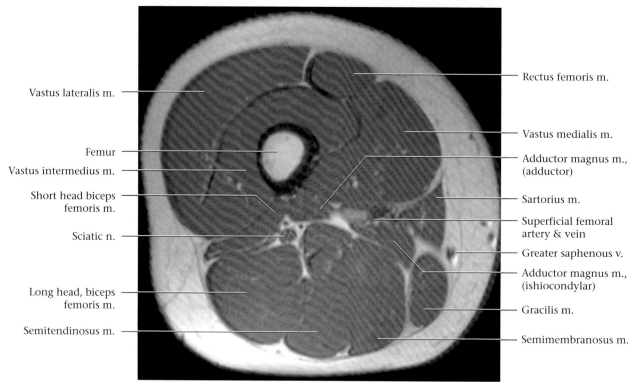

Vastus lateralis m.

Femur

Vastus intermedius m.

Short head biceps femoris m.

Sciatic n.

Long head, biceps femoris m.

Semitendinosus m.

Rectus femoris m.

Vastus medialis m.

Adductor magnus m., (adductor)

Sartorius m.

Superficial femoral artery & vein

Greater saphenous v.

Adductor magnus m., (ishiocondylar)

Gracilis m.

Semimembranosus m.

(Top) The muscle bellies of the rectus femoris and semitendinosus muscle decrease in size in the distal thigh. The short head of the biceps femoris muscle has a long origin from the posterior femur. **(Bottom)** The vastus medialis muscle becomes quite large in the distal thigh. The sciatic nerve continues to reside along the deep surface of the long head of the biceps femoris muscle.

THIGH OVERVIEW

Rectus femoris m. — Vastus lateralis m.

Vastus medialis m. — Femur

Adductor magnus m., (adductor) — Vastus intermedius m.

Sartorius m. — Short head biceps femoris m.

Superficial femoral artery & vein — Sciatic n.

Greater saphenous v.

Adductor magnus m., (ischiocondylar) — Long head, biceps femoris m.

Gracilis m. — Semitendinosus m.

Semimembranosus m.

Rectus femoris m. — Vastus lateralis m.

Vastus medialis m. — Femur

Adductor magnus m., (adductor) — Vastus intermedius m.

Sartorius m. — Short head biceps femoris m.

Superficial femoral artery & vein — Sciatic n.

Greater saphenous v.

Adductor magnus m., (ischiocondylar) — Long head, biceps femoris m.

Gracilis m. — Semitendinosus m.

Semimembranosus m.

(Top) The muscle bellies of the rectus femoris and semitendinosus muscle decrease in size in the distal thigh. The short head of the biceps femoris muscle has a long origin from the posterior femur. (Bottom) The vastus medialis muscle becomes quite large in the distal thigh. The sciatic nerve continues to reside along the deep surface of the long head of the biceps femoris muscle.

AXIAL T1 MR, MID RIGHT THIGH

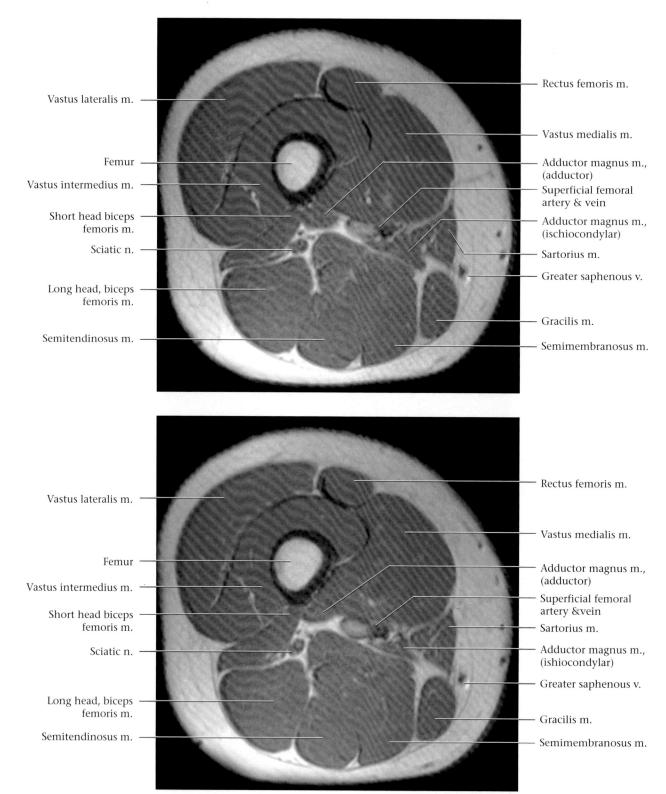

Vastus lateralis m.

Femur

Vastus intermedius m.

Short head biceps femoris m.

Sciatic n.

Long head, biceps femoris m.

Semitendinosus m.

Rectus femoris m.

Vastus medialis m.

Adductor magnus m., (adductor)

Superficial femoral artery & vein

Adductor magnus m., (ischiocondylar)

Sartorius m.

Greater saphenous v.

Gracilis m.

Semimembranosus m.

Vastus lateralis m.

Femur

Vastus intermedius m.

Short head biceps femoris m.

Sciatic n.

Long head, biceps femoris m.

Semitendinosus m.

Rectus femoris m.

Vastus medialis m.

Adductor magnus m., (adductor)

Superficial femoral artery &vein

Sartorius m.

Adductor magnus m., (ishiocondylar)

Greater saphenous v.

Gracilis m.

Semimembranosus m.

(Top) Note the thickening of the posterior cortex of the femur at this level and throughout the thigh. This thickening is the linea aspera which serves as a site of origin and insertion for multiple muscles. The sartorius and gracilis muscles are now within the posterior 1/2 of the medial aspect of the thigh. The semitendinosus muscle is becoming quite small. **(Bottom)** The separation of the adductor and ischiocondylar portions of the adductor magnus muscle forms the adductor hiatus. The superficial femoral vessels pass through the adductor hiatus to enter the popliteal fossa. Upon passing through the hiatus they become the popliteal vessels.

THIGH OVERVIEW

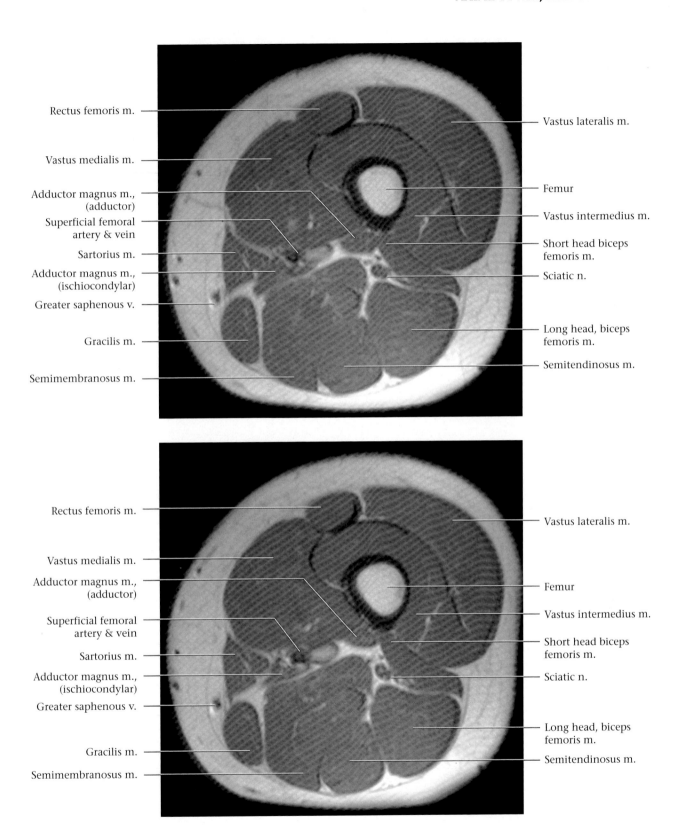

Rectus femoris m.

Vastus medialis m.

Adductor magnus m., (adductor)

Superficial femoral artery & vein

Sartorius m.

Adductor magnus m., (ischiocondylar)

Greater saphenous v.

Gracilis m.

Semimembranosus m.

Vastus lateralis m.

Femur

Vastus intermedius m.

Short head biceps femoris m.

Sciatic n.

Long head, biceps femoris m.

Semitendinosus m.

Rectus femoris m.

Vastus medialis m.

Adductor magnus m., (adductor)

Superficial femoral artery & vein

Sartorius m.

Adductor magnus m., (ischiocondylar)

Greater saphenous v.

Gracilis m.

Semimembranosus m.

Vastus lateralis m.

Femur

Vastus intermedius m.

Short head biceps femoris m.

Sciatic n.

Long head, biceps femoris m.

Semitendinosus m.

(Top) Note the thickening of the posterior cortex of the femur at this level and throughout the thigh. This thickening is the linea aspera which serves as a site of origin and insertion for multiple muscles. The sartorius and gracilis muscles are now within the posterior 1/2 of the medial aspect of the thigh. The semitendinosus muscle is becoming quite small. **(Bottom)** The separation of the adductor and ischiocondylar portions of the adductor magnus muscle forms the adductor hiatus. The superficial femoral vessels pass through the adductor hiatus to enter the popliteal fossa. Upon passing through the hiatus they become the popliteal vessels.

Hip and Pelvis

V

AXIAL T1 MR, MID RIGHT THIGH

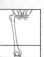

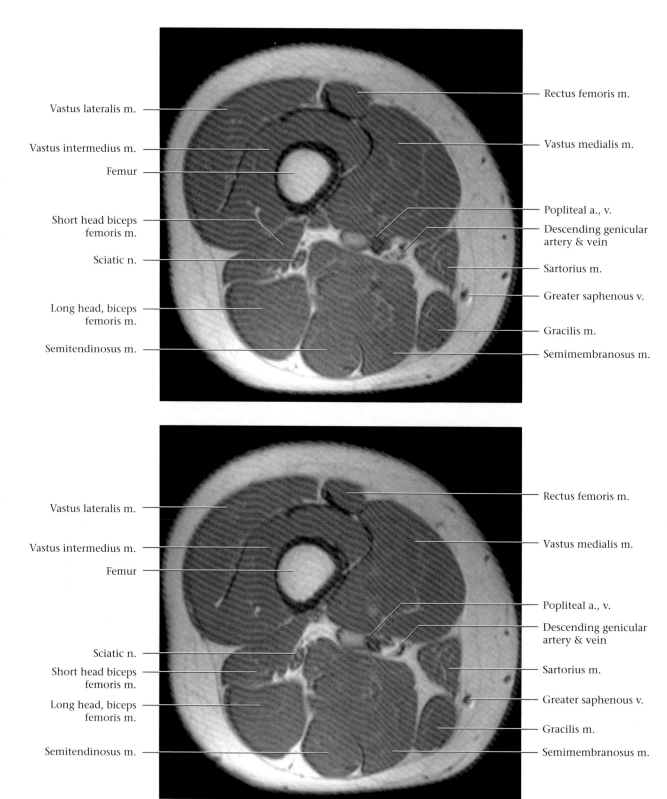

Vastus lateralis m.

Vastus intermedius m.

Femur

Short head biceps femoris m.

Sciatic n.

Long head, biceps femoris m.

Semitendinosus m.

Rectus femoris m.

Vastus medialis m.

Popliteal a., v.

Descending genicular artery & vein

Sartorius m.

Greater saphenous v.

Gracilis m.

Semimembranosus m.

Vastus lateralis m.

Vastus intermedius m.

Femur

Sciatic n.

Short head biceps femoris m.

Long head, biceps femoris m.

Semitendinosus m.

Rectus femoris m.

Vastus medialis m.

Popliteal a., v.

Descending genicular artery & vein

Sartorius m.

Greater saphenous v.

Gracilis m.

Semimembranosus m.

(Top) The superficial femoral vessels upon passing through the adductor hiatus have become the popliteal vessels. Just before this transition the descending genicular artery branches from the superficial femoral artery. The sciatic nerve begins a slightly anterior course along the medial aspect of the short head of the biceps femoris muscle. **(Bottom)** At this inferior level the semimembranosus muscle has a large muscle belly. The distal tendon of the semitendinosus muscle is seen along the posterior surface of the muscle belly.

THIGH OVERVIEW

AXIAL T1 MR, MID LEFT THIGH

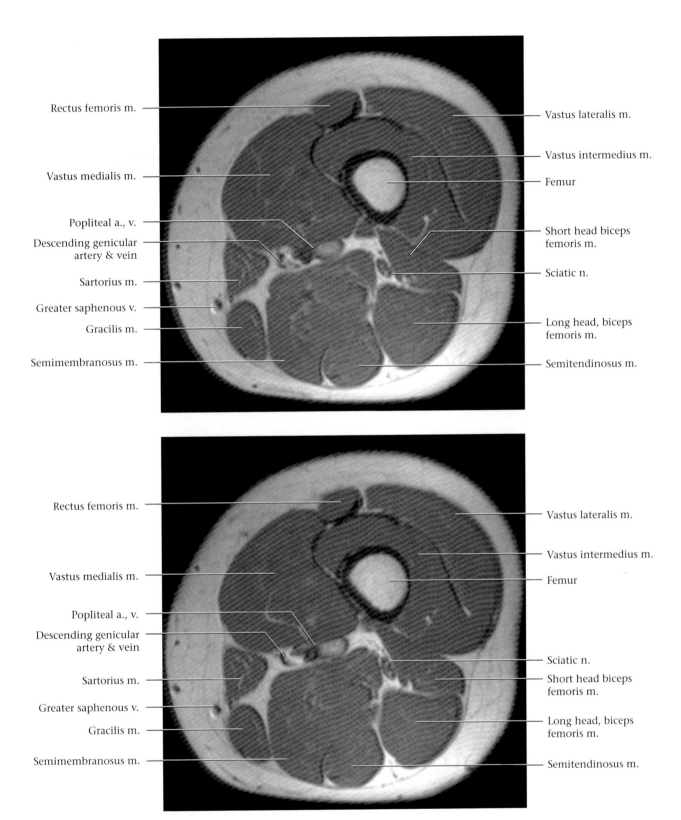

Top image labels:
- Rectus femoris m.
- Vastus medialis m.
- Popliteal a., v.
- Descending genicular artery & vein
- Sartorius m.
- Greater saphenous v.
- Gracilis m.
- Semimembranosus m.
- Vastus lateralis m.
- Vastus intermedius m.
- Femur
- Short head biceps femoris m.
- Sciatic n.
- Long head, biceps femoris m.
- Semitendinosus m.

Bottom image labels:
- Rectus femoris m.
- Vastus medialis m.
- Popliteal a., v.
- Descending genicular artery & vein
- Sartorius m.
- Greater saphenous v.
- Gracilis m.
- Semimembranosus m.
- Vastus lateralis m.
- Vastus intermedius m.
- Femur
- Sciatic n.
- Short head biceps femoris m.
- Long head, biceps femoris m.
- Semitendinosus m.

(Top) The superficial femoral vessels upon passing through the adductor hiatus have become the popliteal vessels. Just before this transition the descending genicular artery branches from the superficial femoral artery. The sciatic nerve begins a slightly anterior course along the medial aspect of the short head of the biceps femoris muscle. **(Bottom)** At this inferior level the semimembranosus muscle has a large muscle belly. The distal tendon of the semitendinosus muscle is seen along the posterior surface of the muscle belly.

Hip and Pelvis

V

245

THIGH OVERVIEW

AXIAL T1 MR, DISTAL RIGHT THIGH

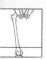

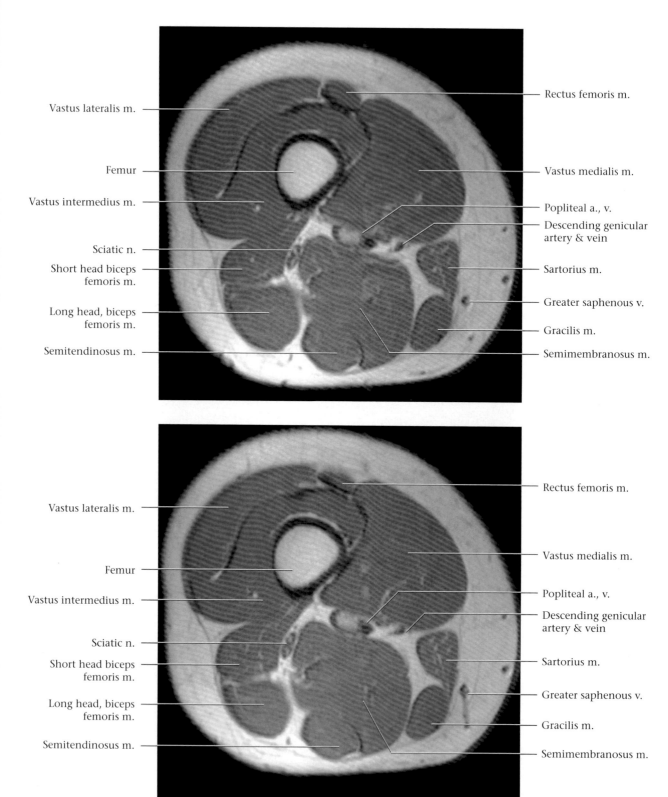

(Top) The popliteal vessels course deep to the semimembranosus muscle as they travel to the popliteal fossa. The sciatic nerve continues to travel anteriorly. **(Bottom)** The short and long heads of the biceps femoris muscle join. The separation of the semimembranosus and semitendinous muscles from the biceps femoris muscle is beginning as images approach the superior aspect of the popliteal fossa.

THIGH OVERVIEW

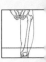

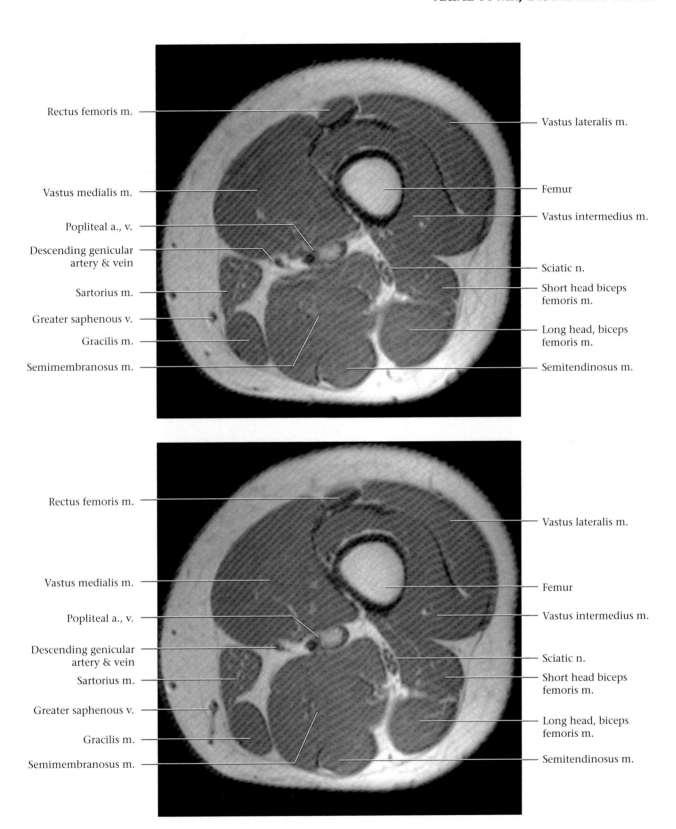

Rectus femoris m.

Vastus medialis m.

Popliteal a., v.

Descending genicular artery & vein

Sartorius m.

Greater saphenous v.

Gracilis m.

Semimembranosus m.

Vastus lateralis m.

Femur

Vastus intermedius m.

Sciatic n.

Short head biceps femoris m.

Long head, biceps femoris m.

Semitendinosus m.

Rectus femoris m.

Vastus medialis m.

Popliteal a., v.

Descending genicular artery & vein

Sartorius m.

Greater saphenous v.

Gracilis m.

Semimembranosus m.

Vastus lateralis m.

Femur

Vastus intermedius m.

Sciatic n.

Short head biceps femoris m.

Long head, biceps femoris m.

Semitendinosus m.

(Top) The popliteal vessels course deep to the semimembranosus muscle as they travel to the popliteal fossa. The sciatic nerve continues to travel anteriorly. **(Bottom)** The short and long heads of the biceps femoris muscle join. The separation of the semimembranosus and semitendinous muscles from the biceps femoris muscle is beginning as images approach the superior aspect of the popliteal fossa.

Hip and Pelvis

V

247

AXIAL T1 MR, DISTAL RIGHT THIGH

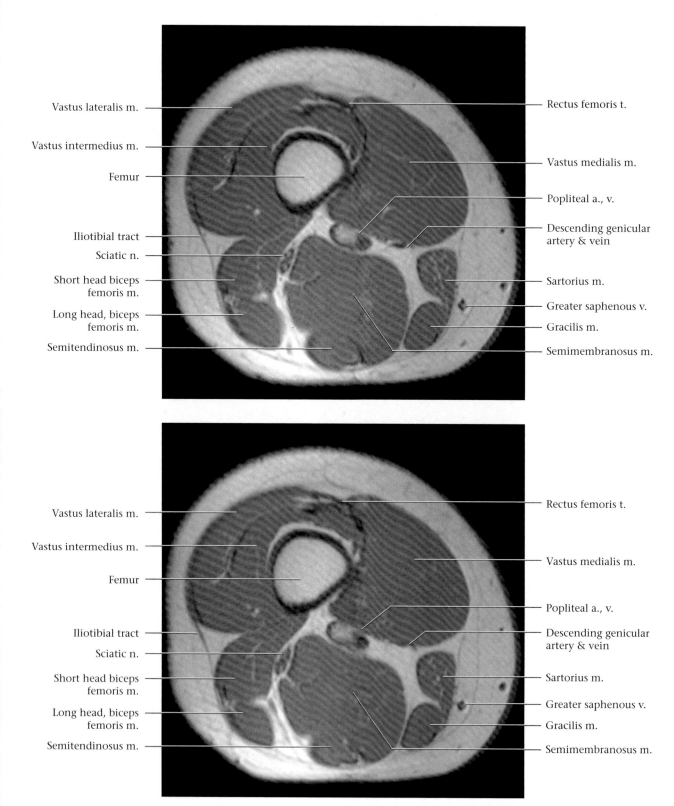

Labels (top image, left): Vastus lateralis m. · Vastus intermedius m. · Femur · Iliotibial tract · Sciatic n. · Short head biceps femoris m. · Long head, biceps femoris m. · Semitendinosus m.

Labels (top image, right): Rectus femoris t. · Vastus medialis m. · Popliteal a., v. · Descending genicular artery & vein · Sartorius m. · Greater saphenous v. · Gracilis m. · Semimembranosus m.

Labels (bottom image, left): Vastus lateralis m. · Vastus intermedius m. · Femur · Iliotibial tract · Sciatic n. · Short head biceps femoris m. · Long head, biceps femoris m. · Semitendinosus m.

Labels (bottom image, right): Rectus femoris t. · Vastus medialis m. · Popliteal a., v. · Descending genicular artery & vein · Sartorius m. · Greater saphenous v. · Gracilis m. · Semimembranosus m.

(Top) The rectus femoris muscle is now a flat tendinous band which forms the central portion of the quadriceps tendon. The tendon of the vastus intermedius muscle is deep to the rectus femoris tendon. The vastus medialis and vastus lateralis tendons are also visible. **(Bottom)** The sciatic nerve has assumed a bilobed appearance as it begins its separation into common peroneal and tibial nerves. On this image the popliteal vein is lateral to the popliteal artery. The veins and arteries can be identified because a vein will always be larger than its companion artery. The more typical position of the artery is deep to the vein.

AXIAL T1 MR, DISTAL LEFT THIGH

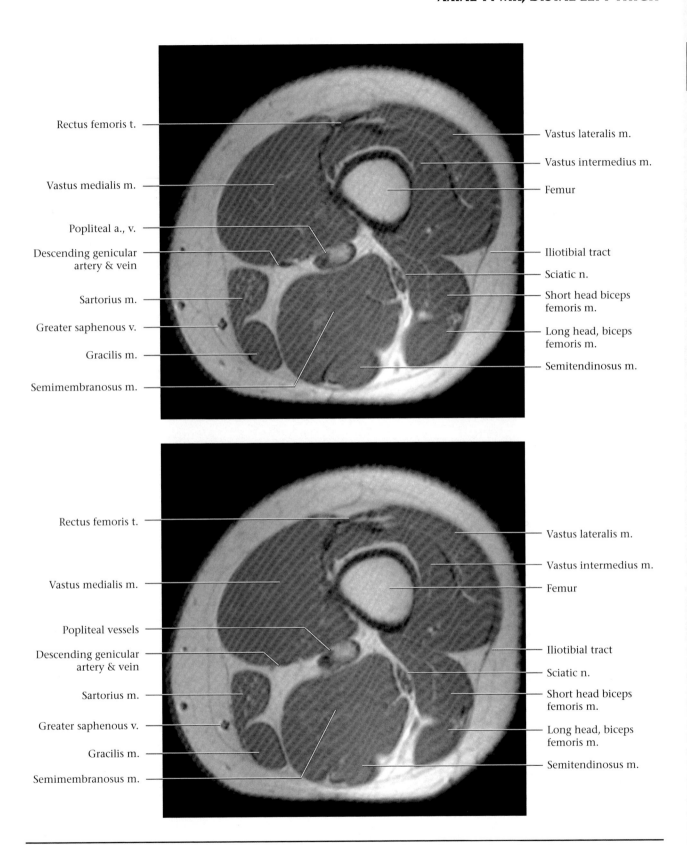

Rectus femoris t.

Vastus medialis m.

Popliteal a., v.

Descending genicular artery & vein

Sartorius m.

Greater saphenous v.

Gracilis m.

Semimembranosus m.

Vastus lateralis m.

Vastus intermedius m.

Femur

Iliotibial tract

Sciatic n.

Short head biceps femoris m.

Long head, biceps femoris m.

Semitendinosus m.

Rectus femoris t.

Vastus medialis m.

Popliteal vessels

Descending genicular artery & vein

Sartorius m.

Greater saphenous v.

Gracilis m.

Semimembranosus m.

Vastus lateralis m.

Vastus intermedius m.

Femur

Iliotibial tract

Sciatic n.

Short head biceps femoris m.

Long head, biceps femoris m.

Semitendinosus m.

(Top) The rectus femoris muscle is now a flat tendinous band which forms the central portion of the quadriceps tendon. The tendon of the vastus intermedius muscle is deep to the rectus femoris tendon. The vastus medialis and vastus lateralis tendons are also visible. **(Bottom)** The sciatic nerve has assumed a bilobed appearance as it begins its separation into common peroneal and tibial nerves. On this image the popliteal vein is lateral to the popliteal artery. The veins and arteries can be identified because a vein will always be larger than its companion artery. The more typical position of the artery is deep to the vein.

Hip and Pelvis

V

AXIAL T1 MR, DISTAL RIGHT THIGH

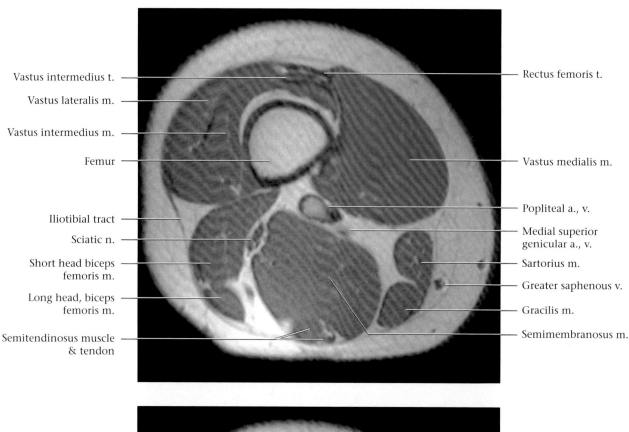

Vastus intermedius t.

Vastus lateralis m.

Vastus intermedius m.

Femur

Iliotibial tract

Sciatic n.

Short head biceps femoris m.

Long head, biceps femoris m.

Semitendinosus muscle & tendon

Rectus femoris t.

Vastus medialis m.

Popliteal a., v.

Medial superior genicular a., v.

Sartorius m.

Greater saphenous v.

Gracilis m.

Semimembranosus m.

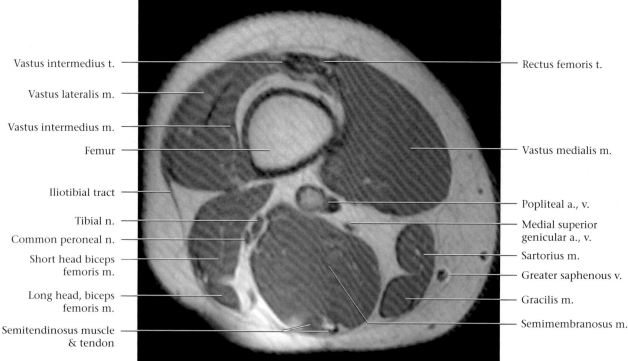

Vastus intermedius t.

Vastus lateralis m.

Vastus intermedius m.

Femur

Iliotibial tract

Tibial n.

Common peroneal n.

Short head biceps femoris m.

Long head, biceps femoris m.

Semitendinosus muscle & tendon

Rectus femoris t.

Vastus medialis m.

Popliteal a., v.

Medial superior genicular a., v.

Sartorius m.

Greater saphenous v.

Gracilis m.

Semimembranosus m.

(Top) The semitendinosus is tendinous through the distal thigh. Here the tendon is seen along the medial aspect of the residual muscle belly. The sartorius and gracilis muscle are now adjacent to one another. **(Bottom)** The sartorius muscle begins to wrap around the gracilis muscle. The medial superior genicular vessels are visible; they are branches of the popliteal vessels. The two divisions of the sciatic nerve are now distinct.

THIGH OVERVIEW

AXIAL T1 MR, DISTAL LEFT THIGH

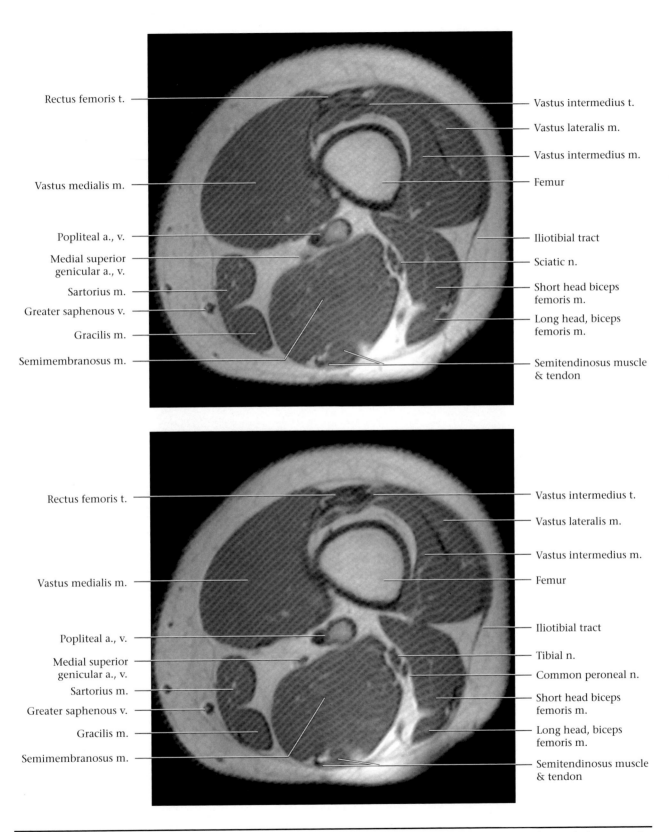

Rectus femoris t. — — Vastus intermedius t.

— Vastus lateralis m.

— Vastus intermedius m.

Vastus medialis m. — — Femur

Popliteal a., v. — — Iliotibial tract

Medial superior genicular a., v. — — Sciatic n.

Sartorius m. — — Short head biceps femoris m.

Greater saphenous v. — — Long head, biceps femoris m.

Gracilis m. —

Semimembranosus m. — — Semitendinosus muscle & tendon

Rectus femoris t. — — Vastus intermedius t.

— Vastus lateralis m.

— Vastus intermedius m.

Vastus medialis m. — — Femur

Popliteal a., v. — — Iliotibial tract

Medial superior genicular a., v. — — Tibial n.

Sartorius m. — — Common peroneal n.

Greater saphenous v. — — Short head biceps femoris m.

Gracilis m. — — Long head, biceps femoris m.

Semimembranosus m. — — Semitendinosus muscle & tendon

(Top) The semitendinosus is tendinous through the distal thigh. Here the tendon is seen along the medial aspect of the residual muscle belly. The sartorius and gracilis muscle are now adjacent to one another. **(Bottom)** The sartorius muscle begins to wrap around the gracilis muscle. The medial superior genicular vessels are visible; they are branches of the popliteal vessels. The two divisions of the sciatic nerve are now distinct.

Hip and Pelvis

V

251

THIGH OVERVIEW

AXIAL T1 MR, DISTAL RIGHT THIGH

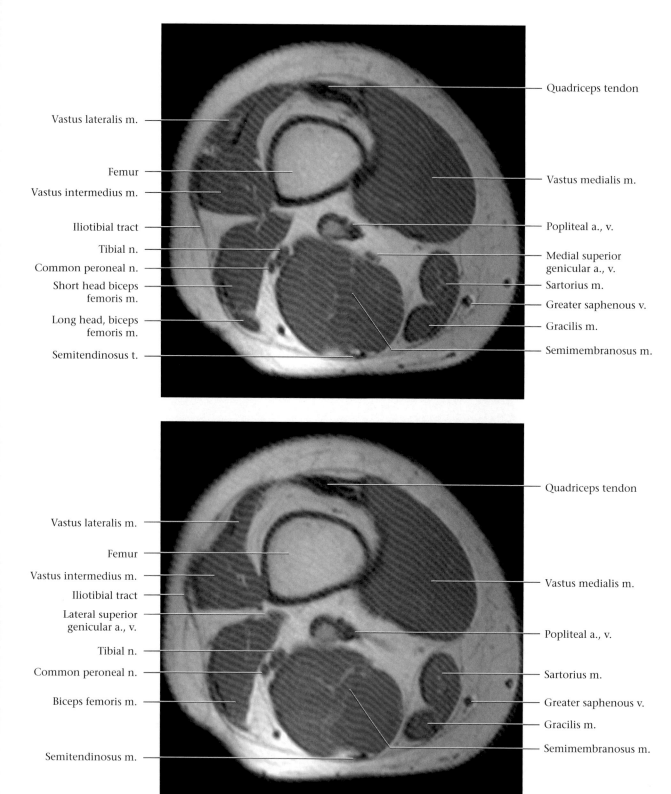

Vastus lateralis m.

Femur

Vastus intermedius m.

Iliotibial tract

Tibial n.

Common peroneal n.

Short head biceps femoris m.

Long head, biceps femoris m.

Semitendinosus t.

Quadriceps tendon

Vastus medialis m.

Popliteal a., v.

Medial superior genicular a., v.

Sartorius m.

Greater saphenous v.

Gracilis m.

Semimembranosus m.

Vastus lateralis m.

Femur

Vastus intermedius m.

Iliotibial tract

Lateral superior genicular a., v.

Tibial n.

Common peroneal n.

Biceps femoris m.

Semitendinosus m.

Quadriceps tendon

Vastus medialis m.

Popliteal a., v.

Sartorius m.

Greater saphenous v.

Gracilis m.

Semimembranosus m.

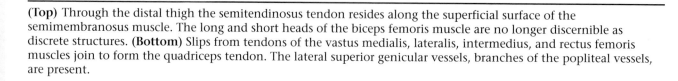

(Top) Through the distal thigh the semitendinosus tendon resides along the superficial surface of the semimembranosus muscle. The long and short heads of the biceps femoris muscle are no longer discernible as discrete structures. **(Bottom)** Slips from tendons of the vastus medialis, lateralis, intermedius, and rectus femoris muscles join to form the quadriceps tendon. The lateral superior genicular vessels, branches of the popliteal vessels, are present.

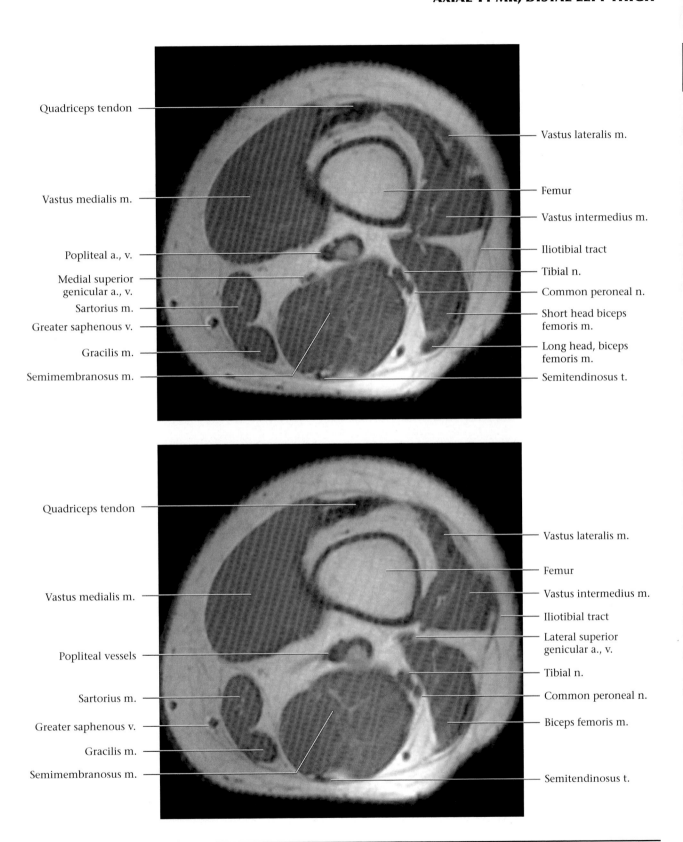

Quadriceps tendon

Vastus medialis m.

Popliteal a., v.

Medial superior genicular a., v.

Sartorius m.

Greater saphenous v.

Gracilis m.

Semimembranosus m.

Vastus lateralis m.

Femur

Vastus intermedius m.

Iliotibial tract

Tibial n.

Common peroneal n.

Short head biceps femoris m.

Long head, biceps femoris m.

Semitendinosus t.

Quadriceps tendon

Vastus medialis m.

Popliteal vessels

Sartorius m.

Greater saphenous v.

Gracilis m.

Semimembranosus m.

Vastus lateralis m.

Femur

Vastus intermedius m.

Iliotibial tract

Lateral superior genicular a., v.

Tibial n.

Common peroneal n.

Biceps femoris m.

Semitendinosus t.

(Top) Through the distal thigh the semitendinosus tendon resides along the superficial surface of the semimembranosus muscle. The long and short heads of the biceps femoris muscle are no longer discernible as discrete structures. **(Bottom)** Slips from tendons of the vastus medialis, lateralis, intermedius, and rectus femoris muscles join to form the quadriceps tendon. The lateral superior genicular vessels, branches of the popliteal vessels, are present.

Hip and Pelvis

V

AXIAL T1 MR, DISTAL RIGHT THIGH

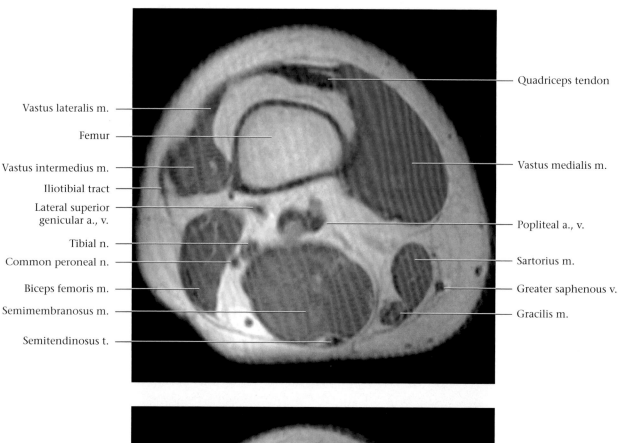

Vastus lateralis m. — Quadriceps tendon

Femur —

Vastus intermedius m. — Vastus medialis m.

Iliotibial tract —

Lateral superior genicular a., v. — Popliteal a., v.

Tibial n. —

Common peroneal n. — Sartorius m.

Biceps femoris m. — Greater saphenous v.

Semimembranosus m. — Gracilis m.

Semitendinosus t. —

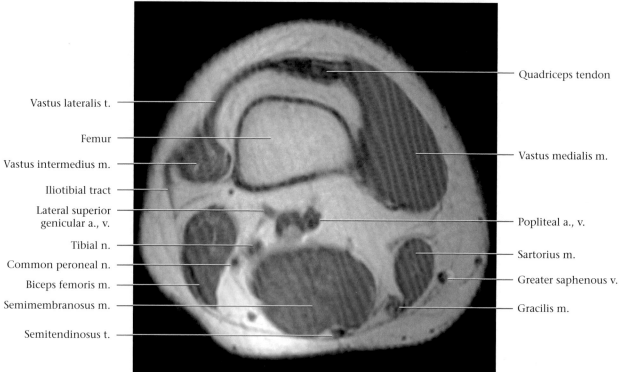

Vastus lateralis t. — Quadriceps tendon

Femur —

Vastus intermedius m. — Vastus medialis m.

Iliotibial tract —

Lateral superior genicular a., v. — Popliteal a., v.

Tibial n. — Sartorius m.

Common peroneal n. —

Biceps femoris m. — Greater saphenous v.

Semimembranosus m. — Gracilis m.

Semitendinosus t. —

(Top) The femur broadens distally during the transition from diaphysis to metaphysis and the supracondylar portion (that portion just above the femoral condyles). **(Bottom)** The gracilis muscle is now extremely small and only the tendon extends inferiorly from this point. The origin of the lateral superior genicular vessels is inferior to the vessels consistent with the lateral and superior course of those vessels.

Hip and Pelvis

AXIAL T1 MR, DISTAL LEFT THIGH

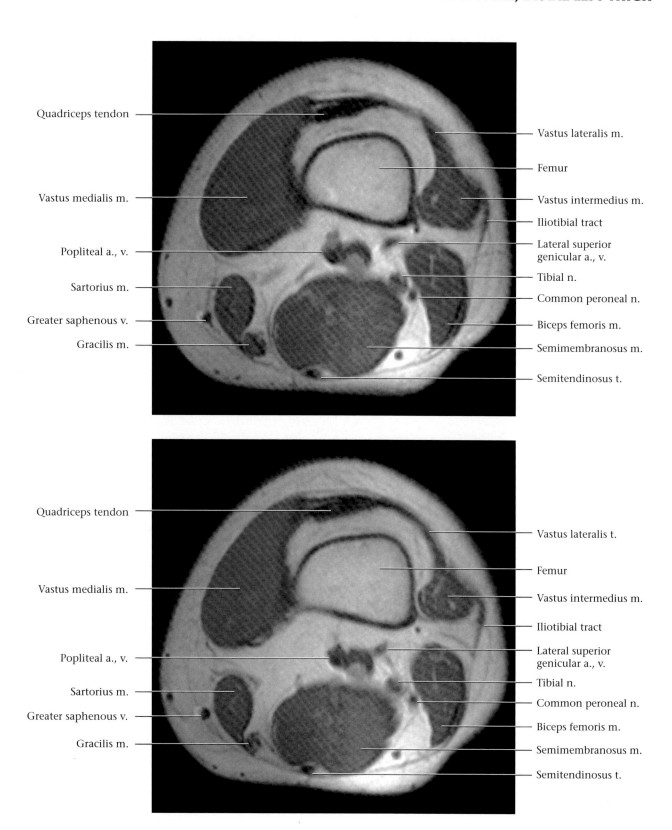

Quadriceps tendon — Vastus lateralis m.

Femur

Vastus medialis m. — Vastus intermedius m.

Iliotibial tract

Popliteal a., v. — Lateral superior genicular a., v.

Sartorius m. — Tibial n.

Greater saphenous v. — Common peroneal n.

Gracilis m. — Biceps femoris m.

Semimembranosus m.

Semitendinosus t.

Quadriceps tendon — Vastus lateralis t.

Femur

Vastus medialis m. — Vastus intermedius m.

Iliotibial tract

Popliteal a., v. — Lateral superior genicular a., v.

Sartorius m. — Tibial n.

Greater saphenous v. — Common peroneal n.

Gracilis m. — Biceps femoris m.

Semimembranosus m.

Semitendinosus t.

(**Top**) The femur broadens distally during the transition from diaphysis to metaphysis and the supracondylar portion (that portion just above the femoral condyles). (**Bottom**) The gracilis muscle is now extremely small and only the tendon extends inferiorly from this point. The origin of the lateral superior genicular vessels is inferior to the vessels consistent with the lateral and superior course of those vessels.

Hip and Pelvis

V

AXIAL T1 MR, DISTAL RIGHT THIGH

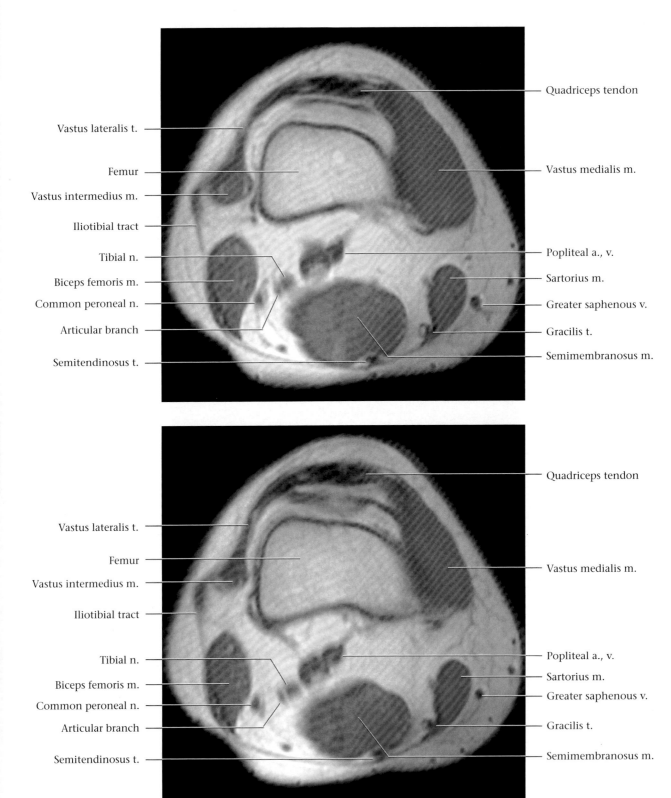

Quadriceps tendon

Vastus lateralis t.

Femur

Vastus intermedius m.

Iliotibial tract

Tibial n.

Biceps femoris m.

Common peroneal n.

Articular branch

Semitendinosus t.

Vastus medialis m.

Popliteal a., v.

Sartorius m.

Greater saphenous v.

Gracilis t.

Semimembranosus m.

Quadriceps tendon

Vastus lateralis t.

Femur

Vastus intermedius m.

Iliotibial tract

Tibial n.

Biceps femoris m.

Common peroneal n.

Articular branch

Semitendinosus t.

Vastus medialis m.

Popliteal a., v.

Sartorius m.

Greater saphenous v.

Gracilis t.

Semimembranosus m.

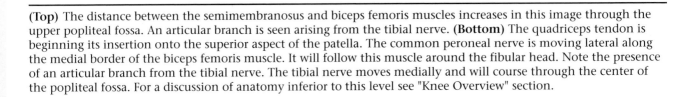

(Top) The distance between the semimembranosus and biceps femoris muscles increases in this image through the upper popliteal fossa. An articular branch is seen arising from the tibial nerve. **(Bottom)** The quadriceps tendon is beginning its insertion onto the superior aspect of the patella. The common peroneal nerve is moving lateral along the medial border of the biceps femoris muscle. It will follow this muscle around the fibular head. Note the presence of an articular branch from the tibial nerve. The tibial nerve moves medially and will course through the center of the popliteal fossa. For a discussion of anatomy inferior to this level see "Knee Overview" section.

AXIAL T1 MR, DISTAL LEFT THIGH

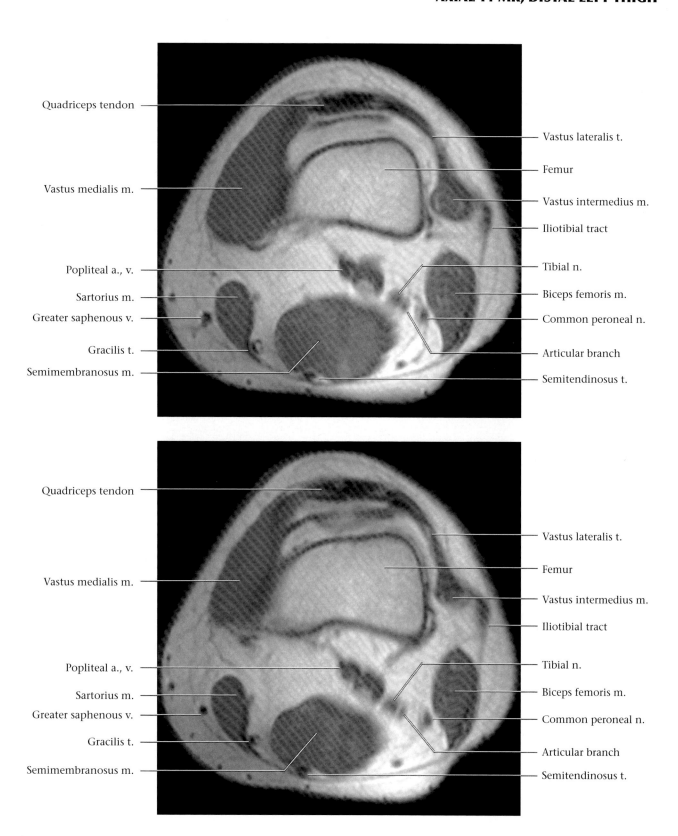

Quadriceps tendon

Vastus medialis m.

Popliteal a., v.

Sartorius m.

Greater saphenous v.

Gracilis t.

Semimembranosus m.

Vastus lateralis t.

Femur

Vastus intermedius m.

Iliotibial tract

Tibial n.

Biceps femoris m.

Common peroneal n.

Articular branch

Semitendinosus t.

Quadriceps tendon

Vastus medialis m.

Popliteal a., v.

Sartorius m.

Greater saphenous v.

Gracilis t.

Semimembranosus m.

Vastus lateralis t.

Femur

Vastus intermedius m.

Iliotibial tract

Tibial n.

Biceps femoris m.

Common peroneal n.

Articular branch

Semitendinosus t.

(Top) The distance between the semimembranosus and biceps femoris muscles increases in this image through the upper popliteal fossa. An articular branch is seen arising from the tibial nerve. **(Bottom)** The quadriceps tendon is beginning its insertion onto the superior aspect of the patella. The common peroneal nerve is moving lateral along the medial border of the biceps femoris muscle. It will follow this muscle around the fibular head. Note the presence of an articular branch from the tibial nerve. The tibial nerve moves medially and will course through the center of the popliteal fossa. For a discussion of anatomy inferior to this level see "Knee Overview" section.

Hip and Pelvis

V

CORONAL T1 MR, POSTERIOR THIGH

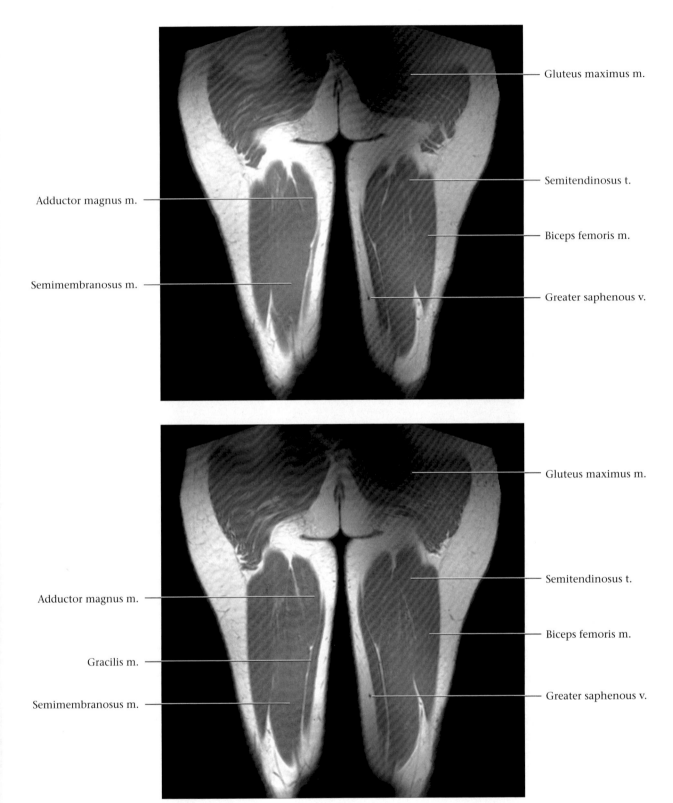

Gluteus maximus m.

Semitendinosus t.

Biceps femoris m.

Greater saphenous v.

Adductor magnus m.

Semimembranosus m.

Gluteus maximus m.

Semitendinosus t.

Biceps femoris m.

Adductor magnus m.

Gracilis m.

Semimembranosus m.

Greater saphenous v.

(Top) First in series of T1 weighted coronal images from posterior to anterior. Superiorly in the posterior thigh the semitendinosus muscle is more prominent while inferiorly the semimembranosus muscle is larger and more prominent. **(Bottom)** A long segment of the gracilis muscle is visible. It is the most medial muscle in the thigh. The semimembranosus and biceps femoris muscles follow diverging courses in the lower thigh at the superior aspect of the popliteal fossa.

THIGH OVERVIEW

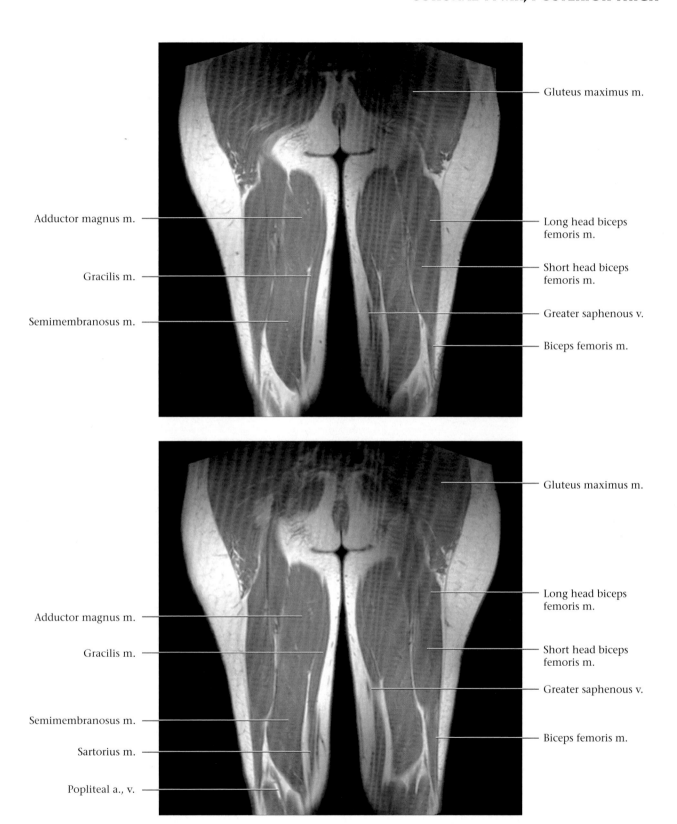

Gluteus maximus m.

Adductor magnus m.

Gracilis m.

Semimembranosus m.

Long head biceps femoris m.

Short head biceps femoris m.

Greater saphenous v.

Biceps femoris m.

Gluteus maximus m.

Adductor magnus m.

Gracilis m.

Semimembranosus m.

Sartorius m.

Popliteal a., v.

Long head biceps femoris m.

Short head biceps femoris m.

Greater saphenous v.

Biceps femoris m.

(Top) In this plane the adductor magnus and semimembranosus muscles are difficult to separate. They can be identified by following their courses more anteriorly. The adductor muscle is more prominent superiorly, the semimembranosus more inferiorly. The greater saphenous vein is the most superficial structure in the medial thigh. **(Bottom)** In the distal thigh the sartorius muscle and the gracilis muscle are closely approximated and the sartorius muscle is located more anteriorly. On this image they appear to be continuous. Each muscle is identified by following it on adjacent images.

THIGH OVERVIEW

CORONAL T1 MR, POSTERIOR THIGH

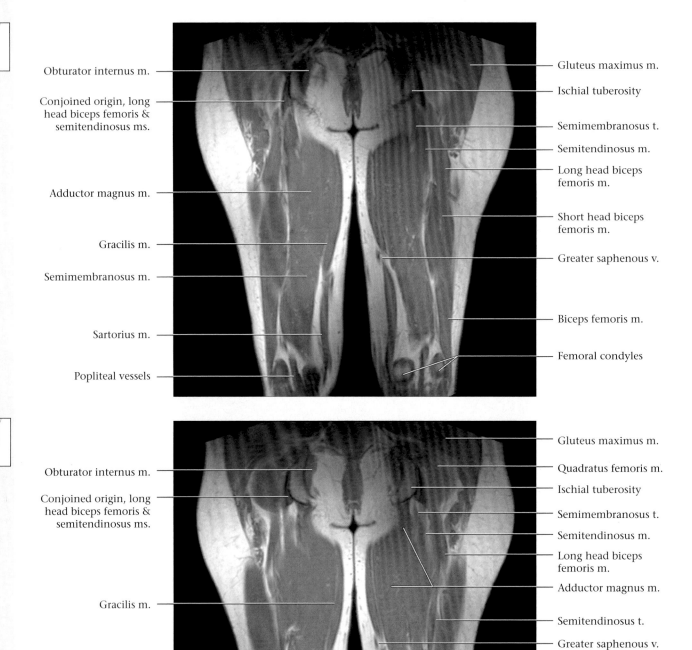

Obturator internus m.

Conjoined origin, long head biceps femoris & semitendinosus ms.

Adductor magnus m.

Gracilis m.

Semimembranosus m.

Sartorius m.

Popliteal vessels

Gluteus maximus m.

Ischial tuberosity

Semimembranosus t.

Semitendinosus m.

Long head biceps femoris m.

Short head biceps femoris m.

Greater saphenous v.

Biceps femoris m.

Femoral condyles

Obturator internus m.

Conjoined origin, long head biceps femoris & semitendinosus ms.

Gracilis m.

Semimembranosus m.

Sartorius m.

Popliteal vessels

Gluteus maximus m.

Quadratus femoris m.

Ischial tuberosity

Semimembranosus t.

Semitendinosus m.

Long head biceps femoris m.

Adductor magnus m.

Semitendinosus t.

Greater saphenous v.

Long head biceps femoris m.

Popliteal fossa

Femoral condyles

(Top) Although the origin of the semimembranosus tendon is immediately proximal and lateral to that of the conjoined long head biceps and semitendinosus tendons, the semimembranosus fairly immediately moves to a more anterior, and then medial position relative to the conjoined tendon. The labeled semimembranosus in this image is of the membranous portion, seen just medial to the conjoined origin of the long head of the biceps femoris and semitendinosus muscles. **(Bottom)** The origin of the ischiocondylar portion of the adductor magnus muscle from the ischial tuberosity is visible. This muscle is the most medial hamstring. The distinction between the gracilis and sartorius muscles is apparent on this image. The quadratus femoris muscle is a flat muscle along the deep surface of the gluteus maximus muscle.

THIGH OVERVIEW

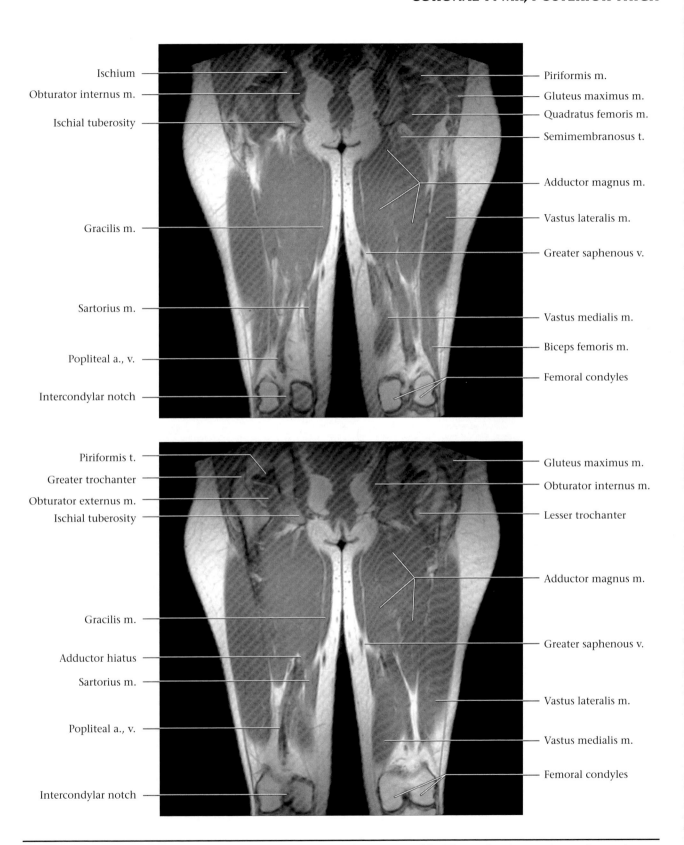

Ischium

Obturator internus m.

Ischial tuberosity

Gracilis m.

Sartorius m.

Popliteal a., v.

Intercondylar notch

Piriformis m.

Gluteus maximus m.

Quadratus femoris m.

Semimembranosus t.

Adductor magnus m.

Vastus lateralis m.

Greater saphenous v.

Vastus medialis m.

Biceps femoris m.

Femoral condyles

Piriformis t.

Greater trochanter

Obturator externus m.

Ischial tuberosity

Gracilis m.

Adductor hiatus

Sartorius m.

Popliteal a., v.

Intercondylar notch

Gluteus maximus m.

Obturator internus m.

Lesser trochanter

Adductor magnus m.

Greater saphenous v.

Vastus lateralis m.

Vastus medialis m.

Femoral condyles

(Top) The course of the piriformis tendon to the greater trochanter is visible. The tendon is superior to the tendons of the other external rotators of the hip. For further details of this anatomy see the "Lateral Hip" section. **(Bottom)** The separation of the adductor and ischiocondylar portions of the adductor magnus muscle creates the adductor hiatus. The superficial femoral vessels transition to popliteal vessels at this point.

CORONAL T1 MR, MID THIGH

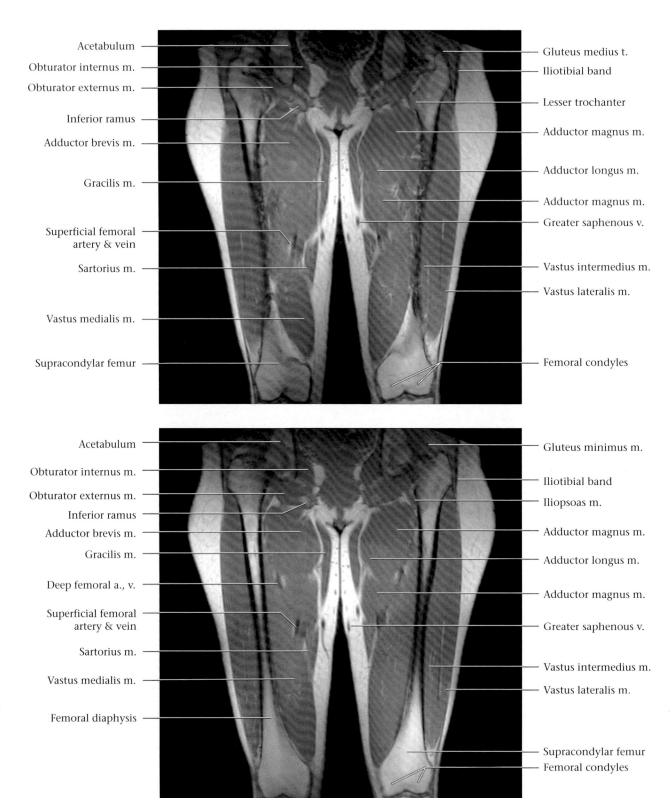

Acetabulum
Obturator internus m.
Obturator externus m.
Inferior ramus
Adductor brevis m.
Gracilis m.
Superficial femoral artery & vein
Sartorius m.
Vastus medialis m.
Supracondylar femur

Gluteus medius t.
Iliotibial band
Lesser trochanter
Adductor magnus m.
Adductor longus m.
Adductor magnus m.
Greater saphenous v.
Vastus intermedius m.
Vastus lateralis m.
Femoral condyles

Acetabulum
Obturator internus m.
Obturator externus m.
Inferior ramus
Adductor brevis m.
Gracilis m.
Deep femoral a., v.
Superficial femoral artery & vein
Sartorius m.
Vastus medialis m.
Femoral diaphysis

Gluteus minimus m.
Iliotibial band
Iliopsoas m.
Adductor magnus m.
Adductor longus m.
Adductor magnus m.
Greater saphenous v.
Vastus intermedius m.
Vastus lateralis m.
Supracondylar femur
Femoral condyles

(Top) The inferior (ischiopubic) ramus is seen in cross section. These rami are rather small and should not be confused with fat deposits. The gluteus medius tendon is seen inserting onto the greater trochanter. **(Bottom)** The deep and superficial femoral vessels are visualized. The obturator internus and externus muscles are visible on either side of the obturator membrane. The adductor longus muscle is difficult to separate from the adductor magnus muscle.

THIGH OVERVIEW

CORONAL T1 MR, MID THIGH

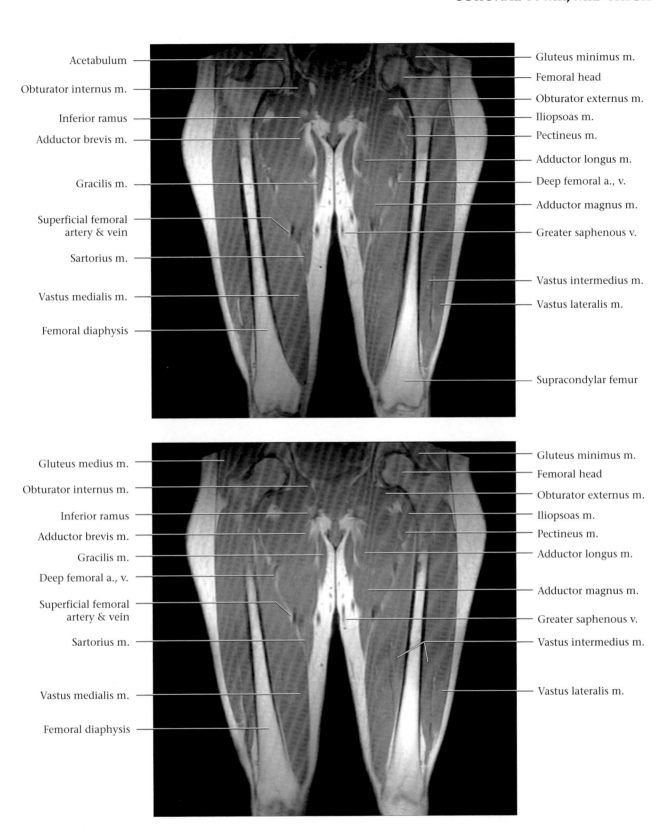

Top image labels (left):
- Acetabulum
- Obturator internus m.
- Inferior ramus
- Adductor brevis m.
- Gracilis m.
- Superficial femoral artery & vein
- Sartorius m.
- Vastus medialis m.
- Femoral diaphysis

Top image labels (right):
- Gluteus minimus m.
- Femoral head
- Obturator externus m.
- Iliopsoas m.
- Pectineus m.
- Adductor longus m.
- Deep femoral a., v.
- Adductor magnus m.
- Greater saphenous v.
- Vastus intermedius m.
- Vastus lateralis m.
- Supracondylar femur

Bottom image labels (left):
- Gluteus medius m.
- Obturator internus m.
- Inferior ramus
- Adductor brevis m.
- Gracilis m.
- Deep femoral a., v.
- Superficial femoral artery & vein
- Sartorius m.
- Vastus medialis m.
- Femoral diaphysis

Bottom image labels (right):
- Gluteus minimus m.
- Femoral head
- Obturator externus m.
- Iliopsoas m.
- Pectineus m.
- Adductor longus m.
- Adductor magnus m.
- Greater saphenous v.
- Vastus intermedius m.
- Vastus lateralis m.

(Top) Within the anterior thigh the adductor longus, brevis and pectineus muscles are most pronounced. The adductor magnus is a more posterior structure within the compartment. The origin of the gracilis muscle from the inferior pubic ramus is visible. The more lateral position of the deep femoral vessels relative to the superficial femoral vessels is evident. **(Bottom)** The iliopsoas muscle hugs the medial aspect of the joint as it nears its insertion onto the lesser trochanter. The vastus intermedius muscle is seen both medial and lateral to the femoral diaphysis. The muscle wraps around a significant portion of the anterior femur in the distal thigh.

THIGH OVERVIEW

CORONAL T1 MR, ANTERIOR THIGH

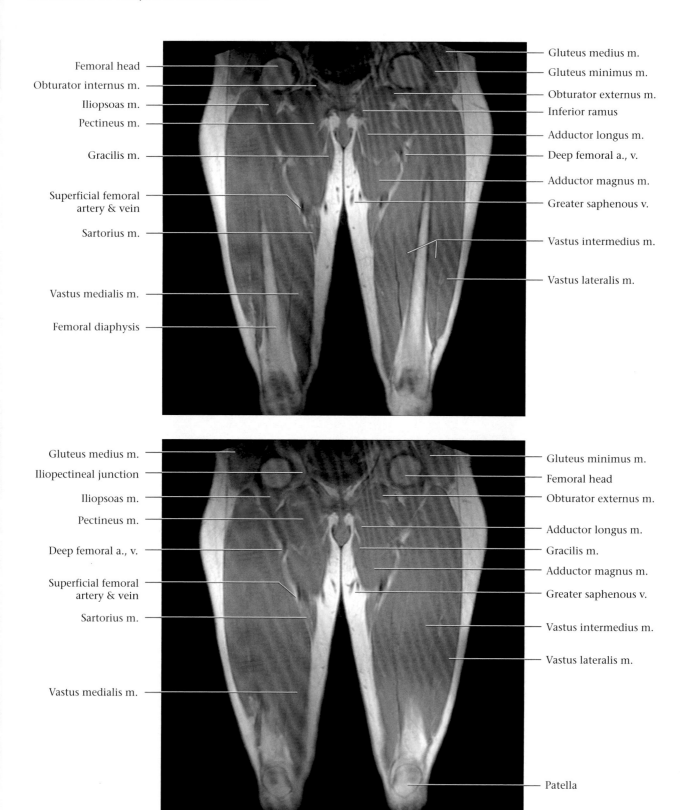

Femoral head
Obturator internus m.
Iliopsoas m.
Pectineus m.

Gracilis m.

Superficial femoral artery & vein

Sartorius m.

Vastus medialis m.

Femoral diaphysis

Gluteus medius m.
Gluteus minimus m.
Obturator externus m.
Inferior ramus
Adductor longus m.
Deep femoral a., v.
Adductor magnus m.
Greater saphenous v.

Vastus intermedius m.

Vastus lateralis m.

Gluteus medius m.
Iliopectineal junction
Iliopsoas m.
Pectineus m.

Deep femoral a., v.

Superficial femoral artery & vein

Sartorius m.

Vastus medialis m.

Gluteus minimus m.
Femoral head
Obturator externus m.

Adductor longus m.
Gracilis m.
Adductor magnus m.
Greater saphenous v.

Vastus intermedius m.

Vastus lateralis m.

Patella

(Top) The pectineus and adductor longus muscles lie in the same coronal plane and the adductor longus is the more inferior muscle. **(Bottom)** The adductor canal is visible. Its boundaries are the sartorius, vastus medialis and adductor magnus muscles. The superficial femoral vessels are within the canal.

THIGH OVERVIEW

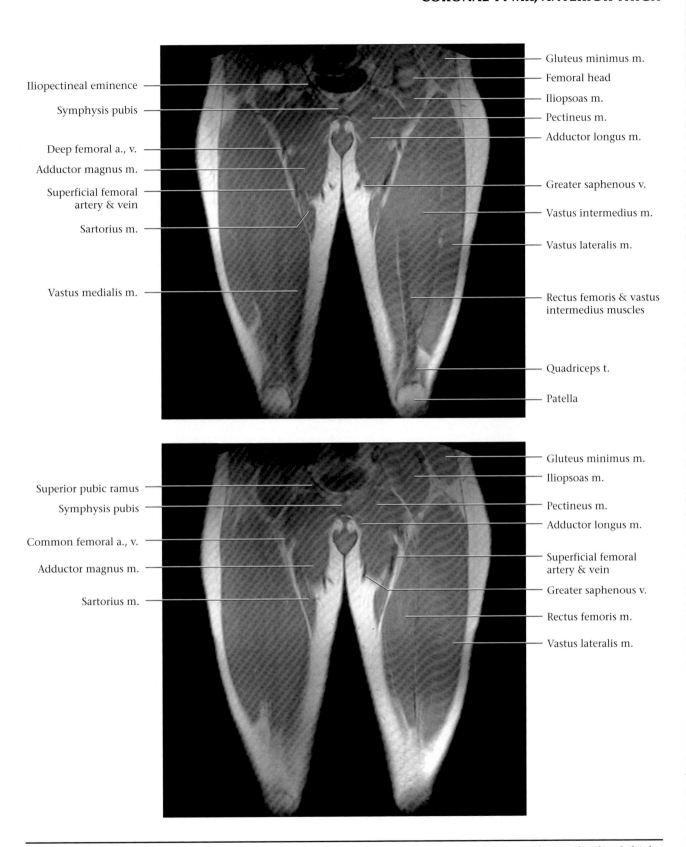

Top image labels (left):
- Iliopectineal eminence
- Symphysis pubis
- Deep femoral a., v.
- Adductor magnus m.
- Superficial femoral artery & vein
- Sartorius m.
- Vastus medialis m.

Top image labels (right):
- Gluteus minimus m.
- Femoral head
- Iliopsoas m.
- Pectineus m.
- Adductor longus m.
- Greater saphenous v.
- Vastus intermedius m.
- Vastus lateralis m.
- Rectus femoris & vastus intermedius muscles
- Quadriceps t.
- Patella

Bottom image labels (left):
- Superior pubic ramus
- Symphysis pubis
- Common femoral a., v.
- Adductor magnus m.
- Sartorius m.

Bottom image labels (right):
- Gluteus minimus m.
- Iliopsoas m.
- Pectineus m.
- Adductor longus m.
- Superficial femoral artery & vein
- Greater saphenous v.
- Rectus femoris m.
- Vastus lateralis m.

(Top) The rectus femoris tendon and the tendon of the vastus intermedius tendon blend together in the distal thigh in the plane between the two muscles. More distally, with the addition of tendons from the vastus medialis and vastus lateralis muscle the quadriceps tendon is formed. **(Bottom)** The symphysis pubis and superior pubic ramus are seen at the anterior aspect of the pelvis. This anatomy is presented in greater detail in the "Anterior Pelvis and Thigh" section. The iliopsoas muscle is seen as it travels from the pelvis to the lower extremity over the iliopectineal eminence. Note the anterior extent of the gluteus minimus muscle.

CORONAL T1 MR, ANTERIOR THIGH

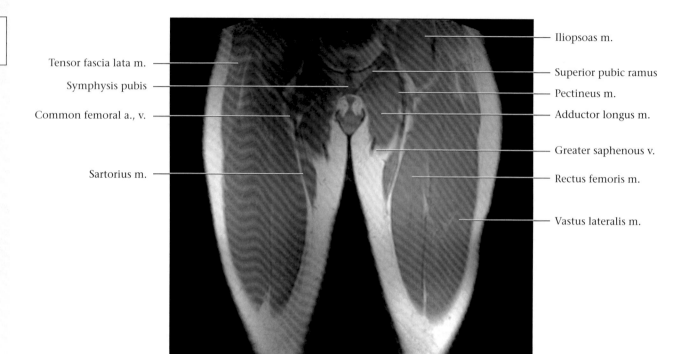

Tensor fascia lata m.
Symphysis pubis
Common femoral a., v.
Sartorius m.

Iliopsoas m.
Superior pubic ramus
Pectineus m.
Adductor longus m.
Greater saphenous v.
Rectus femoris m.
Vastus lateralis m.

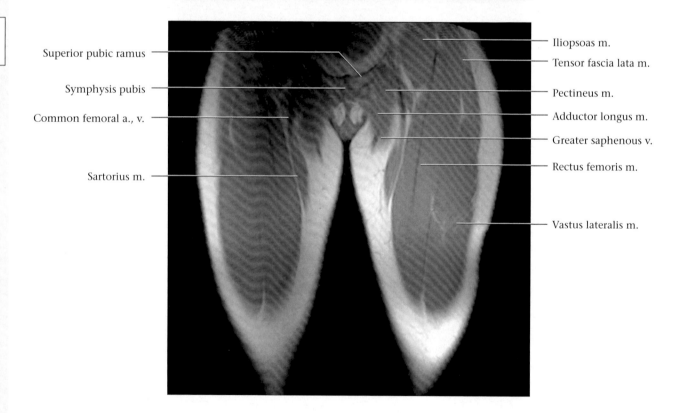

Superior pubic ramus
Symphysis pubis
Common femoral a., v.
Sartorius m.

Iliopsoas m.
Tensor fascia lata m.
Pectineus m.
Adductor longus m.
Greater saphenous v.
Rectus femoris m.
Vastus lateralis m.

(Top) The common femoral vessels are anterior structures entering the thigh just deep to the inguinal ligament. The medial position of the vessels relative to the iliopsoas muscle is well visualized. **(Bottom)** In the upper thigh the tendon of the rectus femoris muscle is located along the anterior aspect of the muscle belly.

CORONAL T1 MR, ANTERIOR THIGH

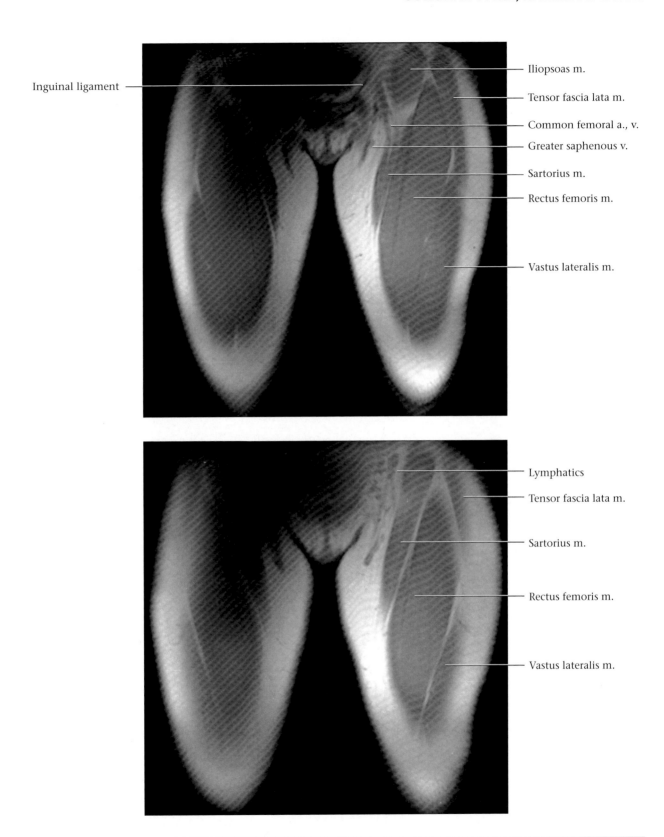

Inguinal ligament

Iliopsoas m.

Tensor fascia lata m.

Common femoral a., v.

Greater saphenous v.

Sartorius m.

Rectus femoris m.

Vastus lateralis m.

Lymphatics

Tensor fascia lata m.

Sartorius m.

Rectus femoris m.

Vastus lateralis m.

(Top) The medial edge of the inguinal ligament is nicely seen. The passage of the vessels deep to the ligaments can be visualized. **(Bottom)** The lymphatics of the inguinal region are well demonstrated, with a series of lymphatic channels traversing between normal sized lymph nodes. The anterior most muscles of the thigh are the sartorius, rectus femoris and vastus lateralis muscles. Note their oblique orientation.

SAGITTAL T1 MR, MEDIAL THIGH

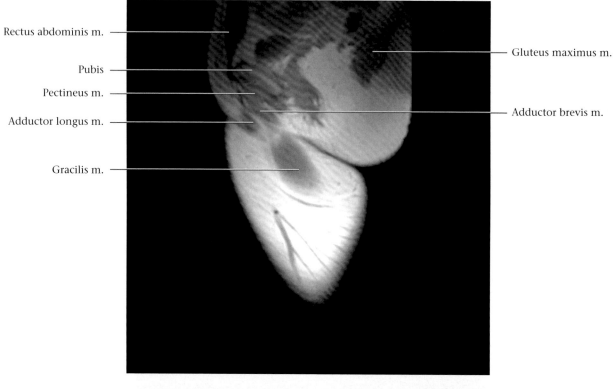

Rectus abdominis m. — Gluteus maximus m.

Pubis —

Pectineus m. —

Adductor longus m. — Adductor brevis m.

Gracilis m. —

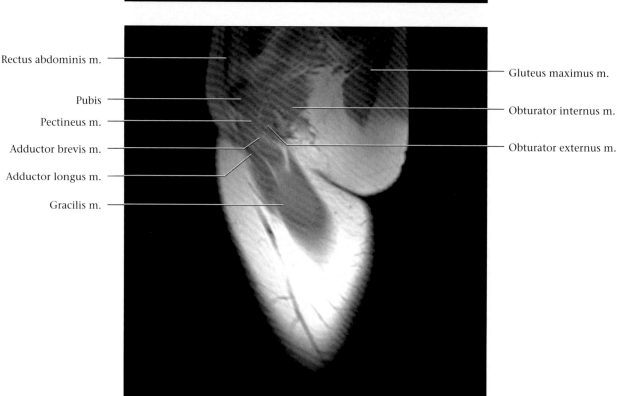

Rectus abdominis m. — Gluteus maximus m.

Pubis —

Pectineus m. — Obturator internus m.

Adductor brevis m. — Obturator externus m.

Adductor longus m. —

Gracilis m. —

(Top) Sagittal images of the thigh from medial to lateral. In the midline the rectus abdominis muscles are present. The gluteus maximus muscle is the only posterior muscle. The gracilis muscle is a thin strip of muscle; the majority of this muscle is only visible on this most medial image. **(Bottom)** The obturator internus muscle is seen en face. The long tendinous origin of the adductor longus muscle is well depicted on this image. Many muscles are present in the medial compartment in the upper thigh. The adductor brevis muscle is deep to the pectineus and adductor longus muscles.

Hip and Pelvis

THIGH OVERVIEW

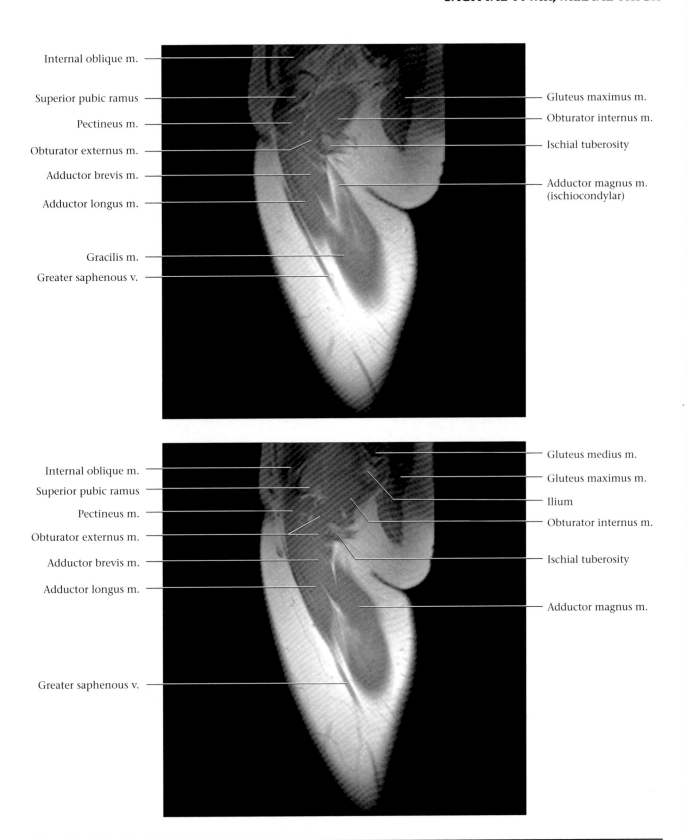

Internal oblique m.

Superior pubic ramus

Pectineus m.

Obturator externus m.

Adductor brevis m.

Adductor longus m.

Gracilis m.

Greater saphenous v.

Gluteus maximus m.

Obturator internus m.

Ischial tuberosity

Adductor magnus m. (ischiocondylar)

Internal oblique m.

Superior pubic ramus

Pectineus m.

Obturator externus m.

Adductor brevis m.

Adductor longus m.

Greater saphenous v.

Gluteus medius m.

Gluteus maximus m.

Ilium

Obturator internus m.

Ischial tuberosity

Adductor magnus m.

(Top) Due to their curved course around the anterior abdominal wall the internal oblique and transversus muscles are obliquely profiled. The long axis of the ischiocondylar portion of the adductor magnus muscle is well visualized. **(Bottom)** A long segment of the greater saphenous vein is evident. The adductor brevis muscle lies deep to the adductor longus muscle. The origin of the pectineus muscle from the superior pubic ramus is nicely seen on this image.

THIGH OVERVIEW

SAGITTAL T1 MR, MEDIAL THIGH

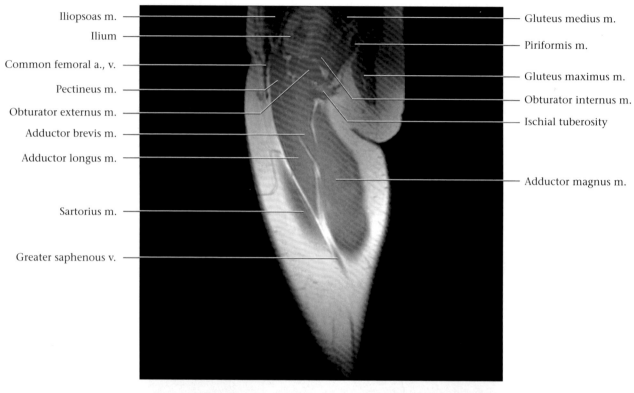

Iliopsoas m. — Gluteus medius m.

Ilium — Piriformis m.

Common femoral a., v. — Gluteus maximus m.

Pectineus m. — Obturator internus m.

Obturator externus m. — Ischial tuberosity

Adductor brevis m.

Adductor longus m. — Adductor magnus m.

Sartorius m.

Greater saphenous v.

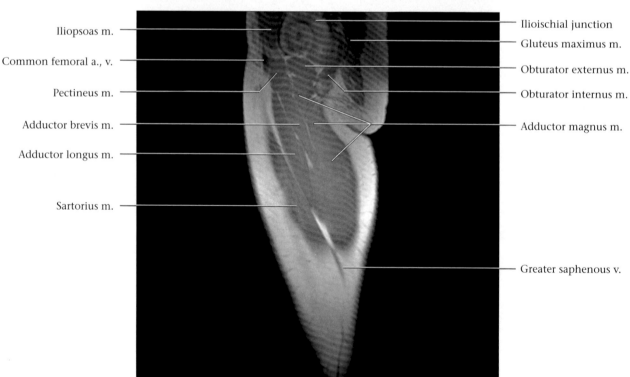

Iliopsoas m. — Ilioischial junction

Common femoral a., v. — Gluteus maximus m.

— Obturator externus m.

Pectineus m. — Obturator internus m.

Adductor brevis m. — Adductor magnus m.

Adductor longus m.

Sartorius m.

Greater saphenous v.

(Top) The obturator internus and externus muscles are separated by the obturator membrane. The pectineus and adductor longus muscle lie in the same coronal plane. The adductor longus muscle is inferior to the pectineus muscle. **(Bottom)** A long segment of the sartorius muscle is seen on the anterior aspect of this medial image. Its distal course is similar to the gracilis muscle. The iliopsoas muscle travels from the pelvis to the thigh over the iliopectineal junction.

THIGH OVERVIEW

SAGITTAL T1 MR, MEDIAL THIGH

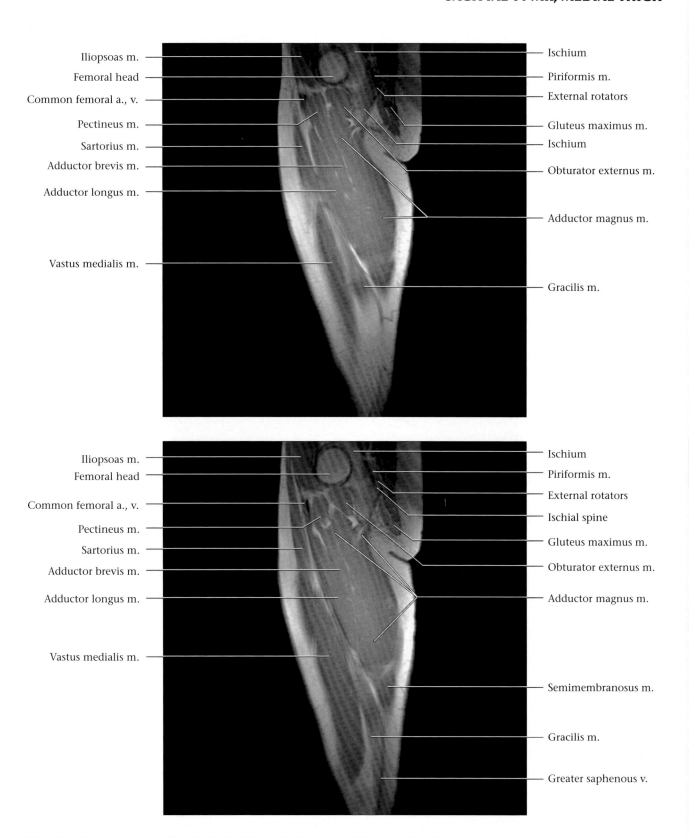

Top image labels (left): Iliopsoas m.; Femoral head; Common femoral a., v.; Pectineus m.; Sartorius m.; Adductor brevis m.; Adductor longus m.; Vastus medialis m.

Top image labels (right): Ischium; Piriformis m.; External rotators; Gluteus maximus m.; Ischium; Obturator externus m.; Adductor magnus m.; Gracilis m.

Bottom image labels (left): Iliopsoas m.; Femoral head; Common femoral a., v.; Pectineus m.; Sartorius m.; Adductor brevis m.; Adductor longus m.; Vastus medialis m.

Bottom image labels (right): Ischium; Piriformis m.; External rotators; Ischial spine; Gluteus maximus m.; Obturator externus m.; Adductor magnus m.; Semimembranosus m.; Gracilis m.; Greater saphenous v.

(Top) The adductor magnus muscle occupies a large portion of the medial thigh. **(Bottom)** The two origins of the adductor magnus muscle are visible. The ischiocondylar portion arises from the ischial tuberosity while the adductor portion of the muscle originates from the ischiopubic ramus. The vastus medialis muscle is also a large muscle along the medial thigh. The external rotators of the hip are present at the level of the ischial spine. Their anatomy is presented in greater detail in the "Lateral Hip" section.

THIGH OVERVIEW

SAGITTAL T1 MR, MEDIAL THIGH

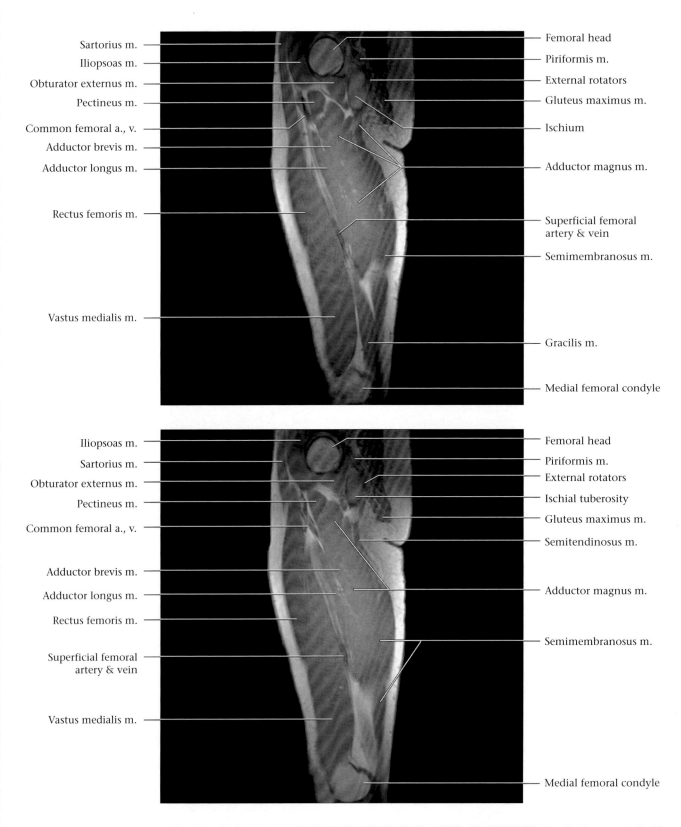

Sartorius m. — Femoral head
Iliopsoas m. — Piriformis m.
Obturator externus m. — External rotators
Pectineus m. — Gluteus maximus m.
Common femoral a., v. — Ischium
Adductor brevis m.
Adductor longus m. — Adductor magnus m.
Rectus femoris m. — Superficial femoral artery & vein
— Semimembranosus m.
Vastus medialis m.
— Gracilis m.
— Medial femoral condyle

Iliopsoas m. — Femoral head
Sartorius m. — Piriformis m.
Obturator externus m. — External rotators
Pectineus m. — Ischial tuberosity
Common femoral a., v. — Gluteus maximus m.
— Semitendinosus m.
Adductor brevis m.
Adductor longus m. — Adductor magnus m.
Rectus femoris m.
Superficial femoral artery & vein — Semimembranosus m.
Vastus medialis m.
— Medial femoral condyle

(Top) The inferior course of the gracilis muscle is seen as it nears it insertion onto the tibia. The course of the superficial femoral vessels in the mid thigh is easily appreciated. **(Bottom)** The semimembranosus muscle belly is a large structure occupying a significant portion of the posterior aspect of the distal thigh. The semitendinosus tendon takes origin from the superior and medial aspect of the inferomedial external surface of the ischial tuberosity.

SAGITTAL T1 MR, MEDIAL THIGH

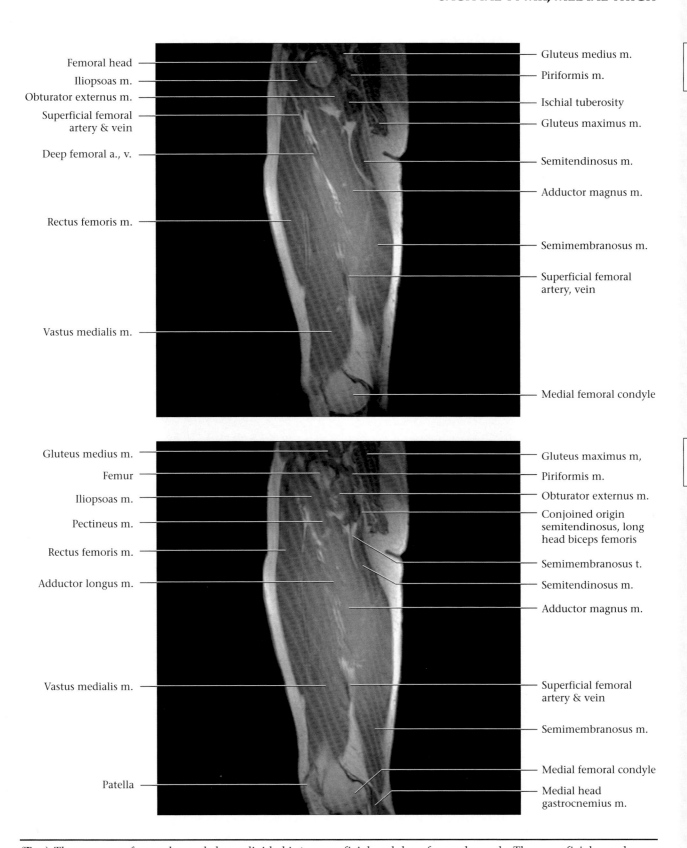

Femoral head

Iliopsoas m.

Obturator externus m.

Superficial femoral artery & vein

Deep femoral a., v.

Rectus femoris m.

Vastus medialis m.

Gluteus medius m.

Piriformis m.

Ischial tuberosity

Gluteus maximus m.

Semitendinosus m.

Adductor magnus m.

Semimembranosus m.

Superficial femoral artery, vein

Medial femoral condyle

Gluteus medius m.

Femur

Iliopsoas m.

Pectineus m.

Rectus femoris m.

Adductor longus m.

Vastus medialis m.

Patella

Gluteus maximus m,

Piriformis m.

Obturator externus m.

Conjoined origin semitendinosus, long head biceps femoris

Semimembranosus t.

Semitendinosus m.

Adductor magnus m.

Superficial femoral artery & vein

Semimembranosus m.

Medial femoral condyle

Medial head gastrocnemius m.

(Top) The common femoral vessels have divided into superficial and deep femoral vessels. The superficial vessels course medially while the deep femoral vessels are seen on this image as they head more laterally. **(Bottom)** The rectus femoris muscle occupies the anterior aspect of the thigh. The membranous origin of the semimembranosus muscle from the superior and lateral aspect of the external surface of the ischial tuberosity is nicely demonstrated on this image. The long head of the biceps femoris muscle and the semitendinosus muscle share a common origin from the ischial tuberosity.

Hip and Pelvis

∨

THIGH OVERVIEW

SAGITTAL T1 MR, MEDIAL THIGH

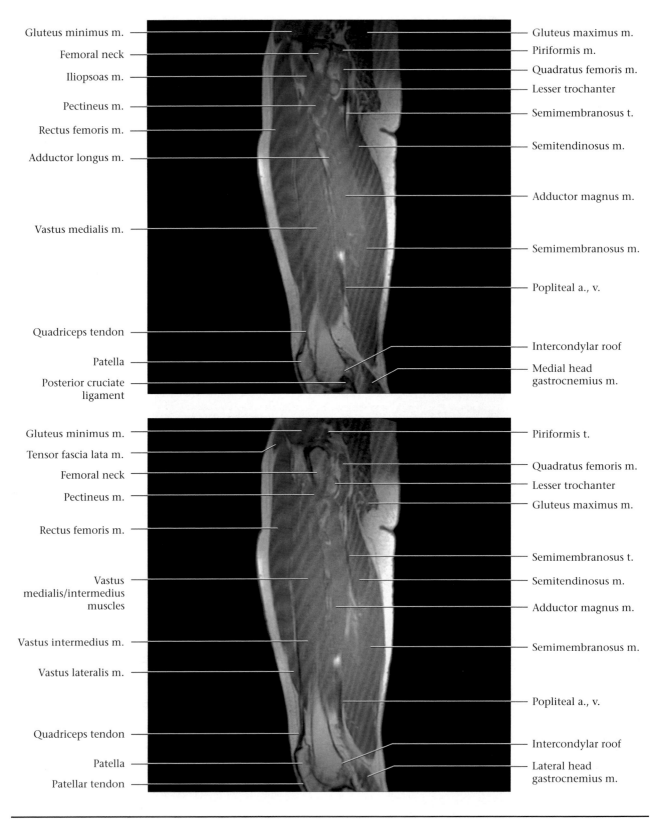

Gluteus minimus m.
Femoral neck
Iliopsoas m.
Pectineus m.
Rectus femoris m.
Adductor longus m.
Vastus medialis m.
Quadriceps tendon
Patella
Posterior cruciate ligament

Gluteus maximus m.
Piriformis m.
Quadratus femoris m.
Lesser trochanter
Semimembranosus t.
Semitendinosus m.
Adductor magnus m.
Semimembranosus m.
Popliteal a., v.
Intercondylar roof
Medial head gastrocnemius m.

Gluteus minimus m.
Tensor fascia lata m.
Femoral neck
Pectineus m.
Rectus femoris m.
Vastus medialis/intermedius muscles
Vastus intermedius m.
Vastus lateralis m.
Quadriceps tendon
Patella
Patellar tendon

Piriformis t.
Quadratus femoris m.
Lesser trochanter
Gluteus maximus m.
Semimembranosus t.
Semitendinosus m.
Adductor magnus m.
Semimembranosus m.
Popliteal a., v.
Intercondylar roof
Lateral head gastrocnemius m.

(Top) The iliopsoas muscle inserts onto the lesser trochanter. Near the iliac wing the 3 gluteus muscles are seen. From anterior to posterior they are gluteus minimus, medius and maximus. **(Bottom)** The transition from vastus medialis to vastus intermedius is difficult to appreciate and is mostly recognized by anatomic position. The vastus intermedius originates from the anterior surface of the mid to distal femur. The junction of the membranous portion of the semimembranous muscle and its muscle belly is well seen on this image.

THIGH OVERVIEW

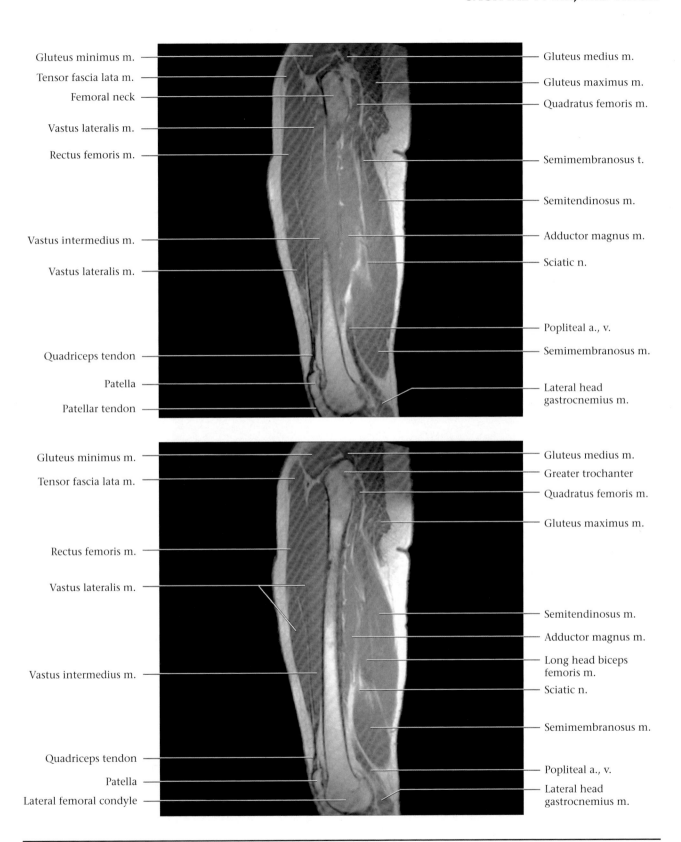

Gluteus minimus m.

Tensor fascia lata m.

Femoral neck

Vastus lateralis m.

Rectus femoris m.

Vastus intermedius m.

Vastus lateralis m.

Quadriceps tendon

Patella

Patellar tendon

Gluteus medius m.

Gluteus maximus m.

Quadratus femoris m.

Semimembranosus t.

Semitendinosus m.

Adductor magnus m.

Sciatic n.

Popliteal a., v.

Semimembranosus m.

Lateral head gastrocnemius m.

Gluteus minimus m.

Tensor fascia lata m.

Rectus femoris m.

Vastus lateralis m.

Vastus intermedius m.

Quadriceps tendon

Patella

Lateral femoral condyle

Gluteus medius m.

Greater trochanter

Quadratus femoris m.

Gluteus maximus m.

Semitendinosus m.

Adductor magnus m.

Long head biceps femoris m.

Sciatic n.

Semimembranosus m.

Popliteal a., v.

Lateral head gastrocnemius m.

(Top) At the anterolateral aspect of the upper thigh the tensor fascia lata muscle is visible. The quadratus femoris muscle is horizontally oriented and travels deep to the gluteus maximus muscle. (Bottom) Note the reciprocal relationship between semimembranosus and semitendinosus muscles. As one muscle belly enlarges the other decreases in size. The medial margin of the popliteal fossa, the semimembranosus muscle, is visible on this image. The insertion of the gluteus medius muscle onto the greater trochanter is seen. For more details see the "Lateral Hip" section.

SAGITTAL T1 MR, MID THIGH

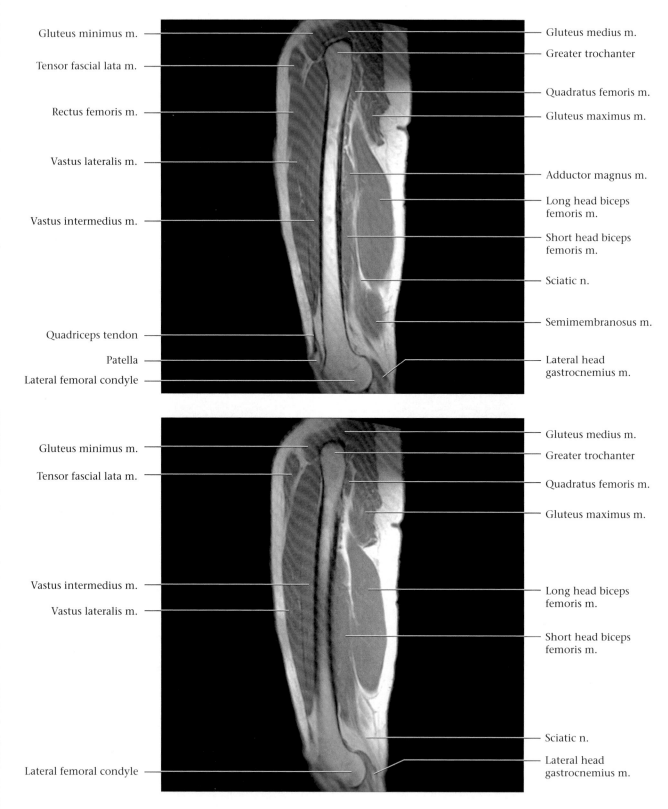

Gluteus minimus m.
Tensor fascial lata m.
Rectus femoris m.
Vastus lateralis m.
Vastus intermedius m.
Quadriceps tendon
Patella
Lateral femoral condyle

Gluteus medius m.
Greater trochanter
Quadratus femoris m.
Gluteus maximus m.
Adductor magnus m.
Long head biceps femoris m.
Short head biceps femoris m.
Sciatic n.
Semimembranosus m.
Lateral head gastrocnemius m.

Gluteus minimus m.
Tensor fascial lata m.
Vastus intermedius m.
Vastus lateralis m.
Lateral femoral condyle

Gluteus medius m.
Greater trochanter
Quadratus femoris m.
Gluteus maximus m.
Long head biceps femoris m.
Short head biceps femoris m.
Sciatic n.
Lateral head gastrocnemius m.

(Top) The sciatic nerve is present along the deep surface of the long head of the biceps femoris muscle. On most images it is not discernible as separate from the muscle. **(Bottom)** The extensive inferior margin of the gluteus maximus muscle can be appreciated on this image. The sciatic nerve is seen bisecting the popliteal fossa.

THIGH OVERVIEW

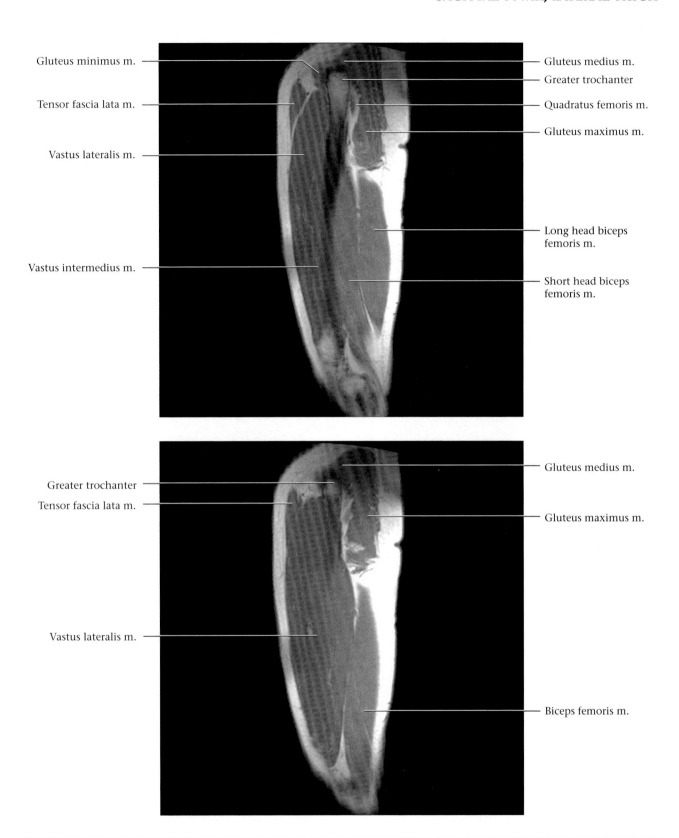

Gluteus minimus m.

Tensor fascia lata m.

Vastus lateralis m.

Vastus intermedius m.

Gluteus medius m.

Greater trochanter

Quadratus femoris m.

Gluteus maximus m.

Long head biceps femoris m.

Short head biceps femoris m.

Greater trochanter

Tensor fascia lata m.

Vastus lateralis m.

Gluteus medius m.

Gluteus maximus m.

Biceps femoris m.

(Top) The origin of the vastus lateralis muscle from the superior most aspect of the femoral diaphysis can be easily seen on this image. The biceps femoris muscle is now visible at the lateral border of the popliteal fossa. **(Bottom)** The broad insertion of the gluteus medius muscle onto the lateral aspect of the superior greater trochanter is easily appreciated. For details see the "Lateral Hip" section.

Hip and Pelvis

∨

THIGH OVERVIEW

SAGITTAL T1 MR, LATERAL THIGH

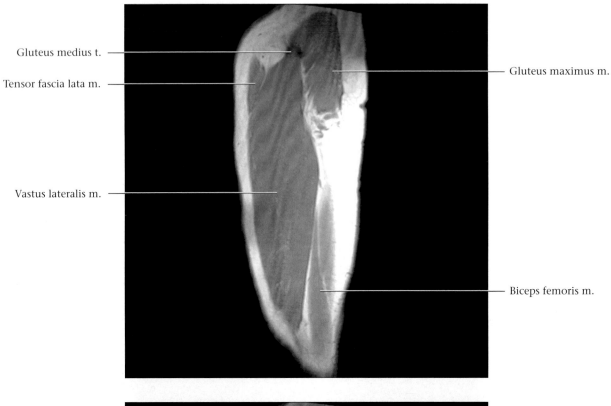

Gluteus medius t.

Tensor fascia lata m.

Vastus lateralis m.

Gluteus maximus m.

Biceps femoris m.

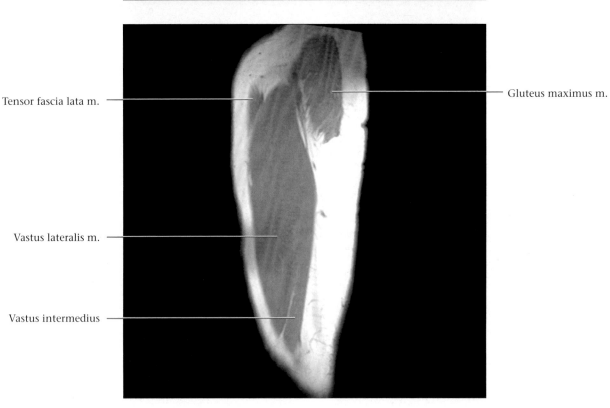

Tensor fascia lata m.

Vastus lateralis m.

Vastus intermedius

Gluteus maximus m.

(Top) Note the tendon of the gluteus medius as it travels along the lateral aspect of the greater trochanter. (Bottom) The most lateral muscles of the thigh are the vastus lateralis and gluteus maximus muscles.

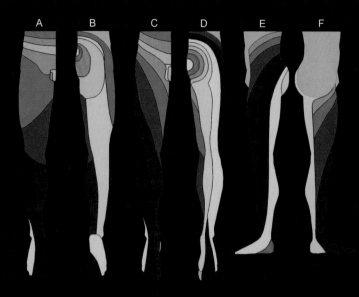

T10	
T11	
T12	
L1	
L2	
L3	
L4	
L5	
S1	
S2	
S3	
S4	
S5	
Co	

(Top) Dermatomes of the anterior (A, C), posterior (B, D), lateral (E) and medial (F) thigh. Two different patterns are recognized for the anterior and posterior thigh as represented by the two diagrams. **(Bottom)** Legend for dermatome diagram.

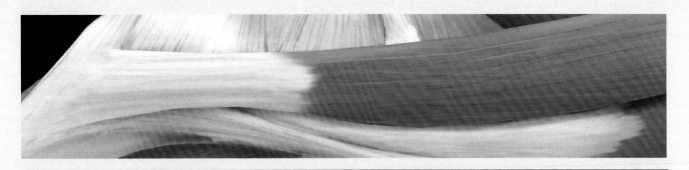

SECTION VI: Knee

KNEE OVERVIEW

Terminology

Abbreviations
- Anterior cruciate ligament (ACL)
- Posterior cruciate ligament (PCL)
- Medial (tibial) collateral ligament (MCL)
- Lateral (fibular) collateral ligament (LCL)

Gross Anatomy

Overview
- Largest and most complex joint
  - Hinge joint throughout its greatest range of motion
  - In all positions, femur in contact with tibia, with large areas of contact
  - In all positions, patella in contact with femur
  - Bones do not interlock; stability maintained by ligaments, tendons, capsule, and menisci
- **Motion** of knee and relationship of osseous structures
  - In full flexion
    - Posterior surfaces of femoral condyles articulate with posterior tibial condyles
    - Lateral facet of patella in contact with lateral femoral condyle
    - Supporting ligaments are not taut, and rotation of leg is allowed
  - During motion of extension
    - Patella slides upwards on femur, passing first on to its middle facet and then its lower facets
    - Femoral condyles roll forward on tibial condyles and menisci
    - Lateral femoral condyle shorter anteroposteriorly than medial and reaches full extension earlier
    - Medial femoral condyle continues to slide after lateral stops, and rotates slightly medially on tibia and medial meniscus ("screwing it home"), and tightens ACL, collateral ligaments, and posterior capsular ligaments, turning knee into a rigid pillar
  - Initiating flexion from fully extended knee
    - Requires slight medial rotation of tibia, produced by popliteus
    - "Unlocks" joint, allowing remainder of motion to take place
- **Muscles acting on knee joint**
  - **Extensors:** Four parts of quadriceps femoris
    - Rectus femoris (origin anterior inferior iliac spine, insertion patella; crosses both hip and knee joints, flexing hip and extending knee)
    - Vastus lateralis (origin lateral shaft of femur, insertion patella)
    - Vastus medialis (origin medial shaft of femur, insertion patella)
    - Vastus intermedius (origin anterior shaft of femur, insertion patella)
  - **Flexors**
    - Biceps femoris (origin ischial tuberosity, insertion fibular head and tibia; crosses both hip and knee joints, extending hip and flexing knee)
    - Sartorius: Origin anterior superior iliac spine, insertion anteromedial tibia, crosses both hip and knee joints, flexes both hip and knee joints, rotating thigh laterally to bring limbs into position adopted by the cross-legged tailor; sartor = a tailor
    - Gracilis (origin pubis, insertion anteromedial tibia; crosses both hip and knee joints, adducts thigh, flexes knee, and rotates flexed leg medially)
    - Semitendinosus (origin ischial tuberosity, insertion anteromedial tibia; crosses both hip and knee joints, extends hip, flexes knee, medially rotates flexed leg)
    - Semimembranosus (origin ischial tuberosity, insertion posterior medial condyle tibia; crosses both hip and knee joints, extends hip, flexes knee, medially rotates flexed knee)
    - Popliteus (arises as tendon from popliteal groove at lateral femoral condyle, inserts onto posterior surface tibia; flexes knee and medially rotates tibia at beginning of flexion
  - **Internal rotators** of leg: Popliteus, gracilis, sartorius, semitendinosus, semimembranosus
  - **External rotator** of leg: Biceps femoris
- **Nerves** of knee joint
  - **Femoral nerve** supplies
    - 3 branches, one to each of the vasti, and to anterosuperior part of joint
    - Largest is nerve to vastus medialis which accompanies descending genicular artery
  - **Common peroneal nerve** supplies
    - Superior lateral genicular nerve descends into popliteal fossa and supplies superolateral part of joint, passing deep to biceps, through lateral intermuscular septum above femoral condyle
    - Inferior lateral genicular nerve: Small & sometimes absent; arises with superior lateral genicular nerve & curves downwards & forwards over lateral head of gastrocnemius, passing between the capsule & fibular collateral ligament
    - Recurrent genicular nerve: Small twigs reaching the anteroinferior part of joint
  - **Tibial nerve** supplies
    - Superior medial genicular nerve: Runs medially around femur above medial condyle, deep to adductor magnus, then through vastus medialis to superomedial part of joint
    - Middle genicular nerve: Runs forwards through fibrous capsule to cruciate ligaments
    - Inferior medial genicular nerve: Largest, running along upper border of popliteus, passing forwards between shaft of tibia and medial collateral ligament, curving superiorly to inferomedial part of capsule
  - **Obturator nerve:** Sends a genicular branch through adductor magnus to join popliteal artery, running to posterior aspect of joint
- **Vessels** of knee joint: 8 arteries supply a large anastomosis
  - **Popliteal** artery supplies 5 genicular branches
  - **Anterior tibial** artery supplies 2 recurrent branches
  - **Femoral** artery supplies descending genicular branch

- o **Lateral circumflex** artery supplies descending genicular branch

Imaging Anatomy

Overview
- Multiple specific anatomic relationships must be maintained in order to assure stability & full function

Osseous Anatomy
- **Distal femur**
  - o **Osseous features**
    - Distal femoral metaphysis flares into medial and lateral epicondyles
    - Osseous irregularity may be seen at posteromedial femoral metaphysis: "Tug" at adductor or medial gastrocnemius insertion, termed "cortical desmoid"
    - Medial femoral condyle larger than lateral
    - Lateral femoral condyle has an indentation in its anterior weight-bearing surface (lateral femoral condylar recess); measures < 2 mm
    - Intercondylar notch accommodates cruciate ligaments; seen as Blumensaat line on radiograph
    - Anteriorly, trochlear groove accommodates patella and is generally V-shaped
  - o **Possible sites of avulsion**
    - Posterolateral intercondylar notch (ACL origin)
    - Medial epicondyle (MCL origin)
  - o **Cartilage**
    - Thicker over posterior condyles than normal weight-bearing surface
    - Focally thin at lateral femoral condylar recess
- **Proximal tibia**
  - o **Osseous features**
    - Posterior tilt of tibial surface 10°
    - Tibial tubercle (apophysis) anterior and slightly lateral, several cm distal to joint
    - Gerdy tubercle anterolateral just distal to joint
  - o **Possible sites of avulsion**
    - Tibial spine (ACL insertion)
    - Posterior mid tibia at joint line (PCL insertion)
    - Medial joint line (coronary ligament insertion)
    - Lateral joint line (capsular insertion; may avulse with valgus twist): Segond
    - Gerdy tubercle (iliotibial band)
    - Tibial apophysis (patellar tendon insertion): In skeletally immature patient
  - o **Cartilage**: Uniformly thin
- **Proximal fibula**
  - o **Osseous features**
    - Posterolateral relative to tibia
    - Fibular styloid process
  - o **Tibiofibular joint**
    - True synovial joint; subject to any arthritic process
    - Connects to knee joint in 20%
  - o **Possible sites of avulsion**
    - Lateral fibular head (insertion of conjoint tendon)
    - Thin fragment medial styloid (insertion of arcuate ligament)
- **Patella**
  - o **Osseous features**
    - Triangular sesamoid
    - Wider at base superiorly than at apex inferiorly
    - Articular surface divided by vertical ridge into lateral and medial facets
    - Lateral facet long and shallow angle
    - Medial facet short and more strongly angulated
    - Several other facets described but not of imaging importance
    - Lower 25% non-articular
    - Non-articular outer surface may develop prominent enthesopathy where quadriceps tendon insertion blends into origin of inferior patellar tendon
    - Bipartite (multipartite) patella: Always upper outer quadrant; osseous fragments may not appear to "match", but cartilage is continuous over defect
  - o **Cartilage**
    - Thickest cartilage in body (3-4 mm)
    - Uniform thickness
    - May have dorsal patellar defect as normal variant

Articular Capsule
- Highly complex, noncontiguous structure
- Contributions from multiple muscles, tendons, and ligaments
- Some structures may be intra-articular but extra-synovial
- Also see sections: "Extensor Mechanism", "Cruciate Ligaments and Posterior Capsule", "Medial Supporting Structures", "Lateral Supporting Structures"

Extensor Mechanism
- Quadriceps tendon converges on patella
- Fibers of rectus femoris course over patella to form inferior patellar tendon
- Fibers of vastus lateralis and medialis contribute to lateral and medial retinacula, respectively
- See also section: "Extensor Mechanism"

Internal Structures
- **Menisci**
  - o Cushion, lubricate, and stabilize knee
  - o Fibrocartilage
  - o Only peripheral portion vascularized
  - o Attached by anterior and posterior roots to tibial surface
  - o Medial attached to capsule throughout extent
  - o Lateral attached to capsule at anterior horn and far posteriorly, but by fascicles to popliteus at body and posterior horn
  - o Lateral has constant size and shape
  - o Medial has elongated posterior horn and small body
  - o See also section: "Menisci"
- **Cruciate ligaments**
  - o Intra-articular but extra-synovial
  - o Major stabilizing structures to anteroposterior motion
  - o ACL originates at posterolateral intercondylar notch, crosses anteromedially, and inserts at medial tibial spine/tibial surface
  - o PCL originates at mid medial intercondylar notch, crosses posteriorly and slightly laterally, and inserts extra-articularly at posterior center of tibia below joint line

- Injury generally intrasubstance, but avulsions may indicate injury (origin and insertion, respectively)
  - ACL: Posterolateral Blumensaat line or medial tibial spine
  - PCL: Mid medial intercondylar notch or posterior central tibia
- Normal variants could possibly be confusing
  - ACL: Infrapatellar plica, meniscocruciate ligament, meniscomeniscal ligament
  - PCL: Meniscofemoral ligaments
- See section: "Cruciate Ligaments"

Medial Supporting Structures

- Superficial (layer 1)
  - Pes anserinus: Anteromedial tibial insertion
    - Sartorius embedded in crural fascia
    - Gracilis immediately deep to sartorius
    - Semitendinosus immediately deep to gracilis
- Middle (layer 2)
  - Superficial medial collateral ligament (longitudinal and oblique components)
    - Origin medial epicondyle; runs slightly anteromedially to insert on tibia 5 cm distal to joint line
    - Anteriorly, longitudinal component fascia blends with layer 1
    - Posteriorly, oblique component blends with layer 3 as posterior oblique ligament
- Deep (layer 3)
  - Capsular layers (sometimes termed deep fibers of MCL) at mid portion of knee
    - Meniscofemoral ligament
    - Meniscotibial (coronary) ligament
  - More posteriorly, superficial MCL blends with capsular layers MCL
  - Posterior oblique ligament arises from superficial MCL
    - Blends with posteromedial meniscus
    - Receives fibers from semimembranosus tendon
    - Envelops posterior aspect femoral condyle, termed oblique popliteal ligament
- See section: "Medial Supporting Structures"

Lateral Supporting Structures

- Superficial (layer 1)
  - Iliotibial band anteriorly, inserting on Gerdy tubercle
  - Superficial portion biceps femoris posterolaterally, inserting on fibular styloid
- Middle (layer 2)
  - Quadriceps retinaculum anteriorly
  - Posteriorly, 2 ligamentous thickenings which originate from lateral patella
    - Proximal one terminates at lateral intermuscular septum on femur
    - Distal one terminates at femoral insertion of posterolateral capsule and lateral head of gastrocnemius
- Deep (layer 3): Several thickening in lateral part of capsule function as discrete structures
  - Lateral (fibular) collateral ligament originates lateral femoral epicondyle, extends posterolaterally to insert on lateral fibular head

- Arcuate ligament originates from styloid process fibular head, interdigitates with popliteus, and inserts into posterior capsule near oblique popliteal ligament
- Several other small and inconstant structures located posterolaterally which are difficult to differentiate by imaging
- See section: "Lateral Supporting Structures"

Anatomy-Based Imaging Issues

Imaging Recommendations

- Radiographs: AP standing, lateral, axial patella with 20° flexion
- MR
  - T1 in one plane to evaluate marrow and anatomy
  - PD is most accurate sequence to evaluate menisci
  - Fluid sensitive sequence to evaluate location and tracking of fluid collections
- MR arthrography (indirect)
  - Clinical indications
    - Articular processes (synovitis)
    - Post surgical (meniscal re-tear)
    - Evaluation of osteochondral defect (for intact cartilage or loose body)
  - Technique
    - Exercise following IV injection
    - Image 20-30 minutes following injection
- MR arthrography (direct)
  - Clinical indications
    - Rarely required; indications similar as for indirect arthrography, but when no effusion is present
  - Technique
    - Knee flexed, either medial or lateral subpatellar needle placement
    - Stay below mid pole of patella (otherwise may inject into pre-femoral fat pad)
    - Aspirate all fluid in knee so that injected fluid is not diluted; inject volume of 40 cc
- CT arthrography
  - Clinical indications: Same as above, if MR contraindicated
  - Technique: Same as above, dilute contrast of choice 50/50 with bacteriostatic saline
  - Acquire sub-millimeter sections; reformat

Imaging Pitfalls

- Variants: Listed above and in sections
- Loose bodies on MR: Easily missed
- Partial voluming over convex surfaces: Morphology of trochlea, femoral condyles, and patella makes them particularly difficult to evaluate in 3 standard planes
- Malpositioning
  - AP radiograph: Flexion obscures joint space
  - Axial patella: Flexion > 20° may reduce subluxation or tilt
- Imaging cartilage
  - T2 underestimates cartilage thickness since cortex and cartilage have similar signal
  - PD may have similar signal for cartilage and adjacent joint fluid, obscuring defects; fat-saturation solves this

KNEE OVERVIEW

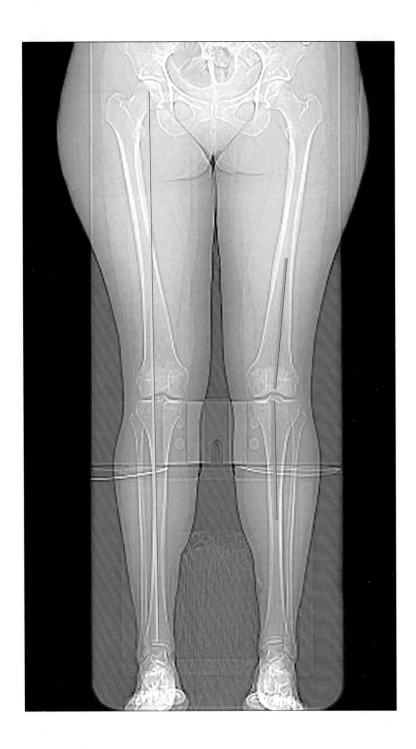

The yellow line drawn on the right lower extremity depicts the mechanical axis, drawn from the center of the femoral head to the center of the tibial plafond. The normal mechanical axis traverses the center of the knee joint. The green lines bisecting the distal femur and proximal tibia shows the normal valgus angulation of the knee (average 6°).

AP & AXIAL RADIOGRAPHS

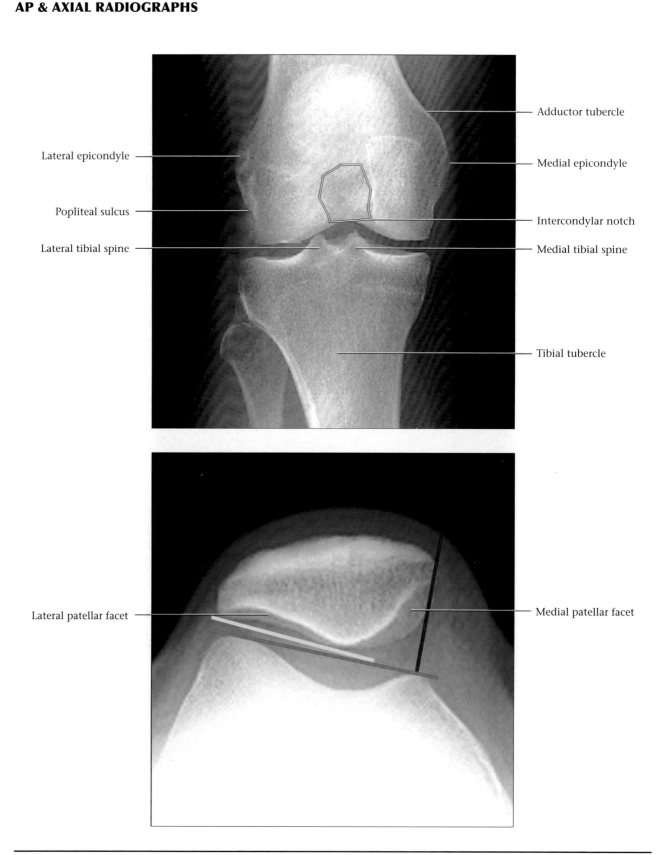

Adductor tubercle

Lateral epicondyle

Medial epicondyle

Popliteal sulcus

Intercondylar notch

Lateral tibial spine

Medial tibial spine

Tibial tubercle

Lateral patellar facet

Medial patellar facet

(Top) AP radiograph of the knee, shows its osseous features. The depth of the intercondylar notch is not appreciated on an AP radiograph. **(Bottom)** Axial radiograph of the knee, obtained with the knee flexed 20° (allows maximal subluxation of patella). Note that the lateral patellar facet is elongated and less sharply angled than the medial. The angle formed by the line through the condylar peaks (green) and lateral patellar facet (yellow) is normally open laterally; reversal of this angle constitutes patellar tilt. A line drawn perpendicular (red) to the condylar peaks line (green), 1 mm lateral to the medial condylar peak should intersect the patella. If the patella lies lateral to this line, it is laterally subluxed. The angle of the sulcus is normally 136 +/- 6°; values > 140° are associated with instability and condylar/lateral trochlear dysplasia.

KNEE OVERVIEW

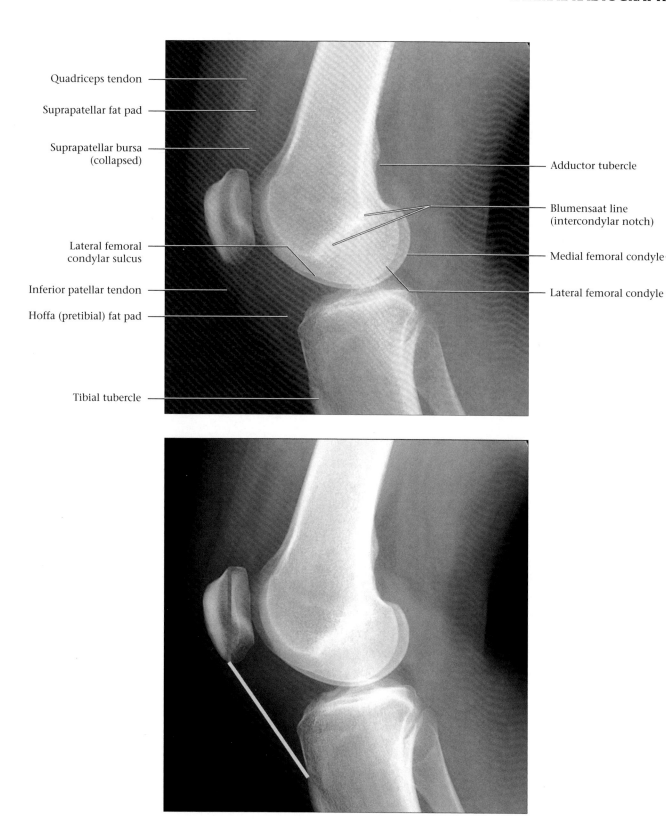

Quadriceps tendon

Suprapatellar fat pad

Suprapatellar bursa (collapsed)

Lateral femoral condylar sulcus

Inferior patellar tendon

Hoffa (pretibial) fat pad

Tibial tubercle

Adductor tubercle

Blumensaat line (intercondylar notch)

Medial femoral condyle

Lateral femoral condyle

(Top) Lateral radiograph of the knee. Note that the intercondylar notch is delineated by Blumensaat line. The medial femoral condyle is slightly larger than the lateral; the lateral femoral condyle can also be identified by the presence of the lateral femoral sulcus at its anterior weight-bearing portion. **(Bottom)** Patellar position on lateral radiograph. the length of the patellar tendon (yellow line) and the greatest length of the patella (green line) form a ratio that averages 1.17 (range 0.8-1.3).

AXIAL CT, FEMORAL TORSION

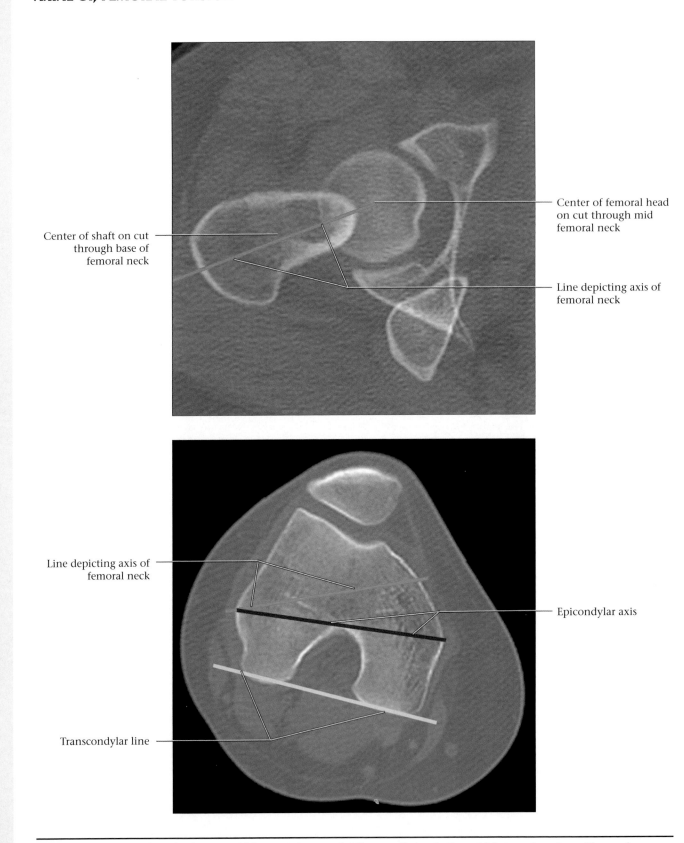

Center of shaft on cut through base of femoral neck

Center of femoral head on cut through mid femoral neck

Line depicting axis of femoral neck

Line depicting axis of femoral neck

Epicondylar axis

Transcondylar line

(Top) Axis of femoral neck, determined by superimposed CT scans through the mid femoral neck and base of femoral neck. The line connecting the center of the head in the superior cut and the center of shaft in the lower cut determines the femoral neck axis; this line makes an angle with the transischial line; in this case there is 15° femoral neck anteversion. **(Bottom)** Femoral torsion, measured by CT. Angle formed by the axis of the femoral neck (green line from previous image) & the transcondylar line (yellow) gives the degree of femoral torsion. In the normal situation, the distal femur is internally rotated relative to the femoral neck, which is termed femoral anteversion or femoral antetorsion; different studies show average anteversion to be 15-24° in adults (range 3-48). The epicondylar/posterior condylar angle should be 5.7 +/- 1.7°. Epicondylar axis (red line) is another useful landmark.

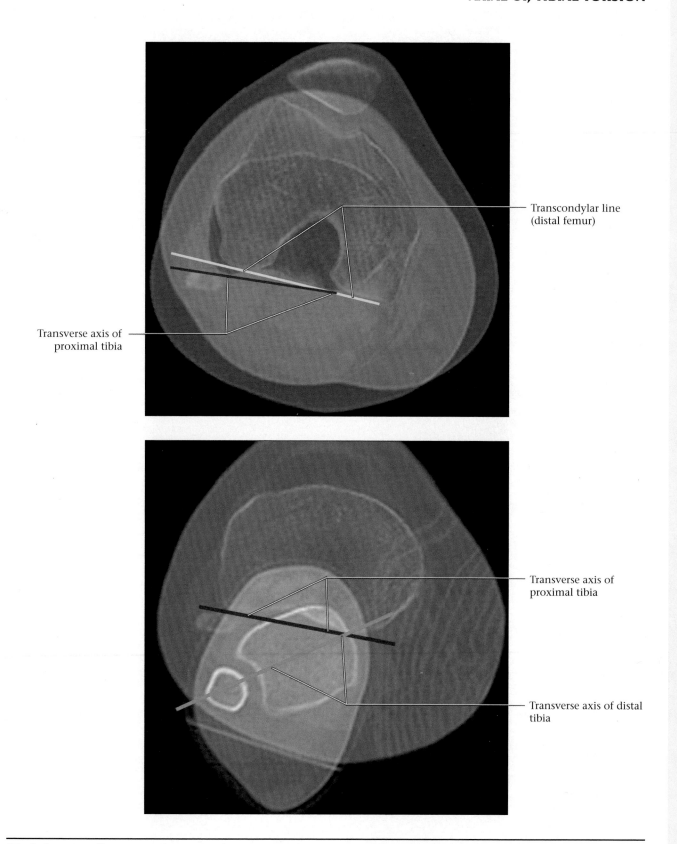

Transcondylar line (distal femur)

Transverse axis of proximal tibia

Transverse axis of proximal tibia

Transverse axis of distal tibia

(Top) Occasionally one may be required to measure the rotation of the proximal tibia on the distal femur. There is usually slightly external rotation of the tibia relative to the femur and is measured by the angle formed by the transcondylar line of the distal femur (yellow) and the transverse axis of the proximal tibia (red line). **(Bottom)** Tibial torsion is measured by the angle formed by the proximal tibial transverse axis (red line) and distal tibial transverse axis (blue line). There is normally external rotation (torsion) of the distal tibia measuring 30° in adults (range 20-50°), as shown by several CT studies. Tibial torsion greater than 40° shows an increased incidence of adverse patellar mechanics and malalignment syndrome.

3D RECONSTRUCTION CT

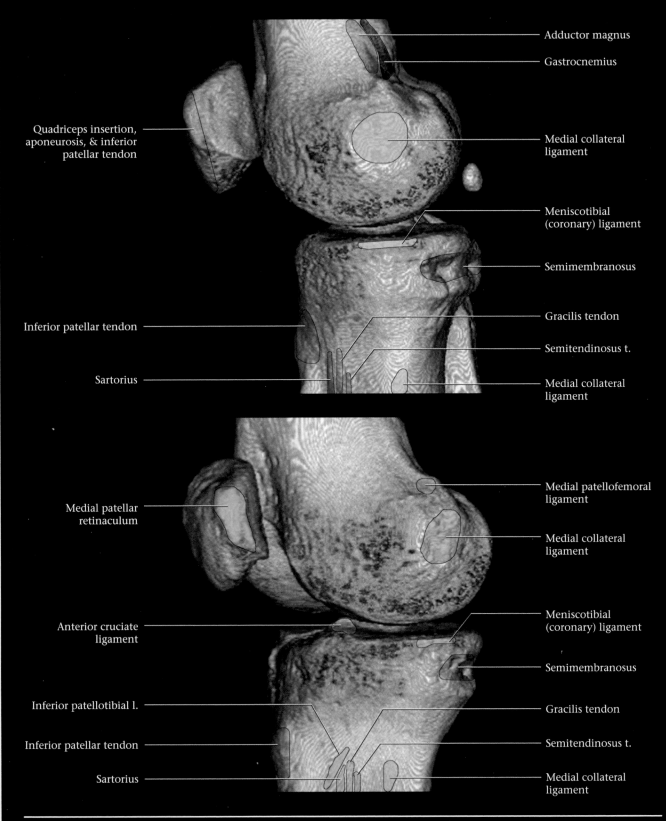

Adductor magnus

Gastrocnemius

Quadriceps insertion, aponeurosis, & inferior patellar tendon

Medial collateral ligament

Meniscotibial (coronary) ligament

Semimembranosus

Inferior patellar tendon

Gracilis tendon

Semitendinosus t.

Sartorius

Medial collateral ligament

Medial patellar retinaculum

Medial patellofemoral ligament

Medial collateral ligament

Meniscotibial (coronary) ligament

Anterior cruciate ligament

Semimembranosus

Inferior patellotibial l.

Gracilis tendon

Inferior patellar tendon

Semitendinosus t.

Sartorius

Medial collateral ligament

(Top) First of eight volume rendered topographic CT images. Image shows the medial aspect of the knee, with associated muscle, tendon, and ligament origins/insertions. **(Bottom)** Anteromedial knee, shows medial stabilizers of knee (primarily medial collateral ligament, superficial and deep fibers, secondarily pes anserinus), as well as medial stabilizers of patella (superiorly medial patellofemoral ligament, mid medial retinaculum, inferiorly patellotibial ligament).

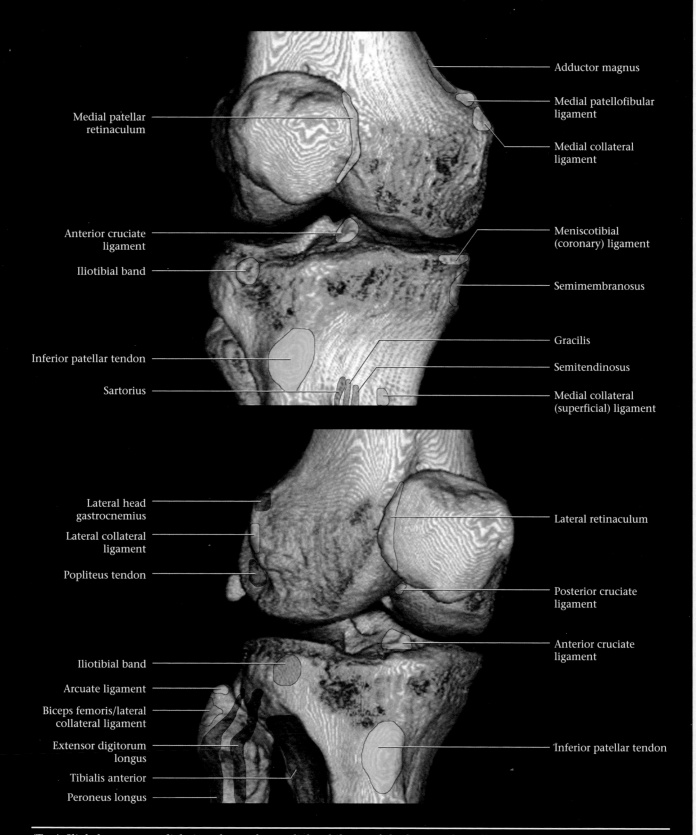

Adductor magnus

Medial patellofibular ligament

Medial collateral ligament

Medial patellar retinaculum

Meniscotibial (coronary) ligament

Anterior cruciate ligament

Semimembranosus

Iliotibial band

Gracilis

Inferior patellar tendon

Semitendinosus

Sartorius

Medial collateral (superficial) ligament

Lateral head gastrocnemius

Lateral retinaculum

Lateral collateral ligament

Popliteus tendon

Posterior cruciate ligament

Anterior cruciate ligament

Iliotibial band

Arcuate ligament

Biceps femoris/lateral collateral ligament

Extensor digitorum longus

Inferior patellar tendon

Tibialis anterior

Peroneus longus

(Top) Slightly anteromedial view shows the medial stabilizers of the knee and patella. Note that only the uppermost portion of the insertions of the pes anserinus (sartorius, gracilis, and semitendinosus) as well as superficial medial collateral ligament are shown; these insertions actually extend several cm more distally on the tibia. **(Bottom)** Slightly anterolateral view, showing the lateral stabilizers of the knee and patella. These consist primarily of lateral collateral ligament, arcuate ligament, popliteal tendon, iliotibial band, and biceps femoris. Origins of several leg muscles are seen; the tibialis anterior, extensor digitorum longus, and peroneus longus origins extend several cm distally beyond the regions indicated here.

3D RECONSTRUCTION CT

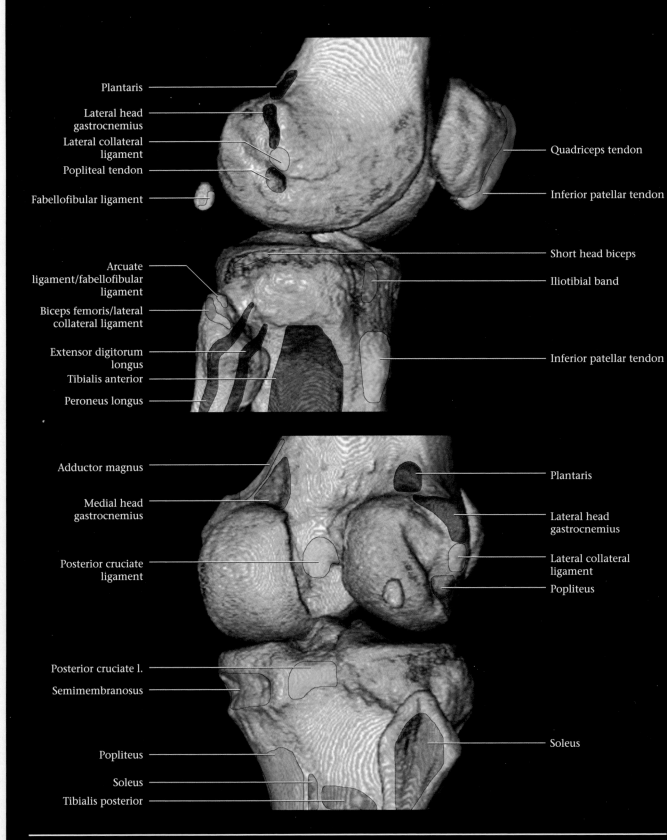

Plantaris

Lateral head gastrocnemius

Lateral collateral ligament

Popliteal tendon

Fabellofibular ligament

Quadriceps tendon

Inferior patellar tendon

Short head biceps

Iliotibial band

Arcuate ligament/fabellofibular ligament

Biceps femoris/lateral collateral ligament

Extensor digitorum longus

Tibialis anterior

Peroneus longus

Inferior patellar tendon

Adductor magnus

Medial head gastrocnemius

Posterior cruciate ligament

Plantaris

Lateral head gastrocnemius

Lateral collateral ligament

Popliteus

Posterior cruciate l.

Semimembranosus

Popliteus

Soleus

Tibialis posterior

Soleus

(**Top**) Lateral view of knee, shows lateral stabilizing structures. Origins of anterior and lateral leg muscles are seen as well. (**Bottom**) Posterior (slightly obliqued) view of the knee. The attachments of the posterior structures are shown. Note that fibular origin of soleus is more proximal than tibial origin.

KNEE OVERVIEW

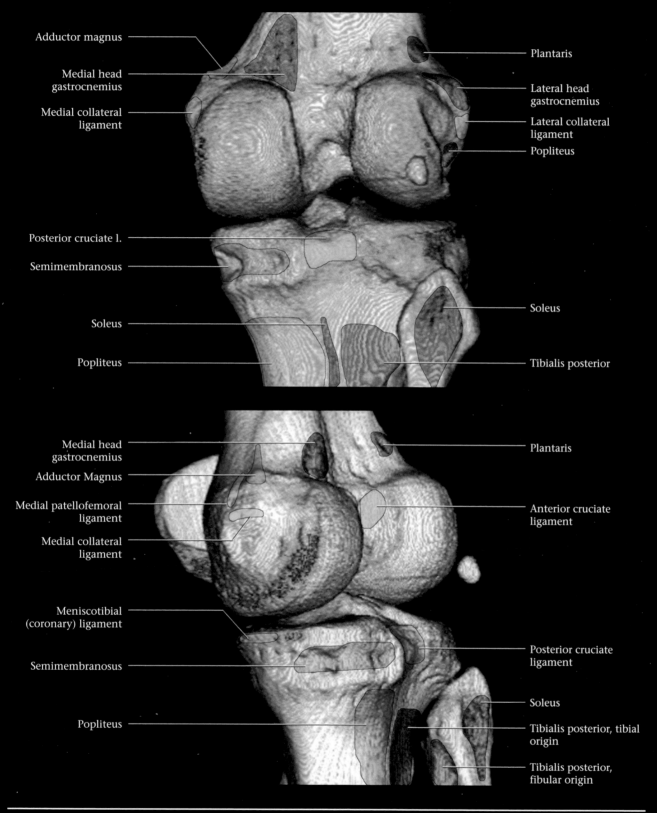

Adductor magnus

Medial head gastrocnemius

Medial collateral ligament

Plantaris

Lateral head gastrocnemius

Lateral collateral ligament

Popliteus

Posterior cruciate l.

Semimembranosus

Soleus

Popliteus

Soleus

Tibialis posterior

Medial head gastrocnemius

Adductor Magnus

Medial patellofemoral ligament

Medial collateral ligament

Meniscotibial (coronary) ligament

Semimembranosus

Popliteus

Plantaris

Anterior cruciate ligament

Posterior cruciate ligament

Soleus

Tibialis posterior, tibial origin

Tibialis posterior, fibular origin

(Top) Direct posterior view. Note that PCL insertion is extra-articular, on the posterior central tibia. **(Bottom)** Posterior, obliqued to medial. Note the extensive insertions of both semimembranosus and popliteus on the posteromedial tibia.

CT ARTHROGRAM, AXIAL & SAGITTAL REFORMATS

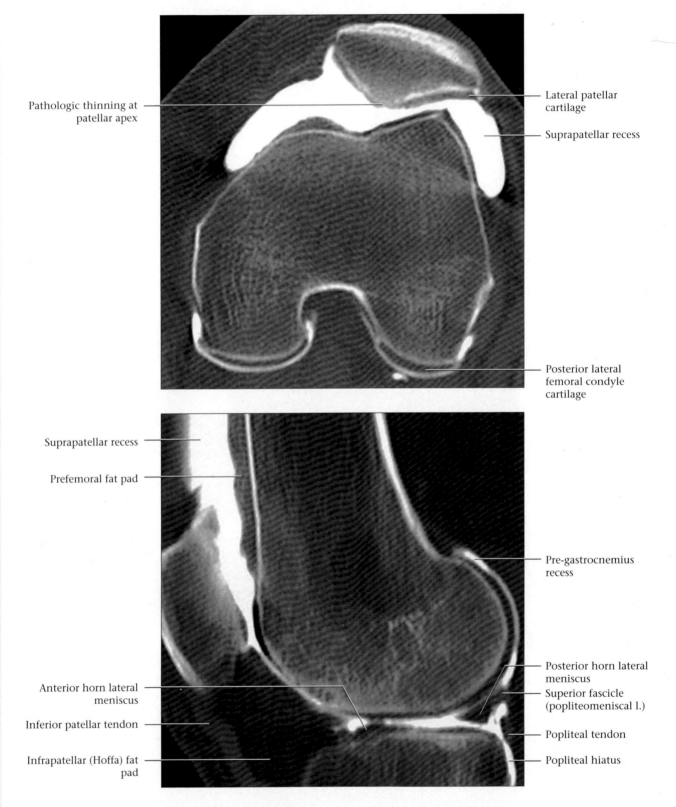

Pathologic thinning at patellar apex

Lateral patellar cartilage

Suprapatellar recess

Posterior lateral femoral condyle cartilage

Suprapatellar recess

Prefemoral fat pad

Pre-gastrocnemius recess

Anterior horn lateral meniscus

Inferior patellar tendon

Infrapatellar (Hoffa) fat pad

Posterior horn lateral meniscus

Superior fascicle (popliteomeniscal l.)

Popliteal tendon

Popliteal hiatus

(Top) Axial direct CT scan through femoral condyles post arthrogram. The contrast distends the joint, filling recesses and outlining cartilage and all intra-articular structures. CT arthrogram may be substituted if there is a contraindication to MR in a patient. **(Bottom)** Sagittal reformat, CT arthrogram, through the lateral compartment. The suprapatellar bursa is distended, outlining patellar cartilage defects. The menisci are outlined, showing them to be intact. The superior fascicle of posterior horn is well seen, as is popliteal tendon in its hiatus.

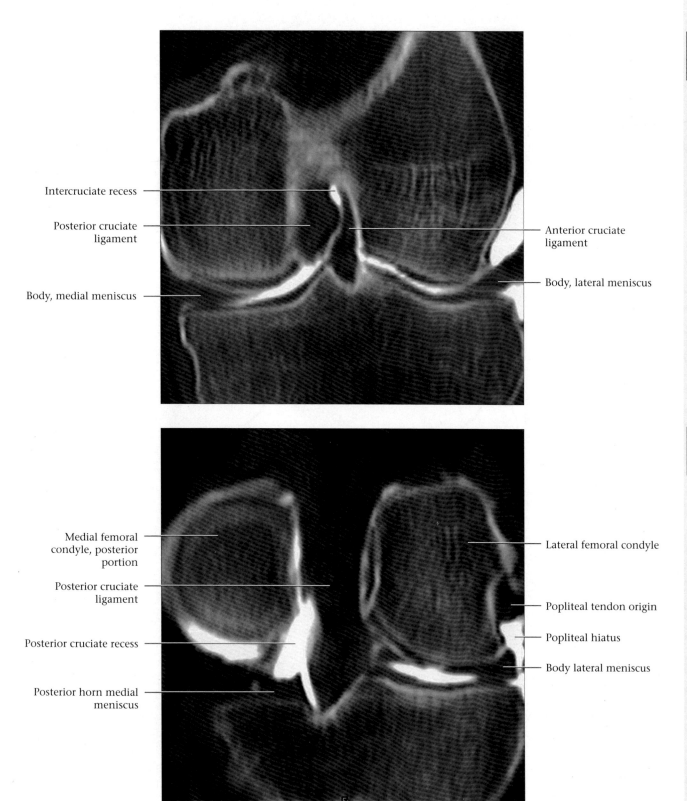

Intercruciate recess

Posterior cruciate ligament

Body, medial meniscus

Anterior cruciate ligament

Body, lateral meniscus

Medial femoral condyle, posterior portion

Posterior cruciate ligament

Posterior cruciate recess

Posterior horn medial meniscus

Lateral femoral condyle

Popliteal tendon origin

Popliteal hiatus

Body lateral meniscus

(Top) Coronal reformat through the mid joint, CT arthrogram. This section outlines the bodies of the menisci well, as well as the cruciate ligaments. **(Bottom)** Coronal reformat, CT arthrogram, in the posterior portion of the knee. The posterior cruciate is outlined, with the adjacent bursa distended. The menisci again are well seen.

GRAPHIC, ANTEROMEDIAL VIEW OF VESSELS

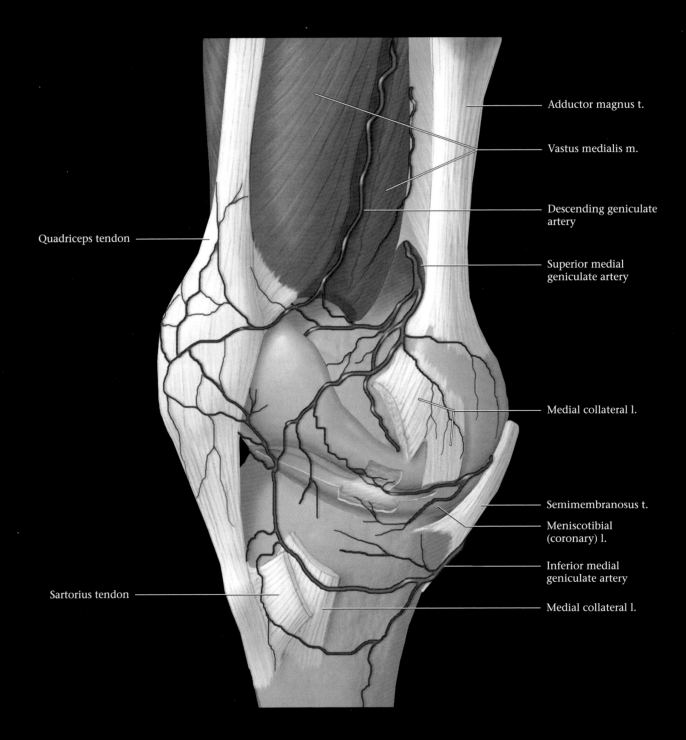

Quadriceps tendon

Sartorius tendon

Adductor magnus t.

Vastus medialis m.

Descending geniculate artery

Superior medial geniculate artery

Medial collateral l.

Semimembranosus t.

Meniscotibial (coronary) l.

Inferior medial geniculate artery

Medial collateral l.

Graphic of the anteromedial knee shows the rich anastomotic vascular network around the knee. There are two named geniculate branches of the popliteal artery in each side (superior and inferior); only those on the medial side are shown here. Additionally, there are two supplementary arteries. The descending geniculate artery (a branch of the femoral artery) descends superomedially. There is also an anterior recurrent branch of the anterior tibial artery which runs inferolaterally, not shown here.

KNEE OVERVIEW

GRAPHIC, POSTERIOR VIEW OF VESSELS

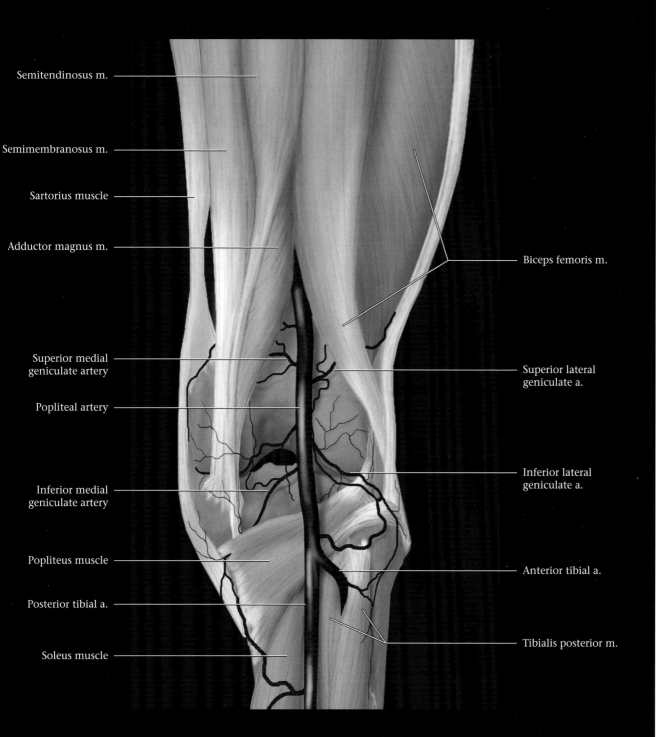

Semitendinosus m.

Semimembranosus m.

Sartorius muscle

Adductor magnus m.

Biceps femoris m.

Superior medial geniculate artery

Popliteal artery

Superior lateral geniculate a.

Inferior lateral geniculate a.

Inferior medial geniculate artery

Popliteus muscle

Anterior tibial a.

Posterior tibial a.

Tibialis posterior m.

Soleus muscle

Graphic shows the anastomoses around the knee, posteriorly. The popliteal artery is seen throughout its course, from the hiatus in adductor magnus proximally to the lower border of popliteus distally. At this point, the popliteal artery bifurcates into anterior and posterior tibial arteries. The anterior tibial is the smaller branch which extends through a slit in tibialis posterior and on through the interosseous membrane to descend along the interosseous membrane down the anterior compartment. Note the 3 ventral relations of the artery: The femur (with fat between them), the joint capsule, and the popliteus. There are 4 named geniculate branches, a superior and inferior both medially and laterally.

GRAPHIC, POSTERIOR SUPERFICIAL MUSCLES & NERVES

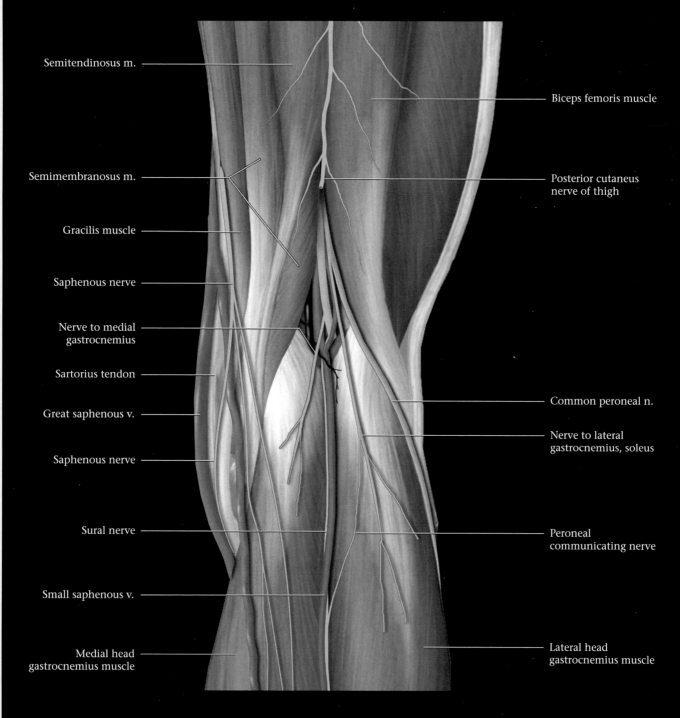

Semitendinosus m.

Biceps femoris muscle

Semimembranosus m.

Posterior cutaneus nerve of thigh

Gracilis muscle

Saphenous nerve

Nerve to medial gastrocnemius

Sartorius tendon

Common peroneal n.

Great saphenous v.

Nerve to lateral gastrocnemius, soleus

Saphenous nerve

Sural nerve

Peroneal communicating nerve

Small saphenous v.

Medial head gastrocnemius muscle

Lateral head gastrocnemius muscle

Graphic shows the superficial posterior muscles and nerves. Note that the common peroneal nerve is part of the deeper nerve system, but travels more superficially, following the posterior biceps femoris muscle and tendon until it wraps around the fibular neck.

GRAPHIC, POSTERIOR DEEP MUSCLES & NERVES

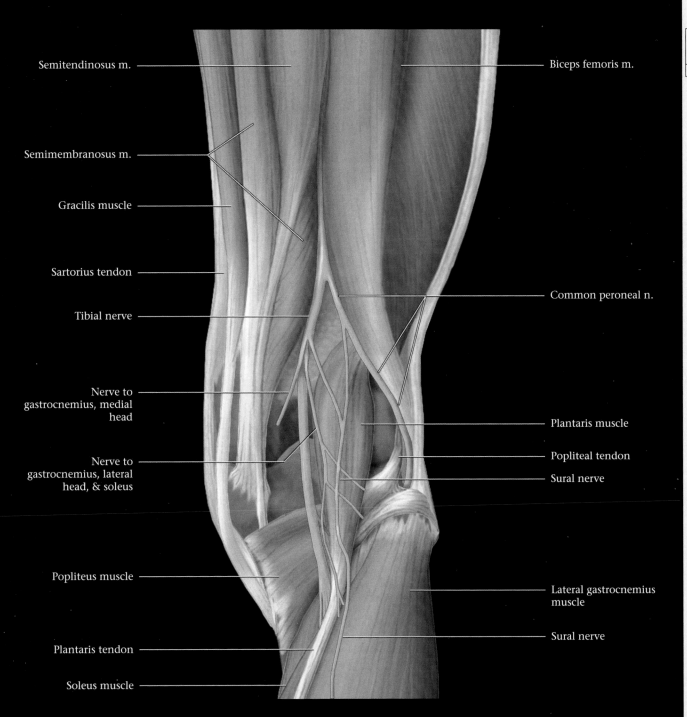

Semitendinosus m.

Biceps femoris m.

Semimembranosus m.

Gracilis muscle

Sartorius tendon

Tibial nerve

Common peroneal n.

Nerve to gastrocnemius, medial head

Nerve to gastrocnemius, lateral head, & soleus

Plantaris muscle

Popliteal tendon

Sural nerve

Popliteus muscle

Lateral gastrocnemius muscle

Sural nerve

Plantaris tendon

Soleus muscle

Graphic shows the relationship of the common peroneal nerve to the posterior biceps femoris tendon. It also shows the tibial nerve with the numerous muscular branches. Note the plantaris muscle, coursing over the popliteus (and popliteal vessels, not shown), and becoming tendinous at the level of the popliteus-soleus muscle junction. The plantaris tendon then courses downward and slightly medially between soleus and medial head gastrocnemius (not shown). The sural nerve arises from branches of both common peroneal and tibial nerves, and courses down superficial to the junction of the two gastrocnemius heads. The tibial nerve travels downward in a deeper position, just posterior to the posterior tibial vessels.

AXIAL T1 MR, RIGHT KNEE

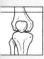

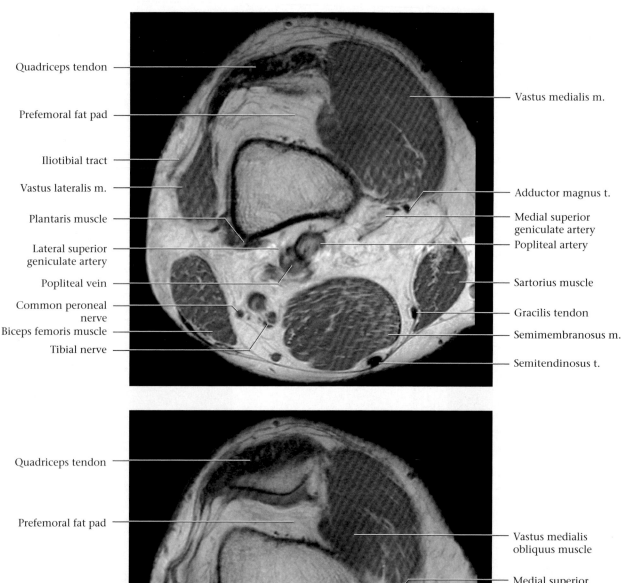

Quadriceps tendon

Prefemoral fat pad

Iliotibial tract

Vastus lateralis m.

Plantaris muscle

Lateral superior geniculate artery

Popliteal vein

Common peroneal nerve

Biceps femoris muscle

Tibial nerve

Vastus medialis m.

Adductor magnus t.

Medial superior geniculate artery

Popliteal artery

Sartorius muscle

Gracilis tendon

Semimembranosus m.

Semitendinosus t.

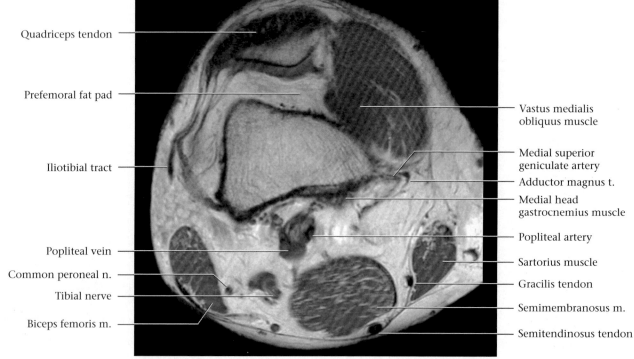

Quadriceps tendon

Prefemoral fat pad

Iliotibial tract

Popliteal vein

Common peroneal n.

Tibial nerve

Biceps femoris m.

Vastus medialis obliquus muscle

Medial superior geniculate artery

Adductor magnus t.

Medial head gastrocnemius muscle

Popliteal artery

Sartorius muscle

Gracilis tendon

Semimembranosus m.

Semitendinosus tendon

(Top) First in series of axial T1 MR images of the right knee. The cut is above the patella and at the proximal portion of the femoral metaphysis. At this level, the origin of plantaris muscle is seen, but it is still proximal to the adductor tubercle. **(Bottom)** This cut is immediately above the adductor tubercle. The vastus medialis obliquus is seen, serving as medial support for the superior portion of the patella.

KNEE OVERVIEW

AXIAL T1 MR, LEFT KNEE

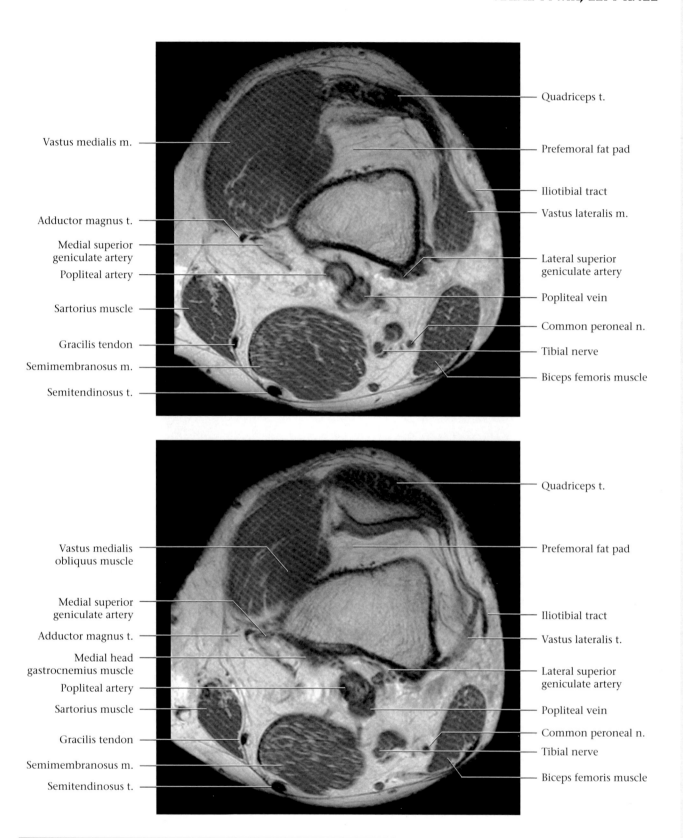

Top image labels:
- Vastus medialis m.
- Adductor magnus t.
- Medial superior geniculate artery
- Popliteal artery
- Sartorius muscle
- Gracilis tendon
- Semimembranosus m.
- Semitendinosus t.
- Quadriceps t.
- Prefemoral fat pad
- Iliotibial tract
- Vastus lateralis m.
- Lateral superior geniculate artery
- Popliteal vein
- Common peroneal n.
- Tibial nerve
- Biceps femoris muscle

Bottom image labels:
- Vastus medialis obliquus muscle
- Medial superior geniculate artery
- Adductor magnus t.
- Medial head gastrocnemius muscle
- Popliteal artery
- Sartorius muscle
- Gracilis tendon
- Semimembranosus m.
- Semitendinosus t.
- Quadriceps t.
- Prefemoral fat pad
- Iliotibial tract
- Vastus lateralis t.
- Lateral superior geniculate artery
- Popliteal vein
- Common peroneal n.
- Tibial nerve
- Biceps femoris muscle

(Top) First in series of axial T1 MR images of the left knee. The cut is above the patella and at the proximal portion of the femoral metaphysis. At this level, the origin of plantaris muscle is seen, but it is still proximal to the adductor tubercle. **(Bottom)** This cut is immediately above the adductor tubercle. The vastus medialis obliquus is seen, serving as medial support for the superior portion of the patella.

AXIAL T1 MR, RIGHT KNEE

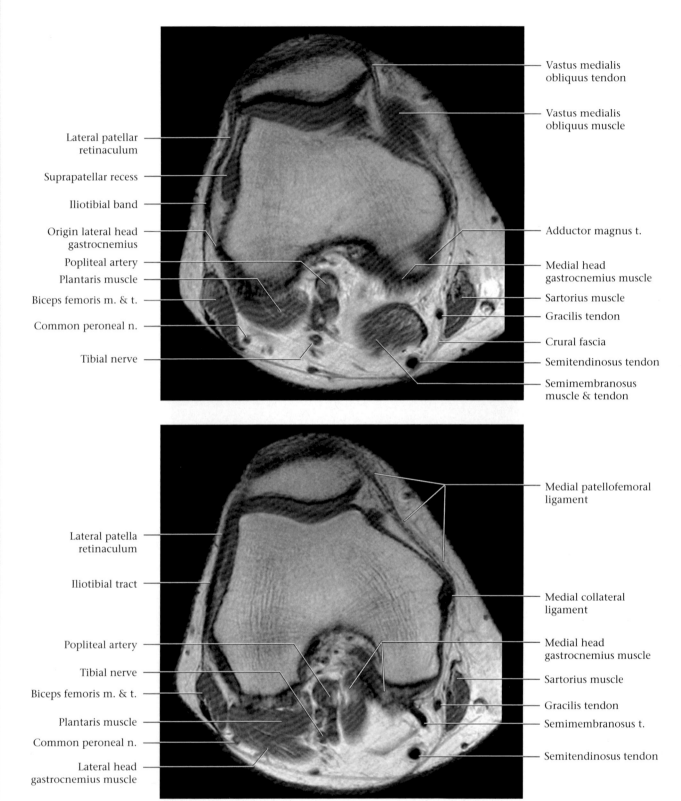

Lateral patellar retinaculum

Suprapatellar recess

Iliotibial band

Origin lateral head gastrocnemius

Popliteal artery

Plantaris muscle

Biceps femoris m. & t.

Common peroneal n.

Tibial nerve

Vastus medialis obliquus tendon

Vastus medialis obliquus muscle

Adductor magnus t.

Medial head gastrocnemius muscle

Sartorius muscle

Gracilis tendon

Crural fascia

Semitendinosus tendon

Semimembranosus muscle & tendon

Lateral patella retinaculum

Iliotibial tract

Popliteal artery

Tibial nerve

Biceps femoris m. & t.

Plantaris muscle

Common peroneal n.

Lateral head gastrocnemius muscle

Medial patellofemoral ligament

Medial collateral ligament

Medial head gastrocnemius muscle

Sartorius muscle

Gracilis tendon

Semimembranosus t.

Semitendinosus tendon

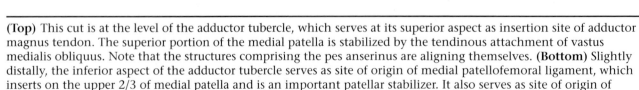

(Top) This cut is at the level of the adductor tubercle, which serves at its superior aspect as insertion site of adductor magnus tendon. The superior portion of the medial patella is stabilized by the tendinous attachment of vastus medialis obliquus. Note that the structures comprising the pes anserinus are aligning themselves. **(Bottom)** Slightly distally, the inferior aspect of the adductor tubercle serves as site of origin of medial patellofemoral ligament, which inserts on the upper 2/3 of medial patella and is an important patellar stabilizer. It also serves as site of origin of superficial medial collateral ligament fibers.

KNEE OVERVIEW

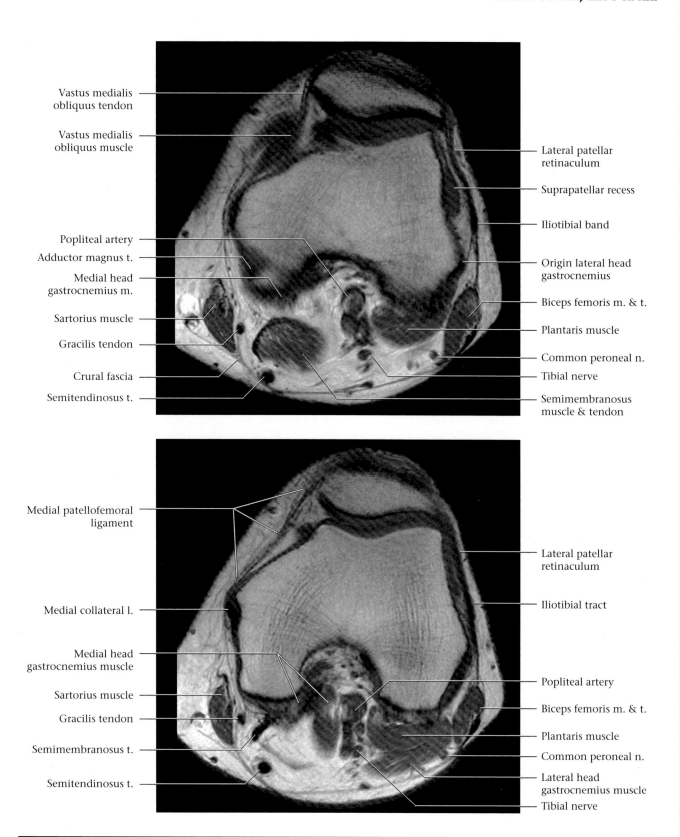

Top image labels (left):
- Vastus medialis obliquus tendon
- Vastus medialis obliquus muscle
- Popliteal artery
- Adductor magnus t.
- Medial head gastrocnemius m.
- Sartorius muscle
- Gracilis tendon
- Crural fascia
- Semitendinosus t.

Top image labels (right):
- Lateral patellar retinaculum
- Suprapatellar recess
- Iliotibial band
- Origin lateral head gastrocnemius
- Biceps femoris m. & t.
- Plantaris muscle
- Common peroneal n.
- Tibial nerve
- Semimembranosus muscle & tendon

Bottom image labels (left):
- Medial patellofemoral ligament
- Medial collateral l.
- Medial head gastrocnemius muscle
- Sartorius muscle
- Gracilis tendon
- Semimembranosus t.
- Semitendinosus t.

Bottom image labels (right):
- Lateral patellar retinaculum
- Iliotibial tract
- Popliteal artery
- Biceps femoris m. & t.
- Plantaris muscle
- Common peroneal n.
- Lateral head gastrocnemius muscle
- Tibial nerve

(Top) This cut is at the level of the adductor tubercle, which serves at its superior aspect as insertion site of adductor magnus tendon. The superior portion of the medial patella is stabilized by the tendinous attachment of vastus medialis obliquus. Note that the structures comprising the pes anserinus are aligning themselves. **(Bottom)** Slightly distally, the inferior aspect of the adductor tubercle serves as site of origin of medial patellofemoral ligament, which inserts on the upper 2/3 of medial patella and is an important patellar stabilizer. It also serves as site of origin of superficial medial collateral ligament fibers.

KNEE OVERVIEW

AXIAL T1 MR, RIGHT KNEE

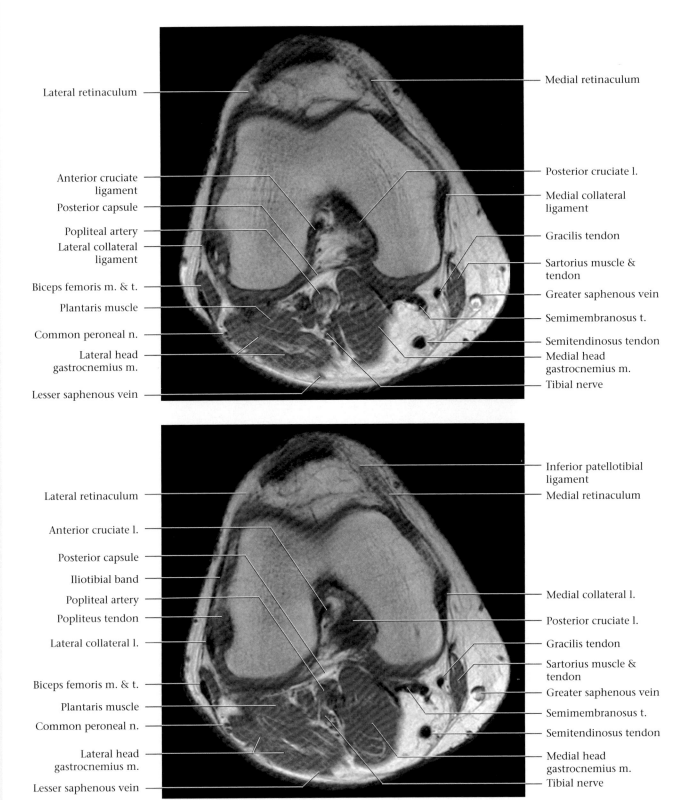

Lateral retinaculum — Medial retinaculum

Anterior cruciate ligament — Posterior cruciate l.

Posterior capsule — Medial collateral ligament

Popliteal artery — Gracilis tendon

Lateral collateral ligament — Sartorius muscle & tendon

Biceps femoris m. & t. — Greater saphenous vein

Plantaris muscle — Semimembranosus t.

Common peroneal n. — Semitendinosus tendon

Lateral head gastrocnemius m. — Medial head gastrocnemius m.

Lesser saphenous vein — Tibial nerve

Inferior patellotibial ligament

Lateral retinaculum — Medial retinaculum

Anterior cruciate l.

Posterior capsule — Medial collateral l.

Iliotibial band — Posterior cruciate l.

Popliteal artery — Gracilis tendon

Popliteus tendon — Sartorius muscle & tendon

Lateral collateral l. — Greater saphenous vein

Biceps femoris m. & t. — Semimembranosus t.

Plantaris muscle — Semitendinosus tendon

Common peroneal n. — Medial head gastrocnemius m.

Lateral head gastrocnemius m. — Tibial nerve

Lesser saphenous vein

(Top) This cut is through the intercondylar notch; origins of both anterior and posterior cruciate ligaments are seen. The hamstrings are nearly completely tendinous, about to cross medially to the knee joint. The origins of both collateral ligaments are now seen. **(Bottom)** At the lower end of patella, the medial support is from the inferior patellotibial ligament. The C-shaped semimembranosus tendon is distinctly different from the elements of pes anserinus (sartorius, gracilis, semitendinosus). The biceps femoris and lateral collateral ligament begin to approach one another as they extend to their insertion on the fibular head; the popliteus tendon arises from its sulcus on the lateral femoral condyle.

KNEE OVERVIEW

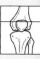

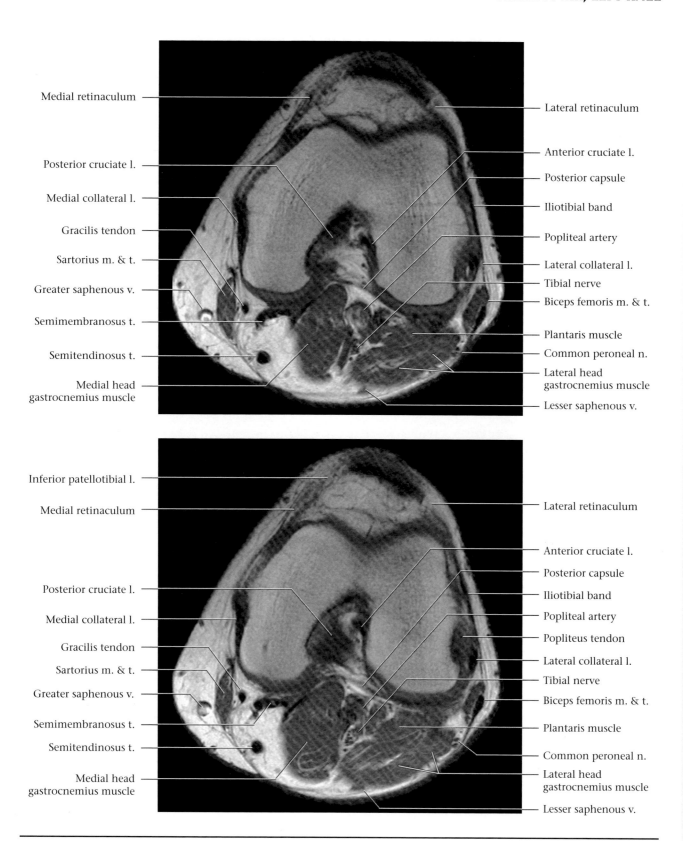

Medial retinaculum — Lateral retinaculum

Posterior cruciate l. — Anterior cruciate l.

Medial collateral l. — Posterior capsule

Gracilis tendon — Iliotibial band

Sartorius m. & t. — Popliteal artery

Greater saphenous v. — Lateral collateral l.

Semimembranosus t. — Tibial nerve

Semitendinosus t. — Biceps femoris m. & t.

Medial head gastrocnemius muscle — Plantaris muscle

Common peroneal n.

Lateral head gastrocnemius muscle

Lesser saphenous v.

Inferior patellotibial l. — Lateral retinaculum

Medial retinaculum — Anterior cruciate l.

Posterior cruciate l. — Posterior capsule

Medial collateral l. — Iliotibial band

Gracilis tendon — Popliteal artery

Sartorius m. & t. — Popliteus tendon

Greater saphenous v. — Lateral collateral l.

Semimembranosus t. — Tibial nerve

Semitendinosus t. — Biceps femoris m. & t.

Medial head gastrocnemius muscle — Plantaris muscle

Common peroneal n.

Lateral head gastrocnemius muscle

Lesser saphenous v.

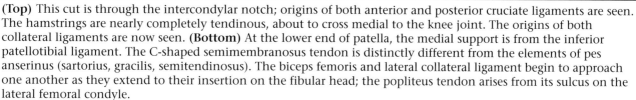

(Top) This cut is through the intercondylar notch; origins of both anterior and posterior cruciate ligaments are seen. The hamstrings are nearly completely tendinous, about to cross medial to the knee joint. The origins of both collateral ligaments are now seen. **(Bottom)** At the lower end of patella, the medial support is from the inferior patellotibial ligament. The C-shaped semimembranosus tendon is distinctly different from the elements of pes anserinus (sartorius, gracilis, semitendinosus). The biceps femoris and lateral collateral ligament begin to approach one another as they extend to their insertion on the fibular head; the popliteus tendon arises from its sulcus on the lateral femoral condyle.

Knee

VI

AXIAL T1 MR, RIGHT KNEE

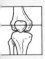

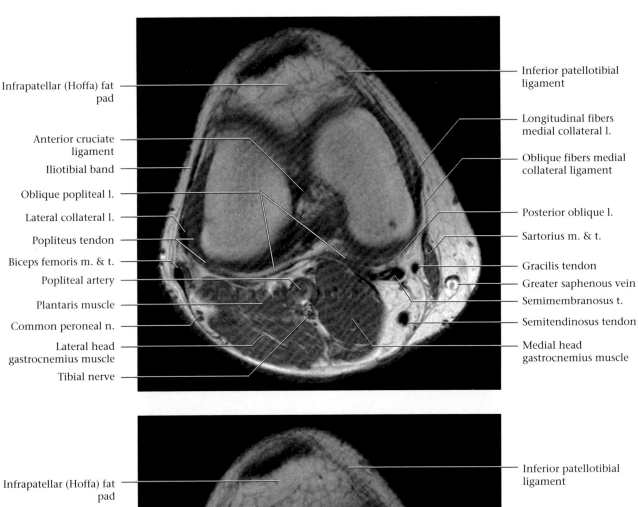

Infrapatellar (Hoffa) fat pad

Anterior cruciate ligament

Iliotibial band

Oblique popliteal l.

Lateral collateral l.

Popliteus tendon

Biceps femoris m. & t.

Popliteal artery

Plantaris muscle

Common peroneal n.

Lateral head gastrocnemius muscle

Tibial nerve

Inferior patellotibial ligament

Longitudinal fibers medial collateral l.

Oblique fibers medial collateral ligament

Posterior oblique l.

Sartorius m. & t.

Gracilis tendon

Greater saphenous vein

Semimembranosus t.

Semitendinosus tendon

Medial head gastrocnemius muscle

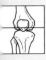

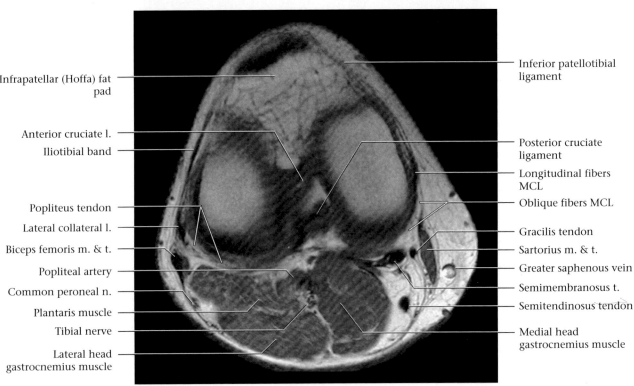

Infrapatellar (Hoffa) fat pad

Anterior cruciate l.

Iliotibial band

Popliteus tendon

Lateral collateral l.

Biceps femoris m. & t.

Popliteal artery

Common peroneal n.

Plantaris muscle

Tibial nerve

Lateral head gastrocnemius muscle

Inferior patellotibial ligament

Posterior cruciate ligament

Longitudinal fibers MCL

Oblique fibers MCL

Gracilis tendon

Sartorius m. & t.

Greater saphenous vein

Semimembranosus t.

Semitendinosus tendon

Medial head gastrocnemius muscle

(Top) This cut is 1.5 cm above the knee joint. The posterolateral structures now include the popliteus tendon, extending posteromedially around the lateral femoral condyle within the popliteal hiatus. Additionally, the posterior oblique ligament, arising from fibers of the medial collateral ligament, joins fibers from semimembranosus to supplement the posterior capsule as the oblique popliteal ligament. **(Bottom)** This cut is immediately above the knee joint. The posterior cruciate is approaching its insertion on posterior tibia and anterior cruciate spreads out towards its insertion on the plateau.

KNEE OVERVIEW

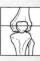

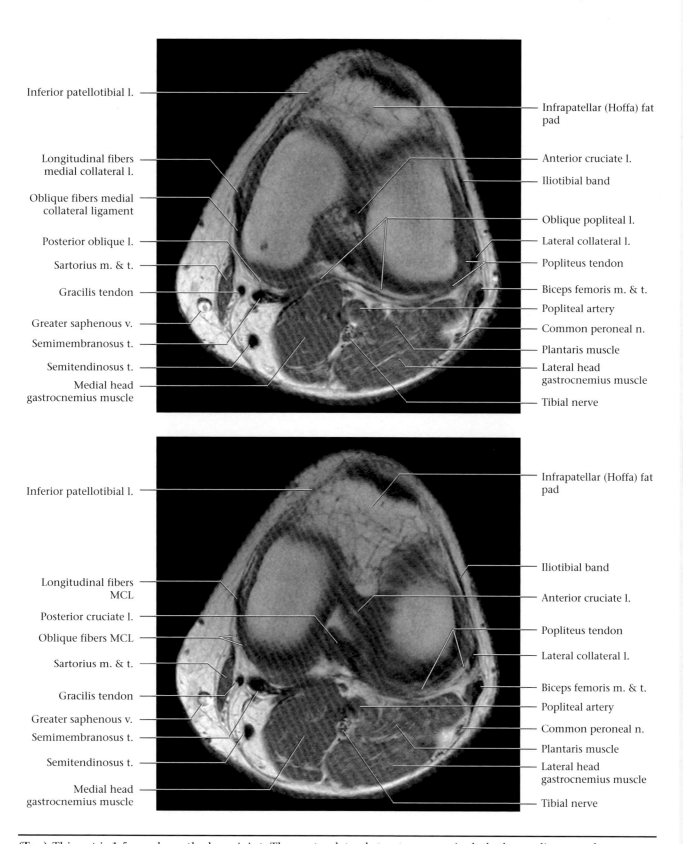

Inferior patellotibial l.

Longitudinal fibers medial collateral l.

Oblique fibers medial collateral ligament

Posterior oblique l.

Sartorius m. & t.

Gracilis tendon

Greater saphenous v.

Semimembranosus t.

Semitendinosus t.

Medial head gastrocnemius muscle

Infrapatellar (Hoffa) fat pad

Anterior cruciate l.

Iliotibial band

Oblique popliteal l.

Lateral collateral l.

Popliteus tendon

Biceps femoris m. & t.

Popliteal artery

Common peroneal n.

Plantaris muscle

Lateral head gastrocnemius muscle

Tibial nerve

Inferior patellotibial l.

Longitudinal fibers MCL

Posterior cruciate l.

Oblique fibers MCL

Sartorius m. & t.

Gracilis tendon

Greater saphenous v.

Semimembranosus t.

Semitendinosus t.

Medial head gastrocnemius muscle

Infrapatellar (Hoffa) fat pad

Iliotibial band

Anterior cruciate l.

Popliteus tendon

Lateral collateral l.

Biceps femoris m. & t.

Popliteal artery

Common peroneal n.

Plantaris muscle

Lateral head gastrocnemius muscle

Tibial nerve

(Top) This cut is 1.5 cm above the knee joint. The posterolateral structures now include the popliteus tendon, extending posteromedially around the lateral femoral condyle within the popliteal hiatus. Additionally, the posterior oblique ligament, arising from fibers of the medial collateral ligament, joins fibers from semimembranosus to supplement the posterior capsule as the oblique popliteal ligament. **(Bottom)** This cut is immediately above the knee joint. The posterior cruciate is approaching its insertion on posterior tibia and anterior cruciate spreads out towards its insertion on the plateau.

Knee

VI

AXIAL T1 MR, RIGHT KNEE

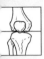

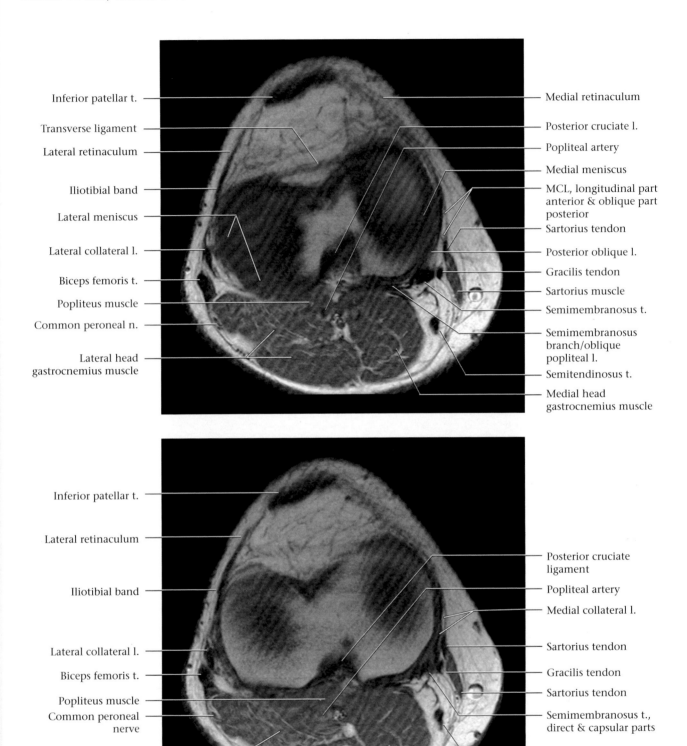

Inferior patellar t. — Medial retinaculum

Transverse ligament — Posterior cruciate l.

Lateral retinaculum — Popliteal artery

Iliotibial band — Medial meniscus

Lateral meniscus — MCL, longitudinal part anterior & oblique part posterior

Lateral collateral l. — Sartorius tendon

— Posterior oblique l.

Biceps femoris t. — Gracilis tendon

Popliteus muscle — Sartorius muscle

Common peroneal n. — Semimembranosus t.

— Semimembranosus branch/oblique popliteal l.

Lateral head gastrocnemius muscle — Semitendinosus t.

— Medial head gastrocnemius muscle

Inferior patellar t. —

Posterior cruciate ligament

Lateral retinaculum — Popliteal artery

Iliotibial band — Medial collateral l.

Lateral collateral l. — Sartorius tendon

Biceps femoris t. — Gracilis tendon

Popliteus muscle — Sartorius tendon

Common peroneal nerve — Semimembranosus t., direct & capsular parts

Lateral head gastrocnemius muscle — Semitendinosus t.

— Medial head gastrocnemius muscle

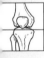

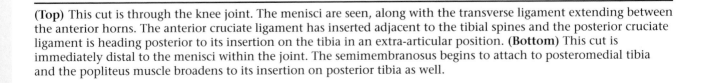

(Top) This cut is through the knee joint. The menisci are seen, along with the transverse ligament extending between the anterior horns. The anterior cruciate ligament has inserted adjacent to the tibial spines and the posterior cruciate ligament is heading posterior to its insertion on the tibia in an extra-articular position. **(Bottom)** This cut is immediately distal to the menisci within the joint. The semimembranosus begins to attach to posteromedial tibia and the popliteus muscle broadens to its insertion on posterior tibia as well.

KNEE OVERVIEW

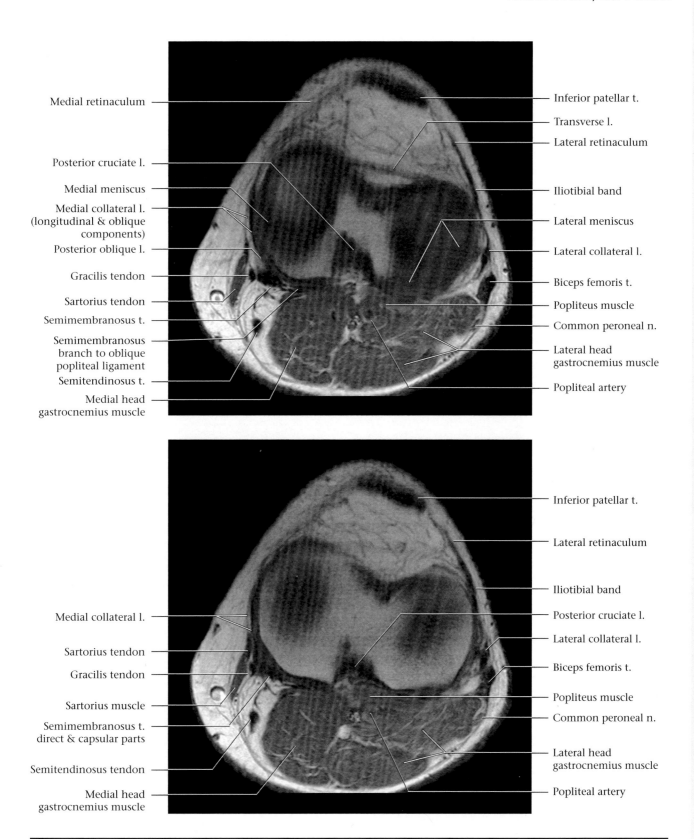

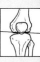

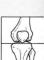

Top image labels:

Medial retinaculum

Posterior cruciate l.

Medial meniscus

Medial collateral l. (longitudinal & oblique components)

Posterior oblique l.

Gracilis tendon

Sartorius tendon

Semimembranosus t.

Semimembranosus branch to oblique popliteal ligament

Semitendinosus t.

Medial head gastrocnemius muscle

Inferior patellar t.

Transverse l.

Lateral retinaculum

Iliotibial band

Lateral meniscus

Lateral collateral l.

Biceps femoris t.

Popliteus muscle

Common peroneal n.

Lateral head gastrocnemius muscle

Popliteal artery

Bottom image labels:

Medial collateral l.

Sartorius tendon

Gracilis tendon

Sartorius muscle

Semimembranosus t. direct & capsular parts

Semitendinosus tendon

Medial head gastrocnemius muscle

Inferior patellar t.

Lateral retinaculum

Iliotibial band

Posterior cruciate l.

Lateral collateral l.

Biceps femoris t.

Popliteus muscle

Common peroneal n.

Lateral head gastrocnemius muscle

Popliteal artery

(Top) This cut is through the knee joint. The menisci are seen, along with the transverse ligament extending between the anterior horns. The anterior cruciate ligament has inserted adjacent to the tibial spines and the posterior cruciate ligament is heading posterior to its insertion on the tibia in an extra-articular position. **(Bottom)** This cut is immediately distal to the menisci within the joint. The semimembranosus begins to attach to posteromedial tibia and the popliteus muscle broadens to its insertion on posterior tibia as well.

Knee

VI

AXIAL T1 MR, RIGHT KNEE

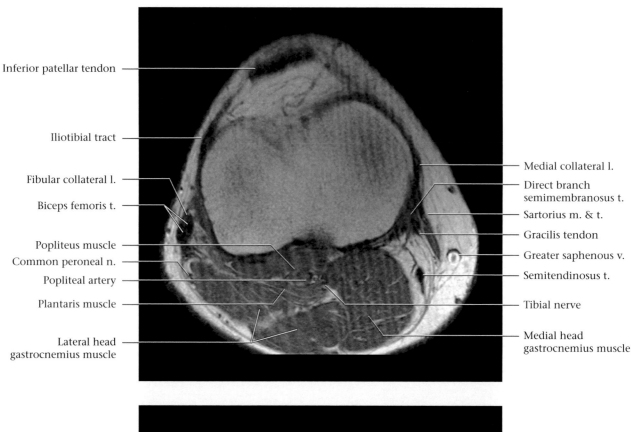

Inferior patellar tendon

Iliotibial tract

Fibular collateral l.

Biceps femoris t.

Popliteus muscle
Common peroneal n.
Popliteal artery
Plantaris muscle

Lateral head
gastrocnemius muscle

Medial collateral l.
Direct branch
semimembranosus t.
Sartorius m. & t.
Gracilis tendon
Greater saphenous v.
Semitendinosus t.
Tibial nerve
Medial head
gastrocnemius muscle

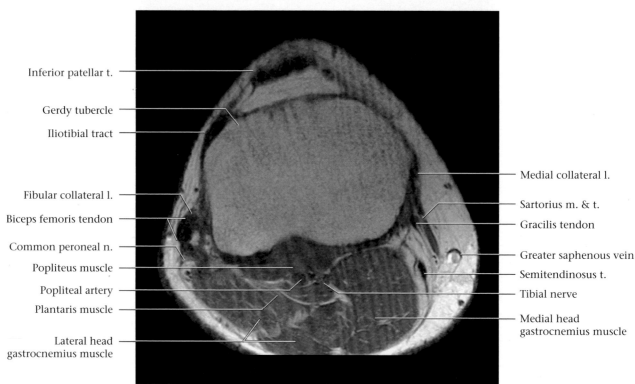

Inferior patellar t.

Gerdy tubercle
Iliotibial tract

Fibular collateral l.
Biceps femoris tendon

Common peroneal n.
Popliteus muscle
Popliteal artery
Plantaris muscle

Lateral head
gastrocnemius muscle

Medial collateral l.
Sartorius m. & t.
Gracilis tendon
Greater saphenous vein
Semitendinosus t.
Tibial nerve
Medial head
gastrocnemius muscle

(Top) This cut is through the tibial plateau. The tendons of pes anserinus (sartorius, gracilis, and semitendinosus) are lining up, extending towards their insertion on the anteromedial tibia. The popliteus muscle is still broad, with the tibial nerve and popliteal vessels interposed between it and the superficial muscles of the leg. **(Bottom)** This cut is through the lower portion of the tibial plateau, immediately proximal to the fibular head. Note the common peroneal nerve, located posterior to the biceps femoris tendon.

KNEE OVERVIEW

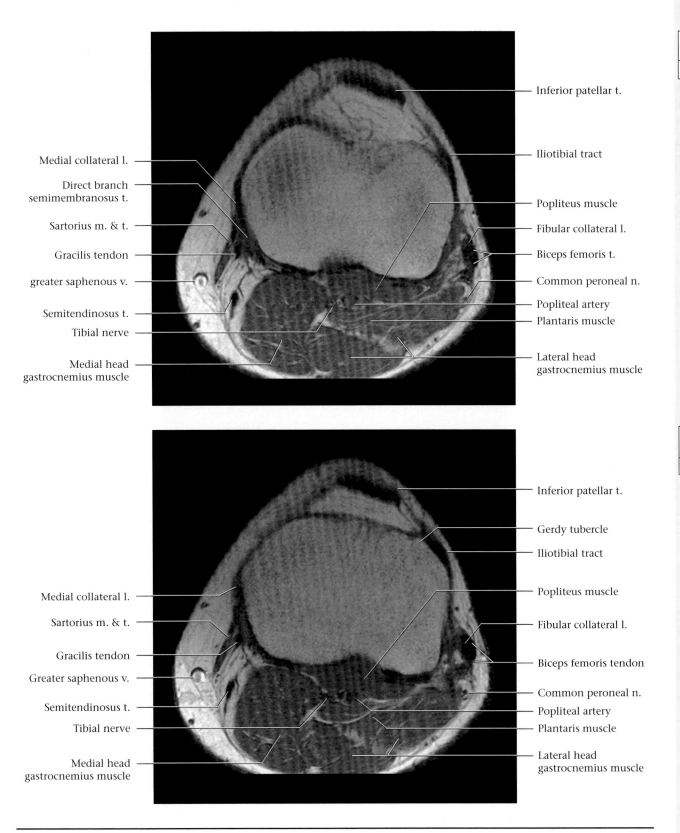

Inferior patellar t.

Iliotibial tract

Medial collateral l.

Direct branch semimembranosus t.

Popliteus muscle

Sartorius m. & t.

Fibular collateral l.

Gracilis tendon

Biceps femoris t.

greater saphenous v.

Common peroneal n.

Semitendinosus t.

Popliteal artery

Tibial nerve

Plantaris muscle

Medial head gastrocnemius muscle

Lateral head gastrocnemius muscle

Inferior patellar t.

Gerdy tubercle

Iliotibial tract

Medial collateral l.

Popliteus muscle

Sartorius m. & t.

Fibular collateral l.

Gracilis tendon

Biceps femoris tendon

Greater saphenous v.

Common peroneal n.

Semitendinosus t.

Popliteal artery

Tibial nerve

Plantaris muscle

Medial head gastrocnemius muscle

Lateral head gastrocnemius muscle

(Top) This cut is through the tibial plateau. The tendons of pes anserinus (sartorius, gracilis, and semitendinosus) are lining up, extending towards their insertion on the anteromedial tibia. The popliteus muscle is still broad, with the tibial nerve and popliteal vessels interposed between it and the superficial muscles of the leg. **(Bottom)** This cut is through the lower portion of the tibial plateau, immediately proximal to the fibular head. Note the common peroneal nerve, located posterior to the biceps femoris tendon.

AXIAL T1 MR, RIGHT KNEE

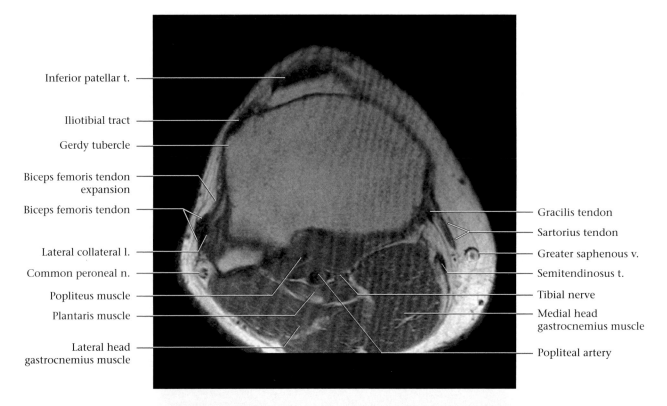

Inferior patellar t.

Iliotibial tract

Gerdy tubercle

Biceps femoris tendon expansion

Biceps femoris tendon

Lateral collateral l.

Common peroneal n.

Popliteus muscle

Plantaris muscle

Lateral head gastrocnemius muscle

Gracilis tendon

Sartorius tendon

Greater saphenous v.

Semitendinosus t.

Tibial nerve

Medial head gastrocnemius muscle

Popliteal artery

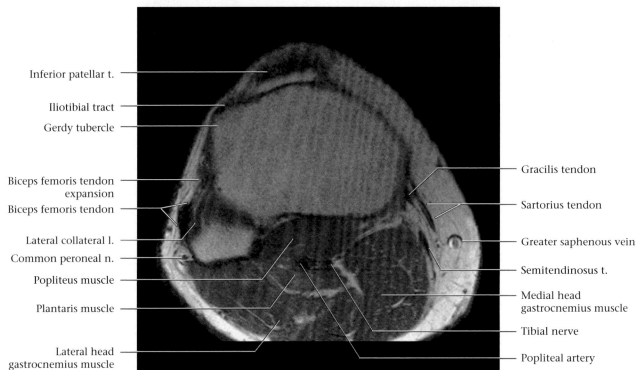

Inferior patellar t.

Iliotibial tract

Gerdy tubercle

Biceps femoris tendon expansion

Biceps femoris tendon

Lateral collateral l.

Common peroneal n.

Popliteus muscle

Plantaris muscle

Lateral head gastrocnemius muscle

Gracilis tendon

Sartorius tendon

Greater saphenous vein

Semitendinosus t.

Medial head gastrocnemius muscle

Tibial nerve

Popliteal artery

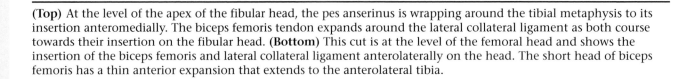

(Top) At the level of the apex of the fibular head, the pes anserinus is wrapping around the tibial metaphysis to its insertion anteromedially. The biceps femoris tendon expands around the lateral collateral ligament as both course towards their insertion on the fibular head. **(Bottom)** This cut is at the level of the femoral head and shows the insertion of the biceps femoris and lateral collateral ligament anterolaterally on the head. The short head of biceps femoris has a thin anterior expansion that extends to the anterolateral tibia.

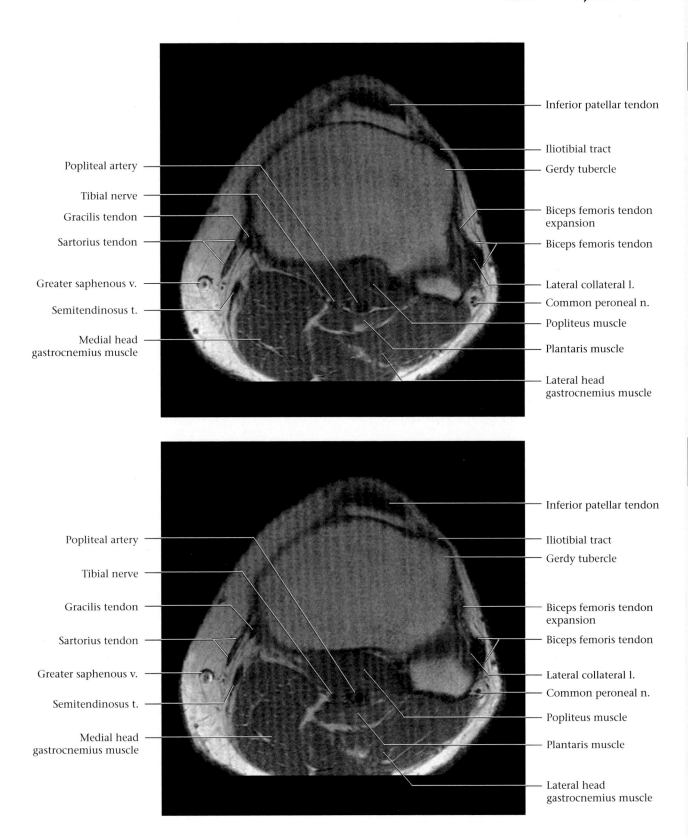

Inferior patellar tendon

Iliotibial tract

Gerdy tubercle

Biceps femoris tendon expansion

Biceps femoris tendon

Lateral collateral l.

Common peroneal n.

Popliteus muscle

Plantaris muscle

Lateral head gastrocnemius muscle

Popliteal artery

Tibial nerve

Gracilis tendon

Sartorius tendon

Greater saphenous v.

Semitendinosus t.

Medial head gastrocnemius muscle

Inferior patellar tendon

Iliotibial tract

Gerdy tubercle

Biceps femoris tendon expansion

Biceps femoris tendon

Lateral collateral l.

Common peroneal n.

Popliteus muscle

Plantaris muscle

Lateral head gastrocnemius muscle

Popliteal artery

Tibial nerve

Gracilis tendon

Sartorius tendon

Greater saphenous v.

Semitendinosus t.

Medial head gastrocnemius muscle

(Top) At the level of the apex of the fibular head, the pes anserinus is wrapping around the tibial metaphysis to its insertion anteromedially. The biceps femoris tendon expands around the lateral collateral ligament as both course towards their insertion on the fibular head. **(Bottom)** This cut is at the level of the femoral head and shows the insertion of the biceps femoris and lateral collateral ligament anterolaterally on the head. The short head of biceps femoris has a thin anterior expansion that extends to the anterolateral tibia.

KNEE OVERVIEW

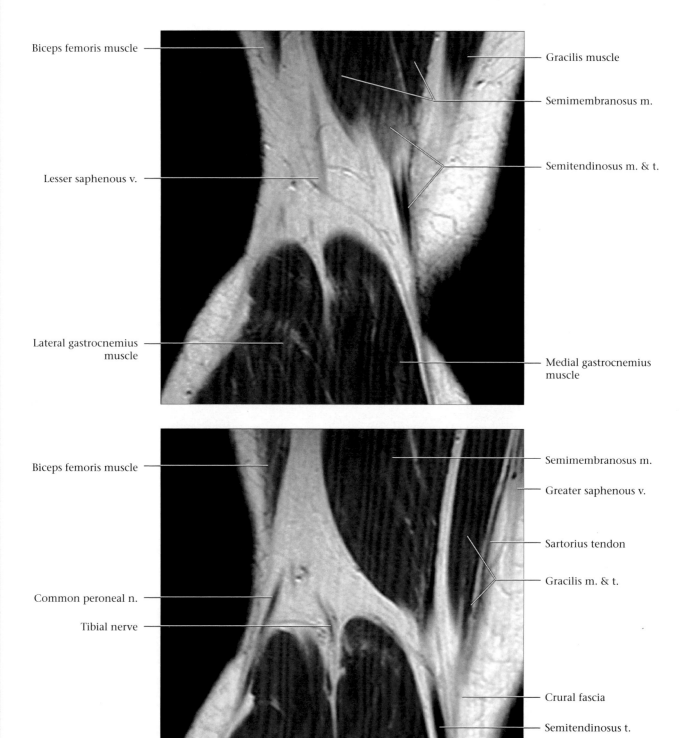

Biceps femoris muscle — Gracilis muscle

Semimembranosus m.

Semitendinosus m. & t.

Lesser saphenous v.

Lateral gastrocnemius muscle — Medial gastrocnemius muscle

Biceps femoris muscle — Semimembranosus m.

Greater saphenous v.

Sartorius tendon

Gracilis m. & t.

Common peroneal n.

Tibial nerve

Crural fascia

Semitendinosus t.

Lateral gastrocnemius muscle — Medial gastrocnemius muscle

(Top) First in series of posterior coronal T1 MR images of the right knee, displayed from posterior to anterior, shows the semitendinosus muscle as well as tendon. We are also posterior enough to see lesser saphenous vein. More distally in the leg, the sural nerve accompanies this structure. **(Bottom)** Slightly more anterior, the courses of common peroneal and tibial nerves can be seen. Semitendinosus tendon is distinctly seen as the posterior portion of the pes anserinus.

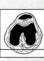

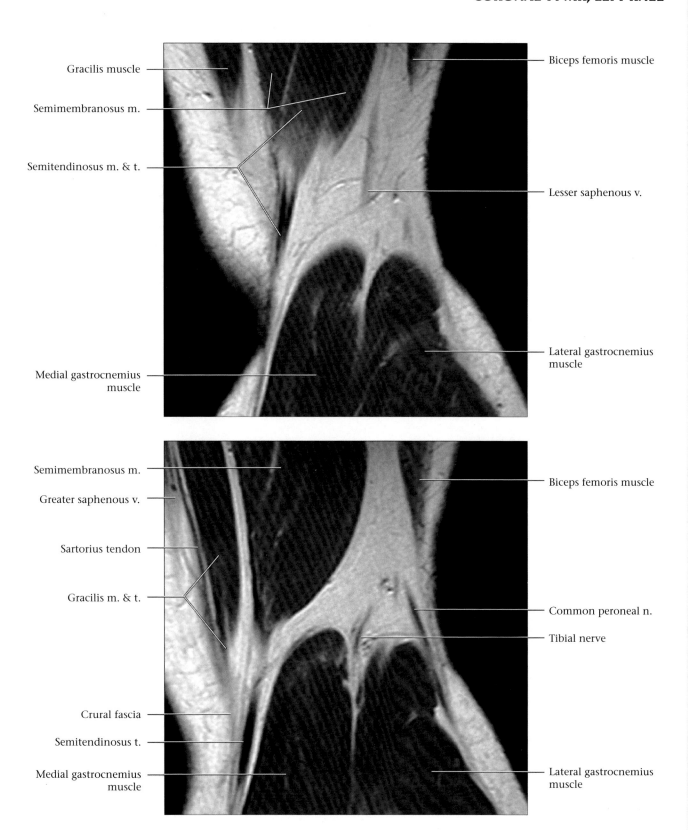

Gracilis muscle

Semimembranosus m.

Semitendinosus m. & t.

Medial gastrocnemius muscle

Biceps femoris muscle

Lesser saphenous v.

Lateral gastrocnemius muscle

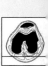

Semimembranosus m.

Greater saphenous v.

Sartorius tendon

Gracilis m. & t.

Crural fascia

Semitendinosus t.

Medial gastrocnemius muscle

Biceps femoris muscle

Common peroneal n.

Tibial nerve

Lateral gastrocnemius muscle

(Top) First in series of posterior coronal T1 MR images of the left knee, displayed from posterior to anterior, shows the semitendinosus muscle as well as tendon. We are also posterior enough to see lesser saphenous vein. More distally in the leg, the sural nerve accompanies this structure. **(Bottom)** Slightly more anterior, the courses of common peroneal and tibial nerves can be seen. Semitendinosus tendon is distinctly seen as the posterior portion of the pes anserinus.

CORONAL T1 MR, RIGHT KNEE

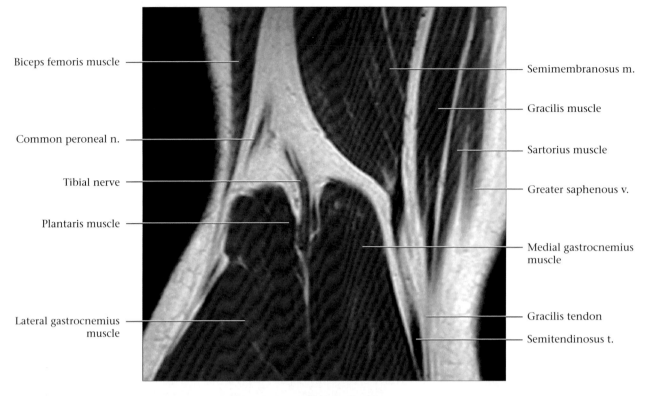

Biceps femoris muscle

Common peroneal n.

Tibial nerve

Plantaris muscle

Lateral gastrocnemius muscle

Semimembranosus m.

Gracilis muscle

Sartorius muscle

Greater saphenous v.

Medial gastrocnemius muscle

Gracilis tendon

Semitendinosus t.

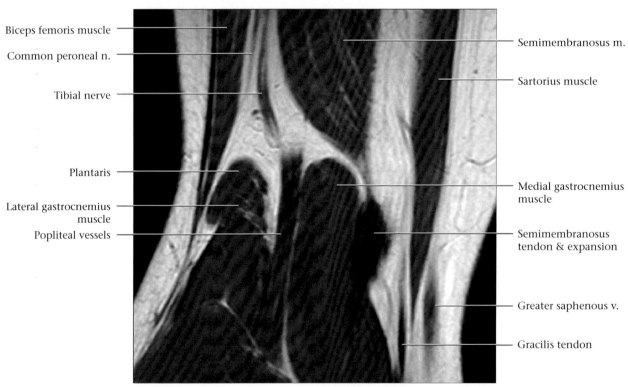

Biceps femoris muscle

Common peroneal n.

Tibial nerve

Plantaris

Lateral gastrocnemius muscle

Popliteal vessels

Semimembranosus m.

Sartorius muscle

Medial gastrocnemius muscle

Semimembranosus tendon & expansion

Greater saphenous v.

Gracilis tendon

(Top) In this slightly more anterior cut, the course of common peroneal nerve is seen following posterior biceps femoris tendon. The elements of pes anserinus are distinctly seen, with gracilis and sartorius muscles in this plane posterior to their tendons (seen in slightly more anterior cuts). Semitendinosus tendon, the posterior of the three elements of the pes, is seen in this section; its muscle fibers however are in a more posterior section (prior images). **(Bottom)** In the most anterior cut of this series, we see the division of the tibial and common peroneal nerves, as well as the separate components of the pes anserinus.

KNEE OVERVIEW

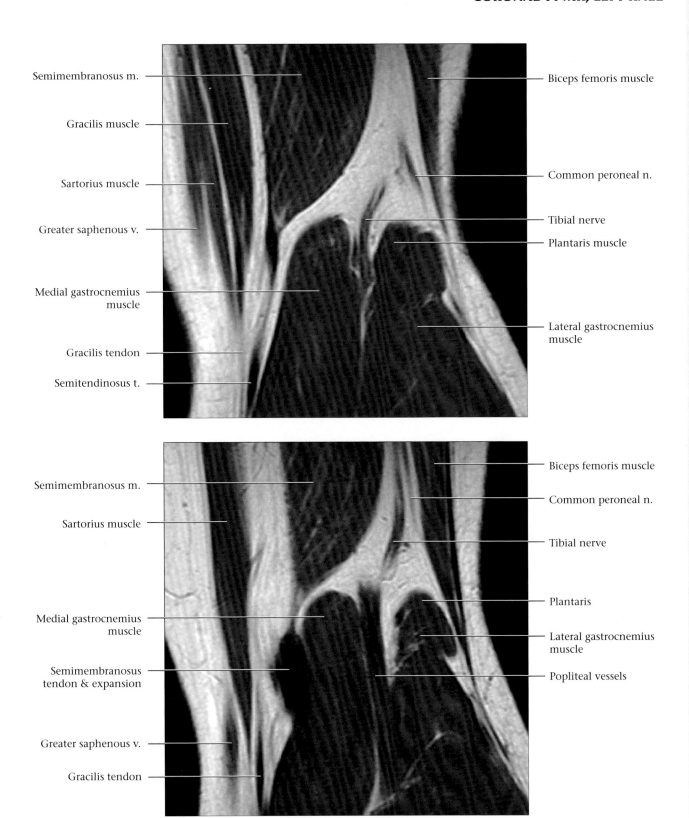

Semimembranosus m.

Gracilis muscle

Sartorius muscle

Greater saphenous v.

Medial gastrocnemius muscle

Gracilis tendon

Semitendinosus t.

Biceps femoris muscle

Common peroneal n.

Tibial nerve

Plantaris muscle

Lateral gastrocnemius muscle

Semimembranosus m.

Sartorius muscle

Medial gastrocnemius muscle

Semimembranosus tendon & expansion

Greater saphenous v.

Gracilis tendon

Biceps femoris muscle

Common peroneal n.

Tibial nerve

Plantaris

Lateral gastrocnemius muscle

Popliteal vessels

(Top) In this slightly more anterior cut, the course of common peroneal nerve is seen following posterior biceps femoris tendon. The elements of pes anserinus are distinctly seen, with gracilis and sartorius muscles in this plane posterior to their tendons (seen in slightly more anterior cuts). Semitendinosus tendon, the posterior of the three elements of the pes, is seen in this section; its muscle fibers however are in a more posterior section (prior images). **(Bottom)** In this most anterior cut of this series, we see the division of the tibial and common peroneal nerves, as well as the separate components of the pes anserinus.

CORONAL T1 MR, RIGHT KNEE

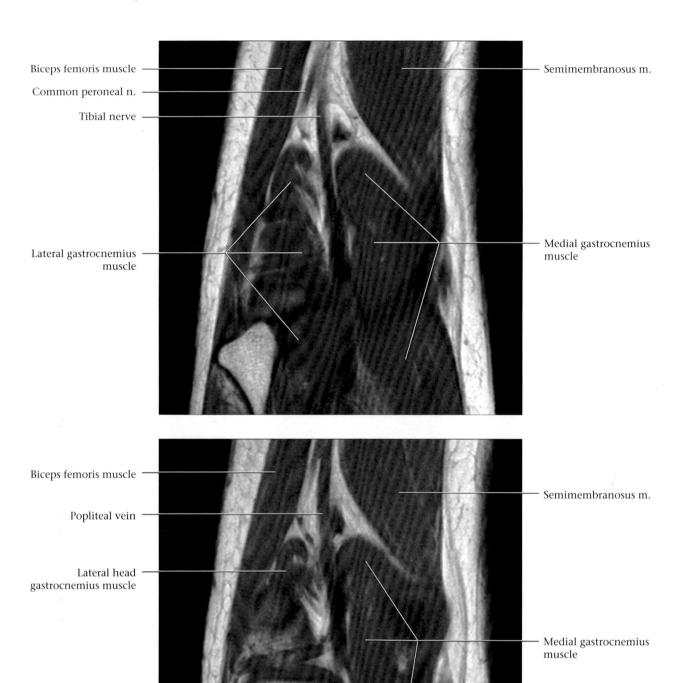

Biceps femoris muscle

Common peroneal n.

Tibial nerve

Lateral gastrocnemius muscle

Semimembranosus m.

Medial gastrocnemius muscle

Biceps femoris muscle

Popliteal vein

Lateral head gastrocnemius muscle

Biceps femoris tendon insertion

Lateral gastrocnemius muscle

Peroneus longus m.

Semimembranosus m.

Medial gastrocnemius muscle

(**Top**) First in series of coronal T1 MR images of the right knee. This series is in a slightly different obliquity than the prior, allowing slightly different combinations of structures to be seen in a single cut. The series is shown from posterior to anterior. The tibial nerve and common peroneal nerve are seen in this cut, as they lie more posterior than the popliteal vessels. (**Bottom**) Slightly more anterior image. The gastrocnemius muscles predominate in the posterior portion of the lower knee; the deeper muscles are smaller at this point. Laterally, the origin of the peroneus longus muscle is seen at the fibula.

KNEE OVERVIEW

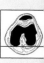

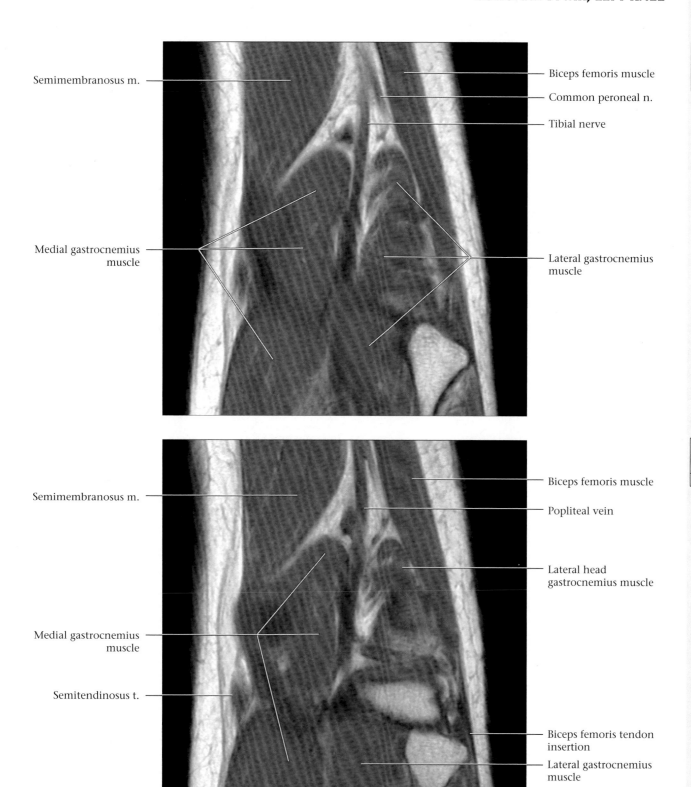

Semimembranosus m.

Biceps femoris muscle

Common peroneal n.

Tibial nerve

Medial gastrocnemius muscle

Lateral gastrocnemius muscle

Semimembranosus m.

Biceps femoris muscle

Popliteal vein

Lateral head gastrocnemius muscle

Medial gastrocnemius muscle

Semitendinosus t.

Biceps femoris tendon insertion

Lateral gastrocnemius muscle

Peroneus longus m.

(Top) First in series of coronal T1 MR images of the left knee. This series is in a slightly different obliquity than the prior, allowing slightly different combinations of structures to be seen in a single cut. The series is shown from posterior to anterior. The tibial nerve and common peroneal nerve are seen in this cut, as they lie more posterior than the popliteal vessels. **(Bottom)** Slightly more anterior image. The gastrocnemius muscles predominate in the posterior portion of the lower knee; the deeper muscles are smaller at this point. Laterally, the origin of the peroneus longus muscle is seen at the fibula.

CORONAL T1 MR, RIGHT KNEE

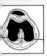

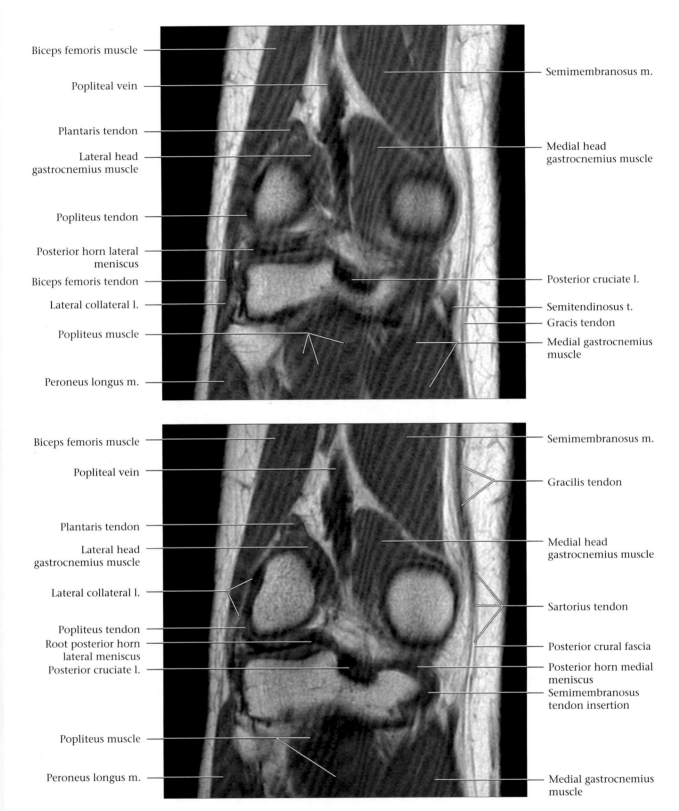

Biceps femoris muscle

Popliteal vein

Plantaris tendon

Lateral head gastrocnemius muscle

Popliteus tendon

Posterior horn lateral meniscus

Biceps femoris tendon

Lateral collateral l.

Popliteus muscle

Peroneus longus m.

Semimembranosus m.

Medial head gastrocnemius muscle

Posterior cruciate l.

Semitendinosus t.

Gracis tendon

Medial gastrocnemius muscle

Biceps femoris muscle

Popliteal vein

Plantaris tendon

Lateral head gastrocnemius muscle

Lateral collateral l.

Popliteus tendon

Root posterior horn lateral meniscus

Posterior cruciate l.

Popliteus muscle

Peroneus longus m.

Semimembranosus m.

Gracilis tendon

Medial head gastrocnemius muscle

Sartorius tendon

Posterior crural fascia

Posterior horn medial meniscus

Semimembranosus tendon insertion

Medial gastrocnemius muscle

(Top) Slightly more anteriorly, and deep to the majority of gastrocnemius muscle mass, the popliteus tendon is seen arising from its notch on the lateral femoral condyle, extending posteriorly and inferiorly to the popliteal hiatus. The individual structures in the posterolateral corner are generally better seen on a fluid sensitive sequence because of the fluid in the popliteal hiatus; for greater detail, see section detailing posterolateral structures. **(Bottom)** The lateral collateral ligament can now be seen arising from lateral femoral condyle, coursing towards its insertion, along with biceps femoris, on the fibular styloid process.

KNEE OVERVIEW

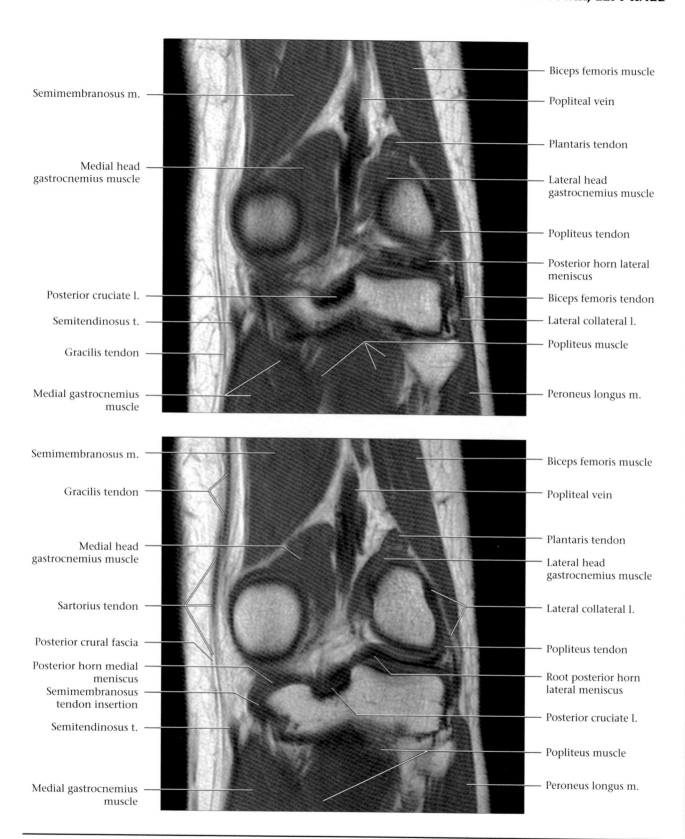

(Top) Top image labels — left side: Semimembranosus m.; Medial head gastrocnemius muscle; Posterior cruciate l.; Semitendinosus t.; Gracilis tendon; Medial gastrocnemius muscle. Right side: Biceps femoris muscle; Popliteal vein; Plantaris tendon; Lateral head gastrocnemius muscle; Popliteus tendon; Posterior horn lateral meniscus; Biceps femoris tendon; Lateral collateral l.; Popliteus muscle; Peroneus longus m.

(Bottom) Bottom image labels — left side: Semimembranosus m.; Gracilis tendon; Medial head gastrocnemius muscle; Sartorius tendon; Posterior crural fascia; Posterior horn medial meniscus; Semimembranosus tendon insertion; Semitendinosus t.; Medial gastrocnemius muscle. Right side: Biceps femoris muscle; Popliteal vein; Plantaris tendon; Lateral head gastrocnemius muscle; Lateral collateral l.; Popliteus tendon; Root posterior horn lateral meniscus; Posterior cruciate l.; Popliteus muscle; Peroneus longus m.

(Top) Slightly more anteriorly, and deep to the majority of gastrocnemius muscle mass, the popliteus tendon is seen arising from its notch on the lateral femoral condyle, extending posteriorly and inferiorly to the popliteal hiatus. The individual structures in the posterolateral corner are generally better seen on a fluid sensitive sequence because of the fluid in the popliteal hiatus; for greater detail, see section detailing posterolateral structures. **(Bottom)** The lateral collateral ligament can now be seen arising from lateral femoral condyle, coursing towards its insertion, along with biceps femoris, on the fibular styloid process.

KNEE OVERVIEW

CORONAL T1 MR, RIGHT KNEE

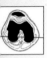

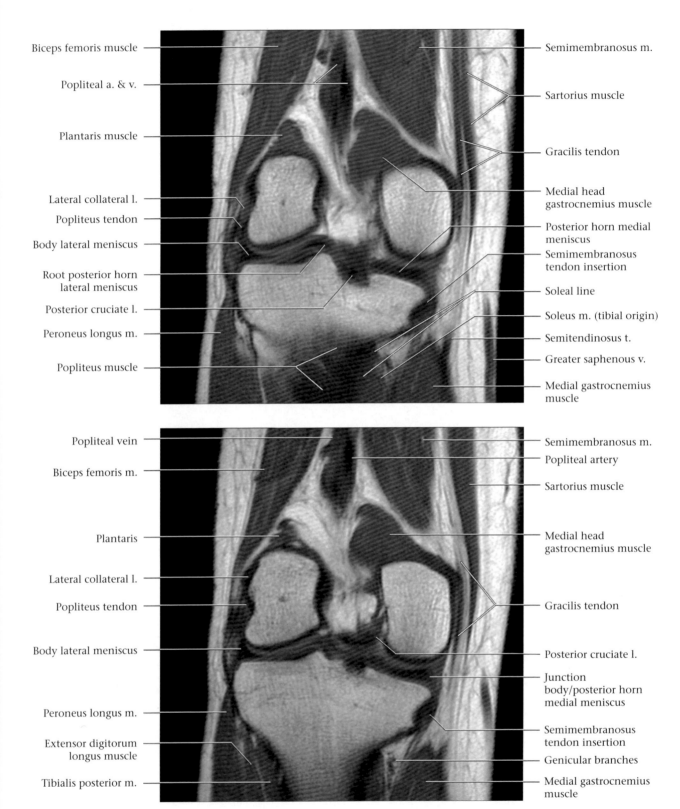

Biceps femoris muscle

Popliteal a. & v.

Plantaris muscle

Lateral collateral l.

Popliteus tendon

Body lateral meniscus

Root posterior horn lateral meniscus

Posterior cruciate l.

Peroneus longus m.

Popliteus muscle

Semimembranosus m.

Sartorius muscle

Gracilis tendon

Medial head gastrocnemius muscle

Posterior horn medial meniscus

Semimembranosus tendon insertion

Soleal line

Soleus m. (tibial origin)

Semitendinosus t.

Greater saphenous v.

Medial gastrocnemius muscle

Popliteal vein

Biceps femoris m.

Plantaris

Lateral collateral l.

Popliteus tendon

Body lateral meniscus

Peroneus longus m.

Extensor digitorum longus muscle

Tibialis posterior m.

Semimembranosus m.

Popliteal artery

Sartorius muscle

Medial head gastrocnemius muscle

Gracilis tendon

Posterior cruciate l.

Junction body/posterior horn medial meniscus

Semimembranosus tendon insertion

Genicular branches

Medial gastrocnemius muscle

(Top) More anteriorly, note the large expanse of insertion of popliteus muscle on posterior tibia. The medial soleus origin arises at its distal edge, along the soleal line. The fibular origin of soleus occurs more proximally. **(Bottom)** Image of the posterior portion of the knee joint, which is more complex than the anterior. The gastrocnemius and posterior vessels are still seen, as well as the hamstring muscles. Inferolaterally, the muscles can be confusing on coronal imaging since in a single plane such as this one, muscles from lateral compartment (peroneus), anterior compartment (extensor digitorum longus), and posterior compartment (tibialis posterior) can be seen. This is because the cut extends obliquely across the interosseous membrane between tibia and fibula.

KNEE OVERVIEW

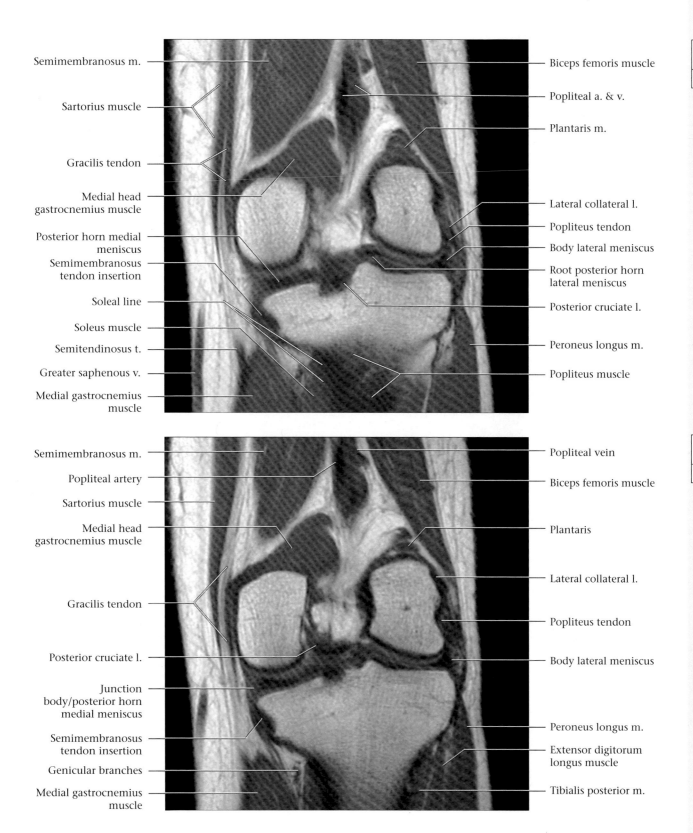

Top image labels (left side):
Semimembranosus m.
Sartorius muscle
Gracilis tendon
Medial head gastrocnemius muscle
Posterior horn medial meniscus
Semimembranosus tendon insertion
Soleal line
Soleus muscle
Semitendinosus t.
Greater saphenous v.
Medial gastrocnemius muscle

Top image labels (right side):
Biceps femoris muscle
Popliteal a. & v.
Plantaris m.
Lateral collateral l.
Popliteus tendon
Body lateral meniscus
Root posterior horn lateral meniscus
Posterior cruciate l.
Peroneus longus m.
Popliteus muscle

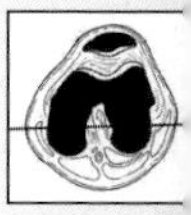

Bottom image labels (left side):
Semimembranosus m.
Popliteal artery
Sartorius muscle
Medial head gastrocnemius muscle
Gracilis tendon
Posterior cruciate l.
Junction body/posterior horn medial meniscus
Semimembranosus tendon insertion
Genicular branches
Medial gastrocnemius muscle

Bottom image labels (right side):
Popliteal vein
Biceps femoris muscle
Plantaris
Lateral collateral l.
Popliteus tendon
Body lateral meniscus
Peroneus longus m.
Extensor digitorum longus muscle
Tibialis posterior m.

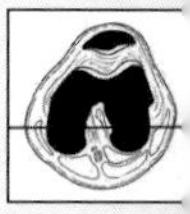

(Top) More anteriorly, note the large expanse of insertion of popliteus muscle on posterior tibia. The medial soleus origin arises at its distal edge, along the soleal line. The fibular origin of soleus occurs more proximally. **(Bottom)** Image of the posterior portion of the knee joint, which is more complex than the anterior. The gastrocnemius and posterior vessels are still seen, as well as the hamstring muscles. Inferolaterally, the muscles can be confusing on coronal imaging since in a single plane such as this one, muscles from lateral compartment (peroneus), anterior compartment (extensor digitorum longus), and posterior compartment (tibialis posterior) can be seen. This is because the cut extends obliquely across the interosseous membrane between tibia and fibula.

CORONAL T1 MR, RIGHT KNEE

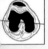

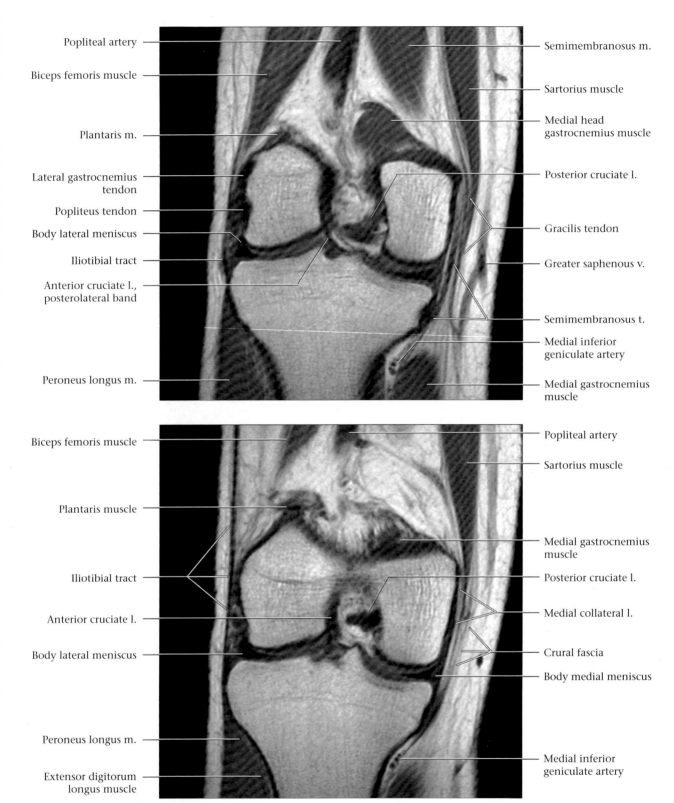

Popliteal artery

Biceps femoris muscle

Plantaris m.

Lateral gastrocnemius tendon

Popliteus tendon

Body lateral meniscus

Iliotibial tract

Anterior cruciate l., posterolateral band

Peroneus longus m.

Semimembranosus m.

Sartorius muscle

Medial head gastrocnemius muscle

Posterior cruciate l.

Gracilis tendon

Greater saphenous v.

Semimembranosus t.

Medial inferior geniculate artery

Medial gastrocnemius muscle

Biceps femoris muscle

Plantaris muscle

Iliotibial tract

Anterior cruciate l.

Body lateral meniscus

Peroneus longus m.

Extensor digitorum longus muscle

Popliteal artery

Sartorius muscle

Medial gastrocnemius muscle

Posterior cruciate l.

Medial collateral l.

Crural fascia

Body medial meniscus

Medial inferior geniculate artery

(Top) As the images become more anterior, one sees the last of the elements of the pes anserinus. Sartorius and gracilis are seen in this image, located more anteriorly at the joint line than the third element of the pes, semitendinosus. The most posterior fibers of knee anterior cruciate ligament are seen as well. **(Bottom)** More anteriorly within the notch, the entire anterior cruciate ligament is seen in its oblique route from the lateral femoral condyle to the insertion adjacent to the medial spines. Note that the deep and superficial fibers of medial collateral ligament are not separable on these T1 images. For more definition of these medial structures, see images and commentary in "Medial Support System" section.

CORONAL T1 MR, LEFT KNEE

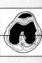

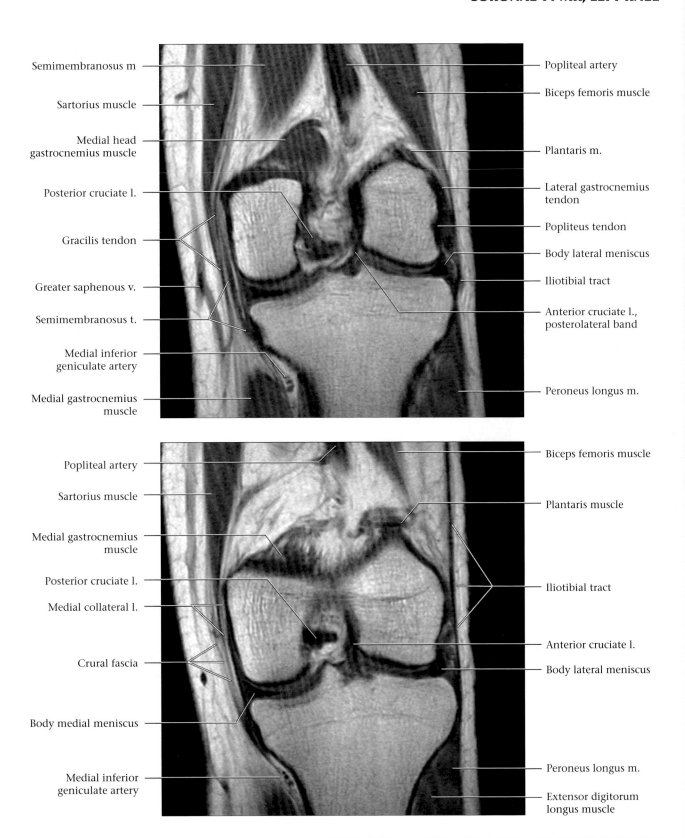

Semimembranosus m

Sartorius muscle

Medial head gastrocnemius muscle

Posterior cruciate l.

Gracilis tendon

Greater saphenous v.

Semimembranosus t.

Medial inferior geniculate artery

Medial gastrocnemius muscle

Popliteal artery

Biceps femoris muscle

Plantaris m.

Lateral gastrocnemius tendon

Popliteus tendon

Body lateral meniscus

Iliotibial tract

Anterior cruciate l., posterolateral band

Peroneus longus m.

Popliteal artery

Sartorius muscle

Medial gastrocnemius muscle

Posterior cruciate l.

Medial collateral l.

Crural fascia

Body medial meniscus

Medial inferior geniculate artery

Biceps femoris muscle

Plantaris muscle

Iliotibial tract

Anterior cruciate l.

Body lateral meniscus

Peroneus longus m.

Extensor digitorum longus muscle

(Top) As the images become more anterior, one sees the last of the elements of the pes anserinus. Sartorius and gracilis are seen in this image, located more anteriorly at the joint line than the third element of the pes, semitendinosus. The most posterior fibers of the anterior cruciate ligament are seen as well. **(Bottom)** More anteriorly within the notch, the entire anterior cruciate ligament is seen in its oblique route from the lateral femoral condyle to the insertion adjacent to the medial spines. Note that the deep and superficial fibers of medial collateral ligament are not separable on these T1 images. For more definition of these medial structures, see images and commentary in "Medial Support System" section.

CORONAL T1 MR, RIGHT KNEE

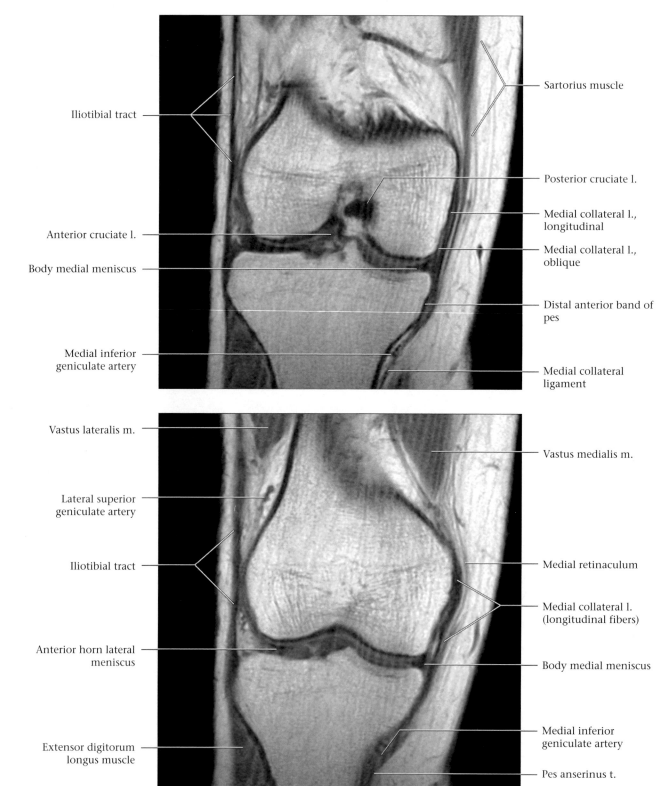

Iliotibial tract

Sartorius muscle

Posterior cruciate l.

Medial collateral l., longitudinal

Anterior cruciate l.

Medial collateral l., oblique

Body medial meniscus

Distal anterior band of pes

Medial inferior geniculate artery

Medial collateral ligament

Vastus lateralis m.

Vastus medialis m.

Lateral superior geniculate artery

Iliotibial tract

Medial retinaculum

Medial collateral l. (longitudinal fibers)

Anterior horn lateral meniscus

Body medial meniscus

Medial inferior geniculate artery

Extensor digitorum longus muscle

Pes anserinus t.

(Top) Note the length of the medial collateral ligament. The origin is intimately associated with the origin of the medial patellofemoral ligament, immediately distal to the adductor tubercle. The insertion is about 5 cm distal to the knee joint and is usually not entirely included in standard knee MR exams. The medial inferior geniculate arterial branches are seen in cross section between the superficial medial collateral ligament and the tibial cortex. **(Bottom)** Anterior cut is through the antero-mid portion of the joint. Because these are T1 images, there is little contrast between hyaline cartilage and menisci. For more detailed images and discussion of menisci, see the "Menisci" section.

KNEE OVERVIEW

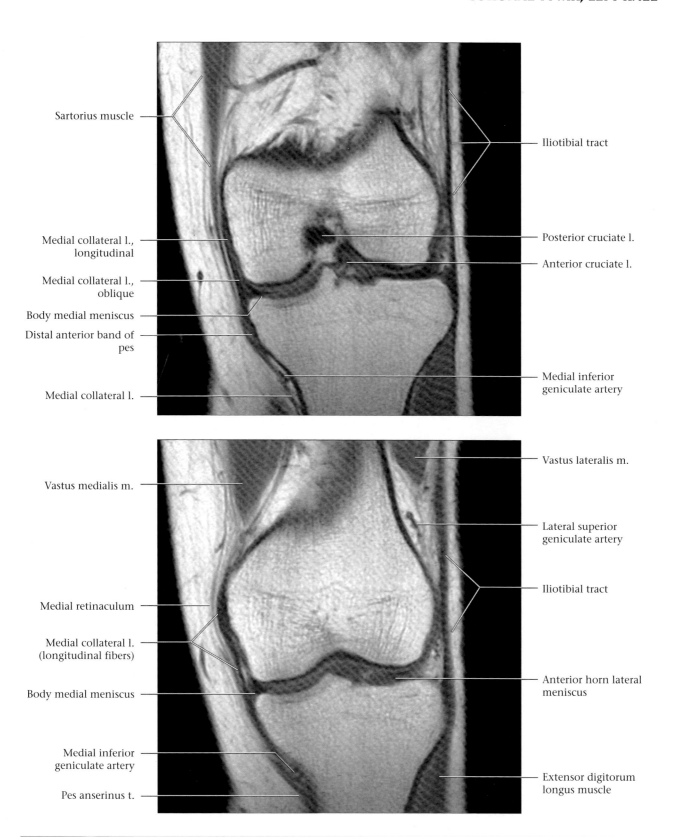

Sartorius muscle

Iliotibial tract

Medial collateral l., longitudinal

Posterior cruciate l.

Anterior cruciate l.

Medial collateral l., oblique

Body medial meniscus

Distal anterior band of pes

Medial inferior geniculate artery

Medial collateral l.

Vastus lateralis m.

Vastus medialis m.

Lateral superior geniculate artery

Medial retinaculum

Iliotibial tract

Medial collateral l. (longitudinal fibers)

Body medial meniscus

Anterior horn lateral meniscus

Medial inferior geniculate artery

Extensor digitorum longus muscle

Pes anserinus t.

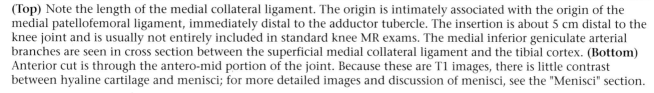

(Top) Note the length of the medial collateral ligament. The origin is intimately associated with the origin of the medial patellofemoral ligament, immediately distal to the adductor tubercle. The insertion is about 5 cm distal to the knee joint and is usually not entirely included in standard knee MR exams. The medial inferior geniculate arterial branches are seen in cross section between the superficial medial collateral ligament and the tibial cortex. **(Bottom)** Anterior cut is through the antero-mid portion of the joint. Because these are T1 images, there is little contrast between hyaline cartilage and menisci; for more detailed images and discussion of menisci, see the "Menisci" section.

CORONAL T1 MR, RIGHT KNEE

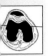

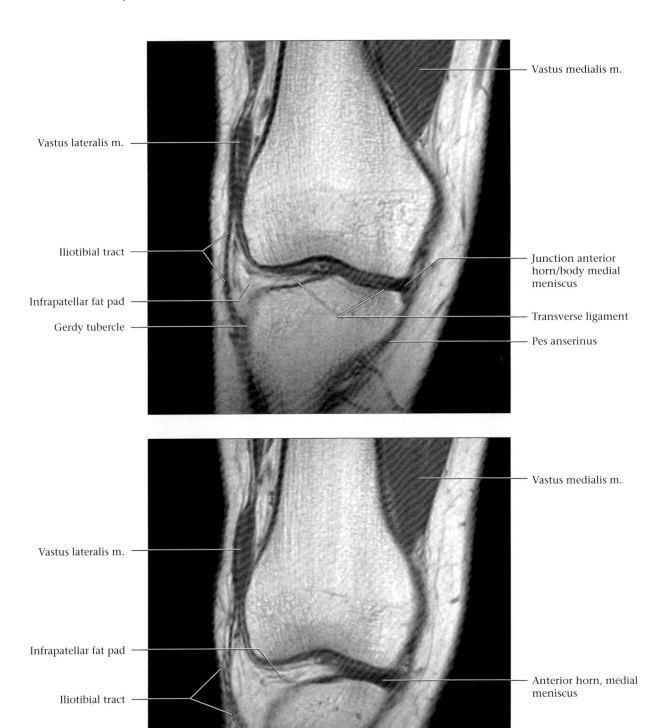

Vastus medialis m.

Vastus lateralis m.

Iliotibial tract

Junction anterior horn/body medial meniscus

Infrapatellar fat pad

Transverse ligament

Gerdy tubercle

Pes anserinus

Vastus medialis m.

Vastus lateralis m.

Infrapatellar fat pad

Anterior horn, medial meniscus

Iliotibial tract

(Top) This far anteriorly, the transverse ligament is seen crossing the anterior joint from the anterior horn medial meniscus towards the anterior horn lateral meniscus. The iliotibial tract is seen inserting on Gerdy tubercle. **(Bottom)** Far anterior cut through the joint space. Note that because of the slightly oblique angle at which coronal knee MR images are obtained, the anterior horn medial meniscus is visualized in far anterior coronal cuts without any portion of the lateral meniscus.

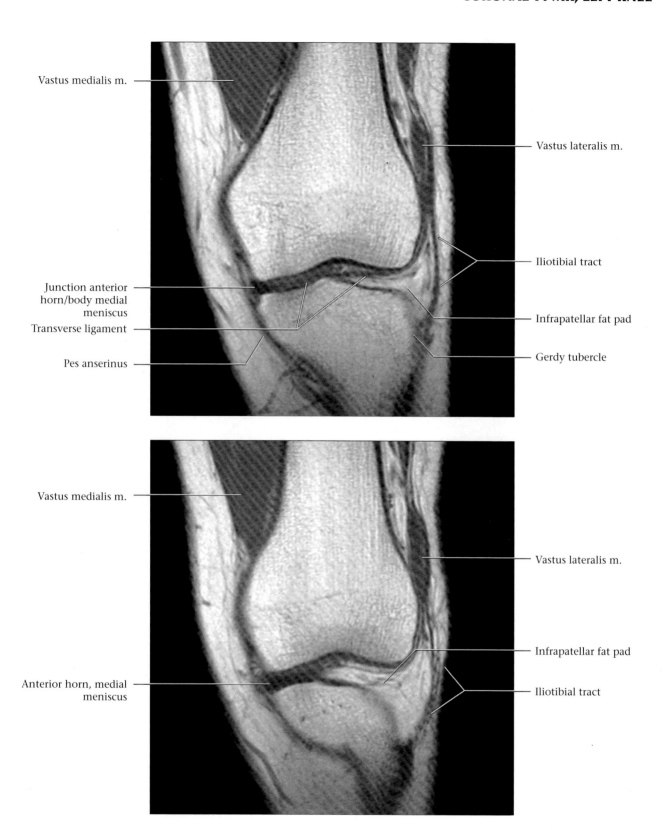

Vastus medialis m.

Vastus lateralis m.

Iliotibial tract

Junction anterior horn/body medial meniscus

Infrapatellar fat pad

Transverse ligament

Pes anserinus

Gerdy tubercle

Vastus medialis m.

Vastus lateralis m.

Infrapatellar fat pad

Anterior horn, medial meniscus

Iliotibial tract

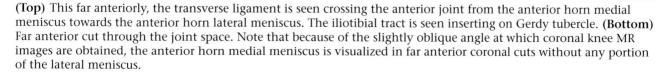

(Top) This far anteriorly, the transverse ligament is seen crossing the anterior joint from the anterior horn medial meniscus towards the anterior horn lateral meniscus. The iliotibial tract is seen inserting on Gerdy tubercle. **(Bottom)** Far anterior cut through the joint space. Note that because of the slightly oblique angle at which coronal knee MR images are obtained, the anterior horn medial meniscus is visualized in far anterior coronal cuts without any portion of the lateral meniscus.

CORONAL T1 MR, RIGHT KNEE

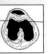

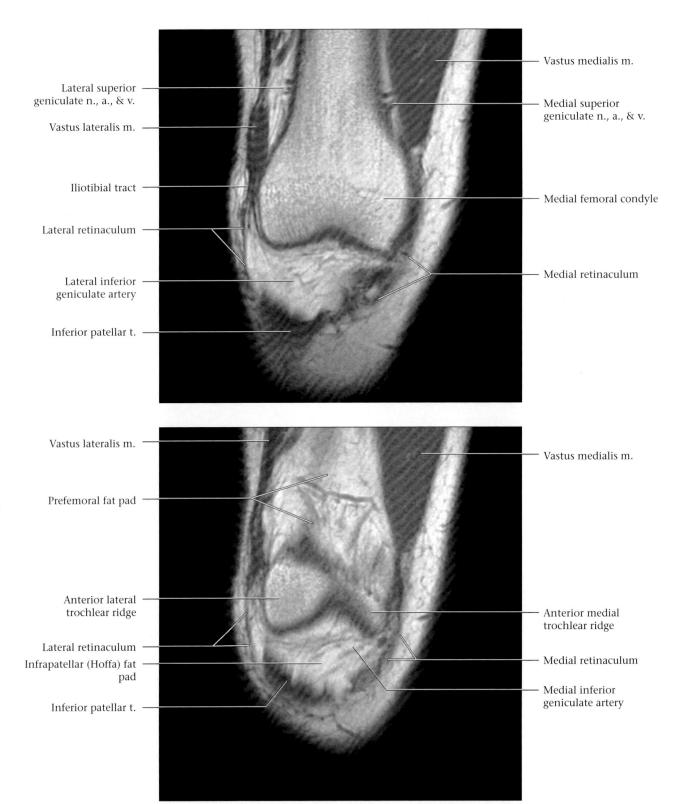

Lateral superior geniculate n., a., & v.

Vastus lateralis m.

Iliotibial tract

Lateral retinaculum

Lateral inferior geniculate artery

Inferior patellar t.

Vastus medialis m.

Medial superior geniculate n., a., & v.

Medial femoral condyle

Medial retinaculum

Vastus lateralis m.

Prefemoral fat pad

Anterior lateral trochlear ridge

Lateral retinaculum

Infrapatellar (Hoffa) fat pad

Inferior patellar t.

Vastus medialis m.

Anterior medial trochlear ridge

Medial retinaculum

Medial inferior geniculate artery

(Top) Coronal cut through the anterior femoral shaft. The joint is fairly featureless, consisting mostly of fat pads and anastomosing vascular structures. **(Bottom)** The cut is through the anterior femoral condyles. Fat pads, both prefemoral and infrapatellar, predominate in the anterior joint. The retinacula are seen as well. Note the multiple geniculate and collateral arteries supplying the knee joint.

KNEE OVERVIEW

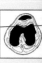

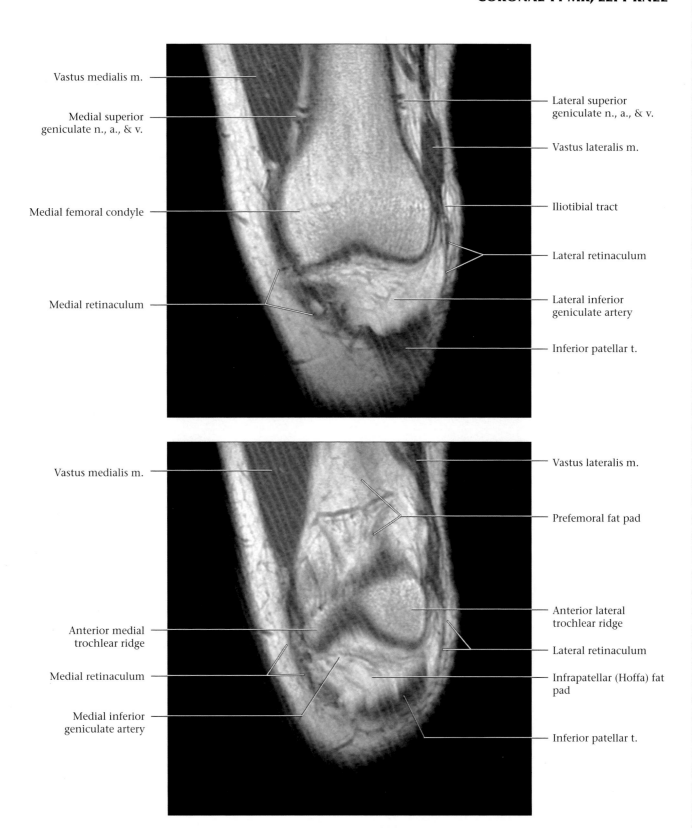

Vastus medialis m.

Medial superior geniculate n., a., & v.

Medial femoral condyle

Medial retinaculum

Lateral superior geniculate n., a., & v.

Vastus lateralis m.

Iliotibial tract

Lateral retinaculum

Lateral inferior geniculate artery

Inferior patellar t.

Vastus medialis m.

Anterior medial trochlear ridge

Medial retinaculum

Medial inferior geniculate artery

Vastus lateralis m.

Prefemoral fat pad

Anterior lateral trochlear ridge

Lateral retinaculum

Infrapatellar (Hoffa) fat pad

Inferior patellar t.

(Top) Coronal cut through the anterior femoral shaft. The joint is fairly featureless, consisting mostly of fat pads and anastomosing vascular structures. **(Bottom)** The cut is through the anterior femoral condyles. Fat pads, both prefemoral and infrapatellar, predominate in the anterior joint. The retinacula are seen as well. Note the multiple geniculate and collateral arteries supplying the knee joint.

KNEE OVERVIEW

CORONAL T1 MR, RIGHT KNEE

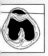

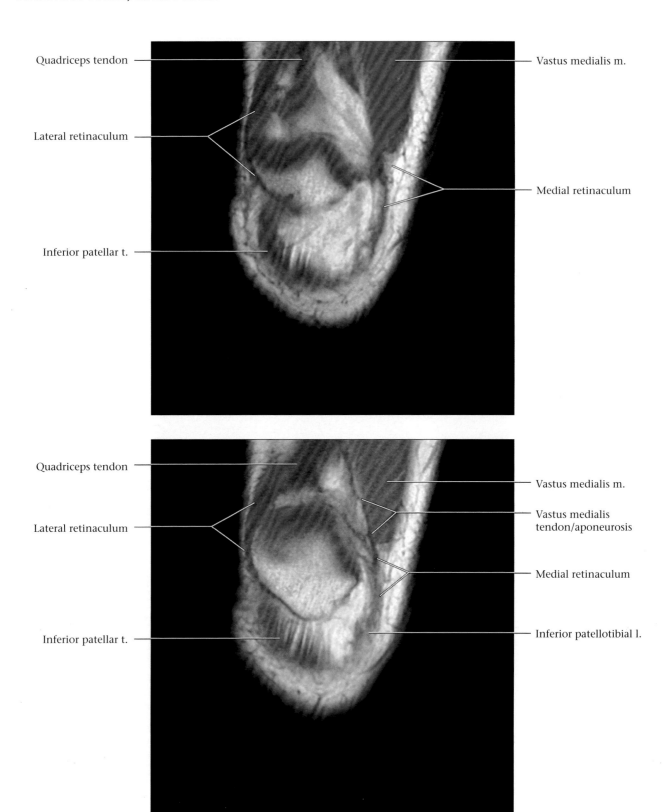

Quadriceps tendon — Vastus medialis m.

Lateral retinaculum —

Medial retinaculum

Inferior patellar t. —

Quadriceps tendon —

Vastus medialis m.

Lateral retinaculum —

Vastus medialis tendon/aponeurosis

Medial retinaculum

Inferior patellar t. —

Inferior patellotibial l.

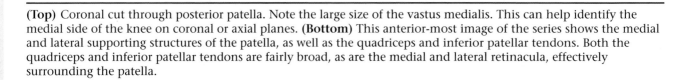

(Top) Coronal cut through posterior patella. Note the large size of the vastus medialis. This can help identify the medial side of the knee on coronal or axial planes. **(Bottom)** This anterior-most image of the series shows the medial and lateral supporting structures of the patella, as well as the quadriceps and inferior patellar tendons. Both the quadriceps and inferior patellar tendons are fairly broad, as are the medial and lateral retinacula, effectively surrounding the patella.

KNEE OVERVIEW

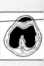

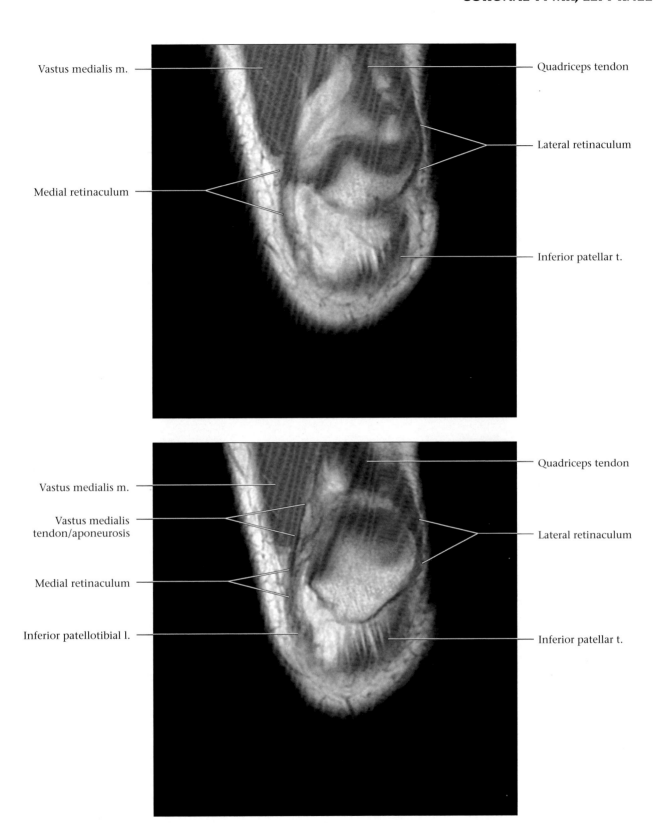

Vastus medialis m. — Quadriceps tendon

Lateral retinaculum

Medial retinaculum

Inferior patellar t.

Quadriceps tendon

Vastus medialis m.

Vastus medialis tendon/aponeurosis

Lateral retinaculum

Medial retinaculum

Inferior patellotibial l.

Inferior patellar t.

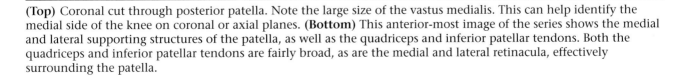

(Top) Coronal cut through posterior patella. Note the large size of the vastus medialis. This can help identify the medial side of the knee on coronal or axial planes. **(Bottom)** This anterior-most image of the series shows the medial and lateral supporting structures of the patella, as well as the quadriceps and inferior patellar tendons. Both the quadriceps and inferior patellar tendons are fairly broad, as are the medial and lateral retinacula, effectively surrounding the patella.

SAGITTAL T1 MR, KNEE

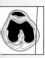

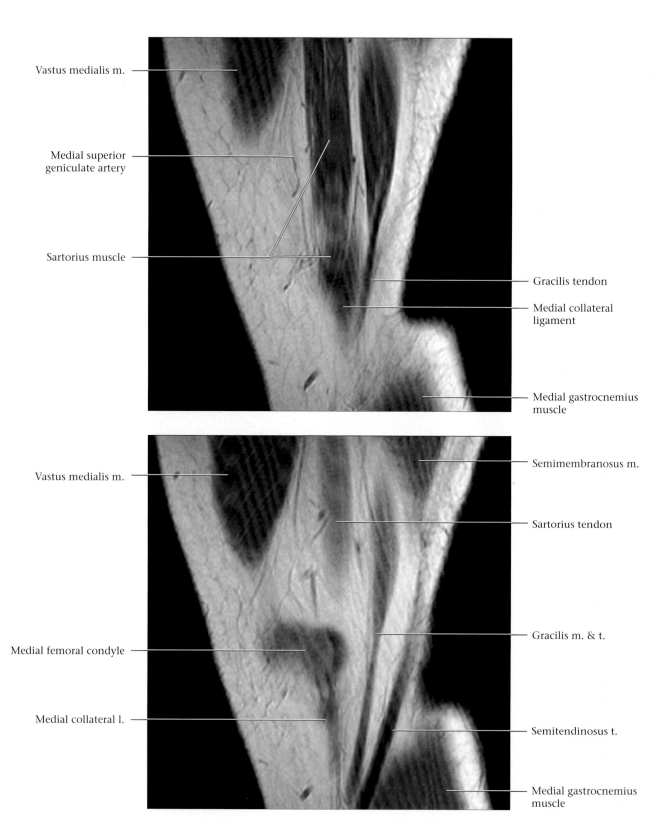

Vastus medialis m.

Medial superior geniculate artery

Sartorius muscle

Gracilis tendon

Medial collateral ligament

Medial gastrocnemius muscle

Vastus medialis m.

Semimembranosus m.

Sartorius tendon

Medial femoral condyle

Gracilis m. & t.

Medial collateral l.

Semitendinosus t.

Medial gastrocnemius muscle

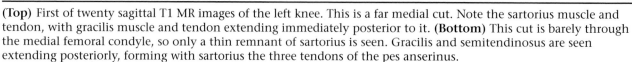

(Top) First of twenty sagittal T1 MR images of the left knee. This is a far medial cut. Note the sartorius muscle and tendon, with gracilis muscle and tendon extending immediately posterior to it. **(Bottom)** This cut is barely through the medial femoral condyle, so only a thin remnant of sartorius is seen. Gracilis and semitendinosus are seen extending posteriorly, forming with sartorius the three tendons of the pes anserinus.

KNEE OVERVIEW

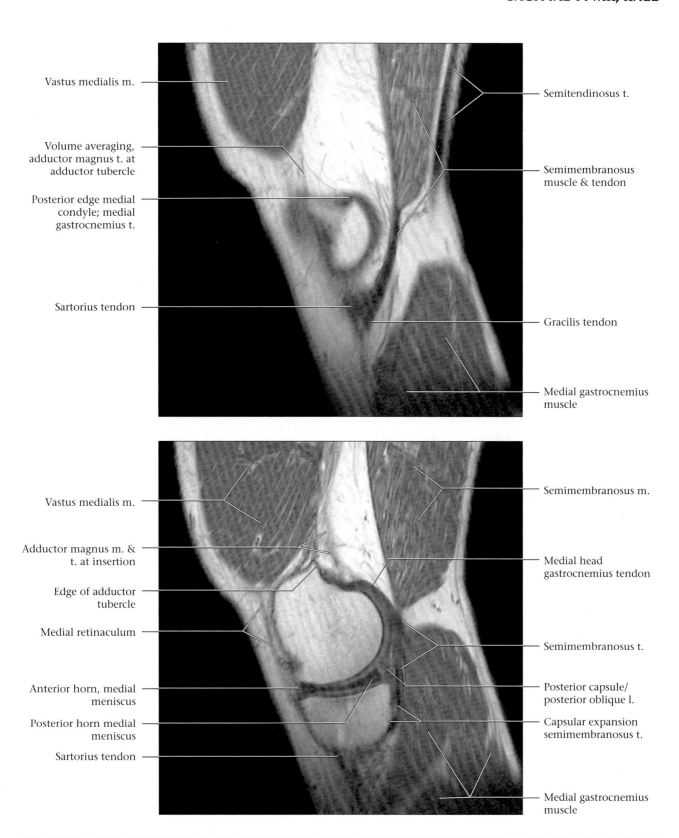

Vastus medialis m.

Volume averaging, adductor magnus t. at adductor tubercle

Posterior edge medial condyle; medial gastrocnemius t.

Sartorius tendon

Semitendinosus t.

Semimembranosus muscle & tendon

Gracilis tendon

Medial gastrocnemius muscle

Vastus medialis m.

Adductor magnus m. & t. at insertion

Edge of adductor tubercle

Medial retinaculum

Anterior horn, medial meniscus

Posterior horn medial meniscus

Sartorius tendon

Semimembranosus m.

Medial head gastrocnemius tendon

Semimembranosus t.

Posterior capsule/ posterior oblique l.

Capsular expansion semimembranosus t.

Medial gastrocnemius muscle

(Top) This is a medial cut through the femoral condyle. Note the large semimembranosus tendon, with its extensive insertion along the posteromedial tibia. **(Bottom)** This cut goes through the medial compartment, near the central edge of body of medial meniscus. This is still slightly a bow tie configuration of the meniscus.

SAGITTAL T1 MR, KNEE

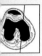

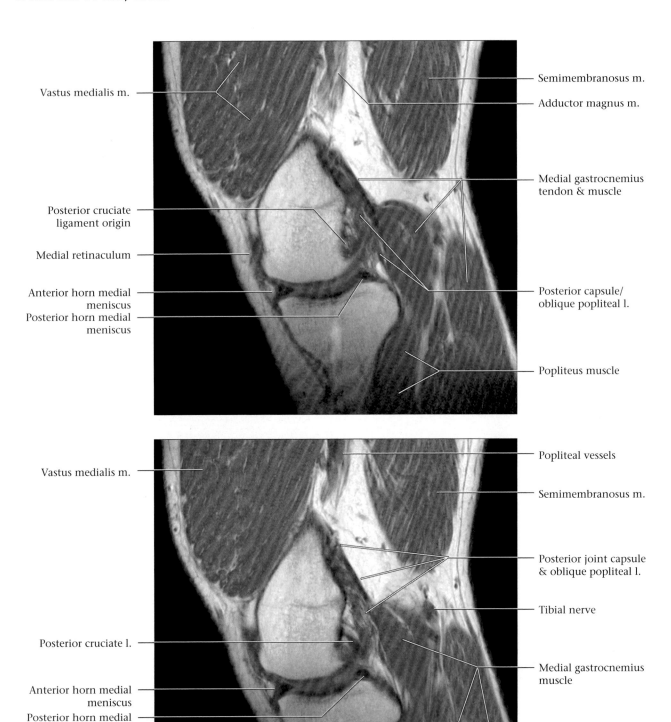

Vastus medialis m.

Semimembranosus m.

Adductor magnus m.

Posterior cruciate ligament origin

Medial retinaculum

Medial gastrocnemius tendon & muscle

Anterior horn medial meniscus

Posterior horn medial meniscus

Posterior capsule/ oblique popliteal l.

Popliteus muscle

Vastus medialis m.

Popliteal vessels

Semimembranosus m.

Posterior joint capsule & oblique popliteal l.

Tibial nerve

Posterior cruciate l.

Anterior horn medial meniscus

Posterior horn medial meniscus

Medial gastrocnemius muscle

Popliteus muscle

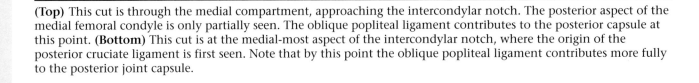

(Top) This cut is through the medial compartment, approaching the intercondylar notch. The posterior aspect of the medial femoral condyle is only partially seen. The oblique popliteal ligament contributes to the posterior capsule at this point. **(Bottom)** This cut is at the medial-most aspect of the intercondylar notch, where the origin of the posterior cruciate ligament is first seen. Note that by this point the oblique popliteal ligament contributes more fully to the posterior joint capsule.

KNEE OVERVIEW

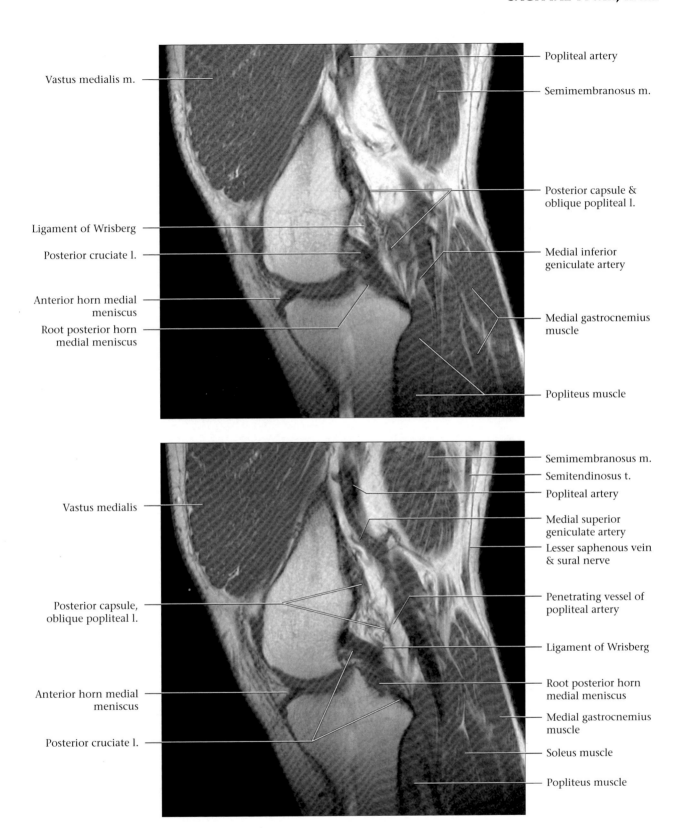

- Vastus medialis m.
- Popliteal artery
- Semimembranosus m.
- Posterior capsule & oblique popliteal l.
- Ligament of Wrisberg
- Posterior cruciate l.
- Medial inferior geniculate artery
- Anterior horn medial meniscus
- Root posterior horn medial meniscus
- Medial gastrocnemius muscle
- Popliteus muscle

- Semimembranosus m.
- Semitendinosus t.
- Popliteal artery
- Vastus medialis
- Medial superior geniculate artery
- Lesser saphenous vein & sural nerve
- Penetrating vessel of popliteal artery
- Posterior capsule, oblique popliteal l.
- Ligament of Wrisberg
- Root posterior horn medial meniscus
- Anterior horn medial meniscus
- Medial gastrocnemius muscle
- Posterior cruciate l.
- Soleus muscle
- Popliteus muscle

(Top) This cut is through the medial aspect of the intercondylar notch. The posterior cruciate ligament is fully seen. **(Bottom)** Mid intercondylar notch. Note that at the posterior intercondylar notch the posterior capsule is penetrated by vessels from the popliteal artery. The capsule is therefore incomplete posteriorly.

SAGITTAL T1 MR, KNEE

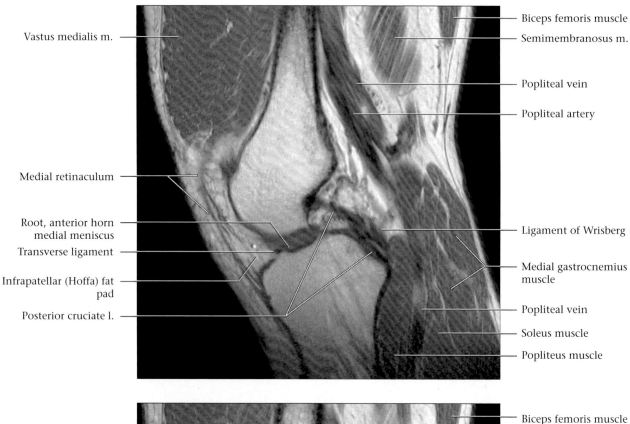

Vastus medialis m.

Medial retinaculum

Root, anterior horn medial meniscus

Transverse ligament

Infrapatellar (Hoffa) fat pad

Posterior cruciate l.

Biceps femoris muscle

Semimembranosus m.

Popliteal vein

Popliteal artery

Ligament of Wrisberg

Medial gastrocnemius muscle

Popliteal vein

Soleus muscle

Popliteus muscle

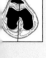

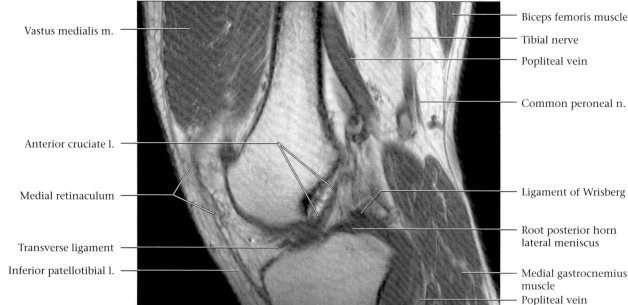

Vastus medialis m.

Anterior cruciate l.

Medial retinaculum

Transverse ligament

Inferior patellotibial l.

Biceps femoris muscle

Tibial nerve

Popliteal vein

Common peroneal n.

Ligament of Wrisberg

Root posterior horn lateral meniscus

Medial gastrocnemius muscle

Popliteal vein

Soleus muscle

Popliteus muscle

(Top) The cut is at the mid intercondylar notch, transitioning from the posterior to anterior cruciate ligament. The posterior capsule is still incomplete, due to penetrating vessels. **(Bottom)** Slightly laterally within the intercondylar notch, the anterior cruciate ligament is most fully seen. In the previous four images, note the pathway of the ligament of Wrisberg (posterior meniscofemoral ligament), arising from the medial aspect of the intercondylar notch, traversing posterior and superior to the posterior cruciate ligament, and inserting on the superior aspect of the root of posterior horn, lateral meniscus.

KNEE OVERVIEW

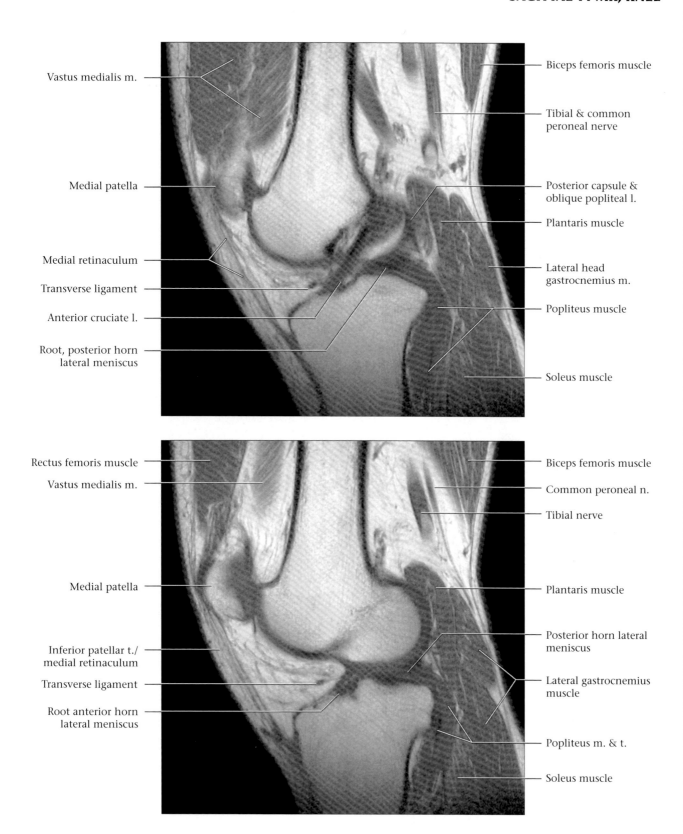

(Top) Laterally within the intercondylar notch, where there is partial voluming of the anterior cruciate/lateral femoral condyle at the ACL insertion. Note the transverse ligament, seen in cross-section, extending across in front of anterior cruciate ligament towards root of anterior horn, lateral meniscus. The anterior horn is not yet seen. **(Bottom)** This cut shows the beginning of the lateral compartment, immediately adjacent to the intercondylar notch. Note the musculotendinous junction of popliteus.

SAGITTAL T1 MR, KNEE

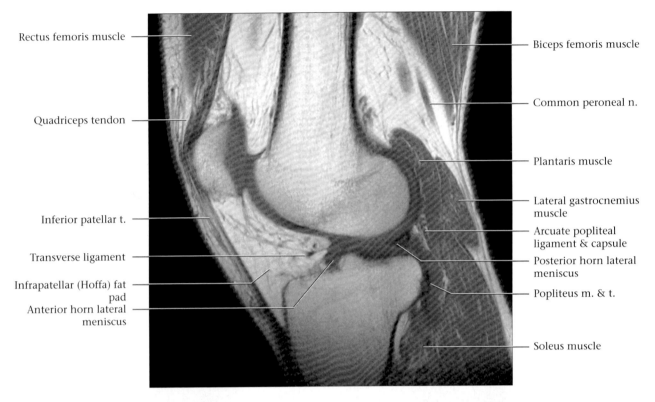

Rectus femoris muscle

Quadriceps tendon

Inferior patellar t.

Transverse ligament

Infrapatellar (Hoffa) fat pad

Anterior horn lateral meniscus

Biceps femoris muscle

Common peroneal n.

Plantaris muscle

Lateral gastrocnemius muscle

Arcuate popliteal ligament & capsule

Posterior horn lateral meniscus

Popliteus m. & t.

Soleus muscle

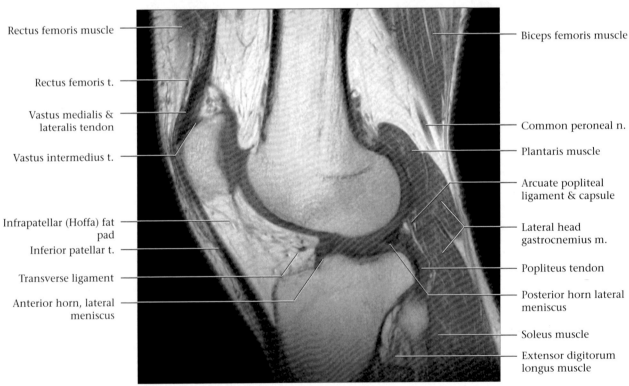

Rectus femoris muscle

Rectus femoris t.

Vastus medialis & lateralis tendon

Vastus intermedius t.

Infrapatellar (Hoffa) fat pad

Inferior patellar t.

Transverse ligament

Anterior horn, lateral meniscus

Biceps femoris muscle

Common peroneal n.

Plantaris muscle

Arcuate popliteal ligament & capsule

Lateral head gastrocnemius m.

Popliteus tendon

Posterior horn lateral meniscus

Soleus muscle

Extensor digitorum longus muscle

(Top) Lateral compartment. Note the path of the common peroneal nerve, anteromedial to the bulk of the biceps femoris muscle. The plantaris muscle is seen, arising on the lateral femoral condyle just medial to the lateral head of gastrocnemius. (Bottom) Because of the obliquity with which sagittals are obtained, the extensor complex is seen in the more lateral sagittal images. The trilaminate nature of the quadriceps tendon is demonstrated here. The transverse ligament has not yet contacted the anterior horn, lateral meniscus. Note the popliteus tendon. Although it is within the popliteal hiatus, it is difficult to distinguish from fluid in the hiatus, as well as the lateral meniscus. This region is better imaged with fluid sensitive sequences. See "Menisci" section for more detail.

KNEE OVERVIEW

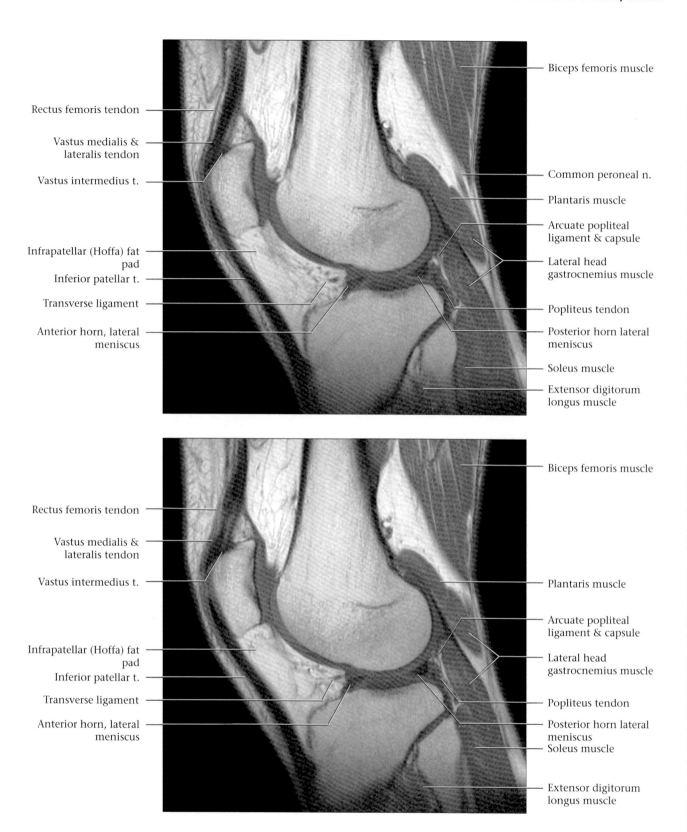

Rectus femoris tendon

Vastus medialis & lateralis tendon

Vastus intermedius t.

Infrapatellar (Hoffa) fat pad

Inferior patellar t.

Transverse ligament

Anterior horn, lateral meniscus

Biceps femoris muscle

Common peroneal n.

Plantaris muscle

Arcuate popliteal ligament & capsule

Lateral head gastrocnemius muscle

Popliteus tendon

Posterior horn lateral meniscus

Soleus muscle

Extensor digitorum longus muscle

Rectus femoris tendon

Vastus medialis & lateralis tendon

Vastus intermedius t.

Infrapatellar (Hoffa) fat pad

Inferior patellar t.

Transverse ligament

Anterior horn, lateral meniscus

Biceps femoris muscle

Plantaris muscle

Arcuate popliteal ligament & capsule

Lateral head gastrocnemius muscle

Popliteus tendon

Posterior horn lateral meniscus

Soleus muscle

Extensor digitorum longus muscle

(Top) In the lateral portion of the knee joint, the popliteus tendon is seen within the popliteal hiatus. It is surrounded by fluid, not easily distinguished on a T1 sequence. Similarly, the fascicles (or popliteomeniscal ligaments) connecting the posterior horn lateral meniscus with popliteus tendon are not easily seen as separate structures. See "Menisci" section for fluid sensitive sequences and greater detail. **(Bottom)** The transverse ligament approaches its insertion site on anterior horn lateral meniscus. The muscles arising from the anterior fibula and anterolateral tibia are seen but not easily distinguished from one another.

KNEE OVERVIEW

SAGITTAL T1 MR, KNEE

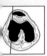

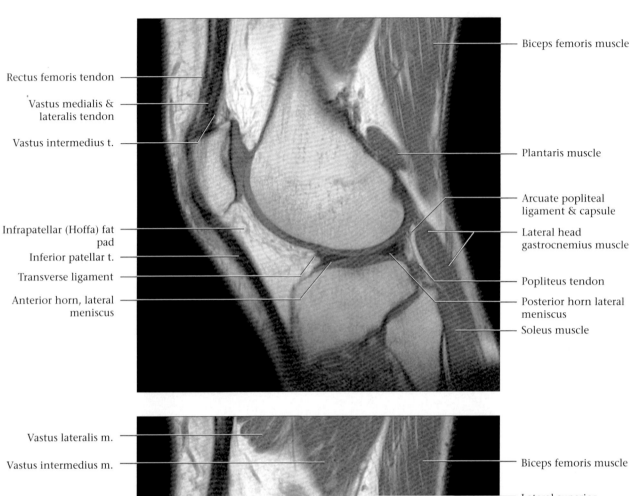

Rectus femoris tendon

Vastus medialis & lateralis tendon

Vastus intermedius t.

Infrapatellar (Hoffa) fat pad

Inferior patellar t.

Transverse ligament

Anterior horn, lateral meniscus

Biceps femoris muscle

Plantaris muscle

Arcuate popliteal ligament & capsule

Lateral head gastrocnemius muscle

Popliteus tendon

Posterior horn lateral meniscus

Soleus muscle

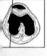

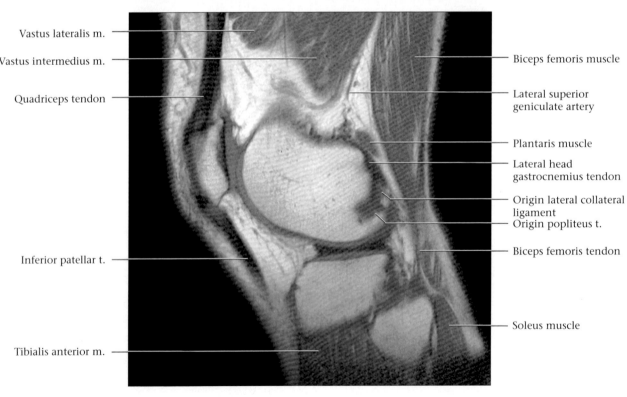

Vastus lateralis m.

Vastus intermedius m.

Quadriceps tendon

Inferior patellar t.

Tibialis anterior m.

Biceps femoris muscle

Lateral superior geniculate artery

Plantaris muscle

Lateral head gastrocnemius tendon

Origin lateral collateral ligament

Origin popliteus t.

Biceps femoris tendon

Soleus muscle

(Top) The transverse ligament inserts on anterior horn lateral meniscus fairly far laterally within this compartment. The popliteus tendon just enters the popliteal hiatus at this posterolateral corner. **(Bottom)** At the lateral aspect of the lateral femoral condyle, one sees the origin of the lateral head of gastrocnemius from the lateral femoral epicondyle, as well as lateral collateral ligament and popliteal tendon.

KNEE OVERVIEW

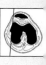

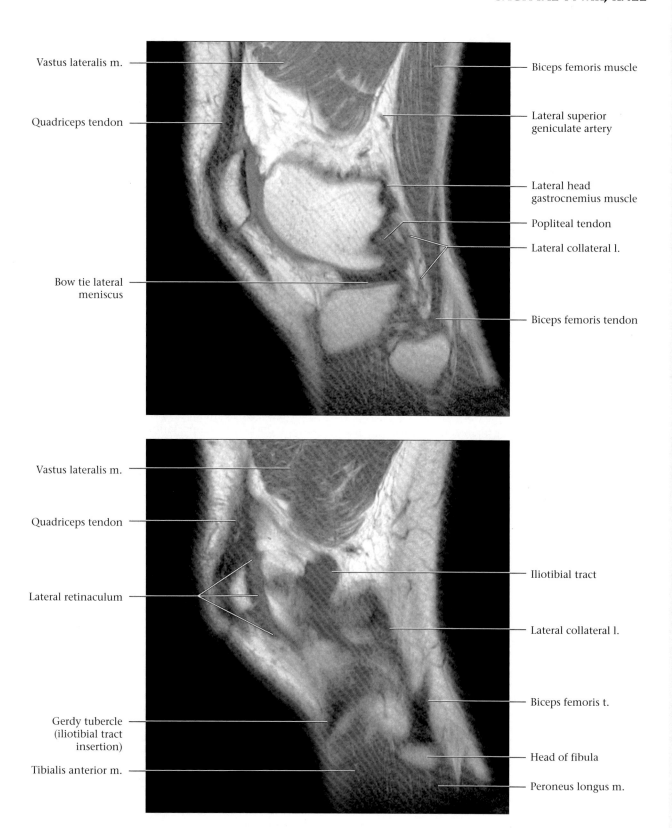

Vastus lateralis m. — Biceps femoris muscle

Quadriceps tendon — Lateral superior geniculate artery

Lateral head gastrocnemius muscle

Popliteal tendon

Lateral collateral l.

Bow tie lateral meniscus

Biceps femoris tendon

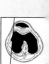

Vastus lateralis m.

Quadriceps tendon

Iliotibial tract

Lateral retinaculum

Lateral collateral l.

Biceps femoris t.

Gerdy tubercle (iliotibial tract insertion)

Tibialis anterior m.

Head of fibula

Peroneus longus m.

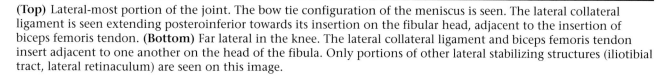

(Top) Lateral-most portion of the joint. The bow tie configuration of the meniscus is seen. The lateral collateral ligament is seen extending posteroinferior towards its insertion on the fibular head, adjacent to the insertion of biceps femoris tendon. **(Bottom)** Far lateral in the knee. The lateral collateral ligament and biceps femoris tendon insert adjacent to one another on the head of the fibula. Only portions of other lateral stabilizing structures (iliotibial tract, lateral retinaculum) are seen on this image.

Knee

VI

EXTENSOR MECHANISM AND RETINACULA

Terminology

Abbreviations
- Vastus medialis obliquus (VMO)
- Medial patellofemoral ligament (MPFL)

Imaging Anatomy

Overview
- Extensor mechanism: Quadriceps muscle and tendon, patella, patellar tendon, and patellar retinacula

Quadriceps
- **Muscles**: Rectus femoris, vastus lateralis, vastus medialis, vastus intermedius
- **Quadriceps tendon**
  - Trilaminar configuration (generally): Fascia of component muscles with interposed fat
    - Superficial (anterior on sagittal): Rectus femoris
    - Middle: Vastus lateralis and vastus medialis
    - Deep (posterior on sagittal): Vastus intermedius
  - May appear as 2 or 4 layers: Medial and lateral components of middle layer merge in different combinations or remain discrete
  - Tendon inserts on non-articular (anterior) portion of patella

Patellar Tendon
- Mainly composed of rectus femoris fibers that course over patella
- Extends from inferior pole of patella to tibial tuberosity
- Length approximates 5 cm
  - Length about equal height of patella
  - Variation by > 20% of craniocaudal length of patella results in patella alta or baja
- 3 cm wide superiorly to 2 cm inferiorly
- 5-6 mm thick
- Solid low signal throughout

Medial Retinaculum Complex
- Medial stabilizer of patellofemoral joint
- Extends from patella to vastus medialis
- Medial retinacular complex divided into superior, mid, and inferior portions, which blend into one another
  - **Superior: VMO and MPFL**
    - VMO: Muscular slip of vastus medialis; arises either from adductor magnus tendon or from adductor tubercle
    - VMO inserts at superior medial border of patella
    - VMO aponeurosis is tightly adherent to underlying MPFL
    - MPFL: Arises from adductor tubercle adjacent to MCL origin and inserts at medial border of patella
  - **Mid portion**: Thin fibers of superficial MCL fascia
  - **Inferior**
    - Patellotibial ligament arises from tibia at level of insertion of gracilis and semitendinosus
    - Patellotibial ligament inserts on inferior aspect patella and patellar tendon
    - Medial patellomeniscal ligament lies deep to patellotibial ligament
- For greater detail, see "Medial Support System" section

Lateral Retinaculum
- Lateral stabilizer of patellofemoral joint
- Extends from patella to vastus lateralis
- 3 layers
  - **I (superficial)**: Iliotibial tract and its anterior expansion, supplemented posteriorly by superficial portion of biceps femoris and its anterior expansion
  - **II (mid)**: Retinaculum of quadriceps (vastus lateralis)
  - **III (deep)**: Lateral part of joint capsule

Anterior Fat Pads
- Each interposed between joint capsule externally and synovium-lined joint cavity (intracapsular but extrasynovial)
- Suprapatellar bursa outlined by anterior suprapatellar (quadriceps) and posterior suprapatellar (pre-femoral) fat pads
- Infrapatellar (Hoffa fat pad)
  - Bordered by
    - Inferior pole patella (superior)
    - Joint capsule and patellar tendon (anterior)
    - Proximal tibia & deep infrapatellar bursa (inferior)
    - Synovial-lined joint capsule (posterior)
  - Can be tethered posteriorly at apex by infrapatellar plica
  - Attached to anterior horns of menisci inferiorly and to tibial periosteum
  - Transverse ligament courses within fat pad
  - Interface between posterior aspect of fat pad and joint space consists of several synovial recesses
  - Anastomotic vessels course through fat pad, seen in cross-section on sagittal images

Plica
- Synovial folds; persistent embryonic remnants
- **Superior** (suprapatellar, superomedial): Common
  - Medial suprapatellar pouch, 2 cm superior to patella
  - Fold or complete septum
  - Runs obliquely downward from synovium at anterior aspect of femoral metaphysis to posterior aspect of quadriceps tendon
  - Inserts above patella; best seen on sagittal
- **Medial** (plica synovialis, patellar shelf, medial intra-articular band)
  - Arises medial wall of synovial pouch or under medial retinaculum & extends obliquely downward to insert on synovium covering infrapatellar fat pad
  - Inserts on synovium covering infrapatellar fat pad, at medial edge of patella; seen on sagittal or axial
  - If large, can impinge on medial facet of trochlea or under medial facet of patella
- **Inferior** (infrapatellar plica/fold/septum, ligamentum mucosa): Common
  - Extends from Hoffa fat pad in intercondylar notch, paralleling and anterior to ACL; best seen on sagittal
  - May be split or fenestrated; dimensions vary
- **Lateral**: Rare
  - Originates from lateral wall superior to popliteal hiatus and extends to infrapatellar fat pad
  - Oblique coronal orientation; thin, 1-2 cm lateral to patella
- Size and morphologic features of a given plica do not reliably indicate whether it is clinically significant

EXTENSOR MECHANISM AND RETINACULA

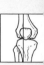

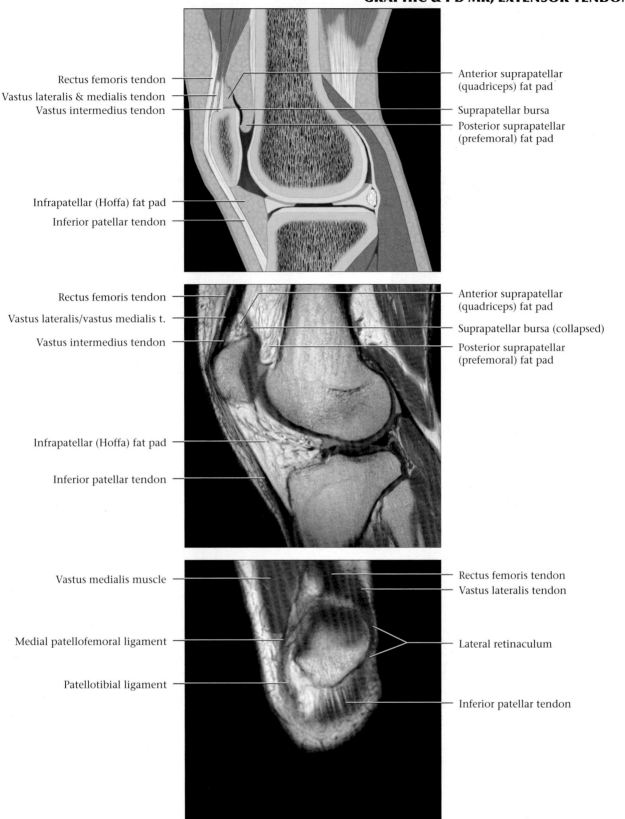

Rectus femoris tendon

Vastus lateralis & medialis tendon

Vastus intermedius tendon

Anterior suprapatellar (quadriceps) fat pad

Suprapatellar bursa

Posterior suprapatellar (prefemoral) fat pad

Infrapatellar (Hoffa) fat pad

Inferior patellar tendon

Rectus femoris tendon

Vastus lateralis/vastus medialis t.

Vastus intermedius tendon

Anterior suprapatellar (quadriceps) fat pad

Suprapatellar bursa (collapsed)

Posterior suprapatellar (prefemoral) fat pad

Infrapatellar (Hoffa) fat pad

Inferior patellar tendon

Vastus medialis muscle

Medial patellofemoral ligament

Patellotibial ligament

Rectus femoris tendon

Vastus lateralis tendon

Lateral retinaculum

Inferior patellar tendon

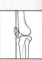

(Top) Graphic shows trilaminar configuration of the quadriceps tendon. The superficial portion is rectus femoris, middle portion is the aponeurosis of vastus medialis and lateralis, and deep portion is vastus intermedius tendon. **(Middle)** Sagittal PD MR shows the trilaminate character of the extensor tendon. The suprapatellar bursa is not distended. The surrounding fat pads are well demonstrated. The infrapatellar fat pad, with anastomosing joint vessels coursing through it, is also seen. **(Bottom)** Anterior coronal T1 MR shows components of patellar attachments. The quadriceps and inferior patellar tendons attach superiorly and inferiorly, respectively. The lateral retinaculum attaches along the entire lateral edge of patella. Vastus medialis obliquus, medial patellofemoral, and inferior patellotibial ligaments contribute to medial retinaculum from superior to inferior.

Knee

VI

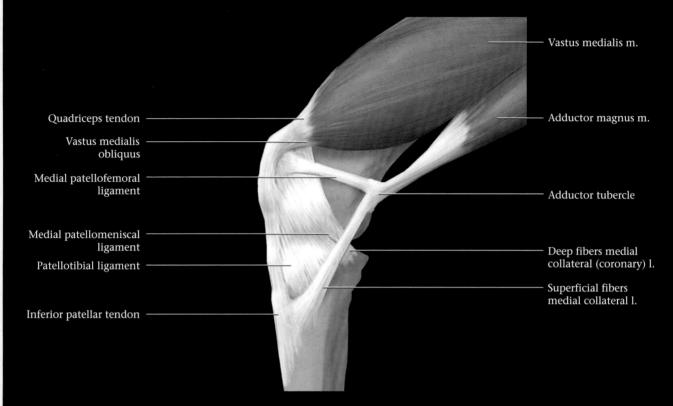

Vastus medialis m.

Adductor magnus m.

Quadriceps tendon

Vastus medialis obliquus

Medial patellofemoral ligament

Adductor tubercle

Medial patellomeniscal ligament

Patellotibial ligament

Deep fibers medial collateral (coronary) l.

Superficial fibers medial collateral l.

Inferior patellar tendon

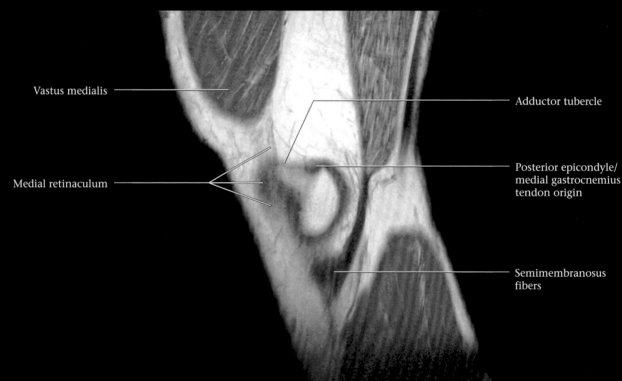

Vastus medialis

Adductor tubercle

Posterior epicondyle/ medial gastrocnemius tendon origin

Medial retinaculum

Semimembranosus fibers

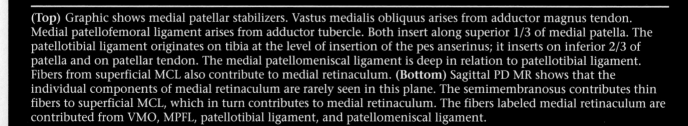

(Top) Graphic shows medial patellar stabilizers. Vastus medialis obliquus arises from adductor magnus tendon. Medial patellofemoral ligament arises from adductor tubercle. Both insert along superior 1/3 of medial patella. The patellotibial ligament originates on tibia at the level of insertion of the pes anserinus; it inserts on inferior 2/3 of patella and on patellar tendon. The medial patellomeniscal ligament is deep in relation to patellotibial ligament. Fibers from superficial MCL also contribute to medial retinaculum. **(Bottom)** Sagittal PD MR shows that the individual components of medial retinaculum are rarely seen in this plane. The semimembranosus contributes thin fibers to superficial MCL, which in turn contributes to medial retinaculum. The fibers labeled medial retinaculum are contributed from VMO, MPFL, patellotibial ligament, and patellomeniscal ligament.

SAGITTAL PD MR, PATELLAR STABILIZERS

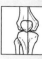

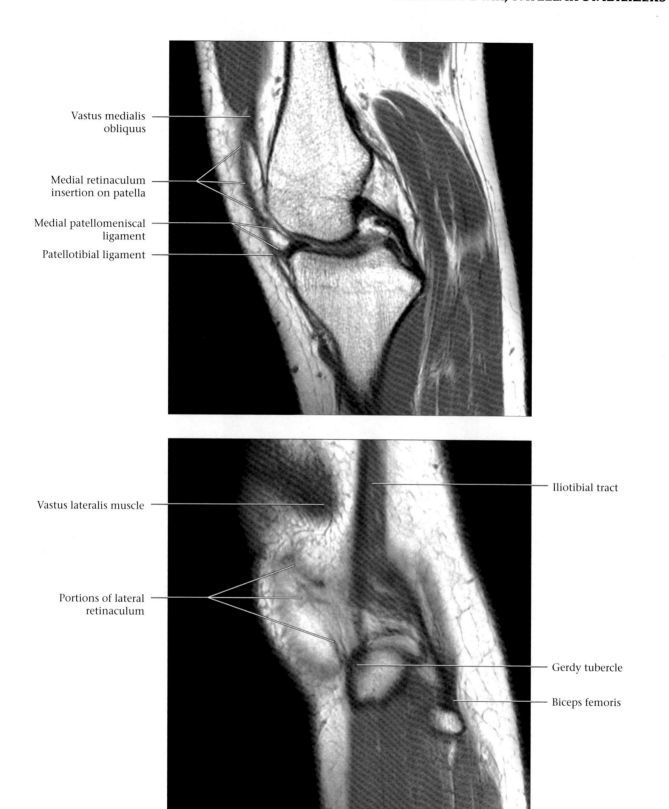

Vastus medialis obliquus

Medial retinaculum insertion on patella

Medial patellomeniscal ligament

Patellotibial ligament

Vastus lateralis muscle

Portions of lateral retinaculum

Iliotibial tract

Gerdy tubercle

Biceps femoris

(Top) Sagittal PD MR image through medial portion of intercondylar notch shows various portions of medial retinaculum, including VMO, medial patellomeniscal ligament, and patellotibial ligament. These, along with medial patellofemoral ligament, blend together to form the medial retinaculum. (Bottom) Sagittal PD MR image, far lateral, shows portions of lateral retinaculum. Contributions come from vastus lateralis, anterior expansion iliotibial tract, anterior expansion superficial biceps femoris, and joint capsule.

AXIAL PD MR, PATELLAR STABILIZERS

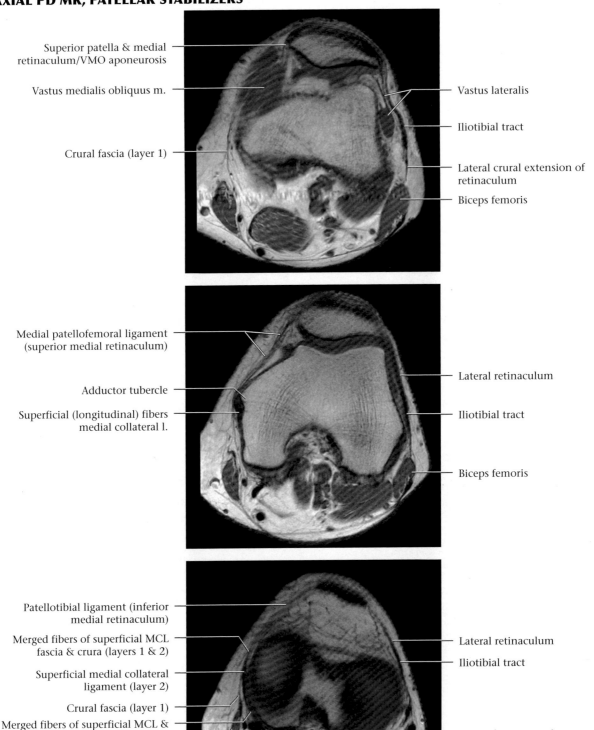

Superior patella & medial retinaculum/VMO aponeurosis

Vastus medialis obliquus m.

Crural fascia (layer 1)

Vastus lateralis

Iliotibial tract

Lateral crural extension of retinaculum

Biceps femoris

Medial patellofemoral ligament (superior medial retinaculum)

Adductor tubercle

Superficial (longitudinal) fibers medial collateral l.

Lateral retinaculum

Iliotibial tract

Biceps femoris

Patellotibial ligament (inferior medial retinaculum)

Merged fibers of superficial MCL fascia & crura (layers 1 & 2)

Superficial medial collateral ligament (layer 2)

Crural fascia (layer 1)

Merged fibers of superficial MCL & deep MCL (layers 2 & 3)

Sartorius

Lateral retinaculum

Iliotibial tract

Biceps femoris tendon

(Top) First of three axial PD MR images, located just above the adductor tubercle, shows vastus medialis obliquus contributing to the superior portion of medial retinaculum. The lateral retinaculum receives fibers from anterior expansions of both iliotibial tract and biceps femoris. **(Middle)** At the level of adductor tubercle, the superficial fibers of MCL and the medial patellofemoral ligament are seen at their origin. The MPFL extends to the patella as the superior portion of medial retinaculum at this level. **(Bottom)** At the level of joint line, the medial retinaculum receives a contribution from the merged fibers of superficial MCL fascia and its overlying crura. The patellotibial ligament is also a major contributor at this level.

EXTENSOR MECHANISM AND RETINACULA

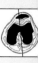

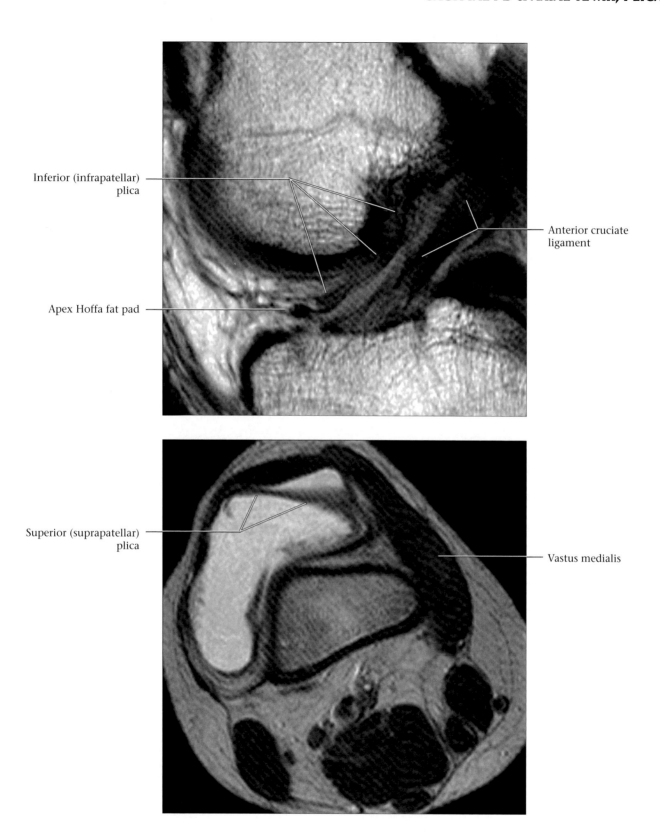

Inferior (infrapatellar) plica

Anterior cruciate ligament

Apex Hoffa fat pad

Superior (suprapatellar) plica

Vastus medialis

(Top) Sagittal PD MR image through the intercondylar notch shows a typical inferior (infrapatellar) plica. This normal variant extends from the inferior pole of the patella, through Hoffa fat pad, parallels the ACL, and attaches to the femoral condyle at the intercondylar notch. It may simulate a meniscocruciate ligament, but the anterior sites of origin are distinctly different. (Bottom) Axial T2 MR image at the level of the distal femur, shows a synovial fold extending across the medial side of the suprapatellar pouch. This is a common form of plica, seen particularly well because of the large effusion. It is termed the superior, or suprapatellar, plica.

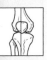

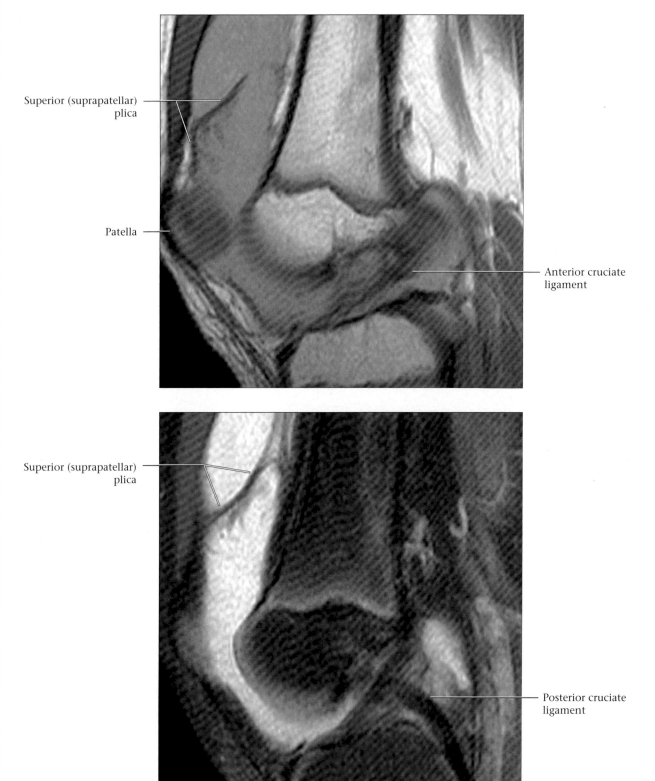

Superior (suprapatellar) plica

Patella

Anterior cruciate ligament

Superior (suprapatellar) plica

Posterior cruciate ligament

(Top) Sagittal PD MR through the intercondylar notch of the same patient seen in the previous image, showing a superior (suprapatellar) plica. The plica extends from just superior to the patella, medially through the suprapatellar pouch. (Bottom) Sagittal PD FS MR image is slightly medial to the previous image (note the posterior cruciate ligament), shows the plica extending further superomedially. This is a common variant which does not have clinical consequences.

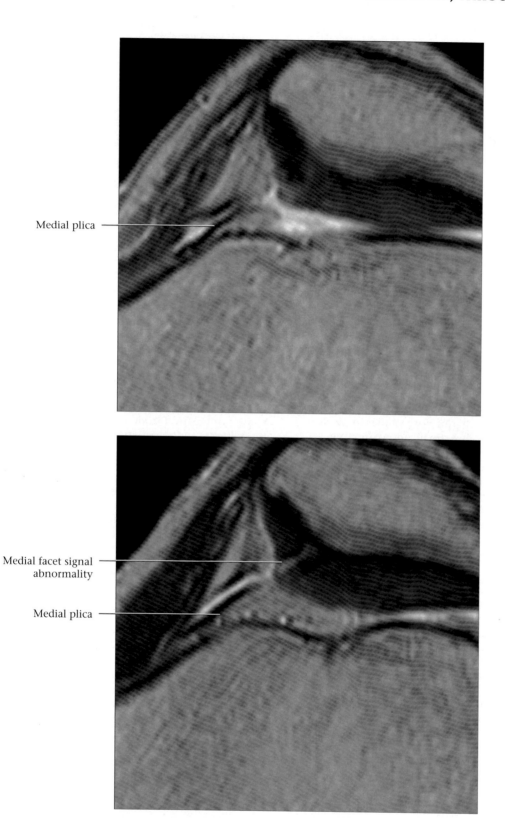

Medial plica —

Medial facet signal abnormality —

Medial plica —

(Top) First of two axial T2 MR images through the mid patella shows a medial plica extending over the medial facet of the trochlea and under the medial facet of the patella. **(Bottom)** Slightly distal image, shows the medial plica, with signal abnormality, approaching the medial facet of the patella, which also shows signal abnormality. The medial plica is more likely to result in symptomatic damage (either at the medial patellar facet or medial trochlea) than the other plicae.

MENISCI

Terminology

Abbreviations
- Anterior/posterior cruciate ligament (ACL/PCL)
- Lateral/medial meniscus (LM/MM)
- Medial collateral ligament (MCL)

Imaging Anatomy

Overview
- Menisci evaluated by morphology, signal and attachments
- All portions taper from height of 3-5 mm peripherally to sharp, thin, central (free) edge
- Normally specific and predictable size/shape
- Morphology variance indicates tear or variant which is at increased risk for tear

Morphology
- **Lateral meniscus**
  - Overall configuration: **Semicircular**
  - **Shape: Uniform**, minimally and gradually enlarging from anterior to posterior
  - Normal recess: Peripheral, located inferiorly at anterior horn
- **Medial meniscus**
  - Overall configuration: **Semilunar (C-shaped)**
  - **Shape non-uniform:** Anterior horn similar in size & shape to LM but midbody is small, approximating an equilateral triangle; MM posterior horn is largest portion of MM, nearly 2x as long as anterior horn
  - Normal recess: Peripheral, located superiorly at posterior horn
- Meniscal "flounce": Buckling of a portion of the meniscus, perhaps related to femorotibial subluxation

Signal
- Generally **uniformly low signal** throughout
- **Exceptions**
  - Children and adolescents may have increased intrameniscal signal that does not extend to surface due to rich vascular supply
  - Adults may develop central degenerative changes seen as linear or globular signal that does not extend to surface
  - Various high signal clefts and dots can normally be seen in anterior horn LM at and near its root attachment, due to immediate adjacency of origin of ACL and divergence of longitudinal fibers at root
  - Peripheral portion of meniscus is quite vascular
    - Outer meniscal margin as seen by MR is usually not true periphery of structure: Meniscus signal in its peripheral vascular portion (10-30%) blends in with gray signal of the capsule
  - "Magic angle" may affect posterior horn of LM in region of intercondylar notch

Meniscal Attachments
- **Osseous attachments: Both menisci are firmly attached to tibia at their roots**
  - LM roots: Located near center of tibial plateau
    - Anterior horn attaches immediately lateral to origin of ACL
    - Posterior horn attaches just posterior to ACL, and anterior to PCL as PCL extends behind tibial plateau to its insertion on posterior tibia
    - Root of posterior horn LM also is anterior to root of posterior horn MM
  - **MM roots:** MM is more semilunar in shape than semicircular LM, so its roots are located at center of tibial plateau, but more anteriorly and posteriorly for anterior horn and posterior horn, respectively than those of LM
    - Root anterior horn MM anterior to origin of ACL
    - Root posterior horn MM immediately anterior to PCL but posterior to root of posterior horn LM
- **Capsular attachments**
  - **MM entirely attached to joint capsule** with exception of small interruption at MCL
    - MM serves as origin of meniscofemoral ligament portion of deep fibers of MCL; this ligament either inserts on the adjacent femur or superficial MCL
    - MM also serves as origin of meniscotibial ligament (coronary ligament) portion of deep fibers of the MCL, which inserts on the adjacent tibia
    - Fibrofatty tissue as well as MCL bursa separate MM and deep fibers of MCL from superficial MCL
  - **LM entirely attached to joint capsule only in anterior and far posterior portions, with attachment being interrupted at body and much of posterior horn by popliteal hiatus**
    - After origination from lateral femoral condyle, popliteus tendon penetrates capsule and takes intra-articular course
    - Intra-articularly, popliteus tendon extends distally in posteromedial direction
    - Popliteus tendon separates LM from its capsular insertion along body & majority of posterior horn
    - Superior and inferior fascicles serve as attachments between LM and popliteal tendon and, in turn, capsule
    - Inferior popliteomeniscal fascicle extends from lateral edge of body of meniscus to inferior portion of popliteus paratenon, forming floor of popliteal hiatus
    - Inferior fascicle complete at level of body of LM, but not posterior horn
    - Superior popliteomeniscal fascicle extends from body/posterior horn LM to superior portion popliteal paratenon and on to capsule, forming ceiling of the popliteal hiatus
    - Superior fascicle incomplete at body, but complete at body/posterior horn LM

Meniscal Variants
- **Transverse ligament:** Connects menisci anteriorly
  - Oblique insertion on LM anterior horn may simulate a tear; may be absent
- **Meniscofemoral ligaments:** Extend from posterior medial femoral condyle to posterior horn LM
  - At insertion on LM, may simulate a tear
- **Oblique menisco-meniscal ligaments:** Cross from anterior horn of one to posterior horn of other meniscus, passing between ACL and PCL
- Various other meniscal variants have been observed, including menisco-ACL ligament

MENISCI

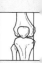

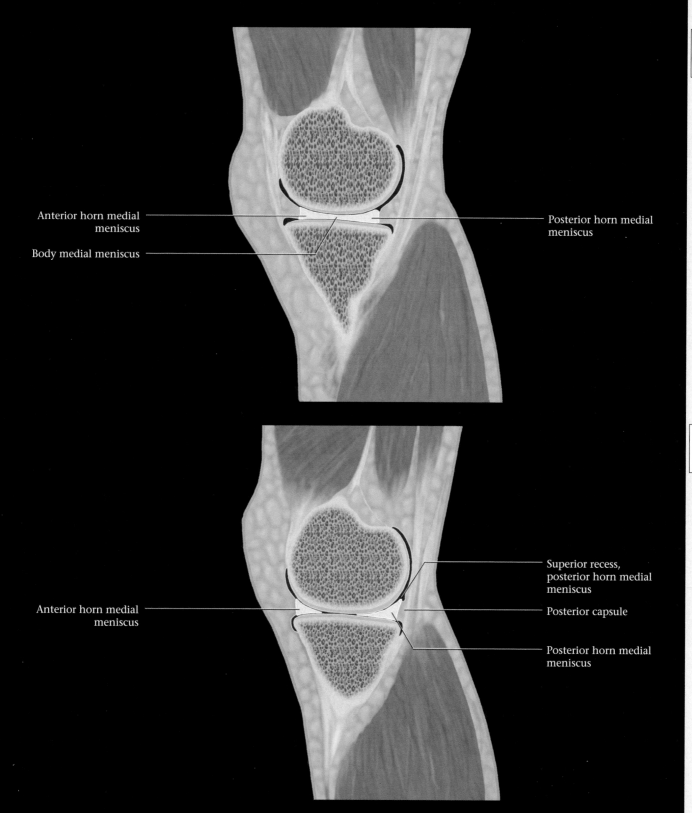

Anterior horn medial meniscus

Body medial meniscus

Posterior horn medial meniscus

Anterior horn medial meniscus

Superior recess, posterior horn medial meniscus

Posterior capsule

Posterior horn medial meniscus

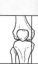

(Top) Sagittal cut through the medial most aspect of the medial meniscus, shows the bowtie configuration. This appearance is due to the cut extending across the full thickness of both the anterior and posterior horns but across only the thinner mid portion of the body. **(Bottom)** Sagittal cut through the mid portion of the medial meniscus, showing the triangular anterior and posterior horns. The posterior horn of the medial meniscus is normally elongated and larger than the anterior horn. There may be a superior recess at the meniscocapsular junction of the posterior horn.

MENISCI

SAGITTAL PD MR, MEDIAL MENISCUS

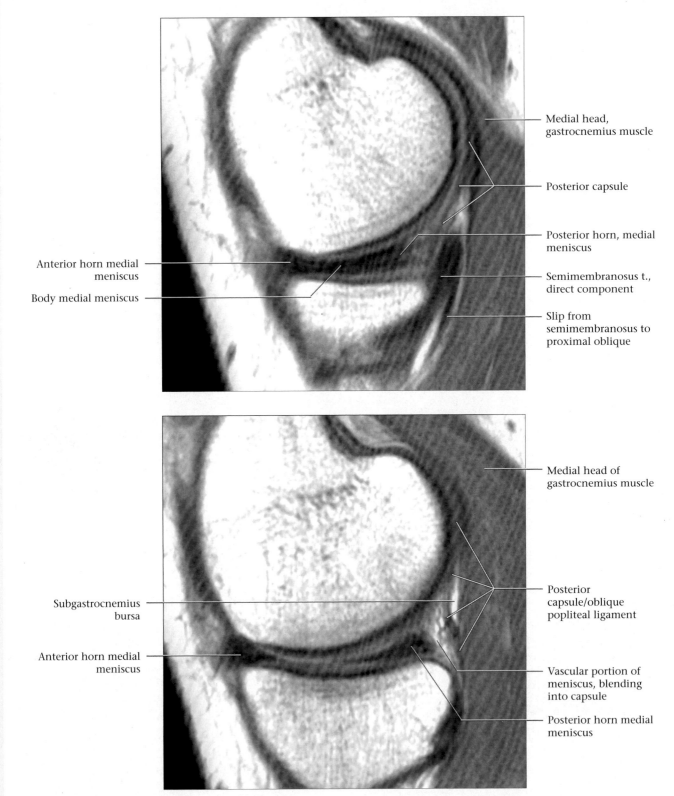

Medial head, gastrocnemius muscle

Posterior capsule

Posterior horn, medial meniscus

Semimembranosus t., direct component

Slip from semimembranosus to proximal oblique

Anterior horn medial meniscus

Body medial meniscus

Medial head of gastrocnemius muscle

Posterior capsule/oblique popliteal ligament

Vascular portion of meniscus, blending into capsule

Posterior horn medial meniscus

Subgastrocnemius bursa

Anterior horn medial meniscus

(Top) First of eight sagittal PD MR images through medial meniscus. Far medial (peripheral) sagittal cut through the medial meniscus, shows the bowtie configuration, encompassing portions of the anterior horn, body, and posterior horn of the medial meniscus. **(Bottom)** Mid sagittal cut through the medial meniscus, shows the differential size and shape of the anterior and posterior horns. This image and previous image show the low signal meniscus blending indistinctly into the gray vascular portion of the meniscus, which in turn blends into the capsule.

MENISCI

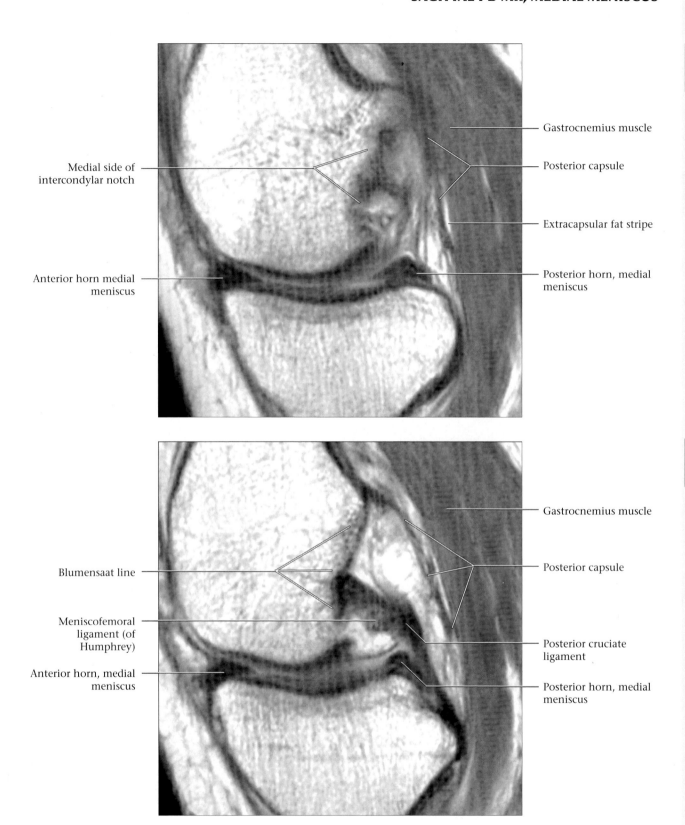

Medial side of intercondylar notch

Anterior horn medial meniscus

Gastrocnemius muscle

Posterior capsule

Extracapsular fat stripe

Posterior horn, medial meniscus

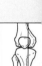

Blumensaat line

Meniscofemoral ligament (of Humphrey)

Anterior horn, medial meniscus

Gastrocnemius muscle

Posterior capsule

Posterior cruciate ligament

Posterior horn, medial meniscus

(Top) Cut through the medial meniscus, approaching the intercondylar notch. The anterior and posterior horns retain their differential size and shape. **(Bottom)** Cut through the medial meniscus as it enters the medial portion of the intercondylar notch. The posterior cruciate ligament is seen, arising from the mid portion of Blumensaat line along the medial femoral condyle. The anteroinferior meniscofemoral ligament (of Humphrey) is seen in cross-section beneath the posterior cruciate ligament. The posterior horn of the medial meniscus is beginning to change its shape as it approaches its root attachment to the tibial plateau. Because of the obliquity at which the knee is scanned for the sagittal images, the anterior horn is not yet approaching its root, but retains its triangular shape.

SAGITTAL PD MR, MEDIAL PORTION OF INTERCONDYLAR NOTCH

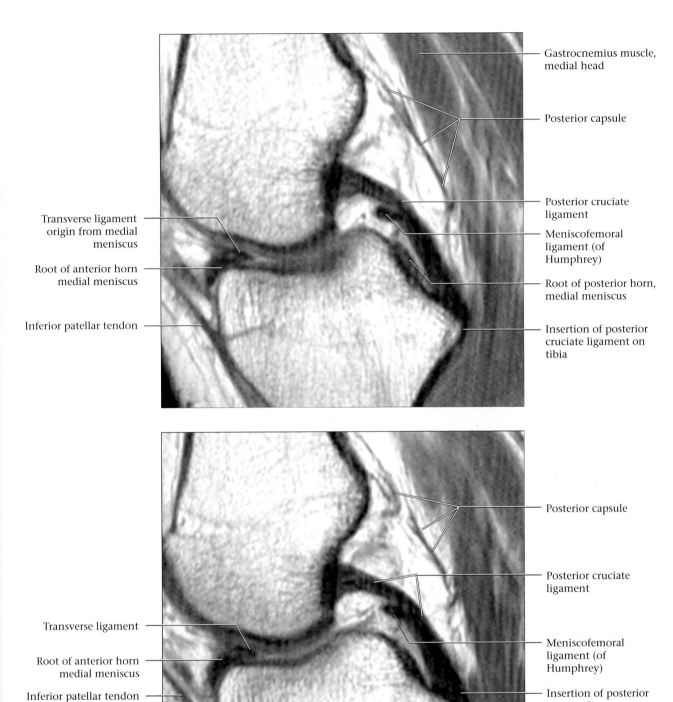

Gastrocnemius muscle, medial head

Posterior capsule

Posterior cruciate ligament

Meniscofemoral ligament (of Humphrey)

Root of posterior horn, medial meniscus

Insertion of posterior cruciate ligament on tibia

Transverse ligament origin from medial meniscus

Root of anterior horn medial meniscus

Inferior patellar tendon

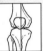

Posterior capsule

Posterior cruciate ligament

Meniscofemoral ligament (of Humphrey)

Insertion of posterior cruciate ligament on tibia

Popliteus muscle

Transverse ligament

Root of anterior horn medial meniscus

Inferior patellar tendon

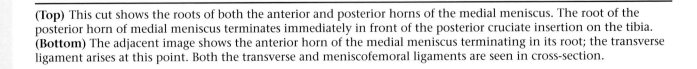

(Top) This cut shows the roots of both the anterior and posterior horns of the medial meniscus. The root of the posterior horn of medial meniscus terminates immediately in front of the posterior cruciate insertion on the tibia. **(Bottom)** The adjacent image shows the anterior horn of the medial meniscus terminating in its root; the transverse ligament arises at this point. Both the transverse and meniscofemoral ligaments are seen in cross-section.

SAGITTAL PD MR, MID INTERCONDYLAR NOTCH

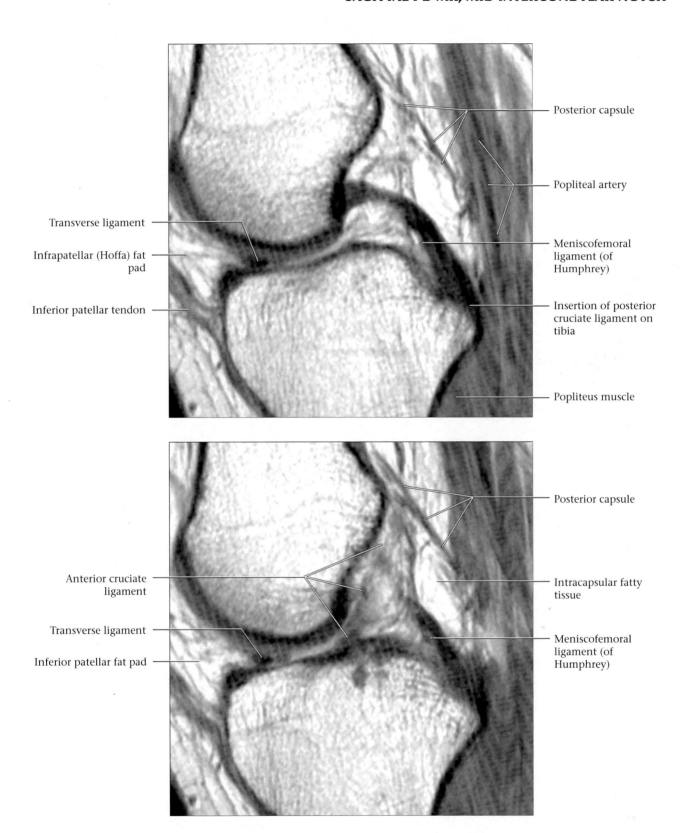

Top image labels:
- Posterior capsule
- Popliteal artery
- Meniscofemoral ligament (of Humphrey)
- Insertion of posterior cruciate ligament on tibia
- Popliteus muscle
- Transverse ligament
- Infrapatellar (Hoffa) fat pad
- Inferior patellar tendon

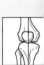

Bottom image labels:
- Posterior capsule
- Intracapsular fatty tissue
- Meniscofemoral ligament (of Humphrey)
- Anterior cruciate ligament
- Transverse ligament
- Inferior patellar fat pad

(Top) This cut shows no menisci; the meniscofemoral ligament is beginning to elongate and parallel the posterior cruciate ligament. Note that the posterior capsule is interrupted, allowing neurovascular structures to enter the joint. **(Bottom)** Cut between the cruciate ligaments shows the transverse ligament in cross-section, continuing across the anterior joint space. The meniscofemoral ligament elongates towards its insertion on the posterior horn of the lateral meniscus; the latter structure is not seen until the next cut towards the lateral side.

GRAPHICS OF THE MENISCI RELATIVE TO THEIR TIBIAL ATTACHMENTS

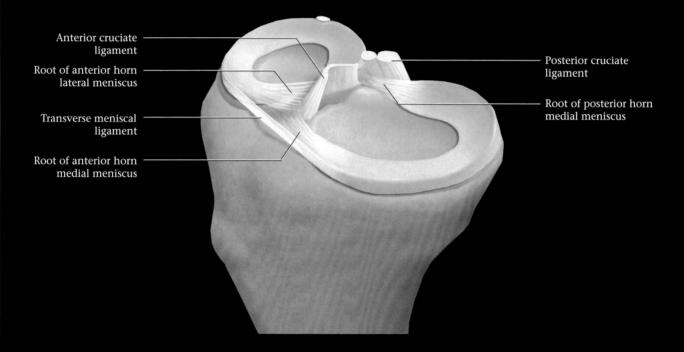

Anterior cruciate ligament

Root of anterior horn lateral meniscus

Transverse meniscal ligament

Root of anterior horn medial meniscus

Posterior cruciate ligament

Root of posterior horn medial meniscus

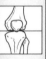

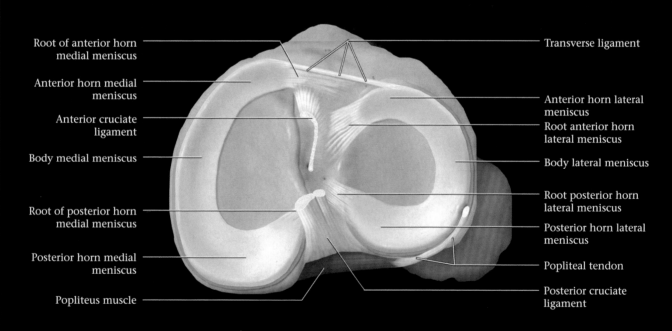

Root of anterior horn medial meniscus

Anterior horn medial meniscus

Anterior cruciate ligament

Body medial meniscus

Root of posterior horn medial meniscus

Posterior horn medial meniscus

Popliteus muscle

Transverse ligament

Anterior horn lateral meniscus

Root anterior horn lateral meniscus

Body lateral meniscus

Root posterior horn lateral meniscus

Posterior horn lateral meniscus

Popliteal tendon

Posterior cruciate ligament

(Top) Oblique axial graphic shows the tibial surface of the knee joint in an external oblique position. It highlights the semilunar medial meniscus, with its anterior and posterior roots located anterior to the ACL and PCL, respectively. The transverse ligament is seen coursing between the anterior horns of the medial and lateral menisci. **(Bottom)** Graphic is an axial view through the joint line. It shows the semilunar MM, with its wider C-shape compared to the more circular LM. The position of the meniscal roots is seen relative to one another as well as to the ACL and PCL. The transverse ligament and popliteal tendon are shown in relation to the menisci. Note also the different size of the various parts of the menisci.

MENISCI

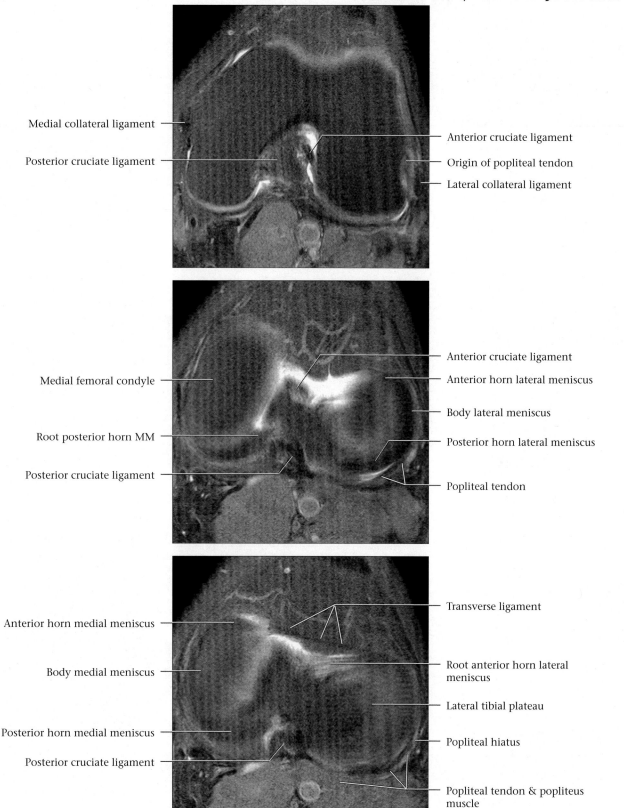

Medial collateral ligament —

Posterior cruciate ligament —

— **Anterior cruciate ligament**

— **Origin of popliteal tendon**

— **Lateral collateral ligament**

Medial femoral condyle —

Root posterior horn MM —

Posterior cruciate ligament —

— **Anterior cruciate ligament**

— **Anterior horn lateral meniscus**

— **Body lateral meniscus**

— **Posterior horn lateral meniscus**

— **Popliteal tendon**

Anterior horn medial meniscus —

Body medial meniscus —

Posterior horn medial meniscus —

Posterior cruciate ligament —

— **Transverse ligament**

— **Root anterior horn lateral meniscus**

— **Lateral tibial plateau**

— **Popliteal hiatus**

— **Popliteal tendon & popliteus muscle**

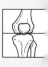

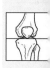

(Top) First of three axial PD FS MR images through the joint line. Image located immediately above the knee joint line. The cruciate ligaments as well as the origins of the medial and lateral collateral ligaments are seen. **(Middle)** Image through the knee joint line, shows parts of the menisci as well as the course of the popliteal tendon through the popliteal hiatus. **(Bottom)** Image through the tibial plateau at the joint line, shows parts of the menisci and their roots. The popliteal tendon is also seen extending to the popliteus muscle. The transverse meniscal ligament bridges between the two anterior horns.

LATERAL GRAPHICS, KNEE JOINT LINE

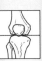

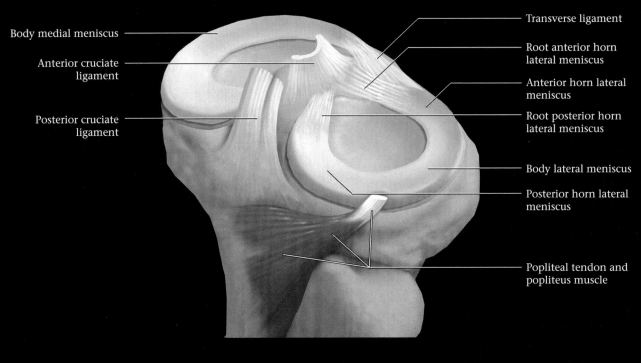

Body medial meniscus

Anterior cruciate ligament

Posterior cruciate ligament

Transverse ligament

Root anterior horn lateral meniscus

Anterior horn lateral meniscus

Root posterior horn lateral meniscus

Body lateral meniscus

Posterior horn lateral meniscus

Popliteal tendon and popliteus muscle

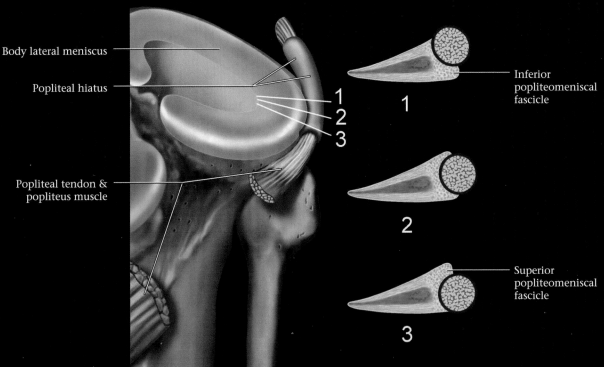

Body lateral meniscus

Popliteal hiatus

Popliteal tendon & popliteus muscle

Inferior popliteomeniscal fascicle

Superior popliteomeniscal fascicle

(Top) Posterolateral oblique view of the knee joint line shows the semicircular lateral meniscus, with its roots located immediately lateral to the anterior cruciate ligament. The popliteal tendon is shown curving around the lateral meniscus. **(Bottom)** Oblique axial graphic shows the course of the popliteal tendon through the knee joint. After the popliteal tendon originates from the lateral femoral condyle, it enters the joint space, interrupting the capsular attachment of the body of the lateral meniscus. It travels posteriorly and downward, curving around the body and posterior horns of the LM. It is bathed in synovial fluid within this space (termed the popliteal hiatus). Note the inferior fascicle which forms the floor of the hiatus at the body of the LM, and the superior fascicle which forms the roof of the hiatus at the LM body/posterior horn.

MENISCI

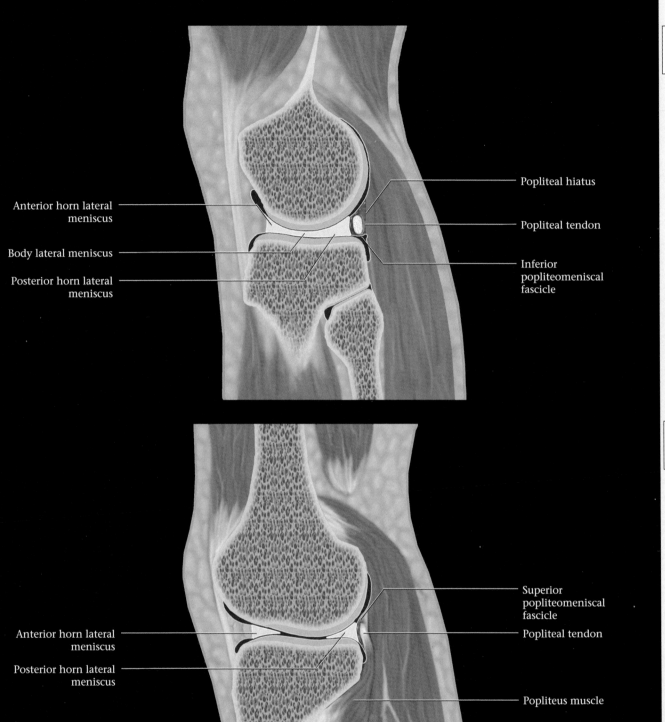

Anterior horn lateral meniscus

Body lateral meniscus

Posterior horn lateral meniscus

Popliteal hiatus

Popliteal tendon

Inferior popliteomeniscal fascicle

Anterior horn lateral meniscus

Posterior horn lateral meniscus

Superior popliteomeniscal fascicle

Popliteal tendon

Popliteus muscle

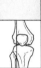

(Top) Sagittal graphic located far laterally in the joint, shows the bowtie configuration of the anterior horn, body, and posterior horn of the LM. The popliteal tendon is seen in the hiatus; at this junction of body and posterior horn of LM, the inferior fascicle can be seen extending from the meniscus towards (but not connecting to) the popliteal tendon. It forms the floor of the popliteal hiatus. (Bottom) In the mid portion of the lateral compartment, the anterior and posterior horns of the LM are nearly equal in size and shape. The popliteal tendon extends into the popliteus muscle. The superior fascicle can be seen extending from the superior portion of the posterior horn to the superior edge of the popliteal tendon (paratenon), continuing to the capsule and forming the roof of the popliteal hiatus.

SAGITTAL PD MR, THROUGH LATERAL PORTION OF INTERCONDYLAR NOTCH

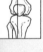

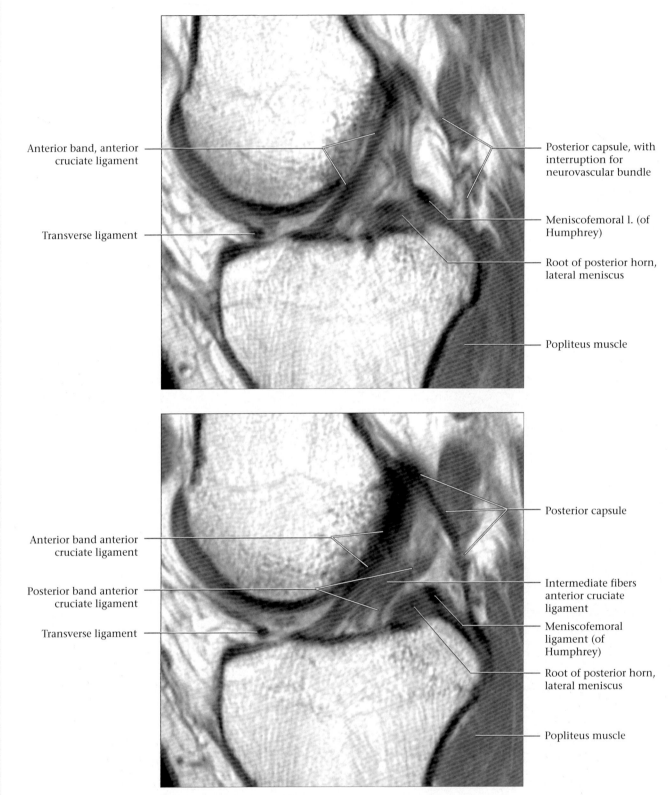

Anterior band, anterior cruciate ligament

Transverse ligament

Posterior capsule, with interruption for neurovascular bundle

Meniscofemoral l. (of Humphrey)

Root of posterior horn, lateral meniscus

Popliteus muscle

Anterior band anterior cruciate ligament

Posterior band anterior cruciate ligament

Transverse ligament

Posterior capsule

Intermediate fibers anterior cruciate ligament

Meniscofemoral ligament (of Humphrey)

Root of posterior horn, lateral meniscus

Popliteus muscle

(Top) First of eight sagittal PD MR images through the lateral compartment shows the mid portion of the intercondylar notch. Note the meniscofemoral ligament approaching the posterior horn lateral meniscus. **(Bottom)** At the lateral aspect of intercondylar notch, the meniscofemoral ligament joins the posterior horn lateral meniscus near its root. This attachment may be misinterpreted as a torn meniscus. Note that, due to the obliquity with which sagittal sequences are routinely obtained, it is not uncommon to see the transverse ligament anteriorly as well as the root of the posterior horn for several cuts before the root of the anterior horn of the lateral meniscus is seen. The root of the lateral meniscal anterior horn arises lateral to the origin of the anterior cruciate ligament from the tibia; therefore we should not expect to see it in these images.

SAGITTAL PD MR, LATERAL COMPARTMENT: ADJACENT TO INTERCONDYLAR NOTCH

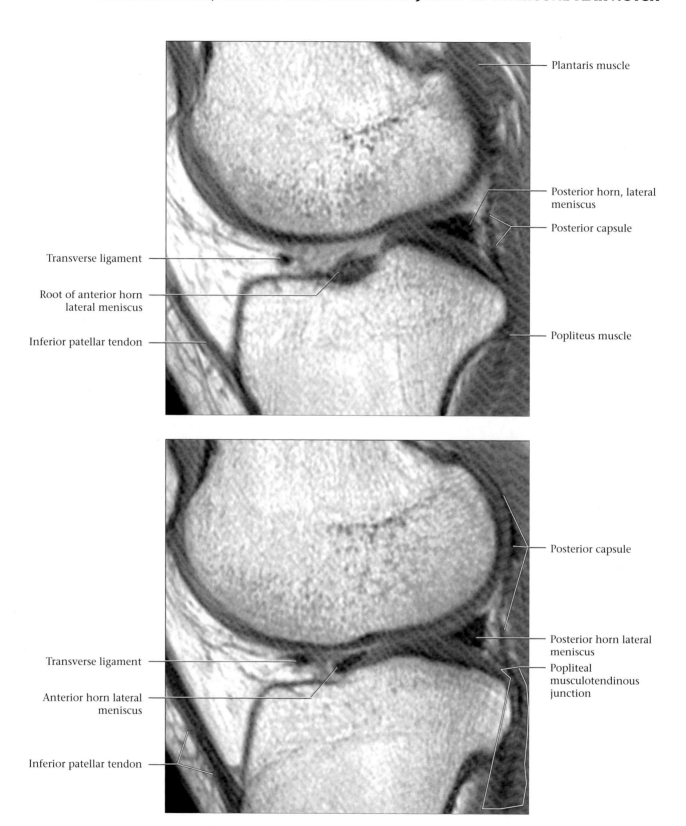

Plantaris muscle

Posterior horn, lateral meniscus

Posterior capsule

Transverse ligament

Root of anterior horn lateral meniscus

Inferior patellar tendon

Popliteus muscle

Posterior capsule

Transverse ligament

Anterior horn lateral meniscus

Posterior horn lateral meniscus

Popliteal musculotendinous junction

Inferior patellar tendon

(Top) In the lateral compartment, adjacent to the intercondylar notch, one sees the root of the anterior horn lateral meniscus, with the transverse ligament approaching it. **(Bottom)** In the adjacent, slightly more lateral, image, the transverse ligament more closely approaches the anterior horn of lateral meniscus. Note that in both of these cuts, the posterior horn of the lateral meniscus blends in directly to the posterior capsule. In these cuts the popliteus muscle (top) and popliteal musculotendinous junction (bottom) are extra-articular. This far posterior region is the only portion of the lateral meniscus which directly attaches to the posterior capsule and is not interrupted by the popliteal hiatus.

SAGITTAL PD MR, MID PORTION OF LATERAL COMPARTMENT

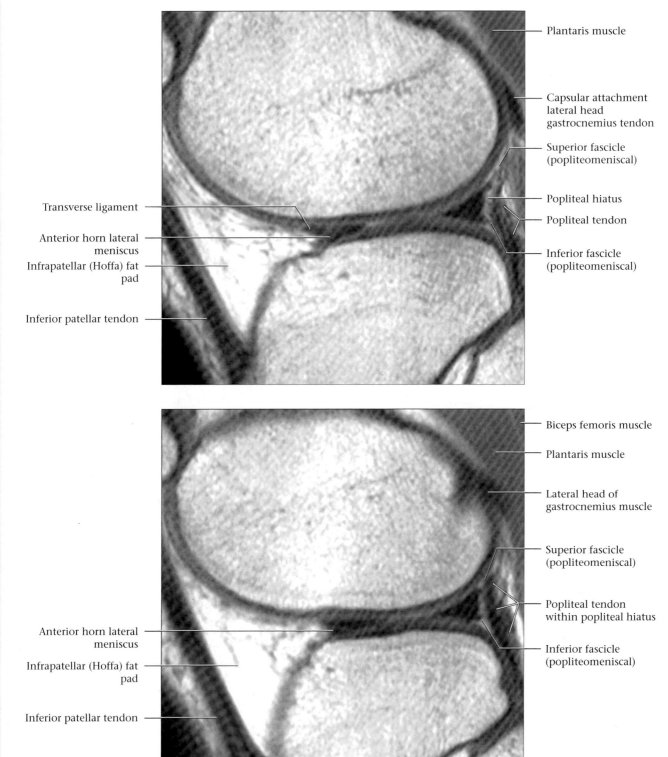

Plantaris muscle

Capsular attachment lateral head gastrocnemius tendon

Superior fascicle (popliteomeniscal)

Transverse ligament

Popliteal hiatus

Popliteal tendon

Anterior horn lateral meniscus

Inferior fascicle (popliteomeniscal)

Infrapatellar (Hoffa) fat pad

Inferior patellar tendon

Biceps femoris muscle

Plantaris muscle

Lateral head of gastrocnemius muscle

Superior fascicle (popliteomeniscal)

Anterior horn lateral meniscus

Popliteal tendon within popliteal hiatus

Infrapatellar (Hoffa) fat pad

Inferior fascicle (popliteomeniscal)

Inferior patellar tendon

(Top) Image through the lateral compartment shows the transverse ligament joining the anterior horn lateral meniscus. Posteriorly, one sees the popliteal tendon within the popliteal hiatus. This structure is intra-articular but extra-synovial. The superior fascicle extends from the superior aspect of the posterior horn lateral meniscus to the paratenon of popliteal tendon and on to the capsule, forming the roof of the popliteal hiatus. The inferior fascicle extends from the inferior aspect of the posterior horn lateral meniscus towards the popliteal tendon but is interrupted by the tendon's passage into the extra-articular position of the musculotendinous junction. **(Bottom)** The adjacent more lateral cut shows a similar relationship of the fascicles, with the superior extending to the popliteal tendon and capsule, and inferior fascicle being interrupted.

MENISCI

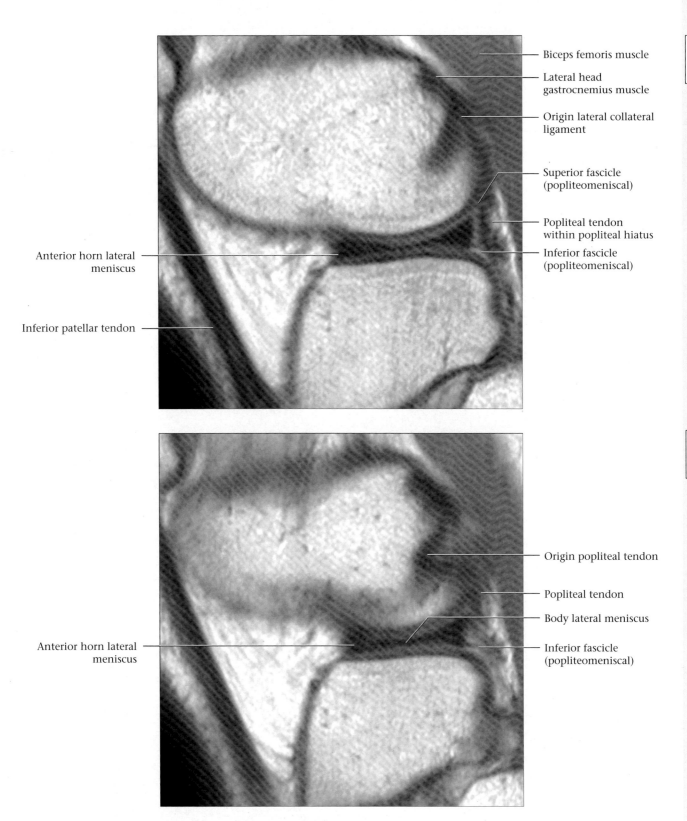

Biceps femoris muscle

Lateral head gastrocnemius muscle

Origin lateral collateral ligament

Superior fascicle (popliteomeniscal)

Popliteal tendon within popliteal hiatus

Inferior fascicle (popliteomeniscal)

Anterior horn lateral meniscus

Inferior patellar tendon

Origin popliteal tendon

Popliteal tendon

Body lateral meniscus

Inferior fascicle (popliteomeniscal)

Anterior horn lateral meniscus

(Top) Cut through the lateral compartment shows the beginning of the bowtie configuration of the meniscus. The popliteal tendon is within the hiatus, outlined superiorly by the superior popliteomeniscal fascicle and inferiorly by the inferior popliteomeniscal fascicle. **(Bottom)** Farther laterally, the bowtie configuration of the lateral meniscus is complete. The origin of the popliteus tendon (located just anteriorly and inferiorly to the origin of the lateral collateral ligament on the lateral femoral condyle) is seen. A portion of the popliteal tendon is seen coursing towards its intra-articular position in the popliteal hiatus. The superior popliteomeniscal fascicle has not yet formed as the popliteal tendon passes the superior portion of the posterior horn but the inferior popliteomeniscal fascicle clearly forms the floor of the hiatus.

MENISCI

CORONAL MID & POSTERIOR KNEE JOINT GRAPHICS

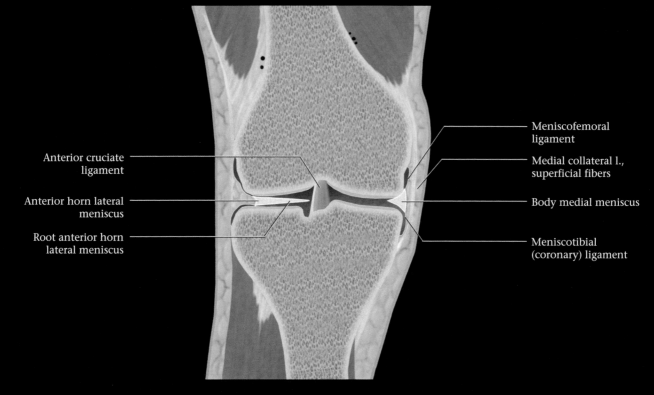

Anterior cruciate
ligament

Anterior horn lateral
meniscus

Root anterior horn
lateral meniscus

Meniscofemoral
ligament

Medial collateral l.,
superficial fibers

Body medial meniscus

Meniscotibial
(coronary) ligament

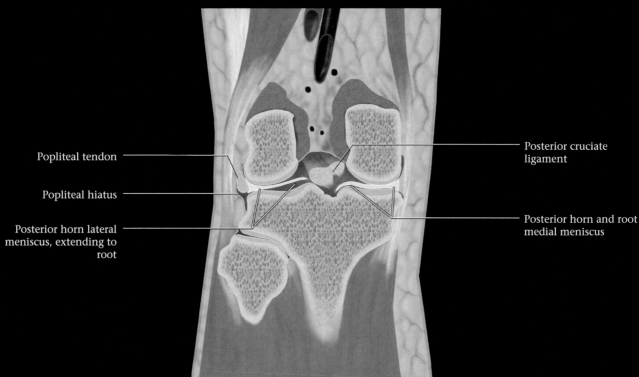

Popliteal tendon

Popliteal hiatus

Posterior horn lateral
meniscus, extending to
root

Posterior cruciate
ligament

Posterior horn and root
medial meniscus

(Top) Coronal graphic through the anterior/mid knee joint, shows the anterior horn and root of the LM. The same cut shows the body of the MM, which is short and shaped as an equilateral triangle. The deep fibers of the medial collateral ligament arise from the body of the MM; the meniscofemoral ligament inserts either on the femoral condyle or the superficial medial collateral ligament while the meniscotibial ligament inserts on the tibia. **(Bottom)** Coronal graphic more posteriorly shows the roots of the posterior horns of both the medial and lateral menisci. The popliteal tendon is also seen coursing through the hiatus adjacent to the body/posterior horn of the LM.

MENISCI

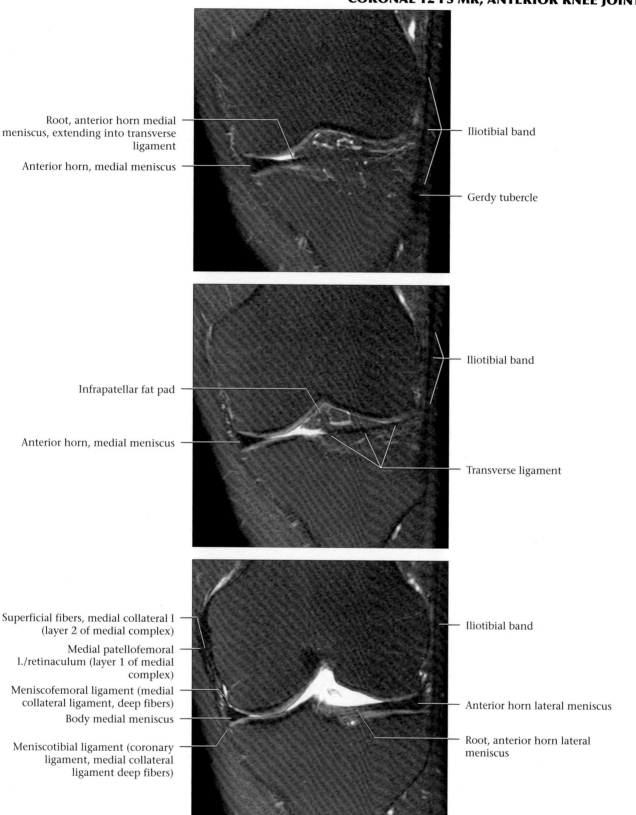

Root, anterior horn medial meniscus, extending into transverse ligament

Anterior horn, medial meniscus

Iliotibial band

Gerdy tubercle

Infrapatellar fat pad

Anterior horn, medial meniscus

Iliotibial band

Transverse ligament

Superficial fibers, medial collateral l. (layer 2 of medial complex)

Medial patellofemoral l./retinaculum (layer 1 of medial complex)

Meniscofemoral ligament (medial collateral ligament, deep fibers)

Body medial meniscus

Meniscotibial ligament (coronary ligament, medial collateral ligament deep fibers)

Iliotibial band

Anterior horn lateral meniscus

Root, anterior horn lateral meniscus

(Top) First of nine coronal T2 FS MR images presented from anterior to posterior. Anterior cut shows that anterior horn medial meniscus is located anterior to anterior horn lateral meniscus. Transverse ligament extends from anterior horn medial meniscus towards anterior horn lateral meniscus **(Middle)** Transverse ligament seen extending towards anterior horn LM. **(Bottom)** Root of anterior horn lateral meniscus is several mm posterior to that of medial meniscus. By this cut, medial meniscus is transforming from anterior horn to body. One can see that in the mid portion of the knee there is separation between layer 2 and 3 of the medial supporting structures (superficial and deep fibers of medial collateral ligament, respectively). Deep fibers consist of the meniscofemoral ligament, extending from body of meniscus to superficial medial collateral ligament, and meniscotibial (coronary) ligament.

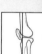

Knee

VI

CORONAL T2 FS MR, MID KNEE JOINT

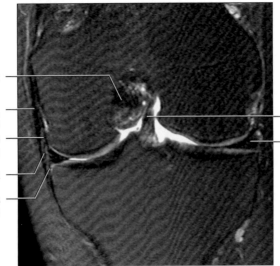

Posterior cruciate ligament

Medial collateral ligament, superficial fibers

Meniscofemoral ligament (deep fibers of medial collateral)

Medial collateral ligament bursa

Meniscotibial ligament (deep fibers of medial collateral)

Anterior cruciate ligament

Anterior horn/body lateral meniscus

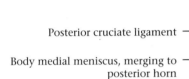

Posterior cruciate ligament

Body medial meniscus, merging to posterior horn

Medial collateral ligament, superficial fibers & oblique fibers

Sartorius tendon

Lateral collateral ligament

Popliteal tendon

Body lateral meniscus

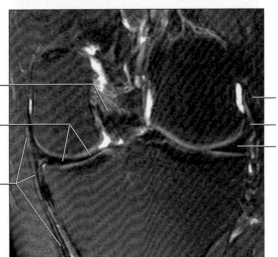

Posterior cruciate ligament

Posterior horn, medial meniscus

Medial collateral ligament

Lateral collateral ligament

Popliteal tendon

Body lateral meniscus

(Top) Coronal cut through the mid joint shows the body of the medial meniscus to be the smallest, approaching an equilateral triangle in shape. The anterior cruciate ligament is reliably seen in this region, as are both the deep and superficial layers of the medial collateral ligament. **(Middle)** In a cut that is slightly more posterior one sees that the deep and superficial layers of the medial collateral ligament merge together. On the lateral side, the popliteal tendon is seen at its origin, extending towards the joint line. The body of the lateral meniscus is still firmly attached to the capsule. **(Bottom)** Even more posteriorly, the medial meniscus is transforming to its posterior horn. On the lateral side, the popliteal tendon is seen entering the joint superiorly to the body of the lateral meniscus, at the beginning of the popliteal hiatus.

MENISCI

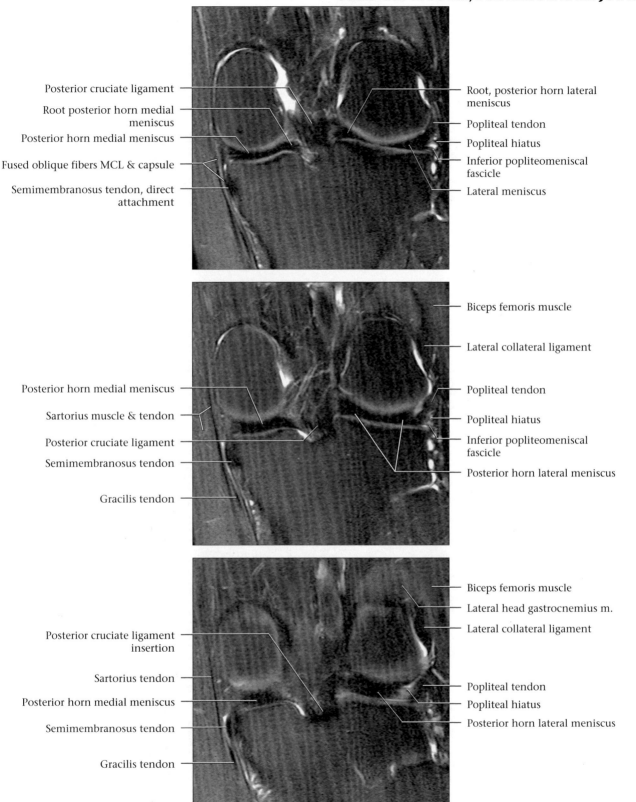

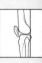

Posterior cruciate ligament

Root posterior horn medial meniscus

Posterior horn medial meniscus

Fused oblique fibers MCL & capsule

Semimembranosus tendon, direct attachment

Root, posterior horn lateral meniscus

Popliteal tendon

Popliteal hiatus

Inferior popliteomeniscal fascicle

Lateral meniscus

Biceps femoris muscle

Lateral collateral ligament

Popliteal tendon

Popliteal hiatus

Inferior popliteomeniscal fascicle

Posterior horn lateral meniscus

Posterior horn medial meniscus

Sartorius muscle & tendon

Posterior cruciate ligament

Semimembranosus tendon

Gracilis tendon

Biceps femoris muscle

Lateral head gastrocnemius m.

Lateral collateral ligament

Popliteal tendon

Popliteal hiatus

Posterior horn lateral meniscus

Posterior cruciate ligament insertion

Sartorius tendon

Posterior horn medial meniscus

Semimembranosus tendon

Gracilis tendon

(Top) Posteriorly in the joint, but anterior to the posterior cruciate ligaments, the posterior meniscal roots are found. Medially, the medial collateral ligament has merged with the capsule. Laterally, the popliteal tendon enters the articular space by way of the popliteal hiatus. **(Middle)** The popliteal hiatus becomes more prominent as the tendon extends posteriorly and downward. The inferior popliteomeniscal fascicle forms the floor of the popliteal hiatus at this point. **(Bottom)** At the posterior extent of the intra-articular portion of the knee joint, the popliteal tendon crosses in its downward and posterior course to its musculotendinous junction. The hiatus is prominent here, and must not be mistaken for a tear in the posterior horn lateral meniscus. Both posterior horns are seen this far posteriorly, beyond their roots.

SAGITTAL PD MR & CORONAL T2 MR, LATERAL COMPARTMENT

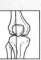

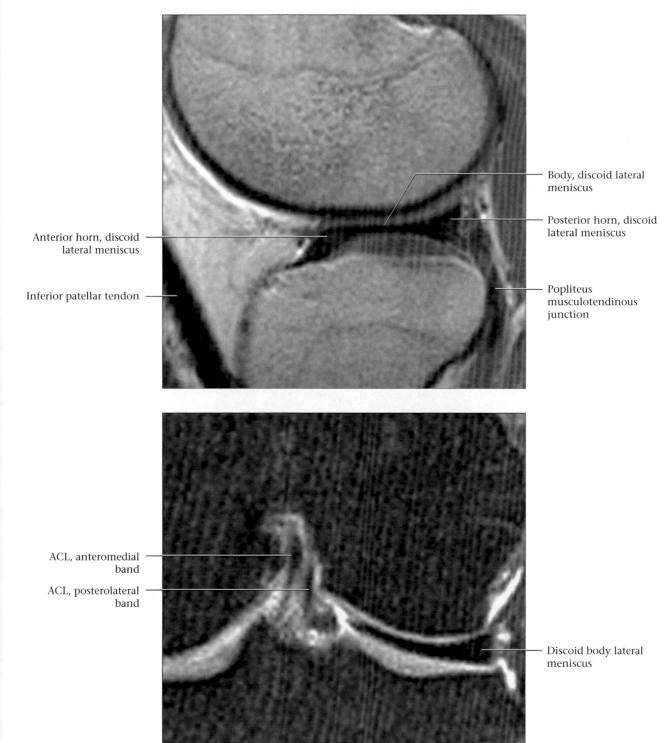

Anterior horn, discoid lateral meniscus

Inferior patellar tendon

Body, discoid lateral meniscus

Posterior horn, discoid lateral meniscus

Popliteus musculotendinous junction

ACL, anteromedial band

ACL, posterolateral band

Discoid body lateral meniscus

(Top) Sagittal image is from the mid portion of the lateral compartment, and shows a discoid lateral meniscus. Note that the meniscus is seen with all three portions, the anterior horn, body, and posterior horn. This bowtie appearance should be seen only in the outer portion of the joint. The fact that the fibula is not seen, as well as that the popliteus musculotendinous junction (rather than just the popliteus tendon) and patellar tendon are both in this image indicates that the location is far too interior in the joint for a normal body of meniscus to be seen. Thus, the body of the meniscus is too large, indicating the discoid variant. (Bottom) Coronal image through the mid portion of the joint (as indicated by the morphology and presence of the ACL) shows the body of the lateral meniscus to be too large, confirming that it is discoid.

MENISCI

SAGITTAL CT ARTHROGRAM, MR ARTHROGRAM: DISTENDED JOINT

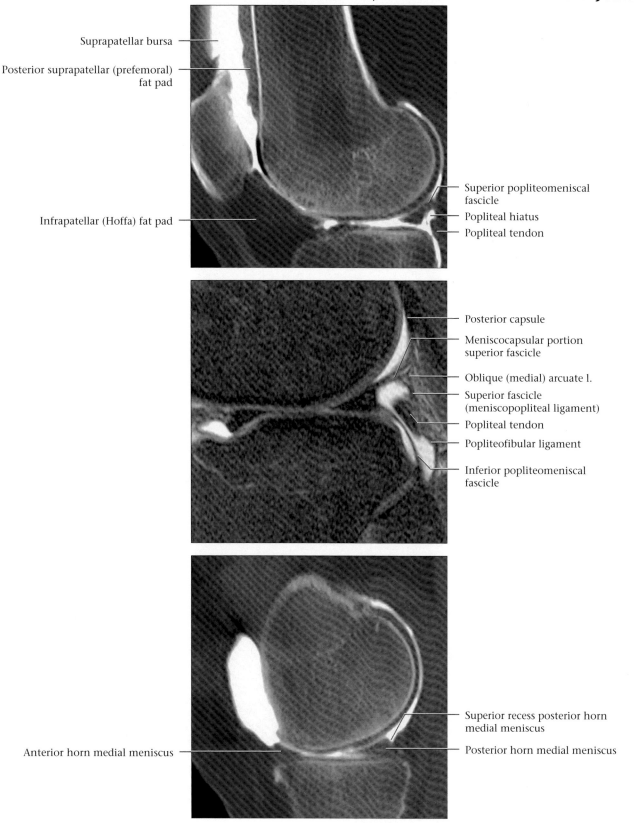

Suprapatellar bursa

Posterior suprapatellar (prefemoral) fat pad

Infrapatellar (Hoffa) fat pad

Superior popliteomeniscal fascicle

Popliteal hiatus

Popliteal tendon

Posterior capsule

Meniscocapsular portion superior fascicle

Oblique (medial) arcuate l.

Superior fascicle (meniscopopliteal ligament)

Popliteal tendon

Popliteofibular ligament

Inferior popliteomeniscal fascicle

Superior recess posterior horn medial meniscus

Posterior horn medial meniscus

Anterior horn medial meniscus

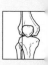
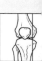

(Top) Reformatted sagittal image through the lateral compartment in a CT arthrogram. Note that with distension of the joint by contrast, continuum of the joint fluid with the popliteal hiatus is readily seen. The superior popliteomeniscal fascicle, extending between the posterior horn lateral meniscus and popliteal tendon, is outlined by fluid. (Middle) MR arthrogram shows distended popliteal hiatus and outlines both the superior and inferior meniscopopliteal fascicles (struts) as well as the popliteal tendon. Popliteofibular and arcuate ligaments are seen well. (Bottom) Reformatted sagittal image through medial compartment in a CT arthrogram shows the superior recess of posterior horn medial meniscus. This should not be mistaken for a peripheral meniscal tear or meniscocapsular separation. Note that cartilage width varies over the femoral condyle (thicker posteriorly).

SAGITTAL PD FS MR & CORONAL PD MR, LIGAMENT OF WRISBERG

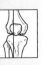

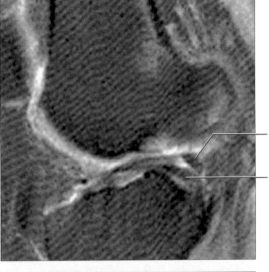

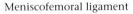

Meniscofemoral ligament

Posterior horn lateral meniscus

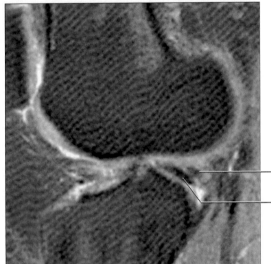

Meniscofemoral ligament

Posterior horn lateral meniscus

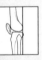

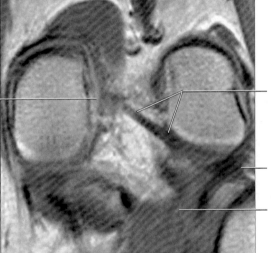

Medial femoral condylar notch origin of meniscofemoral ligament

Meniscofemoral ligament (of Wrisberg)

Posterior horn lateral meniscus

Popliteus muscle

(Top) First of three images depicting the meniscofemoral ligament of Wrisberg. This sagittal image is slightly lateral to the intercondylar notch and root of posterior horn lateral meniscus. Meniscofemoral ligament is distinctly separate from meniscus. (Middle) Approaching intercondylar notch and root of posterior horn lateral meniscus, meniscofemoral ligament more closely approaches lateral meniscus to merge with it. It is at this point that a tear of posterior horn could be mistakenly diagnosed. (Bottom) Coronal image located posteriorly in the joint shows meniscofemoral ligament of Wrisberg over nearly its entire extent, originating at medial femoral condyle in the intertrochanteric notch and merging with posterior horn lateral meniscus.

MENISCI

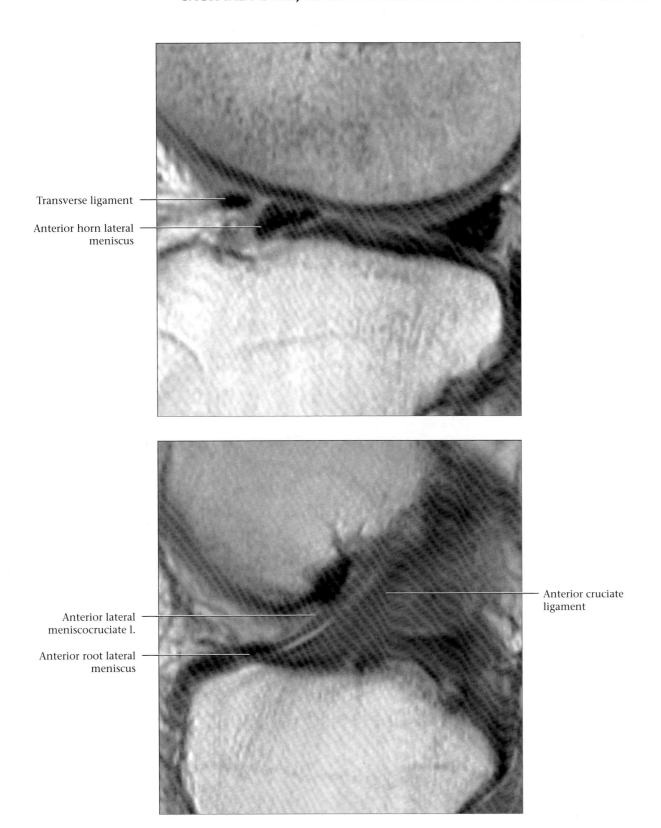

Transverse ligament

Anterior horn lateral meniscus

Anterior cruciate ligament

Anterior lateral meniscocruciate l.

Anterior root lateral meniscus

(Top) First of two sagittal PD MR images near the intercondylar notch, lateral to medial, shows a large transverse ligament. This ligament connects the two anterior meniscal horns and is seen in cross-section on sagittal images. It could possibly be confused for a meniscal tear as it merges with the lateral meniscus, closer to the notch. The ligament is generally smaller than this, or may be absent. (Bottom) Image through the lateral portion of intercondylar notch shows a discrete structure which parallels the anterior cruciate ligament and extends from the root of the anterior horn lateral meniscus to the lateral femoral condyle. This represents the normal variant, anterior lateral meniscocruciate ligament. It is distinguished from infrapatellar plica (which can also parallel the ACL in the same manner) by its site of origin at the meniscus rather than the patella.

AXIAL PD FS & SAGITTAL PD MR, THROUGH INTERCONDYLAR NOTCH: NORMAL VARIANT

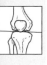

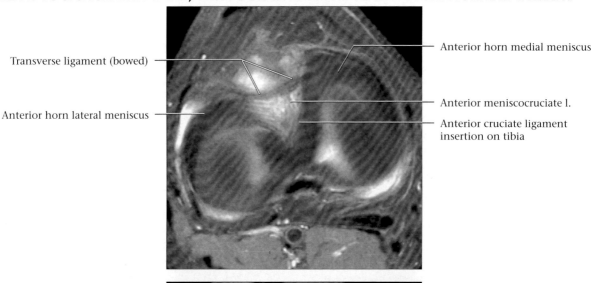

Transverse ligament (bowed)

Anterior horn medial meniscus

Anterior meniscocruciate l.

Anterior horn lateral meniscus

Anterior cruciate ligament insertion on tibia

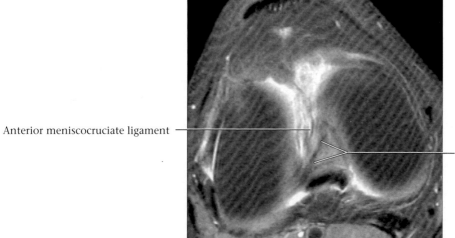

Anterior meniscocruciate ligament

Anterior cruciate ligament

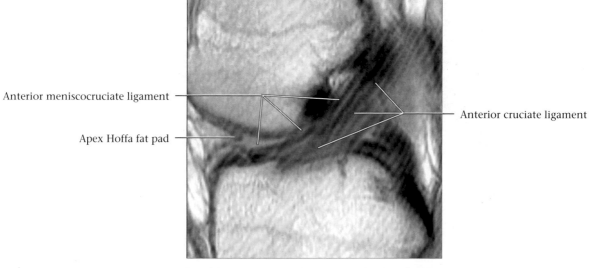

Anterior meniscocruciate ligament

Apex Hoffa fat pad

Anterior cruciate ligament

(Top) First of two axial PD FS MR images at the level of the joint line, shows a slightly tethered transverse ligament, with an anterior meniscocruciate ligament arising from it. Note that the ligament is anterior to the anterior cruciate ligament. **(Middle)** Image slightly higher than the previous image, in the intercondylar notch. The anterior meniscocruciate ligament parallels the anterior cruciate ligament throughout the notch. **(Bottom)** Sagittal PD MR image shows the length of the anterior meniscocruciate ligament, paralleling the anterior cruciate ligament. This normal variant should not be mistaken for an intrasubstance tear of the anterior cruciate. Note that the apex of Hoffa fat pad is free of this ligament (not attached as in an infrapatellar plica).

CORONAL PD FS MR, THROUGH ANTERIOR MID JOINT: NORMAL VARIANT

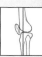

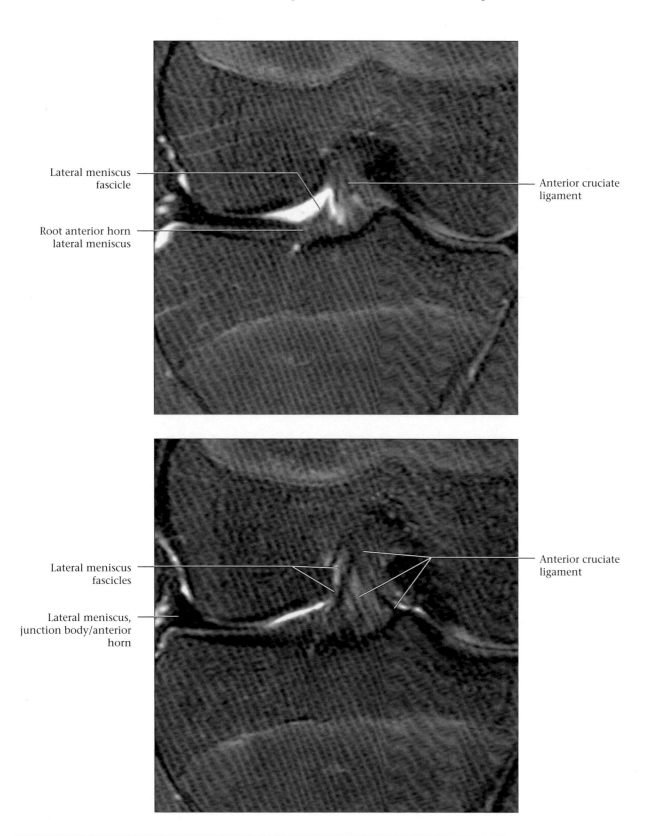

Lateral meniscus fascicle

Root anterior horn lateral meniscus

Anterior cruciate ligament

Lateral meniscus fascicles

Lateral meniscus, junction body/anterior horn

Anterior cruciate ligament

(Top) First of two coronal PD FS MR images in the anterior portion of the joint. The transverse ligament in this patient was absent (more anterior cut not shown). The fibers of the anterior horn lateral meniscus, which normally blend into the transverse ligament, instead form discrete lateral meniscal fascicles which ascend towards the anterior cruciate ligament. **(Bottom)** Coronal image slightly posterior to the previous image shows the lateral meniscal fascicles ascending to intersect the anterior cruciate ligament. These fibers clearly are not part of the anterior cruciate ligament since they ascend at a different angle. This normal variant should not be mistaken for pathology such as a disrupted ACL or a meniscal fragment from a bucket handle tear.

AXIAL PD FS MR, 2 DIFFERENT PATIENTS: NORMAL VARIANTS

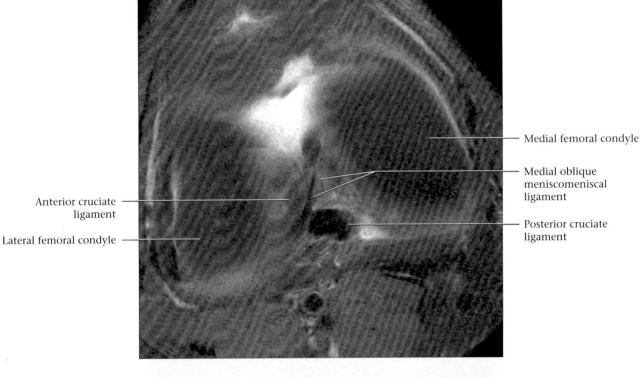

Medial femoral condyle

Medial oblique meniscomeniscal ligament

Anterior cruciate ligament

Posterior cruciate ligament

Lateral femoral condyle

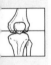

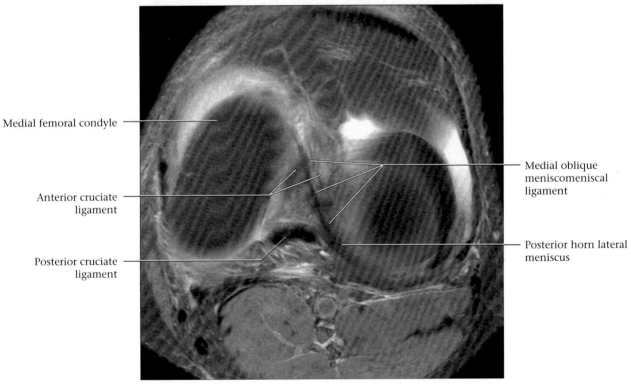

Medial femoral condyle

Medial oblique meniscomeniscal ligament

Anterior cruciate ligament

Posterior cruciate ligament

Posterior horn lateral meniscus

(Top) Single axial image, just above the joint line, shows the normal variant medial oblique meniscomeniscal ligament. It arises from the anterior horn medial meniscus and inserts on the posterior horn lateral meniscus, threading its way between the ACL and PCL. **(Bottom)** First of three images in a different patient, axial PD FS MR through the joint line, shows a normal variant, the medial oblique meniscomeniscal ligament. The ligament extends from the anterior horn medial meniscus across the intercondylar notch to insert on posterior horn lateral meniscus. At this level of the menisci, the variant ligament appears to split the ACL at its insertion on the tibia. It normally extends between the ACL and PCL. The mirror image variant, lateral meniscomeniscal ligament, extends from anterior horn lateral meniscus to posterior horn medial meniscus (not shown here).

MENISCI

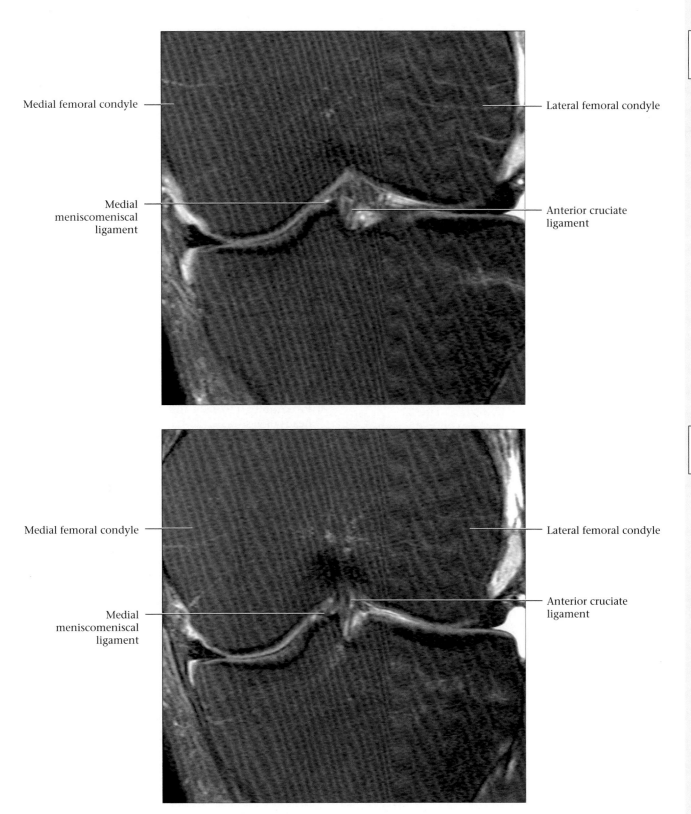

Medial femoral condyle — Lateral femoral condyle

Medial meniscomeniscal ligament — Anterior cruciate ligament

Medial femoral condyle — Lateral femoral condyle

Medial meniscomeniscal ligament — Anterior cruciate ligament

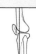

(Top) First of two coronal MR images, at the anterior portion of mid-joint, shows the tiny medial meniscomeniscal ligament in cross section adjacent to the anterior cruciate ligament. This is the same patient as shown on the immediate previous axial image. **(Bottom)** Second coronal image, 3 mm posterior, with the meniscomeniscal ligament giving the appearance of a loose body or fragment adjacent to the ACL. The location and low signal of this normal variant ligament may be misdiagnosed as a meniscal fragment or bucket handle fragment. It is important to correlate it with the appearance on either axial or sagittal images, where the ligament will be seen as a longitudinal structure placed between the ACL and PCL, and angling obliquely across the notch between the two menisci.

CRUCIATE LIGAMENTS/POSTERIOR CAPSULE

Terminology

Abbreviations
- Anterior cruciate ligament (ACL)
- Posterior cruciate ligament (PCL)

Imaging Anatomy

Overview
- Cruciate ligaments are in an **extrasynovial but intracapsular** location
  - Fatty tissue lies between the cruciates
  - Synovial membrane surrounds anterior, medial, and lateral portions of cruciates but is reflected posteriorly from PCL to adjoining parts of joint capsule

ACL
- **Multiple separate fascicles** which spiral laterally from femur to tibia (fibers rotate externally 90°); fatty tissue is seen between fibers
  - Continuum of fibers allows variable tension, with some taut throughout knee range of motion
  - **Anteromedial bundle**: Tight in flexion, lax in extension
  - **Posterolateral bundle**: Tight in extension, lax in flexion
- **Origin of ACL**: Posteriorly from lateral femoral condyle at intercondylar notch (seen on radiograph as junction of posterior femoral cortex and Blumensaat line)
- **Insertion of ACL**: Anteromedial tibial spine and adjacent plateau; bundles fan out at tibial attachment, forming "foot"
- **Function**
  - Primary restraint to anterior tibial translation
  - Major secondary restraint to internal rotation, minor secondary restraint to external rotation
  - Minor secondary restraint to varus/valgus at full extension
- **MR imaging**: Seen well in all three planes, low signal with fat interspersed between bundles
- Blood supply: Middle geniculate artery (pierces posterior capsule from popliteal); lesser supply from fat pad (inferior medial and lateral geniculates)
- Nerve: Posterior articular (branch of posterior tibial)

PCL
- **Appears as a single round ligament** but consists of two major parts; rotates 90° from an antero-posterior alignment at femoral origin to medial-lateral insertion at posterior tibia
  - **Anterolateral bundle**: Bulk of ligament, taut in flexion, lax in extension
  - **Posteromedial (oblique) bundle**: Taut in extension, lax in flexion
- **Origin of PCL**: Mid portion of medial femoral condyle at intercondylar notch
- **Insertion of PCL**: Mid posterior tibia, 1 cm below joint line, where it blends in with posterior capsule
- **Function**: Primary restraint against posterior translation

- **Meniscofemoral ligaments**
  - Both arise from posterior horn lateral meniscus and insert on medial femoral condyle; at least one present 70% of time
  - **Posterior (Wrisberg)** lies posterior to PCL
  - **Anterior (Humphrey)** lies anterior to PCL; intact ligament of Humphrey may mimic an intact PCL
  - May play a role in secondary restraint to posterior instability; may stabilize lateral meniscus during flexion
- **MR imaging**: Seen well in all three planes, solid low signal throughout
- Blood supply: Middle geniculate artery proximal and middle thirds; geniculate and popliteal artery base; capsular vessels through entire length

Posterior Capsule
- **Complex fibrous structure**, augmented by extensions of adjacent tendons
- **Incomplete**, pierced centrally by neurovascular structures
- **Proximal attachment**: Vertical fibers attached to posterior margins of femoral condyles and intercondylar fossae
- **Distal attachment** is to posterior margins of tibial condyles and intercondylar areas
- **Tendons/ligaments** attach to posterior capsule to provide reinforcement
  - **Proximally** (medially and laterally): Tendinous heads of gastrocnemius
  - **Posteromedial corner**: Semimembranosus and posterior oblique ligament
  - **Posterolateral corner**: Arcuate ligament and iliotibial tract
  - **Posterior central**: Oblique popliteal ligament

Spaces Within Cruciate/Posterior Capsule
- Synovial membrane surrounds anterior, medial, and lateral portions of cruciates, but is reflected posteriorly from PCL to adjoining parts of joint capsule
- Results in a potential space (**PCL bursa or recess**)
  - Seen only when fluid-filled, best on coronal and sagittal planes
  - Seen posterior to PCL and adjacent to lateral aspect of medial femoral condyle
  - No contact between PCL recess and the proximal third of the PCL (fat is interposed)
  - Communicates with medial (femorotibial) compartment of knee
  - Does not communicate with lateral compartment
  - If ligament of Wrisberg is present, it lies posterosuperior to PCL recess
- **Intercruciate recess**
  - Localized potential fluid collection between ACL and PCL, best seen on sagittal and axial planes
  - Communicates with either lateral or medial (femorotibial) compartments

Selected References

1. De Maeseneer M et. al: Normal anatomy and pathology of the posterior capsular area of the knee. AJR. 182:955-62, 2004

SAGITTAL T2 FS MR, CRUCIATE LIGAMENTS

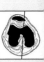

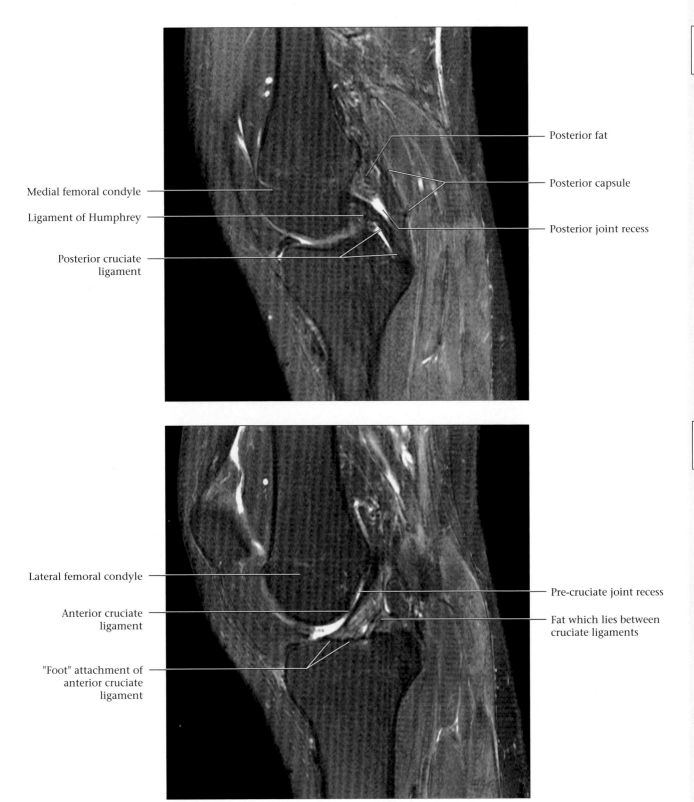

Posterior fat

Posterior capsule

Posterior joint recess

Medial femoral condyle

Ligament of Humphrey

Posterior cruciate ligament

Lateral femoral condyle

Anterior cruciate ligament

"Foot" attachment of anterior cruciate ligament

Pre-cruciate joint recess

Fat which lies between cruciate ligaments

(Top) First of two sagittal T2 FS MR images through the intercondylar notch in the more medial portion of the notch, shows the origin of the PCL from the anterior portion of the medial notch, as well as the insertion posteriorly to the tibia, 1 cm below the joint line. The PCL appears as a thick single band, usually in at least two adjacent images. There is fat located immediately posterior to the proximal portion of the PCL. More distally, the posterior joint recess abuts the PCL. The posterior capsule lies behind this fat and the recess. In this case, the meniscofemoral ligament of Humphrey is present; the ligament of Wrisberg is absent. **(Bottom)** This image is located slightly laterally, within the intercondylar notch. The anterior cruciate ligament arises from the posterior lateral femoral condyle within the notch; the broad insertion on the tibial plateau is seen.

CORONAL T2 FS MR, CRUCIATE LIGAMENTS

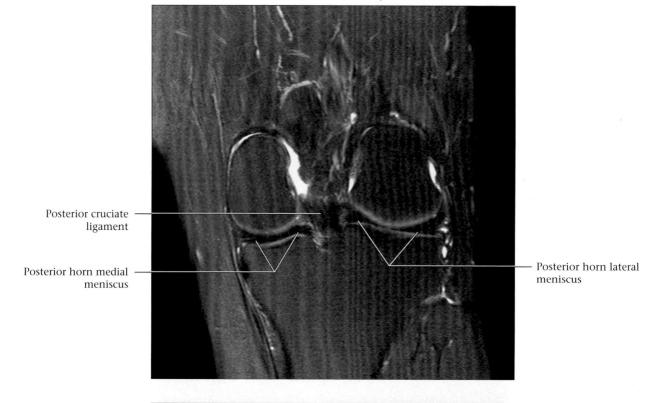

Posterior cruciate ligament

Posterior horn medial meniscus

Posterior horn lateral meniscus

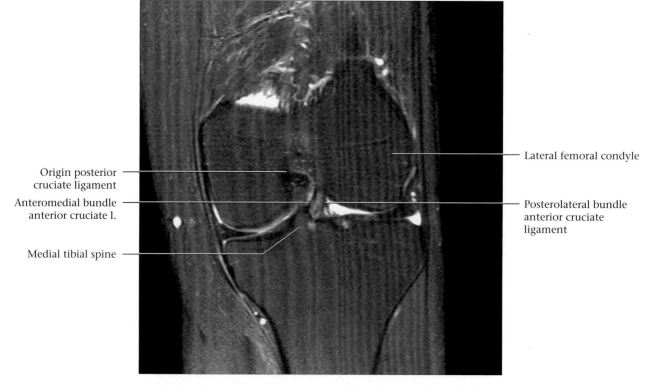

Origin posterior cruciate ligament

Anteromedial bundle anterior cruciate l.

Medial tibial spine

Lateral femoral condyle

Posterolateral bundle anterior cruciate ligament

(Top) First of two coronal T2 FS MR images shows the cruciate ligaments. This more posterior image shows the posterior cruciate ligament approaching its insertion on the posterior aspect of the tibial plateau. No portion of anterior cruciate is seen. Note that while we expect to see the ACL as a complete band on coronal images, the PCL is incompletely seen. **(Bottom)** This more anterior image also shows the cruciate ligaments. The anteromedial bundle and posterolateral bundle of ACL are seen arising from the lateral femoral condyle and inserting on the tibial plateau adjacent to the medial tibial spine. Both are seen on the same cut because of the obliquity at which coronal images are obtained. Because the leg is in extension, the posterolateral bundle is taut.

CRUCIATE LIGAMENTS/POSTERIOR CAPSULE

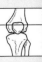
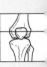

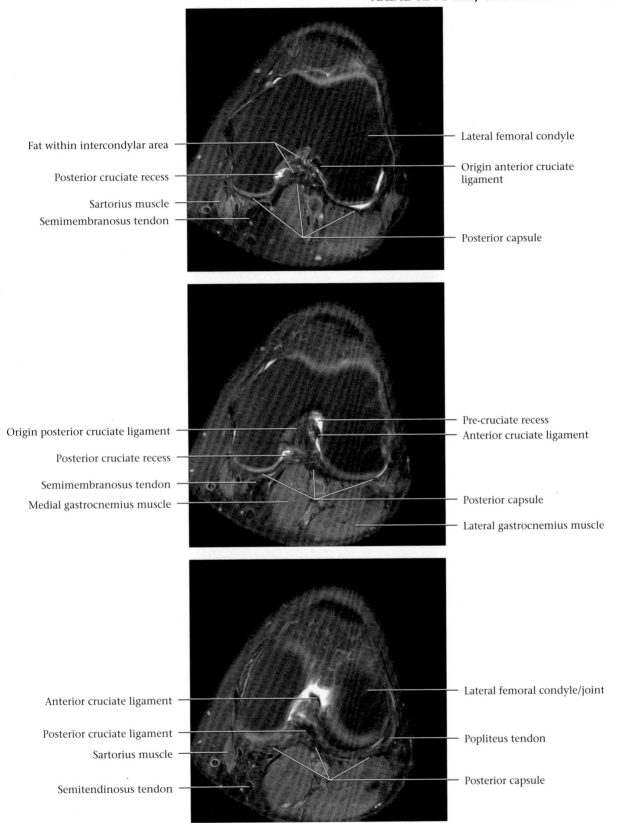

Fat within intercondylar area —

Posterior cruciate recess —

Sartorius muscle —

Semimembranosus tendon —

— Lateral femoral condyle

— Origin anterior cruciate ligament

— Posterior capsule

Origin posterior cruciate ligament —

Posterior cruciate recess —

Semimembranosus tendon —

Medial gastrocnemius muscle —

— Pre-cruciate recess

— Anterior cruciate ligament

— Posterior capsule

— Lateral gastrocnemius muscle

Anterior cruciate ligament —

Posterior cruciate ligament —

Sartorius muscle —

Semitendinosus tendon —

— Lateral femoral condyle/joint

— Popliteus tendon

— Posterior capsule

(Top) First of three axial T2 FS MR images shows the cruciate ligaments within the intercondylar notch. In the upper portion of the notch, the ACL is seen arising from the posterior aspect of the lateral femoral condyle within the notch. The remainder of the notch is filled with fat and a potential space (posterior cruciate bursa). **(Middle)** Axial cut through the mid portion of the intercondylar notch. The ACL extends obliquely towards its insertion on the tibial plateau. The origin of PCL is seen at the anterior medial femoral condyle within the notch. Fluid-filled recesses are seen anterior to the ACL and posteromedial to the PCL. **(Bottom)** Inferior portion of intercondylar notch shows ACL as it approaches insertion on tibial plateau. The PCL is still within capsule, but beginning to blend with it as it approaches insertion on posterior tibia. The cruciates are well seen axially.

Knee

VI

101

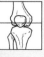

MR, VARIANTS AROUND CRUCIATE LIGAMENTS

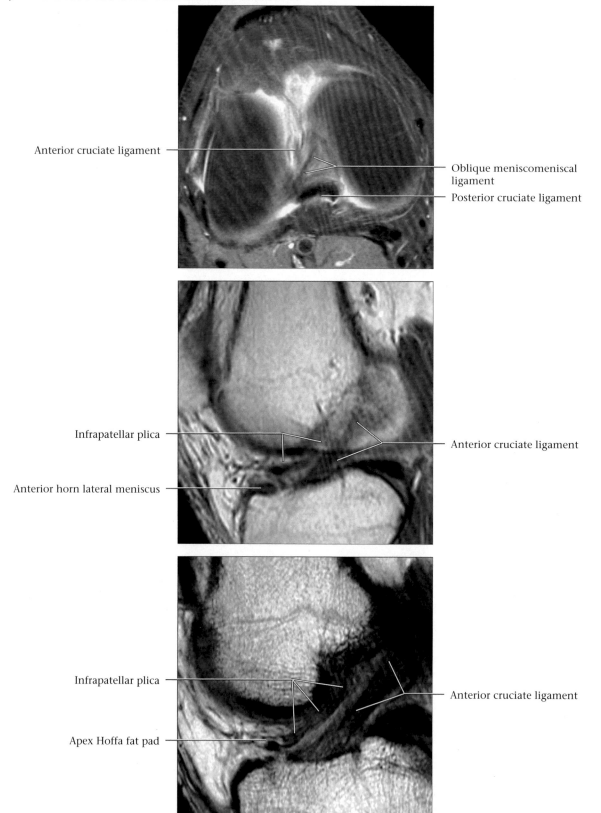

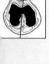

Anterior cruciate ligament

Oblique meniscomeniscal ligament

Posterior cruciate ligament

Infrapatellar plica

Anterior cruciate ligament

Anterior horn lateral meniscus

Infrapatellar plica

Anterior cruciate ligament

Apex Hoffa fat pad

(Top) Axial PD FS MR image through the femoral condyles, shows an oblique meniscomeniscal ligament. This uncommon variant connects the anterior horn of one meniscus with the posterior horn of the contralateral meniscus. It runs between the anterior and posterior cruciate ligaments. **(Middle)** Sagittal PD MR image through the intercondylar notch, shows the variant infrapatellar plica. This plica arises from the patella, extends across Hoffa fat pad, and along the anterior surface of anterior cruciate ligament. **(Bottom)** Sagittal PD MR through the intercondylar notch in another patient, shows an infrapatellar plica. The plica is seen extending through Hoffa fat pad, paralleling the curvature of the femoral condyle, and then paralleling the anterior cruciate ligament.

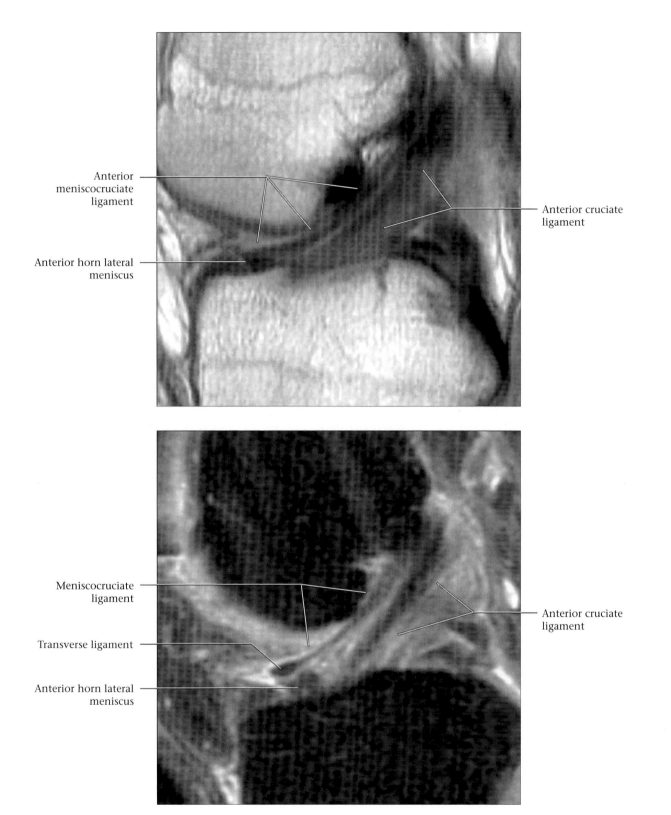

Anterior meniscocruciate ligament

Anterior horn lateral meniscus

Anterior cruciate ligament

Meniscocruciate ligament

Transverse ligament

Anterior horn lateral meniscus

Anterior cruciate ligament

(Top) Sagittal PD MR through the intercondylar notch, shows a meniscocruciate ligament. The ligament arises from the anterior horn medial meniscus and extends along the anterior surface of the anterior cruciate ligament to the femoral condyle. It could possibly be mistaken for a longitudinal tear in the anterior cruciate. (Bottom) Sagittal PD FS image in a different patient, showing another variant meniscocruciate ligament. This ligament is arising from the transverse ligament; as it extends parallel to and anterior to the anterior cruciate ligament, it could simulate a longitudinal or partial tear in this cruciate.

CORONAL PD FS MR IMAGES, VARIANT

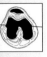

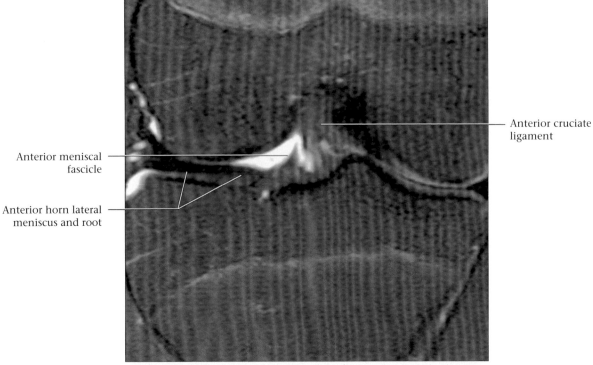

Anterior cruciate ligament

Anterior meniscal fascicle

Anterior horn lateral meniscus and root

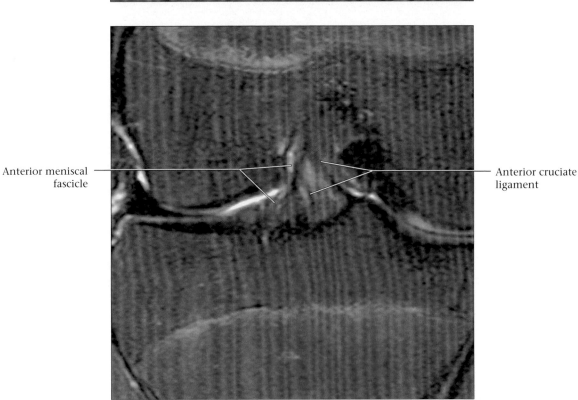

Anterior meniscal fascicle

Anterior cruciate ligament

(Top) First of two coronal PD FS MR images shows a variant anterior meniscal fascicle extending to the anterior cruciate ligament. The fascicle arises from the anterior horn lateral meniscus and its root. It then extends upward to merge with the synovium over the anterior cruciate ligament. In this anterior slice, the fascicle appears as a separate fiber. The anterior cruciate is in its normal position, extending from the lateral femoral condyle to its insertion adjacent to the medial tibial spine. **(Bottom)** Image is located slightly posterior to the previous image. The meniscal fascicle is seen extending from inferolateral to superomedial, an opposite angulation relative to the anterior cruciate. This is a potentially confusing appearance and should not be confused with cruciate pathology.

SAGITTAL & CORONAL MR, LIGAMENT OF WRISBERG

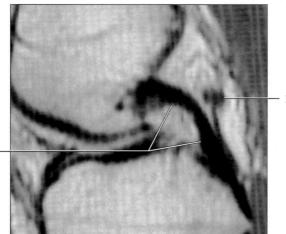

Ligament of Wrisberg

Posterior cruciate ligament

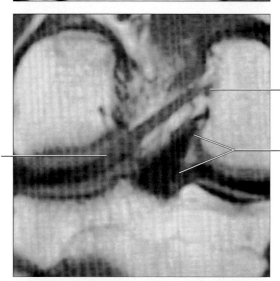

Origin ligament of Wrisberg, medial femoral condyle

Posterior cruciate ligament

Insertion ligament of Wrisberg, posterior horn lateral meniscus

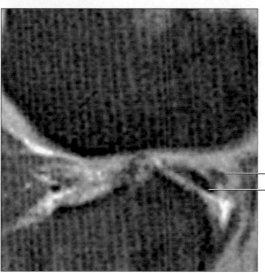

Ligament of Wrisberg

Posterior horn lateral meniscus

(Top) First of three images of the posterior cruciate ligament and the associated posterior meniscofemoral ligament (Wrisberg). Sagittal image through the posterior cruciate shows the ligament of Wrisberg in cross-section as it extends from the medial femoral condyle towards the posterior horn lateral meniscus. **(Middle)** Coronal PD MR image located posteriorly in the joint in the same patient as previous image, shows the ligament of Wrisberg paralleling the posterior cruciate ligament in its path from the medial femoral condyle to the posterior horn lateral meniscus. **(Bottom)** Sagittal PD FS MR image located in the lateral compartment immediately adjacent to the intercondylar notch, at the root of posterior horn lateral meniscus. The ligament of Wrisberg inserts at this point; just prior to the insertion, this appearance could give a false impression of meniscal tear.

AXIAL & CORONAL MR, LIGAMENT OF HUMPHREY

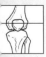

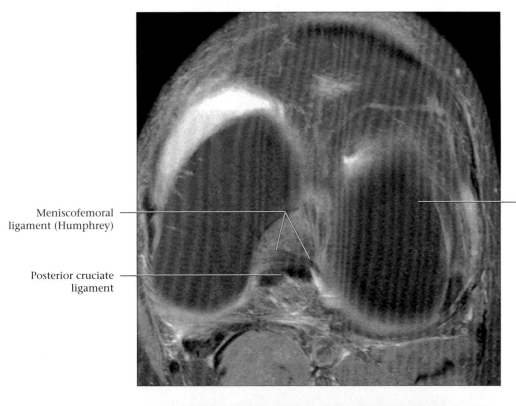

Meniscofemoral ligament (Humphrey) —

Posterior cruciate ligament —

— Lateral femoral condyle

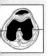

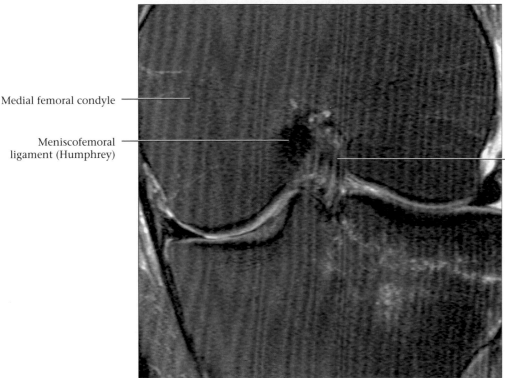

Medial femoral condyle —

Meniscofemoral ligament (Humphrey) —

— Anterior cruciate ligament

(Top) Axial PD FS MR, through the femoral condyles and intercondylar notch. The meniscofemoral ligament of Humphrey extends from the medial femoral condyle across in front of the posterior cruciate ligament towards its insertion on the posterior horn lateral meniscus. (Bottom) Coronal PD FS MR image shows the anterior cruciate ligament extending from the lateral femoral condyle toward the tibial spine. At the same level, there is a ligamentous structure arising from the medial femoral condyle. This is located slightly anteriorly to the origin of the posterior cruciate ligament, and is the meniscofemoral ligament of Humphrey.

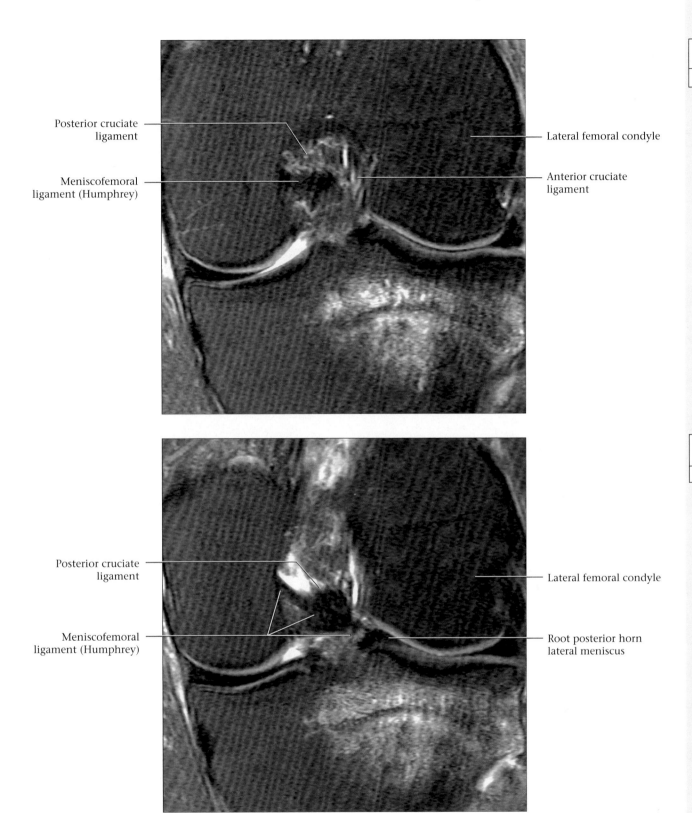

Posterior cruciate ligament — Lateral femoral condyle

Meniscofemoral ligament (Humphrey) — Anterior cruciate ligament

Posterior cruciate ligament — Lateral femoral condyle

Meniscofemoral ligament (Humphrey) — Root posterior horn lateral meniscus

(Top) Coronal PD FS MR image located slightly posterior to previous image. The intercondylar notch is quite full, containing the normally positioned anterior cruciate ligament as well as the origin of posterior cruciate ligament. The origin of meniscofemoral ligament of Humphrey is noted immediately anterior and inferior to that of posterior cruciate. **(Bottom)** This coronal image is located further posteriorly. This shows the meniscofemoral ligament of Humphrey crossing from the medial femoral condyle to insert on the root of posterior horn lateral meniscus. It crosses directly in front of posterior cruciate ligament. It is somewhat unusual to see it in its entirety on a single coronal image. Bone bruise on the lateral tibial plateau is incidentally seen in this example.

SAGITTAL PD MR, KNEE: LIGAMENT OF HUMPHREY

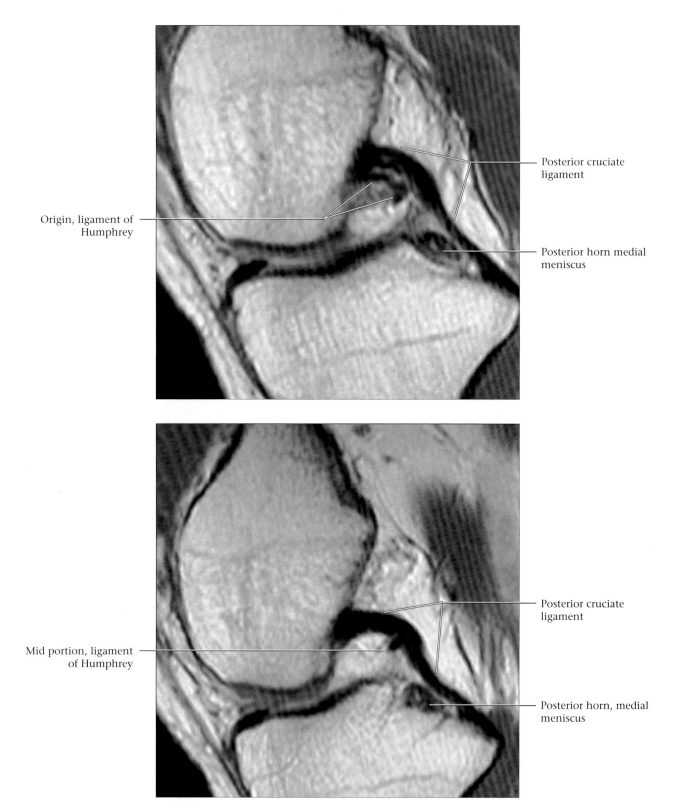

Posterior cruciate ligament

Origin, ligament of Humphrey

Posterior horn medial meniscus

Posterior cruciate ligament

Mid portion, ligament of Humphrey

Posterior horn, medial meniscus

(Top) First of four sagittal PD MR images shows meniscofemoral ligament of Humphrey. Image is medial within the intercondylar notch, at the level of the posterior cruciate ligament. The ligament of Humphrey is seen originating from the medial intercondylar notch, immediately inferior and anterior to the posterior cruciate ligament. **(Bottom)** This image, minimally lateral to the previous image, shows the ligament of Humphrey in cross-section, immediately inferior to the posterior cruciate ligament.

SAGITTAL PD MR, KNEE: LIGAMENT OF HUMPHREY

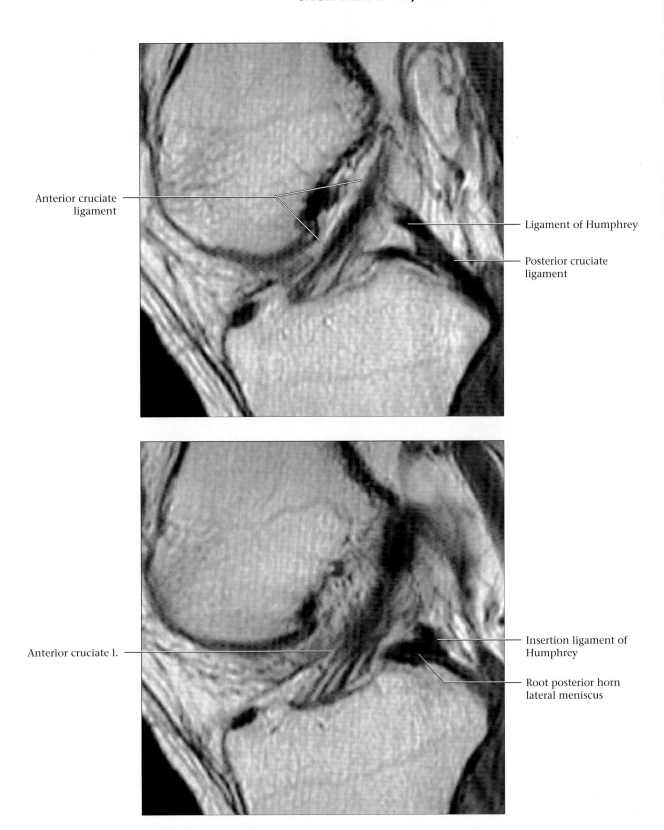

Anterior cruciate ligament

Ligament of Humphrey

Posterior cruciate ligament

Anterior cruciate l.

Insertion ligament of Humphrey

Root posterior horn lateral meniscus

(Top) This image is further lateral within the intercondylar notch compared with the previous two images. Fibers of both anterior and posterior cruciate ligament are seen. The ligament of Humphrey is still located anteroinferior to the posterior cruciate, extending towards the root of posterior horn lateral meniscus. **(Bottom)** Further lateral within the intercondylar notch, this image shows the termination of the ligament of Humphrey as it inserts on the posterior horn lateral meniscus at its root. This insertion may be mistaken for a loose body, meniscal fragment, or other abnormality if it is not correctly identified.

SAGITTAL GRAPHIC & PD MR, POSTERIOR FAR MEDIAL CAPSULE

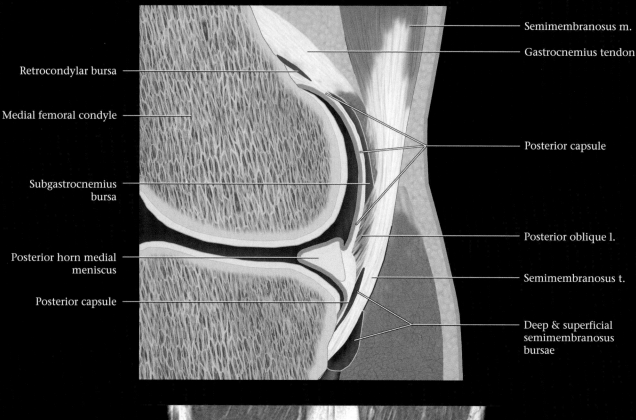

Semimembranosus m.

Gastrocnemius tendon

Retrocondylar bursa

Medial femoral condyle

Posterior capsule

Subgastrocnemius bursa

Posterior oblique l.

Posterior horn medial meniscus

Semimembranosus t.

Posterior capsule

Deep & superficial semimembranosus bursae

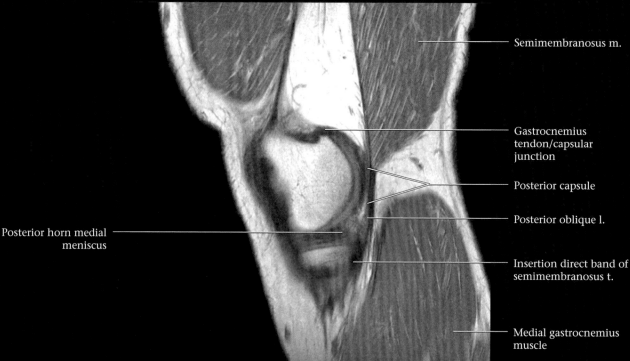

Semimembranosus m.

Gastrocnemius tendon/capsular junction

Posterior capsule

Posterior oblique l.

Posterior horn medial meniscus

Insertion direct band of semimembranosus t.

Medial gastrocnemius muscle

(Top) Graphic of the far medial portion of posterior capsule. The capsule proper is complete and the posterior horn of the meniscus attaches to it. Superiorly the capsule attaches to cortex of posterior femoral condyle, and then fuses with fibers of medial gastrocnemius. A portion of distal semimembranosus tendon contributes fibers to the oblique popliteal ligament; these continue as the posterior oblique ligament, contributing to the posterior capsule. Possible fluid collections in this area include the retrocondylar bursa superiorly, the subgastrocnemius bursa, and deep/superficial bursae on either side of semimembranosus tendon as it inserts on tibia. **(Bottom)** Sagittal PD MR image, located far medially, shows the contribution made by the semimembranosus tendon to posterior capsule. Note that the posterior horn medial meniscus blends directly into the posterior capsule.

SAGITTAL GRAPHIC & PD MR, MEDIAL POSTERIOR CAPSULE

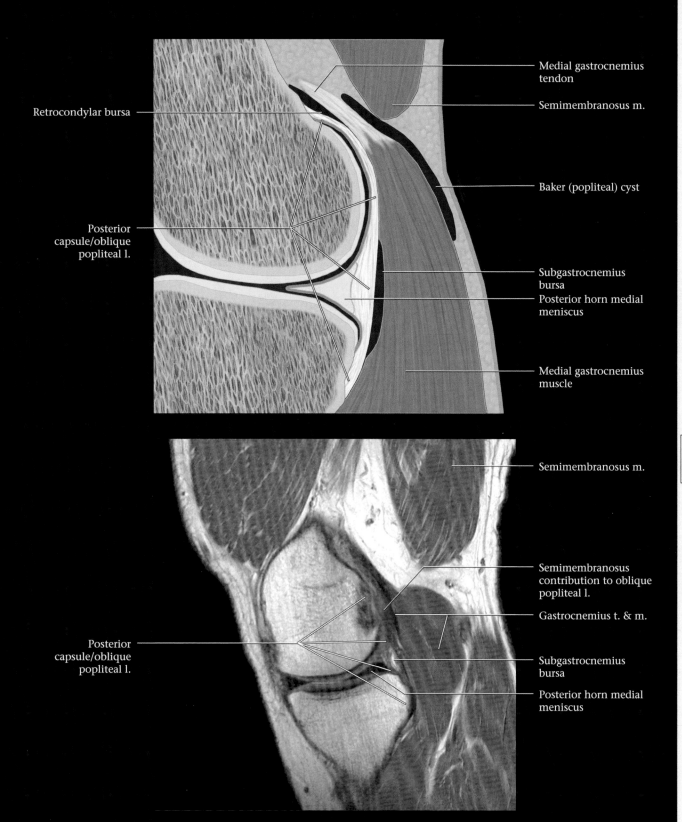

Retrocondylar bursa

Medial gastrocnemius tendon

Semimembranosus m.

Baker (popliteal) cyst

Posterior capsule/oblique popliteal l.

Subgastrocnemius bursa

Posterior horn medial meniscus

Medial gastrocnemius muscle

Semimembranosus m.

Semimembranosus contribution to oblique popliteal l.

Gastrocnemius t. & m.

Posterior capsule/oblique popliteal l.

Subgastrocnemius bursa

Posterior horn medial meniscus

(Top) Sagittal graphic medially in the joint. The capsule is fused superiorly with gastrocnemius tendon. A Baker (popliteal) cyst is shown at the gastrocnemius-semimembranosus bursa. The posterior horn medial meniscus is attached to posterior capsule, reinforced by oblique popliteal ligament. A small subgastrocnemius bursa is between capsule and gastrocnemius muscle; another is more superior between joint capsule and gastrocnemius tendon, the retrocondylar bursa. (Bottom) Sagittal image shows the posterior capsule to be inseparable from medial gastrocnemius tendon proximally. Behind the meniscal attachment to the capsule, however, there is a subgastrocnemius bursa separating the capsule and gastrocnemius muscle. This case does not show a Baker (popliteal) cyst, but if it were present, it would lie between the semimembranosus and gastrocnemius muscle bellies.

SAGITTAL GRAPHIC & PD MR, MID POSTERIOR CAPSULE

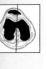

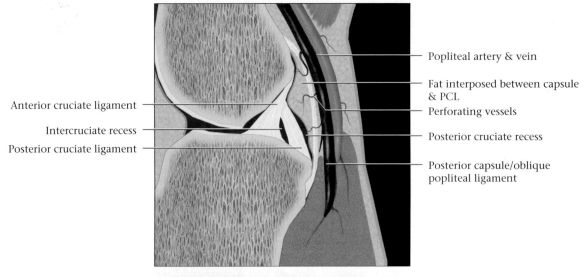

Anterior cruciate ligament

Intercruciate recess

Posterior cruciate ligament

Popliteal artery & vein

Fat interposed between capsule & PCL

Perforating vessels

Posterior cruciate recess

Posterior capsule/oblique popliteal ligament

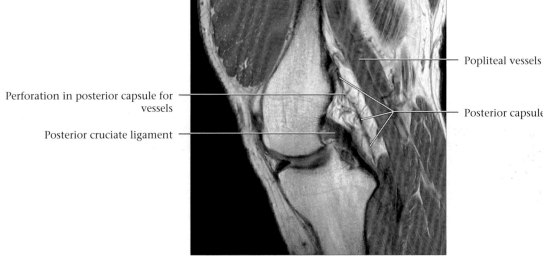

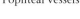

Perforation in posterior capsule for vessels

Posterior cruciate ligament

Popliteal vessels

Posterior capsule

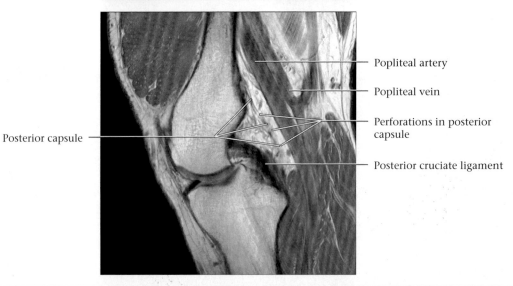

Posterior capsule

Popliteal artery

Popliteal vein

Perforations in posterior capsule

Posterior cruciate ligament

(Top) Graphic at the level of cruciate ligaments. The capsule, strengthened by the oblique popliteal ligament, extends from the posterior margin of femoral condyles to the intercondylar fossa at the tibia. It is incomplete, with several small perforations at its mid portion for vessels extending from the popliteals to the joint. The posterior cruciate recess is found between the capsule and the lower 2/3 of the PCL. There may be a small amount of fluid in the intercruciate recess. **(Middle)** Sagittal image through posterior cruciate, shows posterior capsule with only a small perforation for a vessel; the majority of the capsule appears complete. **(Bottom)** Immediately adjacent, slightly lateral sagittal image shows several more perforations in posterior capsule for vessels. The capsule is incomplete at this point, but is surrounded both anteriorly and posteriorly by fat.

CRUCIATE LIGAMENTS/POSTERIOR CAPSULE

SAGITTAL GRAPHIC & PD MR, LATERAL POSTERIOR CAPSULE

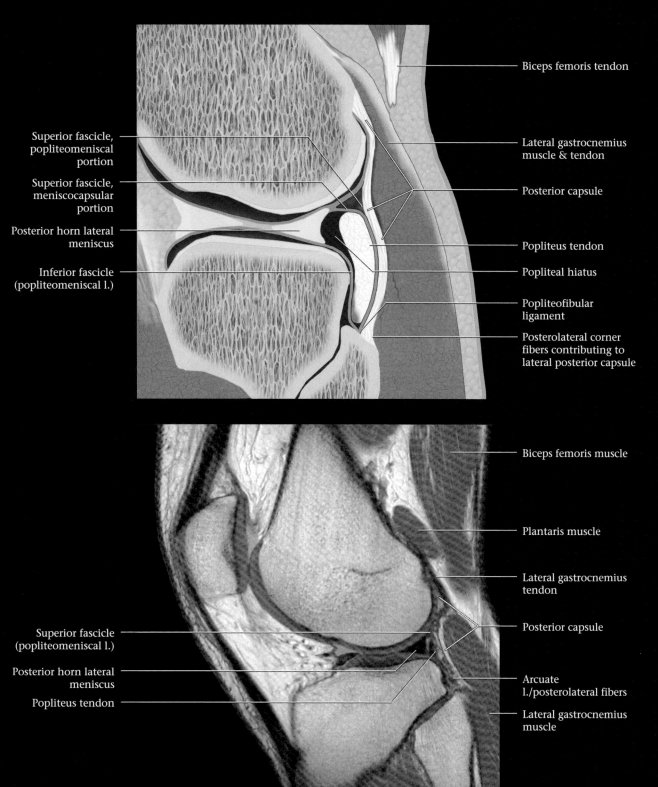

Superior fascicle, popliteomeniscal portion

Superior fascicle, meniscocapsular portion

Posterior horn lateral meniscus

Inferior fascicle (popliteomeniscal l.)

Biceps femoris tendon

Lateral gastrocnemius muscle & tendon

Posterior capsule

Popliteus tendon

Popliteal hiatus

Popliteofibular ligament

Posterolateral corner fibers contributing to lateral posterior capsule

Superior fascicle (popliteomeniscal l.)

Posterior horn lateral meniscus

Popliteus tendon

Biceps femoris muscle

Plantaris muscle

Lateral gastrocnemius tendon

Posterior capsule

Arcuate l./posterolateral fibers

Lateral gastrocnemius muscle

(Top) Graphic of lateral part of posterior capsule shows that it is intimately attached to lateral gastrocnemius muscle. The popliteus tendon is intra-articular but extrasynovial and is attached to capsule. Fibers from posterolateral corner and arcuate ligament originating from fibular head contribute to the lateral portion of the posterior capsule.
(Bottom) Sagittal MR image shows the gastrocnemius tendon contributing to posterior capsule, as well as the arcuate ligament (and fibers from other posterolateral structures). The popliteus tendon and superior fascicle (popliteomeniscal ligament) attach to capsule as well.

GRAPHIC & CT ARTHROGRAM, SPACES WITHIN POSTERIOR CAPSULE REGION

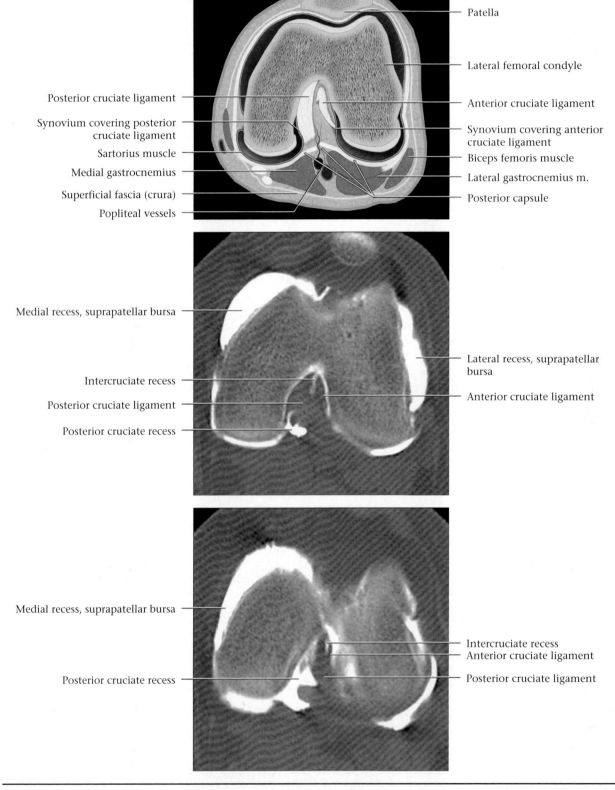

Patella

Lateral femoral condyle

Posterior cruciate ligament

Anterior cruciate ligament

Synovium covering posterior cruciate ligament

Synovium covering anterior cruciate ligament

Sartorius muscle

Biceps femoris muscle

Medial gastrocnemius

Lateral gastrocnemius m.

Superficial fascia (crura)

Posterior capsule

Popliteal vessels

Medial recess, suprapatellar bursa

Lateral recess, suprapatellar bursa

Intercruciate recess

Anterior cruciate ligament

Posterior cruciate ligament

Posterior cruciate recess

Medial recess, suprapatellar bursa

Intercruciate recess
Anterior cruciate ligament

Posterior cruciate recess

Posterior cruciate ligament

(Top) Graphic shows the relationships of the posterior capsule. The most superficial layer is the crural fascia, which envelops the sartorius and otherwise confines all the structures. The posterior capsule (white) is continuous with the synovium (pink, next to purple synovial fluid) both posteromedially and posterolaterally. However, at the intercondylar area, the synovium separates from the capsule and covers the cruciate ligaments. It is this feature that allows us to outline the cruciates with injected fluid; they are intra-articular but extrasynovial. Thus, at this intercondylar area, the posterior capsule has no synovial covering. The capsule continues across the posterior aspect of the joint, anterior to the popliteal vessels, and is interrupted by perforating vessels. (Middle) CT arthrogram, with fluid-filled spaces. (Bottom) Spaces seen more distally.

CRUCIATE LIGAMENTS/POSTERIOR CAPSULE

CT ARTHROGRAM, SPACES WITHIN CRUCIATE/POSTERIOR CAPSULE REGION

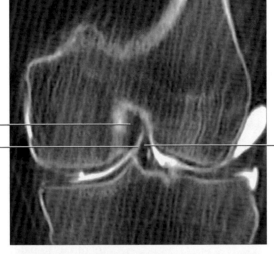

Origin posterior cruciate l.

Intercruciate recess

Anteromedial band anterior cruciate ligament

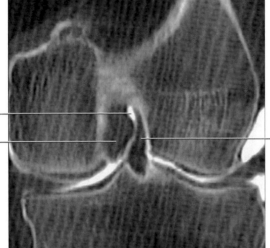

Intercruciate recess

Posterior cruciate ligament

Posterolateral band anterior cruciate ligament

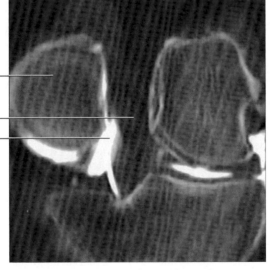

Medial femoral condyle

Posterior cruciate ligament

Posterior cruciate recess

(Top) First of three coronal reformatted images from CT arthrogram. With joint distension, the synovial-lined surfaces of the cruciate ligaments are outlined. In this more anterior cut, the anteromedial band of the ACL is primarily seen; only the origin of PCL is seen at the medial femoral condylar portion of the notch. There is an intercruciate recess that fills with joint distension. Incidental note is made of a focal cartilage defect in the medial femoral weight-bearing surface. **(Middle)** Slightly more posteriorly, both the posterolateral band of ACL and a larger portion of PCL are seen. The menisci are well outlined, and the intercruciate recess is again noted. **(Bottom)** More posteriorly, the PCL is seen approaching its posterior tibial insertion. The posterior cruciate recess contacts the distal 2/3 of PCL and flows into the medial (not lateral) compartment of the knee.

MEDIAL SUPPORT SYSTEM

Terminology

Abbreviations
- Medial (tibial) collateral ligament (MCL)
- Vastus medialis obliquus (VMO)
- Medial patellofemoral ligament (MPFL)

Imaging Anatomy

Overview
- Medial capsuloligamentous complex has **3 layers** that vary from anterior to mid to posterior; highly complex, with layers merging at different sites
- Primary stabilizers of femorotibial joint in valgus motion; secondary stabilizers to rotation
- Primary stabilizer against lateral subluxation/dislocation of patella

Superficial Layer (Layer 1)
- Primarily consists of **crural fascia**
- Anteriorly and superiorly, this crural fascia is continuous with fascia overlying vastus medialis
- **Sartorius** muscle/tendon enveloped by this fascia and is part of superficial layer
- Semimembranosus, semitendinosus, and gracilis are immediately deep to sartorius and superficial fascia
- Tendons of semitendinosus and gracilis blend with fascia of layer 1 and fibers of MCL as they insert distally on tibia
  - This means semitendinosus and gracilis cross just superficial to MCL (layer 2) and are between layers 1 and 2
  - Sartorius, semitendinosus, and gracilis together form pes anserinus at their insertion on anteromedial tibia, approximately 5 cm below joint line
    - Sartorius crosses medial knee joint anterior to gracilis, which in turn is anterior to semitendinosus
    - Sartorius has the broadest and most anterior insertion on tibia
    - Gracilis inserts directly adjacent to sartorius, with semitendinosus directly posterior and slightly inferior to gracilis

Middle Layer (Layer 2)
- **Anteriorly**, superficial (longitudinal) fibers of MCL (layer 2) merge with crural fascia (layer 1)
- **Mid knee**: Superficial fibers of MCL form layer 2
  - Vertical fibers
  - 12 cm long
  - 1-2 cm wide
  - 2-4 mm thick
  - Origin: Medial epicondyle
  - Courses slightly anteriorly to insert on tibia approximately 5 cm below joint line
  - Layer of fat containing medial inferior genicular artery lies between superficial MCL and tibia
- **Posteriorly**, superficial MCL has a posterior oblique component
  - Oblique fibers extend from layer 2 posteriorly and fuse with layer 3

- Attaches closely to posteromedial portion of meniscus; this conjoined structure is termed the posterior oblique ligament

Semimembranosus
- Complex insertion, involving both middle and deep layers
- Main portion inserts on posteromedial tibial plateau
- Other attachments
  - Tibia beneath MCL
  - Posteromedial capsule
  - Oblique popliteal ligament
  - Superficial fibers of MCL

Deep Layer (Layer 3)
- **Anterior**
  - Continuous with capsule along suprapatellar recess
  - Patellomeniscal ligament extends anteriorly from meniscus to patella margin
- **Mid knee**: Capsular layer, sometimes termed deep fibers of MCL
  - Capsule thickens to form these two ligaments
  - **Meniscofemoral**
    - 1-2 cm long
    - Extends from outer superior aspect of body of medial meniscus obliquely and proximally
    - Attaches to either superficial MCL or femur
  - **Meniscotibial (coronary ligament)**
    - Short (1 cm)
    - Extends from outer inferior aspect of body of medial meniscus to tibia just distal to joint line
    - Slightly more posterior than meniscofemoral
  - Capsular layers fuse posteriorly with oblique fibers of superficial MCL (no fat interposed) to form posterior oblique ligament
- **Posteriorly**, primarily capsule, but receives fibers from
  - Semimembranosus
  - Oblique fibers of superficial MCL (in the form of **posterior oblique ligament**)
  - **Oblique popliteal ligament**
    - Receives fibers from semimembranosus, superficial MCL (posterior oblique ligament), and synovial sheath
    - Envelops posterior aspect of femoral condyle to become a posterior structure

Bursa
- Variable amounts of fat between layers 1, 2 and 3
- May see a small bursa (MCL bursa) between superficial and deep layers of MCL
  - Requires fluid (distension) to be seen on MR
  - Bursa can extend to distal extent of superficial MCL, though usually is smaller, lying just over body of meniscus and deep fibers of MCL
  - Delineated anteriorly by anterior margin of superficial MCL
  - Delineated posteriorly by merger of superficial and deep fibers of MCL
- Another bursa separates semimembranosus tendon from posterior capsule

Medial Stabilizers of Patella
- Loosely termed medial retinaculum

- Extends from vastus medialis superiorly to tibia inferiorly
- Inserts along medial edge of patella
- Highly complex, with **3 layers** which differ in superior, mid, and inferior portions
  - **Layer 1** is most superficial, just deep to subcutaneous tissues
    - Deep crural fascia
    - Anterosuperiorly, continuous with fascia overlying vastus medialis
  - **Layer 2** is just deep to layer 1, and just superficial to layer 3 (joint capsule)
  - Within layers 2 and 3, condensations of fibers form ligaments of **medial retinacular complex**
  - Within layer 2, medial retinacular complex ligaments form an inverted triangle in sagittal plane, with a central split which defines 3 separate ligaments
    - MPFL: Superior aspect of triangle
    - Superficial MCL: Posterior aspect of triangle
    - Patellotibial ligament: Anteroinferior aspect of triangle
  - **Layer 3**: Joint capsule
- **Superior** portion of medial patellar stabilizers
  - **Vastus medialis obliquus**
    - Inferior portion of vastus medialis
    - Acts as a dynamic stabilizer, neutralizing the lateralizing forces on patella exerted by vastus lateralis during quadriceps contraction
    - Arises from adductor magnus tendon, medial intermuscular septum, or adductor tubercle
    - Merges with MPFL and inserts on superior 2/3 of medial patella
  - **Medial patellofemoral ligament**
    - Major ligamentous restraint preventing lateral patellar subluxation (50-60% total restraining force)
    - Origin is variable: Adductor tubercle, medial epicondyle, or superficial MCL
    - Runs forward and slightly inferiorly, just deep to VMO, fuses with aponeurosis of VMO
    - Inserts on superior 2/3 of medial patella; seen as distinct structure at insertion
    - Length 4.5-6 cm
    - < 0.5 cm thick
    - Width 1-2 cm at femur, 2-3 cm at patella
    - Merges with layer 2 (medial retinaculum) inferiorly
- **Mid portion** of medial patellar stabilizers
  - Superficial MCL (layer 2), fuses with crural fascia (layer 1) to form medial retinaculum (proper) anteriorly
  - Merges with VMO fascia anteriorly
  - Inserts into medial margin of patella
- **Inferior portion** of medial patellar stabilizers
  - Patellotibial ligament
    - Originates on tibia at level of insertion of gracilis and semitendinosus
    - Joins layer 1 and extends obliquely proximally to insert on inferior aspect of patella and on patellar tendon
  - Medial patellomeniscal ligament

- Deep in relation to patellotibial ligament (anatomically in layer 3)

Posteromedial Capsule

- **Medial side of posterior capsule**: Fibers from several structures merge with and contribute to capsule
  - Fibers from distal semimembranosus tendon, forming oblique popliteal ligament
  - Fibers from superficial MCL, forming posterior oblique ligament, which also contribute to oblique popliteal ligament
  - Capsule attaches to posterior femoral cortex a few cm above the level of the most superior aspect of cartilage
  - Capsule attaches inferiorly to tibia 1-2 cm below joint line
  - A bursa separates capsule and semimembranosus tendon
  - A little more towards center of knee, semimembranosus is replaced by medial gastrocnemius
  - Superiorly, capsule joins gastrocnemius tendon
- **Mid portion of posterior capsule**
  - Capsule is incomplete posteriorly
  - Therefore intraarticular space is not completely separate from extraarticular fat
  - Popliteal artery and vein course behind capsule
    - Perforating vessels extend from these through posterior capsule
    - Perforating nerves accompany vessels

Anatomy-Based Imaging Issues

Imaging Recommendations

- Superficial MCL: Coronal and axial
- Capsular layers (deep MCL): Coronal
- MPFL and VMO best seen on axials immediately inferior to adductor tubercle
  - MPFL seen at its origin in 80%
  - MPFL seen at patellar insertion in 100%
- Medial retinaculum seen just inferior to MPFL/VMO, also on axials
  - Medial retinaculum seen at midsubstance and patellar insertion in 100%
- Patellotibial and medial patellomeniscal meniscal ligaments seen at level of knee joint, on axials
- Oblique popliteal ligament envelops posterior aspect of femoral condyle, best seen on axials
  - Seen 100% on axial MR

Selected References

1. Elias D et al: Acute lateral patellar dislocation at MR imaging: injury patterns of medial patellar soft-tissue restraints and osteochondral injuries of the inferomedial patella. Radiology. 225:736-43, 2002
2. De Maeseneer M et al: Three layers of the medial capsular and supporting structures of the knee: MR imaging-anatomic correlation. Radiographics. 20:S83-S89, 2000
3. Spritzer C et al: Medial retinacular complex injury in acute patellar dislocation: MR findings. AJR. 168:117-22, 1997

GRAPHIC & SAGITTAL T1 MR, MEDIAL KNEE: PES ANSERINUS

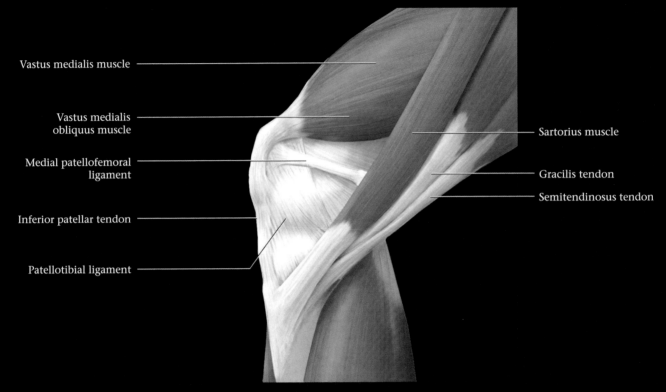

Vastus medialis muscle

Vastus medialis obliquus muscle

Medial patellofemoral ligament

Inferior patellar tendon

Patellotibial ligament

Sartorius muscle

Gracilis tendon

Semitendinosus tendon

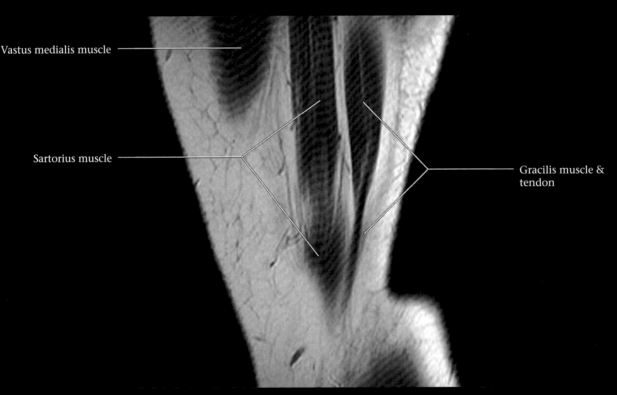

Vastus medialis muscle

Sartorius muscle

Gracilis muscle & tendon

(Top) Graphic shows the anteromedial attachment of the pes anserinus tendons. Sartorius is most anterior & superficial. Gracilis inserts directly adjacent & deep to sartorius & semitendinosus inserts directly posterior & slightly inferior to gracilis. These tendons & their crural fascia compprise the superficial layer of the medial capsuloligamentous complex. **(Bottom)** First of four sagittal T1 MR images, starting far medially, shows the components of pes anserinus. The sartorius has a straight course above the knee joint, directly medial to the knee. Sartorius is invested by the crural fascia to form layer 1 of the medial capsuloligamentous complex. Gracilis maintains its position slightly posterior and deep to sartorius.

MEDIAL SUPPORT SYSTEM

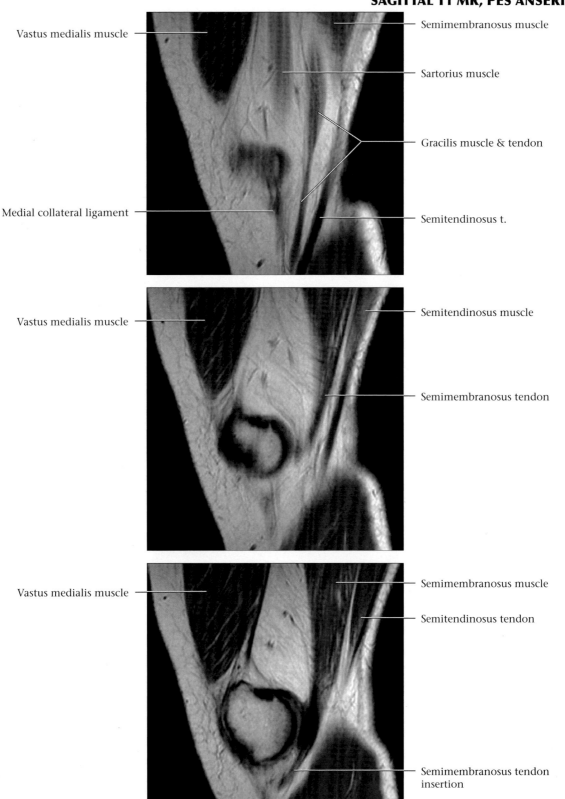

Vastus medialis muscle — Semimembranosus muscle

— Sartorius muscle

— Gracilis muscle & tendon

Medial collateral ligament — Semitendinosus t.

Vastus medialis muscle — Semitendinosus muscle

— Semimembranosus tendon

Vastus medialis muscle — Semimembranosus muscle

— Semitendinosus tendon

— Semimembranosus tendon insertion

(Top) Slightly more medial cut shows a remnant of sartorius. Gracilis tendon is immediately posterior and deep to sartorius. Semitendinosus tendon follows even more posteriorly and medially. **(Middle)** Further medially, the semimembranosus muscle and tendon are seen, with semitendinosus muscle and tendon remain behind them. While the semitendinosus continues its course, following gracilis towards its anteromedial tibial insertion, semimembranosus inserts at the proximal tibia posteriorly and medially. **(Bottom)** Approaching the tibia with a more medial section, semimembranosus is seen to broaden at its tendinous insertion on the posterior as well as medial tibia, immediately below the joint line. The slips from semimembranosus to medial collateral ligament and posterior capsule via the posterior oblique ligament are not seen as separate structures here.

Knee

VI

CORONAL T1 MR, PES ANSERINUS

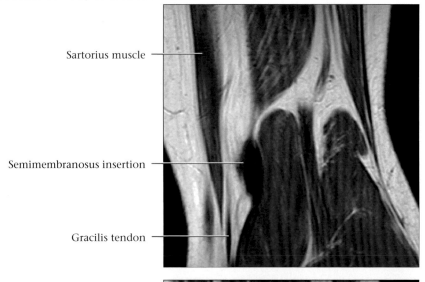

Sartorius muscle

Semimembranosus insertion

Gracilis tendon

Semimembranosus muscle

Gracilis muscle

Sartorius tendon

Semitendinosus tendon

Gracilis muscle

Semimembranosus muscle

Semitendinosus muscle & tendon

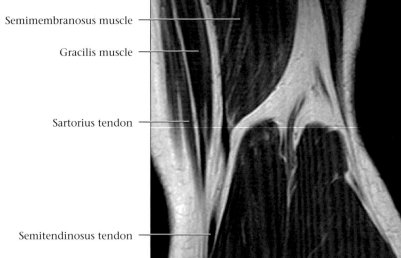

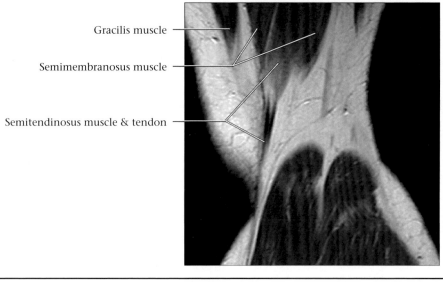

(Top) First of three coronal T1 MR images through the posterior portion of the joint, shows the medial-lateral relationships of the tendons comprising the pes anserinus. At the level of the popliteal vessels, just posterior to the tibia, the semimembranosus spreads out into its insertion, which is wide at the posterior as well as posteromedial tibia. The sartorius muscle is seen at this level, with its tendon curving anteriorly out of the plane. A porion of gracilis tendon is seen paralleling and deep to sartorius tendon. (Middle) Slightly more posteriorly, a remnant of sartorius is seen, but gracilis muscle & tendon are more completely seen. A very small portion of semitendinosus tendon is seen distally, behind & medial to gracilis. (Bottom) Even more posteriorly, semitendinosus muscle & tendon are shown posterior to the muscle belly of semimembranosus.

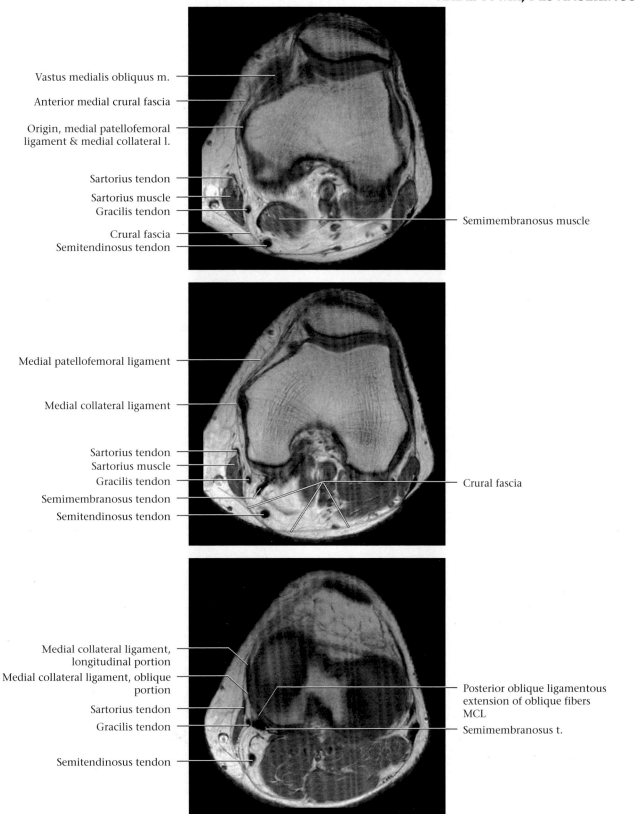

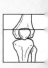
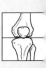

(Top) First of three axial T1 MR images shows the anatomy of pes anserinus. Sartorius is the most superficial. It is invested by crural fascia to form layer 1. Gracilis tendon is medial to sartorius and follows its tendon in a slightly posterior position. Semitendinosus is posterior to semimembranosus, and distinctly posterior and medial to gracilis tendon. **(Middle)** Superficial MCL arises distal to adductor tubercle and forms layer 2. **(Bottom)** At the level of the joint line, the elements of the pes line up in order (sartorius, gracilis, semitendinosus) of their insertion on the anteromedial tibia. Anteriorly, layers 1 (sartorius) and 2 (superficial MCL) merge to contribute to medial retinaculum. Gracilis & semitendinosus lie between layers 1 & 2. Posteriorly, layers 2 & 3 (superficial & deep MCL, respectively) merge to form the posterior oblique ligament, contributing to capsule.

Knee

VI

GRAPHIC, POSTEROMEDIAL STRUCTURES

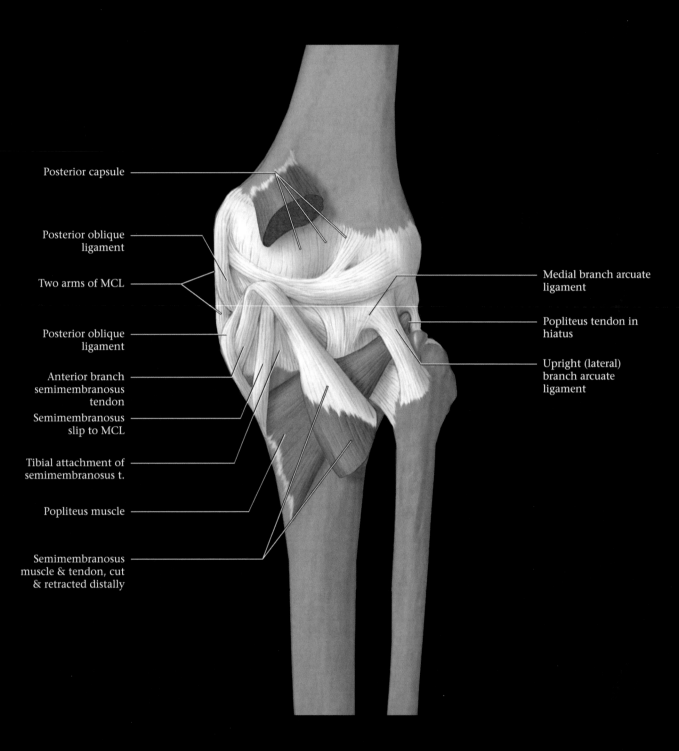

Posterior capsule

Posterior oblique ligament

Two arms of MCL

Posterior oblique ligament

Anterior branch semimembranosus tendon

Semimembranosus slip to MCL

Tibial attachment of semimembranosus t.

Popliteus muscle

Semimembranosus muscle & tendon, cut & retracted distally

Medial branch arcuate ligament

Popliteus tendon in hiatus

Upright (lateral) branch arcuate ligament

The semimembranosus tendon has a complex insertion, both at the posteromedial tibia and more anteriorly at the medial tibia. Semimembranosus also provides slips to the posterior aspect of MCL, as well as providing an expansion to the oblique popliteal ligament. The posterior oblique ligament arises from several arms of the superficial MCL, both superiorly and inferiorly, as well as from the posterior aspect of the deep MCL (therefore both layers 2 and 3 contribute to it). The posterior oblique ligament then extends from its posteromedial position to contribute to the oblique popliteal ligament, which in turn strengthens the posterior capsule. On the lateral side, fibers from the arcuate ligament blend into and contribute to oblique popliteal ligament as well.

MEDIAL SUPPORT SYSTEM

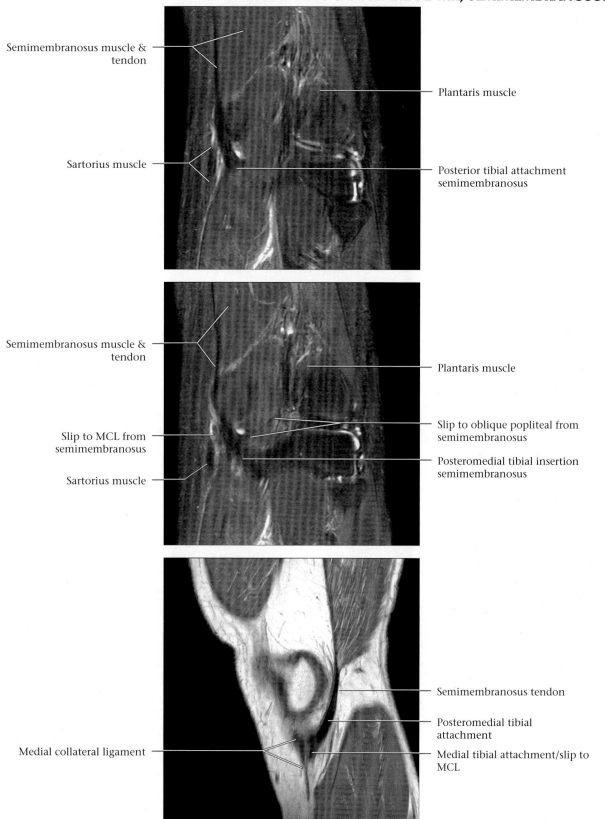

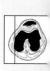

Semimembranosus muscle & tendon

Plantaris muscle

Sartorius muscle

Posterior tibial attachment semimembranosus

Semimembranosus muscle & tendon

Plantaris muscle

Slip to MCL from semimembranosus

Slip to oblique popliteal from semimembranosus

Posteromedial tibial insertion semimembranosus

Sartorius muscle

Semimembranosus tendon

Posteromedial tibial attachment

Medial collateral ligament

Medial tibial attachment/slip to MCL

(Top) First of two posterior coronal T2 FS images shows semimembranosus insertion at the posteromedial tibia. **(Middle)** Slightly more anterior cut shows the multiple slips of semimembranosus. These include insertions at the posteromedial tibia, and another more directly medially. Additionally, there are slips extending from semimembranosus to the oblique popliteal and medial collateral ligaments. **(Bottom)** Sagittal PD MR image shows semimembranosus insertion on the posteromedial tibia, along with its slip extending to the medial collateral ligament.

CORONAL GRAPHIC AT JOINT LINE & CORONAL PD FS MR, MEDIAL COLLATERAL LIGAMENT

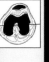

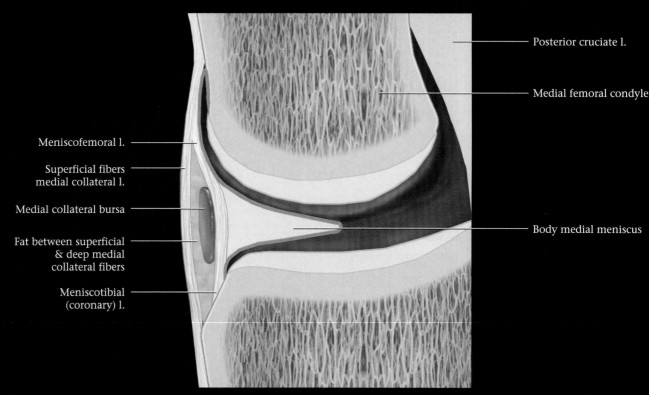

Posterior cruciate l.

Medial femoral condyle

Meniscofemoral l.

Superficial fibers medial collateral l.

Medial collateral bursa

Fat between superficial & deep medial collateral fibers

Meniscotibial (coronary) l.

Body medial meniscus

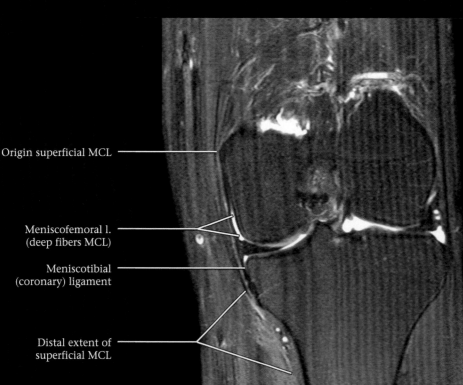

Origin superficial MCL

Meniscofemoral l. (deep fibers MCL)

Meniscotibial (coronary) ligament

Distal extent of superficial MCL

(Top) Coronal graphic at mid joint, shows the relationship of deep & superficial fibers of medial collateral ligament. Superficial fibers extend from adjacent to adductor tubercle to approximately 5 cm distal to joint line. Deep fibers are much shorter: Meniscotibial (coronary) ligament extends from meniscus to tibia adjacent to joint line & meniscofemoral ligament extends from meniscus to either femur or superficial MCL. A variable amount of fat and a small bursa may be seen between deep & superficial fibers. (Bottom) Coronal shows the deep medial collateral fibers, outlined by joint fluid. The meniscofemoral ligament inserts on the femur; it may also normally insert on the superficial MCL at the same level above the joint. The short coronary (meniscotibial) ligament is seen. Superficial MCL is only faintly seen due to the fat-saturation. There is no bursal fluid.

GRAPHIC & AXIAL T1 MR, MEDIAL CAPSULOLIGAMENTOUS COMPLEX

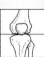

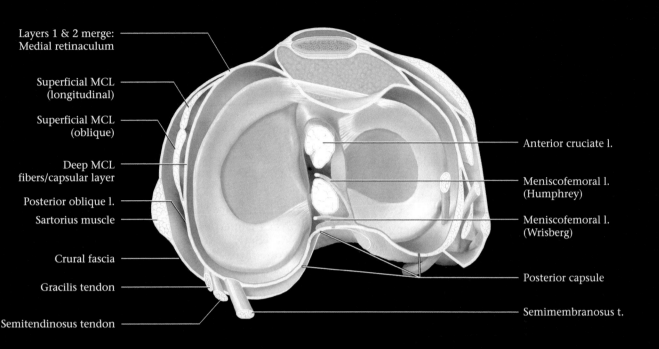

Layers 1 & 2 merge:
Medial retinaculum

Superficial MCL
(longitudinal)

Superficial MCL
(oblique)

Deep MCL
fibers/capsular layer

Posterior oblique l.

Sartorius muscle

Crural fascia

Gracilis tendon

Semitendinosus tendon

Anterior cruciate l.

Meniscofemoral l.
(Humphrey)

Meniscofemoral l.
(Wrisberg)

Posterior capsule

Semimembranosus t.

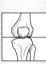

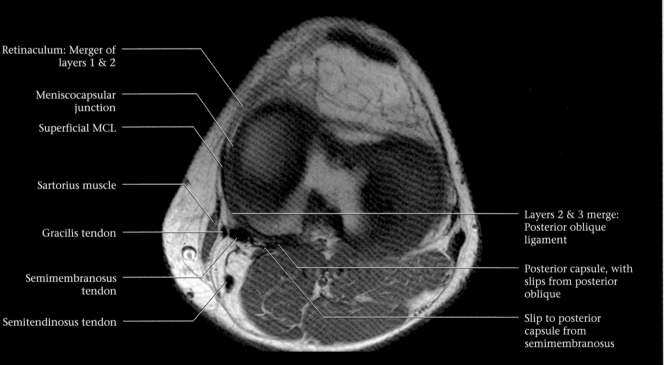

Retinaculum: Merger of
layers 1 & 2

Meniscocapsular
junction

Superficial MCL

Sartorius muscle

Gracilis tendon

Semimembranosus
tendon

Semitendinosus tendon

Layers 2 & 3 merge:
Posterior oblique
ligament

Posterior capsule, with
slips from posterior
oblique

Slip to posterior
capsule from
semimembranosus

(Top) Graphic shows 3 layers of medial capsuloligamentous complex. Layer 1 consists of crural fascia, which envelops sartorius. Superficial fibers of MCL form layer 2. Layers 1 & 2 merge anteriorly to contribute to medial retinaculum. Gracilis & semitendinosus lie between suyers 1 & 2. Posteriorly, superficial MCL fibers (layer 2) fuse with deep MCL fibers (layer 3) to form posterior oblique ligament; this ligament contributes to the posterior capsule at its posteromedial aspect. **(Bottom)** Axial T1 MR shows some of the complexity of the posteromedial structures, including the elements of the pes anserinus as well as the various attachments and slips of the semimembranosus tendon. Note in this example the slip from semimembranosus extending to the posterior oblique ligament & posterior capsule.

LATERAL SUPPORTING STRUCTURES

Terminology

Abbreviations
- Iliotibial (IT) tract
- Lateral (fibular) collateral ligament (LCL)

Synonyms
- Popliteofibular = short external lateral ligament = fibular origin of popliteus = popliteofibular fascicles

Imaging Anatomy

Overview
- Combination of muscles, tendons, and ligaments which contribute to lateral stability of knee

Muscles Contributing to Lateral Stability
- **Iliotibial tract**
  - **Origin**: Strong band of deep fascia composed of the fusion of aponeurotic coverings of
    - Tensor fascia lata
    - Gluteus maximus
    - Gluteus minimus
  - Above knee, IT tract has insertion arms to
    - Supracondylar tubercle of lateral femoral condyle
    - Blends with intermuscular septum
  - **Main insertion**
    - Gerdy tubercle (anterolateral tibia near plateau)
    - Small other attachments to patella and patellar ligament
- **Biceps femoris**
  - Long head joined by short head above knee
  - **Main insertion** site is head and styloid process fibula
  - Several tendinous and fascial insertional components, including a portion that inserts on posterior edge of IT tract
  - Anterior oblique fibers of conjoined tendon arise from anterior bundle of short head biceps and insert on tibia
- **Popliteus**
  - Tendinous attachment at **popliteal sulcus** of lateral femoral condyle
    - Inferior and deep to origin of LCL
  - Extends posteromedially through **popliteal hiatus** (runs deep to fabellofibular and arcuate ligaments)
  - **Superior popliteomeniscal fascicle** extends from posterior horn lateral meniscus to paratenon tissues of popliteus tendon
    - Superior popliteomeniscal fascicle and arcuate ligament form **roof of popliteal hiatus**
  - **Inferior popliteomeniscal fascicle** extends from posterior horn lateral meniscus to paratenon tissues of popliteus tendon
    - Inferior popliteomeniscal fascicle forms **floor of popliteal hiatus**
  - Superior and inferior fascicles join and insert on fibular styloid as **popliteofibular ligament**
  - **Popliteus muscle** attaches to posteromedial aspect of proximal tibial metaphysis
  - **Function** of popliteus muscle
    - Assist with flexion of knee
    - Internally rotates tibia on femur (at initiation of flexion of knee)
    - Protects posterior horn lateral meniscus by withdrawing it from joint space during flexion and rotation
    - Stabilizes posterolateral corner from rotatory instability

Posterolateral Capsule
- Arcuate ligament fibers contribute to capsule laterally
- Popliteal tendon (intraarticular but extrasynovial) firmly attached to posterior capsule
- Popliteal recess may extend deeply behind tibia (in front of capsule); may have continuity with proximal tibiofibular joint
- Lateral gastrocnemius muscle contributes fibers to capsule

Lateral Support System Consists of 3 Layers
- **Layer 1 (superficial)**
  - Anteriorly, IT tract
  - Posterolaterally, superficial portion of biceps
- **Layer 2 (middle)**
  - Anteriorly, lateral retinaculum
  - 2 ligamentous thickenings originate from lateral patella
    - Proximal one terminates at lateral intermuscular septum
    - Distal one terminates at femoral insertion of posterolateral capsule and lateral head of gastrocnemius tendon
- **Layer 3 (deep)**
  - Forms lateral part of capsule
  - Contains several thickenings that function as discrete structures
    - Lateral (fibular) collateral ligament
    - Arcuate complex, consisting of multiple ligaments
  - Posterolateral corner ligament anatomy is extremely complex

Posterolateral Corner Structures
- All insert on fibular head and provide posterolateral support
- Not all are seen with equal reliability on imaging (see "Anatomy-Based Imaging Issues" below)
- Posterolateral corner structures may be divided into superficial and deep
  - Superficial: Long and short heads of biceps femoris, and LCL
  - Deep: Posterolateral reinforcements of fibrous capsule, including fabellofibular, arcuate, oblique popliteal, and popliteofibular ligaments
- **Long head of biceps femoris**
  - 2 major tendinous components
    - Direct arm inserts on fibular head
    - Anterior arm inserts just anterior to direct arm on fibular head and continues distally as the anterior aponeurosis that extends anterolaterally around leg
- **Short head of biceps femoris**
  - 2 tendinous components
    - Direct arm inserts on fibular head anterior to styloid process and medial to long head biceps

- ■ Anterior arm passes medial to lateral collateral ligament and inserts into superolateral edge of lateral tibial condyle, approaching Gerdy tubercle
- Lateral collateral ligament
  - ○ Proximal attachment at distal femur just proximal and posterior to lateral epicondyle
  - ○ Proximal attachment is slightly proximal and anterior to sulcus for origin of popliteus tendon
  - ○ LCL extends posterolaterally to insert on upper facet of fibular head
    - ■ Anterolateral to attachment of fabellofibular and arcuate ligaments
- Fabellofibular ligament
  - ○ Originates at fabella (or proximal to it)
  - ○ Inserts at lateral aspect of apex of fibular head (styloid process)
  - ○ Inserts just anterolateral to insertion of popliteofibular ligament on fibular head
  - ○ Fabellofibular ligament may be dominant when arcuate is diminutive
- Arcuate ligament
  - ○ Y-shaped
  - ○ Arises from fibular styloid process, just deep to fabellofibular ligament
  - ○ Lateral limb courses straight upward along lateral knee capsule to reach lateral femoral condyle
  - ○ Medial limb crosses over posterior surface of popliteal tendon and attaches to posterior knee capsule
    - ■ Medial limb, along with superior popliteomeniscal fascicle, forms bowed roof of popliteal hiatus
    - ■ At insertion on posterior knee capsule, medial limb arcuate merges with fibers from oblique popliteal ligament
  - ○ Arcuate may be dominant when fabellofibular is absent (or may contain fibers of fabellofibular ligament)
  - ○ Inferior lateral geniculate artery passes anterior relative to arcuate
- Oblique popliteal ligament
  - ○ Arises medially from slips of semimembranosus and medial tibial condyle, courses superolaterally; see "Medial Support System" section
  - ○ Joins arcuate ligament posterolaterally at its femoral insertion (margin of intercondylar fossa and posterior surface of lateral femoral condyle)
- Popliteofibular ligament
  - ○ Arises from confluence of superior & inferior fascicles
  - ○ Inserts on fibular head (see "popliteus" above)
  - ○ Popliteofibular ligament may be dominant, with neither arcuate or fabellofibular ligaments present

Anatomy-Based Imaging Issues

Imaging Recommendations

- Crucial posterolateral structures seen on axial and routine oblique sagittal imaging (generally prescribed on axial, obliqued along course of anterior cruciate l.)
- Coronal oblique suggested to increase probability of visualizing posterolateral structures
  - ○ Prescribed off sagittal image

- ○ Obliquity runs anterosuperior to posteroinferior, generally parallel to popliteal tendon as seen on sagittals

Imaging "Sweet Spots"

- Statistics below based on 1.5T MR imaging
- Biceps seen well in all 3 planes, 100%
  - ○ Individual components may be seen separately on axials near fibular attachment
    - ■ Short head biceps, direct arm 70%
    - ■ Long head biceps, direct and anterior arms 70%
- LCL seen well in all 3 planes, 100%
- Superior popliteomeniscal fascicle seen best on sagittal fluid sensitive sequence, at level of posterior horn lateral meniscus; 100%
- Inferior popliteomeniscal fascicle seen best on coronal fluid sensitive sequence, at level of body lateral meniscus; 100%
- Arcuate ligament
  - ○ In cadaver study, at least 1 limb seen in 70% on sagittal or coronal MR
    - ■ Lateral limb arcuate seen 57% (better when fabella absent)
    - ■ Medial limb arcuate seen 57% (better when fabella present)
  - ○ Coronal oblique MR may increase likelihood
- Fabellofibular ligament rarely seen as separate entity (coronal or sagittal)
- Popliteofibular ligament
  - ○ In cadaver study, seen 57% using coronal oblique (38% with standard planes)
- Oblique popliteal ligament 100%, axial

Avulsion Fractures at Posterolateral Corner

- "Arcuate sign"
  - ○ Thin sliver avulsion at posterosuperior portion of fibular styloid
  - ○ Site of (near) common insertion of fabellofibular, popliteofibular, and arcuate ligaments
  - ○ Marrow edema may also indicate injury at this site
  - ○ Posterior cruciate ligament injury is often associated
- Anterolateral femoral head avulsion (not fibular styloid)
  - ○ LCL/biceps avulsion

Clinical Implications

Clinical Importance

- Posterolateral structures act primarily as static constraints to varus angulation and external rotation of knee
- Secondary restraint against posterior translation of tibia

Biomechanical Selective Cutting Study

- Major structures preventing posterolateral instability are LCL and popliteus tendon
- Popliteofibular ligament also important in providing static stability
- Surgery primarily focuses on restoring these ligaments
- Identifying popliteofibular on MR is variable (even with coronal oblique)
  - ○ Limitation in assessing posterolateral corner injuries

GRAPHIC & AXIAL T1 MR, POSTEROLATERAL CORNER

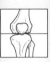

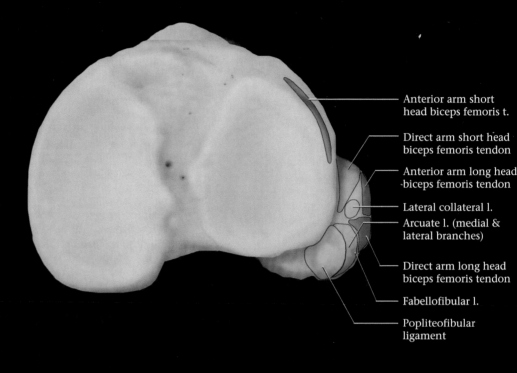

Anterior arm short head biceps femoris t.

Direct arm short head biceps femoris tendon

Anterior arm long head biceps femoris tendon

Lateral collateral l.

Arcuate l. (medial & lateral branches)

Direct arm long head biceps femoris tendon

Fabellofibular l.

Popliteofibular ligament

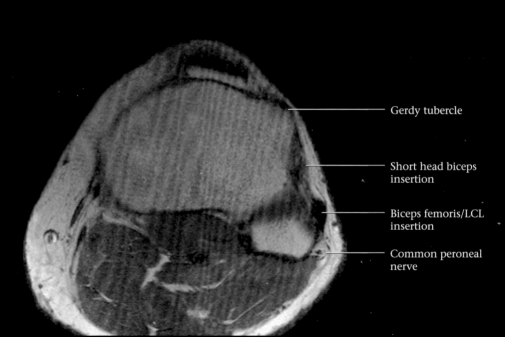

Gerdy tubercle

Short head biceps insertion

Biceps femoris/LCL insertion

Common peroneal nerve

(Top) Graphic shows insertion sites of posterolateral structures on the proximal fibula. Note that the 2 heads of short head biceps femoris insert most anteriorly, with lateral collateral ligament and 2 heads long head biceps femoris directly posterior to that. The arcuate, fabellofibular, and popliteofibular stigaments insert more posteriorly, at the apex of the fibular head. (Bottom) Axial T1 MR at the head of the fibula, biceps femoris/LCL tendon insert laterally. The arcuate and popliteofibular ligaments have already inserted on the fibular styloid apex slightly more proximally (not shown).

GRAPHIC & AXIAL T2 MR, POSTEROLATERAL CORNER STRUCTURES

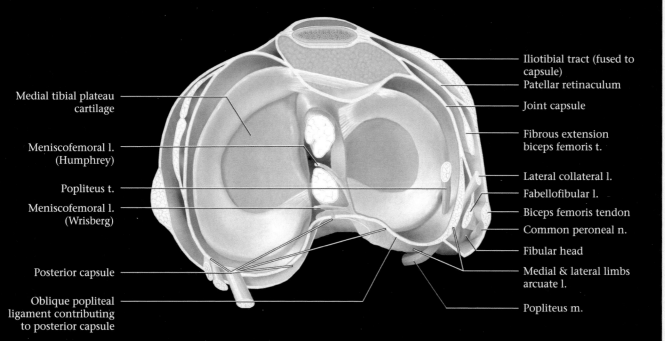

Medial tibial plateau cartilage

Meniscofemoral l. (Humphrey)

Popliteus t.

Meniscofemoral l. (Wrisberg)

Posterior capsule

Oblique popliteal ligament contributing to posterior capsule

Iliotibial tract (fused to capsule)

Patellar retinaculum

Joint capsule

Fibrous extension biceps femoris t.

Lateral collateral l.

Fabellofibular l.

Biceps femoris tendon

Common peroneal n.

Fibular head

Medial & lateral limbs arcuate l.

Popliteus m.

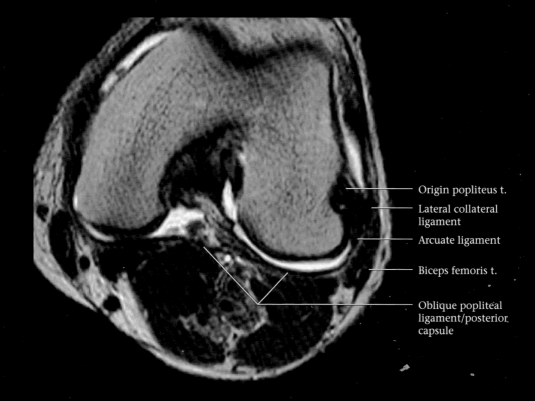

Origin popliteus t.

Lateral collateral ligament

Arcuate ligament

Biceps femoris t.

Oblique popliteal ligament/posterior capsule

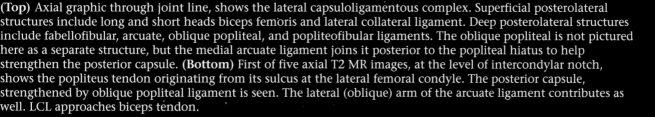

(Top) Axial graphic through joint line, shows the lateral capsuloligamentous complex. Superficial posterolateral structures include long and short heads biceps femoris and lateral collateral ligament. Deep posterolateral structures include fabellofibular, arcuate, oblique popliteal, and popliteofibular ligaments. The oblique popliteal is not pictured here as a separate structure, but the medial arcuate ligament joins it posterior to the popliteal hiatus to help strengthen the posterior capsule. **(Bottom)** First of five axial T2 MR images, at the level of intercondylar notch, shows the popliteus tendon originating from its sulcus at the lateral femoral condyle. The posterior capsule, strengthened by oblique popliteal ligament is seen. The lateral (oblique) arm of the arcuate ligament contributes as well. LCL approaches biceps tendon.

AXIAL T2 MR, POSTEROLATERAL STRUCTURES

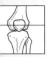

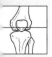

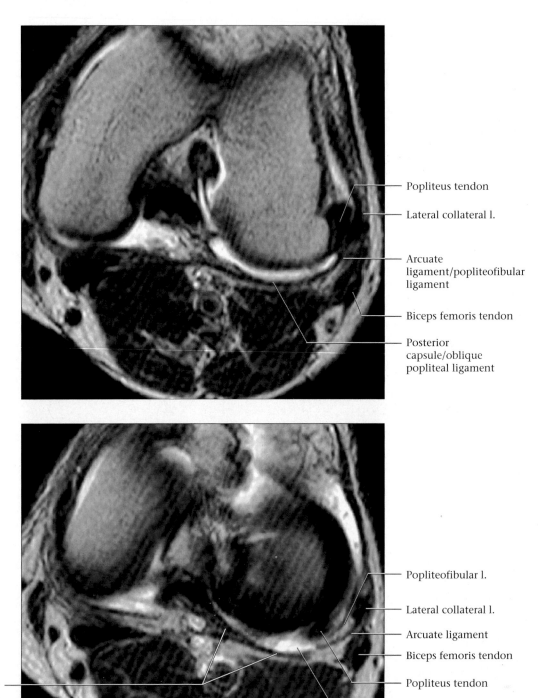

Popliteus tendon

Lateral collateral l.

Arcuate ligament/popliteofibular ligament

Biceps femoris tendon

Posterior capsule/oblique popliteal ligament

Popliteofibular l.

Lateral collateral l.

Arcuate ligament

Biceps femoris tendon

Popliteus tendon

Popliteal hiatus

Posterior capsule/oblique popliteal ligament

(Top) Slightly distally, the popliteus tendon enters the popliteal hiatus as it travels posteriorly and inferiorly around the lateral femoral condyle towards the joint line. **(Bottom)** Approaching the joint line, the popliteus tendon curves posteriorly within the popliteal hiatus. Both the arcuate and popliteofibular ligaments are seen extending from their origin at the fibular styloid process proximally to contribute to the posterior capsule and popliteus paratenon, respectively. More superficially, the lateral collateral ligament approaches biceps femoris as they head towards their insertion on the lateral fibular head.

LATERAL SUPPORTING STRUCTURES

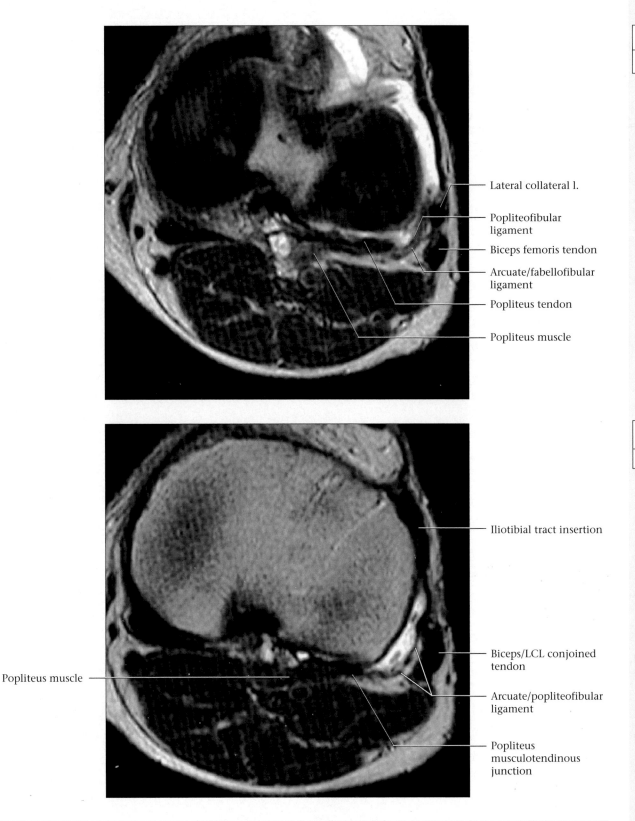

Top image labels:
- Lateral collateral l.
- Popliteofibular ligament
- Biceps femoris tendon
- Arcuate/fabellofibular ligament
- Popliteus tendon
- Popliteus muscle

Bottom image labels:
- Iliotibial tract insertion
- Biceps/LCL conjoined tendon
- Arcuate/popliteofibular ligament
- Popliteus musculotendinous junction
- Popliteus muscle

(Top) At the level of the joint line, the biceps and LCL approach merger to become a conjoined tendon prior to insertion on fibular head; this occurs fairly often. The tissue lying between the conjoined tendon and posterolateral tibia consists of the popliteofibular ligament (deep) and arcuate & fabellofibular ligaments (more superficial). The popliteus continues in the hiatus towards its musculotendinous junction. **(Bottom)** Approaching the fibular head, the same relationships maintain except that popliteus tendon now reaches the musculotendinous junction and popliteus muscle is seen posterior to the tibia. Anterolaterally, iliotibial band has inserted on Gerdy tubercle.

GRAPHIC & MR ARTHROGRAM, RELATIONSHIP OF POPLITEUS & ITS ATTACHMENTS

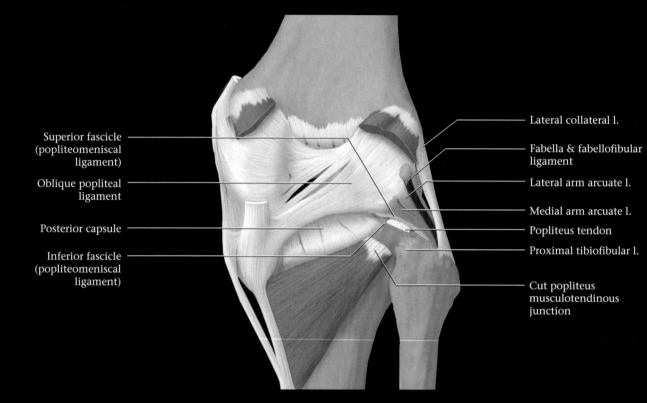

Superior fascicle (popliteomeniscal ligament)

Oblique popliteal ligament

Posterior capsule

Inferior fascicle (popliteomeniscal ligament)

Lateral collateral l.

Fabella & fabellofibular ligament

Lateral arm arcuate l.

Medial arm arcuate l.

Popliteus tendon

Proximal tibiofibular l.

Cut popliteus musculotendinous junction

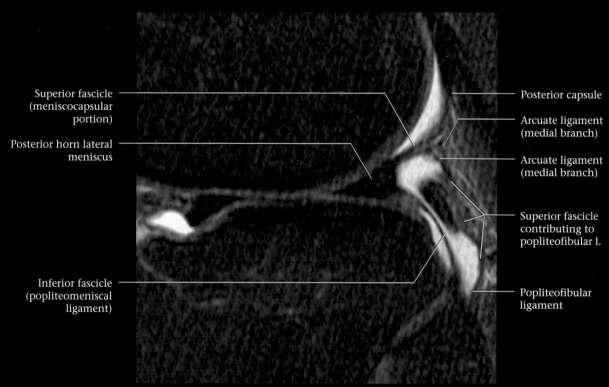

Superior fascicle (meniscocapsular portion)

Posterior horn lateral meniscus

Inferior fascicle (popliteomeniscal ligament)

Posterior capsule

Arcuate ligament (medial branch)

Arcuate ligament (medial branch)

Superior fascicle contributing to popliteofibular l.

Popliteofibular ligament

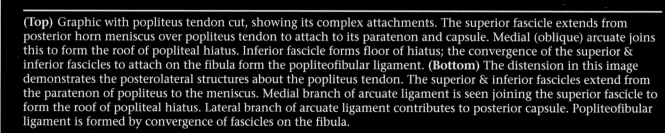

(Top) Graphic with popliteus tendon cut, showing its complex attachments. The superior fascicle extends from posterior horn meniscus over popliteus tendon to attach to its paratenon and capsule. Medial (oblique) arcuate joins this to form the roof of popliteal hiatus. Inferior fascicle forms floor of hiatus; the convergence of the superior & inferior fascicles to attach on the fibula form the popliteofibular ligament. **(Bottom)** The distension in this image demonstrates the posterolateral structures about the popliteus tendon. The superior & inferior fascicles extend from the paratenon of popliteus to the meniscus. Medial branch of arcuate ligament is seen joining the superior fascicle to form the roof of popliteal hiatus. Lateral branch of arcuate ligament contributes to posterior capsule. Popliteofibular ligament is formed by convergence of fascicles on the fibula.

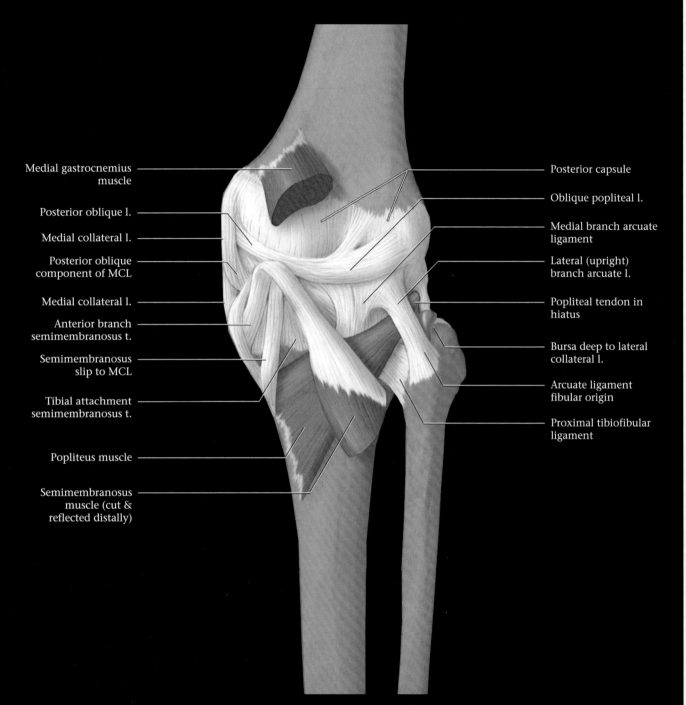

Medial gastrocnemius muscle

Posterior oblique l.

Medial collateral l.

Posterior oblique component of MCL

Medial collateral l.

Anterior branch semimembranosus t.

Semimembranosus slip to MCL

Tibial attachment semimembranosus t.

Popliteus muscle

Semimembranosus muscle (cut & reflected distally)

Posterior capsule

Oblique popliteal l.

Medial branch arcuate ligament

Lateral (upright) branch arcuate l.

Popliteal tendon in hiatus

Bursa deep to lateral collateral l.

Arcuate ligament fibular origin

Proximal tibiofibular ligament

Graphic shows posterior stabilizing structures of knee. Posterolateral structures include popliteus tendon and muscle, with the fascicles' insertion on fibular head (popliteofibular ligament). The arcuate ligament arises from posterior fibular head; both the lateral and medial branches contribute to the oblique popliteal ligament, which strengthens the posterior capsule. The semimembranosus insertion is complex, and does not have such distinct structures as are shown in the graphic. These attachments include: Posteromedial tibial plateau, anterior branch to tibia beneath medial collateral ligament (MCL), posteromedial capsule (not shown as separate structure), and slips to oblique popliteal ligament (not shown as separate structure). The posterior oblique ligament, originating from posterior fibers of MCL, blends posteriorly into capsule and oblique popliteal ligament.

Knee

VI

CORONAL & SAGITTAL T1 MR, FABELLOFIBULAR LIGAMENT

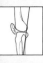

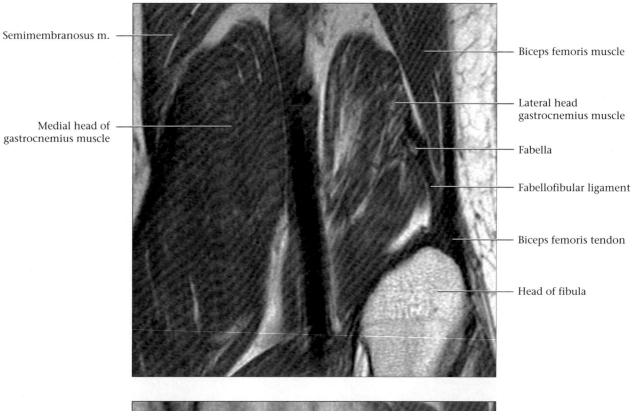

Semimembranosus m.

Medial head of gastrocnemius muscle

Biceps femoris muscle

Lateral head gastrocnemius muscle

Fabella

Fabellofibular ligament

Biceps femoris tendon

Head of fibula

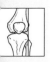

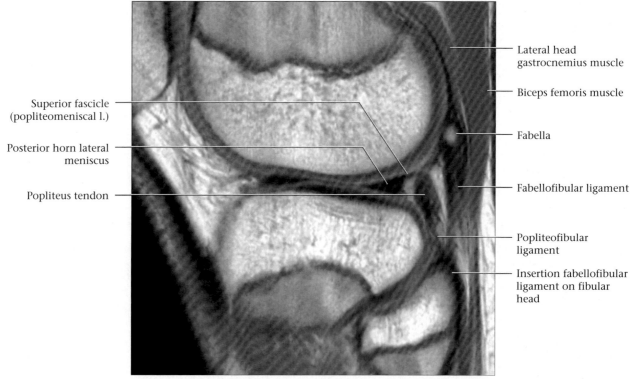

Superior fascicle (popliteomeniscal l.)

Posterior horn lateral meniscus

Popliteus tendon

Lateral head gastrocnemius muscle

Biceps femoris muscle

Fabella

Fabellofibular ligament

Popliteofibular ligament

Insertion fabellofibular ligament on fibular head

(Top) This far posterior coronal cut shows a fabella within the lateral head of the gastrocnemius. There is a prominent fabellofibular ligament, extending from the fabella to the posterior aspect of the head of the fibula, immediately posteromedial to long head biceps tendon insertion. This ligament is hypertrophied; it is not usually seen this well. **(Bottom)** Sagittal cut located laterally shows the hypertrophied fabellofibular ligament in the same patient as previous image. The fabella is distinctly seen, with the fabellofibular ligament investing it and extending to the apex of fibular styloid. The popliteus tendon is within the popliteal hiatus; the superior fascicle extends from posterior horn lateral meniscus to the superior paratenon of popliteus. The thin popliteofibular ligament is seen extending from fibular head to popliteus as well.

SAGITTAL T1 MR, BICEPS FEMORIS INSERTION, FABELLOFIBULAR, & ARCUATE LIGAMENTS

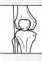

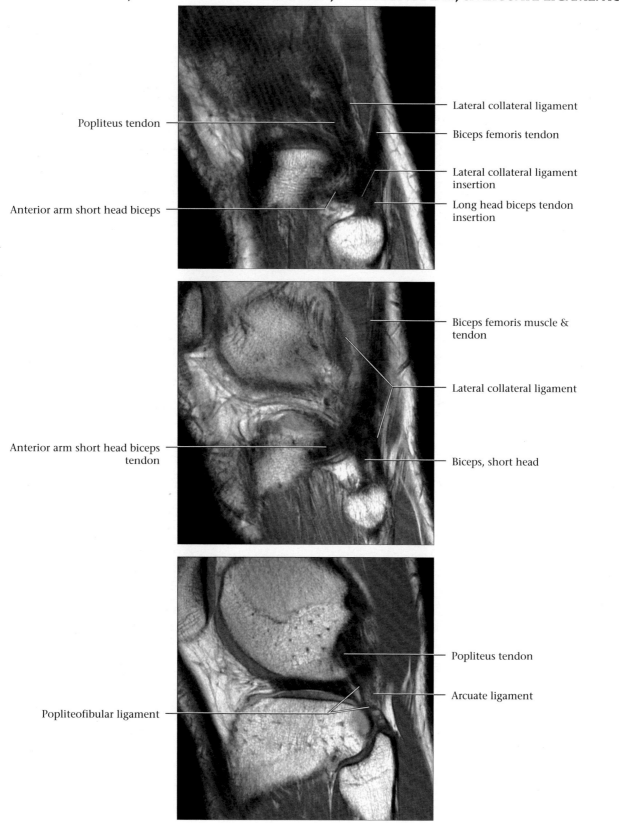

Popliteus tendon

Anterior arm short head biceps

Lateral collateral ligament

Biceps femoris tendon

Lateral collateral ligament insertion

Long head biceps tendon insertion

Anterior arm short head biceps tendon

Biceps femoris muscle & tendon

Lateral collateral ligament

Biceps, short head

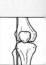

Popliteofibular ligament

Popliteus tendon

Arcuate ligament

(Top) First of three sagittal T1 MR images, far lateral, showing the complex set of insertions of long and short heads of biceps femoris. Although they are not often discerned as separate on MR imaging, the long head of biceps has two insertions on the posterolateral portion of fibular head. The short head of biceps has one insertion on the fibular head immediately anterior to the long head & a second broad insertion on anterolateral tibia. The LCL inserts immediately medial to long head biceps. **(Middle)** Slightly medial, one sees a remnant of lateral collateral ligament. Short head of biceps is still seen inserting on anterolateral tibia, with a branch inserting on fibular head. **(Bottom)** Image at the level of bowtie of meniscus, shows popliteus tendon extending to hiatus, popliteofibular ligament extending from paratenon to fibula, and posteriorly, the arcuate ligament.

SAGITTAL PD MR, POPLITEUS TENDON

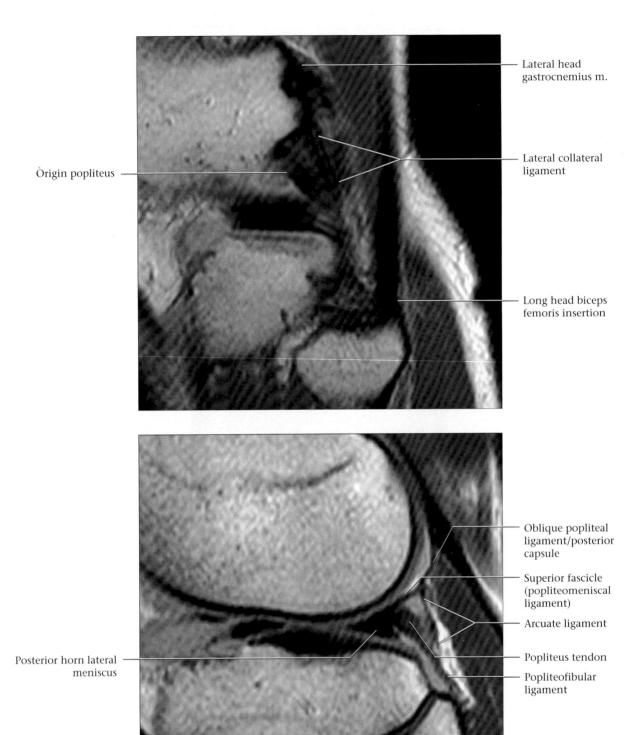

Origin popliteus

Lateral head gastrocnemius m.

Lateral collateral ligament

Long head biceps femoris insertion

Oblique popliteal ligament/posterior capsule

Superior fascicle (popliteomeniscal ligament)

Arcuate ligament

Popliteus tendon

Popliteofibular ligament

Posterior horn lateral meniscus

(Top) First of five sagittal PD MR images following the course of the popliteus tendon. In this far lateral image, the biceps femoris is seen inserting on fibular head. A hint of origin of popliteus tendon in its sulcus in lateral femoral condyle is seen, along with the origin of lateral collateral ligament. **(Bottom)** Slightly medially, the popliteus tendon enters the joint and its hiatus. The lateral (oblique) head of arcuate ligament is seen arising along with popliteofibular ligament from the fibular styloid; the arcuate ligament continues towards the oblique popliteal ligament and capsule of the joint.

LATERAL SUPPORTING STRUCTURES

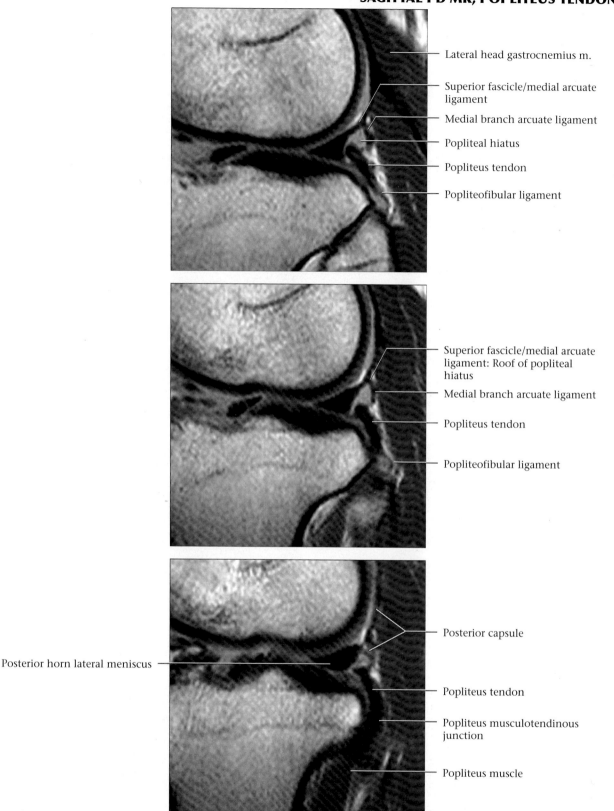

- Lateral head gastrocnemius m.
- Superior fascicle/medial arcuate ligament
- Medial branch arcuate ligament
- Popliteal hiatus
- Popliteus tendon
- Popliteofibular ligament

- Superior fascicle/medial arcuate ligament: Roof of popliteal hiatus
- Medial branch arcuate ligament
- Popliteus tendon
- Popliteofibular ligament

Posterior horn lateral meniscus —

- Posterior capsule
- Popliteus tendon
- Popliteus musculotendinous junction
- Popliteus muscle

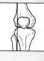

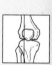

(**Top**) Slightly more medially, the popliteus elongates downward; the popliteofibular ligament merges with its paratenon. By this point, the medial branch of arcuate ligament has joined the superior fascicle to form the roof of the popliteal hiatus. (**Middle**) The popliteus tendon approaches its musculotendinous junction. Note the arched roof of popliteal hiatus formed by the superior fascicle and the medial branch of the arcuate ligament. (**Bottom**) Approaching, but not yet in the intercondylar notch, the popliteus tendon is at its musculotendinous junction. The muscle can be seen extending distally toward its insertion on posterior tibia. By this point, the posterior horn lateral meniscus has rejoined the posterior capsule.

Knee

VI

CORONAL T1 MR, POSTEROLATERAL STRUCTURES

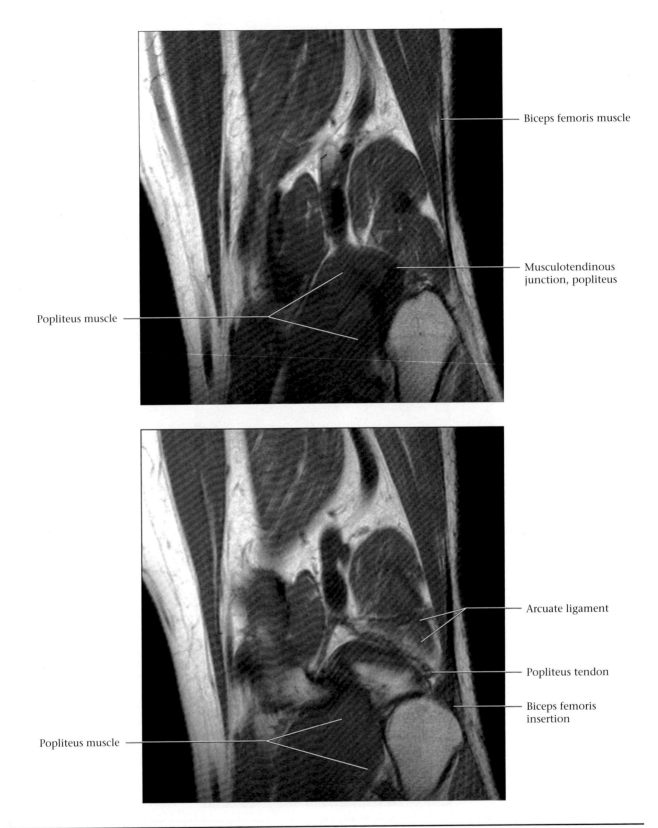

Biceps femoris muscle

Musculotendinous junction, popliteus

Popliteus muscle

Arcuate ligament

Popliteus tendon

Biceps femoris insertion

Popliteus muscle

(Top) First of two coronal T1 MR images, far posterior, shows structures in the posterior-most aspect of posterolateral corner. The musculotendinous junction of popliteus is seen, extending into popliteus muscle. **(Bottom)** Slightly more anteriorly, the long head of biceps femoris inserts on the outer aspect of fibular head. A corner of popliteus tendon is seen extending around the posterolateral tibia towards its musculotendinous junction. Arcuate ligament is seen joining posterior capsule.

CORONAL PD MR, POSTEROLATERAL STRUCTURES

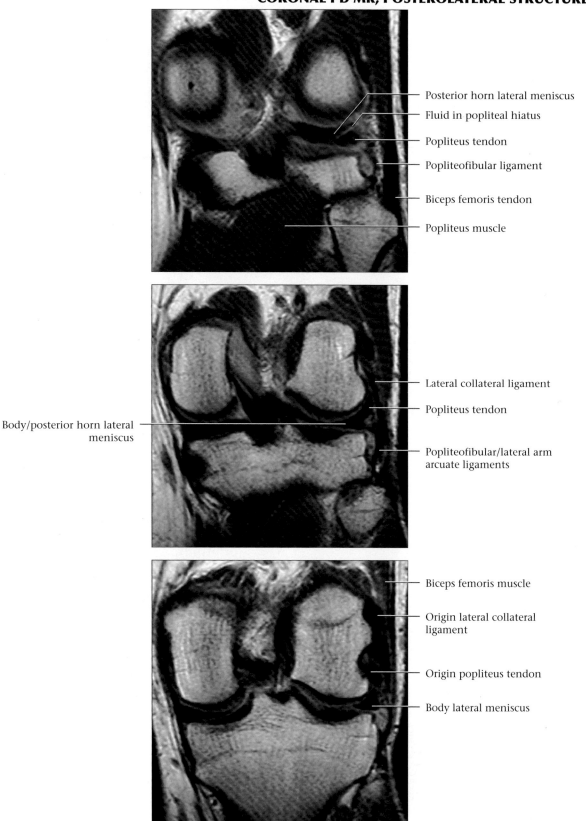

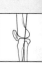

Top image labels:
- Posterior horn lateral meniscus
- Fluid in popliteal hiatus
- Popliteus tendon
- Popliteofibular ligament
- Biceps femoris tendon
- Popliteus muscle

Middle image labels:
- Body/posterior horn lateral meniscus
- Lateral collateral ligament
- Popliteus tendon
- Popliteofibular/lateral arm arcuate ligaments

Bottom image labels:
- Biceps femoris muscle
- Origin lateral collateral ligament
- Origin popliteus tendon
- Body lateral meniscus

(Top) First of three coronal PD MR images, following the popliteus tendon, outlined by fluid within the popliteal hiatus. This more posterior of the three shows the popliteus muscle, as well as the popliteus tendon as it traverses the hiatus, with fluid separating the tendon from the posterior horn lateral meniscus. Biceps femoris tendon inserts laterally on fibular head. **(Middle)** Slightly more anteriorly, the mid portion of lateral collateral ligament is seen extending towards its insertion on lateral femoral head. Popliteus tendon is just entering the hiatus at the level of junction posterior horn/body of lateral meniscus. **(Bottom)** At a mid-coronal cut, the origins of both lateral collateral ligament and popliteus tendon are seen. At this point, the body of lateral meniscus is directly attached to capsule since popliteus has not yet entered the hiatus.

Knee

VI

CORONAL OBLIQUE T1 MR, POSTEROLATERAL STRUCTURES

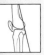

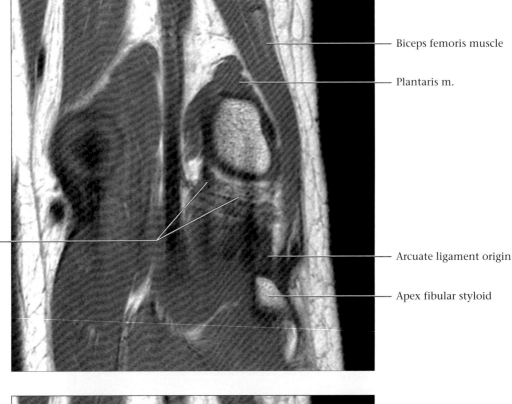

Biceps femoris muscle

Plantaris m.

Medial arm arcuate ligament, blending into posterior capsule

Arcuate ligament origin

Apex fibular styloid

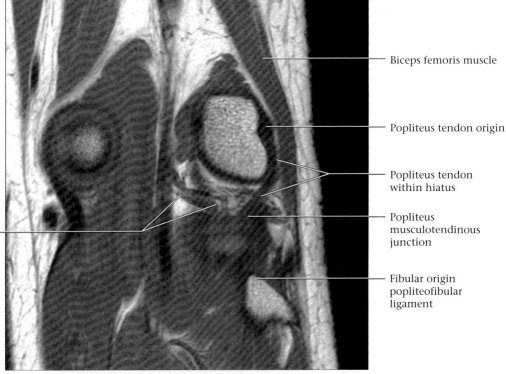

Biceps femoris muscle

Popliteus tendon origin

Popliteus tendon within hiatus

Popliteus musculotendinous junction

Lateral geniculate nerve & vein

Fibular origin popliteofibular ligament

(Top) First of four coronal oblique T1 MR images of posterolateral structures. The images are prescribed off a sagittal, angling from anterosuperior to posteroinferior, following the popliteus tendon. Thus, in this image we see more of the lateral femoral condyle than fibula. It allows visualization of oblique posterior structures such as the fabellofibular ligament and arcuate ligament. This image is too far posterior to include much popliteus tendon. (Bottom) Slightly anterior to the previous image, this lays the popliteus tendon out such that it is seen from its origin to musculotendinous junction. The fibular origin of the popliteofibular ligament is seen, with fibers stretching up to meet the popliteal paratenon. Portions of the arcuate ligament may be present but are not well seen. Since we are at the apex of the fibula, the biceps has not yet inserted.

CORONAL OBLIQUE T1 MR, POSTEROLATERAL STRUCTURES

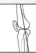

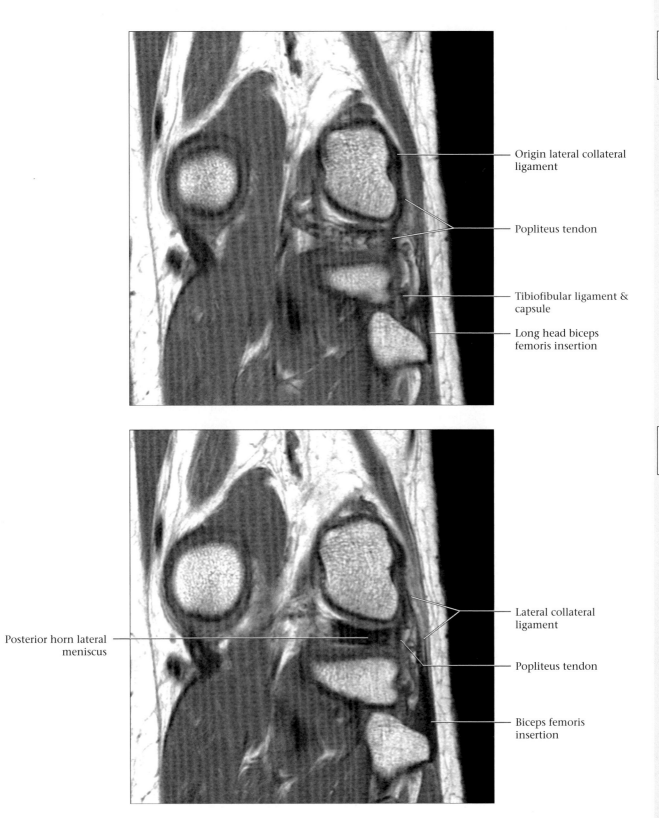

Origin lateral collateral ligament

Popliteus tendon

Tibiofibular ligament & capsule

Long head biceps femoris insertion

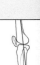

Posterior horn lateral meniscus

Lateral collateral ligament

Popliteus tendon

Biceps femoris insertion

(Top) Slightly anterior image continues to show more of the origin of popliteus tendon. The origin of LCL is seen, and the long head of biceps femoris inserts on the mid portion of the fibula laterally. **(Bottom)** More anteriorly, popliteus tendon is seen separated from posterior horn lateral meniscus by fluid in the popliteal hiatus. The biceps more fully inserts on fibula, with lateral collateral ligament inserting immediately medial to it.

Knee

VI

LEG OVERVIEW

Gross Anatomy

Osseous Anatomy
- **Tibia**
  - Proximal tibiofibular joint
    - Head of fibula and lateral condyle tibia joined by fibrous capsule
    - May communicate with knee joint
    - Posterolaterally located
    - Synovial; at risk for any articular process
  - Anterolateral tibia: Origin of anterior muscles of leg
  - Anterior border (shin): Sharp ridge running from tibial tuberosity proximally to anterior margin of medial malleolus
  - Medial tibial surface
    - Wide and flat
    - Proximally, covered by pes anserinus
    - Remainder is subcutaneous
  - Medial border of tibia: Saphenous nerve and great saphenous vein run along it
  - Posterior tibia: Origin of deep posterior muscles of leg
  - Lateral border of tibia: Ridge for attachment of interosseous membrane
  - Medial malleolus: 2 colliculi, anterior longer than posterior
  - Distal tibiofibular joint
    - Fibula articulates with tibia at fibular notch; joined by interosseous ligament
    - Strengthened by anterior and posterior tibiofibular ligaments
    - Posterolaterally located
- **Fibula**
  - Anterior fibula
    - Origin of lateral muscles of leg
  - Medial fibula
    - Origin of deep posterior muscles of leg
  - Posterolateral fibula
    - Origin of posterior muscles of leg
  - Lateral malleolus: 1 cm longer than medial malleolus

Interosseous Membrane
- Stretches across interval between tibia and fibula
- Greatly extends surface for origin of muscles
- Strong, oblique fibers run downwards and laterally from tibia to fibula
- In upper part, below lateral condyle of tibia, there is an opening for passage of anterior tibial vessels
- Distally, an opening allows passage of perforating branch of peroneal artery
- Tibialis posterior and flexor hallucis longus take partial origin from the back of membrane
- Tibialis anterior, long extensors of toes, and peroneus tertius take partial origin from front of membrane

Retinacula
- Discussed in greater detail in "Ankle Overview" section
- Superior extensor retinaculum
  - Strong, broad band
  - Stretches across front of leg from tibia to fibula, immediately above ankle joint
  - Ends attached to anterior borders of tibia and fibula
  - Long extensors, peroneus tertius, anterior tibial vessels, and deep peroneal nerve pass behind it
  - Medial part splits to enclose tendon of tibialis anterior, forming a sling for it
- Inferior extensor retinaculum: Distal to ankle joint except for attachment of one band to anterior part of medial malleolus
- Superior peroneal retinaculum
  - Thickened deep fascia securing peroneal tendons to back of lateral malleolus, peroneus longus superficial to brevis
  - Retinaculum attached to back of lateral malleolus and to lateral retrotrochlear tubercle of calcaneus
- Flexor retinaculum: Posteroinferior to medial malleolus

Muscles of Leg
- Compartments separated by deep fascia, which give partial origin to several muscles
- **Posterior compartment: Superficial muscles**
  - **Gastrocnemius**
    - Origin: Medial from posterior femoral metaphysis; lateral from posterior edge of lateral epicondyle
    - Heads separated from posterior capsule by a bursa
    - 2 heads unite to form main bulk of muscle
    - Join in a thin aponeurotic tendon near mid leg
    - Joins soleus aponeurosis to form Achilles tendon; concave in cross section; musculotendinous junction 5 cm above calcaneal insertion
    - Nerve supply: Tibial nerve
    - Action: Plantar flexor of ankle and flexor of knee
  - **Plantaris**
    - Origin: Superior and medial to lateral head of gastrocnemius origin, as well as from oblique popliteal ligament
    - Continues deep to lateral head gastrocnemius
    - Myotendinous junction at level of origin of soleus (muscle is 5-10 cm long)
    - Tendon then lies between medial head gastrocnemius and soleus
    - Follows medial side of Achilles to insert either anteromedially on Achilles or on calcaneus
    - Plantaris absent 7-10%
    - Nerve supply: Tibial nerve
    - Action: Acts with gastrocnemius
  - **Soleus**
    - Origin: Extensive, from back of fibular head and upper 1/3 of posterior surface of shaft of fibula, from soleal line and middle 1/3 of medial border of tibia, and from tendinous arch joining these across the popliteal vessels
    - Flat, thick, powerful muscle ends in strong tendon
    - Joins with tendon of gastrocnemius to form Achilles tendon
    - Nerve supply: Tibial nerve
    - Action: Stabilizes ankle in standing, plantarflexes ankle
    - Accessory soleus: Rare variant, arises from anterior surface of soleus or from fibula and soleal line of tibia; inserts into Achilles or onto calcaneus anteromedially to Achilles; presents as mass
- **Posterior compartment: Deep muscles**

LEG OVERVIEW

- **Popliteus**
  - Origin: Tendon from popliteal groove of lateral femoral condyle
  - Passes through popliteal hiatus posteriorly and medially, pierces posterior capsule of knee
  - M. fibers directed medially & downwards to insert on posterior surface of tibia above soleal line
  - Nerve supply: Tibial nerve
  - Action: Flexes knee and medially rotates leg at onset of flexion (unlocking extension "screwing home" mechanism)
- **Tibialis Posterior**
  - Origin: Interosseous membrane and adjoining parts of posterior surfaces of tibia and fibula
  - Superior end bifid; anterior tibial vessels pass forward between the 2 attachments
  - Distally it inclines medially, under flexor digitorum longus
  - Grooves and curves around medial malleolus
  - Nerve supply: Tibial nerve
  - Action: Plantarflexes and inverts foot
- **Flexor digitorum longus**
  - Origin: Posterior surface of tibia, below popliteus, and medial to the vertical ridge
  - Crosses superficial to distal part of tibialis posterior
  - Tendon grooves lower end of tibia lateral to that of the tibialis posterior, passes around medial malleolus to foot
  - Nerve supply: Tibial nerve
  - Action: Flexes interphalangeal and metatarsophalangeal joints of lateral 4 toes; plantarflexes and inverts foot
- **Flexor hallucis longus**
  - Origin: Posterior surface of fibula, below origin of soleus
  - Passes medially, descends down posterior to mid tibia
  - Associated with os trigonum posterior to talus
  - Tendon occupies deep groove on posterior surface of talus, passes around medial malleolus, to great toe
  - Nerve supply: Tibial nerves
  - Action: Flexes the interphalangeal and metatarsophalangeal joints of great toe; plantarflexes foot
- **Lateral compartment**
  - Peroneals separated from extensors by anterior intermuscular septum and from posterior muscles by posterior septum
  - **Peroneus longus**
    - Origin upper 2/3 lateral surface of fibula and intermuscular septa and adjacent muscular fascia
    - Becomes tendinous a few cm above lateral malleolus
    - Curves forward behind lateral malleolus, posterior to peroneus brevis
    - Nerve supply: Superficial peroneal
    - Action: Everts foot and secondarily plantarflexes foot
  - **Peroneus brevis**
    - Origin lower 2/3 lateral surface of fibula and intermuscular septa and adjacent muscular fascia
    - Muscle is medial to peroneus longus at origin but overlaps peroneus longus in middle 1/3
    - Tendon curves forward behind lateral malleolus, in front of peroneus longus tendon
    - Nerve supply: Superficial peroneal
    - Action: Everts foot and secondarily plantarflexes foot
  - Synovial sheath for peroneals begins 5 cm above tip of lateral malleolus and envelops both tendons; divides into 2 sheaths at level of calcaneus
  - Peroneus tertius (see anterior compartment)
  - **Peroneus quartus**: Accessory muscle with prevalence of 10%; originates from distal leg, frequently from peroneal muscles, with variable insertion sites at foot; at level of malleolus, located medial or posterior to both peroneal tendons
  - **Peroneus digiti minimi**: Accessory with prevalence of 15-36%; extends from peroneus brevis muscle around medial malleolus to foot; tiny tendinous slip
- **Anterior compartment**
  - **Tibialis anterior**
    - Origin upper half of lateral surface of tibia and interosseous membrane
    - Tendon originates in distal 1/3; passes through retinacula
    - Nerve supply: Deep peroneal and recurrent genicular
    - Action: Dorsiflexor and invertor of foot
  - **Extensor digitorum longus**
    - Origin from upper 3/4 anterior surface fibula
    - Descends behind extensor retinacula to ankle
    - Nerve supply: Deep peroneal
    - Action: Extends interphalangeal and metatarsophalangeal joints of lateral 4 toes, dorsiflexes foot
  - **Peroneus tertius**
    - Small, not always present
    - Origin: Continuous with extensor digitorum longus, arising from distal 1/4 of anterior surface of fibula and interosseous membrane
    - Inserts into dorsal surface base 5th metatarsal
    - Nerve supply: Deep peroneal
    - Action: Dorsiflexes ankle and everts foot
  - **Extensor hallucis**
    - Thin muscle hidden between tibialis anterior and extensor digitorum longus
    - Origin: Middle 2/4 of anterior surface of fibula and interosseous membrane
    - Tendon passes deep to retinacula to great toe
    - Nerve supply: Deep peroneal
    - Action: Extends phalanges of great toe and dorsiflexes foot

Vessels of Leg

- **Popliteal artery**
  - Ends at distal border of popliteus in two branches: Anterior and posterior tibial arteries
  - Paired venae comitantes of anterior and posterior tibial arteries join to form popliteal vein
- **Anterior tibial artery**
  - Smaller of the 2 terminal branches of popliteal
  - Origin in back of leg, at distal border of popliteus m.
  - Passes through upper part of interosseous membrane

- o Straight course down front of leg to become dorsalis pedis
- o Muscular branches along length
- o Malleolar branches ramify over malleoli; lateral one anastomoses with perforating branch of peroneal artery
- **Posterior tibial artery**
  - o Larger of the 2 terminal branches of popliteal
  - o Main blood supply to foot
  - o Passes downwards and slightly medially along with tibial nerve to end in space between medial malleolus and calcaneus
  - o Divides into lateral and medial plantar arteries
  - o Branches
    - Circumflex fibular (may arise from anterior tibial), runs laterally around neck of fibula
    - Nutrient artery to tibia
    - Muscular branches
    - **Peroneal artery**: Largest branch of posterior tibial artery; runs obliquely downwards and laterally beneath soleus to fibula, along which it descends deep to flexor hallucis longus
- **Great saphenous vein**
  - o Begins at medial border of foot
  - o Ascends in front of medial malleolus
  - o Passes obliquely upwards and backwards across medial surface of distal 1/3 of tibia
  - o Passes vertically upward along medial border of tibia to posterior part of medial side of knee
- **Small saphenous vein**
  - o Extends behind lateral malleolus, ascends lateral to Achilles
  - o At midline of calf in lower popliteal region, pierces popliteal fascia and terminates in popliteal vein

Nerves of Leg

- **Common peroneal**
  - o Smaller of 2 terminal divisions of sciatic nerve
  - o Arises mid thigh, runs downwards laterally along medial border of biceps femoris
  - o Crosses plantaris and lateral head of gastrocnemius, passes posterior and superficial to head of fibula
  - o This location at fibular head/neck put peroneal nerve at risk in multiple clinical situations
    - Fibular neck fracture may result in foot drop
    - Total knee replacement in a patient who had been in chronic valgus may damage nerve with realignment of knee
  - o Ends between lateral side of neck of fibula and peroneus longus by dividing into 2 terminal branches
  - o **Deep peroneal nerve**: One of 2 terminal branches
    - Arises on lateral side of neck of fibula, under peroneus longus
    - Pierces anterior intermuscular septum & extensor digitorum longus to enter anterior compartment
    - Extends down to ankle between tibialis anterior and long extensors
    - Near ankle, crossed by extensor hallucis and passes to ankle midway between malleoli
    - Muscular branches to anterior compartment and articular twig to ankle joint
    - Medial terminal branch to dorsum of foot

- Lateral terminal branch to lateral dorsum of ankle
  - o **Superficial peroneal nerve**: 2nd of 2 terminal branches
    - Descends in substance of peroneus longus until it reaches peroneus brevis
    - Passes obliquely over anterior border of brevis and descends in groove between peroneus brevis and extensor digitorum longus
    - In distal 1/3 of leg, pierces deep fascia and divides into medial and lateral branches to foot
- **Tibial nerve**
  - o Descends under fascial septum which separates deep and superficial posterior muscle compartments
  - o In upper 2/3, lies on fascia of tibialis posterior and on flexor digitorum longus
  - o In lower 1/3, located midway between Achilles tendon and medial border of tibia
  - o Crosses posterior surfaces of tibia and ankle joint
  - o Posterior tibial vessels run with it, crossing in front of it from lateral to medial side
  - o At ankle, under flexor retinaculum, divides into lateral and medial plantar nerves
- **Saphenous nerve**
  - o Longest branch of femoral nerve, arising 2 cm below inguinal ligament and descending via adductor canal
  - o Passes posterior to sartorius, descends posteromedial to knee where it pierces the deep fascia
  - o In leg, accompanies great saphenous vein
- **Sural nerve**
  - o Arises in popliteal fossa from tibial nerve
  - o Descends between 2 heads of gastrocnemius
  - o Pierces deep fascia midway between knee and ankle
  - o Accompanies small saphenous vein to lateral border of foot

Imaging Anatomy

Anatomy Relationships

- Critical variant: Third head of gastrocnemius
  - o Muscular anomalies of gastrocnemius are numerous
  - o 2% show anomalous third head of gastrocnemius
    - Originate from posterior distal femoral metaphysis either medially or at mid portion
    - Courses laterally to join lateral head of gastrocnemius
    - Popliteal vessels located between third head and medial head of gastrocnemius
  - o These anomalies have potential for causing popliteal compression, and should be sought (axial images), but may be asymptomatic
- Critical variant: Hypertrophy of short head biceps
  - o May cause encroachment on fat surrounding common peroneal nerve
  - o Abnormalities which may cause peroneal neuropathy
    - Hypertrophied short head biceps
    - Distal extension of long head of biceps
    - Prominent lateral head of gastrocnemius
    - Diabetics may accumulate excess fat around peroneal nerve at fibular neck

3D CT RECONSTRUCTION, MEDIAL LEG

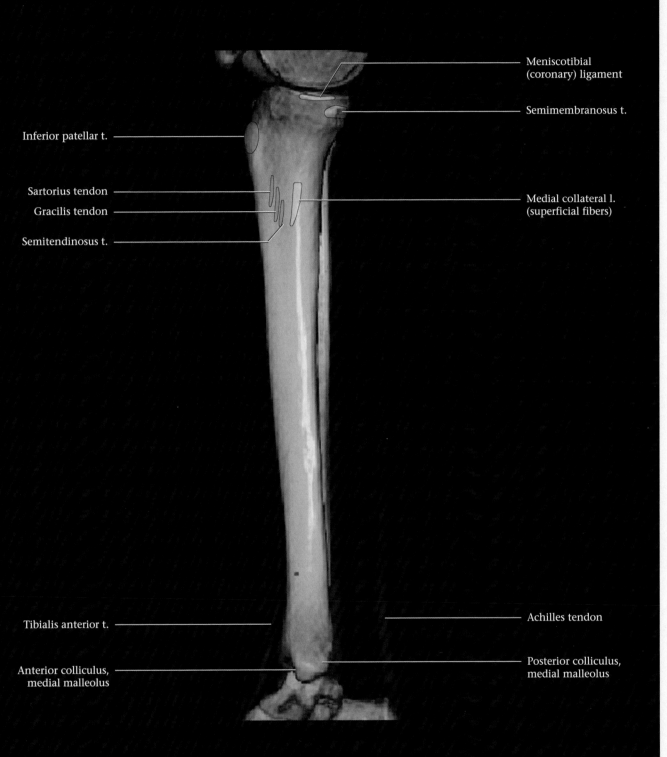

Meniscotibial
(coronary) ligament

Semimembranosus t.

Inferior patellar t.

Sartorius tendon

Gracilis tendon

Semitendinosus t.

Medial collateral l.
(superficial fibers)

Tibialis anterior t.

Achilles tendon

Anterior colliculus,
medial malleolus

Posterior colliculus,
medial malleolus

View of the medial leg. Other than insertions of the pes anserinus and medial collateral ligament proximally, the medial tibial surface is subcutaneous.

3D CT RECONSTRUCTION, POSTERIOR LEG

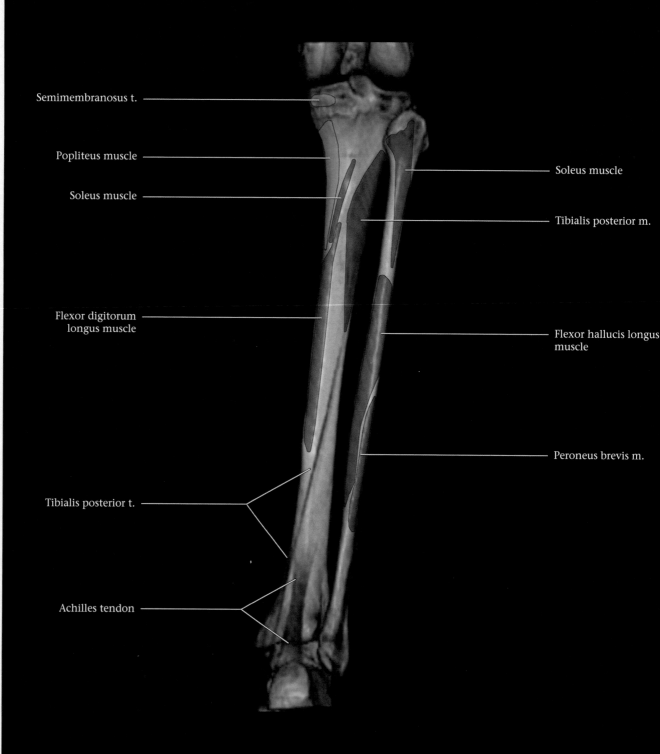

Semimembranosus t.

Popliteus muscle

Soleus muscle

Flexor digitorum longus muscle

Tibialis posterior t.

Achilles tendon

Soleus muscle

Tibialis posterior m.

Flexor hallucis longus muscle

Peroneus brevis m.

Posterior view of the leg. Note the large surface area which serves as origin of muscles from the tibia and fibula. The interosseous septum extends this surface area.

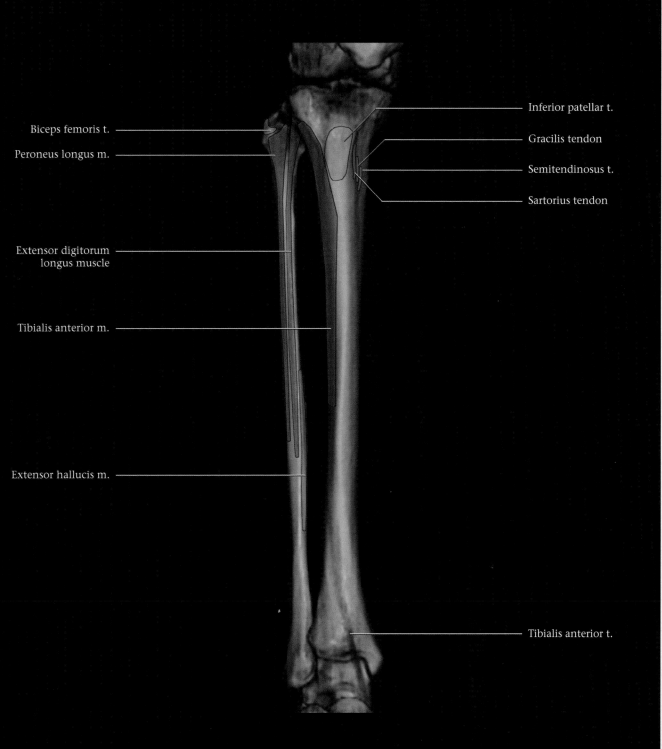

Biceps femoris t.

Peroneus longus m.

Extensor digitorum longus muscle

Tibialis anterior m.

Extensor hallucis m.

Inferior patellar t.

Gracilis tendon

Semitendinosus t.

Sartorius tendon

Tibialis anterior t.

Anterior view of the leg, showing the extensive origins of the tibialis anterior from the anterolateral aspect of the tibia and the long origins of the peroneus longus, extensor hallucis, and extensor digitorum longus from the fibula. These muscles also all have extensive origin from the interosseous membrane.

3D CT RECONSTRUCTION, ANTERIOR INTERNAL OBLIQUE LEG

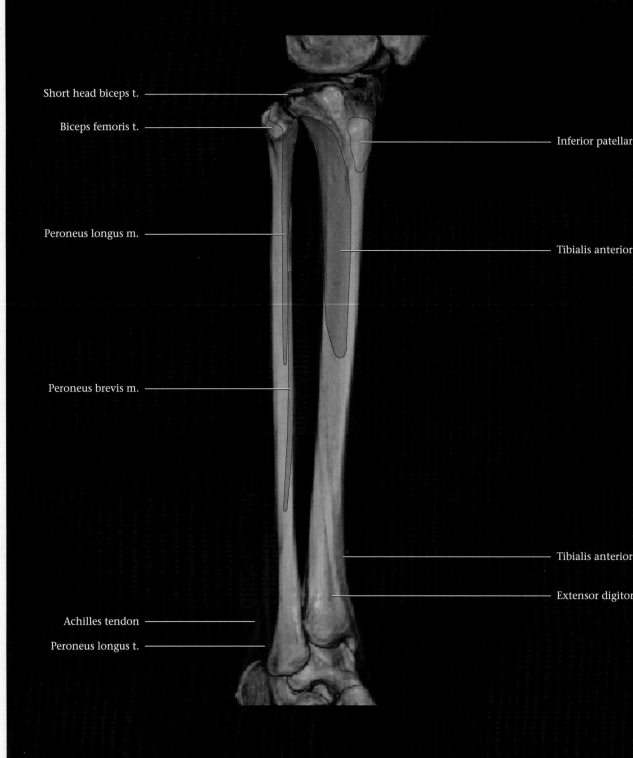

Short head biceps t.

Biceps femoris t.

Peroneus longus m.

Peroneus brevis m.

Achilles tendon

Peroneus longus t.

Inferior patellar

Tibialis anterior

Tibialis anterior

Extensor digitor

Anterior view of leg, internally rotated, showing the extensive origins of tibialis anterior, peroneus longus, and peroneus brevis.

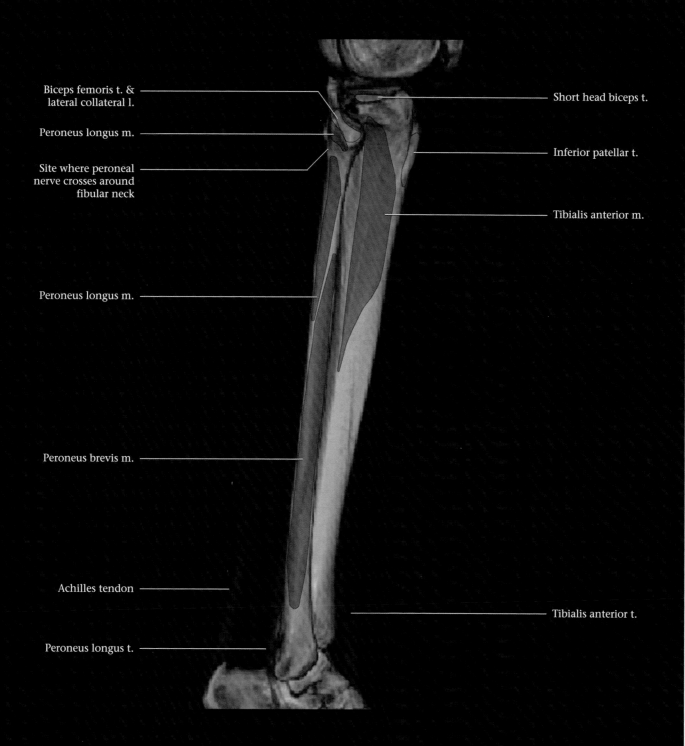

Biceps femoris t. & lateral collateral l.

Peroneus longus m.

Site where peroneal nerve crosses around fibular neck

Peroneus longus m.

Peroneus brevis m.

Achilles tendon

Peroneus longus t.

Short head biceps t.

Inferior patellar t.

Tibialis anterior m.

Tibialis anterior t.

Lateral view of the leg. Note that the peroneus longus is shown as having two separate origins, so that the site of passage of the common peroneal nerve around the neck of the fibula is seen. Also note that there is some overlap of sites of origin of the peroneus longus and brevis from the anterolateral fibula, with peroneus longus originating in the upper 2/3 and brevis in the lower 2/3 of the bone.

LEG OVERVIEW

RADIOGRAPH, ANTEROPOSTERIOR

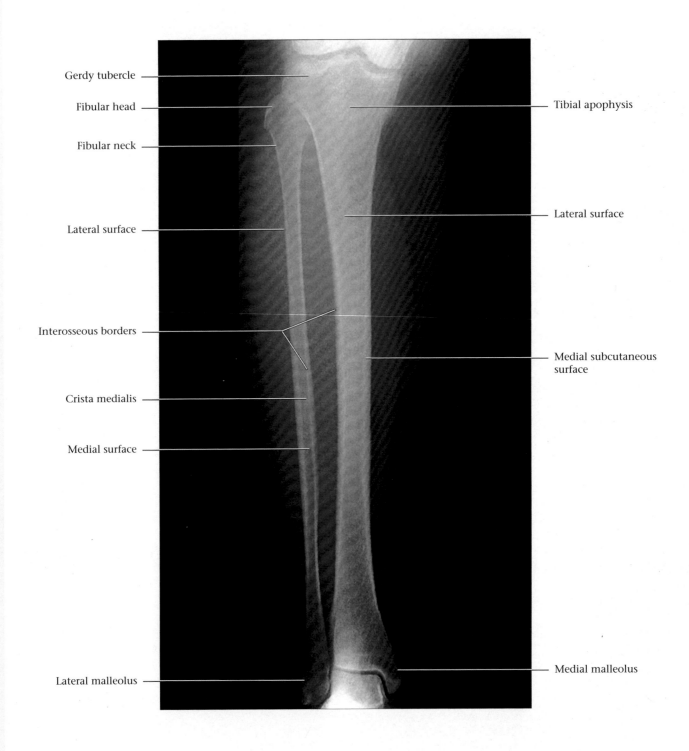

Gerdy tubercle

Fibular head

Fibular neck

Lateral surface

Interosseous borders

Crista medialis

Medial surface

Lateral malleolus

Tibial apophysis

Lateral surface

Medial subcutaneous surface

Medial malleolus

Anteroposterior radiograph of the leg. Note that the fibula is slightly posterolateral to the tibia, and that there is expected overlap at the proximal and distal tibiofibular joints. The interosseous borders of both long bones are often irregular; this relates to the insertion of the strong interosseous membrane and is not periosteal reaction. The lateral malleolus extends 1 cm farther distal than the medial.

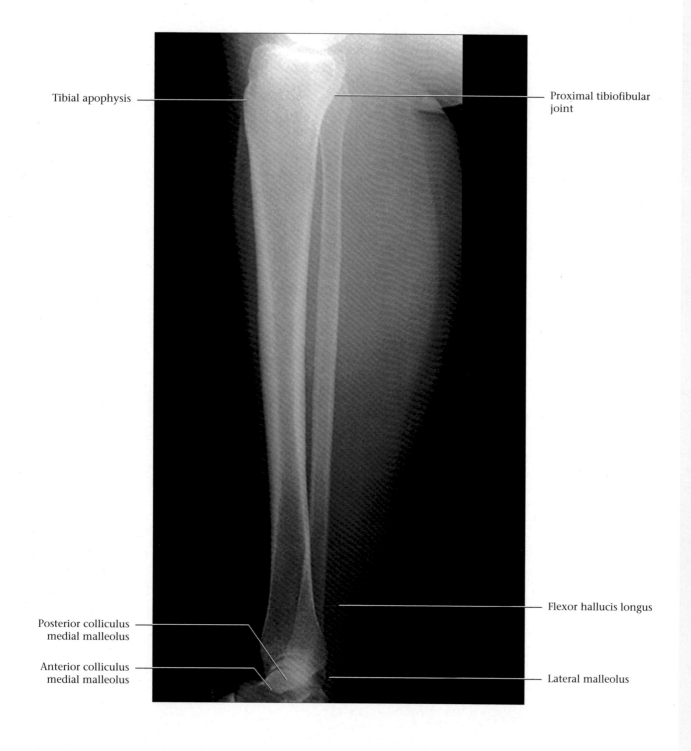

Tibial apophysis

Proximal tibiofibular joint

Posterior colliculus medial malleolus

Anterior colliculus medial malleolus

Flexor hallucis longus

Lateral malleolus

Lateral radiograph of the leg. As on the anteroposterior view, there is overlap of the bones at both the proximal and distal tibiofibular joints. At the ankle, both the colliculi of the medial malleolus can be seen, along with the slightly longer lateral malleolus.

LEG OVERVIEW

GRAPHIC, POSTERIOR SUPERFICIAL MUSCLES

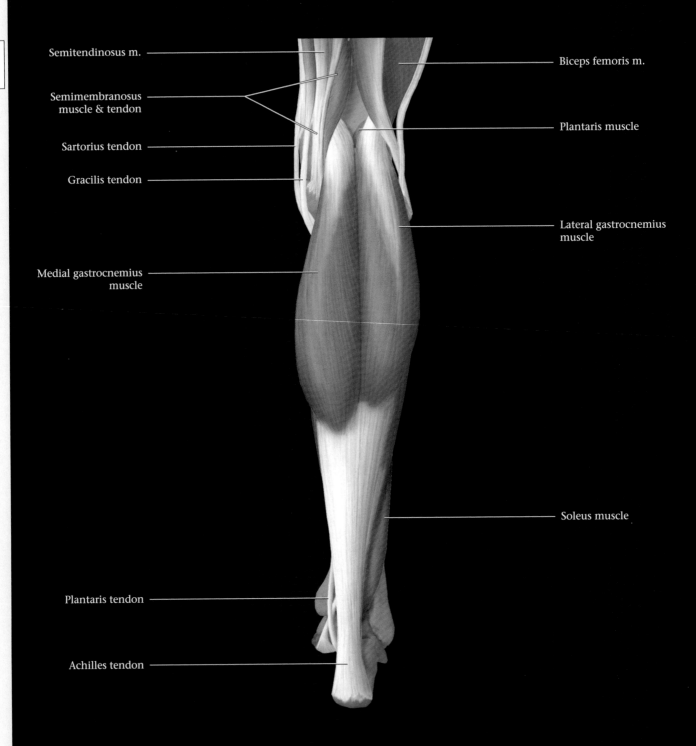

Semitendinosus m.

Semimembranosus muscle & tendon

Sartorius tendon

Gracilis tendon

Medial gastrocnemius muscle

Plantaris tendon

Achilles tendon

Biceps femoris m.

Plantaris muscle

Lateral gastrocnemius muscle

Soleus muscle

Posterior view of superficial muscles and tendons of the leg. The gastrocnemius muscles are bulky in the proximal half of the leg and taper to an aponeurosis which blends with the soleus more distally to become the Achilles tendon. The plantaris muscle is superficial only at its origin from the lateral femoral metaphysis, just medial to the origin of the lateral head of gastrocnemius. The muscle extends only a few centimeters before becoming tendinous, extending distally between the soleus and medial gastrocnemius; eventually, the plantaris tendon merges with the medial side of Achilles or inserts on the calcaneus medial to the Achilles insertion.

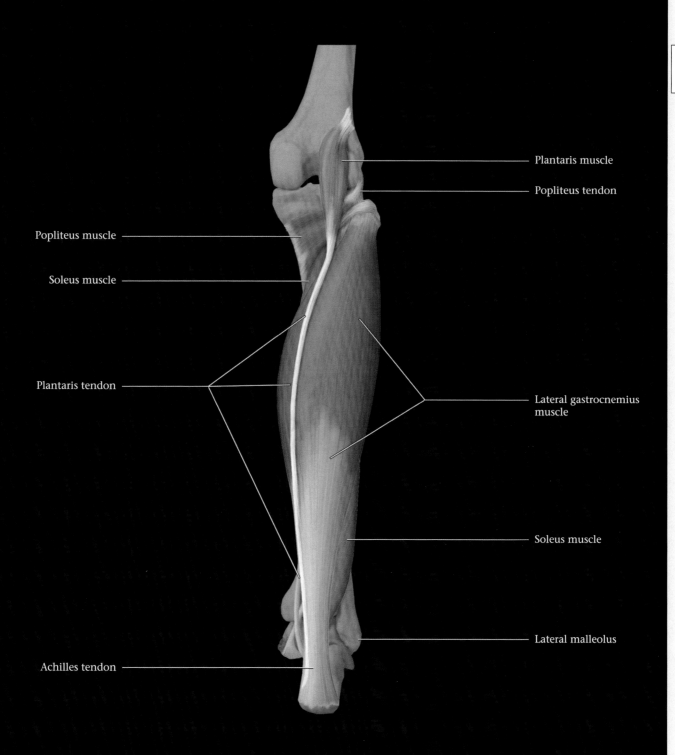

Plantaris muscle

Popliteus tendon

Popliteus muscle

Soleus muscle

Plantaris tendon

Lateral gastrocnemius muscle

Soleus muscle

Lateral malleolus

Achilles tendon

Graphic of posterior leg, with medial gastrocnemius peeled away. Additionally, the origin of lateral head of gastrocnemius has been removed. This allows visualization of the course of plantaris muscle and tendon. The origin of plantaris on the lateral femoral metaphysis is superficial, adjacent to the origin of lateral gastrocnemius. The muscle is fleshy over a short distance, becoming tendinous once the soleus originates from the tibia. The tendon then continues to course distally, located between soleus (anterior to it) and medial gastrocnemius (posterior to it). The plantaris tendon moves slightly medially over this course. It becomes superficial ponce the soleus joins the Achilles tendon, and inserts either on the Achilles or the calcaneus, medial to Achilles. Note that the tibial origin of soleus is adjacent to the distal insertion of popliteus muscle on the tibia.

GRAPHIC & CORONAL T1 MR, POPLITEUS MUSCLE

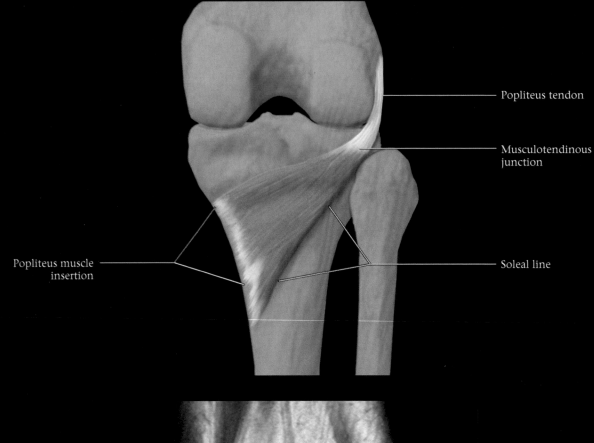

Popliteus tendon

Musculotendinous junction

Popliteus muscle insertion

Soleal line

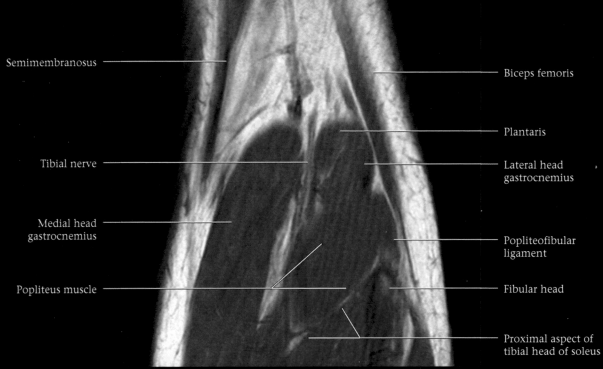

Semimembranosus

Biceps femoris

Plantaris

Tibial nerve

Lateral head gastrocnemius

Medial head gastrocnemius

Popliteofibular ligament

Popliteus muscle

Fibular head

Proximal aspect of tibial head of soleus

(Top) Graphic shows the complicated path of the popliteus tendon and muscle. After the popliteus tendon arises from the sulcus at the lateral femoral condyle, it passes through the popliteal hiatus and then expands to the musculotendinous junction. The muscle broadens over a large area of the proximal posterior tibia to insert at the posteromedial tibia, immediately proximal to the tibial origin of the tibial head of the soleus. (Bottom) Posterior coronal T1 MR image shows the large popliteus muscle, which is found deep to the popliteal vessels and gastrocnemius muscles. Note that in this example the popliteus muscle fibers are oriented superolateral to inferomedial, as opposed to the portion of gastrocnemius seen which runs supero-inferior. The proximal aspect of the tibial head of soleus is located at the distal aspect of popliteus insertion on tibia.

LEG OVERVIEW

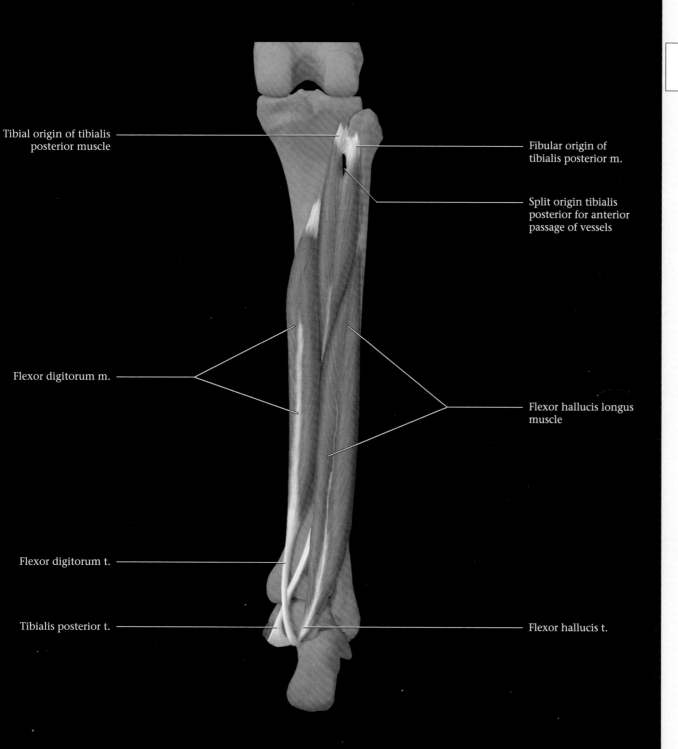

Tibial origin of tibialis posterior muscle

Fibular origin of tibialis posterior m.

Split origin tibialis posterior for anterior passage of vessels

Flexor digitorum m.

Flexor hallucis longus muscle

Flexor digitorum t.

Tibialis posterior t.

Flexor hallucis t.

Graphic of deep muscles of leg, with gastrocnemius, soleus, and plantaris peeled away. Flexor hallucis longus is the largest of the muscles, and its muscular portion extends far distal to the others, becoming tendinous at the level of talus. Tibialis posterior originates from interosseous membrane and adjoining parts of posterior surfaces of tibia and fibula; its tendon crosses anteriorly to the tendon of flexor digitorum longus, so that it is the most medial of the three tendons coursing around medial malleolus. Remember the mnemonic "Tom, Dick, & Harry" for the order of the tendons of the deep muscles of the leg at the level of the ankle joint, from medial to lateral.

GRAPHIC, ANTERIOR LEG MUSCLES

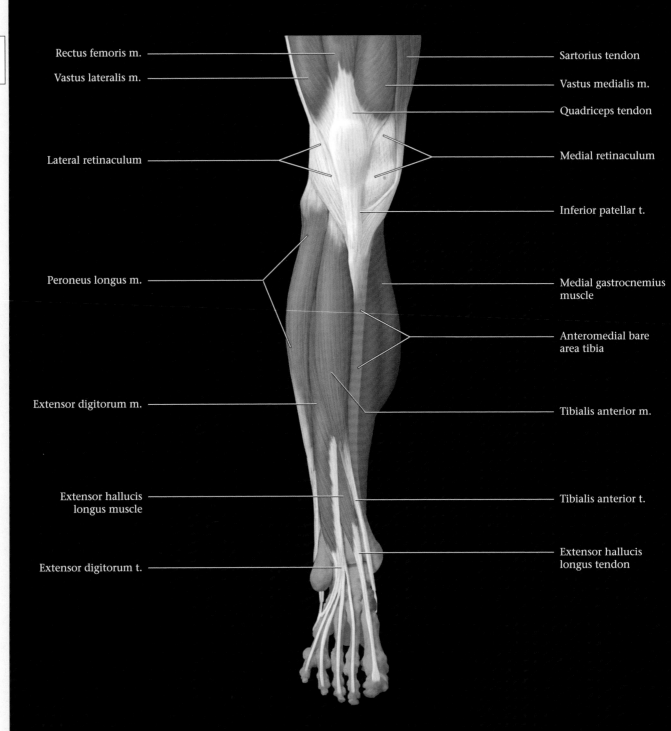

Rectus femoris m.

Vastus lateralis m.

Lateral retinaculum

Peroneus longus m.

Extensor digitorum m.

Extensor hallucis
longus muscle

Extensor digitorum t.

Sartorius tendon

Vastus medialis m.

Quadriceps tendon

Medial retinaculum

Inferior patellar t.

Medial gastrocnemius
muscle

Anteromedial bare
area tibia

Tibialis anterior m.

Tibialis anterior t.

Extensor hallucis
longus tendon

Graphic of anterior leg muscles. Note that nearly the entire anteromedial tibialis bare of muscle; it is thus poorly vascularized, resulting in slow fracture healing. The tibialis anterior has an extensive origin from both tibia and interosseous membrane and is the most substantial muscle of the anterior compartment. Extensor digitorum originates from fibula. Extensor hallucis longus originates between the two, from fibula and interosseous membrane. These three muscles retain the same orientation as they become tendinous anterior to the ankle. The mnemonic "Tom, Harry, & Dick" applies to the tendon order, from medial to lateral. The retinacula, which stabilize the tendons as they course over the anterior ankle, are not shown on this graphic.

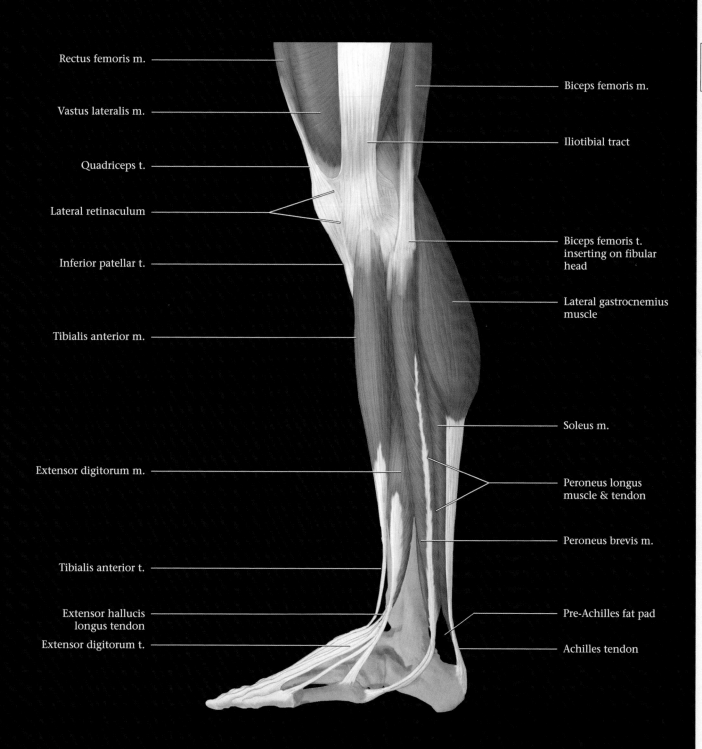

Rectus femoris m.

Vastus lateralis m.

Quadriceps t.

Lateral retinaculum

Inferior patellar t.

Tibialis anterior m.

Extensor digitorum m.

Tibialis anterior t.

Extensor hallucis longus tendon

Extensor digitorum t.

Biceps femoris m.

Iliotibial tract

Biceps femoris t. inserting on fibular head

Lateral gastrocnemius muscle

Soleus m.

Peroneus longus muscle & tendon

Peroneus brevis m.

Pre-Achilles fat pad

Achilles tendon

Graphic of the lateral leg, showing the anterior compartment (extensors), lateral compartment (peroneals), and superficial muscles of the posterior compartment.

LEG OVERVIEW

GRAPHIC, POSTERIOR VESSELS & NERVES

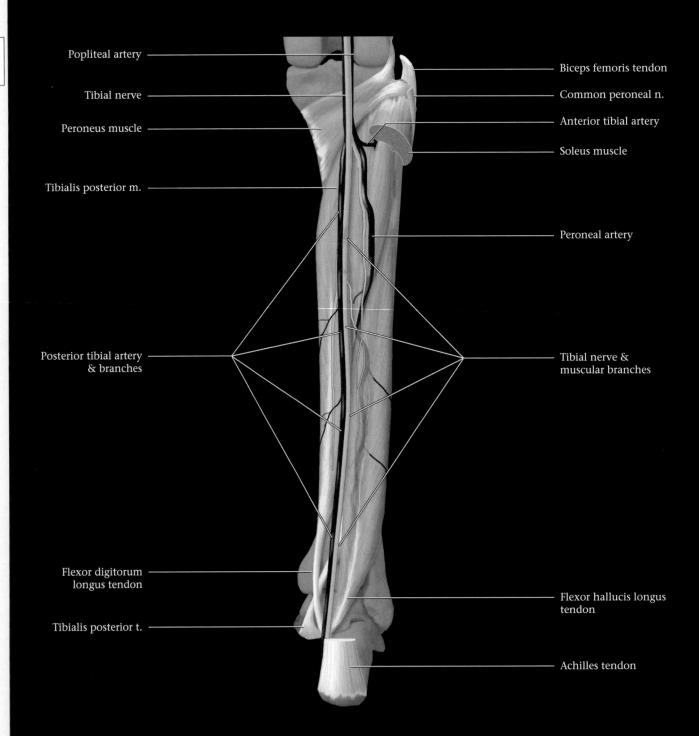

Popliteal artery

Tibial nerve

Peroneus muscle

Tibialis posterior m.

Posterior tibial artery & branches

Flexor digitorum longus tendon

Tibialis posterior t.

Biceps femoris tendon

Common peroneal n.

Anterior tibial artery

Soleus muscle

Peroneal artery

Tibial nerve & muscular branches

Flexor hallucis longus tendon

Achilles tendon

The popliteal artery ends at the distal border of popliteus in two branches: 1) anterior tibial artery passes through a slit in tibialis posterior muscle and the interosseous membrane to the anterior compartment, and 2) posterior tibial artery passes downwards and slightly medially adjacent to tibial nerve to end in space between medial malleolus and calcaneus. The largest branch of posterior tibial artery is the peroneal, which runs obliquely downwards and laterally beneath soleus to fibula. The sciatic nerve divides into common peroneal and tibial branches at the mid thigh. The common peroneal nerve follows posterior to biceps and around the lateral fibular neck; its course and branches are more completely described in graphics later in this section. The tibial nerve descends between the deep and superficial posterior leg muscles, paralleling the posterior tibial artery.

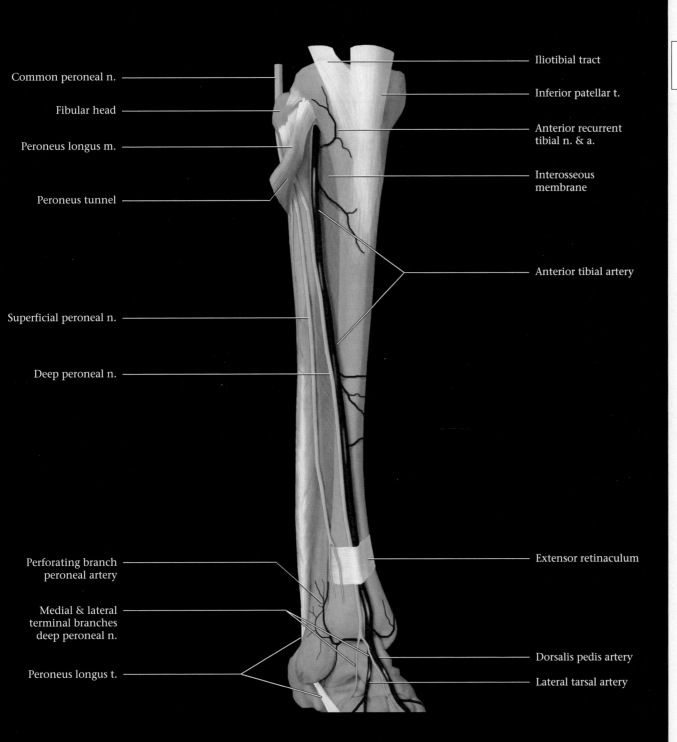

Common peroneal n.

Fibular head

Peroneus longus m.

Peroneus tunnel

Superficial peroneal n.

Deep peroneal n.

Perforating branch peroneal artery

Medial & lateral terminal branches deep peroneal n.

Peroneus longus t.

Iliotibial tract

Inferior patellar t.

Anterior recurrent tibial n. & a.

Interosseous membrane

Anterior tibial artery

Extensor retinaculum

Dorsalis pedis artery

Lateral tarsal artery

Graphic of anterior leg shows anterior tibial artery perforating the interosseous septum proximally and descending along this membrane down the front of leg to terminate as dorsalis pedis. It gives off muscular branches along its length. Distally one sees a perforating branch of the peroneal artery, which in a variant situation may provide the major blood supply to the dorsum of the foot. The common peroneal nerve is seen extending through the peroneal tunnel (between peroneus longus tendon and fibular neck), branching into deep and superficial components. Both have muscular branches along their length; the deep peroneal nerve parallels the anterior tibial artery and terminates in medial and lateral branches to the dorsum of the foot and ankle, respectively.

AXIAL T1 MR, RIGHT LEG

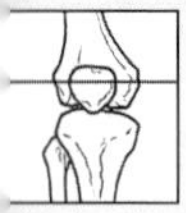

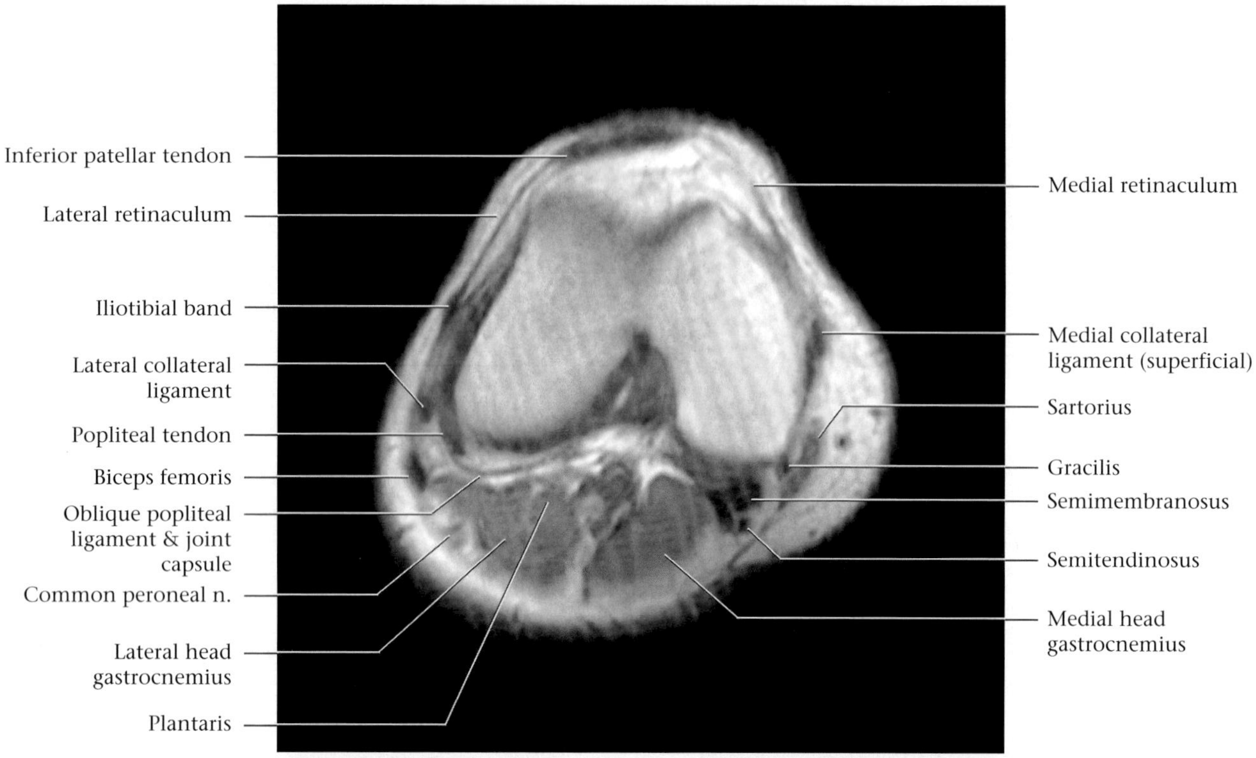
Inferior patellar tendon
Lateral retinaculum
Iliotibial band
Lateral collateral ligament
Popliteal tendon
Biceps femoris
Oblique popliteal ligament & joint capsule
Common peroneal n.
Lateral head gastrocnemius
Plantaris
Medial retinaculum
Medial collateral ligament (superficial)
Sartorius
Gracilis
Semimembranosus
Semitendinosus
Medial head gastrocnemius

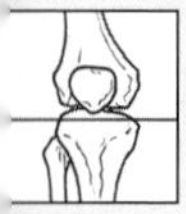

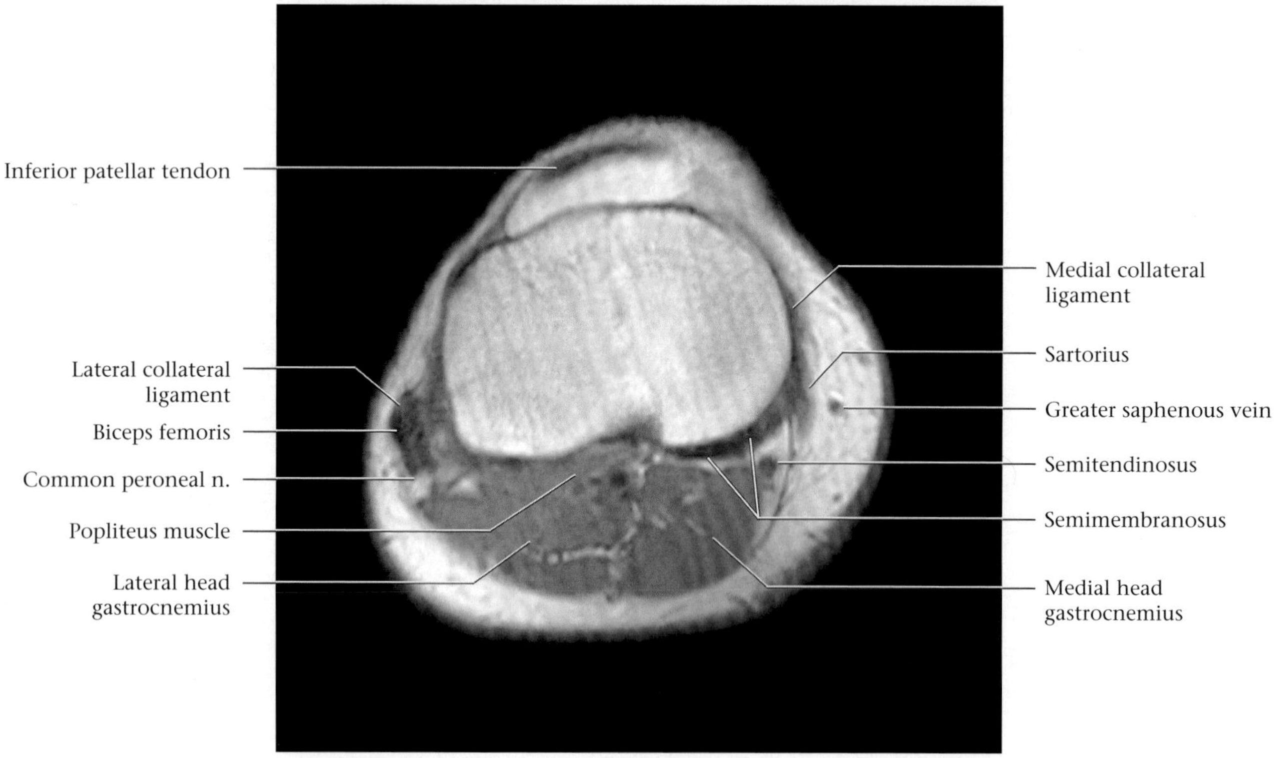
Inferior patellar tendon
Lateral collateral ligament
Biceps femoris
Common peroneal n.
Popliteus muscle
Lateral head gastrocnemius
Medial collateral ligament
Sartorius
Greater saphenous vein
Semitendinosus
Semimembranosus
Medial head gastrocnemius

(Top) First in series of axial T1 MR images of the right leg; this is just above the knee joint, included for continuity of structures. **(Bottom)** Axial T1 MR image of right leg, just below the knee joint. For greater detail about the knee joint, see "Knee Overview" section.

LEG OVERVIEW

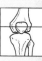

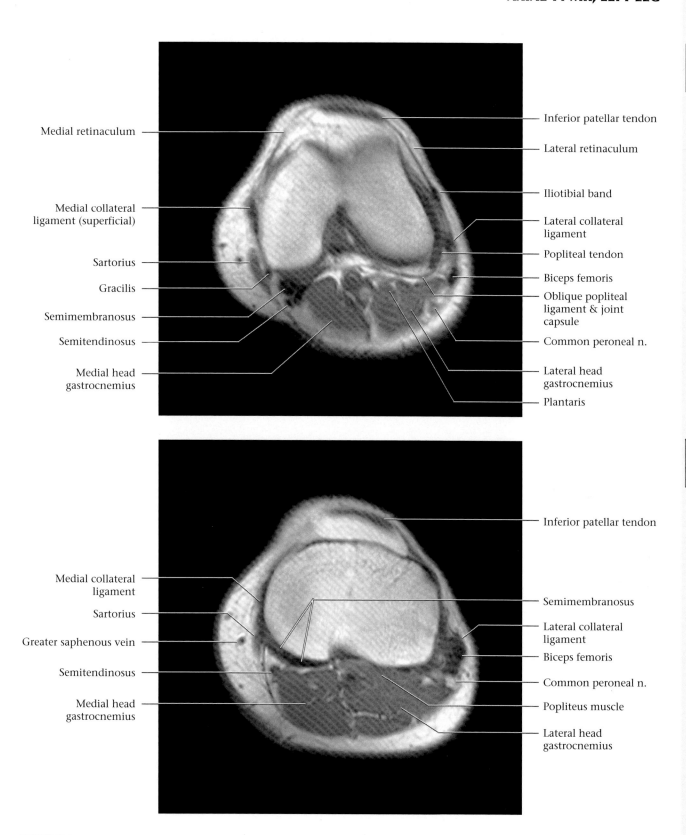

Medial retinaculum

Medial collateral ligament (superficial)

Sartorius

Gracilis

Semimembranosus

Semitendinosus

Medial head gastrocnemius

Inferior patellar tendon

Lateral retinaculum

Iliotibial band

Lateral collateral ligament

Popliteal tendon

Biceps femoris

Oblique popliteal ligament & joint capsule

Common peroneal n.

Lateral head gastrocnemius

Plantaris

Medial collateral ligament

Sartorius

Greater saphenous vein

Semitendinosus

Medial head gastrocnemius

Inferior patellar tendon

Semimembranosus

Lateral collateral ligament

Biceps femoris

Common peroneal n.

Popliteus muscle

Lateral head gastrocnemius

(Top) First in series of axial T1 MR images of the left leg; this is just above the knee joint, included for continuity of structures **(Bottom)** Axial MR image of left leg, just below the knee joint. For greater detail about the knee joint, see "Knee Overview" section.

AXIAL T1 MR, RIGHT LEG

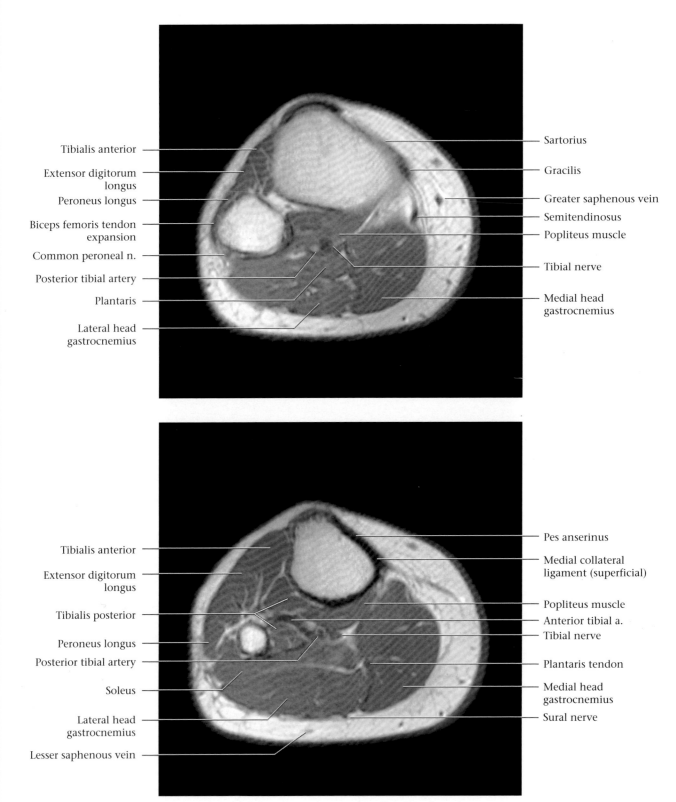

Tibialis anterior

Extensor digitorum longus

Peroneus longus

Biceps femoris tendon expansion

Common peroneal n.

Posterior tibial artery

Plantaris

Lateral head gastrocnemius

Sartorius

Gracilis

Greater saphenous vein

Semitendinosus

Popliteus muscle

Tibial nerve

Medial head gastrocnemius

Tibialis anterior

Extensor digitorum longus

Tibialis posterior

Peroneus longus

Posterior tibial artery

Soleus

Lateral head gastrocnemius

Lesser saphenous vein

Pes anserinus

Medial collateral ligament (superficial)

Popliteus muscle

Anterior tibial a.

Tibial nerve

Plantaris tendon

Medial head gastrocnemius

Sural nerve

(Top) Axial T1 MR image of right leg at the proximal tibiofibular joint. Note that the plantaris is still muscular, lying in front of the lateral head of the gastrocnemius. **(Bottom)** Axial T1 MR image of right leg at the proximal metaphysis. By this point, the soleus has arisen from the fibula; the section is too proximal to see the tibial origin of soleus since the popliteal muscle is still present. The plantaris is now tendinous, lying between the soleus and medial head of gastrocnemius. At this level, one sees the tibialis posterior arising as a bifid structure from both tibia and fibula; the anterior tibial vessels are seen coursing forward towards the anterior compartment, between these two attachments.

AXIAL T1 MR, LEFT LEG

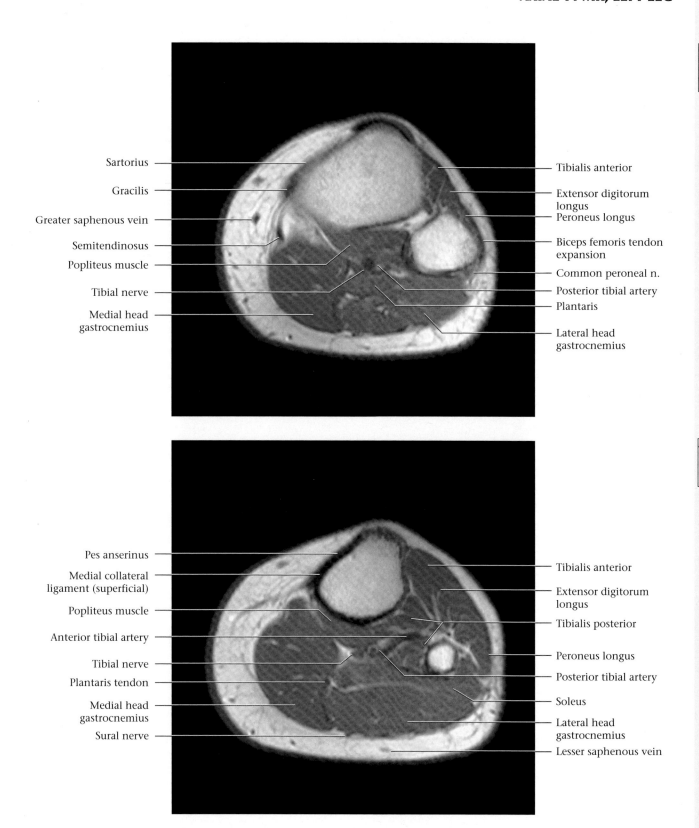

Sartorius

Gracilis

Greater saphenous vein

Semitendinosus

Popliteus muscle

Tibial nerve

Medial head gastrocnemius

Tibialis anterior

Extensor digitorum longus

Peroneus longus

Biceps femoris tendon expansion

Common peroneal n.

Posterior tibial artery

Plantaris

Lateral head gastrocnemius

Pes anserinus

Medial collateral ligament (superficial)

Popliteus muscle

Anterior tibial artery

Tibial nerve

Plantaris tendon

Medial head gastrocnemius

Sural nerve

Tibialis anterior

Extensor digitorum longus

Tibialis posterior

Peroneus longus

Posterior tibial artery

Soleus

Lateral head gastrocnemius

Lesser saphenous vein

(Top) Axial T1 MR image of left leg at the proximal tibiofemoral joint. Note that the plantaris is still muscular, lying in front of the lateral head of the gastrocnemius. **(Bottom)** Axial T1 MR image of left leg at the proximal metaphysis. By this point, the soleus has arisen from the fibula; the section is too proximal to see the tibial origin of soleus since the popliteal muscle is still present. The plantaris is now tendinous, lying between the soleus and medial head of gastrocnemius. At this level, one sees the tibialis posterior arising as a bifid structure from both tibia and fibula; the anterior tibial vessels are seen coursing forward towards the anterior compartment, between these two attachments.

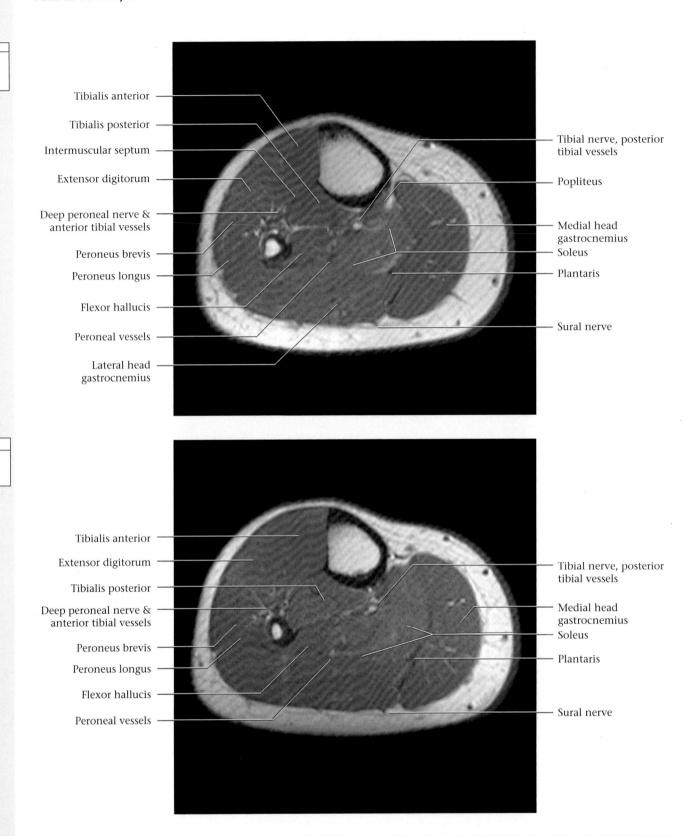

LEG OVERVIEW

AXIAL T1 MR, RIGHT LEG

Labels (Top image):
- Tibialis anterior
- Tibialis posterior
- Intermuscular septum
- Extensor digitorum
- Deep peroneal nerve & anterior tibial vessels
- Peroneus brevis
- Peroneus longus
- Flexor hallucis
- Peroneal vessels
- Lateral head gastrocnemius
- Tibial nerve, posterior tibial vessels
- Popliteus
- Medial head gastrocnemius
- Soleus
- Plantaris
- Sural nerve

Labels (Bottom image):
- Tibialis anterior
- Extensor digitorum
- Tibialis posterior
- Deep peroneal nerve & anterior tibial vessels
- Peroneus brevis
- Peroneus longus
- Flexor hallucis
- Peroneal vessels
- Tibial nerve, posterior tibial vessels
- Medial head gastrocnemius
- Soleus
- Plantaris
- Sural nerve

(Top) Axial T1 MR image of right leg at the proximal diaphysis. Note that by this point, peroneus brevis and flexor hallucis begin to originate from the fibula. There remains a slip of popliteus at the posterior tibia. The major vessels of the leg have trifurcated. **(Bottom)** Axial T1 MR image of right leg, slightly distal. Note that the popliteus insertion on the tibia has ended, and the soleus gains its tibial origin. The lateral head of gastrocnemius has become entirely tendinous.

Knee

VI

LEG OVERVIEW

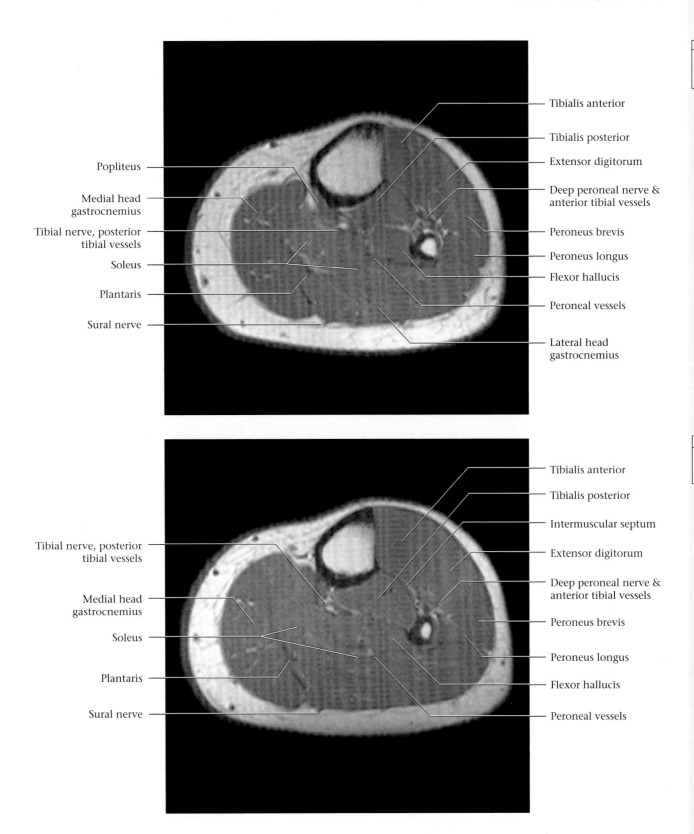

Top image labels:

- Popliteus
- Medial head gastrocnemius
- Tibial nerve, posterior tibial vessels
- Soleus
- Plantaris
- Sural nerve
- Tibialis anterior
- Tibialis posterior
- Extensor digitorum
- Deep peroneal nerve & anterior tibial vessels
- Peroneus brevis
- Peroneus longus
- Flexor hallucis
- Peroneal vessels
- Lateral head gastrocnemius

Bottom image labels:

- Tibial nerve, posterior tibial vessels
- Medial head gastrocnemius
- Soleus
- Plantaris
- Sural nerve
- Tibialis anterior
- Tibialis posterior
- Intermuscular septum
- Extensor digitorum
- Deep peroneal nerve & anterior tibial vessels
- Peroneus brevis
- Peroneus longus
- Flexor hallucis
- Peroneal vessels

(Top) Axial T1 MR image of left leg at the proximal diaphysis. Note that by this point, peroneus brevis and flexor hallucis begin to originate from the fibula. There remains a slip of popliteus at the posterior tibia. The major vessels of the leg have trifurcated. **(Bottom)** Axial T1 MR image of left leg, slightly distal. Note that the popliteus insertion on the tibia has ended, and the soleus gains its tibial origin. The lateral head of gastrocnemius has become entirely tendinous.

AXIAL T1 MR, RIGHT LEG

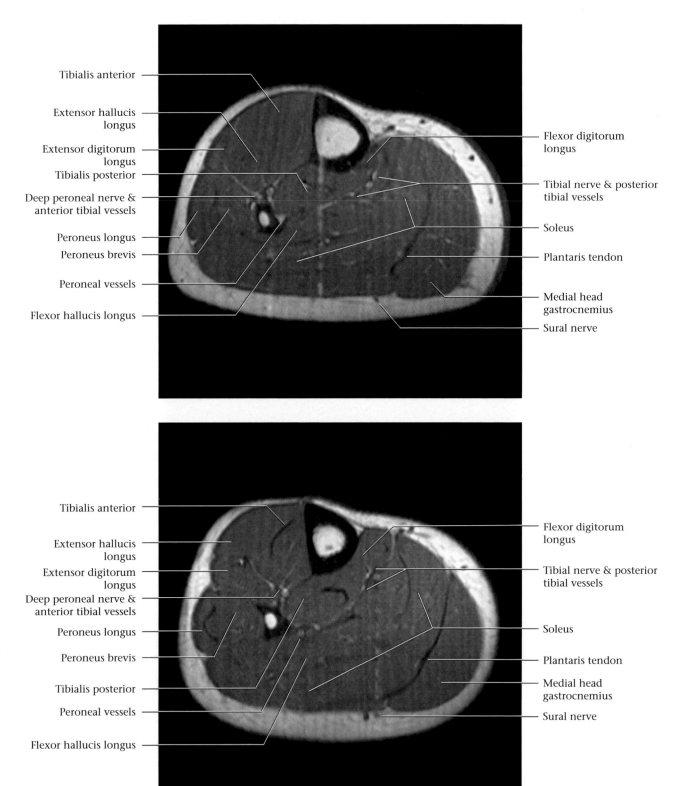

Top image labels:

Tibialis anterior
Extensor hallucis longus
Extensor digitorum longus
Tibialis posterior
Deep peroneal nerve & anterior tibial vessels
Peroneus longus
Peroneus brevis
Peroneal vessels
Flexor hallucis longus

Flexor digitorum longus
Tibial nerve & posterior tibial vessels
Soleus
Plantaris tendon
Medial head gastrocnemius
Sural nerve

Bottom image labels:

Tibialis anterior
Extensor hallucis longus
Extensor digitorum longus
Deep peroneal nerve & anterior tibial vessels
Peroneus longus
Peroneus brevis
Tibialis posterior
Peroneal vessels
Flexor hallucis longus

Flexor digitorum longus
Tibial nerve & posterior tibial vessels
Soleus
Plantaris tendon
Medial head gastrocnemius
Sural nerve

(Top) Axial T1 MR image of the right leg at the junction of proximal and middle thirds. At this point, the extensor hallucis longus makes its appearance, arising from the anterior fibula and interosseous membrane. Flexor digitorum longus also is now seen, arising from the posterior tibia. The lateral head of gastrocnemius has become tendinous, with soleus making up the bulk of the posterior muscles. **(Bottom)** Slightly distal axial T1 MR image of the right leg. At this point, the extensor hallucis longus is located between tibialis anterior and extensor digitorum longus and is not easily distinguished from them. Similarly, the peroneal muscle/tendons are not easily distinguished because of poorly visualized fat planes in the leg. Note also that the plantaris tendon still lies between medial head of gastrocnemius and soleus, but is tracking medially.

AXIAL T1 MR, LEFT LEG

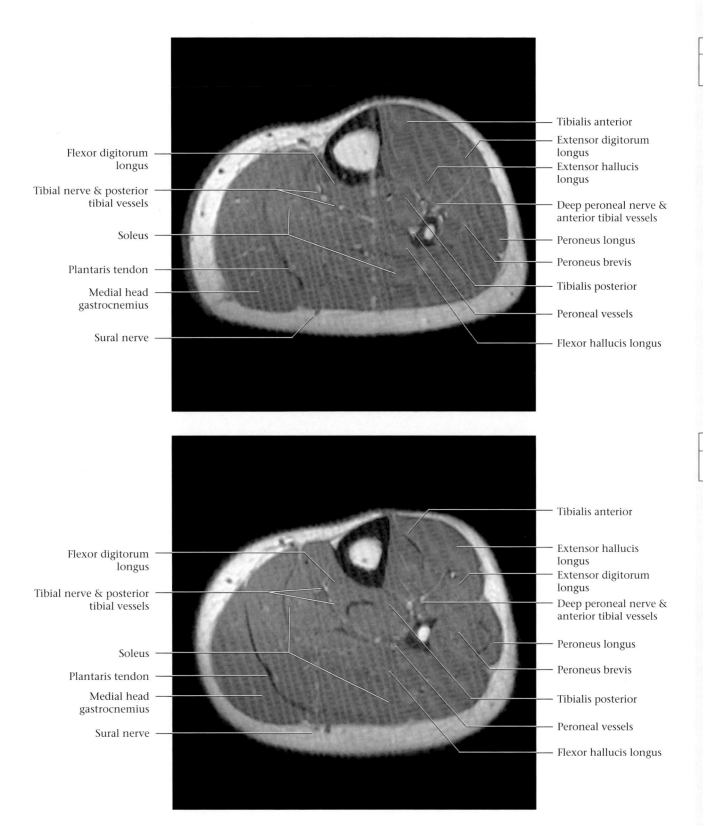

Flexor digitorum longus

Tibial nerve & posterior tibial vessels

Soleus

Plantaris tendon

Medial head gastrocnemius

Sural nerve

Tibialis anterior

Extensor digitorum longus

Extensor hallucis longus

Deep peroneal nerve & anterior tibial vessels

Peroneus longus

Peroneus brevis

Tibialis posterior

Peroneal vessels

Flexor hallucis longus

Flexor digitorum longus

Tibial nerve & posterior tibial vessels

Soleus

Plantaris tendon

Medial head gastrocnemius

Sural nerve

Tibialis anterior

Extensor hallucis longus

Extensor digitorum longus

Deep peroneal nerve & anterior tibial vessels

Peroneus longus

Peroneus brevis

Tibialis posterior

Peroneal vessels

Flexor hallucis longus

(Top) Axial T1 MR image of the left leg at the junction of proximal and middle thirds. At this point, the extensor hallucis longus makes its appearance, arising from the anterior fibula and interosseous membrane. Flexor digitorum longus also is now seen, arising from the posterior tibia. The lateral head of gastrocnemius has become tendinous, with soleus making up the bulk of the posterior muscles. **(Bottom)** Slightly distal axial T1 MR image of the left leg. At this point, the extensor hallucis longus is located between tibialis anterior and extensor digitorum longus and is not easily distinguished from them. Similarly, the peroneal muscle/tendons are not easily distinguished because lef poorly visualized fat planes in the leg. Note also that the plantaris tendon still lies between medial head of gastrocnemius and soleus, but is tracking medially.

Knee

VI

AXIAL T1 MR, RIGHT LEG

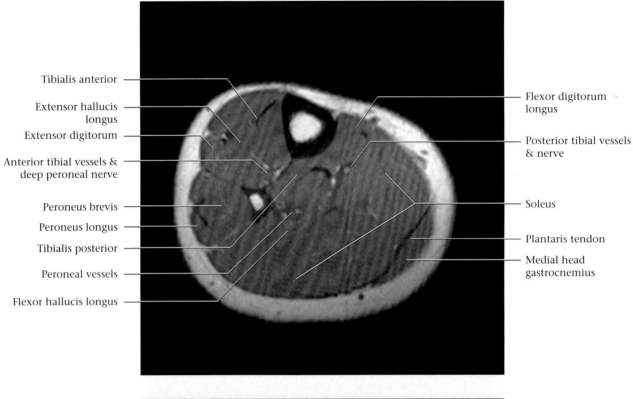

Tibialis anterior

Extensor hallucis longus

Extensor digitorum

Anterior tibial vessels & deep peroneal nerve

Peroneus brevis

Peroneus longus

Tibialis posterior

Peroneal vessels

Flexor hallucis longus

Flexor digitorum longus

Posterior tibial vessels & nerve

Soleus

Plantaris tendon

Medial head gastrocnemius

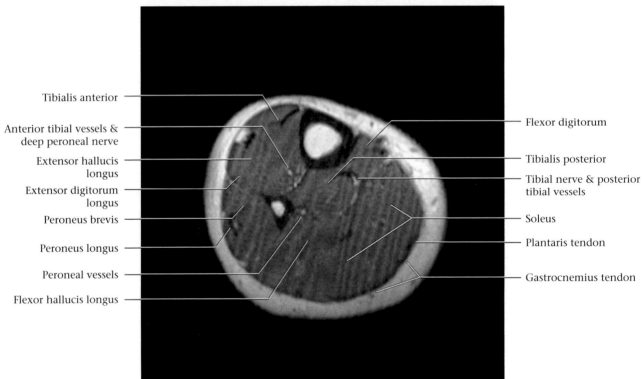

Tibialis anterior

Anterior tibial vessels & deep peroneal nerve

Extensor hallucis longus

Extensor digitorum longus

Peroneus brevis

Peroneus longus

Peroneal vessels

Flexor hallucis longus

Flexor digitorum

Tibialis posterior

Tibial nerve & posterior tibial vessels

Soleus

Plantaris tendon

Gastrocnemius tendon

(Top) Axial T1 MR image of the right leg at the mid diaphysis. At this point, in the mid leg, the gastrocnemius muscle has become nearly completely tendinous. **(Bottom)** Slightly distal axial T1 MR image of the right leg. The gastrocnemius is now entirely tendinous, and the plantaris tendon lies subcutaneously adjacent to the medial aspect of the gastrocnemius tendon.

LEG OVERVIEW

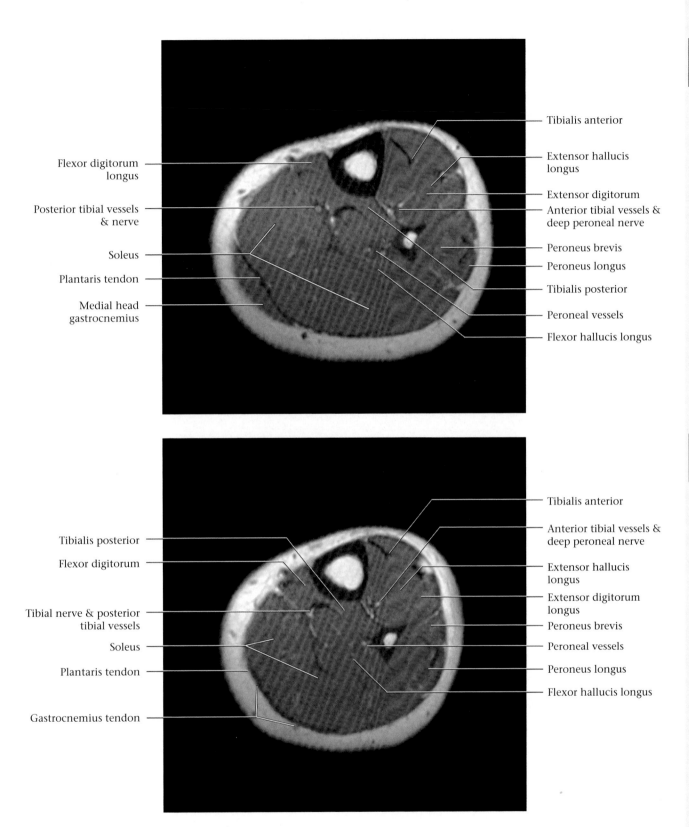

(Top) Axial T1 MR image of the left leg at the mid diaphysis. At this point, in the mid leg, the gastrocnemius muscle has become nearly completely tendinous. **(Bottom)** Slightly distal axial T1 MR image of the left leg. The gastrocnemius is now entirely tendinous, and the plantaris tendon lies subcutaneously adjacent to the medial aspect of the gastrocnemius tendon.

AXIAL T1 MR, RIGHT LEG

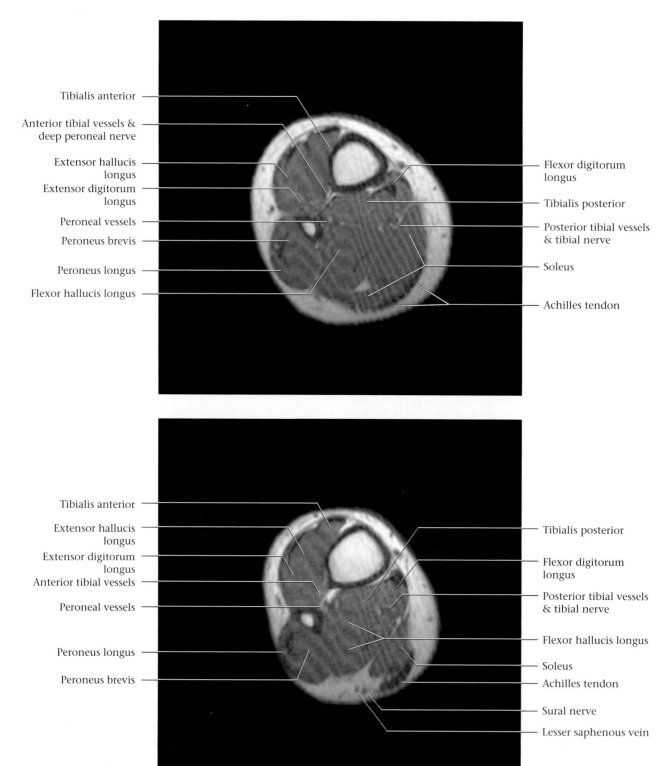

Tibialis anterior
Anterior tibial vessels & deep peroneal nerve
Extensor hallucis longus
Extensor digitorum longus
Peroneal vessels
Peroneus brevis
Peroneus longus
Flexor hallucis longus

Flexor digitorum longus
Tibialis posterior
Posterior tibial vessels & tibial nerve
Soleus
Achilles tendon

Tibialis anterior
Extensor hallucis longus
Extensor digitorum longus
Anterior tibial vessels
Peroneal vessels
Peroneus longus
Peroneus brevis

Tibialis posterior
Flexor digitorum longus
Posterior tibial vessels & tibial nerve
Flexor hallucis longus
Soleus
Achilles tendon
Sural nerve
Lesser saphenous vein

(Top) Axial T1 MR image of the right leg at the junction of middle and distal thirds. The deep muscles of the posterior compartment are now more prominent than the superficial. **(Bottom)** Slightly distal axial T1 MR images of the right leg, with the compartments more distinctly seen.

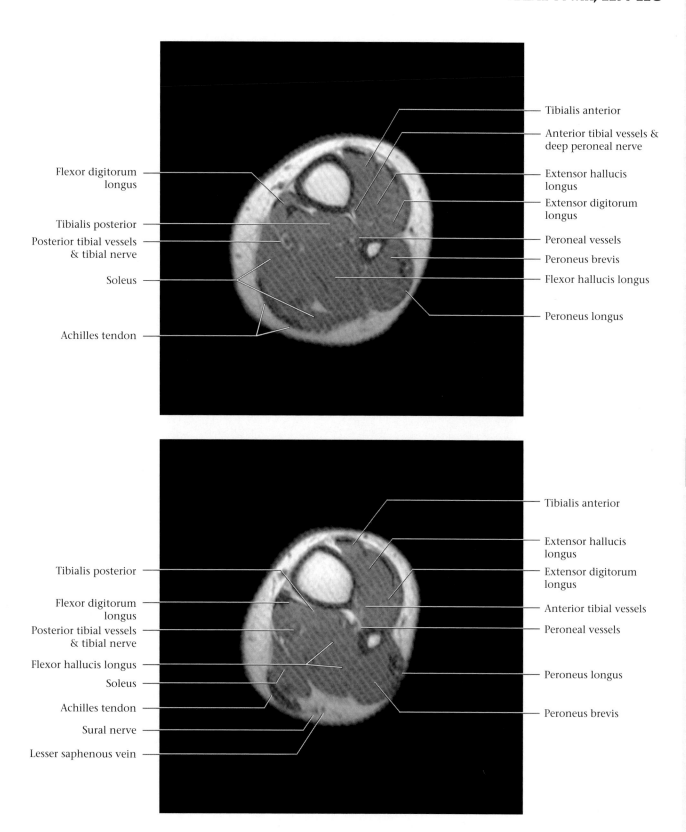

Flexor digitorum longus

Tibialis posterior

Posterior tibial vessels & tibial nerve

Soleus

Achilles tendon

Tibialis anterior

Anterior tibial vessels & deep peroneal nerve

Extensor hallucis longus

Extensor digitorum longus

Peroneal vessels

Peroneus brevis

Flexor hallucis longus

Peroneus longus

Tibialis posterior

Flexor digitorum longus

Posterior tibial vessels & tibial nerve

Flexor hallucis longus

Soleus

Achilles tendon

Sural nerve

Lesser saphenous vein

Tibialis anterior

Extensor hallucis longus

Extensor digitorum longus

Anterior tibial vessels

Peroneal vessels

Peroneus longus

Peroneus brevis

(Top) Axial T1 MR images of the left leg at the junction of the middle and distal thirds. The deep muscles of the posterior compartment are now more prominent than the superficial. **(Bottom)** Slightly distal axial T1 MR images of the left leg, with the compartments more distinctly seen.

AXIAL T1 MR, RIGHT LEG

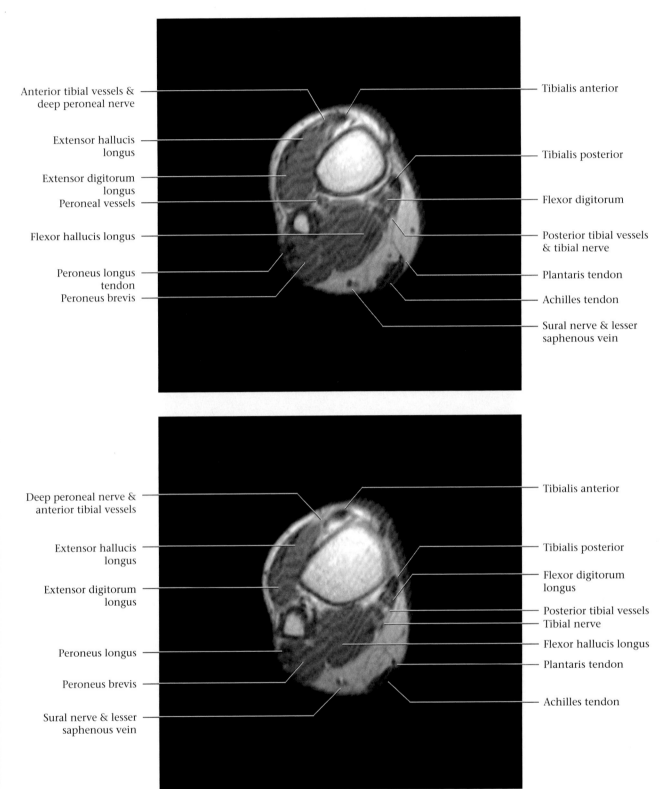

Anterior tibial vessels & deep peroneal nerve

Extensor hallucis longus

Extensor digitorum longus
Peroneal vessels

Flexor hallucis longus

Peroneus longus tendon
Peroneus brevis

Tibialis anterior

Tibialis posterior

Flexor digitorum

Posterior tibial vessels & tibial nerve

Plantaris tendon

Achilles tendon

Sural nerve & lesser saphenous vein

Deep peroneal nerve & anterior tibial vessels

Extensor hallucis longus

Extensor digitorum longus

Peroneus longus

Peroneus brevis

Sural nerve & lesser saphenous vein

Tibialis anterior

Tibialis posterior

Flexor digitorum longus

Posterior tibial vessels
Tibial nerve

Flexor hallucis longus

Plantaris tendon

Achilles tendon

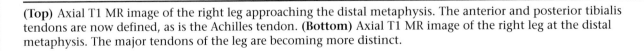

(Top) Axial T1 MR image of the right leg approaching the distal metaphysis. The anterior and posterior tibialis tendons are now defined, as is the Achilles tendon. **(Bottom)** Axial T1 MR image of the right leg at the distal metaphysis. The major tendons of the leg are becoming more distinct.

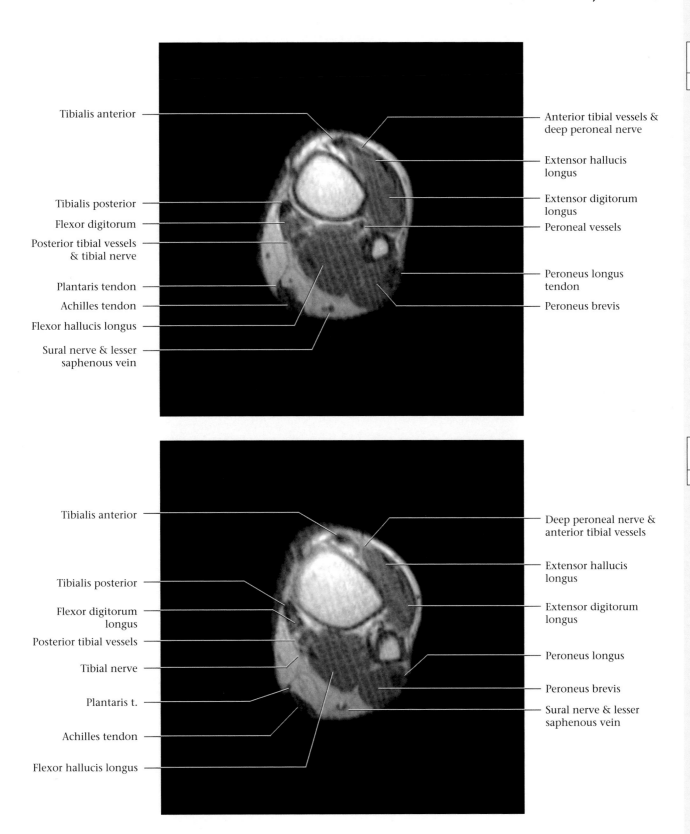

Tibialis anterior

Anterior tibial vessels & deep peroneal nerve

Extensor hallucis longus

Tibialis posterior

Extensor digitorum longus

Flexor digitorum

Peroneal vessels

Posterior tibial vessels & tibial nerve

Plantaris tendon

Peroneus longus tendon

Achilles tendon

Peroneus brevis

Flexor hallucis longus

Sural nerve & lesser saphenous vein

Tibialis anterior

Deep peroneal nerve & anterior tibial vessels

Extensor hallucis longus

Tibialis posterior

Flexor digitorum longus

Extensor digitorum longus

Posterior tibial vessels

Tibial nerve

Peroneus longus

Plantaris t.

Peroneus brevis

Achilles tendon

Sural nerve & lesser saphenous vein

Flexor hallucis longus

(Top) Axial T1 MR image of the left leg approaching the distal metaphysis. The anterior and posterior tibialis tendons are now defined, as is the Achilles tendon. **(Bottom)** Axial T1 MR image of the left leg at the distal metaphysis. The major tendons of the leg are becoming more distinct.

AXIAL T1 MR, RIGHT LEG

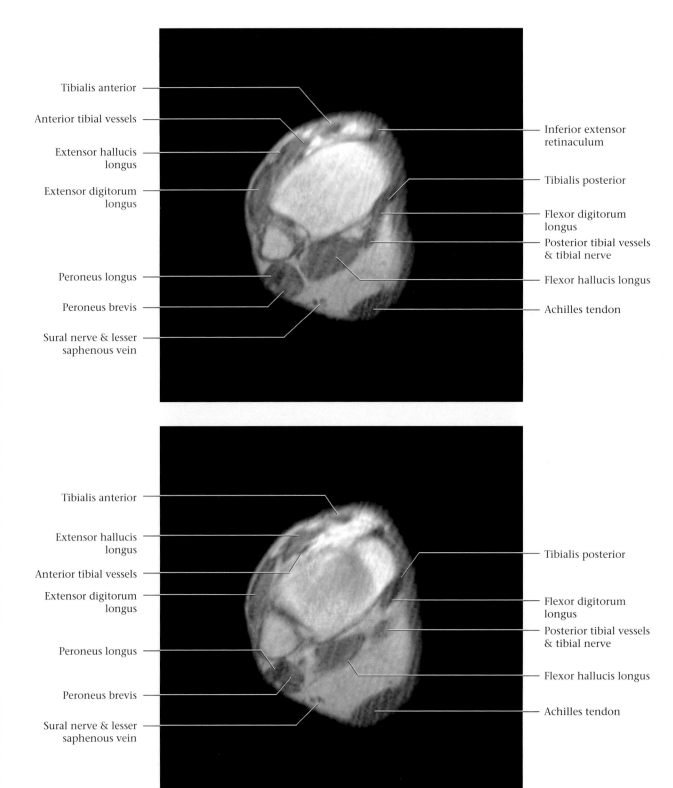

Tibialis anterior

Anterior tibial vessels

Extensor hallucis longus

Extensor digitorum longus

Peroneus longus

Peroneus brevis

Sural nerve & lesser saphenous vein

Inferior extensor retinaculum

Tibialis posterior

Flexor digitorum longus

Posterior tibial vessels & tibial nerve

Flexor hallucis longus

Achilles tendon

Tibialis anterior

Extensor hallucis longus

Anterior tibial vessels

Extensor digitorum longus

Peroneus longus

Peroneus brevis

Sural nerve & lesser saphenous vein

Tibialis posterior

Flexor digitorum longus

Posterior tibial vessels & tibial nerve

Flexor hallucis longus

Achilles tendon

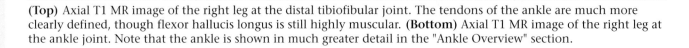

(Top) Axial T1 MR image of the right leg at the distal tibiofibular joint. The tendons of the ankle are much more clearly defined, though flexor hallucis longus is still highly muscular. **(Bottom)** Axial T1 MR image of the right leg at the ankle joint. Note that the ankle is shown in much greater detail in the "Ankle Overview" section.

LEG OVERVIEW

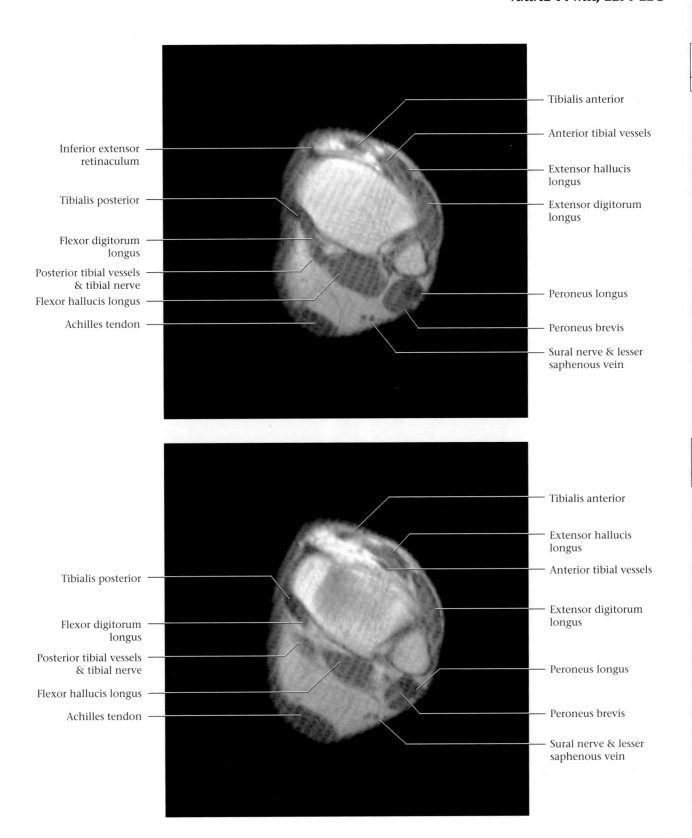

Inferior extensor retinaculum

Tibialis posterior

Flexor digitorum longus

Posterior tibial vessels & tibial nerve

Flexor hallucis longus

Achilles tendon

Tibialis anterior

Anterior tibial vessels

Extensor hallucis longus

Extensor digitorum longus

Peroneus longus

Peroneus brevis

Sural nerve & lesser saphenous vein

Tibialis posterior

Flexor digitorum longus

Posterior tibial vessels & tibial nerve

Flexor hallucis longus

Achilles tendon

Tibialis anterior

Extensor hallucis longus

Anterior tibial vessels

Extensor digitorum longus

Peroneus longus

Peroneus brevis

Sural nerve & lesser saphenous vein

(Top) Axial T1 MR image of the left leg at the distal tibiofibular joint. The tendons of the ankle are much more clearly defined, though flexor hallucis longus is still highly muscular. **(Bottom)** Axial T1 MR image of the left leg at the ankle joint. Note that the ankle is shown in much greater detail in the "Ankle Overview" section.

CORONAL T1 MR, BILATERAL LEGS

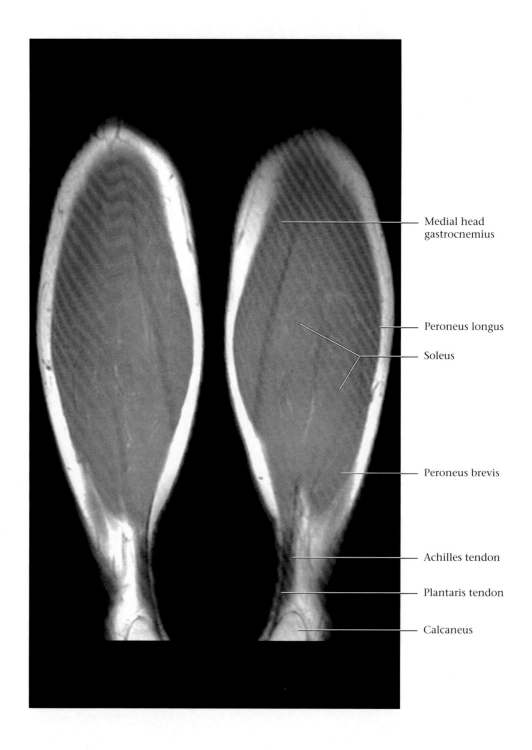

Medial head gastrocnemius

Peroneus longus

Soleus

Peroneus brevis

Achilles tendon

Plantaris tendon

Calcaneus

First of four coronal images of the legs. This is the most posterior image, largely through the posterior superficial muscles. Note the plantaris tendon which is seen well in the left leg, traveling and inserting medially to the Achilles tendon.

LEG OVERVIEW

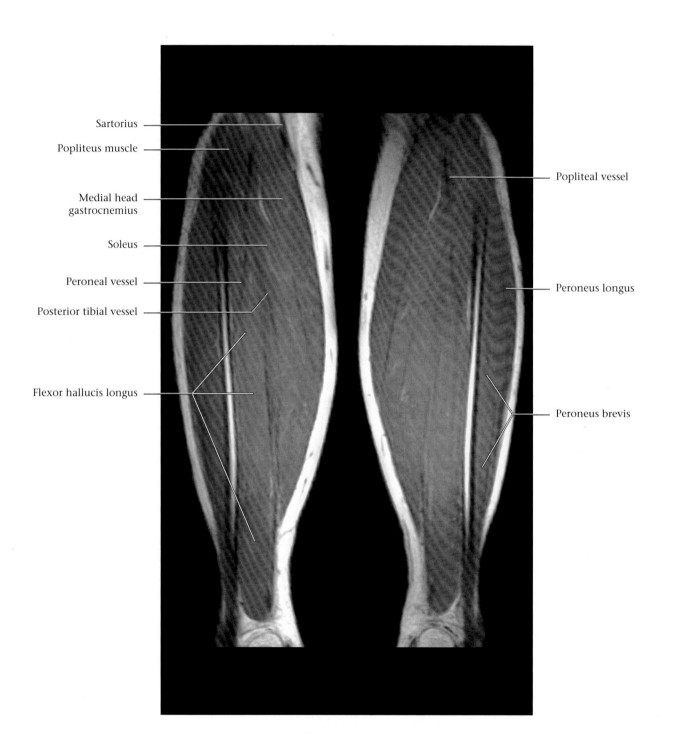

Sartorius

Popliteus muscle

Medial head gastrocnemius

Soleus

Peroneal vessel

Posterior tibial vessel

Flexor hallucis longus

Popliteal vessel

Peroneus longus

Peroneus brevis

Slightly more anterior coronal image of the legs, located posteriorly, through the fibula. Portions of the deep and superficial posterior compartment are seen, along with the lateral compartment.

CORONAL T1 MR, BILATERAL LEGS

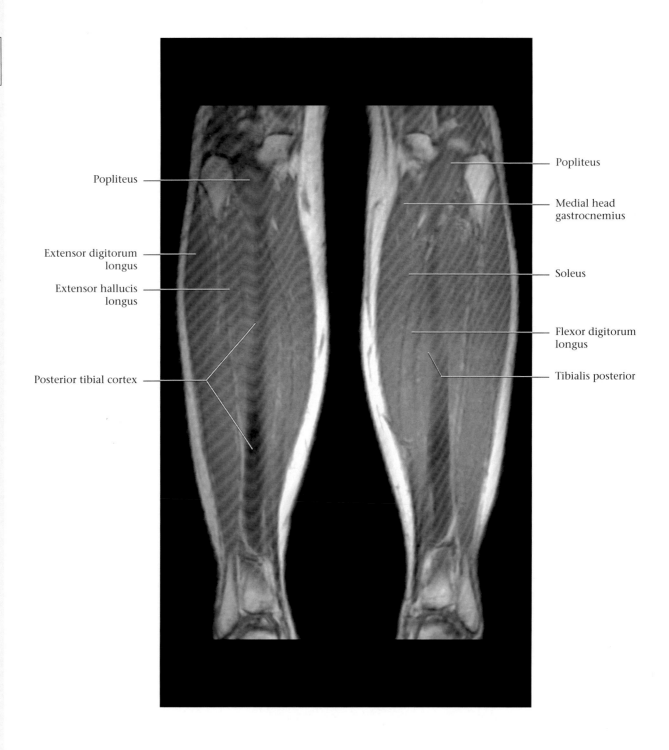

Popliteus

Extensor digitorum
longus

Extensor hallucis
longus

Posterior tibial cortex

Popliteus

Medial head
gastrocnemius

Soleus

Flexor digitorum
longus

Tibialis posterior

Coronal image of the legs, through the posterior tibial cortex. The more complex deep and superficial posterior compartments are partially seen.

CORONAL T1 MR, BILATERAL LEGS

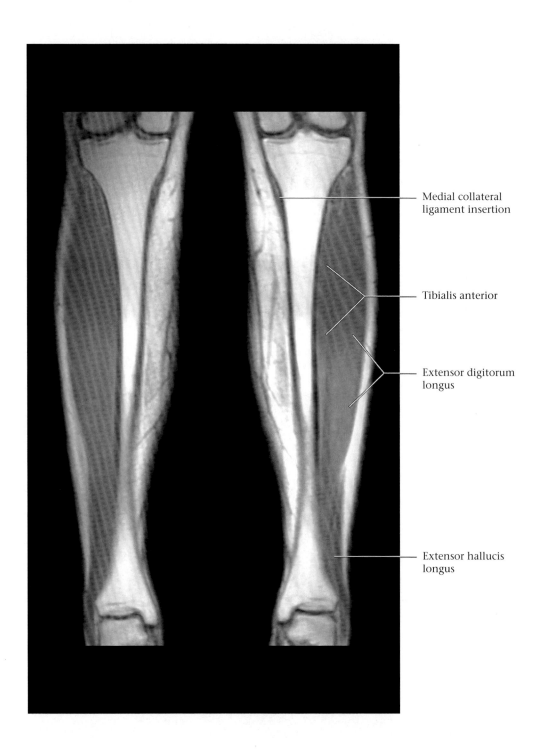

Medial collateral ligament insertion

Tibialis anterior

Extensor digitorum longus

Extensor hallucis longus

Coronal image of the legs, located anteriorly. Note the bare anteromedial aspect of the tibia. Because there is no overlying muscle, the blood supply is easily compromised when the tibia is fractured.

SAGITTAL T1 MR, LEG

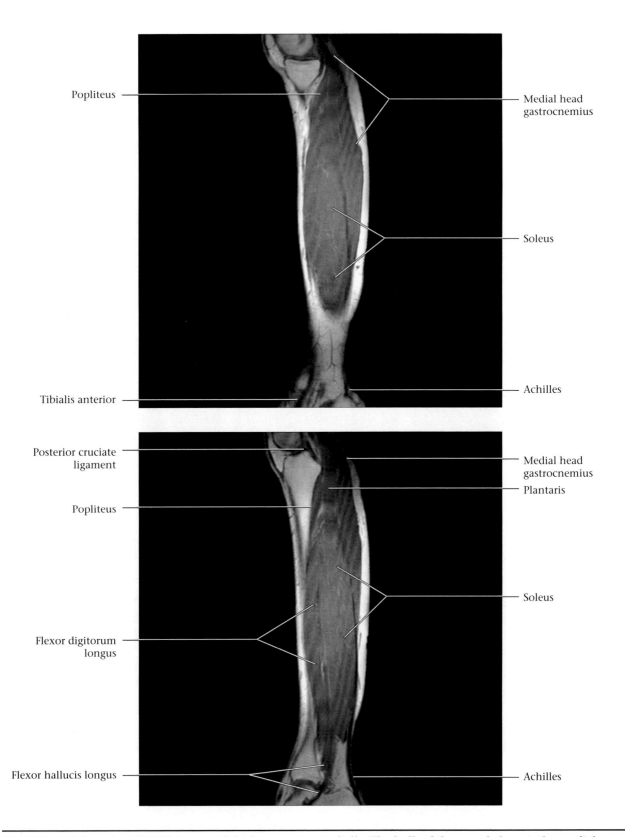

Popliteus

Medial head
gastrocnemius

Soleus

Achilles

Tibialis anterior

Posterior cruciate
ligament

Medial head
gastrocnemius

Plantaris

Popliteus

Flexor digitorum
longus

Soleus

Flexor hallucis longus

Achilles

(Top) First of six sagittal T1 MR images of the leg, starting medially. The bulk of the muscle here is the medial superficial posterior muscles, soleus and gastrocnemius. **(Bottom)** Sagittal T1 MR image, medial leg. A portion of the deep posterior muscles is now seen, including the distal tendon of flexor hallucis longus. Note the distal extent of popliteus muscle, and the fact that the tibial origin of soleus is from the soleal line, along the distal site of insertion of popliteus.

LEG OVERVIEW

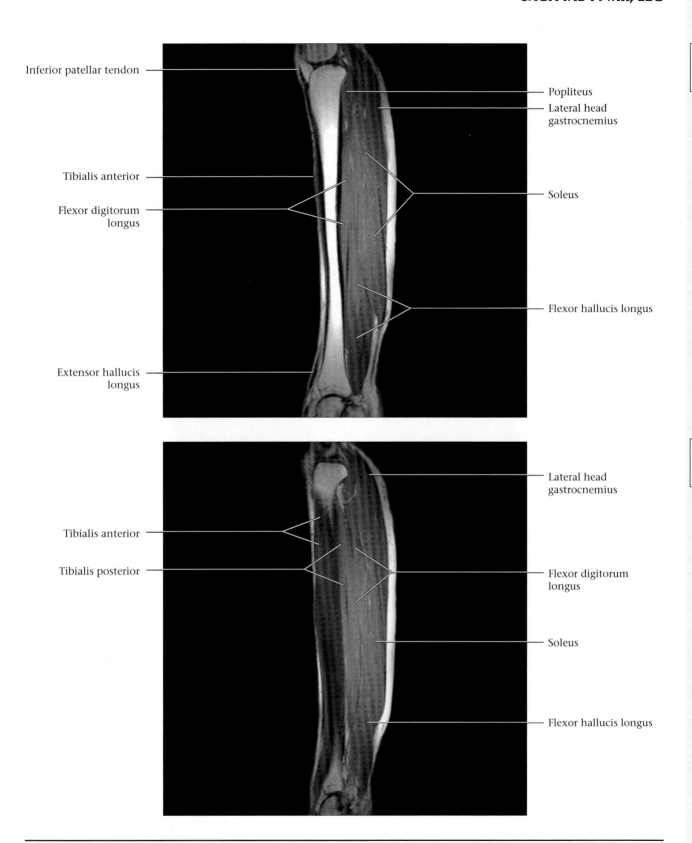

Inferior patellar tendon

Popliteus

Lateral head gastrocnemius

Tibialis anterior

Flexor digitorum longus

Soleus

Flexor hallucis longus

Extensor hallucis longus

Lateral head gastrocnemius

Tibialis anterior

Tibialis posterior

Flexor digitorum longus

Soleus

Flexor hallucis longus

(Top) Sagittal T1 MR image, mid leg. The bulkiness of flexor hallucis longus can be appreciated, along with the pre-Achilles fat pad separating it from Achilles tendon. Note also the bare medial aspect of the shaft of tibia.
(Bottom) Sagittal T1 MR image, slightly lateral in the leg. Tibialis anterior is seen arising from the lateral aspect of the shaft of tibia.

SAGITTAL T1 MR, LEG

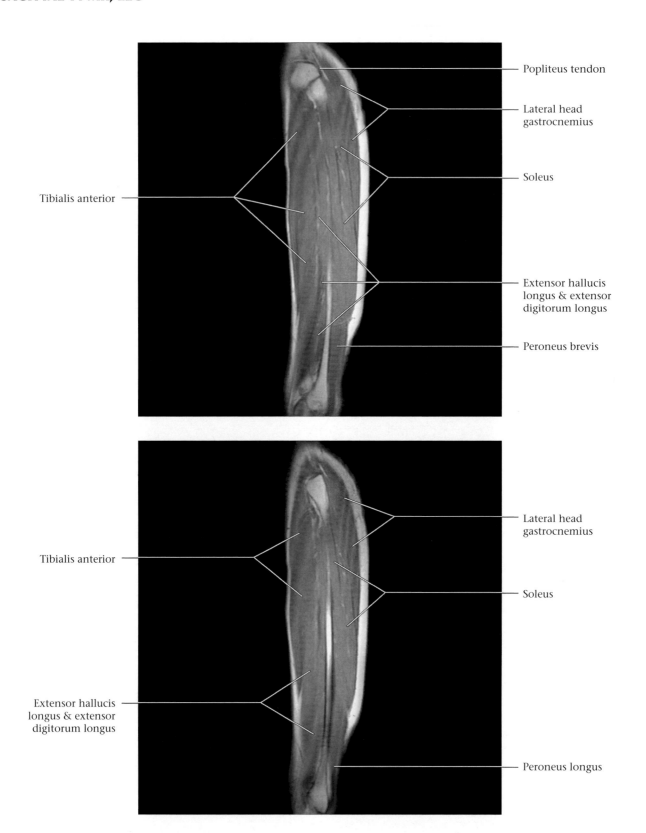

Popliteus tendon

Lateral head gastrocnemius

Soleus

Tibialis anterior

Extensor hallucis longus & extensor digitorum longus

Peroneus brevis

Lateral head gastrocnemius

Tibialis anterior

Soleus

Extensor hallucis longus & extensor digitorum longus

Peroneus longus

(Top) Sagittal T1 MR image, level of fibula. The fibular origin of the soleus, as well as peroneus and extensor digitorum is seen. **(Bottom)** Sagittal T1 MR image, level of fibula. Given the bulky muscles arising from the fibula, it is not surprising that the fibular surface is irregular. This should not be mistaken for periosteal reaction.

AXIAL T2 MR OF KNEE, VARIANT GASTROCNEMIUS

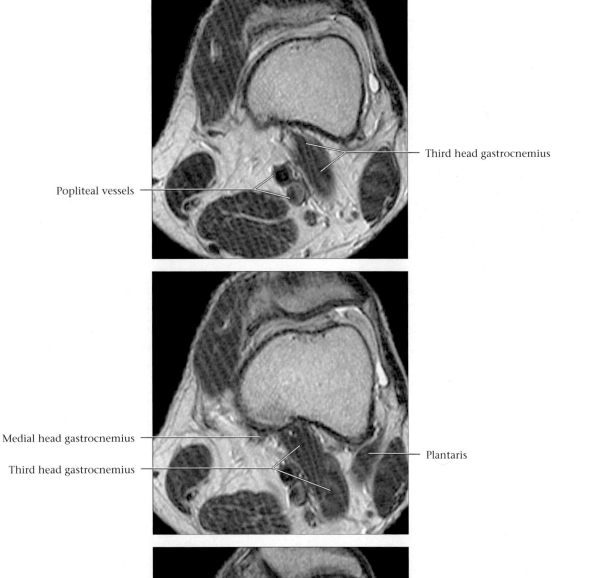

Popliteal vessels

Third head gastrocnemius

Medial head gastrocnemius

Third head gastrocnemius

Plantaris

Lateral head gastrocnemius m.

Medial head gastrocnemius

Plantaris muscle

Third head gastrocnemius

Popliteal vessels

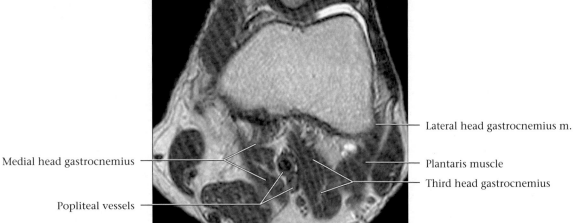

(Top) First of three axial T2 MR images showing a variant, third head of gastrocnemius. The aberrant head arises from the medial femoral metaphysis, adjacent to the normal medial head gastrocnemius. However, it deviates laterally, forming a muscular sling around the popliteal vessels. **(Middle)** Image in series is slightly more distal, showing the aberrant third head as well as the normal medial and lateral heads of gastrocnemius. **(Bottom)** Final axial image, slightly more distal towards knee joint, shows the popliteal vessels surrounded by the normal medial head and the third head of the gastrocnemius. This may result in symptoms of claudication. However, the variant is more likely to cause symptoms if it splits the popliteal artery and vein.

GRAPHIC, ANTERIOR LEG SHOWING PATH OF COMMON PERONEAL NERVE

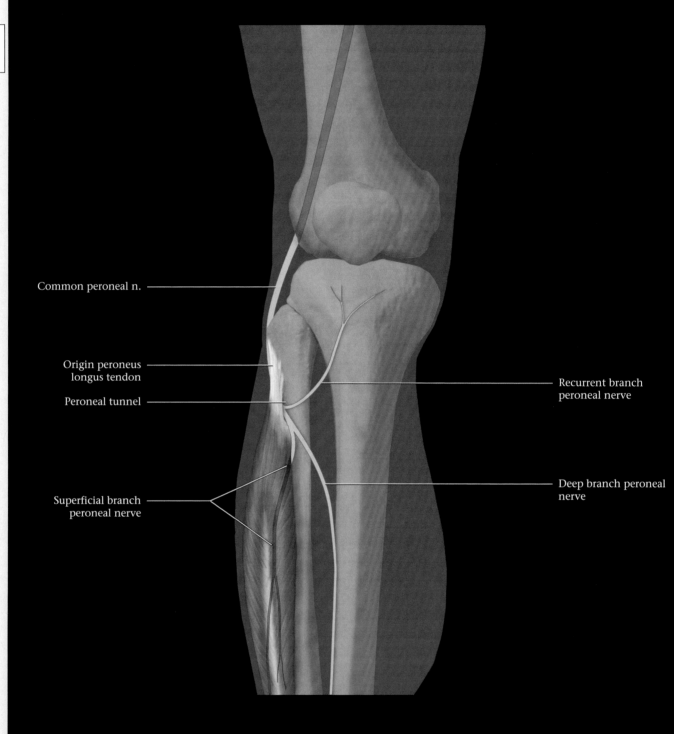

Common peroneal n.

Origin peroneus
longus tendon

Peroneal tunnel

Superficial branch
peroneal nerve

Recurrent branch
peroneal nerve

Deep branch peroneal
nerve

The common peroneal nerve branches from the sciatic nerve in the proximal popliteal fossa. It courses anterolaterally, posterior to biceps femoris muscle, then winds around the fibular head. As it curves around the anterior surface of the fibula, the nerve enters the peroneal (fibular) tunnel. Within the tunnel, the nerve runs deep to the tendinous origin of peroneus longus and rests against the surface of the fibular neck, where it divides into deep, superficial, and recurrent peroneal nerves. Peroneal nerve compression may occur at the peroneal tunnel, either from repetitive activity involving inversion or pronation of the foot, fibular neck fractures, or total knee arthroplasty with correction of a significant valgus angulation of the knee. Fat hypertrophy within the tunnel has been reported to relate to peroneal nerve compression in diabetic patients.

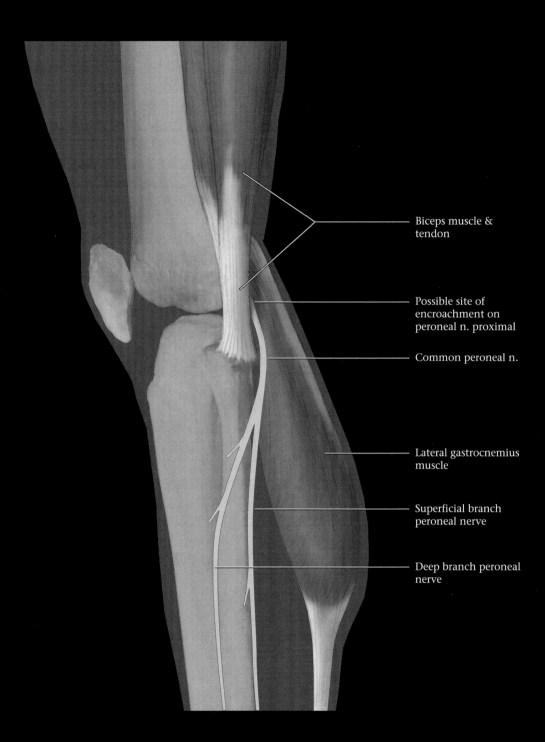

Biceps muscle & tendon

Possible site of encroachment on peroneal n. proximal

Common peroneal n.

Lateral gastrocnemius muscle

Superficial branch peroneal nerve

Deep branch peroneal nerve

Lateral graphic with the peroneus longus muscle peeled away. This demonstrates the site at which the common peroneal nerve can be compressed proximal to the fibular head. Such compression may be due to one of the following 3 etiologies: 1) hypertrophied short head of biceps femoris; 2) distal extension of long head of biceps femoris; 3) prominent lateral head of gastrocnemius.

AXIAL T1 MR, VARIANT, HYPERTROPHIED BICEPS FEMORIS

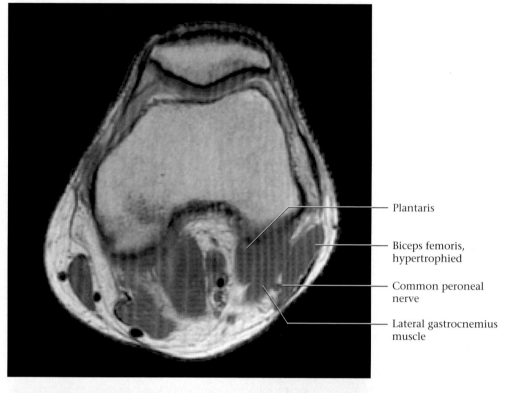

Plantaris

Biceps femoris, hypertrophied

Common peroneal nerve

Lateral gastrocnemius muscle

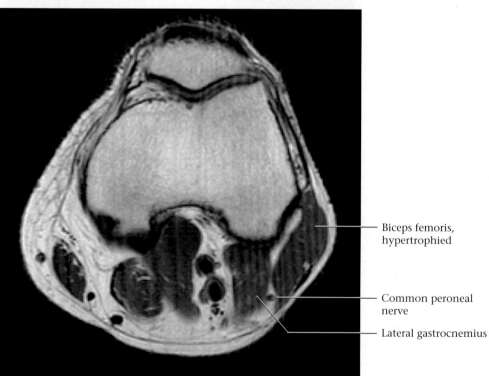

Biceps femoris, hypertrophied

Common peroneal nerve

Lateral gastrocnemius

(Top) First of two images, this one at the top of the intercondylar notch. These two axial T1 MR images show compression of the common peroneal nerve between a hypertrophied biceps femoris muscle and the lateral gastrocnemius. Normally the biceps is more gracile in this location, with the common peroneal nerve located more posteriorly. This variant may cause nerve compression and may be symptomatic. (Bottom) Slightly more distal axial T1 MR image shows persistence of the relationship of the hypertrophied biceps, compressing the common peroneal nerve against the gastrocnemius muscle.

AXIAL & SAGITTAL MR, VARIANT: ACCESSORY SOLEUS

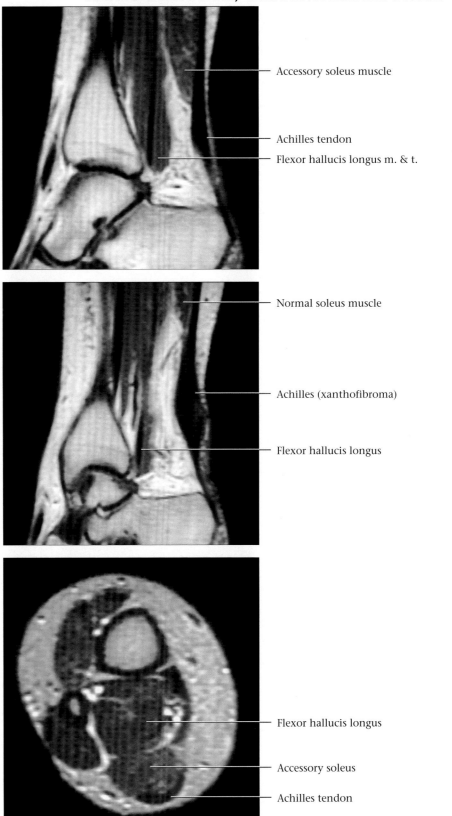

Accessory soleus muscle

Achilles tendon

Flexor hallucis longus m. & t.

Normal soleus muscle

Achilles (xanthofibroma)

Flexor hallucis longus

Flexor hallucis longus

Accessory soleus

Achilles tendon

(Top) Sagittal T2 MR image shows a bulky soleus muscle extending more distally than expected. This is an accessory soleus and presents clinically as a mass. (Middle) Opposite leg in same patient as previous image, showing the normal soleus for comparison. It happens that this patient has an abnormal Achilles tendon on this side (xanthofibroma). (Bottom) Axial T2 MR of the first imaged leg, showing the accessory soleus. At this level, on the opposite leg, there was no soleus muscle remaining (not shown).

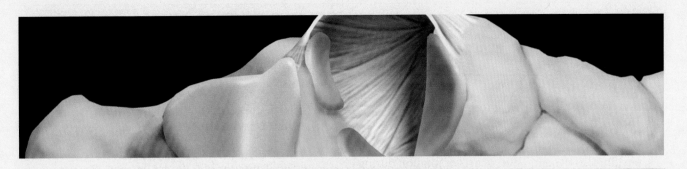

SECTION VII: Ankle

Gross Anatomy

Osseous Anatomy

- **Ankle (talocrural) joint**
  - Tibia, fibula & talus form synovial joint
  - Supported by lateral & medial collateral ligaments
  - Mainly uniaxial hinge joint, dorsiflexion, plantar flexion, also dynamic shift of axis of rotation during dorsi & plantar flexion
- **Distal tibiofibular joint**
  - Fibrous joint
  - Supported by syndesmotic ligaments
  - Synovial recess from ankle joint extends into joint
  - May have articular cartilage far distally
  - Minimal stretch ("give") during dorsiflexion: Allows increase in malleolar gap & slight fibular lateral rotation
- **Hindfoot: Talus & calcaneus**
  - Posterior, middle & anterior subtalar joints between talus & calcaneus
  - Middle & anterior subtalar joints often confluent
  - Aids in inversion, eversion, adduction, abduction
  - **Talus**
    - Affords plantarflexion & dorsiflexion of ankle
    - Keystone of medial longitudinal arch
    - Proximal body (trochlea) articulates with tibia
    - Trochlea broader anteriorly than posteriorly
    - Body articulates with medial & lateral malleoli
    - Posterior process: Groove between medial & lateral tubercles for flexor hallucis longus tendon
    - 3 inferior facets articulate with calcaneus
    - Head articulates with navicular bone, spring ligament & sustentaculum tali
    - No muscle attachments, 2/3 covered by cartilage, dominant blood supply enters neck
  - **Calcaneus**
    - Talar articulations: Anterior, middle & posterior facets
    - Weight-bearing, springboard for locomotion
    - Anterior process articulates with cuboid
    - Sustentaculum tali: Medial protuberance, middle facet
    - Tuberosity: Achilles tendon insertion, posterior subtalar facet
    - Plantar surface: Anterior, medial & lateral tubercles
    - Critical angle of Gissane: Junction of posterior facet & anterior calcaneal process
- **Sinus tarsi**
  - Lateral, funnel shaped space between talar neck & calcaneus
  - Base is tarsal canal, between posterior subtalar joint & sustentaculum tali
  - Traversed by: Medial, lateral & intermediate roots of inferior extensor retinaculum, cervical & talocalcaneal interosseous ligaments, fat, neurovascular anastomosis
  - Talocalcaneal interosseous ligament: Most medial, extends from talar sulcus to calcaneus between posterior & middle calcaneal facets, taut in eversion
  - Cervical ligament: Anterior & lateral, extends from talar neck to calcaneus, taut in inversion

Ligaments

- 3 sets bind ankle: Distal tibiofibular syndesmotic complex, lateral collateral & deltoid ligaments
- **4 tibiofibular syndesmotic ligaments**
  - **Anterior & posterior tibiofibular ligaments**
    - Extend obliquely between anterior & posterior tibial & fibular tubercles respectively
    - Distal anterior tibiofibular ligament: Bassett ligament
  - **Inferior transverse ligament**: Distal part of posterior tibiofibular ligament
  - **Interosseous ligament**: Distal thickening of syndesmotic membrane
- **3 lateral collateral ligaments**
  - **Anterior talofibular ligament**
    - Originates 1 cm proximal to lateral malleolar tip, inserts on talar neck
    - Stabilizes talus against anterior displacement, internal rotation & inversion
    - Weakest, first to tear
  - **Calcaneofibular ligament**
    - Originates from lateral malleolar tip, inserts on calcaneal trochlear eminence
    - Deep to peroneal tendons
    - Lateral restraint of subtalar joint, often tears with anterior talofibular ligament
  - **Posterior talofibular ligament**
    - Extends from lateral malleolar fossa to lateral talar tubercle
    - Strongest, rarely tears
- **Deltoid ligament (medial collateral ligament)**
  - Fan shaped, originates from anterior, apex & posterior medial malleolus, inserts on talus, sustentaculum tali, spring ligament & navicular
  - Deep: Posterior & anterior tibiotalar bands
  - Superficial: Tibiocalcaneal, tibiospring, tibionavicular & posterior tibiotalar (variable) bands
- **Spring ligament (plantar calcaneonavicular ligament)**
  - Binds calcaneus to navicular, 3 components
  - Superomedial - **origin**: Sustentaculum tali, **insertion**: Superomedial navicular, tibiospring band of deltoid
  - Medioplantar oblique - **origin**: Calcaneal coronoid fossa, **insertion**: Plantar navicular
  - Inferoplantar longitudinal - **origin**: Coronoid fossa, **insertion**: Navicular beak

Retinacula

- Focal thickening of deep fascia
- Prevents bowstringing, binds tendons down
- **Superior extensor retinaculum**
  - A few cm above ankle joint
  - Attaches to anterior fibula laterally, tibia medially
  - Proximally continues with fascia cruris
  - Distally attaches to inferior extensor retinaculum
  - Binds down anterior compartment muscles
- **Inferior extensor retinaculum**
  - At ankle joint, Y shaped, stem laterally, proximal & distal bands medially
  - Stem attaches laterally to upper calcaneus
    - Loops around extensor tendons

- Roots extend into sinus tarsi
  - Proximal medial band has deep & superficial layers, loop around extensor hallus longus tendon & occasionally tibialis anterior tendon
  - Distal medial band superficial to extensor hallucis longus & tibialis anterior tendons
    - Attaches to plantar aponeurosis
  - Dorsalis pedis vessels, deep peroneal nerve: Deep to all layers of inferior extensor retinaculum
- **Flexor retinaculum**
  - Attaches to medial malleolus
  - Proximally continuous with deep fascia of leg
  - Distally continuous with plantar aponeurosis
  - Abductor hallucis partly attached to it
  - Binds deep flexor tendons to tibial & calcaneal grooves
  - Lateral border of tarsal tunnel
- **Superior peroneal retinaculum**
  - Origin: Lateral malleolus, insertions vary, most commonly to deep fascia of leg & calcaneus
  - Binds peroneal tendons into retrofibular groove
- **Inferior peroneal retinaculum**
  - Continuous with inferior extensor retinaculum
  - Inserts on lateral calcaneus, peroneal tubercle (trochlea)
  - Binds peroneus brevis, peroneus longus tendons to calcaneus

Tendons
- Muscles discussed in greater detail in leg module
- **Anterior (extensor) compartment**
  - **Tibialis anterior tendon**
    - Most medial & largest tendon in anterior compartment
    - Inserts on medial cuneiform, base of 1st metatarsal
    - Dorsiflexes ankle, inverts foot, tightens plantar aponeurosis
    - Supports medial longitudinal arch during walking
  - **Extensor hallucis longus tendon**
    - Inserts on dorsal base of 1st distal phalanx
    - Extends 1st phalanges, dorsiflexes foot
  - **Extensor digitorum longus tendon**
    - Divides into four slips on dorsum of foot
    - Slips receive tendinous contributions from extensor digitorum brevis, lumbricals & interosseous muscles
    - Each slip divides into 3: Central one inserts on dorsal base of middle phalanx & 2 collateral ones which reunite & insert on bases of 2nd-5th distal phalanges
    - Dorsiflexes ankle, extends toes, tightens plantar aponeurosis
  - **Peroneus tertius tendon**
    - Typically part of extensor digitorum longus tendon
    - Inserts on dorsal base of 5th metatarsal
- **Lateral compartment**
  - **Peroneus longus tendon**
    - Posterolateral to peroneus brevis tendon in retrofibular groove, deep to superior peroneal retinaculum

- Proximally has common tendon sheath with peroneus brevis
- Second tendon sheath at sole of foot
- Descends behind peroneal tubercle, deep to inferior peroneal retinaculum
- Curves under cuboid deep to long plantar ligament
- Inserts on plantar base of 1st metatarsal, medial cuneiform
- Plantarflexes ankle, everts foot, supports longitudinal & transverse arches during walking
- Os peroneum always present, ossified in about 20% of individuals
  - **Peroneus brevis tendon**
    - Anteromedial to peroneus longus tendon in retrofibular groove, deep to superior peroneal retinaculum
    - Descends anterior to peroneal tubercle of calcaneus, deep to inferior peroneal retinaculum
    - Inserts into base of 5th metatarsal
    - Everts foot, limits foot inversion
- **Superficial posterior compartment**
  - **Achilles tendon**
    - Largest & strongest tendon in body
    - Conjoined tendon of medial & lateral gastrocnemius & soleus muscles
    - Approximately 15 cm long
    - Lacks tendon sheath, enclosed by paratenon
    - Inserts on posterior calcaneal tuberosity
    - Retrocalcaneal bursa between distal tendon & calcaneal tuberosity
    - Main plantarflexor of ankle, foot
- **Plantaris tendon**
  - Vestigial, slender tendon, medial to Achilles tendon
  - Inserts on or medial to Achilles tendon
- **Deep posterior (flexor) compartment**
  - **Tibialis posterior tendon**
    - Crosses flexor digitorum longus tendon above ankle joint to become most posteromedial tendon
    - Shares tibial groove with flexor digitorum longus tendon
    - Inserts on navicular tuberosity, cuneiforms, sustentaculum tali, bases of 2nd-4th metatarsals
    - Main invertor of foot, aids in plantar flexion
    - Supports medial longitudinal arch
  - **Flexor digitorum longus tendon**
    - Lateral to tibialis posterior tendon in tibial groove
    - Crosses flexor hallucis longus tendon at master knot of Henry
    - Divides into 4 slips which give origin to lumbricals
    - Slips pass through openings in corresponding tendons of flexor digitorum brevis
    - Slips insert on bases of 2nd-5th distal phalanges
    - Flexes distal phalanges, assists in plantar flexion of ankle
    - When foot on ground: Maintains pads of toes on ground
    - When foot off ground: Plantar flexes 2nd-5th phalanges, aids in maintaining longitudinal arches
  - **Flexor hallucis longus tendon**

- Passes 3 fibro-osseous tunnels: 1) between medial & lateral talar tubercles, 2) under sustentaculum tali, 3) between 1st medial & lateral sesamoids
- Crosses & sends slip to flexor digitorum longus at master knot of Henry
- Inserts on base of 1st distal phalanx
- When foot on ground: Maintains pad of 1st toe on ground
- When foot off ground: Plantar flexes 1st phalanges, aids in maintaining medial longitudinal arch
- Weak plantar flexor of ankle
- Innervated by tibial nerve

Vessels (For Detail, See Leg & Foot Sections)
- **Anterior tibial artery** becomes **dorsalis pedis** at ankle joint
- **Posterior tibial artery** divides into medial & lateral plantar arteries in tarsal tunnel

Nerves
- **Posterior tibial nerve**
  - Traverses tarsal tunnel
  - **Tarsal tunnel:** Deep to flexor retinaculum, traversed by tibialis posterior, flexor digitorum & flexor hallucis tendons & posterior tibial neurovascular bundle
  - Posterior tibial nerve divides proximal or at tarsal tunnel into: Medial calcaneal nerve, medial & lateral plantar nerves
    - 1st branch of lateral plantar nerve is inferior calcaneal nerve (Baxter nerve)
  - **Medial calcaneal nerve**
    - Sensory to medial heel
  - **Medial plantar nerve**
    - Sensory to medial 2/3 of plantar foot
    - Motor to abductor hallucis, flexor digitorum brevis, flexor hallucis brevis, 1st lumbrical
  - **Lateral plantar nerve**
    - Sensory to lateral mid foot & forefoot
    - Supplies most plantar muscles of foot
- **Deep peroneal nerve**
  - Deep to extensor retinacula, in anterior tarsal tunnel
  - Predominantly motor
  - Divides just above ankle into medial (mainly sensory), lateral (mainly motor) branches
    - **Medial branch** continues dorsal to talonavicular joint, middle cuneiform & in between 1st & 2nd metatarsals
    - **Lateral branch** ends at extensor digitorum brevis
  - In leg: Motor to anterior tibial, extensor digitorum longus, extensor hallucis longus, peroneus tertius
  - In foot: Motor to extensor digitorum brevis, sensory (& sometimes motor) to 1st web space
- **Superficial peroneal nerve**
  - Exits deep fascia 10-15 cm above ankle joint
  - Subcutaneous 6 cm above ankle, divides into subcutaneous branches
  - In leg motor to peroneus brevis & peroneus longus tendons, sensory to distal 2/3 lateral leg
  - In foot sensory to dorsal foot
- **Sural nerve**
  - Formed by merger of branches from tibial nerve & common peroneal nerve
  - Purely sensory to lateral ankle, foot up to base of 5th metatarsal

Imaging Anatomy

Overview
- **Radiography of ankle joint**
- Routine radiographs: AP, lateral & ankle mortise (15-20° internal oblique) views
  - AP view: Talus overlaps medial aspect of lateral malleolus
  - Ankle mortise view taken in dorsiflexion to avoid overlap of fibula on calcaneus
  - Talus should be equidistant from tibial plafond on AP & mortise views
    - May appear asymmetric in joint when AP taken in plantarflexion
    - Talar tilt of up to 5° considered normal by many
  - Transverse line across medial malleolus: Base of posterior colliculus
  - Convex line within tip of lateral malleolus: Attachment of posterior talofibular ligament
  - Syndesmotic tibiofibular clear space (TFC), tibiofibular overlap (TFO), medial clear space (MC): Assess ligamentous integrity, measured on AP & mortise views
  - TFC: Distance between peroneal groove (or anterior tibial cortex) & medial fibular cortex
  - TFO: Overlap between posterior tibial cortex and fibula
  - TFC, TFO measured 1 cm above tibial plafond, range varies with gender
  - Normal TFC same on AP & mortise views: 4 mm, (up to 6 mm considered normal by some), < 44% of fibular width
  - Normal TFO: > 6 mm, > 24% of fibular width on AP, > 1 mm on mortise
  - Normal MC: Measured 1/2 cm below tibial plafond, 4 mm or equal to superior tibiotalar space
- Poor lateral view (5 cm heel lift), 45° internal and external AP views: Better visualization of posterior, medial, lateral malleoli & anterior tibial tubercle respectively
- Broden view, os calcis (tangential calcaneal) views depict subtalar joints
- **Computed tomography**
  - Oblique axial images optimal visualization of subtalar joints
  - Superior to MR for detecting small avulsion fragments
  - 3D volume rendering of bones, tendons
- **MR of ankle & hindfoot**
  - Must image in axial, coronal & sagittal planes
  - Coronals parallel to anterior talar margin, based on transverse image
  - Sagittals parallel to longitudinal calcaneal axial, based on transverse image
  - Axials optimal for ankle tendons, ligaments
  - Coronals useful for bones, cartilage, ankle and sinus tarsi ligaments
  - Sagittals optimal for Achilles tendon, bones, cartilage, sinus tarsi ligaments

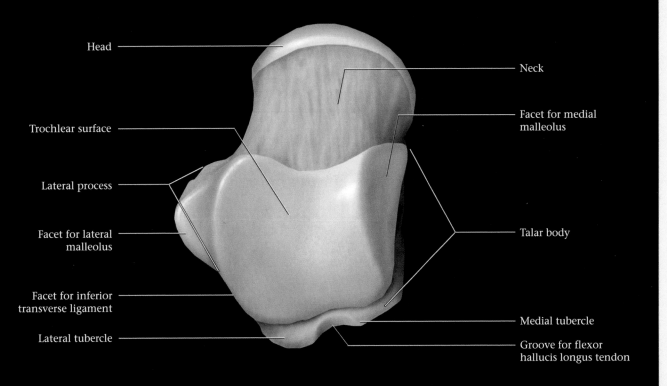

Head

Neck

Trochlear surface

Facet for medial malleolus

Lateral process

Facet for lateral malleolus

Talar body

Facet for inferior transverse ligament

Lateral tubercle

Medial tubercle

Groove for flexor hallucis longus tendon

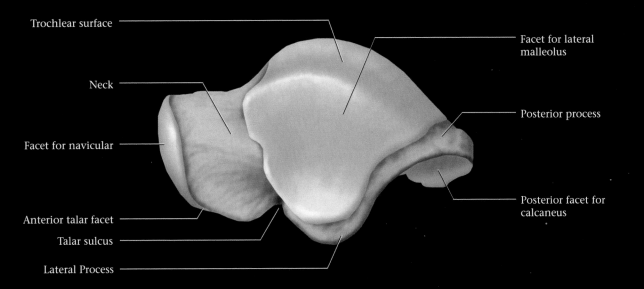

Trochlear surface

Neck

Facet for navicular

Anterior talar facet

Talar sulcus

Lateral Process

Facet for lateral malleolus

Posterior process

Posterior facet for calcaneus

(Top) View of talus from above. The talus is subdivided into the head, neck and body. The body includes the trochlea which forms the talocrural joint with the tibia. It also includes the facets which articulate with the medial & lateral malleoli & posterior, middle and anterior facets articulating with the calcaneus. The talus has no muscles or tendons attaching to it & 2/3 is covered by cartilage (blue), blood supply is therefore tenuous. The flexor hallucis longus tendon traverses in a groove between the medial and lateral tubercles of the posterior process of the talus. **(Bottom)** A lateral view of the talus. The tibia transmits body weight to the talus which then redistributes it to the calcaneus and navicular. The talar sulcus & calcaneal sulcus together form the sinus tarsi space.

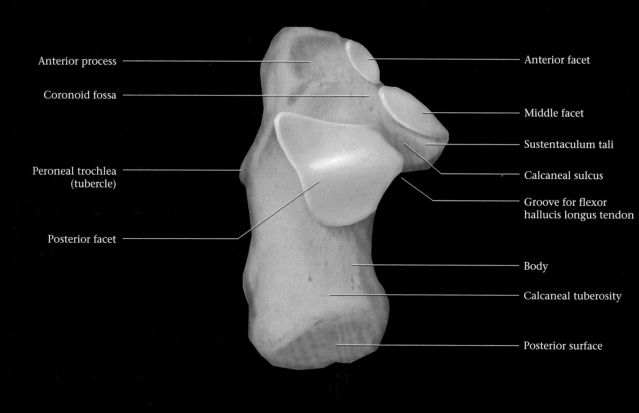

Anterior process

Coronoid fossa

Peroneal trochlea
(tubercle)

Posterior facet

Anterior facet

Middle facet

Sustentaculum tali

Calcaneal sulcus

Groove for flexor
hallucis longus tendon

Body

Calcaneal tuberosity

Posterior surface

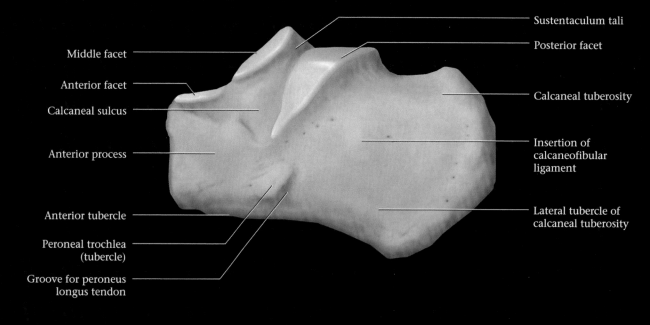

Middle facet

Anterior facet

Calcaneal sulcus

Anterior process

Anterior tubercle

Peroneal trochlea
(tubercle)

Groove for peroneus
longus tendon

Sustentaculum tali

Posterior facet

Calcaneal tuberosity

Insertion of
calcaneofibular
ligament

Lateral tubercle of
calcaneal tuberosity

(Top) View of the calcaneus from above. The calcaneus is subdivided into anterior process, body and tuberosity. The calcaneus articulates with the talus via 3 facets: Anterior, middle and posterior. The anterior and middle facets are often confluent. The anterior process of the calcaneus articulates with the cuboid. **(Bottom)** A lateral view of the calcaneus. The Achilles tendon is the only tendon that inserts into the calcaneus at the superior calcaneal tuberosity. The peroneal tendons descend along the lateral aspect of the calcaneus, separated from one another by the peroneal tubercle (present in 40% of people) & inferior peroneal retinaculum. The flexor hallucis longus tendon descends posterior to the sustentaculum tali of the calcaneus.

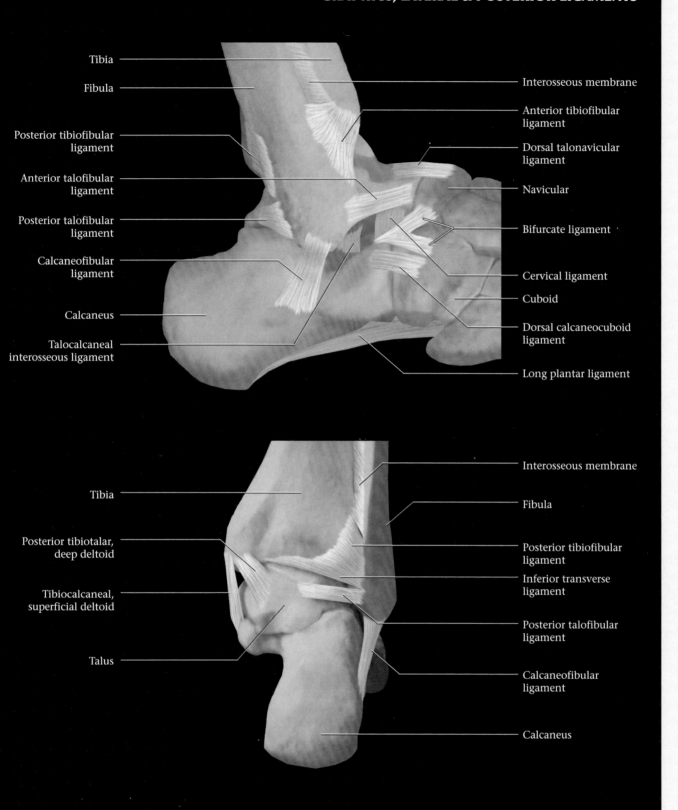

Tibia

Fibula

Posterior tibiofibular ligament

Anterior talofibular ligament

Posterior talofibular ligament

Calcaneofibular ligament

Calcaneus

Talocalcaneal interosseous ligament

Interosseous membrane

Anterior tibiofibular ligament

Dorsal talonavicular ligament

Navicular

Bifurcate ligament

Cervical ligament

Cuboid

Dorsal calcaneocuboid ligament

Long plantar ligament

Tibia

Posterior tibiotalar, deep deltoid

Tibiocalcaneal, superficial deltoid

Talus

Interosseous membrane

Fibula

Posterior tibiofibular ligament

Inferior transverse ligament

Posterior talofibular ligament

Calcaneofibular ligament

Calcaneus

(Top) Lateral view of the ankle. Two groups of lateral ligaments support the ankle: 1) the syndesmotic ligaments, including the anterior tibiofibular, posterior tibiofibular & syndesmotic ligaments, and 2) the lateral collateral ligaments including the anterior talofibular, posterior talofibular & calcaneofibular ligaments. Other ligaments that bind the lateral hindfoot include the talocalcaneal interosseous ligament and cervical ligament in the sinus tarsi. Note the bifurcate ligament which extends from the calcaneus to the navicular and cuboid. **(Bottom)** Posterior view of the ankle. The tibiofibular ligaments are obliquely oriented and their fibular origin is above the fibular fossa. The inferior transverse ligament, which is the inferior aspect of the posterior tibiofibular ligament, extends distal to the tibial posterior surface.

GRAPHICS: DELTOID, SPRING AND BIFURCATE LIGAMENTS

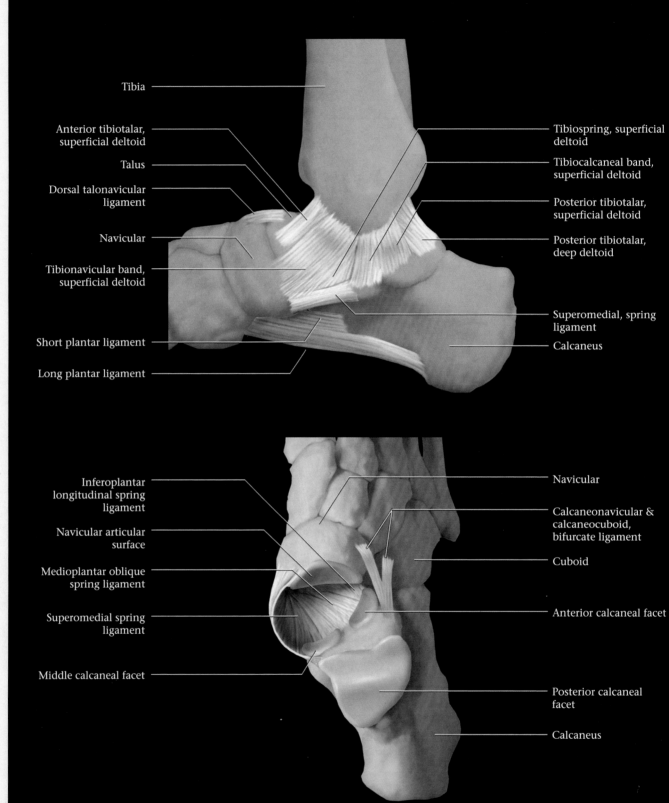

Tibia

Anterior tibiotalar, superficial deltoid

Talus

Dorsal talonavicular ligament

Navicular

Tibionavicular band, superficial deltoid

Short plantar ligament

Long plantar ligament

Tibiospring, superficial deltoid

Tibiocalcaneal band, superficial deltoid

Posterior tibiotalar, superficial deltoid

Posterior tibiotalar, deep deltoid

Superomedial, spring ligament

Calcaneus

Inferoplantar longitudinal spring ligament

Navicular articular surface

Medioplantar oblique spring ligament

Superomedial spring ligament

Middle calcaneal facet

Navicular

Calcaneonavicular & calcaneocuboid, bifurcate ligament

Cuboid

Anterior calcaneal facet

Posterior calcaneal facet

Calcaneus

(Top) Medial view of the ankle. The deltoid ligament is the major supporter of the ankle. It has many variable components but a commonly accepted division includes the deep anterior & posterior tibiotalar & superficial anterior & posterior tibiotalar, tibiocalcaneal, tibiospring & tibionavicular bands. Note that the superficial deltoid is band-like and distinction between its various components relies on the sites of insertion. **(Bottom)** Spring ligament seen from above with the talus removed. The ligament forms a sling supporting the talar head & is composed of the superomedial, medioplantar oblique & inferoplantar longitudinal bands. It originates from the sustentaculum tali, tibiospring & coronoid fossa & inserts onto the plantar navicular. The bifurcate ligament originates more laterally & inserts onto the navicular & cuboid.

GRAPHICS, RETINACULA

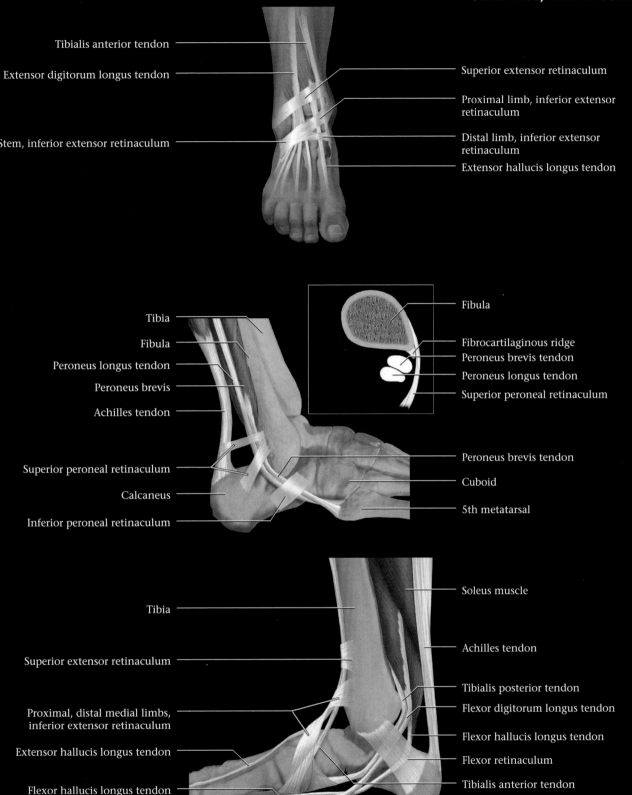

Tibialis anterior tendon

Extensor digitorum longus tendon

Stem, inferior extensor retinaculum

Superior extensor retinaculum

Proximal limb, inferior extensor retinaculum

Distal limb, inferior extensor retinaculum

Extensor hallucis longus tendon

Tibia

Fibula

Peroneus longus tendon

Peroneus brevis

Achilles tendon

Superior peroneal retinaculum

Calcaneus

Inferior peroneal retinaculum

Fibula

Fibrocartilaginous ridge

Peroneus brevis tendon

Peroneus longus tendon

Superior peroneal retinaculum

Peroneus brevis tendon

Cuboid

5th metatarsal

Soleus muscle

Tibia

Superior extensor retinaculum

Proximal, distal medial limbs, inferior extensor retinaculum

Extensor hallucis longus tendon

Flexor hallucis longus tendon

Achilles tendon

Tibialis posterior tendon

Flexor digitorum longus tendon

Flexor hallucis longus tendon

Flexor retinaculum

Tibialis anterior tendon

Flexor digitorum longus tendon

(Top) Extensor retinacula. The superior & inferior extensor retinacula loop over & bind the anterior compartment tendons. The superior extensor retinaculum is above the ankle joint. The inferior extensor retinaculum is Y-shaped & is composed of lateral stem & two medial limbs. The stem originates at the calcaneus & the medial limbs attach to medial malleolus & plantar aponeurosis. **(Middle)** Peroneal retinacula. The superior peroneal retinaculum holds the peroneal tendons in the retrofibular groove. The retinaculum has variable insertions but typically inserts on deep fascia of leg & on the calcaneus. The inferior peroneal retinaculum holds the peroneal tendons against calcaneus. **(Bottom)** Flexor retinaculum. The retinaculum extends from the medial malleolus to the plantar aponeurosis. It binds the posterior compartment tendons & forms lateral border of tarsal tunnel.

GRAPHICS, TENDONS

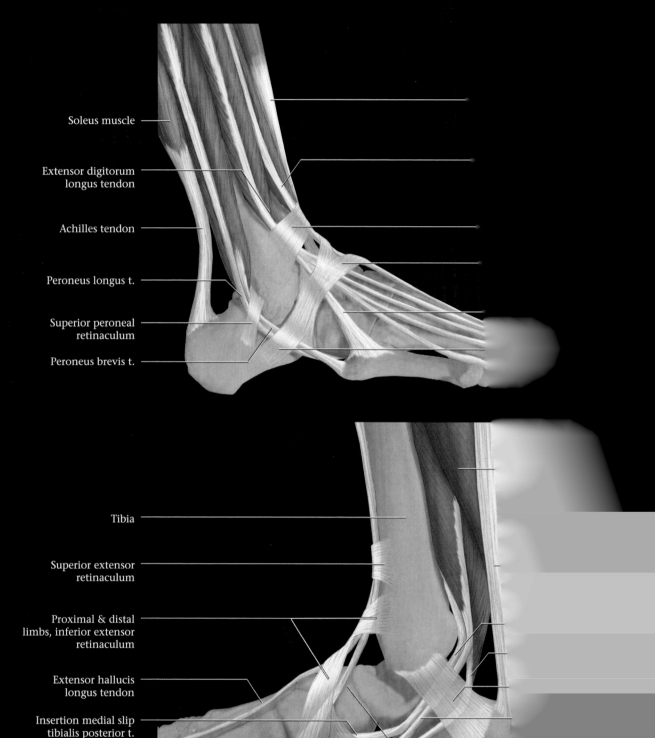

Soleus muscle

Extensor digitorum longus tendon

Achilles tendon

Peroneus longus t.

Superior peroneal retinaculum

Peroneus brevis t.

Tibia

Superior extensor retinaculum

Proximal & distal limbs, inferior extensor retinaculum

Extensor hallucis longus tendon

Insertion medial slip tibialis posterior t.

Flexor hallucis longus tendon

(Top) Lateral view of the tendons of the ankle. The peroneus brevis & peroneus longus tend compartment. They descend posterior to fibula, held by the superior peroneal retinaculum, lateral wall of calcaneus, held by the inferior peroneal retinaculum. Fibers of inferior peronea separate the two tendons. The peroneus longus tendon curves around the cuboid to enter the peroneus brevis and peroneus tertius insert on the 5th metatarsal base. **(Bottom)** Medial view posterior, flexor digitorum longus & flexor hallucis longus tendons traversing beneath the fle the tarsal tunnel. The flexor digitorum longus & flexor hallucis longus tendons cross each oth

ANKLE AND HINDFOOT OVERVIEW

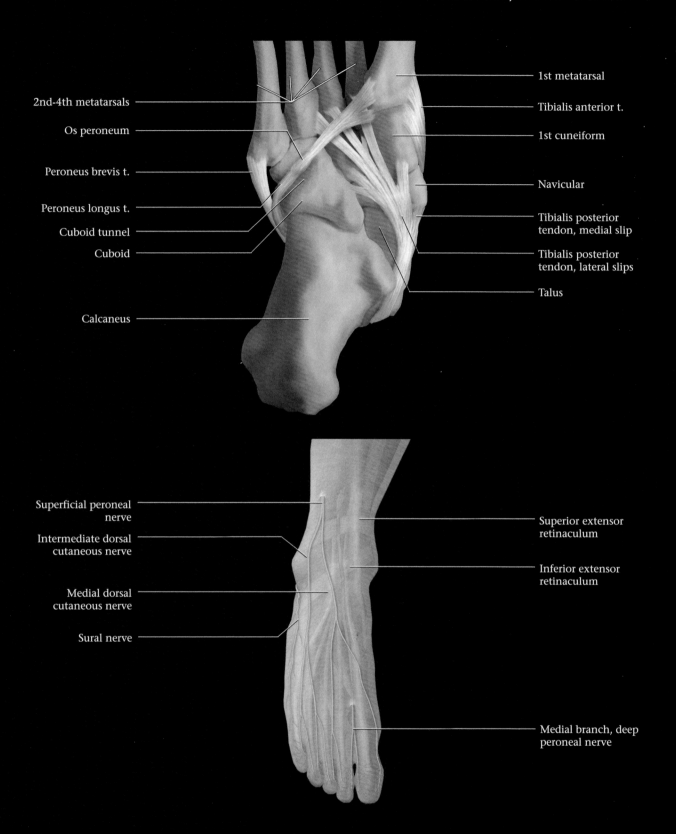

2nd-4th metatarsals

Os peroneum

Peroneus brevis t.

Peroneus longus t.

Cuboid tunnel

Cuboid

Calcaneus

1st metatarsal

Tibialis anterior t.

1st cuneiform

Navicular

Tibialis posterior tendon, medial slip

Tibialis posterior tendon, lateral slips

Talus

Superficial peroneal nerve

Intermediate dorsal cutaneous nerve

Medial dorsal cutaneous nerve

Sural nerve

Superior extensor retinaculum

Inferior extensor retinaculum

Medial branch, deep peroneal nerve

(Top) Tendon insertions on plantar foot. The tibialis posterior tendon inserts on all tarsal bones (excluding talus) & on 2nd-4th metatarsal bases. The medial slip inserts on the plantar-medial aspect of the navicular. The tibialis anterior inserts on the medial plantar aspect of 1st cuneiform & 1st metatarsal. The peroneus longus tendon inserts onto the lateral plantar 1st cuneiform & base of 1st metatarsal. **(Bottom)** Dorsal nerves of ankle & foot. The superficial peroneal nerve pierces deep fascia of distal leg & carries sensation from dorsal skin of all toes, except lateral 5th metatarsal (supplied by sural nerve & 1st web space supplied by medial branch of deep peroneal nerve). The sural nerve is formed by merger of branches of the common peroneal nerve & posterior tibial nerve. It is purely sensory to lateral ankle & foot up to the base of 5th metatarsal.

GRAPHICS, NERVES & TARSAL TUNNEL

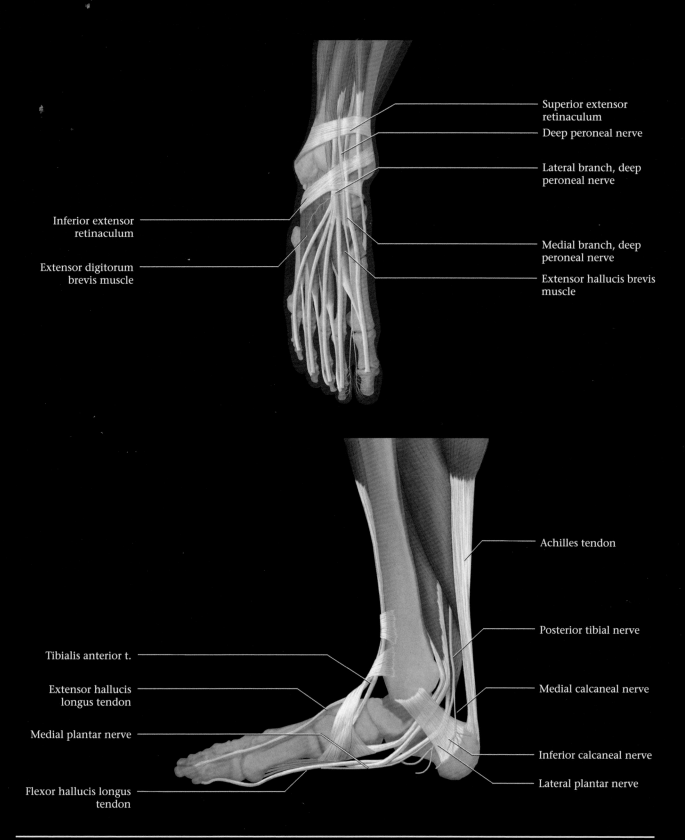

Superior extensor retinaculum

Deep peroneal nerve

Lateral branch, deep peroneal nerve

Inferior extensor retinaculum

Extensor digitorum brevis muscle

Medial branch, deep peroneal nerve

Extensor hallucis brevis muscle

Achilles tendon

Posterior tibial nerve

Tibialis anterior t.

Extensor hallucis longus tendon

Medial calcaneal nerve

Medial plantar nerve

Inferior calcaneal nerve

Lateral plantar nerve

Flexor hallucis longus tendon

(Top) The deep peroneal nerve travels deep to extensor retinacula, in anterior tarsal tunnel, & gives a lateral motor branch to extensor digitorum brevis muscle. The medial branch continues dorsal to talonavicular joint, middle cuneiform & in between 1st & 2nd metatarsal to provide mostly sensory but some motor supply to 1st web space. **(Bottom)** Tarsal tunnel. The tunnel, deep to flexor retinaculum, accommodates the posterior tibial neurovascular bundle. The medial calcaneal nerve supplies skin of medial heel. The medial plantar nerve supplies flexor hallucis brevis, abductor hallucis, flexor digitorum brevis and 1st lumbrical. It carries sensation from medial 2/3 of plantar foot. The lateral plantar nerve supplies all other plantar muscles including 2nd-4th lumbricals and all interossei. It carries sensation from lateral 1/3 of midfoot & forefoot.

AP & OBLIQUE RADIOGRAPHS, RIGHT ANKLE

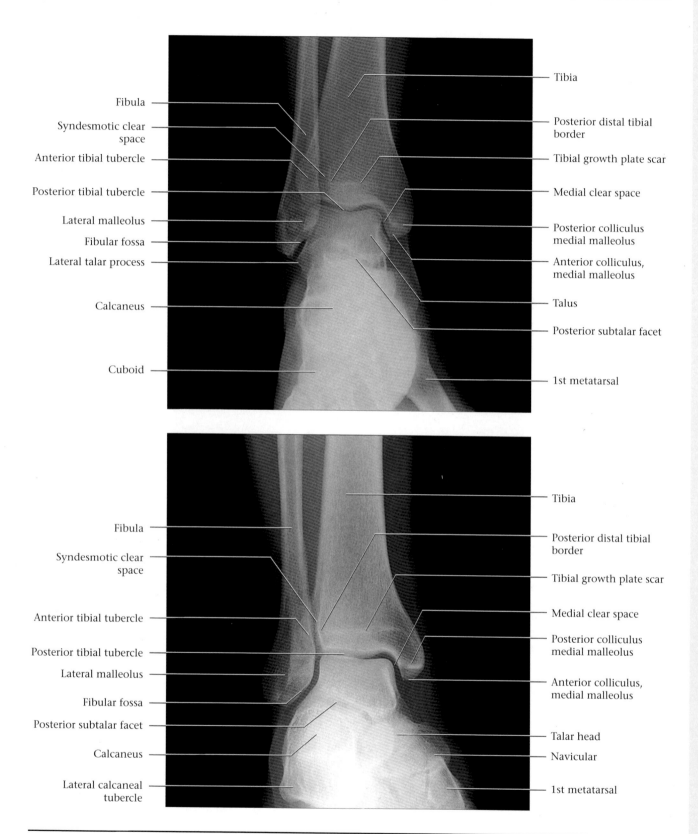

(Top) Routine non weight-bearing AP view of the ankle is obtained with the patient supine, the heel on the cassette and the toes pointed upward. The X-ray beam is directed at the center of the ankle joint. The talus overlaps the distal fibula obscuring the lateral ankle mortise. Note that hinterior margin of the tibia extends further laterally compared to the posterior tibial margin. Similarly the anterior colliculus of the medial malleolus extends more distally than the posterior colliculus. **(Bottom)** Non weight-bearing ankle mortise view (oblique) is obtained with the patient supine and the foot internally rotated until the medial and lateral malleoli are equidistant from the cassette. The lateral ankle mortise is now visualized. The talus should be equidistant from the tibial plafond on both the AP and ankle mortise view.

ANKLE AND HINDFOOT OVERVIEW

LATERAL RADIOGRAPHS, RIGHT ANKLE

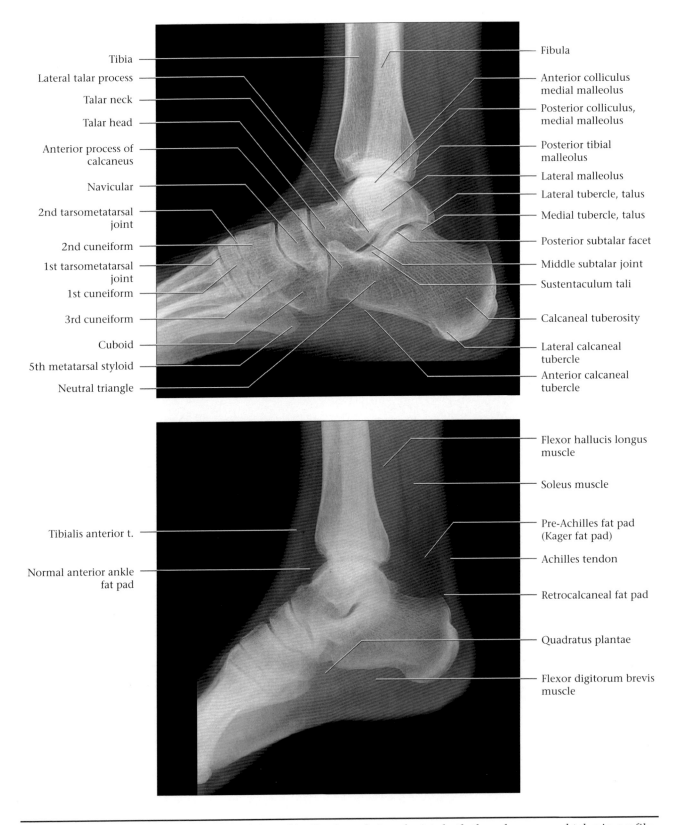

Labels (top radiograph), left side:
- Tibia
- Lateral talar process
- Talar neck
- Talar head
- Anterior process of calcaneus
- Navicular
- 2nd tarsometatarsal joint
- 2nd cuneiform
- 1st tarsometatarsal joint
- 1st cuneiform
- 3rd cuneiform
- Cuboid
- 5th metatarsal styloid
- Neutral triangle

Labels (top radiograph), right side:
- Fibula
- Anterior colliculus medial malleolus
- Posterior colliculus, medial malleolus
- Posterior tibial malleolus
- Lateral malleolus
- Lateral tubercle, talus
- Medial tubercle, talus
- Posterior subtalar facet
- Middle subtalar joint
- Sustentaculum tali
- Calcaneal tuberosity
- Lateral calcaneal tubercle
- Anterior calcaneal tubercle

Labels (bottom radiograph), left side:
- Tibialis anterior t.
- Normal anterior ankle fat pad

Labels (bottom radiograph), right side:
- Flexor hallucis longus muscle
- Soleus muscle
- Pre-Achilles fat pad (Kager fat pad)
- Achilles tendon
- Retrocalcaneal fat pad
- Quadratus plantae
- Flexor digitorum brevis muscle

(Top) A non weight-bearing lateral view of the ankle. The lateral view depicts both the calcaneus and talus in profile. The posterior, medial and lateral malleoli are superimposed over one another and over the talus, potentially obscuring fractures at those locations. The lateral view should include the base of the 5th metatarsal. The middle subtalar joint is typically visualized on a weight-bearing lateral view. **(Bottom)** Lateral view, ankle soft tissues. The Achilles tendon should be uniform in diameter. A small retrocalcaneal fat pad, location of retrocalcaneal bursa, is found between the tendon & calcaneus. A normal pre-Achilles fat pad separates the Achilles tendon from the ankle joint. The tibialis anterior tendon is noted on the dorsal surface of the ankle. Obliteration of a small fat pad anterior to the anterior joint line is consistent with joint effusion.

OS CALCIS & BRODEN RADIOGRAPHS, RIGHT ANKLE

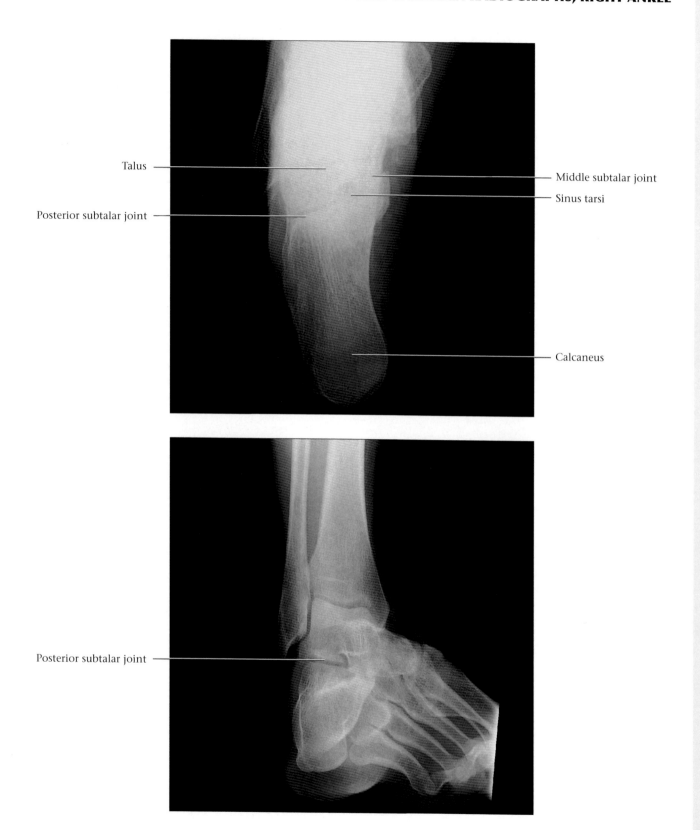

Talus

Posterior subtalar joint

Middle subtalar joint

Sinus tarsi

Calcaneus

Posterior subtalar joint

(Top) The os calcis view is obtained with the patient supine or standing and the foot in maximum dorsiflexion. The view depicts the middle and posterior subtalar joints. (Bottom) Broden views are obtained with the patient supine, foot in 45° of internal rotation and 10, 20, 30 and 40° of tube angulation. The views afford visualization of the posterior subtalar joint but have become somewhat obsolete as computed tomography is used more frequently for problem solving in the ankle.

RADIOGRAPHS, CALCANEAL PITCH & TALAR BASE ANGLES

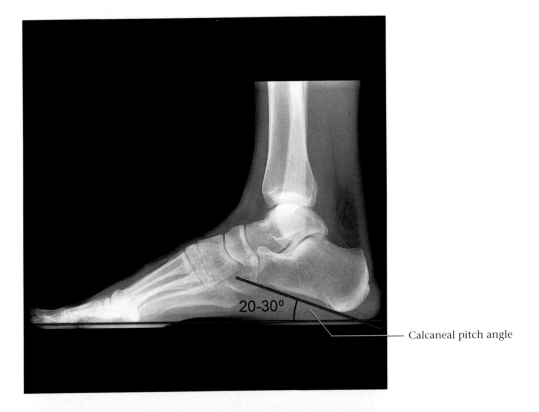

20-30° — Calcaneal pitch angle

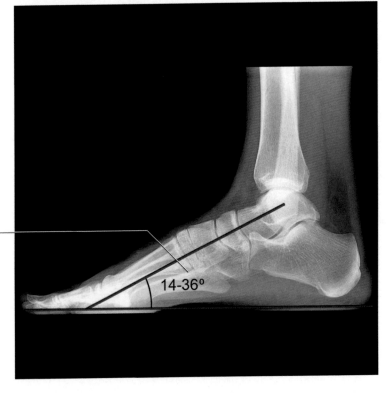

Talar base angle

14-36°

(Top) A weight-bearing lateral view of the foot provides information on the height of the longitudinal arch. The calcaneal pitch is an angle formed by intersection of a line along the plantar aspect of the calcaneus with the floor. It should measure about 20-30°. **(Bottom)** The normal talar-base angle is formed by the intersection of the longitudinal axis of the talus with a line parallel to the floor. It normally measures 14-36°.

RADIOGRAPHS, ANGLES OF THE HINDFOOT

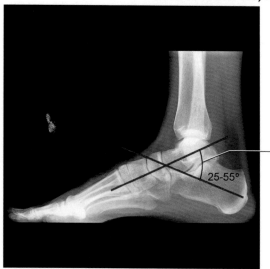

Talocalcaneal angle (Kite angle)

25-55°

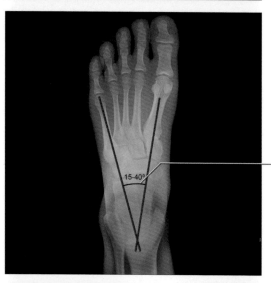

Talocalcaneal angle (Kite angle)

15-40°

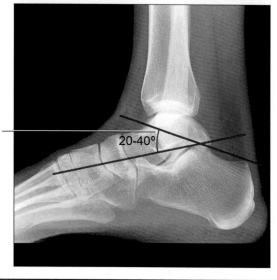

Boehler angle

20-40°

(Top) Normal lateral talocalcaneal angle, (Kite angle), formed by intersection of talar & calcaneal longitudinal axes, measures 25-55°. Decrease in lateral angle is indicative of equinus hindfoot deformity & increase is indicative of calcaneus hindfoot deformity. **(Middle)** Normal AP talocalcaneal angle, measured along longitudinal axes of talus & calcaneus is 15-40°. Decrease in AP angle is indicative of varus hindfoot deformity & increase is indicative of valgus hindfoot deformity. **(Bottom)** Boehler angle reflects integrity of the posterior calcaneal facet & calcaneal height. The angle is formed by the intersection of a line drawn along the apices of anterior calcaneal process & posterior calcaneal facet & a line drawn along the apices of superior calcaneal tuberosity & posterior calcaneal facet. The normal range is 20-40°.

Ankle

VII

17

RADIOGRAPHIC MEASUREMENTS, ANKLE

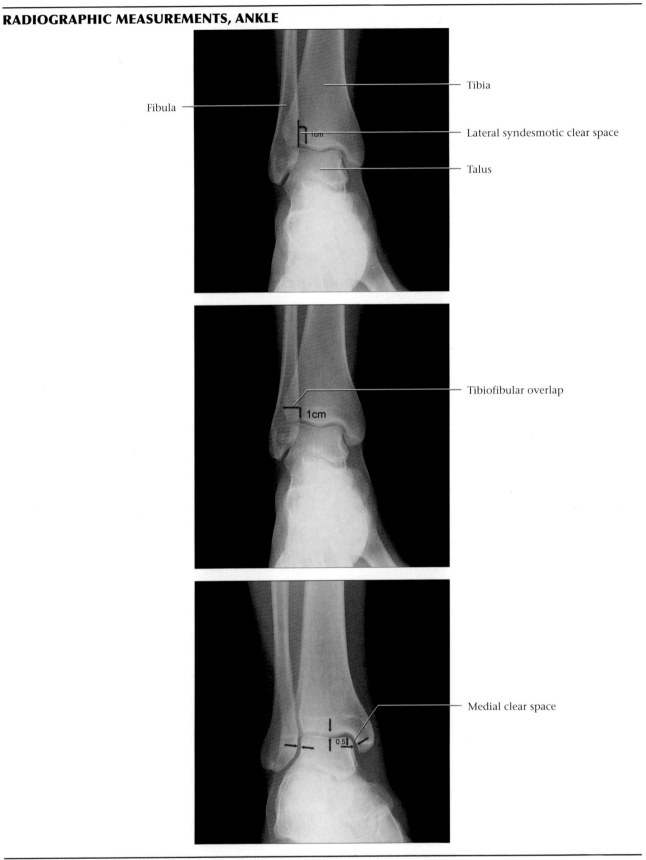

Fibula

Tibia

Lateral syndesmotic clear space

Talus

Tibiofibular overlap

1cm

Medial clear space

0.5

(Top) The lateral syndesmotic clear space & tibiofibular overlap, indicators of the integrity of the tibiofibular syndesmotic joint, are measured approximately 1 cm above the tibial plafond. The lateral syndesmotic clear space is measured from the posterior tibial margin to the medial fibular margin. Normal measurements vary in the literature and range from 4-6 mm on both the AP ankle and ankle mortise views. (Middle) The tibiofibular overlap measurements also vary and range from 6-10 mm in the literature. An overlap of 6 mm, however, on the AP view and 1 mm on the ankle mortise view are considered normal by most. (Bottom) The talus should be equidistant from the tibial plafond on the AP and ankle mortise views. Minimal tilts are within normal. The normal medial clear space, measured 0.5 cm below the talar articular surface, should be 4 mm in size.

AXIAL CT, RIGHT HINDFOOT

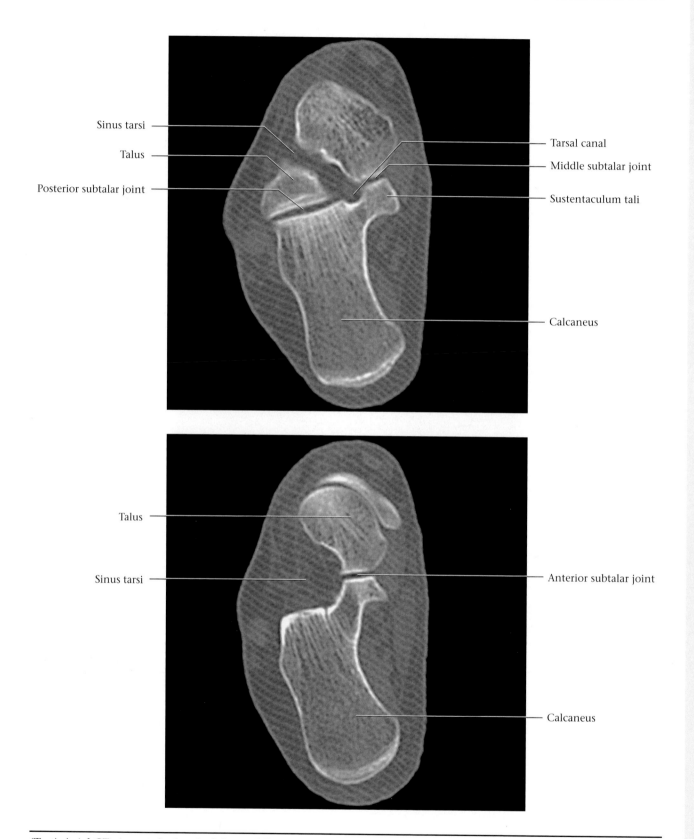

Sinus tarsi

Talus

Posterior subtalar joint

Tarsal canal

Middle subtalar joint

Sustentaculum tali

Calcaneus

Talus

Sinus tarsi

Anterior subtalar joint

Calcaneus

(Top) Axial CT view at the level of the middle and posterior subtalar joint. At this level the posterior and middle subtalar joints are usually parallel to each other. The tarsal canal is a medial space, continuous with the sinus tarsi laterally, which separates the posterior from the middle subtalar joints. **(Bottom)** A more anterior axial CT. The anterior subtalar joint is usually horizontal in orientation. The opening of the sinus tarsi toward the lateral aspect of the ankle is now better visualized.

SAGITTAL CT REFORMATS, RIGHT ANKLE

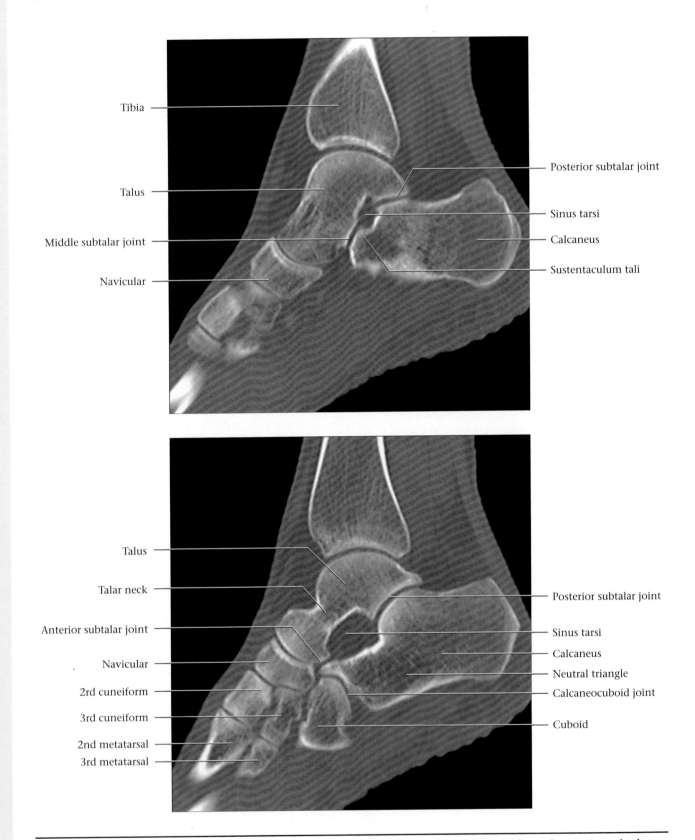

Tibia

Talus

Middle subtalar joint

Navicular

Posterior subtalar joint

Sinus tarsi

Calcaneus

Sustentaculum tali

Talus

Talar neck

Anterior subtalar joint

Navicular

2rd cuneiform

3rd cuneiform

2nd metatarsal

3rd metatarsal

Posterior subtalar joint

Sinus tarsi

Calcaneus

Neutral triangle

Calcaneocuboid joint

Cuboid

(Top) Medial sagittal reconstruction of the ankle. At this fairly medial level both the middle and posterior subtalar joints are visualized. Far medially the posterior subtalar joint tends to be more horizontal than lateral. An area of relative radiolucency in the calcaneus between the hompressile trabeculae that occasionally can mimic a lytic lesion is seen. **(Bottom)** A more lateral sagittal reconstruction. The anterior subtalar joint is more horizontal than the middle one while the posterior subtalar joint is now more obliqued than it was more medially. The neutral triangle is an area of trabecular rarefaction noted in between the posterior and anterior compressile trabeculae of the calcaneus and should not be mistaken for a lytic lesion.

CORONAL CT REFORMATS, RIGHT ANKLE

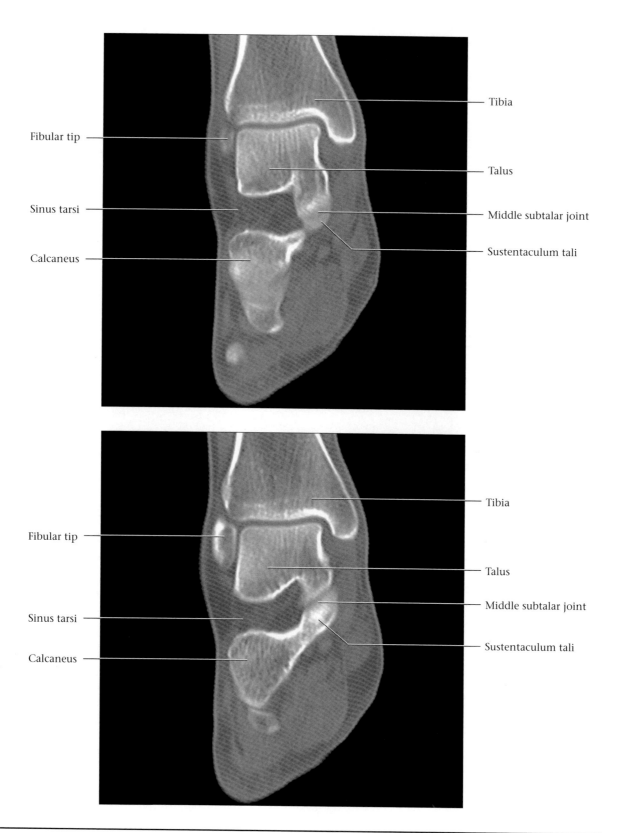

Fibular tip

Sinus tarsi

Calcaneus

Tibia

Talus

Middle subtalar joint

Sustentaculum tali

Fibular tip

Sinus tarsi

Calcaneus

Tibia

Talus

Middle subtalar joint

Sustentaculum tali

(Top) Coronal CT reconstructions at the middle subtalar joint. Note that the middle subtalar joint is often suboptimally seen on coronal reconstructions due to partial volume averaging. This may also be noted on axial CT images and should not be misinterpreted as subtalar coalition. Performing axial images perpendicular to the subtalar joints is advisable when tarsal coalition is suspected. Also, sagittal reconstructions will usually depict the normal relationship between the sustentaculum tali and the talus. **(Bottom)** Coronal reconstruction at the middle subtalar joint. Note that the middle subtalar joint is more clearly seen on this image but, due to partial volume averaging, is still not optimally defined as on the sagittal reconstructions.

AXIAL T1 MR, RIGHT ANKLE

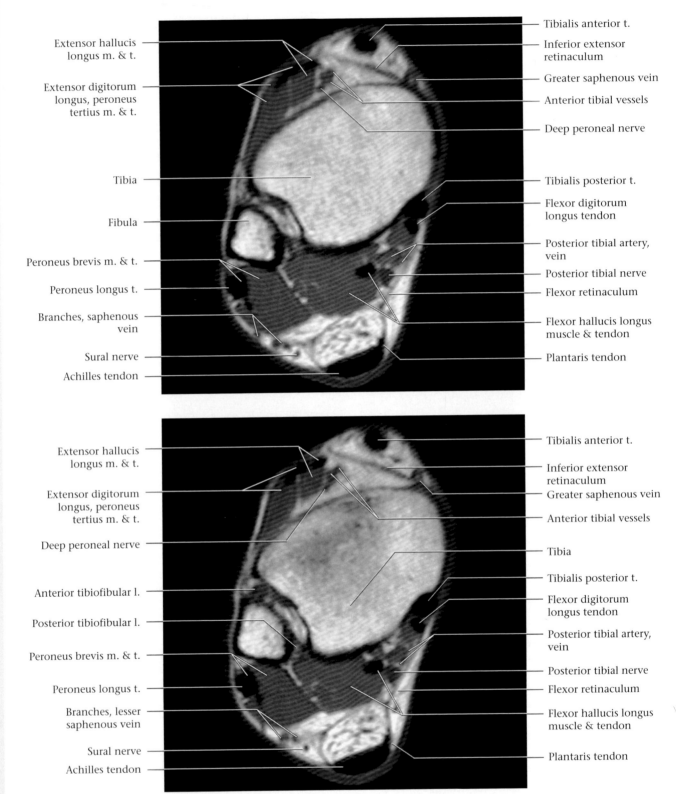

Top image labels (left):
- Extensor hallucis longus m. & t.
- Extensor digitorum longus, peroneus tertius m. & t.
- Tibia
- Fibula
- Peroneus brevis m. & t.
- Peroneus longus t.
- Branches, saphenous vein
- Sural nerve
- Achilles tendon

Top image labels (right):
- Tibialis anterior t.
- Inferior extensor retinaculum
- Greater saphenous vein
- Anterior tibial vessels
- Deep peroneal nerve
- Tibialis posterior t.
- Flexor digitorum longus tendon
- Posterior tibial artery, vein
- Posterior tibial nerve
- Flexor retinaculum
- Flexor hallucis longus muscle & tendon
- Plantaris tendon

Bottom image labels (left):
- Extensor hallucis longus m. & t.
- Extensor digitorum longus, peroneus tertius m. & t.
- Deep peroneal nerve
- Anterior tibiofibular l.
- Posterior tibiofibular l.
- Peroneus brevis m. & t.
- Peroneus longus t.
- Branches, lesser saphenous vein
- Sural nerve
- Achilles tendon

Bottom image labels (right):
- Tibialis anterior t.
- Inferior extensor retinaculum
- Greater saphenous vein
- Anterior tibial vessels
- Tibia
- Tibialis posterior t.
- Flexor digitorum longus tendon
- Posterior tibial artery, vein
- Posterior tibial nerve
- Flexor retinaculum
- Flexor hallucis longus muscle & tendon
- Plantaris tendon

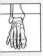
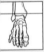

(Top) First in series of axial T1 MR images of the right ankle. The cut is just above the tibial plafond. At this level, excluding the tibialis anterior, tibialis posterior and peroneus longus, all the muscles of the anterior, lateral and deep posterior compartment are still visualized. The posterior tibial nerve, found behind the posterior tibial vessels, has not yet divided into the medial and lateral plantar nerves. The sural nerve is anterolateral to the Achilles tendon.
(Bottom) The anterior and posterior tibiofibular ligaments extend from the distal tibia to the fibula and along with the interosseus ligament, support the distal tibiofibular joint. The anterior surface of the Achilles tendon is flat. The tendon is partially surrounded by a paratenon. The plantaris tendon is found just medial to the Achilles tendon.

ANKLE AND HINDFOOT OVERVIEW

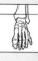

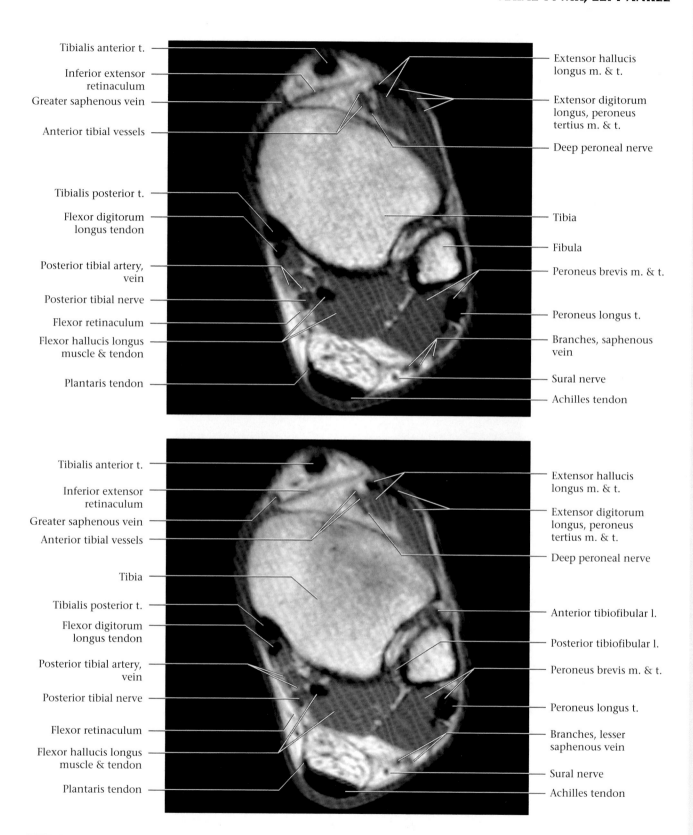

Tibialis anterior t.

Inferior extensor retinaculum

Greater saphenous vein

Anterior tibial vessels

Tibialis posterior t.

Flexor digitorum longus tendon

Posterior tibial artery, vein

Posterior tibial nerve

Flexor retinaculum

Flexor hallucis longus muscle & tendon

Plantaris tendon

Extensor hallucis longus m. & t.

Extensor digitorum longus, peroneus tertius m. & t.

Deep peroneal nerve

Tibia

Fibula

Peroneus brevis m. & t.

Peroneus longus t.

Branches, saphenous vein

Sural nerve

Achilles tendon

Tibialis anterior t.

Inferior extensor retinaculum

Greater saphenous vein

Anterior tibial vessels

Tibia

Tibialis posterior t.

Flexor digitorum longus tendon

Posterior tibial artery, vein

Posterior tibial nerve

Flexor retinaculum

Flexor hallucis longus muscle & tendon

Plantaris tendon

Extensor hallucis longus m. & t.

Extensor digitorum longus, peroneus tertius m. & t.

Deep peroneal nerve

Anterior tibiofibular l.

Posterior tibiofibular l.

Peroneus brevis m. & t.

Peroneus longus t.

Branches, lesser saphenous vein

Sural nerve

Achilles tendon

(Top) First in series of axial T1 MR images of the left ankle. The cut is just above the tibial plafond. At this level, excluding the tibialis anterior, tibialis posterior and peroneus longus, all the muscles of the anterior, lateral and deep posterior compartment are still visualized. The posterior tibial nerve, found behind the posterior tibial vessels, has not yet divided into the medial and lateral plantar nerves. The sural nerve is anterolateral to the Achilles tendon. **(Bottom)** The anterior and posterior tibiofibular ligaments extend from the distal tibia to the fibula and along with the interosseous ligament, support the distal fibrous tibiofibular joint. The anterior surface of the Achilles tendon is flat. The tendon is partially surrounded by a paratenon. The plantaris tendon is found just medial to the Achilles tendon.

Ankle

VII

AXIAL T1 MR, RIGHT ANKLE

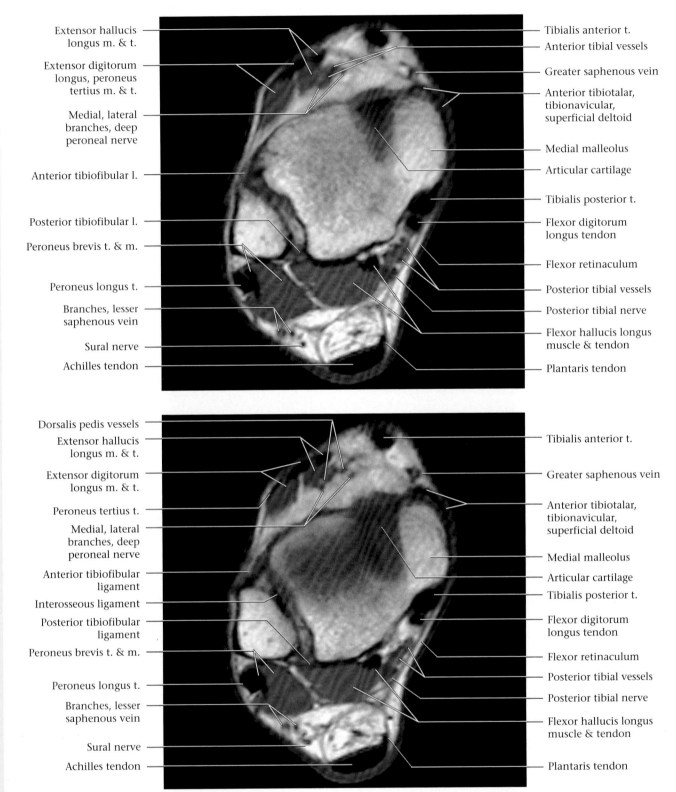

Extensor hallucis longus m. & t.

Extensor digitorum longus, peroneus tertius m. & t.

Medial, lateral branches, deep peroneal nerve

Anterior tibiofibular l.

Posterior tibiofibular l.

Peroneus brevis t. & m.

Peroneus longus t.

Branches, lesser saphenous vein

Sural nerve

Achilles tendon

Tibialis anterior t.

Anterior tibial vessels

Greater saphenous vein

Anterior tibiotalar, tibionavicular, superficial deltoid

Medial malleolus

Articular cartilage

Tibialis posterior t.

Flexor digitorum longus tendon

Flexor retinaculum

Posterior tibial vessels

Posterior tibial nerve

Flexor hallucis longus muscle & tendon

Plantaris tendon

Dorsalis pedis vessels

Extensor hallucis longus m. & t.

Extensor digitorum longus m. & t.

Peroneus tertius t.

Medial, lateral branches, deep peroneal nerve

Anterior tibiofibular ligament

Interosseous ligament

Posterior tibiofibular ligament

Peroneus brevis t. & m.

Peroneus longus t.

Branches, lesser saphenous vein

Sural nerve

Achilles tendon

Tibialis anterior t.

Greater saphenous vein

Anterior tibiotalar, tibionavicular, superficial deltoid

Medial malleolus

Articular cartilage

Tibialis posterior t.

Flexor digitorum longus tendon

Flexor retinaculum

Posterior tibial vessels

Posterior tibial nerve

Flexor hallucis longus muscle & tendon

Plantaris tendon

(Top) The shared groove of the tibialis posterior and flexor digitorum longus tendons is noted posterior to the medial malleolus. The deep peroneal nerve and its accompanying anterior tibial and then dorsalis pedis vessels are located deep to the inferior extensor retinaculum but may be difficult to distinguish from each other. The deep peroneal nerve divides into a lateral, motor branch, supplying the extensor digitorum brevis muscle and a medial branch which carries sensation and occasionally supplies motor innervation to the 1st dorsal web space. **(Bottom)** The interosseous ligament is visualized in between the tibia and fibula. This ligament, a thickening of the interosseous membrane, is variable, & may be perforated or absent. The cross sectional area of the tibialis posterior tendon is greater than the rest of posterior compartment tendons.

AXIAL T1 MR, LEFT ANKLE

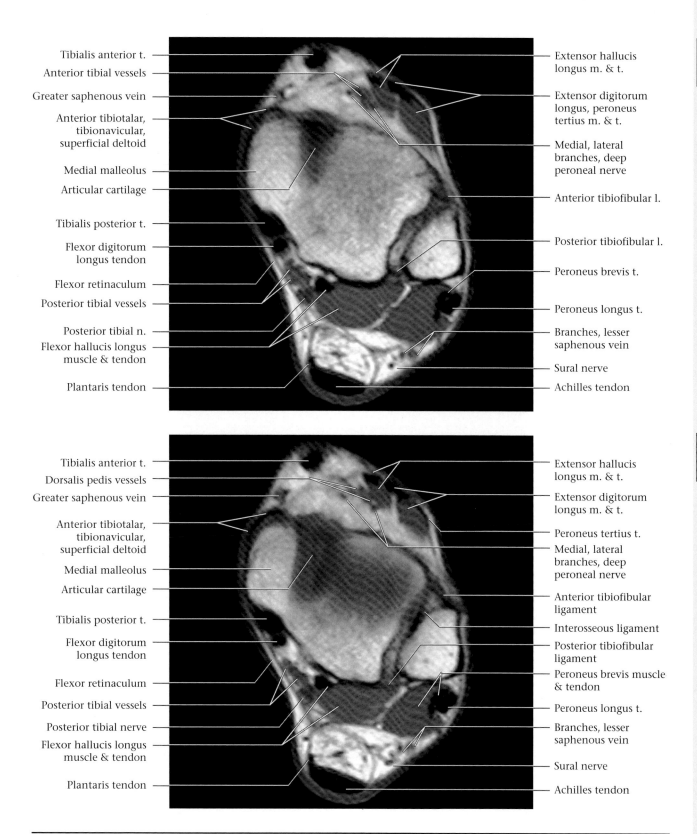

Tibialis anterior t.
Anterior tibial vessels
Greater saphenous vein
Anterior tibiotalar, tibionavicular, superficial deltoid
Medial malleolus
Articular cartilage
Tibialis posterior t.
Flexor digitorum longus tendon
Flexor retinaculum
Posterior tibial vessels
Posterior tibial n.
Flexor hallucis longus muscle & tendon
Plantaris tendon

Extensor hallucis longus m. & t.
Extensor digitorum longus, peroneus tertius m. & t.
Medial, lateral branches, deep peroneal nerve
Anterior tibiofibular l.
Posterior tibiofibular l.
Peroneus brevis t.
Peroneus longus t.
Branches, lesser saphenous vein
Sural nerve
Achilles tendon

Tibialis anterior t.
Dorsalis pedis vessels
Greater saphenous vein
Anterior tibiotalar, tibionavicular, superficial deltoid
Medial malleolus
Articular cartilage
Tibialis posterior t.
Flexor digitorum longus tendon
Flexor retinaculum
Posterior tibial vessels
Posterior tibial nerve
Flexor hallucis longus muscle & tendon
Plantaris tendon

Extensor hallucis longus m. & t.
Extensor digitorum longus m. & t.
Peroneus tertius t.
Medial, lateral branches, deep peroneal nerve
Anterior tibiofibular ligament
Interosseous ligament
Posterior tibiofibular ligament
Peroneus brevis muscle & tendon
Peroneus longus t.
Branches, lesser saphenous vein
Sural nerve
Achilles tendon

(Top) The shared groove of the tibialis posterior and flexor digitorum longus tendons is noted posterior to the medial malleolus. The deep peroneal nerve and its accompanying anterior tibial and then dorsalis pedis vessels are located deep to the inferior extensor retinaculum but may be difficult to distinguish from each other. The deep peroneal nerve divides into a lateral, motor branch, supplying the extensor digitorum brevis muscle and a medial branch which carries sensation and occasionally supplies motor innervation to the 1st dorsal web space. **(Bottom)** The interosseous ligament is visualized in between the tibia and fibula. This ligament, a thickening of the interosseous membrane, is variable, & may be perforated or absent. The cross sectional area of the tibialis posterior tendon is greater than the rest of posterior compartment tendons.

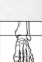

Ankle

VII

AXIAL T1 MR, RIGHT ANKLE

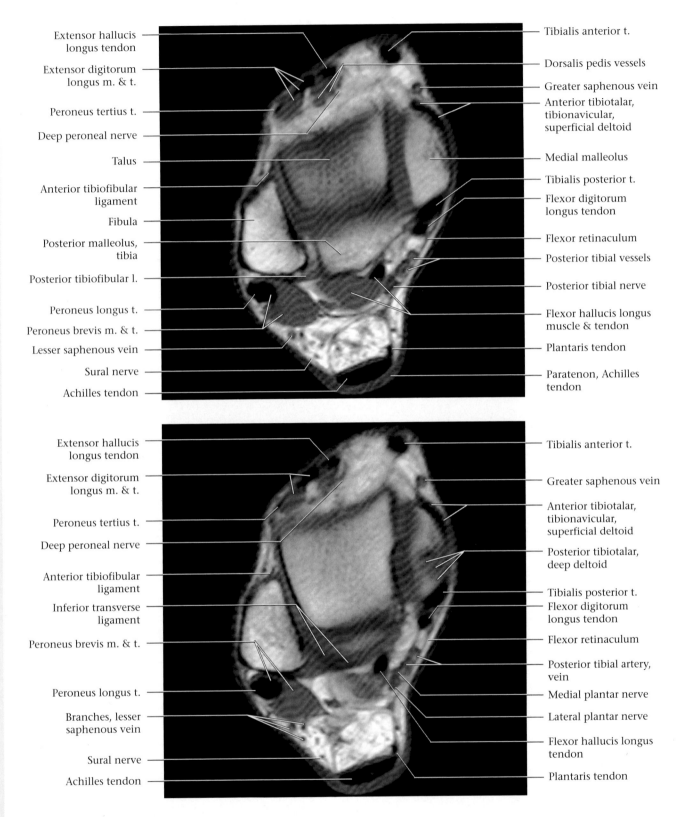

Extensor hallucis longus tendon

Extensor digitorum longus m. & t.

Peroneus tertius t.

Deep peroneal nerve

Talus

Anterior tibiofibular ligament

Fibula

Posterior malleolus, tibia

Posterior tibiofibular l.

Peroneus longus t.

Peroneus brevis m. & t.

Lesser saphenous vein

Sural nerve

Achilles tendon

Tibialis anterior t.

Dorsalis pedis vessels

Greater saphenous vein

Anterior tibiotalar, tibionavicular, superficial deltoid

Medial malleolus

Tibialis posterior t.

Flexor digitorum longus tendon

Flexor retinaculum

Posterior tibial vessels

Posterior tibial nerve

Flexor hallucis longus muscle & tendon

Plantaris tendon

Paratenon, Achilles tendon

Extensor hallucis longus tendon

Extensor digitorum longus m. & t.

Peroneus tertius t.

Deep peroneal nerve

Anterior tibiofibular ligament

Inferior transverse ligament

Peroneus brevis m. & t.

Peroneus longus t.

Branches, lesser saphenous vein

Sural nerve

Achilles tendon

Tibialis anterior t.

Greater saphenous vein

Anterior tibiotalar, tibionavicular, superficial deltoid

Posterior tibiotalar, deep deltoid

Tibialis posterior t.

Flexor digitorum longus tendon

Flexor retinaculum

Posterior tibial artery, vein

Medial plantar nerve

Lateral plantar nerve

Flexor hallucis longus tendon

Plantaris tendon

(Top) Only the muscles of the flexor hallucis longus & peroneus brevis are seen while the other muscles have become tendinous. The anterior tibiotalar & tibionavicular bands of the superficial deltoid originate from the anterior colliculus of medial malleolus. Note that the fibula is round at the level of syndesmotic ligaments. **(Bottom)** The deep posterior tibiotalar component of the deltoid ligament originates from the posterior colliculus & is typically striated. The very tip of the anterior tibiofibular ligament is noted at the level of the talar dome (talus is square at this level). The inferior transverse ligament, the very inferior aspect of the posterior tibiofibular ligament, extends distal to the tibial posterior surface. It can insert into the tibia quite far medially, as seen here.

AXIAL T1 MR, LEFT ANKLE

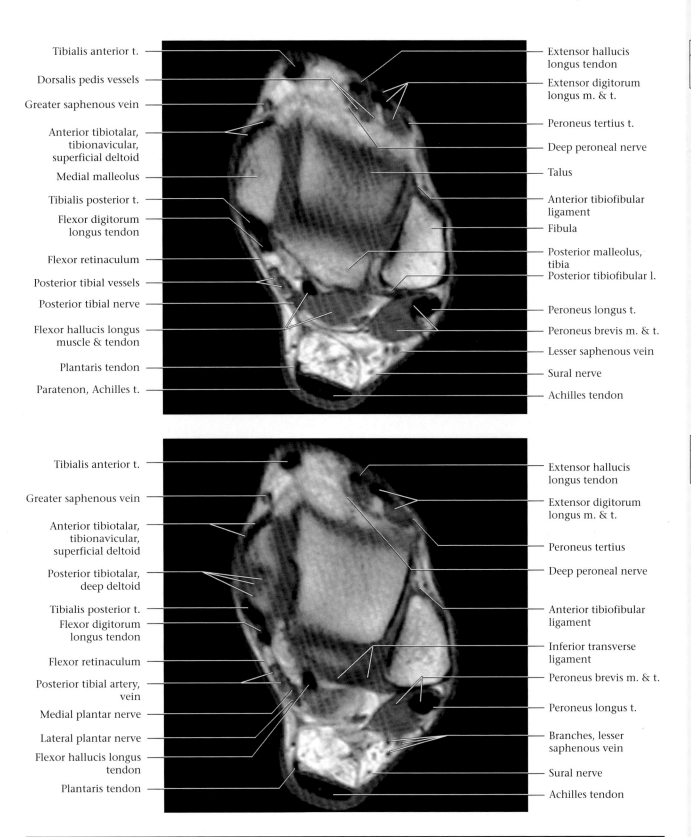

Tibialis anterior t.

Dorsalis pedis vessels

Greater saphenous vein

Anterior tibiotalar, tibionavicular, superficial deltoid

Medial malleolus

Tibialis posterior t.

Flexor digitorum longus tendon

Flexor retinaculum

Posterior tibial vessels

Posterior tibial nerve

Flexor hallucis longus muscle & tendon

Plantaris tendon

Paratenon, Achilles t.

Extensor hallucis longus tendon

Extensor digitorum longus m. & t.

Peroneus tertius t.

Deep peroneal nerve

Talus

Anterior tibiofibular ligament

Fibula

Posterior malleolus, tibia

Posterior tibiofibular l.

Peroneus longus t.

Peroneus brevis m. & t.

Lesser saphenous vein

Sural nerve

Achilles tendon

Tibialis anterior t.

Greater saphenous vein

Anterior tibiotalar, tibionavicular, superficial deltoid

Posterior tibiotalar, deep deltoid

Tibialis posterior t.

Flexor digitorum longus tendon

Flexor retinaculum

Posterior tibial artery, vein

Medial plantar nerve

Lateral plantar nerve

Flexor hallucis longus tendon

Plantaris tendon

Extensor hallucis longus tendon

Extensor digitorum longus m. & t.

Peroneus tertius

Deep peroneal nerve

Anterior tibiofibular ligament

Inferior transverse ligament

Peroneus brevis m. & t.

Peroneus longus t.

Branches, lesser saphenous vein

Sural nerve

Achilles tendon

(Top) Only the muscles of the flexor hallucis longus & peroneus brevis are seen while the other muscles have become tendinous. The anterior tibiotalar & tibionavicular bands of the superficial deltoid originate from the anterior colliculus of medial malleolus. Note that the fibula is round at the level of syndesmotic ligaments. **(Bottom)** The deep posterior tibiotalar component of the deltoid ligament originates from the posterior colliculus & is typically striated. The very tip of the anterior tibiofibular ligament is noted at the level of the talar dome (talus is square at this level). The inferior transverse ligament, the very inferior aspect of the posterior tibiofibular ligament, extends distal to the tibial posterior surface. It can insert into the tibia quite far medially, as seen here.

Ankle

VII

AXIAL T1 MR, RIGHT ANKLE

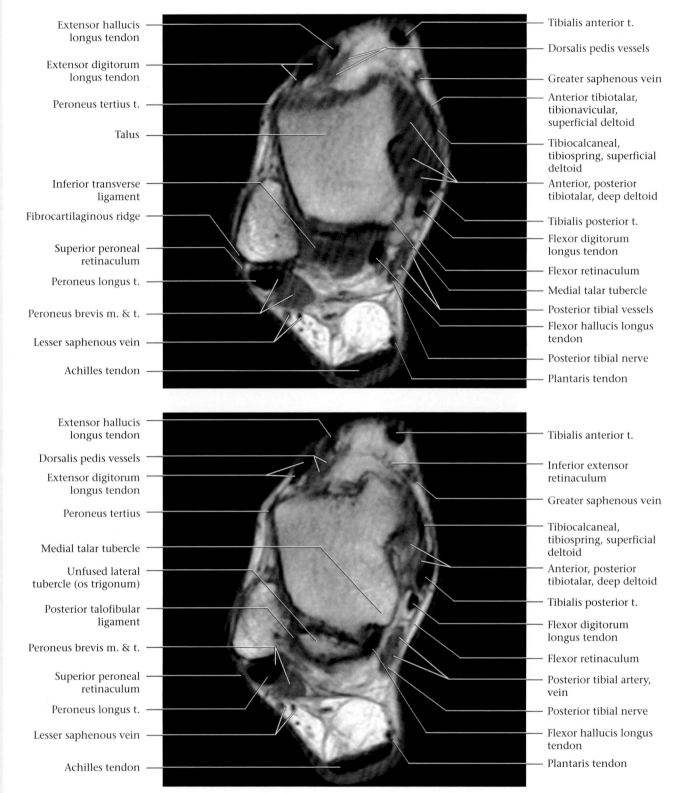

Extensor hallucis longus tendon

Extensor digitorum longus tendon

Peroneus tertius t.

Talus

Inferior transverse ligament

Fibrocartilaginous ridge

Superior peroneal retinaculum

Peroneus longus t.

Peroneus brevis m. & t.

Lesser saphenous vein

Achilles tendon

Tibialis anterior t.

Dorsalis pedis vessels

Greater saphenous vein

Anterior tibiotalar, tibionavicular, superficial deltoid

Tibiocalcaneal, tibiospring, superficial deltoid

Anterior, posterior tibiotalar, deep deltoid

Tibialis posterior t.

Flexor digitorum longus tendon

Flexor retinaculum

Medial talar tubercle

Posterior tibial vessels

Flexor hallucis longus tendon

Posterior tibial nerve

Plantaris tendon

Extensor hallucis longus tendon

Dorsalis pedis vessels

Extensor digitorum longus tendon

Peroneus tertius

Medial talar tubercle

Unfused lateral tubercle (os trigonum)

Posterior talofibular ligament

Peroneus brevis m. & t.

Superior peroneal retinaculum

Peroneus longus t.

Lesser saphenous vein

Achilles tendon

Tibialis anterior t.

Inferior extensor retinaculum

Greater saphenous vein

Tibiocalcaneal, tibiospring, superficial deltoid

Anterior, posterior tibiotalar, deep deltoid

Tibialis posterior t.

Flexor digitorum longus tendon

Flexor retinaculum

Posterior tibial artery, vein

Posterior tibial nerve

Flexor hallucis longus tendon

Plantaris tendon

(Top) The talus is wider anteriorly than posteriorly. Its posterior process is subdivided into medial and lateral tubercles, thus providing a tunnel for the flexor hallucis longus tendon. The deep deltoid ligament is subdivided into an anterior and posterior tibiotalar bands. The superficial deltoid components form a triangular band which is divided into its various ligaments based on their respective insertion sites. The fibula at the level of the syndesmotic ligaments is round and the talus is square. (Bottom) The flexor hallucis longus tendon descends between the medial and lateral tubercles of the posterior talar process. In this instance the lateral tubercle is unfused, and is termed an os trigonum. The peroneus brevis tendon often has a mild crescentic shape as it accommodates to the fibula anteriorly and the peroneus longus tendon posteriorly.

ANKLE AND HINDFOOT OVERVIEW

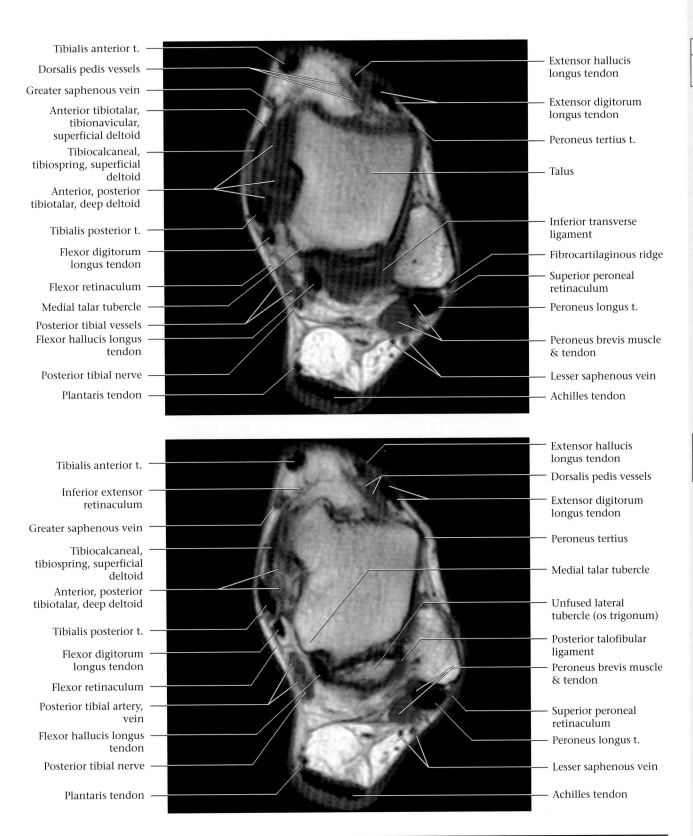

Tibialis anterior t.

Dorsalis pedis vessels

Greater saphenous vein

Anterior tibiotalar, tibionavicular, superficial deltoid

Tibiocalcaneal, tibiospring, superficial deltoid

Anterior, posterior tibiotalar, deep deltoid

Tibialis posterior t.

Flexor digitorum longus tendon

Flexor retinaculum

Medial talar tubercle

Posterior tibial vessels

Flexor hallucis longus tendon

Posterior tibial nerve

Plantaris tendon

Extensor hallucis longus tendon

Extensor digitorum longus tendon

Peroneus tertius t.

Talus

Inferior transverse ligament

Fibrocartilaginous ridge

Superior peroneal retinaculum

Peroneus longus t.

Peroneus brevis muscle & tendon

Lesser saphenous vein

Achilles tendon

Tibialis anterior t.

Inferior extensor retinaculum

Greater saphenous vein

Tibiocalcaneal, tibiospring, superficial deltoid

Anterior, posterior tibiotalar, deep deltoid

Tibialis posterior t.

Flexor digitorum longus tendon

Flexor retinaculum

Posterior tibial artery, vein

Flexor hallucis longus tendon

Posterior tibial nerve

Plantaris tendon

Extensor hallucis longus tendon

Dorsalis pedis vessels

Extensor digitorum longus tendon

Peroneus tertius

Medial talar tubercle

Unfused lateral tubercle (os trigonum)

Posterior talofibular ligament

Peroneus brevis muscle & tendon

Superior peroneal retinaculum

Peroneus longus t.

Lesser saphenous vein

Achilles tendon

(Top) The talus is wider anteriorly than posteriorly. Its posterior process is subdivided into medial and lateral tubercles, thus providing a tunnel for the flexor hallucis longus tendon. The deep deltoid ligament is subdivided into an anterior and posterior tibiotalar bands. The superficial deltoid components form a triangular band which is divided into its various ligaments based on their respective insertion sites. The fibula at the level of the syndesmotic ligaments is round and the talus is square. **(Bottom)** The flexor hallucis longus tendon descends between the medial and lateral tubercles of the posterior talar process. In this instance the lateral tubercle is unfused, and is termed an os trigonum. The peroneus brevis tendon often has a mild crescentic shape as it accommodates to the fibula anteriorly and the peroneus longus tendon posteriorly.

Ankle

VII

ANKLE AND HINDFOOT OVERVIEW

AXIAL T1 MR, RIGHT ANKLE

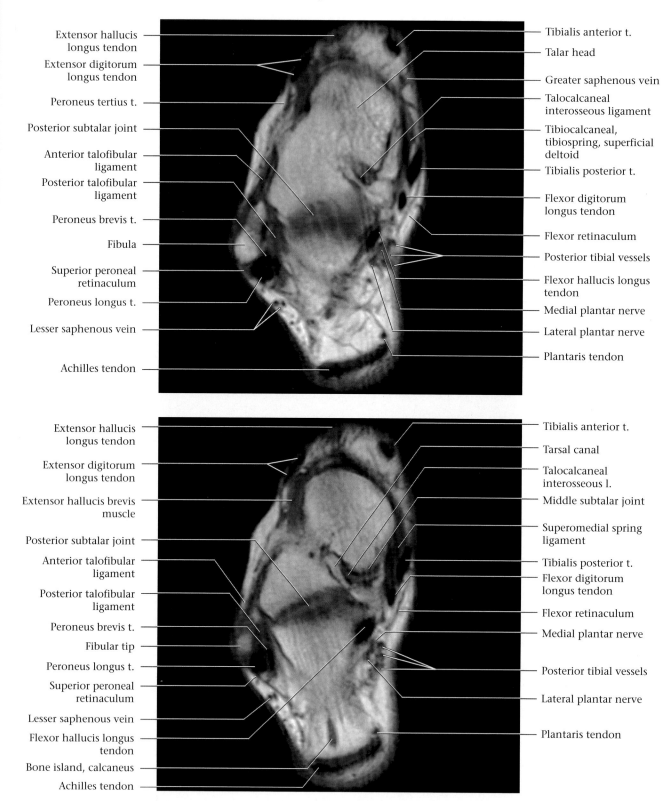

Top image labels (left):
- Extensor hallucis longus tendon
- Extensor digitorum longus tendon
- Peroneus tertius t.
- Posterior subtalar joint
- Anterior talofibular ligament
- Posterior talofibular ligament
- Peroneus brevis t.
- Fibula
- Superior peroneal retinaculum
- Peroneus longus t.
- Lesser saphenous vein
- Achilles tendon

Top image labels (right):
- Tibialis anterior t.
- Talar head
- Greater saphenous vein
- Talocalcaneal interosseous ligament
- Tibiocalcaneal, tibiospring, superficial deltoid
- Tibialis posterior t.
- Flexor digitorum longus tendon
- Flexor retinaculum
- Posterior tibial vessels
- Flexor hallucis longus tendon
- Medial plantar nerve
- Lateral plantar nerve
- Plantaris tendon

Bottom image labels (left):
- Extensor hallucis longus tendon
- Extensor digitorum longus tendon
- Extensor hallucis brevis muscle
- Posterior subtalar joint
- Anterior talofibular ligament
- Posterior talofibular ligament
- Peroneus brevis t.
- Fibular tip
- Peroneus longus t.
- Superior peroneal retinaculum
- Lesser saphenous vein
- Flexor hallucis longus tendon
- Bone island, calcaneus
- Achilles tendon

Bottom image labels (right):
- Tibialis anterior t.
- Tarsal canal
- Talocalcaneal interosseous l.
- Middle subtalar joint
- Superomedial spring ligament
- Tibialis posterior t.
- Flexor digitorum longus tendon
- Flexor retinaculum
- Medial plantar nerve
- Posterior tibial vessels
- Lateral plantar nerve
- Plantaris tendon

(Top) The extensor hallucis longus tendon is barely visualized due to magic angle effect. The anterior and posterior talofibular ligaments are visualized distal to the talar dome. Note that the fibula has a medial indentation, the malleolar fossa, and that the talus has lost its square shape at this level. **(Bottom)** The superomedial component of the spring ligament extends from the sustentaculum tali of the calcaneus to the plantar navicular, forming a sling around the talar head. It also inserts on the tibiospring component of the deltoid ligament. The superomedial component of the spring ligament is seen on coronal images as well as on axial images, as it hugs the talar head, deep to the tibialis posterior tendon. The posterior tibial nerve has now split into its two major branches, the medial and lateral plantar nerves.

ANKLE AND HINDFOOT OVERVIEW

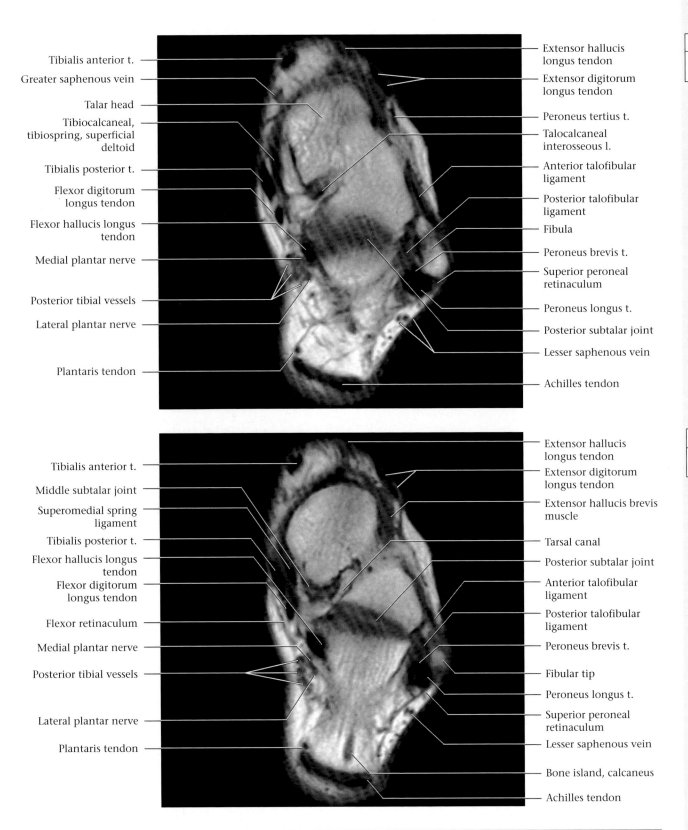

Top image labels (left):
- Tibialis anterior t.
- Greater saphenous vein
- Talar head
- Tibiocalcaneal, tibiospring, superficial deltoid
- Tibialis posterior t.
- Flexor digitorum longus tendon
- Flexor hallucis longus tendon
- Medial plantar nerve
- Posterior tibial vessels
- Lateral plantar nerve
- Plantaris tendon

Top image labels (right):
- Extensor hallucis longus tendon
- Extensor digitorum longus tendon
- Peroneus tertius t.
- Talocalcaneal interosseous l.
- Anterior talofibular ligament
- Posterior talofibular ligament
- Fibula
- Peroneus brevis t.
- Superior peroneal retinaculum
- Peroneus longus t.
- Posterior subtalar joint
- Lesser saphenous vein
- Achilles tendon

Bottom image labels (left):
- Tibialis anterior t.
- Middle subtalar joint
- Superomedial spring ligament
- Tibialis posterior t.
- Flexor hallucis longus tendon
- Flexor digitorum longus tendon
- Flexor retinaculum
- Medial plantar nerve
- Posterior tibial vessels
- Lateral plantar nerve
- Plantaris tendon

Bottom image labels (right):
- Extensor hallucis longus tendon
- Extensor digitorum longus tendon
- Extensor hallucis brevis muscle
- Tarsal canal
- Posterior subtalar joint
- Anterior talofibular ligament
- Posterior talofibular ligament
- Peroneus brevis t.
- Fibular tip
- Peroneus longus t.
- Superior peroneal retinaculum
- Lesser saphenous vein
- Bone island, calcaneus
- Achilles tendon

(Top) The extensor hallucis longus tendon is barely visualized due to magic angle effect. The anterior and posterior talofibular ligaments are visualized distal to the talar dome. Note that the fibula has a medial indentation, the malleolar fossa, and that the talus has lost its square shape at this level. **(Bottom)** The superomedial component of the spring ligament extends from the sustentaculum tali of the calcaneus to the plantar navicular, forming a sling around the talar head. It also inserts on the tibiospring component of the deltoid ligament. The superomedial component of the spring ligament is seen on coronal images as well as on axial images, as it hugs the talar head, deep to the tibialis posterior tendon. The posterior tibial nerve has now split into its two major branches, the medial and lateral plantar nerves.

AXIAL T1 MR, RIGHT ANKLE

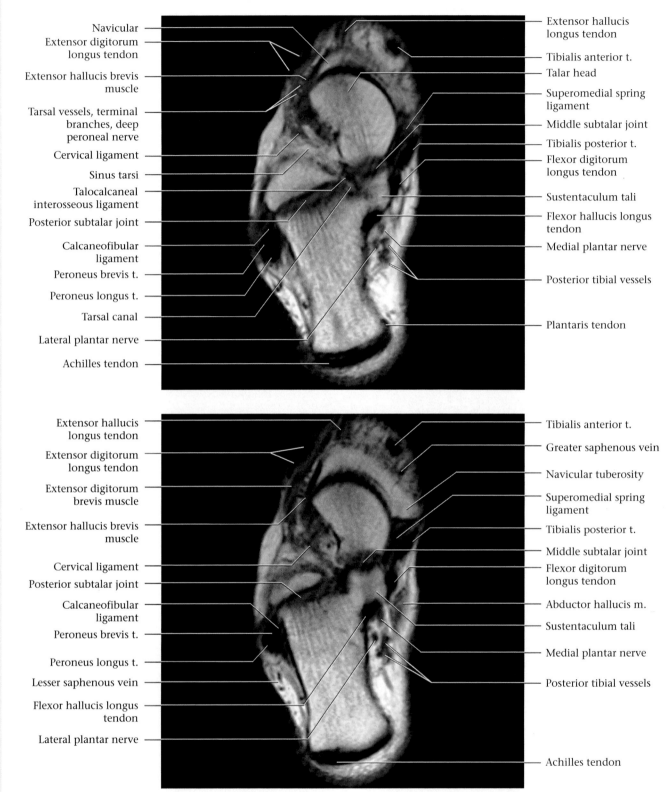

Navicular
Extensor digitorum longus tendon
Extensor hallucis brevis muscle
Tarsal vessels, terminal branches, deep peroneal nerve
Cervical ligament
Sinus tarsi
Talocalcaneal interosseous ligament
Posterior subtalar joint
Calcaneofibular ligament
Peroneus brevis t.
Peroneus longus t.
Tarsal canal
Lateral plantar nerve
Achilles tendon

Extensor hallucis longus tendon
Tibialis anterior t.
Talar head
Superomedial spring ligament
Middle subtalar joint
Tibialis posterior t.
Flexor digitorum longus tendon
Sustentaculum tali
Flexor hallucis longus tendon
Medial plantar nerve
Posterior tibial vessels
Plantaris tendon

Extensor hallucis longus tendon
Extensor digitorum longus tendon
Extensor digitorum brevis muscle
Extensor hallucis brevis muscle
Cervical ligament
Posterior subtalar joint
Calcaneofibular ligament
Peroneus brevis t.
Peroneus longus t.
Lesser saphenous vein
Flexor hallucis longus tendon
Lateral plantar nerve

Tibialis anterior t.
Greater saphenous vein
Navicular tuberosity
Superomedial spring ligament
Tibialis posterior t.
Middle subtalar joint
Flexor digitorum longus tendon
Abductor hallucis m.
Sustentaculum tali
Medial plantar nerve
Posterior tibial vessels
Achilles tendon

(Top) The posterior and middle subtalar joint are now seen. The anterior subtalar joint is often confluent with the middle subtalar joint and may not be seen as a distinct joint. The posterior tibial nerve has split into the medial and lateral plantar nerves. The flexor hallucis longus tendon is now traveling within its second fibro-osseous tunnel under the sustentaculum tali. The tarsal canal is a narrow space in between the middle and posterior subtalar joints, traversed by the interosseous talocalcaneal ligament and contiguous laterally with the sinus tarsi space. **(Bottom)** The sinus tarsi is a fat-filled space traversed by the cervical ligament and by the medial, intermediate and lateral roots of the inferior extensor retinaculum. The calcaneofibular ligament is seen adjacent to the lateral calcaneal wall and deep to the peroneus brevis and peroneus longus tendons.

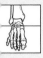

ANKLE AND HINDFOOT OVERVIEW

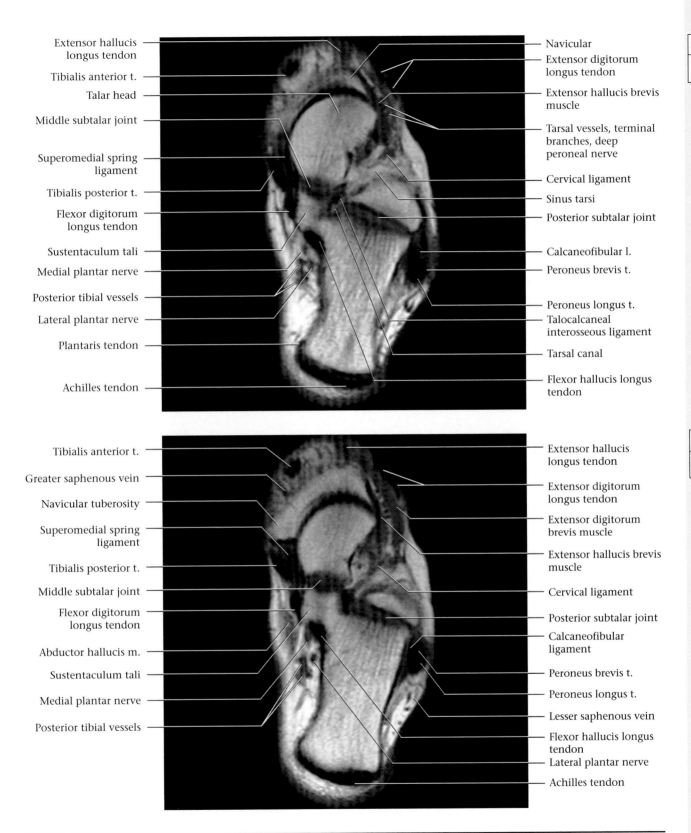

AXIAL T1 MR, LEFT ANKLE

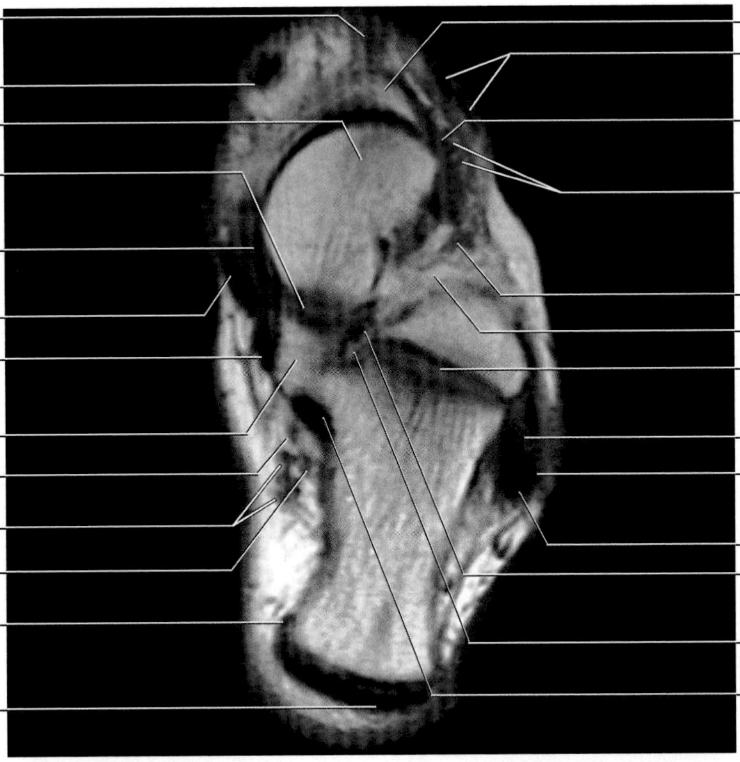

Extensor hallucis longus tendon
Tibialis anterior t.
Talar head
Middle subtalar joint
Superomedial spring ligament
Tibialis posterior t.
Flexor digitorum longus tendon
Sustentaculum tali
Medial plantar nerve
Posterior tibial vessels
Lateral plantar nerve
Plantaris tendon
Achilles tendon
Navicular
Extensor digitorum longus tendon
Extensor hallucis brevis muscle
Tarsal vessels, terminal branches, deep peroneal nerve
Cervical ligament
Sinus tarsi
Posterior subtalar joint
Calcaneofibular l.
Peroneus brevis t.
Peroneus longus t.
Talocalcaneal interosseous ligament
Tarsal canal
Flexor hallucis longus tendon

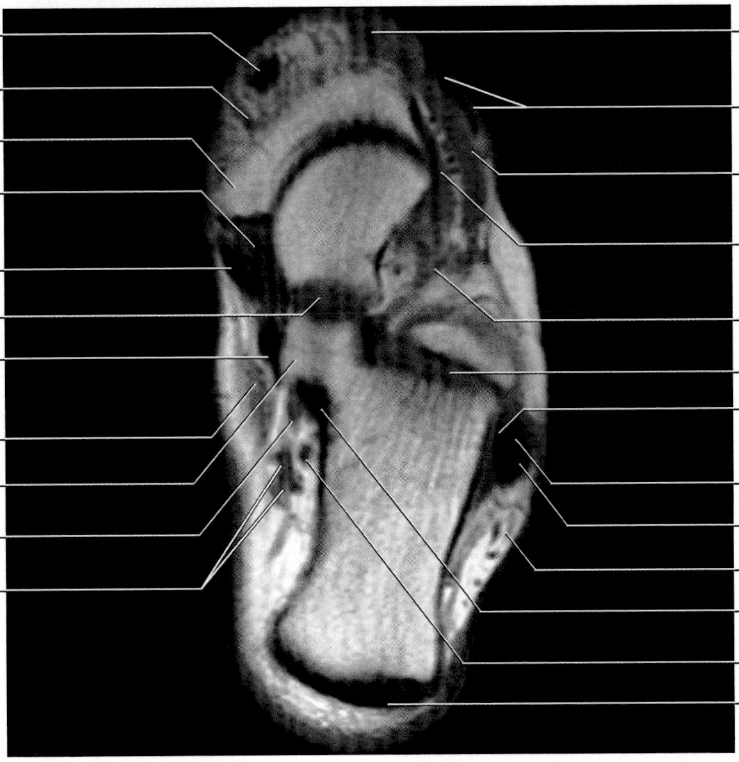

Tibialis anterior t.
Greater saphenous vein
Navicular tuberosity
Superomedial spring ligament
Tibialis posterior t.
Middle subtalar joint
Flexor digitorum longus tendon
Abductor hallucis m.
Sustentaculum tali
Medial plantar nerve
Posterior tibial vessels
Extensor hallucis longus tendon
Extensor digitorum longus tendon
Extensor digitorum brevis muscle
Extensor hallucis brevis muscle
Cervical ligament
Posterior subtalar joint
Calcaneofibular ligament
Peroneus brevis t.
Peroneus longus t.
Lesser saphenous vein
Flexor hallucis longus tendon
Lateral plantar nerve
Achilles tendon

(Top) The posterior and middle subtalar joint are now seen. The anterior subtalar joint is often confluent with the middle subtalar joint and may not be seen as a distinct joint. The posterior tibial nerve has split into the medial and lateral plantar nerves. The flexor hallucis longus tendon is now traveling within its second fibro-osseous tunnel under the sustentaculum tali. The tarsal canal is a narrow space in between the middle and posterior subtalar joints, traversed by the interosseous talocalcaneal ligament and contiguous laterally with the sinus tarsi space. **(Bottom)** The sinus tarsi is a fat-filled space traversed by the cervical ligament and by the medial, intermediate and lateral roots of the inferior extensor retinaculum. The calcaneofibular ligament is seen adjacent to the lateral calcaneal wall and deep to the peroneus brevis and peroneus longus tendons.

AXIAL T1 MR, RIGHT ANKLE

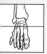

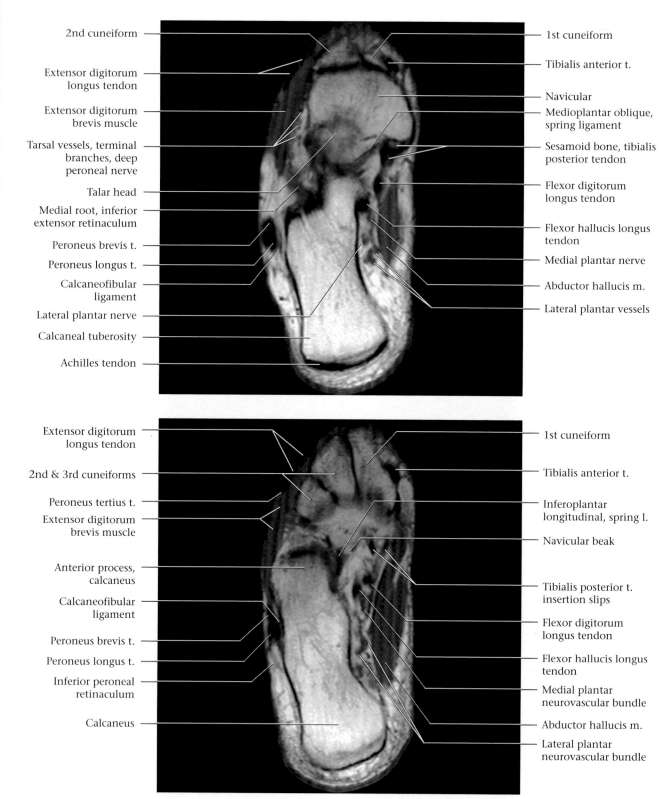

2nd cuneiform

Extensor digitorum longus tendon

Extensor digitorum brevis muscle

Tarsal vessels, terminal branches, deep peroneal nerve

Talar head

Medial root, inferior extensor retinaculum

Peroneus brevis t.

Peroneus longus t.

Calcaneofibular ligament

Lateral plantar nerve

Calcaneal tuberosity

Achilles tendon

1st cuneiform

Tibialis anterior t.

Navicular

Medioplantar oblique, spring ligament

Sesamoid bone, tibialis posterior tendon

Flexor digitorum longus tendon

Flexor hallucis longus tendon

Medial plantar nerve

Abductor hallucis m.

Lateral plantar vessels

Extensor digitorum longus tendon

2nd & 3rd cuneiforms

Peroneus tertius t.

Extensor digitorum brevis muscle

Anterior process, calcaneus

Calcaneofibular ligament

Peroneus brevis t.

Peroneus longus t.

Inferior peroneal retinaculum

Calcaneus

1st cuneiform

Tibialis anterior t.

Inferoplantar longitudinal, spring l.

Navicular beak

Tibialis posterior t. insertion slips

Flexor digitorum longus tendon

Flexor hallucis longus tendon

Medial plantar neurovascular bundle

Abductor hallucis m.

Lateral plantar neurovascular bundle

(Top) The medioplantar oblique band of the spring ligament originates from coronoid fossa of calcaneus, between the middle and anterior calcaneal facets and inserts on the navicular, lateral to the tibialis posterior tendon. It is often striated and is best seen on axial images. A small sesamoid bone in the tibialis posterior tendon should not be misinterpreted as a tendon tear. The insertion of the calcaneofibular ligament to the calcaneus is seen deep to the peroneal tendons. (Bottom) The inferoplantar longitudinal component of the spring ligament is short and straight and inserts into the navicular beak. The tibialis posterior tendon, distal to its navicular insertion, continues toward its various insertion sites into the remainder of the tarsal bones and the 2nd-4th metatarsal bases. The abductor hallucis muscle forms the medial border of the tarsal tunnel.

ANKLE AND HINDFOOT OVERVIEW

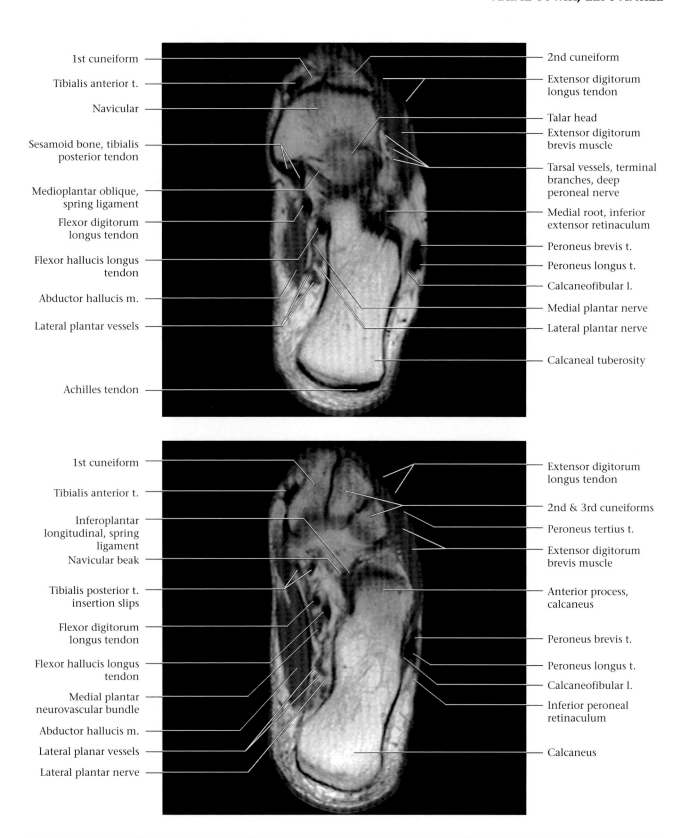

Top image labels (left): 1st cuneiform · Tibialis anterior t. · Navicular · Sesamoid bone, tibialis posterior tendon · Medioplantar oblique, spring ligament · Flexor digitorum longus tendon · Flexor hallucis longus tendon · Abductor hallucis m. · Lateral plantar vessels · Achilles tendon

Top image labels (right): 2nd cuneiform · Extensor digitorum longus tendon · Talar head · Extensor digitorum brevis muscle · Tarsal vessels, terminal branches, deep peroneal nerve · Medial root, inferior extensor retinaculum · Peroneus brevis t. · Peroneus longus t. · Calcaneofibular l. · Medial plantar nerve · Lateral plantar nerve · Calcaneal tuberosity

Bottom image labels (left): 1st cuneiform · Tibialis anterior t. · Inferoplantar longitudinal, spring ligament · Navicular beak · Tibialis posterior t. insertion slips · Flexor digitorum longus tendon · Flexor hallucis longus tendon · Medial plantar neurovascular bundle · Abductor hallucis m. · Lateral planar vessels · Lateral plantar nerve

Bottom image labels (right): Extensor digitorum longus tendon · 2nd & 3rd cuneiforms · Peroneus tertius t. · Extensor digitorum brevis muscle · Anterior process, calcaneus · Peroneus brevis t. · Peroneus longus t. · Calcaneofibular l. · Inferior peroneal retinaculum · Calcaneus

(Top) The medioplantar oblique band of the spring ligament originates from coronoid fossa of calcaneus, between the middle and anterior calcaneal facets and inserts on the navicular, lateral to the tibialis posterior tendon. It is often striated and is best seen on axial images. A small sesamoid bone in the tibialis posterior tendon should not be misinterpreted as a tendon tear. The insertion of the calcaneofibular ligament to the calcaneus is seen deep to the peroneal tendons. (Bottom) The inferoplantar longitudinal component of the spring ligament is short and straight and inserts into the navicular beak. The tibialis posterior tendon, distal to its navicular insertion, continues toward its various insertion sites into the remainder of the tarsal bones and the 2nd-4th metatarsal bases. The abductor hallucis muscle forms the medial border of the tarsal tunnel.

AXIAL T1 MR, RIGHT ANKLE

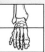

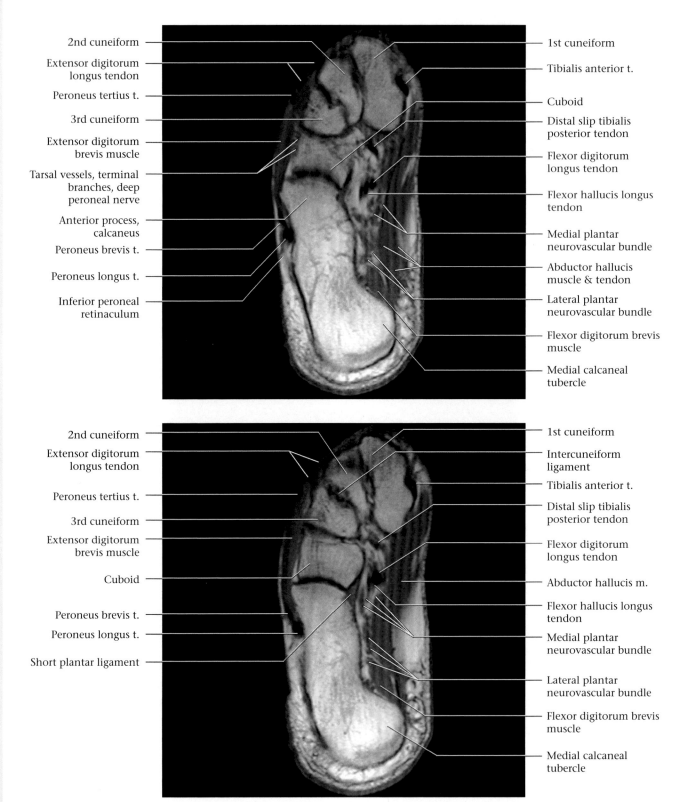

2nd cuneiform

Extensor digitorum longus tendon

Peroneus tertius t.

3rd cuneiform

Extensor digitorum brevis muscle

Tarsal vessels, terminal branches, deep peroneal nerve

Anterior process, calcaneus

Peroneus brevis t.

Peroneus longus t.

Inferior peroneal retinaculum

1st cuneiform

Tibialis anterior t.

Cuboid

Distal slip tibialis posterior tendon

Flexor digitorum longus tendon

Flexor hallucis longus tendon

Medial plantar neurovascular bundle

Abductor hallucis muscle & tendon

Lateral plantar neurovascular bundle

Flexor digitorum brevis muscle

Medial calcaneal tubercle

2nd cuneiform

Extensor digitorum longus tendon

Peroneus tertius t.

3rd cuneiform

Extensor digitorum brevis muscle

Cuboid

Peroneus brevis t.

Peroneus longus t.

Short plantar ligament

1st cuneiform

Intercuneiform ligament

Tibialis anterior t.

Distal slip tibialis posterior tendon

Flexor digitorum longus tendon

Abductor hallucis m.

Flexor hallucis longus tendon

Medial plantar neurovascular bundle

Lateral plantar neurovascular bundle

Flexor digitorum brevis muscle

Medial calcaneal tubercle

(Top) The flexor digitorum longus and flexor hallucis longus tendons are just about to cross each other at the knot of Henry, plantar to the navicular (not seen). A distal insertion slip of the tibialis posterior tendon, approaching the cuneiforms, is seen. The tibialis anterior tendon inserts to the medioplantar aspect of the 1st cuneiform and to the base of the 1st metatarsal. The medial plantar nerve continues in the plantar aspect of the foot in close proximity to the flexor hallucis longus tendon. The plantar nerves and their associated vessels may be difficult to distinguish from one another. **(Bottom)** The short and long plantar ligaments bind the cuboid to the calcaneus. The short plantar ligament is a thicker band that is deeper and more medial than the long plantar ligament. The intercuneiform ligaments bind the cuneiforms to one another.

AXIAL T1 MR, LEFT ANKLE

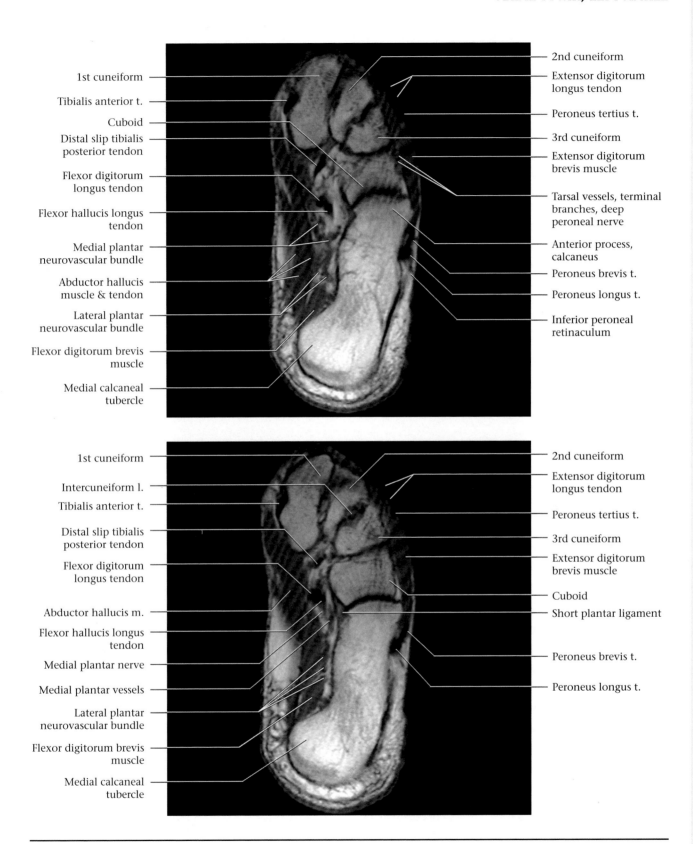

1st cuneiform

Tibialis anterior t.

Cuboid

Distal slip tibialis posterior tendon

Flexor digitorum longus tendon

Flexor hallucis longus tendon

Medial plantar neurovascular bundle

Abductor hallucis muscle & tendon

Lateral plantar neurovascular bundle

Flexor digitorum brevis muscle

Medial calcaneal tubercle

2nd cuneiform

Extensor digitorum longus tendon

Peroneus tertius t.

3rd cuneiform

Extensor digitorum brevis muscle

Tarsal vessels, terminal branches, deep peroneal nerve

Anterior process, calcaneus

Peroneus brevis t.

Peroneus longus t.

Inferior peroneal retinaculum

1st cuneiform

Intercuneiform l.

Tibialis anterior t.

Distal slip tibialis posterior tendon

Flexor digitorum longus tendon

Abductor hallucis m.

Flexor hallucis longus tendon

Medial plantar nerve

Medial plantar vessels

Lateral plantar neurovascular bundle

Flexor digitorum brevis muscle

Medial calcaneal tubercle

2nd cuneiform

Extensor digitorum longus tendon

Peroneus tertius t.

3rd cuneiform

Extensor digitorum brevis muscle

Cuboid

Short plantar ligament

Peroneus brevis t.

Peroneus longus t.

(Top) The flexor digitorum longus and flexor hallucis longus tendons are just about to cross each other at the knot of Henry, plantar to the navicular (not seen). A distal insertion slip of the tibialis posterior tendon, approaching the cuneiforms, is seen. The tibialis anterior tendon inserts to the medioplantar aspect of the 1st cuneiform and to the base of the 1st metatarsal. The medial plantar nerve continues in the plantar aspect of the foot in close proximity to the flexor hallucis longus tendon. The plantar nerves and their associated vessels may be difficult to distinguish from one another. (Bottom) The short and long plantar ligaments bind the cuboid to the calcaneus. The short plantar ligament is a thicker band that is deeper and more medial than the long plantar ligament. The intercuneiform ligaments bind the cuneiforms to one another.

AXIAL T1 MR, RIGHT ANKLE

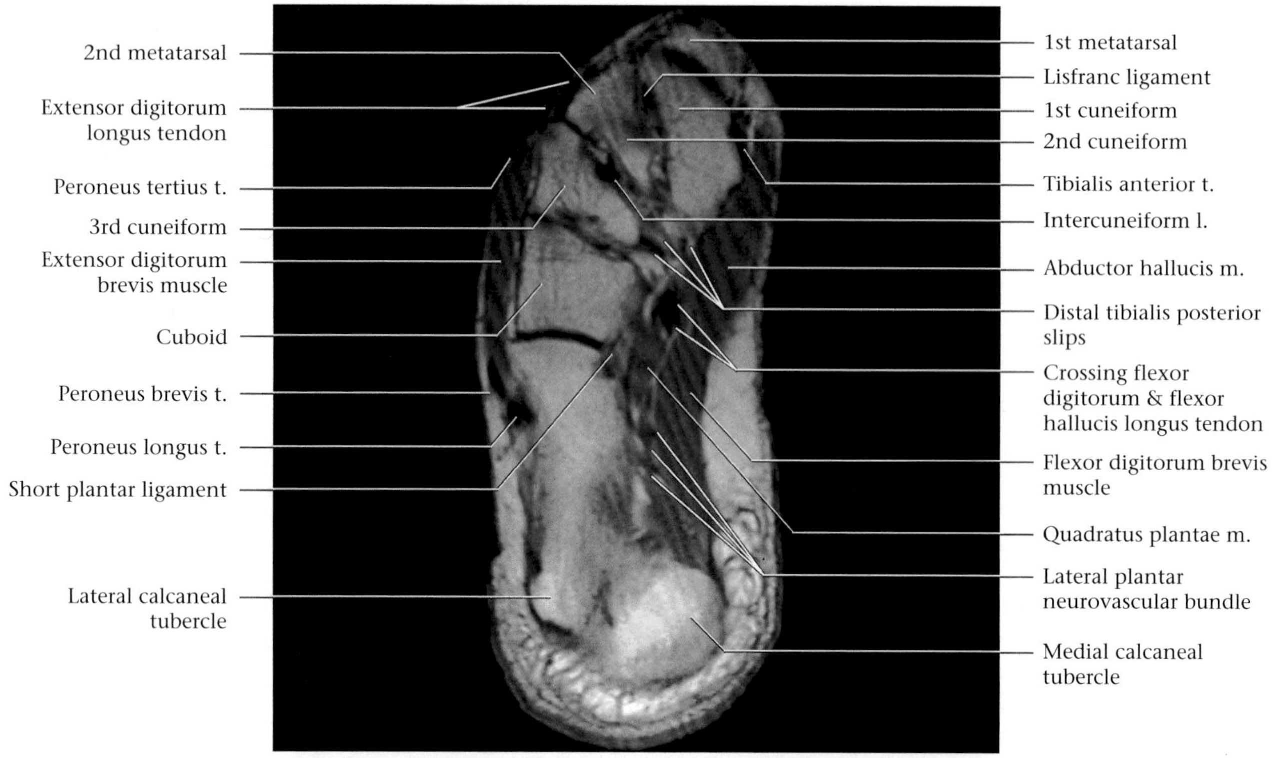
2nd metatarsal
Extensor digitorum longus tendon
Peroneus tertius t.
3rd cuneiform
Extensor digitorum brevis muscle
Cuboid
Peroneus brevis t.
Peroneus longus t.
Short plantar ligament
Lateral calcaneal tubercle
1st metatarsal
Lisfranc ligament
1st cuneiform
2nd cuneiform
Tibialis anterior t.
Intercuneiform l.
Abductor hallucis m.
Distal tibialis posterior slips
Crossing flexor digitorum & flexor hallucis longus tendon
Flexor digitorum brevis muscle
Quadratus plantae m.
Lateral plantar neurovascular bundle
Medial calcaneal tubercle

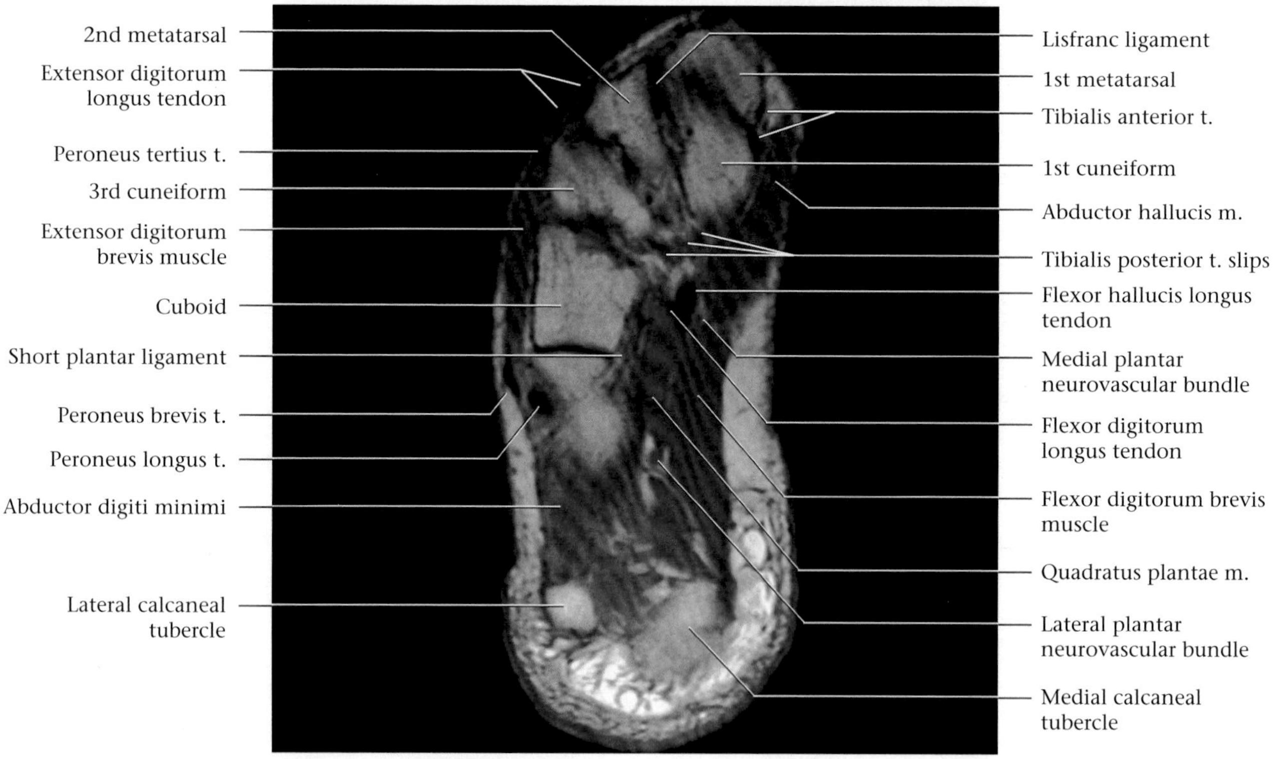
2nd metatarsal
Extensor digitorum longus tendon
Peroneus tertius t.
3rd cuneiform
Extensor digitorum brevis muscle
Cuboid
Short plantar ligament
Peroneus brevis t.
Peroneus longus t.
Abductor digiti minimi
Lateral calcaneal tubercle
Lisfranc ligament
1st metatarsal
Tibialis anterior t.
1st cuneiform
Abductor hallucis m.
Tibialis posterior t. slips
Flexor hallucis longus tendon
Medial plantar neurovascular bundle
Flexor digitorum longus tendon
Flexor digitorum brevis muscle
Quadratus plantae m.
Lateral plantar neurovascular bundle
Medial calcaneal tubercle

(Top) The medial plantar nerve and its accompanying vessels occupy a fat plane in between the abductor hallucis and flexor digitorum brevis muscles. The lateral plantar nerve and its accompanying vessels occupy the fat plane in between the flexor digitorum brevis and quadratus plantae muscles. Lisfranc ligament originates from the 1st cuneiform and extends toward its 2nd metatarsal insertion. **(Bottom)** The calcaneus has two posterior plantar tubercles: The larger medial tubercle and slightly more anterior lateral tubercle. These provide the origin for the 3 muscles of the 1st layer of the foot. The medial tubercle gives origin to all three muscles: Abductor digiti minimi, flexor digitorum brevis and abductor hallucis while the lateral tubercle gives origin only to the abductor digiti minimi muscle.

ANKLE AND HINDFOOT OVERVIEW

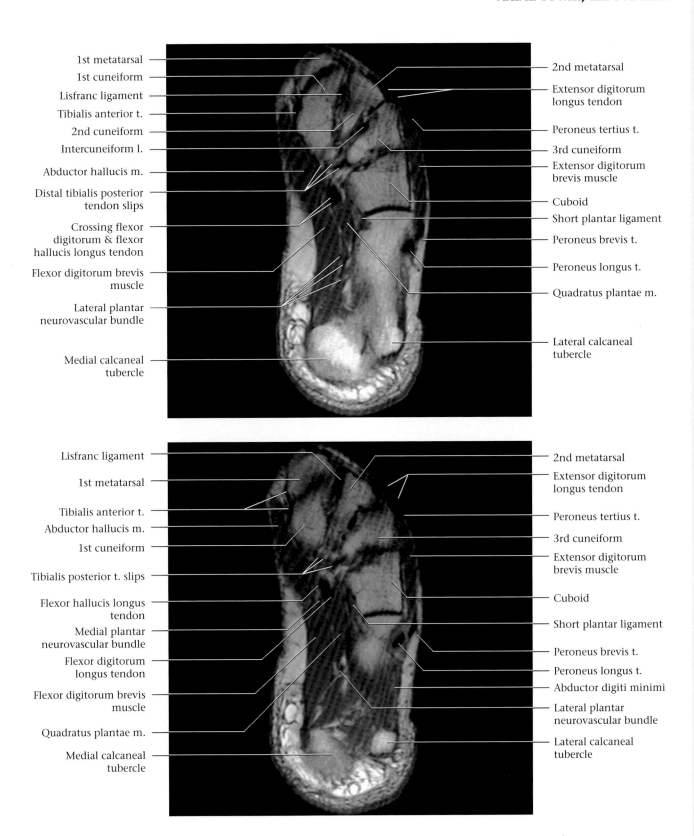
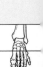

1st metatarsal

1st cuneiform

Lisfranc ligament

Tibialis anterior t.

2nd cuneiform

Intercuneiform l.

Abductor hallucis m.

Distal tibialis posterior tendon slips

Crossing flexor digitorum & flexor hallucis longus tendon

Flexor digitorum brevis muscle

Lateral plantar neurovascular bundle

Medial calcaneal tubercle

2nd metatarsal

Extensor digitorum longus tendon

Peroneus tertius t.

3rd cuneiform

Extensor digitorum brevis muscle

Cuboid

Short plantar ligament

Peroneus brevis t.

Peroneus longus t.

Quadratus plantae m.

Lateral calcaneal tubercle

Lisfranc ligament

1st metatarsal

Tibialis anterior t.

Abductor hallucis m.

1st cuneiform

Tibialis posterior t. slips

Flexor hallucis longus tendon

Medial plantar neurovascular bundle

Flexor digitorum longus tendon

Flexor digitorum brevis muscle

Quadratus plantae m.

Medial calcaneal tubercle

2nd metatarsal

Extensor digitorum longus tendon

Peroneus tertius t.

3rd cuneiform

Extensor digitorum brevis muscle

Cuboid

Short plantar ligament

Peroneus brevis t.

Peroneus longus t.

Abductor digiti minimi

Lateral plantar neurovascular bundle

Lateral calcaneal tubercle

(Top) The medial plantar nerve and its accompanying vessels occupy a fat plane in between the abductor hallucis and flexor digitorum brevis muscles. The lateral plantar nerve and its accompanying vessels occupy the fat plane in between the flexor digitorum brevis and quadratus plantae muscles. Lisfranc ligament originates from the 1st cuneiform and extends toward its 2nd metatarsal insertion. **(Bottom)** The calcaneus has two posterior plantar tubercles which provide origin to the 3 muscles of the 1st layer of the foot: The larger medial tubercle and slightly more anterior lateral tubercle. The medial tubercle gives origin to all three muscles: Abductor digiti minimi, flexor digitorum brevis and abductor hallucis while the lateral tubercle gives origin only to the abductor digiti minimi muscle.

AXIAL T1 MR, RIGHT ANKLE

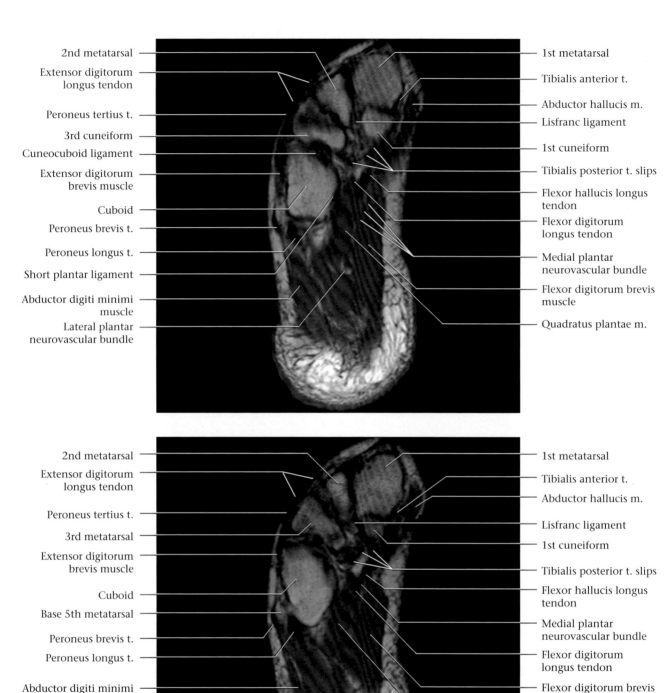

Top image labels (left side):
- 2nd metatarsal
- Extensor digitorum longus tendon
- Peroneus tertius t.
- 3rd cuneiform
- Cuneocuboid ligament
- Extensor digitorum brevis muscle
- Cuboid
- Peroneus brevis t.
- Peroneus longus t.
- Short plantar ligament
- Abductor digiti minimi muscle
- Lateral plantar neurovascular bundle

Top image labels (right side):
- 1st metatarsal
- Tibialis anterior t.
- Abductor hallucis m.
- Lisfranc ligament
- 1st cuneiform
- Tibialis posterior t. slips
- Flexor hallucis longus tendon
- Flexor digitorum longus tendon
- Medial plantar neurovascular bundle
- Flexor digitorum brevis muscle
- Quadratus plantae m.

Bottom image labels (left side):
- 2nd metatarsal
- Extensor digitorum longus tendon
- Peroneus tertius t.
- 3rd metatarsal
- Extensor digitorum brevis muscle
- Cuboid
- Base 5th metatarsal
- Peroneus brevis t.
- Peroneus longus t.
- Abductor digiti minimi muscle

Bottom image labels (right side):
- 1st metatarsal
- Tibialis anterior t.
- Abductor hallucis m.
- Lisfranc ligament
- 1st cuneiform
- Tibialis posterior t. slips
- Flexor hallucis longus tendon
- Medial plantar neurovascular bundle
- Flexor digitorum longus tendon
- Flexor digitorum brevis muscle
- Quadratus plantae m.

(Top) The quadratus plantae muscle originates from the lateral and medial surfaces of the calcaneus. The bases of the cuneiforms and the bases of the metatarsals are wedged, thus forming the transverse arch of the foot. The lateral 3 extensor digitorum brevis tendons join the extensor hidigitorum longus tendons passing to 2nd-4th toes. **(Bottom)** The peroneus longus tendon is just about to curve under the cuboid tunnel toward its insertion into the plantar base of the 1st metatarsal. The roof of the cuboid tunnel is formed by the long plantar ligament. The peroneus brevis tendon becomes more linear in shape as it approaches its insertion into the base of the 5th metatarsal.

ANKLE AND HINDFOOT OVERVIEW

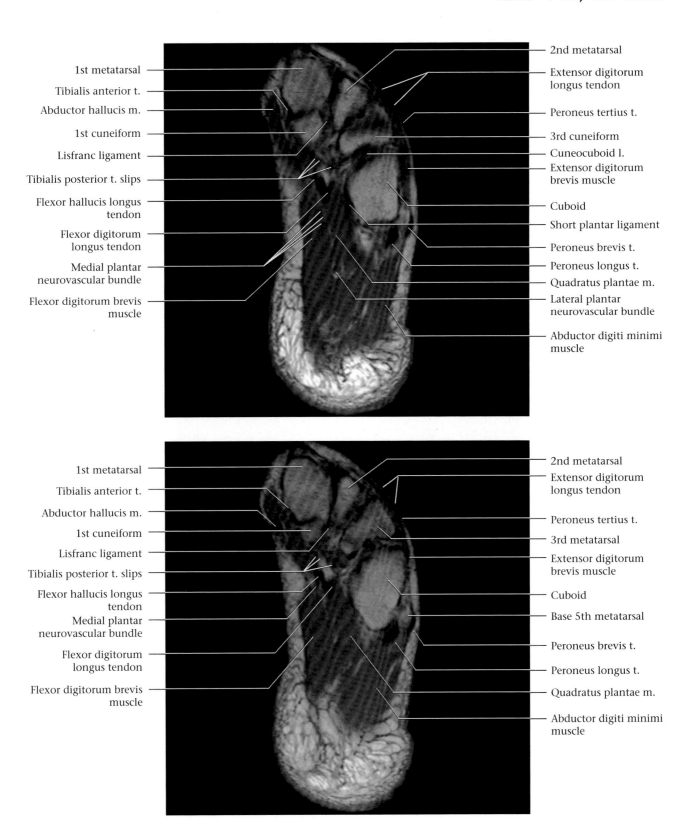

Top image labels (left):
- 1st metatarsal
- Tibialis anterior t.
- Abductor hallucis m.
- 1st cuneiform
- Lisfranc ligament
- Tibialis posterior t. slips
- Flexor hallucis longus tendon
- Flexor digitorum longus tendon
- Medial plantar neurovascular bundle
- Flexor digitorum brevis muscle

Top image labels (right):
- 2nd metatarsal
- Extensor digitorum longus tendon
- Peroneus tertius t.
- 3rd cuneiform
- Cuneocuboid l.
- Extensor digitorum brevis muscle
- Cuboid
- Short plantar ligament
- Peroneus brevis t.
- Peroneus longus t.
- Quadratus plantae m.
- Lateral plantar neurovascular bundle
- Abductor digiti minimi muscle

Bottom image labels (left):
- 1st metatarsal
- Tibialis anterior t.
- Abductor hallucis m.
- 1st cuneiform
- Lisfranc ligament
- Tibialis posterior t. slips
- Flexor hallucis longus tendon
- Medial plantar neurovascular bundle
- Flexor digitorum longus tendon
- Flexor digitorum brevis muscle

Bottom image labels (right):
- 2nd metatarsal
- Extensor digitorum longus tendon
- Peroneus tertius t.
- 3rd metatarsal
- Extensor digitorum brevis muscle
- Cuboid
- Base 5th metatarsal
- Peroneus brevis t.
- Peroneus longus t.
- Quadratus plantae m.
- Abductor digiti minimi muscle

(Top) The quadratus plantae muscle originates from the lateral and medial surfaces of the calcaneus. The bases of the cuneiforms and the bases of the metatarsals are wedged, thus forming the transverse arch of the foot. The lateral 3 extensor digitorum brevis tendons join the extensor digitorum longus tendons passing to 2nd-4th toes. **(Bottom)** The peroneus longus tendon is just about to curve under the cuboid tunnel toward its insertion into the plantar base of the 1st metatarsal. The roof of the cuboid tunnel is formed by the long plantar ligament. The peroneus brevis tendon becomes more linear in shape as it approaches its insertion into the base of the 5th metatarsal.

CORONAL T1 MR, RIGHT ANKLE

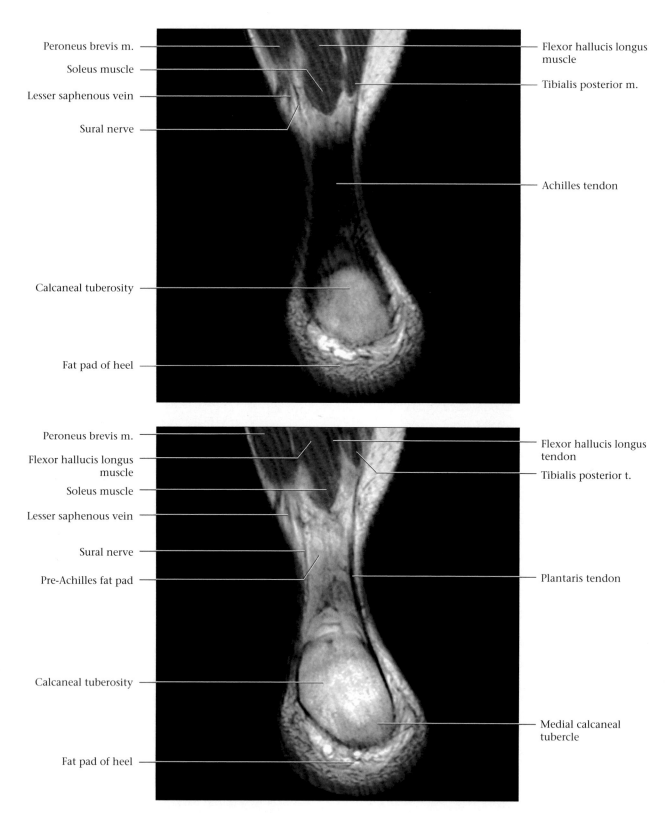

Peroneus brevis m.

Soleus muscle

Lesser saphenous vein

Sural nerve

Flexor hallucis longus muscle

Tibialis posterior m.

Achilles tendon

Calcaneal tuberosity

Fat pad of heel

Peroneus brevis m.

Flexor hallucis longus muscle

Soleus muscle

Lesser saphenous vein

Sural nerve

Pre-Achilles fat pad

Flexor hallucis longus tendon

Tibialis posterior t.

Plantaris tendon

Calcaneal tuberosity

Medial calcaneal tubercle

Fat pad of heel

(Top) First in series of coronal T1 MR images or right ankle. The Achilles tendon is the largest tendon in the body. It inserts into the calcaneal tuberosity slightly below its superior apex. The Achilles tendon is separated from the calcaneus by a small fat pad and the retrocalcaneal bursa. The Achilles tendon does not have a tendon sheath but rather a paratenon. **(Bottom)** The pre-Achilles fat pad, also called Kager fat pad, is found anterior to the calcaneus and is traversed by small vessels. The long and thin plantaris tendon descends to insert on the posterior surface of the calcaneus medial and slightly anterior to the Achilles tendon. The sural nerve and lesser saphenous vein descend together anterior and lateral to the Achilles tendon.

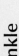

Ankle

CORONAL T1 MR, LEFT ANKLE

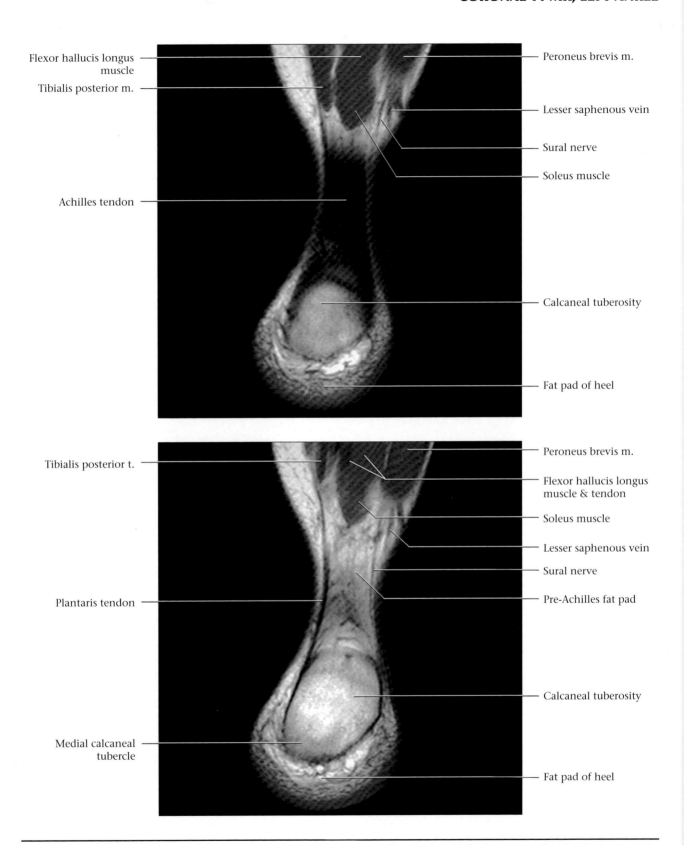

Flexor hallucis longus muscle

Tibialis posterior m.

Achilles tendon

Peroneus brevis m.

Lesser saphenous vein

Sural nerve

Soleus muscle

Calcaneal tuberosity

Fat pad of heel

Tibialis posterior t.

Plantaris tendon

Medial calcaneal tubercle

Peroneus brevis m.

Flexor hallucis longus muscle & tendon

Soleus muscle

Lesser saphenous vein

Sural nerve

Pre-Achilles fat pad

Calcaneal tuberosity

Fat pad of heel

(Top) First in series of coronal T1 MR images of left ankle. The Achilles tendon is the largest tendon in the body and is the strongest plantar flexor of the ankle. It inserts into the calcaneal tuberosity slightly below its superior apex. The Achilles tendon is separated from the calcaneus by a small fat pad and the retrocalcaneal bursa. The Achilles tendon does not have a tendon sheath but rather a paratenon which partially encircles the tendon. (Bottom) The pre-Achilles fat pad, also called Kager fat pad, is anterior to the calcaneus and is traversed by small vessels and septa. The long and thin plantaris tendon descends to insert on the posterior surface of the calcaneus medial and slightly anterior to the Achilles tendon. The sural nerve and lesser saphenous vein descend together anterior and lateral to the Achilles tendon.

Ankle

VII

43

CORONAL T1 MR, RIGHT ANKLE

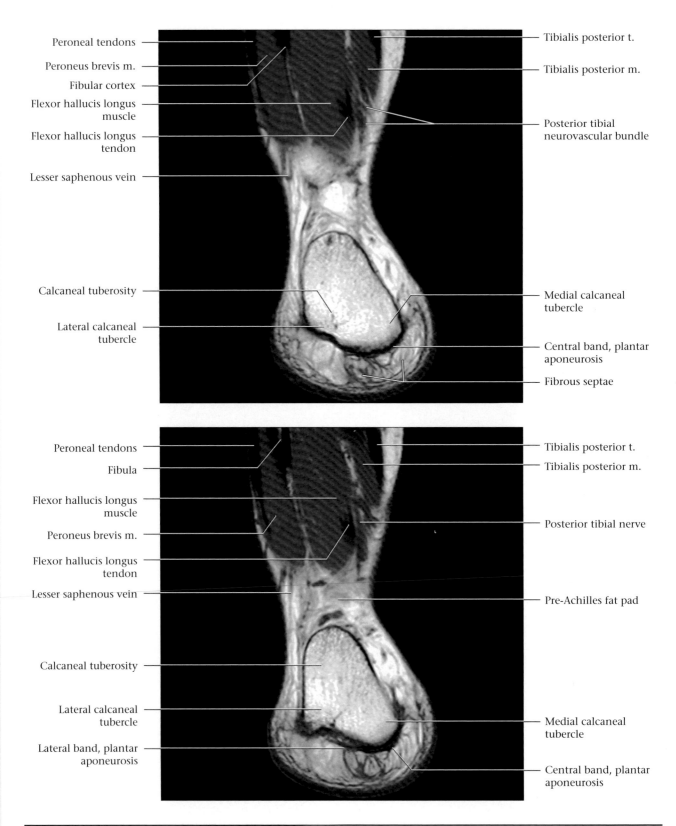

Peroneal tendons
Peroneus brevis m.
Fibular cortex
Flexor hallucis longus muscle
Flexor hallucis longus tendon
Lesser saphenous vein

Tibialis posterior t.
Tibialis posterior m.
Posterior tibial neurovascular bundle

Calcaneal tuberosity
Lateral calcaneal tubercle

Medial calcaneal tubercle
Central band, plantar aponeurosis
Fibrous septae

Peroneal tendons
Fibula
Flexor hallucis longus muscle
Peroneus brevis m.
Flexor hallucis longus tendon
Lesser saphenous vein

Tibialis posterior t.
Tibialis posterior m.
Posterior tibial nerve
Pre-Achilles fat pad

Calcaneal tuberosity
Lateral calcaneal tubercle
Lateral band, plantar aponeurosis

Medial calcaneal tubercle
Central band, plantar aponeurosis

(Top) The flexor hallucis longus muscle is broad and remains muscular more distally than the other muscles of the posterior compartment of the leg; it may be seen down to the ankle joint. The peroneus brevis muscle also descends down to the ankle joint while the peroneus longus muscle is no longer visualized at that level. (Bottom) In the distal leg and ankle the posterior tibial nerve and its accompanying vessels descend within a fat plane anteromedial to the flexor hallucis longus muscle and posterior to the tibialis posterior and flexor digitorum longus muscles. The peroneal tendons can be difficult to separate from one another on coronal images but the peroneus longus is typically more lateral that the peroneus brevis tendon. The tibialis posterior tendon is lateral to the flexor digitorum longus tendon above the ankle joint.

ANKLE AND HINDFOOT OVERVIEW

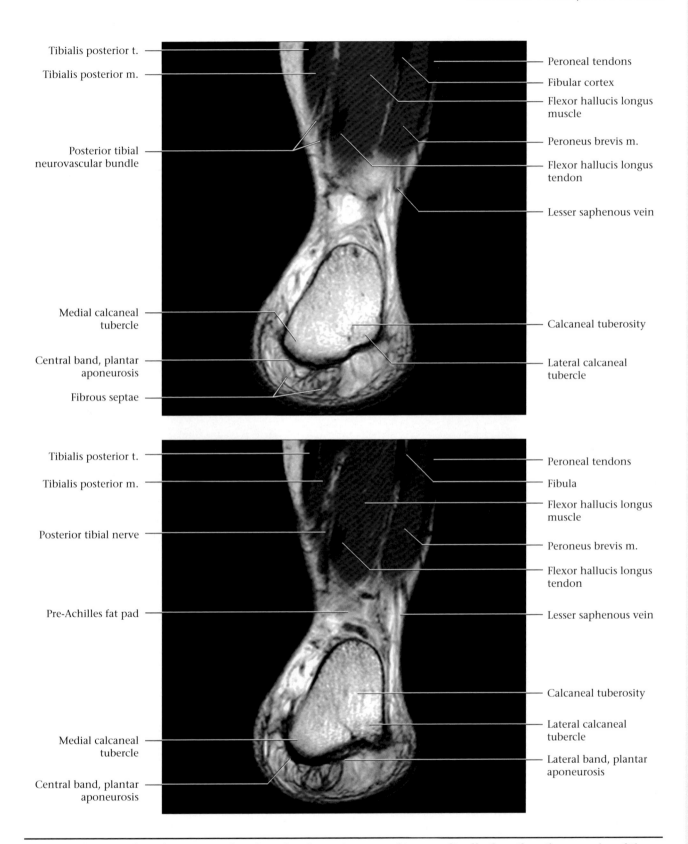

Tibialis posterior t.

Tibialis posterior m.

Posterior tibial neurovascular bundle

Medial calcaneal tubercle

Central band, plantar aponeurosis

Fibrous septae

Peroneal tendons

Fibular cortex

Flexor hallucis longus muscle

Peroneus brevis m.

Flexor hallucis longus tendon

Lesser saphenous vein

Calcaneal tuberosity

Lateral calcaneal tubercle

Tibialis posterior t.

Tibialis posterior m.

Posterior tibial nerve

Pre-Achilles fat pad

Medial calcaneal tubercle

Central band, plantar aponeurosis

Peroneal tendons

Fibula

Flexor hallucis longus muscle

Peroneus brevis m.

Flexor hallucis longus tendon

Lesser saphenous vein

Calcaneal tuberosity

Lateral calcaneal tubercle

Lateral band, plantar aponeurosis

(Top) The flexor hallucis longus muscle is broad and remains muscular more distally than the other muscles of the posterior compartment of the leg; it may be seen down to the ankle joint. The peroneus brevis muscle also descends down to the ankle joint while the peroneus longus muscle is no longer visualized at that level. **(Bottom)** In the distal leg and ankle the posterior tibial nerve and its accompanying vessels descend within a fat plane anteromedial to the flexor hallucis longus muscle and posterior to the tibialis posterior and flexor digitorum longus muscles. The peroneal tendons can be difficult to separate from one another on coronal images but the peroneus longus tendon is typically more lateral that the peroneus brevis tendon. The tibialis posterior tendon is lateral to flexor digitorum longus tendon at distal leg but is more medial to it at the ankle joint.

ANKLE AND HINDFOOT OVERVIEW

CORONAL T1 MR, RIGHT ANKLE

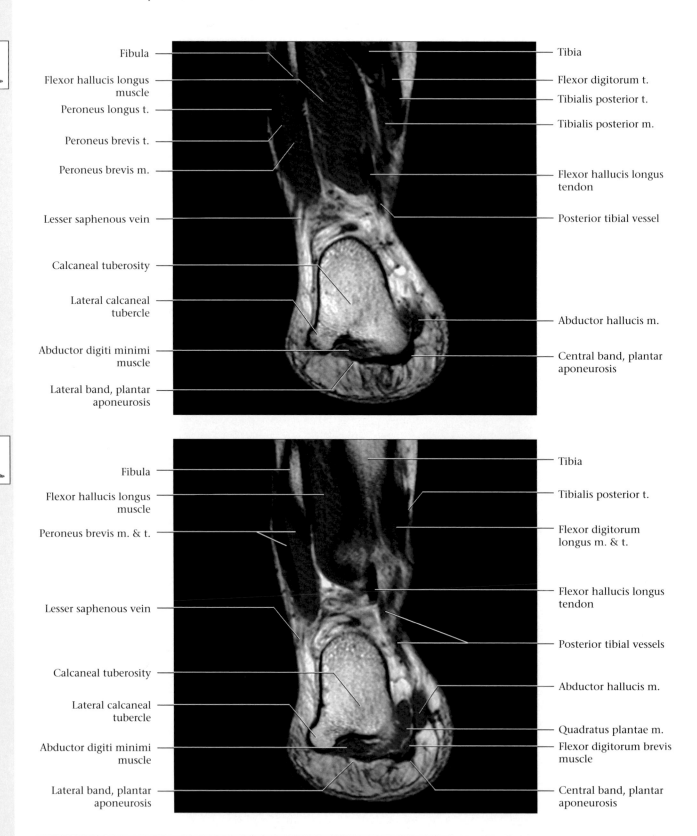

Top image labels (left): Fibula; Flexor hallucis longus muscle; Peroneus longus t.; Peroneus brevis t.; Peroneus brevis m.; Lesser saphenous vein; Calcaneal tuberosity; Lateral calcaneal tubercle; Abductor digiti minimi muscle; Lateral band, plantar aponeurosis

Top image labels (right): Tibia; Flexor digitorum t.; Tibialis posterior t.; Tibialis posterior m.; Flexor hallucis longus tendon; Posterior tibial vessel; Abductor hallucis m.; Central band, plantar aponeurosis

Bottom image labels (left): Fibula; Flexor hallucis longus muscle; Peroneus brevis m. & t.; Lesser saphenous vein; Calcaneal tuberosity; Lateral calcaneal tubercle; Abductor digiti minimi muscle; Lateral band, plantar aponeurosis

Bottom image labels (right): Tibia; Tibialis posterior t.; Flexor digitorum longus m. & t.; Flexor hallucis longus tendon; Posterior tibial vessels; Abductor hallucis m.; Quadratus plantae m.; Flexor digitorum brevis muscle; Central band, plantar aponeurosis

(Top) The medial & lateral tubercles of the calcaneus give origin to the first layer of intrinsic muscles of the foot & to the plantar aponeurosis. The abductor digiti minimi muscle originates from the lateral tubercle & the flexor digitorum brevis, abductor hallucis & abductor digiti minimi muscles originate from the medial tubercle. **(Bottom)** The tibialis posterior tendon crosses the flexor digitorum longus tendon just above the ankle joint to become the most medial tendon of the posterior compartment. The posterior tibial neurovascular bundle descends medial to the flexor hallucis longus tendon. The plantar aponeurosis has 3 proximal parts: A strong, broad and thick central band, a lateral band covering the abductor digiti minimi and a thin band covering the abductor hallucis muscle, and continuous with the flexor retinaculum.

CORONAL T1 MR, LEFT ANKLE

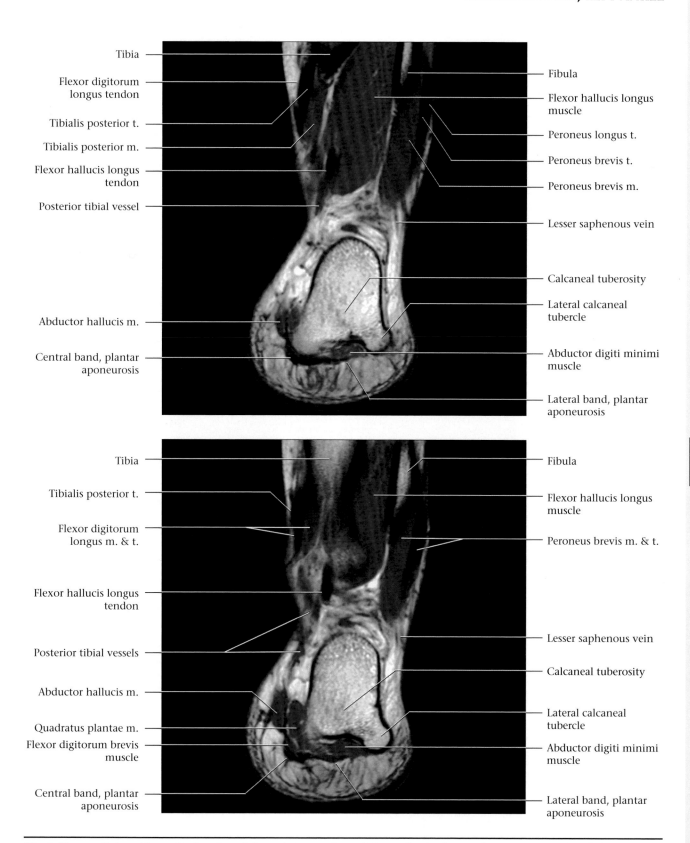

Tibia

Flexor digitorum longus tendon

Tibialis posterior t.

Tibialis posterior m.

Flexor hallucis longus tendon

Posterior tibial vessel

Abductor hallucis m.

Central band, plantar aponeurosis

Fibula

Flexor hallucis longus muscle

Peroneus longus t.

Peroneus brevis t.

Peroneus brevis m.

Lesser saphenous vein

Calcaneal tuberosity

Lateral calcaneal tubercle

Abductor digiti minimi muscle

Lateral band, plantar aponeurosis

Tibia

Tibialis posterior t.

Flexor digitorum longus m. & t.

Flexor hallucis longus tendon

Posterior tibial vessels

Abductor hallucis m.

Quadratus plantae m.

Flexor digitorum brevis muscle

Central band, plantar aponeurosis

Fibula

Flexor hallucis longus muscle

Peroneus brevis m. & t.

Lesser saphenous vein

Calcaneal tuberosity

Lateral calcaneal tubercle

Abductor digiti minimi muscle

Lateral band, plantar aponeurosis

(Top) The medial and lateral tubercles of the calcaneus give origin to the 1st layer of intrinsic muscles of the foot and to the plantar aponeurosis. The abductor digiti minimi muscle originates from the lateral tubercle and the flexor digitorum brevis, abductor hallucis and abductor digiti minimi muscles originate from the medial tubercle. **(Bottom)** The tibialis posterior tendon crosses the flexor digitorum longus tendon above the ankle joint to become the most medial tendon of the posterior compartment. The posterior tibial neurovascular bundle descends medial to the flexor hallucis longus tendon. The plantar aponeurosis has 3 proximal parts: A strong, broad and thick central band, a lateral band covering the abductor digiti minimi and a thin, medial band which covers the abductor hallucis muscle, and continuous with the flexor retinaculum.

Ankle

VII

ANKLE AND HINDFOOT OVERVIEW

CORONAL T1 MR, RIGHT ANKLE

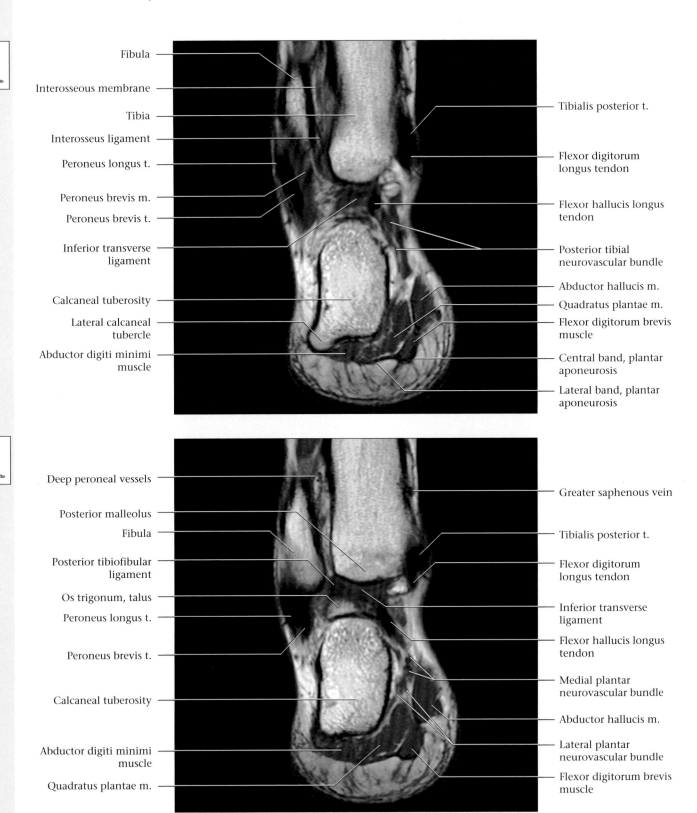

Fibula

Interosseous membrane

Tibia

Interosseus ligament

Peroneus longus t.

Peroneus brevis m.

Peroneus brevis t.

Inferior transverse ligament

Calcaneal tuberosity

Lateral calcaneal tubercle

Abductor digiti minimi muscle

Tibialis posterior t.

Flexor digitorum longus tendon

Flexor hallucis longus tendon

Posterior tibial neurovascular bundle

Abductor hallucis m.

Quadratus plantae m.

Flexor digitorum brevis muscle

Central band, plantar aponeurosis

Lateral band, plantar aponeurosis

Deep peroneal vessels

Posterior malleolus

Fibula

Posterior tibiofibular ligament

Os trigonum, talus

Peroneus longus t.

Peroneus brevis t.

Calcaneal tuberosity

Abductor digiti minimi muscle

Quadratus plantae m.

Greater saphenous vein

Tibialis posterior t.

Flexor digitorum longus tendon

Inferior transverse ligament

Flexor hallucis longus tendon

Medial plantar neurovascular bundle

Abductor hallucis m.

Lateral plantar neurovascular bundle

Flexor digitorum brevis muscle

(Top) The posterior tibial and flexor digitorum tendon share a retrotibial groove and descend in close proximity to one another. The flexor hallucis longus tendon descends posterior to the talus in between the medial and lateral tubercles (best seen on axial images). The interosseus membrane and interosseus ligament are noted in between the tibia and fibula. **(Bottom)** The posterior tibial nerve has split into the medial and lateral plantar nerves. These branches may be difficult to distinguish from their accompanying vessels on coronal images. Typically the nerves are found more lateral than the vessels. The medial plantar nerve travels superior to the lateral plantar nerve and close to the flexor hallucis longus tendon. The posterior tibiofibular ligament and inferior transverse ligament are now seen. The inferior transverse ligament extends distal to the tibia.

ANKLE AND HINDFOOT OVERVIEW

CORONAL T1 MR, LEFT ANKLE

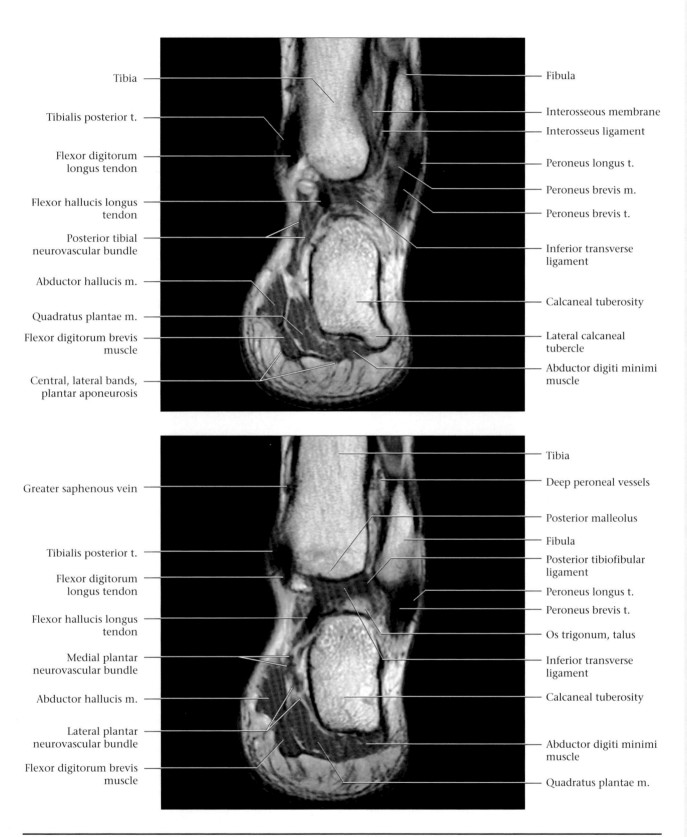

Top image labels (left): Tibia; Tibialis posterior t.; Flexor digitorum longus tendon; Flexor hallucis longus tendon; Posterior tibial neurovascular bundle; Abductor hallucis m.; Quadratus plantae m.; Flexor digitorum brevis muscle; Central, lateral bands, plantar aponeurosis

Top image labels (right): Fibula; Interosseous membrane; Interosseus ligament; Peroneus longus t.; Peroneus brevis m.; Peroneus brevis t.; Inferior transverse ligament; Calcaneal tuberosity; Lateral calcaneal tubercle; Abductor digiti minimi muscle

Bottom image labels (left): Greater saphenous vein; Tibialis posterior t.; Flexor digitorum longus tendon; Flexor hallucis longus tendon; Medial plantar neurovascular bundle; Abductor hallucis m.; Lateral plantar neurovascular bundle; Flexor digitorum brevis muscle

Bottom image labels (right): Tibia; Deep peroneal vessels; Posterior malleolus; Fibula; Posterior tibiofibular ligament; Peroneus longus t.; Peroneus brevis t.; Os trigonum, talus; Inferior transverse ligament; Calcaneal tuberosity; Abductor digiti minimi muscle; Quadratus plantae m.

(Top) The posterior tibial and flexor digitorum tendon share a retrotibial groove and descend in close proximity to one another. The flexor hallucis longus tendon descends posterior to the talus in between the medial and lateral tubercles (best seen on axial images). The interosseus membrane and interosseus ligament are noted in between the tibia and fibula. **(Bottom)** The posterior tibial nerve has split into the medial and lateral plantar nerves. These branches may be difficult to distinguish from their accompanying vessels on coronal images. Typically the nerves are found more lateral than the vessels. The medial plantar nerve travels superior to the lateral plantar nerve and close to the flexor hallucis longus tendon. The posterior tibiofibular ligament and inferior transverse ligament are now seen. The inferior transverse ligament extends distal to the tibia.

Ankle

VII

CORONAL T1 MR, RIGHT ANKLE

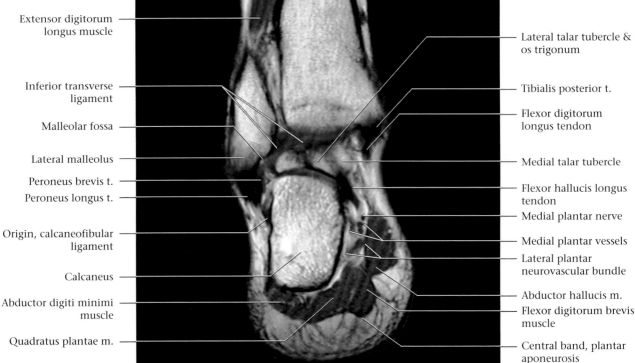

Extensor digitorum longus muscle

Lateral talar tubercle & os trigonum

Inferior transverse ligament

Tibialis posterior t.

Malleolar fossa

Flexor digitorum longus tendon

Lateral malleolus

Medial talar tubercle

Peroneus brevis t.

Flexor hallucis longus tendon

Peroneus longus t.

Medial plantar nerve

Origin, calcaneofibular ligament

Medial plantar vessels

Calcaneus

Lateral plantar neurovascular bundle

Abductor digiti minimi muscle

Abductor hallucis m.

Quadratus plantae m.

Flexor digitorum brevis muscle

Central band, plantar aponeurosis

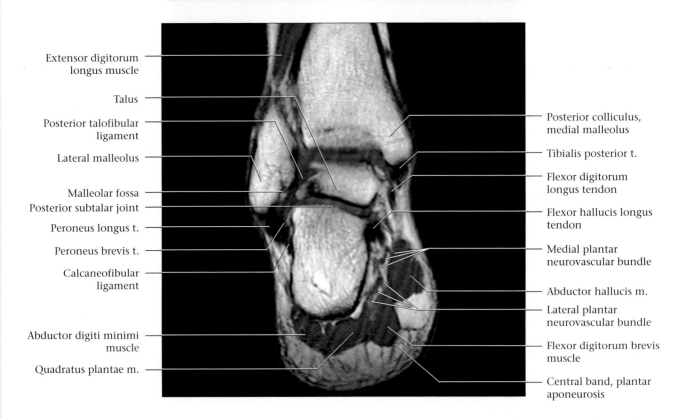

Extensor digitorum longus muscle

Talus

Posterior colliculus, medial malleolus

Posterior talofibular ligament

Tibialis posterior t.

Lateral malleolus

Flexor digitorum longus tendon

Malleolar fossa

Posterior subtalar joint

Flexor hallucis longus tendon

Peroneus longus t.

Peroneus brevis t.

Medial plantar neurovascular bundle

Calcaneofibular ligament

Abductor hallucis m.

Lateral plantar neurovascular bundle

Abductor digiti minimi muscle

Flexor digitorum brevis muscle

Quadratus plantae m.

Central band, plantar aponeurosis

(Top) The calcaneofibular ligament is consistently seen on coronal images of the hindfoot deep to the peroneal tendons and can be followed, in cross section, from its fibular origin to its insertion to the calcaneus. The posterior tibiofibular ligament originates from the inferior tibia and inserts into the fibula above the malleolar fossa. The inferior transverse ligament extends distal to the tibial posterior surface and inserts quite far medially close to the medial malleolus. **(Bottom)** The posterior talofibular ligament originates below the talar dome and inserts into the fibula at the malleolar fossa. The subcutaneous fat between the abductor hallucis and flexor digitorum brevis muscle is typically not traversed by septa and therefore can be mistaken for a lipoma.

CORONAL T1 MR, LEFT ANKLE

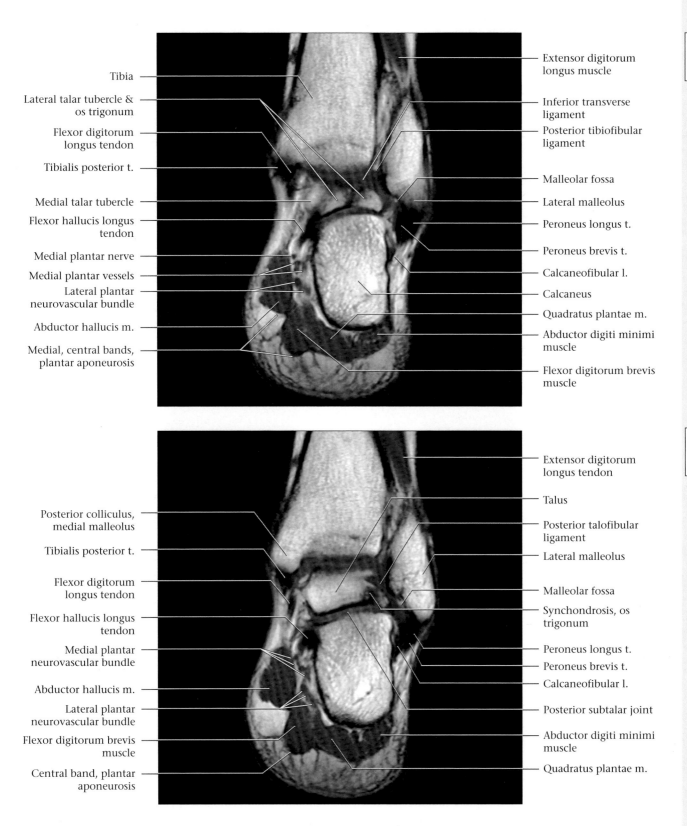

Tibia

Lateral talar tubercle & os trigonum

Flexor digitorum longus tendon

Tibialis posterior t.

Medial talar tubercle

Flexor hallucis longus tendon

Medial plantar nerve

Medial plantar vessels

Lateral plantar neurovascular bundle

Abductor hallucis m.

Medial, central bands, plantar aponeurosis

Extensor digitorum longus muscle

Inferior transverse ligament

Posterior tibiofibular ligament

Malleolar fossa

Lateral malleolus

Peroneus longus t.

Peroneus brevis t.

Calcaneofibular l.

Calcaneus

Quadratus plantae m.

Abductor digiti minimi muscle

Flexor digitorum brevis muscle

Posterior colliculus, medial malleolus

Tibialis posterior t.

Flexor digitorum longus tendon

Flexor hallucis longus tendon

Medial plantar neurovascular bundle

Abductor hallucis m.

Lateral plantar neurovascular bundle

Flexor digitorum brevis muscle

Central band, plantar aponeurosis

Extensor digitorum longus tendon

Talus

Posterior talofibular ligament

Lateral malleolus

Malleolar fossa

Synchondrosis, os trigonum

Peroneus longus t.

Peroneus brevis t.

Calcaneofibular l.

Posterior subtalar joint

Abductor digiti minimi muscle

Quadratus plantae m.

(**Top**) The calcaneofibular ligament is seen on sequential coronal images deep to the peroneal tendons from its fibular origin to its insertion to the calcaneus. The posterior tibiofibular ligament originates from the inferior tibia and inserts into the fibula above the malleolar fossa. The lateral tubercle of the talus may remain unfused to the talus forming an os trigonum. (**Bottom**) The posterior talofibular ligament originates below the talar dome and inserts into the fibula at the malleolar fossa, a medial indentation in the distal fibula. The calcaneus is in minimal valgus orientation relative to the tibial shaft. The medial neurovascular bundle remains plantar to the flexor hallucis longus tendon throughout most of its course in the foot.

Ankle

VII

CORONAL T1 MR, RIGHT ANKLE

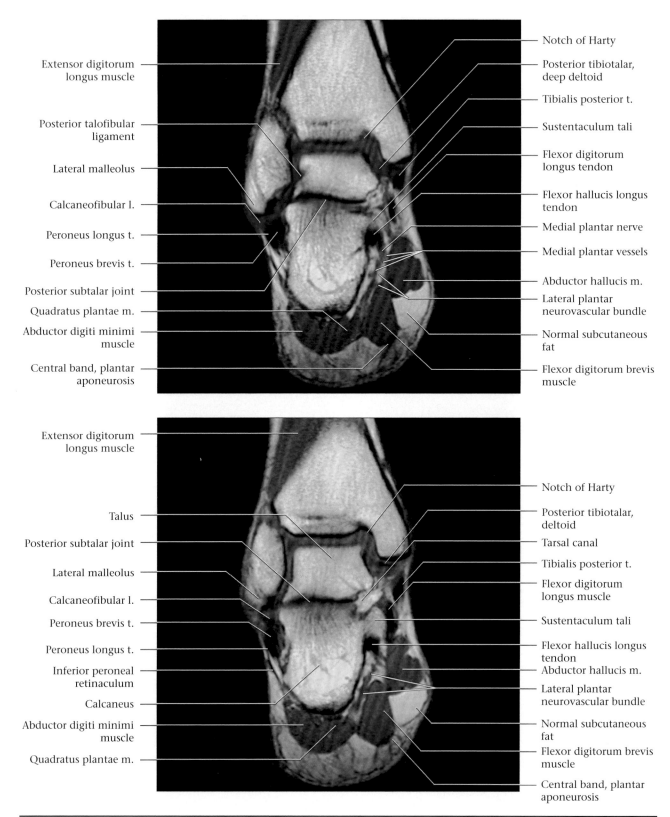

Extensor digitorum longus muscle

Posterior talofibular ligament

Lateral malleolus

Calcaneofibular l.

Peroneus longus t.

Peroneus brevis t.

Posterior subtalar joint

Quadratus plantae m.

Abductor digiti minimi muscle

Central band, plantar aponeurosis

Notch of Harty

Posterior tibiotalar, deep deltoid

Tibialis posterior t.

Sustentaculum tali

Flexor digitorum longus tendon

Flexor hallucis longus tendon

Medial plantar nerve

Medial plantar vessels

Abductor hallucis m.

Lateral plantar neurovascular bundle

Normal subcutaneous fat

Flexor digitorum brevis muscle

Extensor digitorum longus muscle

Talus

Posterior subtalar joint

Lateral malleolus

Calcaneofibular l.

Peroneus brevis t.

Peroneus longus t.

Inferior peroneal retinaculum

Calcaneus

Abductor digiti minimi muscle

Quadratus plantae m.

Notch of Harty

Posterior tibiotalar, deltoid

Tarsal canal

Tibialis posterior t.

Flexor digitorum longus muscle

Sustentaculum tali

Flexor hallucis longus tendon

Abductor hallucis m.

Lateral plantar neurovascular bundle

Normal subcutaneous fat

Flexor digitorum brevis muscle

Central band, plantar aponeurosis

(Top) The sustentaculum tali is a medial protuberance of the calcaneus which accommodates the middle subtalar joint & gives origin to the spring ligament. The flexor hallucis longus tendon has traversed its first tunnel between the lateral and medial talar tubercles and is now traversing its second tunnel under the sustentaculum tali. **(Bottom)** The deep posterior tibiotalar band of the deltoid ligament is an orderly striated structure originating from the posterior colliculus of the medial malleolus. The superficial band of the deltoid is a broad, fan shaped structure whose components (tibiotalar, tibiocalcaneal, tibiospring and tibionavicular) are variable and best identified based on their insertion sites. The subcutaneous fat in between the abductor hallucis and flexor digitorum brevis muscles lacks septa and should not be misinterpreted for a lipoma.

ANKLE AND HINDFOOT OVERVIEW

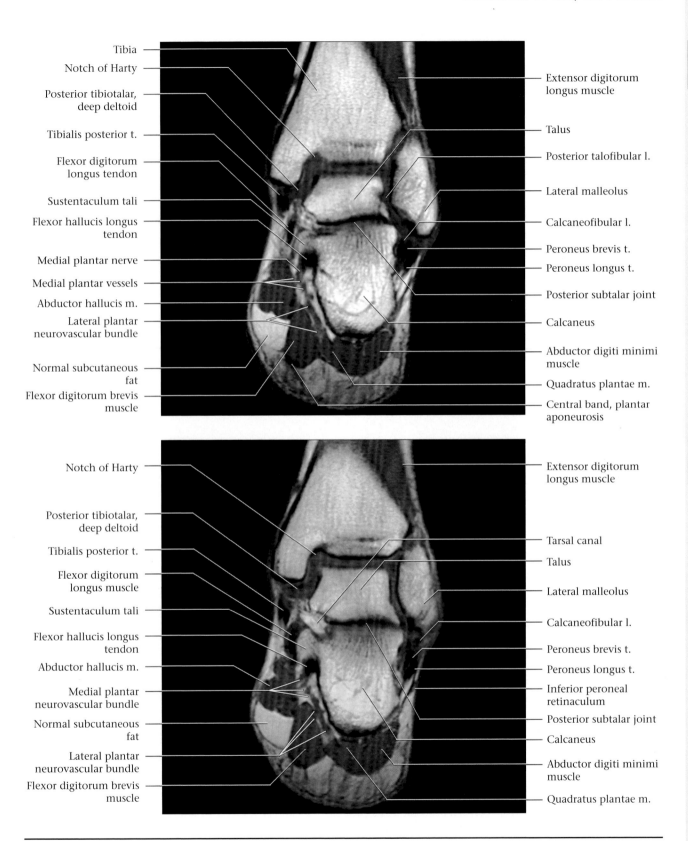

(Top) The sustentaculum tali is a medial protuberance of the calcaneus which accommodates the middle subtalar joint & gives origin to the spring ligament. The flexor hallucis longus tendon has traversed its first tunnel between the lateral and medial talar tubercles and is now traversing its second tunnel under the sustentaculum tali. **(Bottom)** The deep posterior tibiotalar band of the deltoid ligament is an orderly striated structure originating from the posterior colliculus of the medial malleolus. The superficial band of the deltoid is a broad, fan shaped structure whose components (tibiotalar, tibiocalcaneal, tibiospring and tibionavicular) are variable and best identified based on their insertion sites. The subcutaneous fat in between the abductor hallucis and flexor digitorum brevis muscles lacks septa and should not be misinterpreted for a lipoma.

CORONAL T1 MR, RIGHT ANKLE

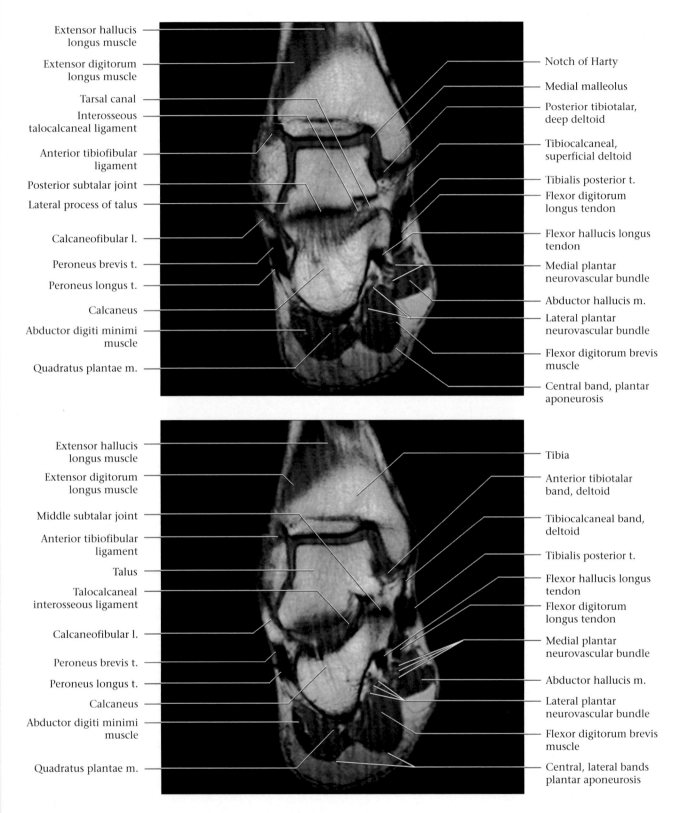

Extensor hallucis longus muscle

Extensor digitorum longus muscle

Tarsal canal

Interosseous talocalcaneal ligament

Anterior tibiofibular ligament

Posterior subtalar joint

Lateral process of talus

Calcaneofibular l.

Peroneus brevis t.

Peroneus longus t.

Calcaneus

Abductor digiti minimi muscle

Quadratus plantae m.

Notch of Harty

Medial malleolus

Posterior tibiotalar, deep deltoid

Tibiocalcaneal, superficial deltoid

Tibialis posterior t.

Flexor digitorum longus tendon

Flexor hallucis longus tendon

Medial plantar neurovascular bundle

Abductor hallucis m.

Lateral plantar neurovascular bundle

Flexor digitorum brevis muscle

Central band, plantar aponeurosis

Extensor hallucis longus muscle

Extensor digitorum longus muscle

Middle subtalar joint

Anterior tibiofibular ligament

Talus

Talocalcaneal interosseous ligament

Calcaneofibular l.

Peroneus brevis t.

Peroneus longus t.

Calcaneus

Abductor digiti minimi muscle

Quadratus plantae m.

Tibia

Anterior tibiotalar band, deltoid

Tibiocalcaneal band, deltoid

Tibialis posterior t.

Flexor hallucis longus tendon

Flexor digitorum longus tendon

Medial plantar neurovascular bundle

Abductor hallucis m.

Lateral plantar neurovascular bundle

Flexor digitorum brevis muscle

Central, lateral bands plantar aponeurosis

(Top) The posterior subtalar joint is quite broad and wide and is seen on multiple images. The posterior subtalar joint is separated from the middle subtalar joint by the tarsal canal. The tibiocalcaneal ligament is the strongest of the superficial deltoid components. It is in continuity anteriorly with the tibiospring ligament. The tibialis posterior tendon crosses the tibiocalcaneal and tibiospring ligaments and its tenosynovial floor is difficult to separate from the ligaments. **(Bottom)** The interosseous talocalcaneal ligament traverses the tarsal canal medially. The middle subtalar joint is often suboptimally seen on coronal MR images & requires correlation with sagittal images to avoid overcalling a subtalar coalition. The fibular insertion of calcaneofibular ligament is visualized. Note atrophy of quadratus plantae muscle in this patient.

CORONAL T1 MR, LEFT ANKLE

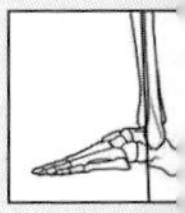

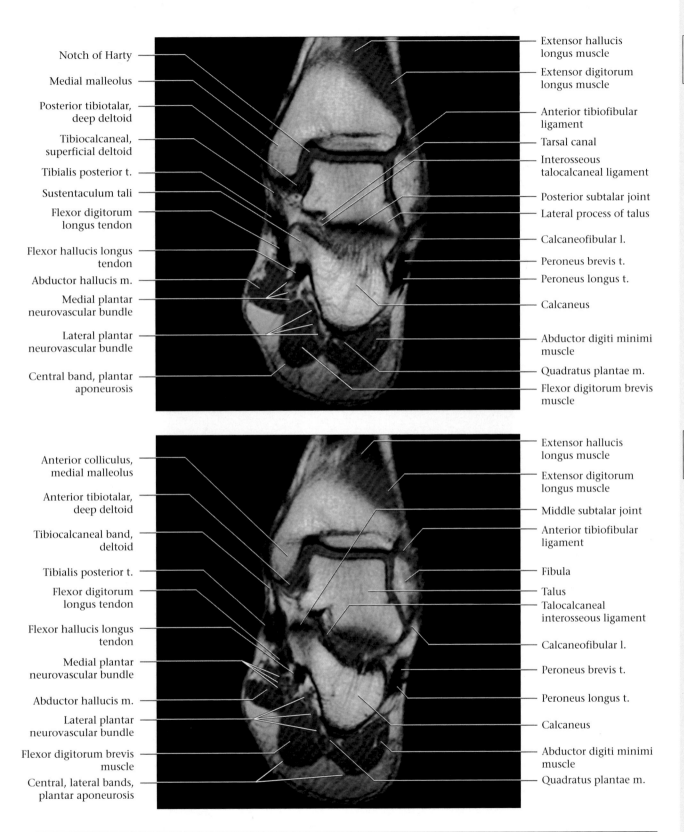

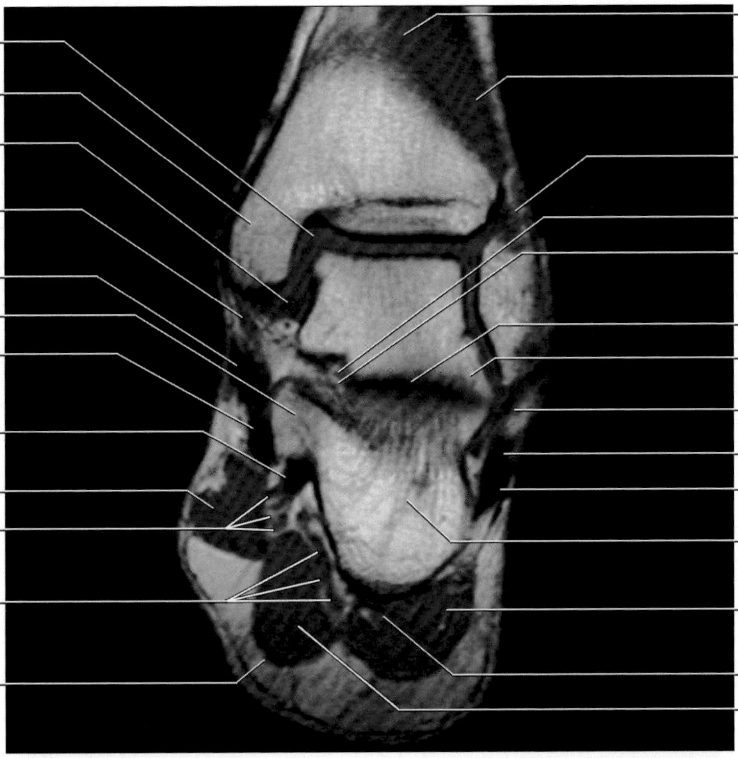
Notch of Harty
Medial malleolus
Posterior tibiotalar, deep deltoid
Tibiocalcaneal, superficial deltoid
Tibialis posterior t.
Sustentaculum tali
Flexor digitorum longus tendon
Flexor hallucis longus tendon
Abductor hallucis m.
Medial plantar neurovascular bundle
Lateral plantar neurovascular bundle
Central band, plantar aponeurosis
Extensor hallucis longus muscle
Extensor digitorum longus muscle
Anterior tibiofibular ligament
Tarsal canal
Interosseous talocalcaneal ligament
Posterior subtalar joint
Lateral process of talus
Calcaneofibular l.
Peroneus brevis t.
Peroneus longus t.
Calcaneus
Abductor digiti minimi muscle
Quadratus plantae m.
Flexor digitorum brevis muscle

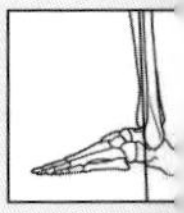

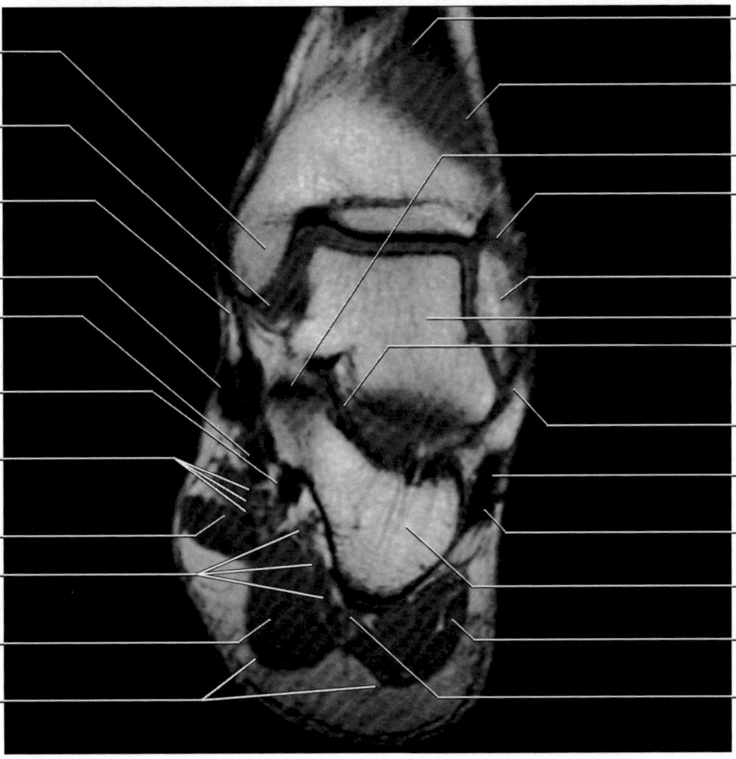
Anterior colliculus, medial malleolus
Anterior tibiotalar, deep deltoid
Tibiocalcaneal band, deltoid
Tibialis posterior t.
Flexor digitorum longus tendon
Flexor hallucis longus tendon
Medial plantar neurovascular bundle
Abductor hallucis m.
Lateral plantar neurovascular bundle
Flexor digitorum brevis muscle
Central, lateral bands, plantar aponeurosis
Extensor hallucis longus muscle
Extensor digitorum longus muscle
Middle subtalar joint
Anterior tibiofibular ligament
Fibula
Talus
Talocalcaneal interosseous ligament
Calcaneofibular l.
Peroneus brevis t.
Peroneus longus t.
Calcaneus
Abductor digiti minimi muscle
Quadratus plantae m.

(Top) The posterior subtalar joint is quite wide and is seen on multiple images. It is separated from the middle subtalar joint by the tarsal canal. The tibiocalcaneal ligament is the strongest of the superficial deltoid components. It inserts into the sustentaculum tali and is in continuity anteriorly with the tibiospring ligament. The tibialis posterior tendon is superficial to the tibiocalcaneal and tibiospring ligaments and its tenosynovial floor is difficult to separate from the ligaments. **(Bottom)** The interosseous talocalcaneal ligament traverses the tarsal canal medially. The middle subtalar joint is often suboptimally seen on coronal MR images & requires correlation with sagittal images to avoid overcalling a subtalar coalition. The fibular insertion of calcaneofibular ligament is visualized. Note atrophy of quadratus plantae muscle in this patient.

ANKLE AND HINDFOOT OVERVIEW

CORONAL T1 MR, RIGHT ANKLE

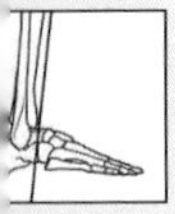

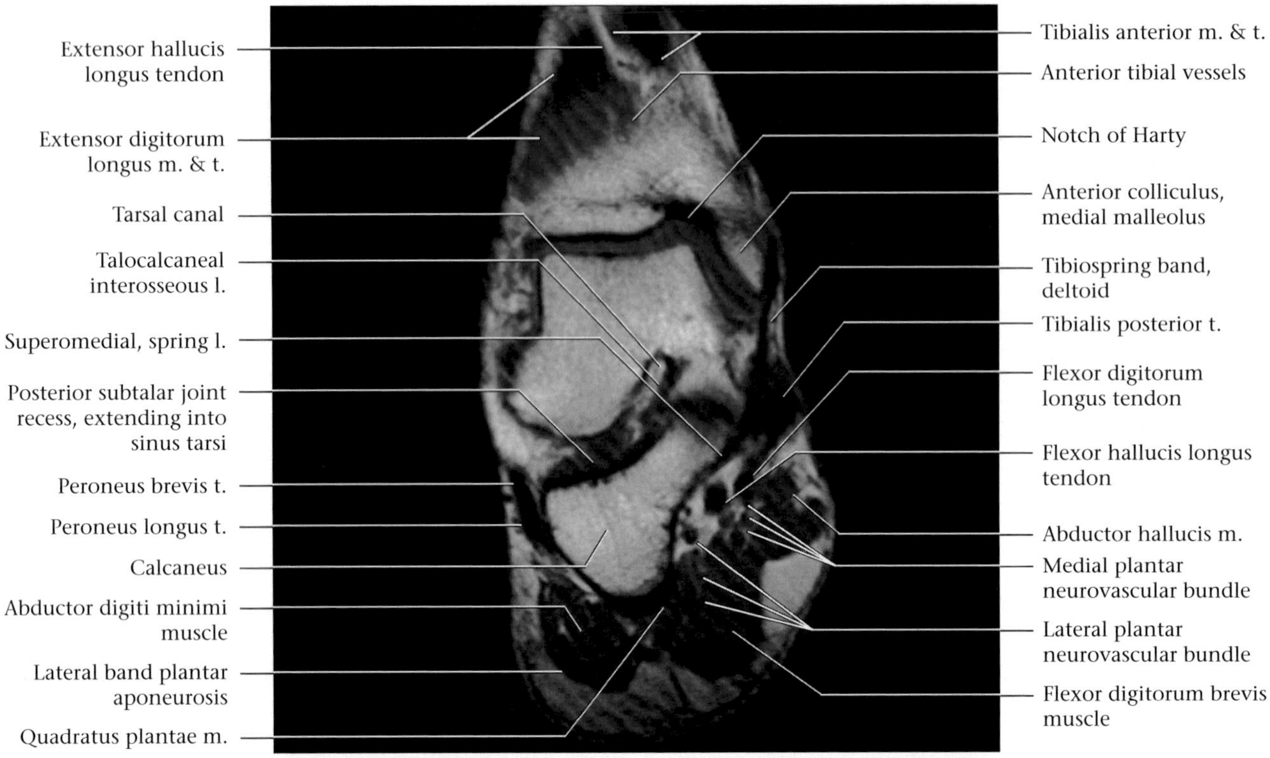

Extensor hallucis longus tendon
Extensor digitorum longus m. & t.
Tarsal canal
Talocalcaneal interosseous l.
Superomedial, spring l.
Posterior subtalar joint recess, extending into sinus tarsi
Peroneus brevis t.
Peroneus longus t.
Calcaneus
Abductor digiti minimi muscle
Lateral band plantar aponeurosis
Quadratus plantae m.
Tibialis anterior m. & t.
Anterior tibial vessels
Notch of Harty
Anterior colliculus, medial malleolus
Tibiospring band, deltoid
Tibialis posterior t.
Flexor digitorum longus tendon
Flexor hallucis longus tendon
Abductor hallucis m.
Medial plantar neurovascular bundle
Lateral plantar neurovascular bundle
Flexor digitorum brevis muscle

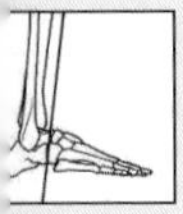

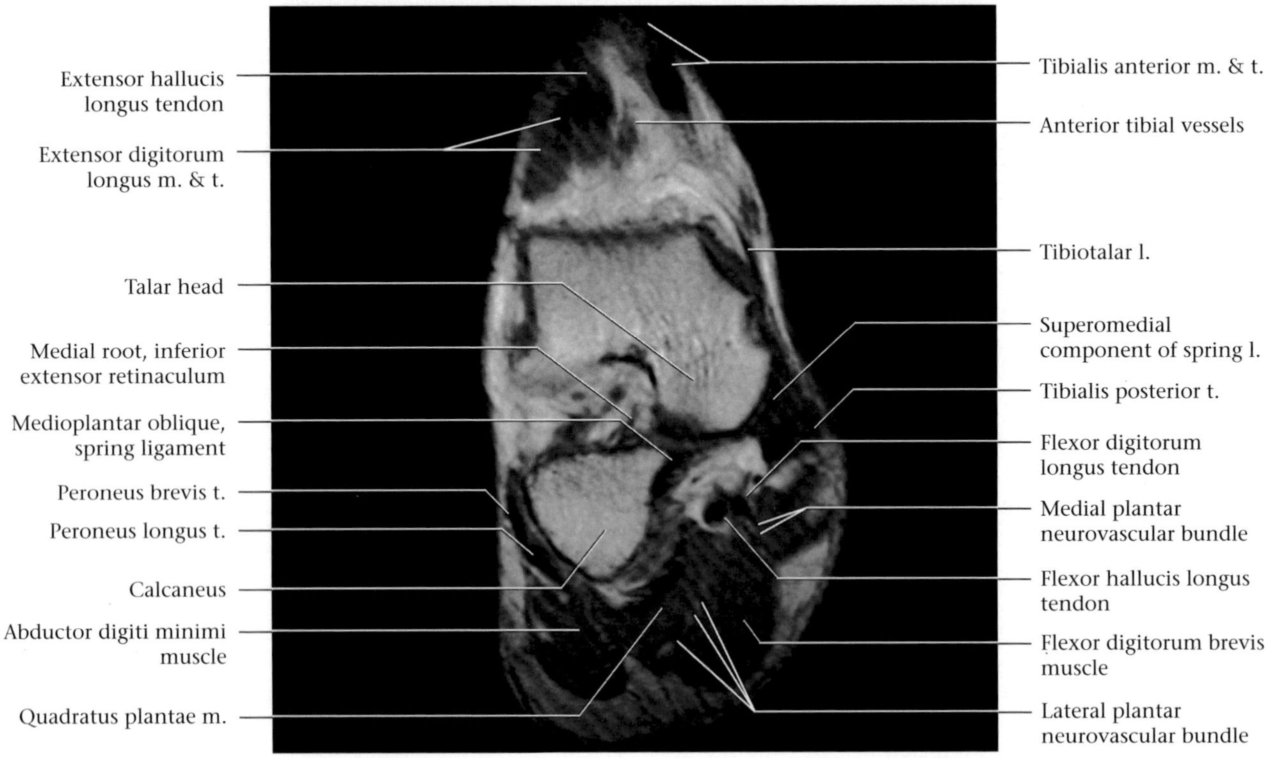

Extensor hallucis longus tendon
Extensor digitorum longus m. & t.
Talar head
Medial root, inferior extensor retinaculum
Medioplantar oblique, spring ligament
Peroneus brevis t.
Peroneus longus t.
Calcaneus
Abductor digiti minimi muscle
Quadratus plantae m.
Tibialis anterior m. & t.
Anterior tibial vessels
Tibiotalar l.
Superomedial component of spring l.
Tibialis posterior t.
Flexor digitorum longus tendon
Medial plantar neurovascular bundle
Flexor hallucis longus tendon
Flexor digitorum brevis muscle
Lateral plantar neurovascular bundle

(Top) The notch of Harty is a small elevation in the tibial medial surface, often associated with low signal sclerosis above it, that should not be mistaken for tibial osteochondral lesion. The tibiospring component of the deltoid descends to join the superomedial component of the spring. Fluid-filled recess may extend from the posterior subtalar joint into the sinus tarsi and should not be interpreted as disease. Note atrophy of the quadratus plantae muscle. **(Bottom)** The tibialis anterior tendon is the largest extensor tendon. It can be followed on sequential coronal images of the hindfoot but its attachment to the 1st cuneiform and base of 1st metatarsal may only be visualized on midfoot images. The sinus tarsi is a lateral, funnel shaped space between the talus and calcaneus which is continuous with the medially located tarsal canal (see previous image).

ANKLE AND HINDFOOT OVERVIEW

CORONAL T1 MR, LEFT ANKLE

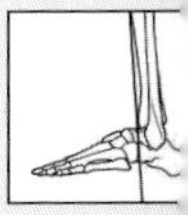

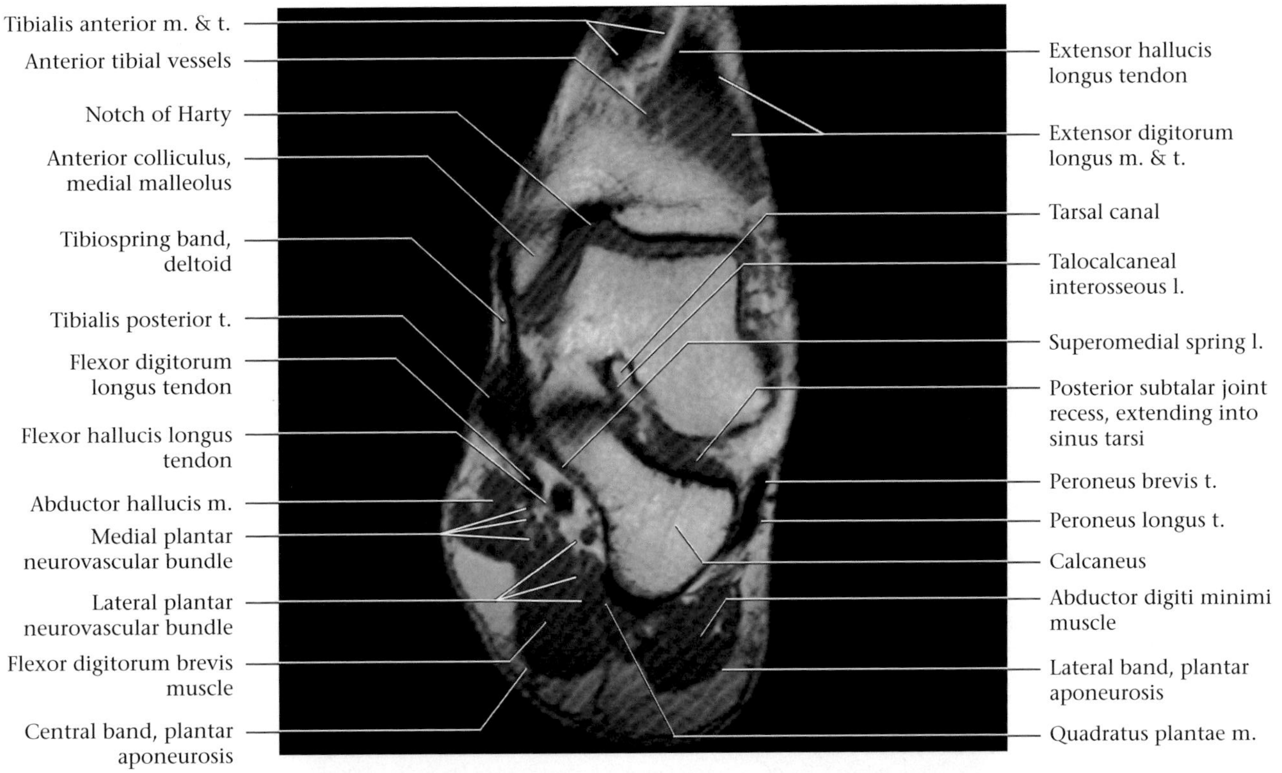

Tibialis anterior m. & t.
Anterior tibial vessels
Notch of Harty
Anterior colliculus, medial malleolus
Tibiospring band, deltoid
Tibialis posterior t.
Flexor digitorum longus tendon
Flexor hallucis longus tendon
Abductor hallucis m.
Medial plantar neurovascular bundle
Lateral plantar neurovascular bundle
Flexor digitorum brevis muscle
Central band, plantar aponeurosis
Extensor hallucis longus tendon
Extensor digitorum longus m. & t.
Tarsal canal
Talocalcaneal interosseous l.
Superomedial spring l.
Posterior subtalar joint recess, extending into sinus tarsi
Peroneus brevis t.
Peroneus longus t.
Calcaneus
Abductor digiti minimi muscle
Lateral band, plantar aponeurosis
Quadratus plantae m.

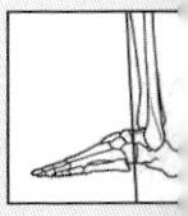

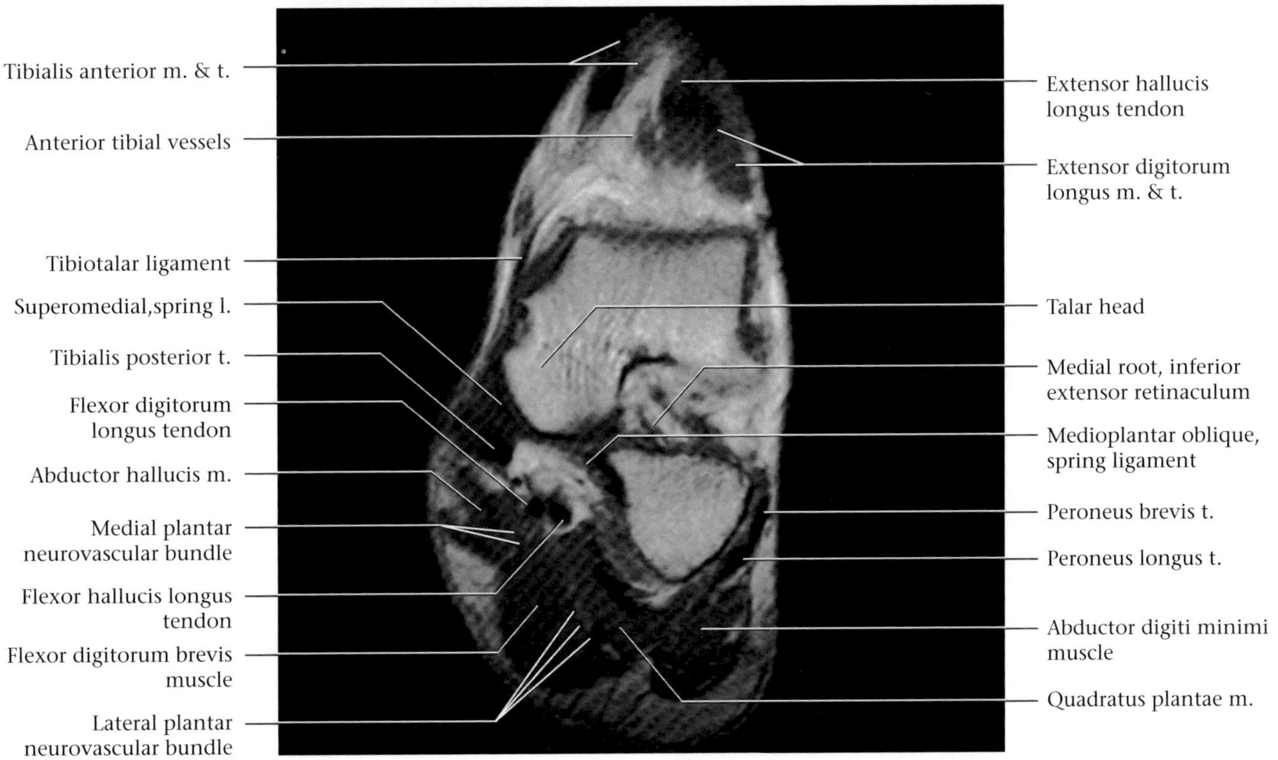

Tibialis anterior m. & t.
Anterior tibial vessels
Tibiotalar ligament
Superomedial,spring l.
Tibialis posterior t.
Flexor digitorum longus tendon
Abductor hallucis m.
Medial plantar neurovascular bundle
Flexor hallucis longus tendon
Flexor digitorum brevis muscle
Lateral plantar neurovascular bundle
Extensor hallucis longus tendon
Extensor digitorum longus m. & t.
Talar head
Medial root, inferior extensor retinaculum
Medioplantar oblique, spring ligament
Peroneus brevis t.
Peroneus longus t.
Abductor digiti minimi muscle
Quadratus plantae m.

(Top) The notch of Harty is a small elevation in the tibial medial surface, often associated with low signal sclerosis above it, that should not be mistaken for tibial osteochondral lesion. The tibiospring component of the deltoid descends to join the superomedial component of the spring. Fluid-filled recess may extend from the posterior subtalar joint into the sinus tarsi and should not be interpreted as disease. Note atrophy of the quadratus plantae muscle. **(Bottom)** The tibialis anterior tendon is the largest extensor tendon. It can be followed on sequential coronal images of the hindfoot but its attachment to the 1st cuneiform and base of 1st metatarsal may only be visualized on midfoot images. The sinus tarsi is a lateral, funnel shaped space between the talus and calcaneus which is continuous with the medially located tarsal canal (see previous image).

ANKLE AND HINDFOOT OVERVIEW

CORONAL T1 MR, RIGHT ANKLE

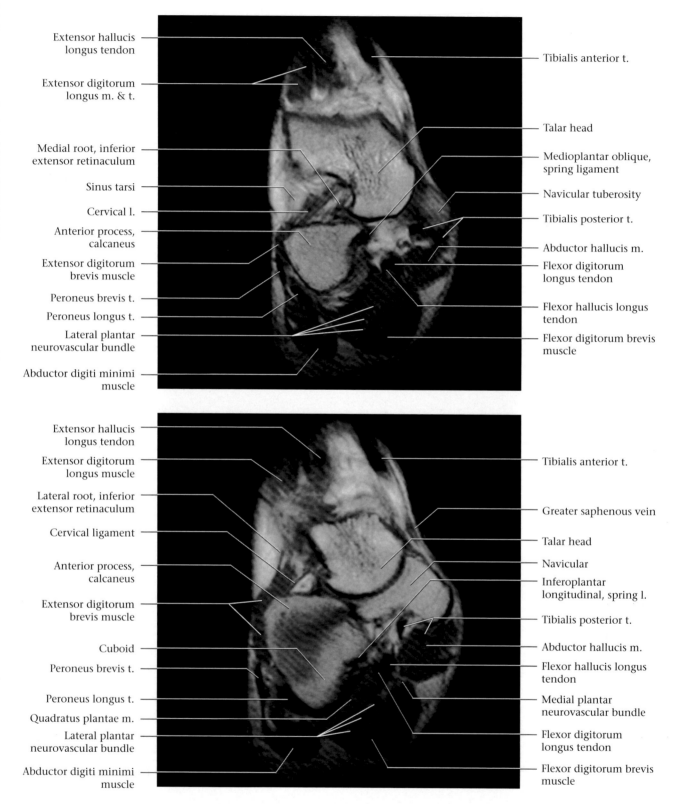

Extensor hallucis longus tendon

Extensor digitorum longus m. & t.

Medial root, inferior extensor retinaculum

Sinus tarsi

Cervical l.

Anterior process, calcaneus

Extensor digitorum brevis muscle

Peroneus brevis t.

Peroneus longus t.

Lateral plantar neurovascular bundle

Abductor digiti minimi muscle

Tibialis anterior t.

Talar head

Medioplantar oblique, spring ligament

Navicular tuberosity

Tibialis posterior t.

Abductor hallucis m.

Flexor digitorum longus tendon

Flexor hallucis longus tendon

Flexor digitorum brevis muscle

Extensor hallucis longus tendon

Extensor digitorum longus muscle

Lateral root, inferior extensor retinaculum

Cervical ligament

Anterior process, calcaneus

Extensor digitorum brevis muscle

Cuboid

Peroneus brevis t.

Peroneus longus t.

Quadratus plantae m.

Lateral plantar neurovascular bundle

Abductor digiti minimi muscle

Tibialis anterior t.

Greater saphenous vein

Talar head

Navicular

Inferoplantar longitudinal, spring l.

Tibialis posterior t.

Abductor hallucis m.

Flexor hallucis longus tendon

Medial plantar neurovascular bundle

Flexor digitorum longus tendon

Flexor digitorum brevis muscle

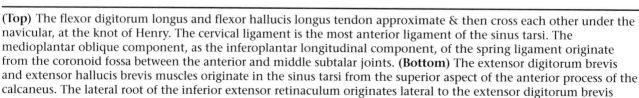

(Top) The flexor digitorum longus and flexor hallucis longus tendon approximate & then cross each other under the navicular, at the knot of Henry. The cervical ligament is the most anterior ligament of the sinus tarsi. The medioplantar oblique component, as the inferoplantar longitudinal component, of the spring ligament originate from the coronoid fossa between the anterior and middle subtalar joints. **(Bottom)** The extensor digitorum brevis and extensor hallucis brevis muscles originate in the sinus tarsi from the superior aspect of the anterior process of the calcaneus. The lateral root of the inferior extensor retinaculum originates lateral to the extensor digitorum brevis muscle. The peroneus longus tendon is beginning to curve under the cuboid toward its insertion into the base of the 1st metatarsal and 1st cuneiform.

ANKLE AND HINDFOOT OVERVIEW

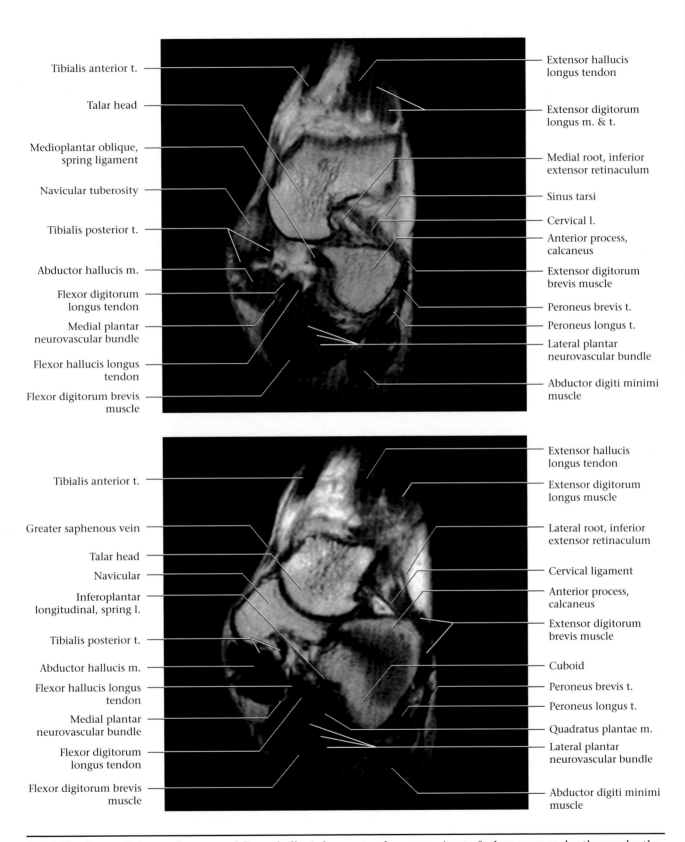

Tibialis anterior t.

Talar head

Medioplantar oblique, spring ligament

Navicular tuberosity

Tibialis posterior t.

Abductor hallucis m.

Flexor digitorum longus tendon

Medial plantar neurovascular bundle

Flexor hallucis longus tendon

Flexor digitorum brevis muscle

Extensor hallucis longus tendon

Extensor digitorum longus m. & t.

Medial root, inferior extensor retinaculum

Sinus tarsi

Cervical l.

Anterior process, calcaneus

Extensor digitorum brevis muscle

Peroneus brevis t.

Peroneus longus t.

Lateral plantar neurovascular bundle

Abductor digiti minimi muscle

Tibialis anterior t.

Greater saphenous vein

Talar head

Navicular

Inferoplantar longitudinal, spring l.

Tibialis posterior t.

Abductor hallucis m.

Flexor hallucis longus tendon

Medial plantar neurovascular bundle

Flexor digitorum longus tendon

Flexor digitorum brevis muscle

Extensor hallucis longus tendon

Extensor digitorum longus muscle

Lateral root, inferior extensor retinaculum

Cervical ligament

Anterior process, calcaneus

Extensor digitorum brevis muscle

Cuboid

Peroneus brevis t.

Peroneus longus t.

Quadratus plantae m.

Lateral plantar neurovascular bundle

Abductor digiti minimi muscle

(Top) The flexor digitorum longus and flexor hallucis longus tendon approximate & then cross each other under the navicular, at the knot of Henry. The cervical ligament is the most anterior ligament of the sinus tarsi. The medioplantar oblique component, as the inferoplantar longitudinal component, of the spring ligament originates from the coronoid fossa in between the anterior and middle subtalar joints. **(Bottom)** The extensor digitorum brevis and extensor hallucis brevis muscles originate in the sinus tarsi from the superior aspect of the anterior process of the calcaneus. The lateral root of the inferior extensor retinaculum originates lateral to the extensor digitorum brevis muscle. The peroneus longus tendon is beginning to curve under the cuboid toward its insertion into the base of the 1st metatarsal and 1st cuneiform.

SAGITTAL T1 MR

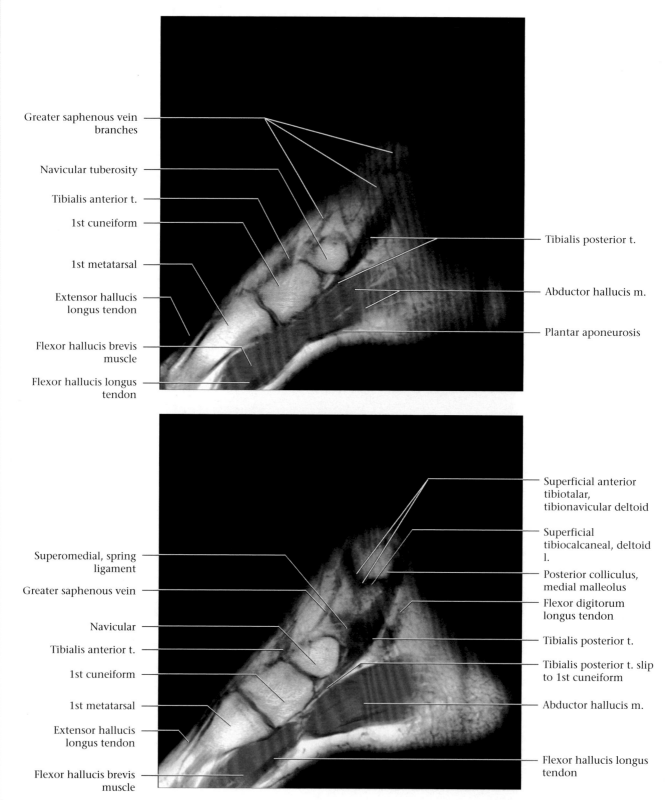

Greater saphenous vein branches

Navicular tuberosity

Tibialis anterior t.

1st cuneiform

1st metatarsal

Extensor hallucis longus tendon

Flexor hallucis brevis muscle

Flexor hallucis longus tendon

Tibialis posterior t.

Abductor hallucis m.

Plantar aponeurosis

Superomedial, spring ligament

Greater saphenous vein

Navicular

Tibialis anterior t.

1st cuneiform

1st metatarsal

Extensor hallucis longus tendon

Flexor hallucis brevis muscle

Superficial anterior tibiotalar, tibionavicular deltoid

Superficial tibiocalcaneal, deltoid l.

Posterior colliculus, medial malleolus

Flexor digitorum longus tendon

Tibialis posterior t.

Tibialis posterior t. slip to 1st cuneiform

Abductor hallucis m.

Flexor hallucis longus tendon

(Top) The most medial sagittal image depicts branches of the greater saphenous vein. Three tendon attachments are present along the 1st metatarsal axis: Tibialis posterior tendon to the navicular tuberosity and 1st cuneiform, anterior tibial tendon to the 1st cuneiform and 1st metatarsal base and the peroneus longus tendon to the lateral plantar base of the 1st metatarsal. Not infrequently small tendinous slips of the tibialis posterior tendon may be visualized as they go under the navicular to their respective insertion sites. (Bottom) The superficial components of the deltoid ligament including the tibiotalar, tibionavicular, tibiospring & tibiocalcaneal ligaments originate from the anterior & posterior colliculi of the medial malleolus. The superomedial component of the spring ligament and tibialis posterior tendon insertion to the cuneiform are also visualized.

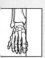

ANKLE AND HINDFOOT OVERVIEW

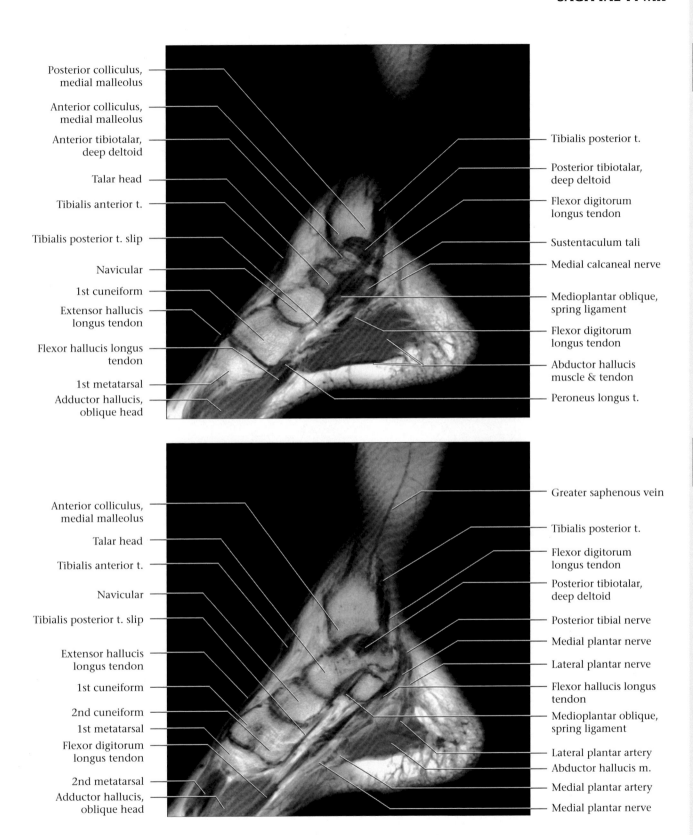

Posterior colliculus, medial malleolus

Anterior colliculus, medial malleolus

Anterior tibiotalar, deep deltoid

Talar head

Tibialis anterior t.

Tibialis posterior t. slip

Navicular

1st cuneiform

Extensor hallucis longus tendon

Flexor hallucis longus tendon

1st metatarsal

Adductor hallucis, oblique head

Tibialis posterior t.

Posterior tibiotalar, deep deltoid

Flexor digitorum longus tendon

Sustentaculum tali

Medial calcaneal nerve

Medioplantar oblique, spring ligament

Flexor digitorum longus tendon

Abductor hallucis muscle & tendon

Peroneus longus t.

Anterior colliculus, medial malleolus

Talar head

Tibialis anterior t.

Navicular

Tibialis posterior t. slip

Extensor hallucis longus tendon

1st cuneiform

2nd cuneiform

1st metatarsal

Flexor digitorum longus tendon

2nd metatarsal

Adductor hallucis, oblique head

Greater saphenous vein

Tibialis posterior t.

Flexor digitorum longus tendon

Posterior tibiotalar, deep deltoid

Posterior tibial nerve

Medial plantar nerve

Lateral plantar nerve

Flexor hallucis longus tendon

Medioplantar oblique, spring ligament

Lateral plantar artery

Abductor hallucis m.

Medial plantar artery

Medial plantar nerve

(Top) The deep tibiotalar component of the deltoid ligament originates from the posterior colliculus of the medial malleolus. The insertion of the peroneus longus tendon on the plantar lateral base of the 1st metatarsal & on the 1st cuneiform is now visualized. The superomedial component of the spring ligament originates from the sustentaculum tali and can sometimes be seen slightly medial to the tibialis posterior tendon insertion on the navicular. **(Bottom)** The talar insertion of the deep tibiotalar deltoid ligament forms a low signal shadow on the medial talar body. The posterior tibial nerve divides into the medial and lateral plantar nerves deep or proximal to the flexor retinaculum. The flexor digitorum longus tendon overlies the sustentaculum tali (see previous image) while the flexor hallucis longus tendon traverses under it.

SAGITTAL T1 MR

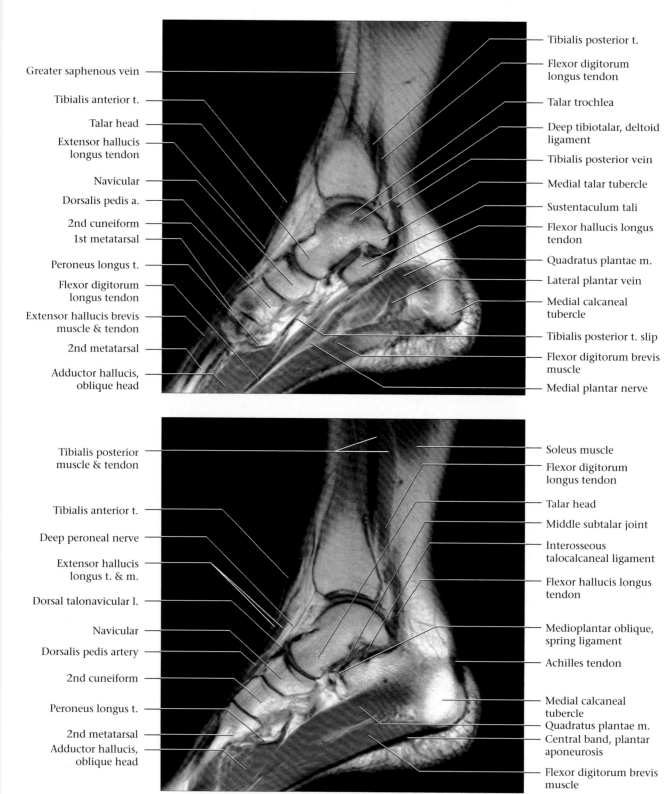

Greater saphenous vein

Tibialis anterior t.

Talar head

Extensor hallucis
longus tendon

Navicular

Dorsalis pedis a.

2nd cuneiform
1st metatarsal

Peroneus longus t.

Flexor digitorum
longus tendon

Extensor hallucis brevis
muscle & tendon

2nd metatarsal

Adductor hallucis,
oblique head

Tibialis posterior t.

Flexor digitorum
longus tendon

Talar trochlea

Deep tibiotalar, deltoid
ligament

Tibialis posterior vein

Medial talar tubercle

Sustentaculum tali

Flexor hallucis longus
tendon

Quadratus plantae m.

Lateral plantar vein

Medial calcaneal
tubercle

Tibialis posterior t. slip

Flexor digitorum brevis
muscle

Medial plantar nerve

Tibialis posterior
muscle & tendon

Tibialis anterior t.

Deep peroneal nerve

Extensor hallucis
longus t. & m.

Dorsal talonavicular l.

Navicular

Dorsalis pedis artery

2nd cuneiform

Peroneus longus t.

2nd metatarsal
Adductor hallucis,
oblique head

Soleus muscle

Flexor digitorum
longus tendon

Talar head

Middle subtalar joint

Interosseous
talocalcaneal ligament

Flexor hallucis longus
tendon

Medioplantar oblique,
spring ligament

Achilles tendon

Medial calcaneal
tubercle
Quadratus plantae m.
Central band, plantar
aponeurosis

Flexor digitorum brevis
muscle

(Top) The flexor digitorum longus tendon travels obliquely and changes positions relative to the rest of the posterior compartment tendons. Proximal to the ankle joint it is first medial and then posterior to the tibialis posterior tendon. More distally it is lateral to the tibialis posterior tendon and medial to the flexor hallucis longus tendon. Under the navicular tuberosity the tendon crosses and becomes lateral to the flexor hallucis longus tendon. (Bottom) The plantar aponeurosis is subdivided into three bands: A thin medial band overlying the abductor hallucis muscle, a strong central band, overlying the flexor digitorum brevis muscle (seen here), and a lateral band overlying the abductor digiti minimi. The medioplantar oblique band of the spring ligament originates from the coronoid fossa, slightly lateral to the sustentaculum tali.

SAGITTAL T1 MR

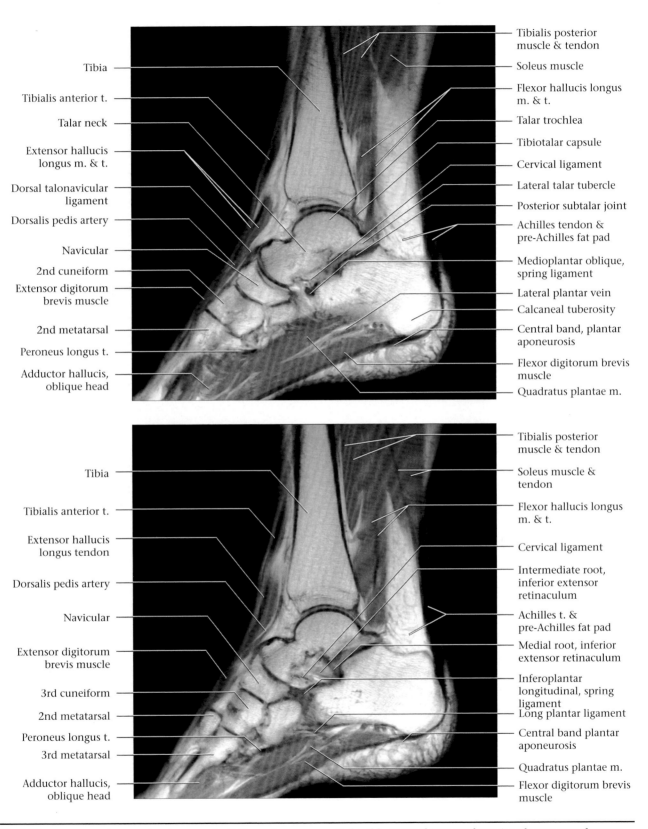

Top image labels (left side):
- Tibia
- Tibialis anterior t.
- Talar neck
- Extensor hallucis longus m. & t.
- Dorsal talonavicular ligament
- Dorsalis pedis artery
- Navicular
- 2nd cuneiform
- Extensor digitorum brevis muscle
- 2nd metatarsal
- Peroneus longus t.
- Adductor hallucis, oblique head

Top image labels (right side):
- Tibialis posterior muscle & tendon
- Soleus muscle
- Flexor hallucis longus m. & t.
- Talar trochlea
- Tibiotalar capsule
- Cervical ligament
- Lateral talar tubercle
- Posterior subtalar joint
- Achilles tendon & pre-Achilles fat pad
- Medioplantar oblique, spring ligament
- Lateral plantar vein
- Calcaneal tuberosity
- Central band, plantar aponeurosis
- Flexor digitorum brevis muscle
- Quadratus plantae m.

Bottom image labels (left side):
- Tibia
- Tibialis anterior t.
- Extensor hallucis longus tendon
- Dorsalis pedis artery
- Navicular
- Extensor digitorum brevis muscle
- 3rd cuneiform
- 2nd metatarsal
- Peroneus longus t.
- 3rd metatarsal
- Adductor hallucis, oblique head

Bottom image labels (right side):
- Tibialis posterior muscle & tendon
- Soleus muscle & tendon
- Flexor hallucis longus m. & t.
- Cervical ligament
- Intermediate root, inferior extensor retinaculum
- Achilles t. & pre-Achilles fat pad
- Medial root, inferior extensor retinaculum
- Inferoplantar longitudinal, spring ligament
- Long plantar ligament
- Central band plantar aponeurosis
- Quadratus plantae m.
- Flexor digitorum brevis muscle

(Top) The peroneus longus tendon can be followed on sequential ankle sagittal images from its plantar attachment to base of 1st metatarsal up to its descent posterior to the fibula. The sinus tarsi is traversed by the lateral, intermediate and medial roots of the extensor retinaculum and by the cervical ligament. The tarsal canal, medial to the sinus tarsi is traversed by the interosseous talocalcaneal ligament. **(Bottom)** The soleus tendon, together with tendons of the gastrocnemius, form the Achilles tendon. The inferoplantar longitudinal band of the spring ligament inserts to the navicular beak & due to its straight course, is often seen on a lateral sagittal image. The cervical ligament is the most anterior ligament traversing the sinus tarsi. The intermediate root of the inferior extensor retinaculum is typically found posterior to it.

SAGITTAL T1 MR

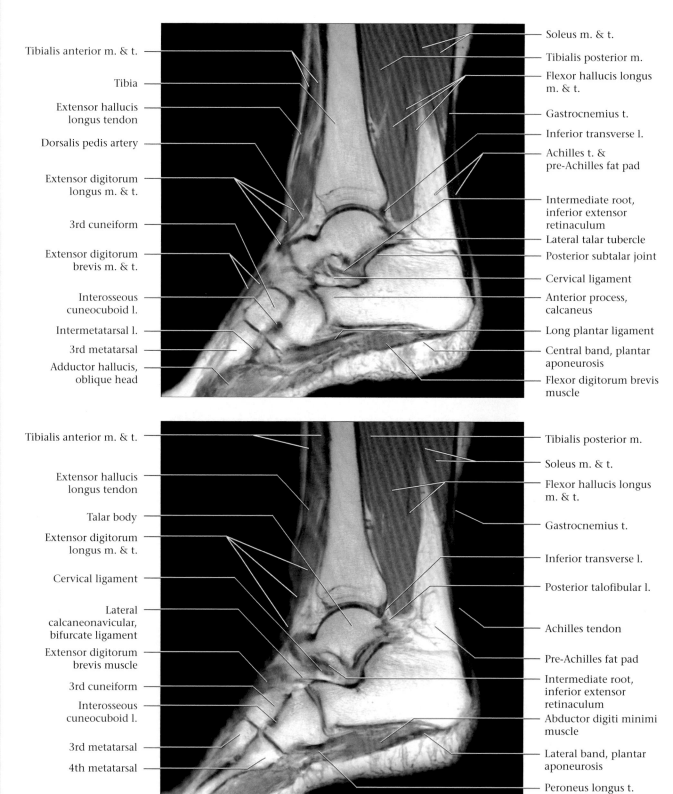

Tibialis anterior m. & t.

Tibia

Extensor hallucis longus tendon

Dorsalis pedis artery

Extensor digitorum longus m. & t.

3rd cuneiform

Extensor digitorum brevis m. & t.

Interosseous cuneocuboid l.

Intermetatarsal l.

3rd metatarsal

Adductor hallucis, oblique head

Soleus m. & t.

Tibialis posterior m.

Flexor hallucis longus m. & t.

Gastrocnemius t.

Inferior transverse l.

Achilles t. & pre-Achilles fat pad

Intermediate root, inferior extensor retinaculum

Lateral talar tubercle

Posterior subtalar joint

Cervical ligament

Anterior process, calcaneus

Long plantar ligament

Central band, plantar aponeurosis

Flexor digitorum brevis muscle

Tibialis anterior m. & t.

Extensor hallucis longus tendon

Talar body

Extensor digitorum longus m. & t.

Cervical ligament

Lateral calcaneonavicular, bifurcate ligament

Extensor digitorum brevis muscle

3rd cuneiform

Interosseous cuneocuboid l.

3rd metatarsal

4th metatarsal

Tibialis posterior m.

Soleus m. & t.

Flexor hallucis longus m. & t.

Gastrocnemius t.

Inferior transverse l.

Posterior talofibular l.

Achilles tendon

Pre-Achilles fat pad

Intermediate root, inferior extensor retinaculum

Abductor digiti minimi muscle

Lateral band, plantar aponeurosis

Peroneus longus t.

(Top) The pre-Achilles fat pad, also called Kager fat pad, separates the Achilles tendon from the posterior compartment muscles. It is typically traversed by fine septa and vascular channels. The peroneus longus tendon curves under the cuboid to travel toward its insertion to the 1st metatarsal base. The long plantar ligament binds the calcaneocuboid joint, extends to the bases of the metatarsals and thus forms the roof of the cubital tunnel. The posterior tibiofibular ligament originates from the posterior tibia. It extends distal to the ankle joint as the inferior transverse ligament. **(Bottom)** The bifurcate ligament originates from the calcaneus just lateral to the spring ligament. Its navicular limb (shown here) inserts into the navicular, dorsal and lateral to the spring ligament insertion. A second limb (not seen) inserts into the cuboid.

SAGITTAL T1 MR

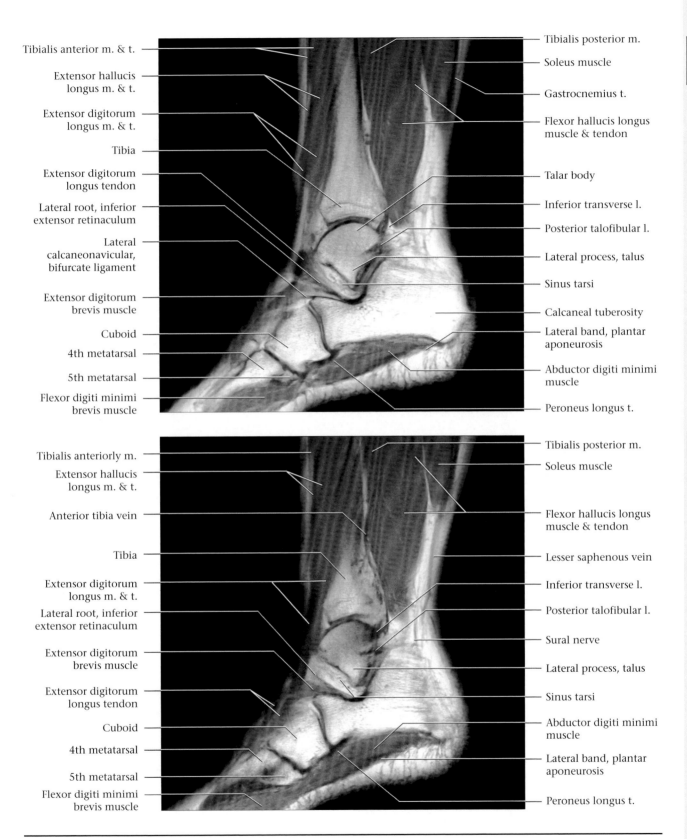

Tibialis anterior m. & t.

Extensor hallucis longus m. & t.

Extensor digitorum longus m. & t.

Tibia

Extensor digitorum longus tendon

Lateral root, inferior extensor retinaculum

Lateral calcaneonavicular, bifurcate ligament

Extensor digitorum brevis muscle

Cuboid

4th metatarsal

5th metatarsal

Flexor digiti minimi brevis muscle

Tibialis posterior m.

Soleus muscle

Gastrocnemius t.

Flexor hallucis longus muscle & tendon

Talar body

Inferior transverse l.

Posterior talofibular l.

Lateral process, talus

Sinus tarsi

Calcaneal tuberosity

Lateral band, plantar aponeurosis

Abductor digiti minimi muscle

Peroneus longus t.

Tibialis anteriorly m.

Extensor hallucis longus m. & t.

Anterior tibia vein

Tibia

Extensor digitorum longus m. & t.

Lateral root, inferior extensor retinaculum

Extensor digitorum brevis muscle

Extensor digitorum longus tendon

Cuboid

4th metatarsal

5th metatarsal

Flexor digiti minimi brevis muscle

Tibialis posterior m.

Soleus muscle

Flexor hallucis longus muscle & tendon

Lesser saphenous vein

Inferior transverse l.

Posterior talofibular l.

Sural nerve

Lateral process, talus

Sinus tarsi

Abductor digiti minimi muscle

Lateral band, plantar aponeurosis

Peroneus longus t.

(Top) The extensor digitorum brevis muscle originates from the superior anterior calcaneus within the lateral sinus tarsi space. The lateral root of the inferior extensor retinaculum enter the sinus tarsi lateral and slightly posterior to the muscle. The talofibular ligament origin from the talus is visualized. The inferior transverse ligament extends beyond the tibial posterior surface. **(Bottom)** The deep peroneal nerve and anterior tibial vessels are optimally visualized on axial images but occasionally may be noted (as seen here) on a sagittal image in a plane between the tibia and fibula. The lateral band of the plantar fascia is superficial to the abductor digiti minimi muscle. The extensor digitorum longus tendon and extensor hallucis longus tendon travel close to each other in the distal leg and may be difficult to distinguish from one another.

Ankle

VII

SAGITTAL T1 MR

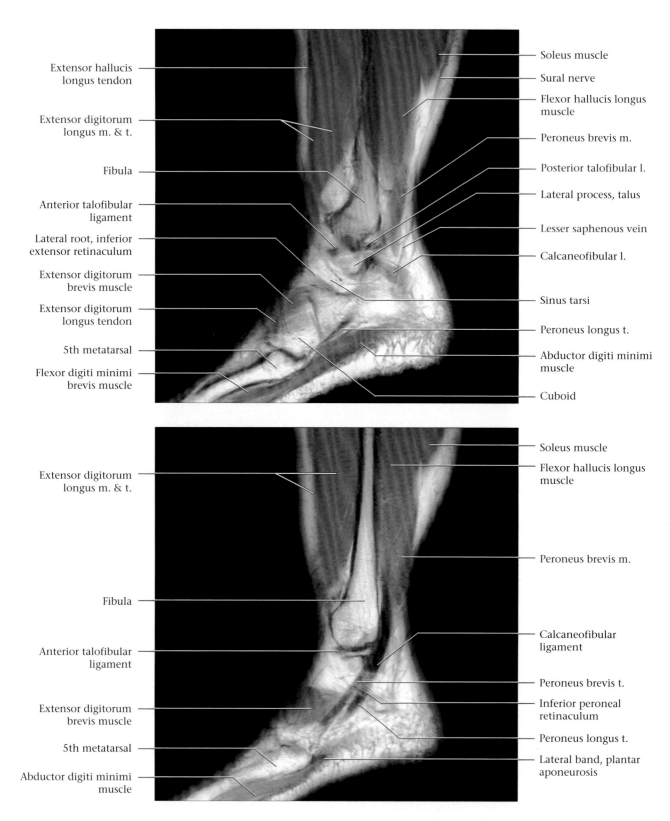

Extensor hallucis longus tendon

Extensor digitorum longus m. & t.

Fibula

Anterior talofibular ligament

Lateral root, inferior extensor retinaculum

Extensor digitorum brevis muscle

Extensor digitorum longus tendon

5th metatarsal

Flexor digiti minimi brevis muscle

Soleus muscle

Sural nerve

Flexor hallucis longus muscle

Peroneus brevis m.

Posterior talofibular l.

Lateral process, talus

Lesser saphenous vein

Calcaneofibular l.

Sinus tarsi

Peroneus longus t.

Abductor digiti minimi muscle

Cuboid

Extensor digitorum longus m. & t.

Fibula

Anterior talofibular ligament

Extensor digitorum brevis muscle

5th metatarsal

Abductor digiti minimi muscle

Soleus muscle

Flexor hallucis longus muscle

Peroneus brevis m.

Calcaneofibular ligament

Peroneus brevis t.

Inferior peroneal retinaculum

Peroneus longus t.

Lateral band, plantar aponeurosis

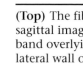

(Top) The fibular origins of the syndesmotic and collateral ligaments are sometime encountered on a far lateral sagittal image. Due to partial volume averaging the calcaneofibular ligament may be seen as an obliquely oriented band overlying the peroneal tendons (see next image also). The peroneus longus tendon is descending along the lateral wall of the calcaneus toward its cuboid tunnel. **(Bottom)** The peroneal tendons descend posterior to the fibula with the peroneus longus tendon posterior to the peroneus brevis tendon. They diverge from each other along the lateral wall of the calcaneus, sometimes separated by a peroneal tubercle. The inferior peroneal retinaculum, difficult to visualize on sagittal images, separates the tendons from one another.

SAGITTAL T1 MR

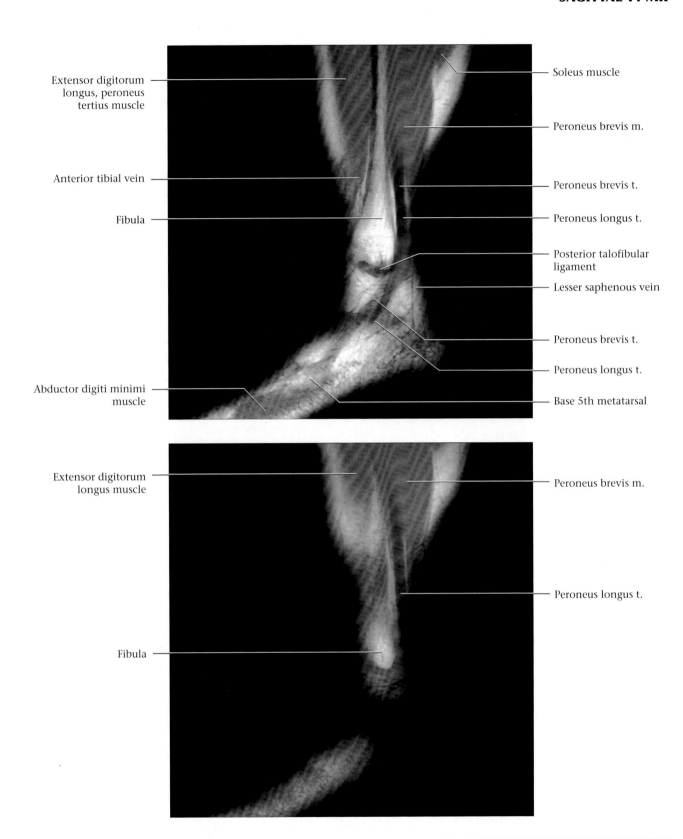

Extensor digitorum longus, peroneus tertius muscle

Anterior tibial vein

Fibula

Abductor digiti minimi muscle

Soleus muscle

Peroneus brevis m.

Peroneus brevis t.

Peroneus longus t.

Posterior talofibular ligament

Lesser saphenous vein

Peroneus brevis t.

Peroneus longus t.

Base 5th metatarsal

Extensor digitorum longus muscle

Fibula

Peroneus brevis m.

Peroneus longus t.

(Top) The peroneus longus tendon is typically posterolateral to the peroneus brevis tendon and is appreciated better posterior to the fibula on far lateral images. The peroneus brevis inserts onto the base of the 5th metatarsal. The anterior tibial vein pierces the intermuscular septum and may be seen anterior to the fibula on far lateral sagittal images. **(Bottom)** The extensor digitorum longus muscle and peroneus brevis muscle are respectively the most anterolateral and posterolateral muscles of the distal leg.

TENDONS OVERVIEW

Imaging Anatomy

Overview

- **Radiographs**
  - **Achilles tendon** visualized on lateral view of ankle
    - Inserts approximately 1 cm distal to superior calcaneal tuberosity
    - Small fat pad separates tendon from calcaneal tuberosity, location of retrocalcaneal bursa
    - Kager fat pad anterior to Achilles tendon
- **Computed tomography**
  - Tendons suboptimally visualized on routine images
  - 3D volume rendering reconstructions can be performed but presently not routinely utilized for assessing tendons except as associated with fracture
- **MR**
  - Tendons are optimally visualized on axial MR images
  - Sagittal images optimal for Achilles tendon
  - Tendons typically low in signal on all pulse sequences
  - **Exceptions to low signal of normal tendons**: Magic angle effect, ossicles, fibrocartilage in tendons
    - **Magic angle effect**
    - All tendons, except for Achilles, are susceptible to magic angle effect as they curve around ankle joint
    - Magic angle effect results in increased tendon signal on low TE sequences
    - Magic angle effect can be avoided by 1: Plantar flexing foot, patient supine 2: Imaging patient prone 3: Correlating tendon's signal alterations on high TE sequences
  - **Tendon sheath**
    - Present in all tendons except Achilles
    - Minimal fluid normal in flexor tendons
    - Low in signal, seen only if distended by fluid
    - Fluid in extensor sheaths usually pathologic
    - Large amount of fluid in flexor hallucis longus sheath can be normal due to normal communication of sheath with ankle joint
  - Achilles tendon has a paratenon, loose connective tissue around tendon, but no tendon sheath
  - **Normal MR of Achilles tendon**
    - Tendon best seen on sagittal images
    - Uniform in diameter on sagittal images
    - Concave or flat anterior surface on axial images
    - Occasional shifting bulge on anterior surface reflects spiraling soleus and gastrocnemius tendon fibers
    - Punctate increased signal on T1, PD, due to infolding paratenon vessels, connective tissue
    - Paratenon: Ring of intermediate signal surrounding medial, posterior, lateral tendon margins
    - Kager fat pad anterior to tendon, typically traversed by vessels
    - Minimal amount of fluid in retrocalcaneal bursa is normal
    - Small tendon medial to Achilles is plantaris
  - **Normal MR of peroneal tendons**
    - Peroneus brevis typically anterior or anteromedial to peroneus longus

- Peroneus brevis typically flat to mildly crescentic in retrofibular groove
- Peroneus brevis tendon may be globular when medial to peroneus longus, may simulate medial subluxation as it descends under the fibular tip
- Muscle of peroneus brevis noted at ankle joint
- Peroneus brevis, peroneus longus share a common tendon sheath proximally
- Retrofibular groove concave/flat in 82% of individuals
- **Superior peroneal retinaculum** holds tendons within retrofibular groove
- **Superior peroneal retinaculum**: Low signal curvilinear structure, best seen on axial images originating from lateral malleolus approximately 1 cm above distal fibular tip
- Fibrous ridge, small low signal triangle, originates from lateral fibular tip, deepens retrofibular groove
- Calcaneofibular ligament deep to peroneal tendons
- Inferior peroneal retinaculum: Low signal, curvilinear structure inserts on peroneal tubercle, separates peroneal tendons lateral to calcaneal wall
  - **Normal MR of the posterior tibial tendon**
    - Most posteromedial tendon
    - Shares groove behind tibia with flexor digitorum longus tendon
    - Held in groove by flexor retinaculum
    - Except Achilles largest posterior tendon, approximately 2-3 times size of adjacent flexor digitorum on axial images
    - May have normal minimal fluid in tendon sheath
    - Often increased signal at navicular attachment due to magic angle effect, fibrocartilage, os
    - No tendon sheath distally; distal peritendinous signal is abnormal
    - Distal insertion slips can be seen on axial images
    - Inhomogeneous signal distally may be related to magic angle effect, fat between the distal tendon slips, presence of type I os naviculare
    - When a type II accessory navicular is present: Typically tendon inserts directly into it and is discontinuous from distal tendon slips
  - **Normal MR of the flexor hallucis longus tendon**
    - Often surrounded by fluid due to normal communication of sheath with ankle joint
    - Can sometimes have a seagull appearance in distal leg as tendinous slips join each other to form a single tendon
    - Muscle extends more distally than all other muscles in ankle
    - Identified on sagittal images as tendon curving posterior to sustentaculum tali
    - Susceptible to magic angle effect at level of sustentaculum tali
  - **Normal MR of extensor tendons**
    - Largest most medial dorsal tendon is anterior tibial tendon
    - Tendon sheath fluid is rare and usually pathologic
    - Very susceptible to magic angle effect

GRAPHICS, TENDONS OF THE ANKLE

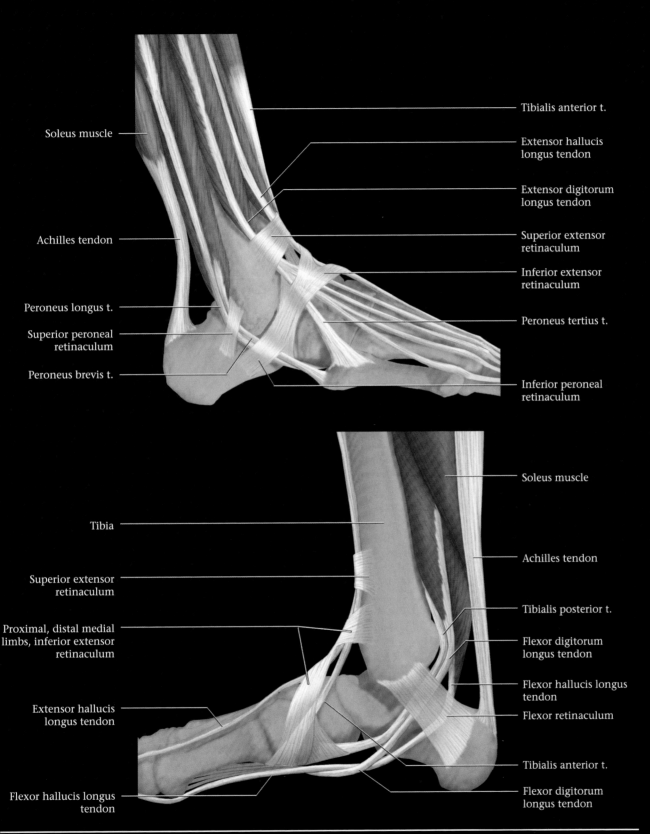

Soleus muscle

Achilles tendon

Peroneus longus t.

Superior peroneal retinaculum

Peroneus brevis t.

Tibialis anterior t.

Extensor hallucis longus tendon

Extensor digitorum longus tendon

Superior extensor retinaculum

Inferior extensor retinaculum

Peroneus tertius t.

Inferior peroneal retinaculum

Tibia

Superior extensor retinaculum

Proximal, distal medial limbs, inferior extensor retinaculum

Extensor hallucis longus tendon

Flexor hallucis longus tendon

Soleus muscle

Achilles tendon

Tibialis posterior t.

Flexor digitorum longus tendon

Flexor hallucis longus tendon

Flexor retinaculum

Tibialis anterior t.

Flexor digitorum longus tendon

(Top) Lateral view. The peroneus brevis & peroneus longus tendons descend posterior to the fibula, maintained within the retromalleolar groove by the superior peroneal retinaculum and continue along the lateral wall of calcaneus, held in place by the inferior peroneal retinaculum. Fibers of the inferior peroneal retinaculum insert and separate the two tendons. The peroneus longus tendon curves around the cuboid to enter the sole of foot. Both the peroneus brevis and peroneus tertius tendons insert on the fifth metatarsal base. **(Bottom)** Medial view. The tibialis posterior, flexor digitorum longus & flexor hallucis longus tendons traverse under the flexor retinaculum within the tarsal tunnel. The flexor digitorum longus & flexor hallucis longus tendons cross each other under the navicular. The extensor tendons descend deep to the extensor retinacula.

TENDONS OVERVIEW

GRAPHICS, TENDONS OF THE ANKLE

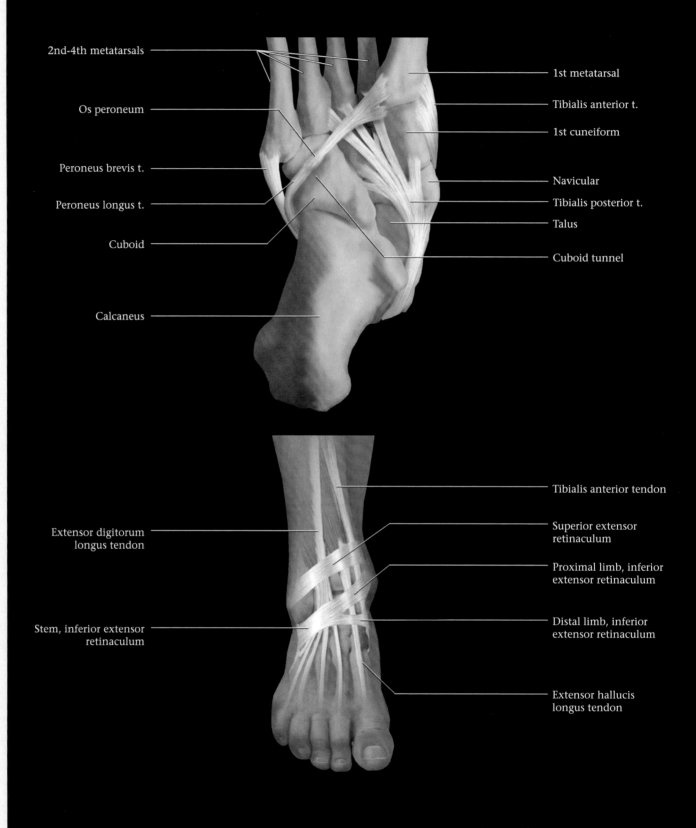

2nd-4th metatarsals

Os peroneum

Peroneus brevis t.

Peroneus longus t.

Cuboid

Calcaneus

1st metatarsal

Tibialis anterior t.

1st cuneiform

Navicular

Tibialis posterior t.

Talus

Cuboid tunnel

Extensor digitorum
longus tendon

Stem, inferior extensor
retinaculum

Tibialis anterior tendon

Superior extensor
retinaculum

Proximal limb, inferior
extensor retinaculum

Distal limb, inferior
extensor retinaculum

Extensor hallucis
longus tendon

(Top) Insertions of long tendons on the plantar foot. The tibialis posterior tendon inserts on all the tarsal bones (excluding talus) & on 2nd-4th metatarsal bases. The tibialis posterior, tibialis anterior & peroneus longus tendons insert onto the medial & lateral plantar 1st cuneiform & base of 1st metatarsal respectively. Together they form a sling supporting the medial longitudinal arch. **(Bottom)** Anterior view. The peroneus tertius and tibialis anterior tendon insert proximally, on the base of the 5th metatarsal and on the medial cuneiform and 1st metatarsal respectively. The rest of the extensor tendons continue distally toward their insertion sites on the digits. The extensor tendons are held in place by the superior and inferior extensor retinacula.

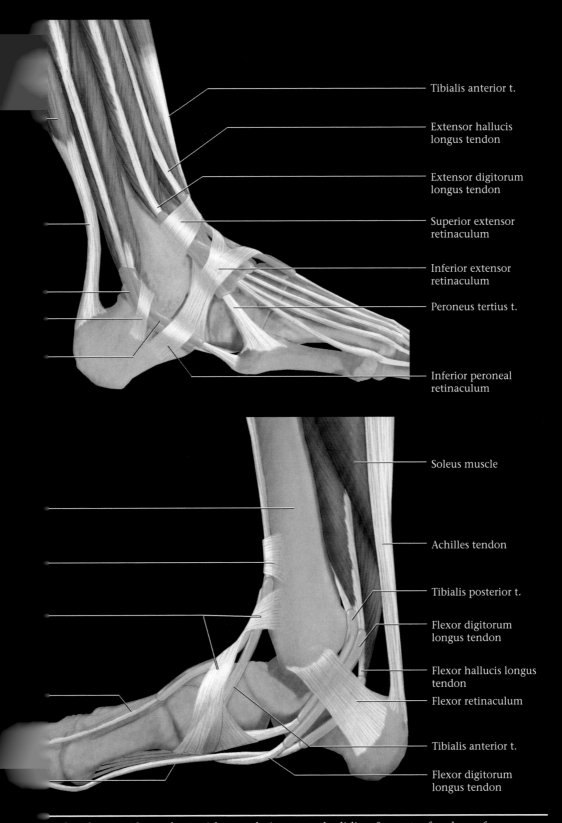

Tibialis anterior t.

Extensor hallucis longus tendon

Extensor digitorum longus tendon

Superior extensor retinaculum

Inferior extensor retinaculum

Peroneus tertius t.

Inferior peroneal retinaculum

Soleus muscle

Achilles tendon

Tibialis posterior t.

Flexor digitorum longus tendon

Flexor hallucis longus tendon

Flexor retinaculum

Tibialis anterior t.

Flexor digitorum longus tendon

n sheaths provide tendons with vascularity, smooth gliding & greater freedom of
endon is only ankle tendon without a tendon sheath; it is surrounded by paratenon. The
common sheath above inferior peroneal retinaculum. More distally each tendon is
ath. The peroneus longus tendon has a second sheath under the sole of foot. **(Bottom)** The
tendon disappears about 1-2 cm proximal to its navicular insertion. Thus, fluid at that
al tendon sheath fluid is normal except in flexor hallucis longus sheath where a large
on due to normal communication with ankle joint. Reactive fluid in sheaths of peroneal &
s seen with calcaneofibular & deltoid ligament injuries respectively.

TENDONS OVERVIEW

LATERAL RADIOGRAPH & COMPUTED TOMOGRAPHIC 3D VOLUME RENDERING

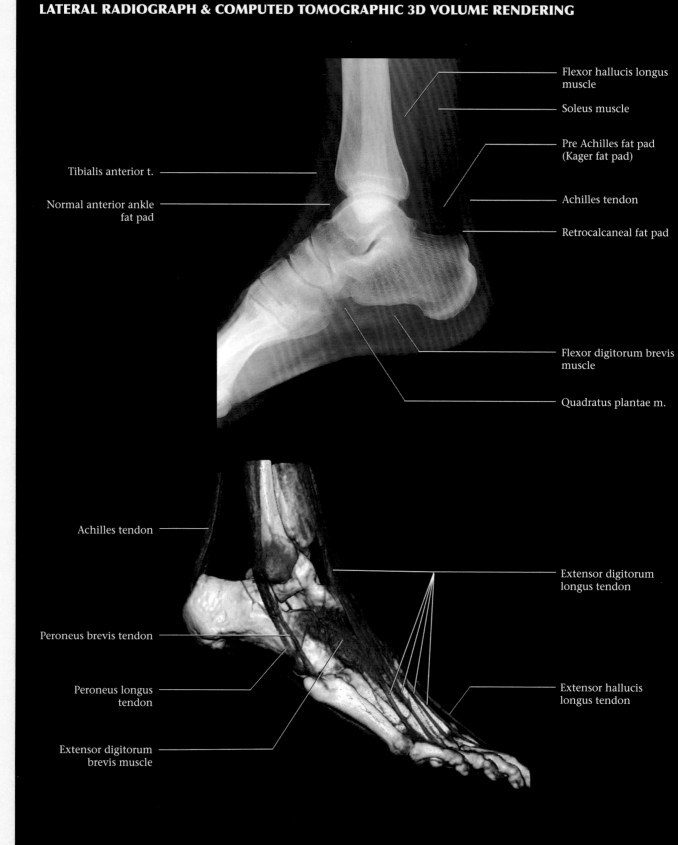

Flexor hallucis longus muscle

Soleus muscle

Pre Achilles fat pad (Kager fat pad)

Achilles tendon

Retrocalcaneal fat pad

Tibialis anterior t.

Normal anterior ankle fat pad

Flexor digitorum brevis muscle

Quadratus plantae m.

Achilles tendon

Peroneus brevis tendon

Peroneus longus tendon

Extensor digitorum brevis muscle

Extensor digitorum longus tendon

Extensor hallucis longus tendon

(Top) Lateral radiograph. The Achilles & tibialis anterior are the only tendons that are visualized on plain radiography (lateral view). The Achilles tendon is the most posterior & superficial tendon. It should be uniform in diameter from its musculotendinous junction to its calcaneal onsertion. A small retrocalcaneal fat pad, location of the retrocalcaneal bursa, is found between the tendon & calcaneus. A normal pre-Achilles fat pad separates the Achilles tendon from the ankle joint. The tibialis anterior tendon is noted on the dorsal surface of ankle. **(Bottom)** 3D volume rendering image of the lateral ankle. Multidetector-row computed tomography (MDCT) allows faster imaging at better resolution. 3D volume rendering images of the tendons, utilizing post processing workstations, can be obtained. Note the high resolution of the visualized tendons.

TENDONS OVERVIEW

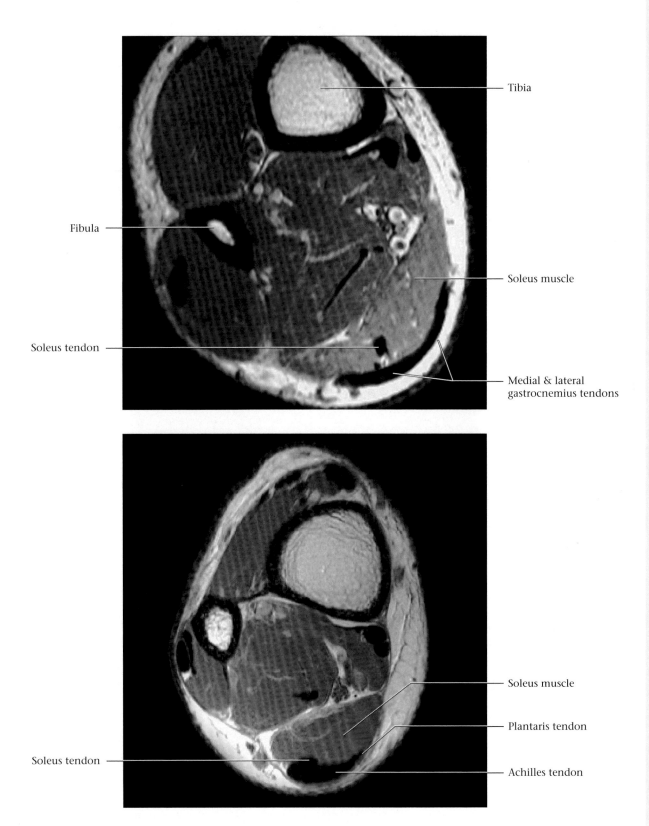

(Top) The Achilles tendon originates at the musculotendinous junction of the soleus and gastrocnemius tendons (aponeurosis) in the middle of the calf. Prior to the merger, the gastrocnemius tendons form a C-shaped aponeurosis along the posterior aspect of the distal leg. The soleus tendon is found anterior to the aponeurosis embedded in its muscle. **(Bottom)** As the soleus joins the gastrocnemius aponeurosis it forms a lateral bump on the anterior surface of the tendon. The Achilles tendon spirals as it descends down the calf so that the gastrocnemius contribution is mainly on the lateral & posterior surface of the tendon. This spiraling, which occurs a few cm above the tendon's insertion to the calcaneus, produces a focal area which is vulnerable to tearing.

AXIAL T1 MR, RIGHT ANKLE: ACHILLES TENDON

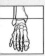

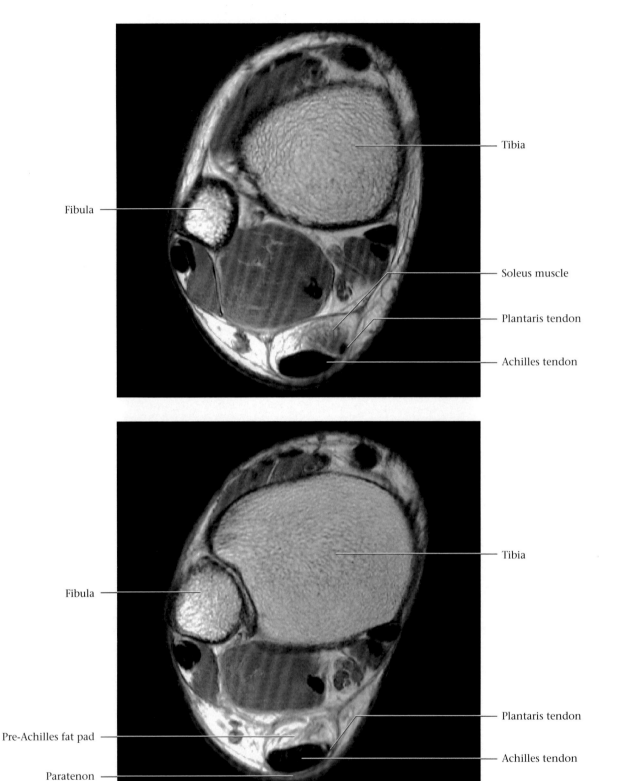

Tibia

Fibula

Soleus muscle

Plantaris tendon

Achilles tendon

Fibula

Tibia

Pre-Achilles fat pad

Plantaris tendon

Achilles tendon

Paratenon

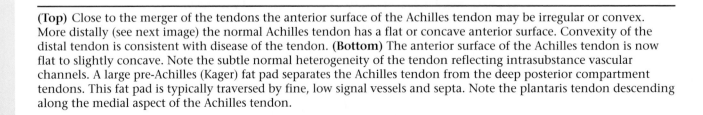

(Top) Close to the merger of the tendons the anterior surface of the Achilles tendon may be irregular or convex. More distally (see next image) the normal Achilles tendon has a flat or concave anterior surface. Convexity of the distal tendon is consistent with disease of the tendon. **(Bottom)** The anterior surface of the Achilles tendon is now flat to slightly concave. Note the subtle normal heterogeneity of the tendon reflecting intrasubstance vascular channels. A large pre-Achilles (Kager) fat pad separates the Achilles tendon from the deep posterior compartment tendons. This fat pad is typically traversed by fine, low signal vessels and septa. Note the plantaris tendon descending along the medial aspect of the Achilles tendon.

Ankle

VII

74

AXIAL T1 MR, RIGHT ANKLE: ACHILLES TENDON

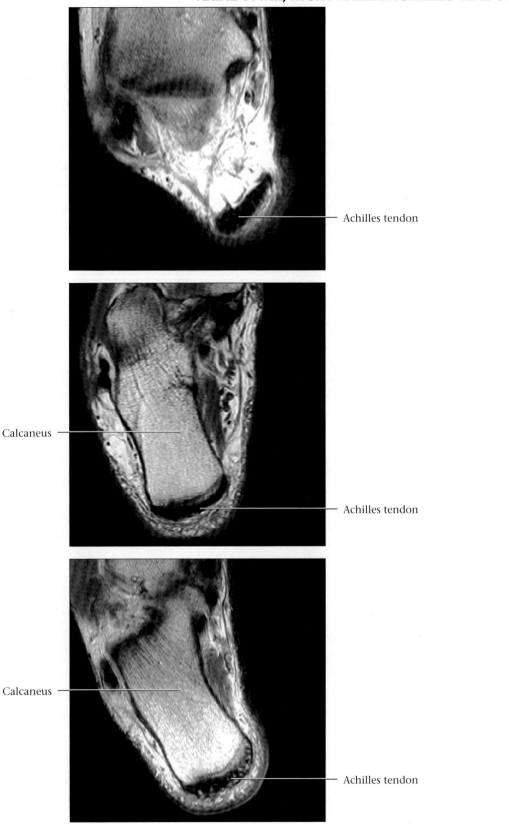

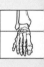

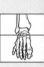

Achilles tendon

Calcaneus

Achilles tendon

Calcaneus

Achilles tendon

(Top) The Achilles tendon inserts into a large rough area on the posterior calcaneus, a few millimeters below the apex of the calcaneal tuberosity. The tendon flattens approximately 4 cm above its insertion as seen in this image. Note normal heterogeneity of the tendon. The tendon may be cartilaginous at its very distal aspect. (Middle) Note broad insertion of the Achilles tendon to calcaneus. (Bottom) Note interdigitation of bone and tendon at the insertion of Achilles tendon to calcaneus.

Ankle

VII

SAGITTAL T1 MR, RIGHT ANKLE: ACHILLES TENDON

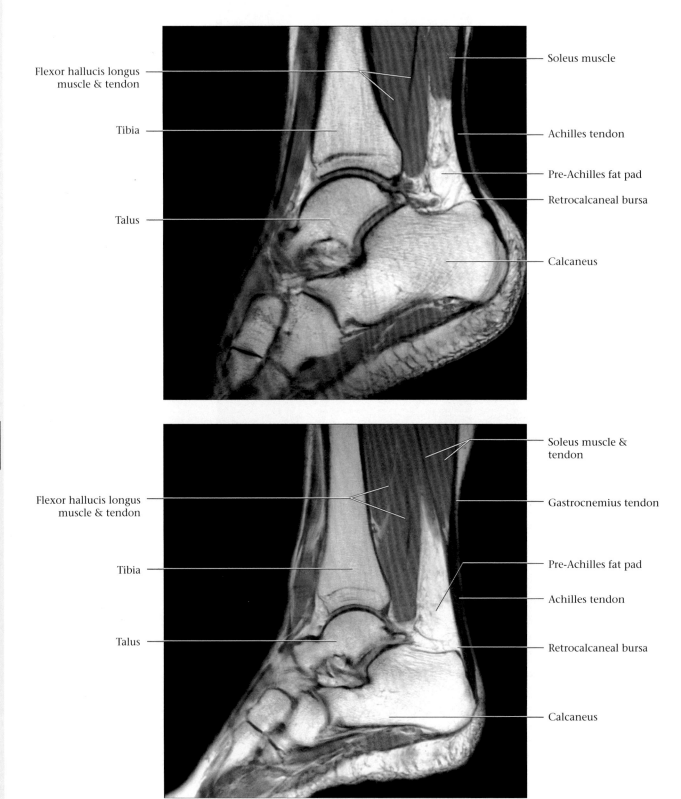

Flexor hallucis longus muscle & tendon

Tibia

Talus

Soleus muscle

Achilles tendon

Pre-Achilles fat pad

Retrocalcaneal bursa

Calcaneus

Flexor hallucis longus muscle & tendon

Tibia

Talus

Soleus muscle & tendon

Gastrocnemius tendon

Pre-Achilles fat pad

Achilles tendon

Retrocalcaneal bursa

Calcaneus

(Top) The Achilles tendon measures approximately 15 cm in length. Unlike most tendons that are best assessed on axial images the Achilles tendon is optimally visualized on sagittal images. The tendon is typically low in signal on all pulse sequences. Its anterior & posterior margins are parallel to one another on sagittal images. **(Bottom)** Note the merger of the soleus tendon with the gastrocnemius tendon/aponeurosis. Tears of the Achilles tendon typically occur 2-6 cm above the insertion of the tendon, an area that is well seen on routine sagittal ankle images. Tears of the Achilles musculotendinous junction, however, may require more proximal imaging of the distal leg.

Ankle

SAGITTAL & AXIAL T2 FS MR, RIGHT ANKLE: ACHILLES TENDON

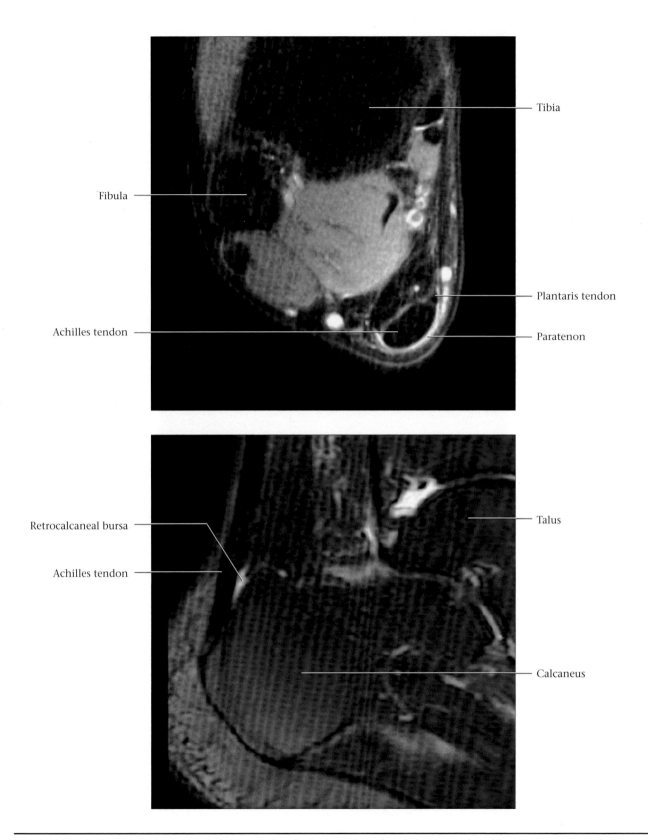

Tibia

Fibula

Achilles tendon

Plantaris tendon

Paratenon

Retrocalcaneal bursa

Achilles tendon

Talus

Calcaneus

(Top) The Achilles paratenon. The Achilles tendon lacks a tendon sheath but is enclosed by a paratenon, a thin gliding membrane of loose areolar tissue which is seen as a ring of bright signal around the tendon on fat suppressed axial images. **(Bottom)** Retrocalcaneal bursa. A small fat pad separates the Achilles tendon from the apex of the calcaneal tuberosity; the retrocalcaneal bursa is found within this fat pad. Minimal amount of fluid within the retrocalcaneal bursa is a normal finding which should not be misinterpreted as disease.

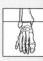

Ankle

AXIAL T1 MR, RIGHT ANKLE: TIBIALIS POSTERIOR TENDON

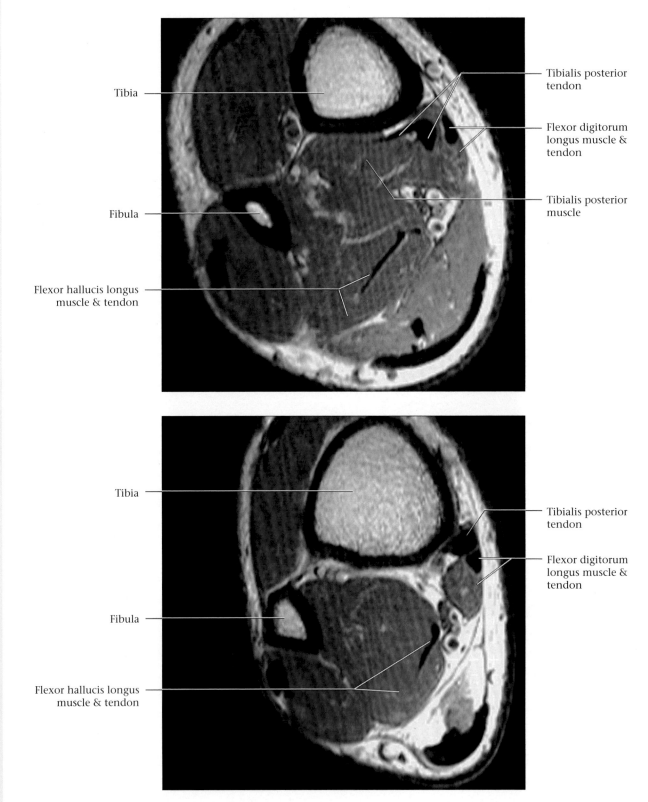

Tibia

Fibula

Flexor hallucis longus muscle & tendon

Tibialis posterior tendon

Flexor digitorum longus muscle & tendon

Tibialis posterior muscle

Tibia

Fibula

Flexor hallucis longus muscle & tendon

Tibialis posterior tendon

Flexor digitorum longus muscle & tendon

(Top) In the distal leg the tibialis posterior muscle lies between the flexor hallucis longus and flexor digitorum longus muscles. Often, the muscle has two tendinous slips (as seen here) which typically fuse into one slip by the time the tendon reaches the ankle joint. Occasionally the two tendon slips are still seen at the ankle joint and should not be mistaken for a torn tendon. **(Bottom)** A few cm above ankle joint the tibialis posterior tendon crosses deep to the flexor digitorum longus tendon to become the most medial tendon of the deep posterior compartment. Note that the muscle of the tibialis posterior has disappeared while the rest of the deep posterior compartment muscles are still visualized.

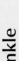

TENDONS OVERVIEW

AXIAL T1 MR, RIGHT ANKLE: TIBIALIS POSTERIOR TENDON

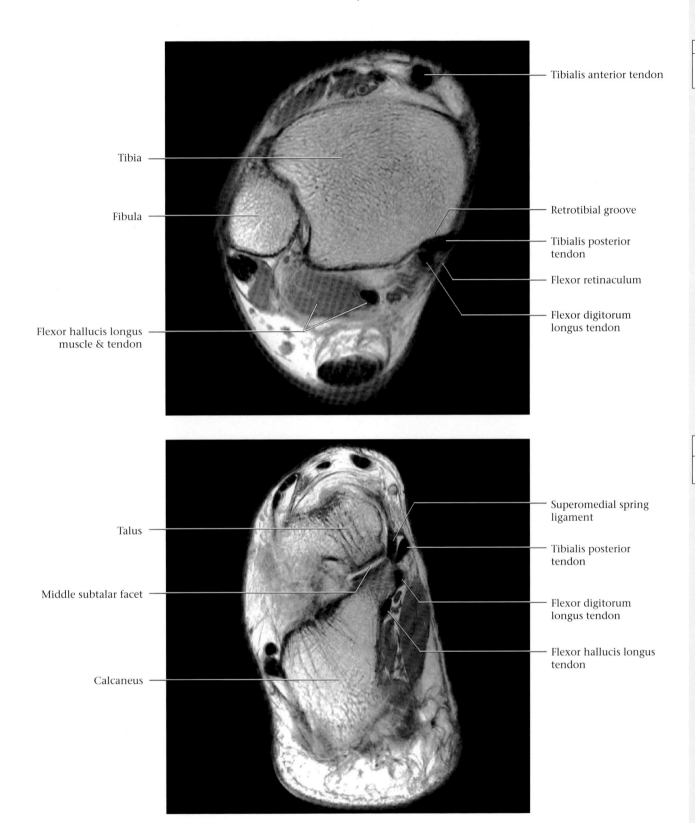

Tibialis anterior tendon

Tibia

Fibula

Retrotibial groove

Tibialis posterior tendon

Flexor retinaculum

Flexor hallucis longus muscle & tendon

Flexor digitorum longus tendon

Talus

Superomedial spring ligament

Tibialis posterior tendon

Middle subtalar facet

Flexor digitorum longus tendon

Flexor hallucis longus tendon

Calcaneus

(Top) Just above the ankle joint the tibialis posterior & the more laterally located flexor digitorum longus tendon descend together, deep to the flexor retinaculum, within a common retrotibial groove posterior to the tibia & medial malleolus. Each tendon, however, is enclosed within its own operate tendon sheath. The flexor retinaculum holds the tendons in place within the retrotibial groove. The tibialis posterior tendon at this level is uniformly low in signal. Its size should be approximately 2-3 times the size of the adjacent flexor digitorum longus tendon. **(Bottom)** As the tibialis posterior tendon descends medial to the talar head, it lies superficial to the deltoid ligament and then superficial to the superomedial component of the spring ligament.

AXIAL T1 MR, RIGHT ANKLE: TIBIALIS POSTERIOR TENDON

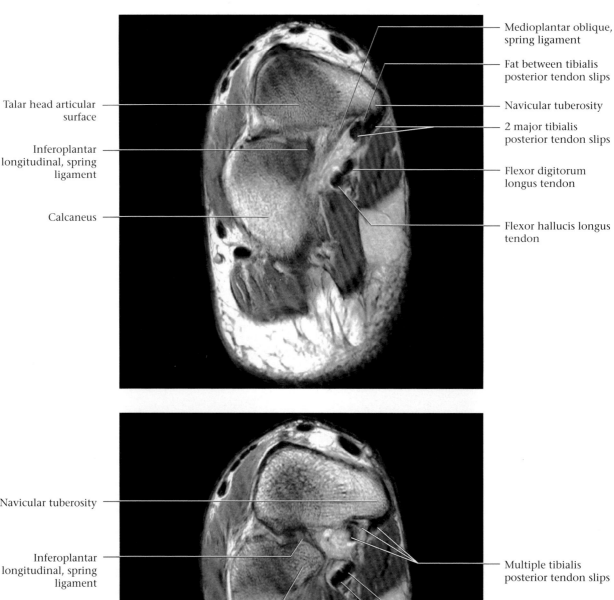

Talar head articular surface

Inferoplantar longitudinal, spring ligament

Calcaneus

Medioplantar oblique, spring ligament

Fat between tibialis posterior tendon slips

Navicular tuberosity

2 major tibialis posterior tendon slips

Flexor digitorum longus tendon

Flexor hallucis longus tendon

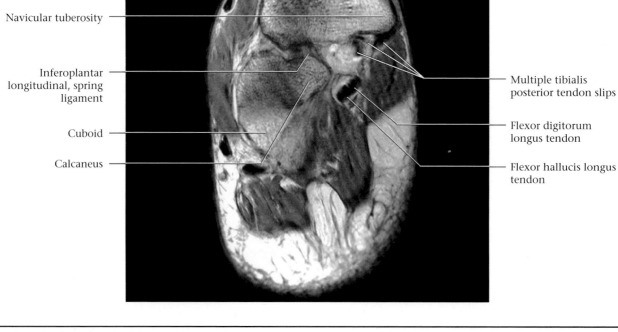

Navicular tuberosity

Inferoplantar longitudinal, spring ligament

Cuboid

Calcaneus

Multiple tibialis posterior tendon slips

Flexor digitorum longus tendon

Flexor hallucis longus tendon

(Top) In the foot the tibialis posterior tendon divides into two major components as seen in this image: 1) larger, more medial division inserts directly into the navicular tuberosity, 2) lateral, smaller division inserts to all other tarsal bones, (excluding talus), & 2nd-4th metatarsal bases. The tibialis posterior tendon may appear heterogeneous at its navicular insertion for the following reasons: 1) magic angle effect, can be minimized by imaging in mild plantar flexion (supine) or in prone position (uncomfortable to patient), 2) fat in between the various tendon slips (seen here), 3) presence of an fibrocartilage/type I os naviculare, 4) heterogeneity related to adjacent deltoid & spring ligaments. (Bottom) An image slightly more distal depicts further splitting of the tibialis posterior tendon.

TENDONS OVERVIEW

AXIAL T1 MR, RIGHT ANKLE: TIBIALIS POSTERIOR TENDON

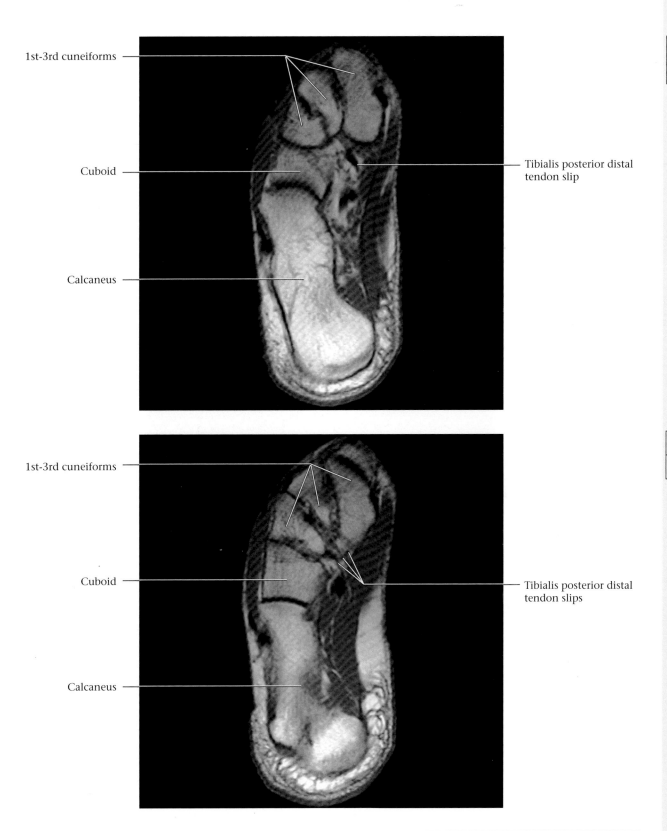

1st-3rd cuneiforms

Cuboid

Calcaneus

Tibialis posterior distal tendon slip

1st-3rd cuneiforms

Cuboid

Calcaneus

Tibialis posterior distal tendon slips

(Top) A single, prominent distal tibialis posterior tendon slip is seen approaching the bases of the cuneiforms. **(Bottom)** More distal axial image depicts a number of tibialis posterior tendon slips. The most lateral & most prominent one inserts on the plantar base of the 3rd cuneiform. Two other slips are seen approaching the plantar surfaces of 1st & 2nd cuneiforms. The numerous plantar insertion sites of the tibialis posterior tendon make it the most powerful invertor of the foot. The tendon is also a major contributor to maintaining the medial longitudinal arch.

AXIAL T1 & T2 FS MR, RIGHT ANKLE: TIBIALIS POSTERIOR TENDON

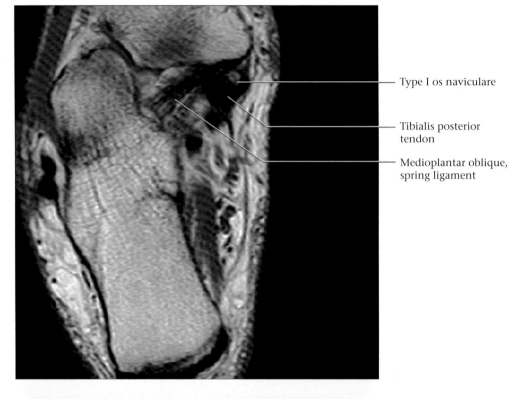

Type I os naviculare

Tibialis posterior tendon

Medioplantar oblique, spring ligament

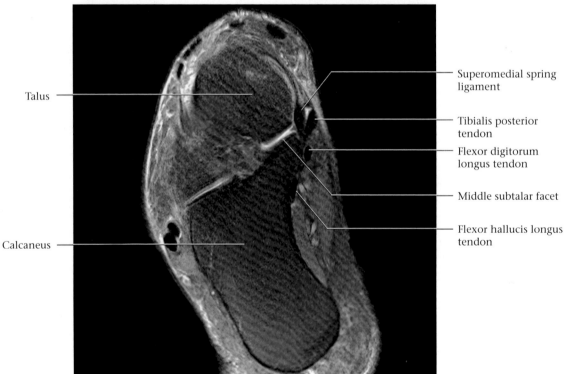

Talus

Calcaneus

Superomedial spring ligament

Tibialis posterior tendon

Flexor digitorum longus tendon

Middle subtalar facet

Flexor hallucis longus tendon

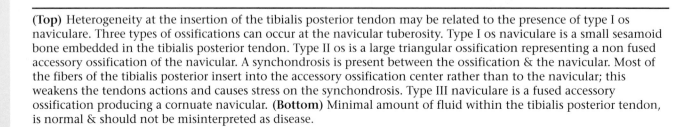

(Top) Heterogeneity at the insertion of the tibialis posterior tendon may be related to the presence of type I os naviculare. Three types of ossifications can occur at the navicular tuberosity. Type I os naviculare is a small sesamoid bone embedded in the tibialis posterior tendon. Type II os is a large triangular ossification representing a non fused accessory ossification of the navicular. A synchondrosis is present between the ossification & the navicular. Most of the fibers of the tibialis posterior insert into the accessory ossification center rather than to the navicular; this weakens the tendons actions and causes stress on the synchondrosis. Type III naviculare is a fused accessory ossification producing a cornuate navicular. **(Bottom)** Minimal amount of fluid within the tibialis posterior tendon, is normal & should not be misinterpreted as disease.

TENDONS OVERVIEW

SAGITTAL T1 MR, RIGHT ANKLE: TIBIALIS POSTERIOR TENDON

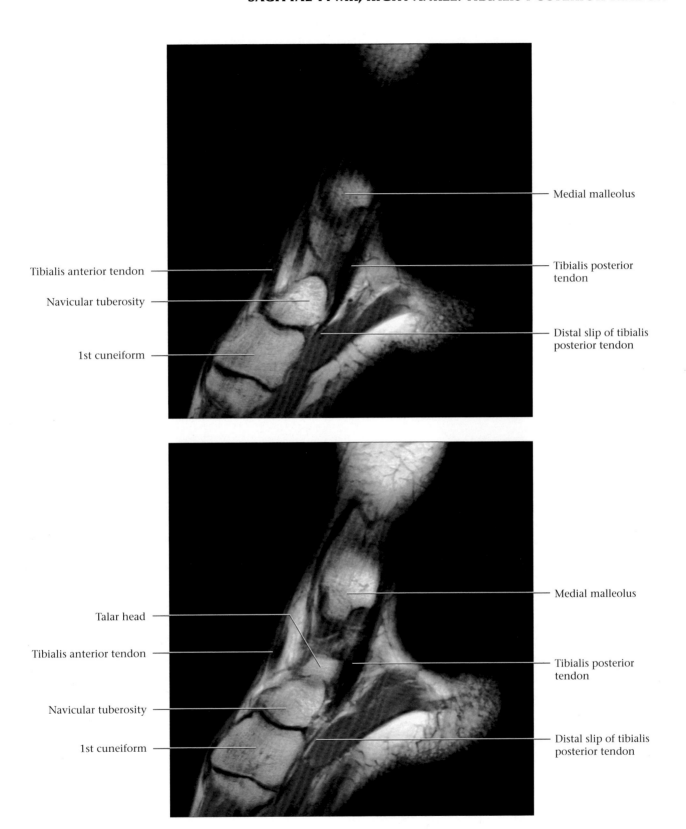
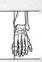

Tibialis anterior tendon — (top image)

Navicular tuberosity —

1st cuneiform —

Medial malleolus

Tibialis posterior tendon

Distal slip of tibialis posterior tendon

Talar head —

Tibialis anterior tendon —

Navicular tuberosity —

1st cuneiform —

Medial malleolus

Tibialis posterior tendon

Distal slip of tibialis posterior tendon

(Top) The tibialis posterior tendon is optimally assessed on axial images. The distal insertion of the tendon, however, is often better assessed on sagittal images. The synovial sheath of the tendon terminates 1-2 cm above the navicular insertion. Therefore, fluid at the navicular insertion of the tendon is pathologic. Sagittal images often depict the more distal slips of the tibialis posterior tendon. Incidentally noted is the tibialis anterior tendon coursing toward its 1st cuneiform, 1st metatarsal insertion. **(Bottom)** A distal slip of the tibialis posterior tendon to the cuneiform is noted.

TENDONS OVERVIEW

AXIAL T1 MR, RIGHT ANKLE: FLEXOR HALLUCIS LONGUS TENDON

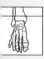

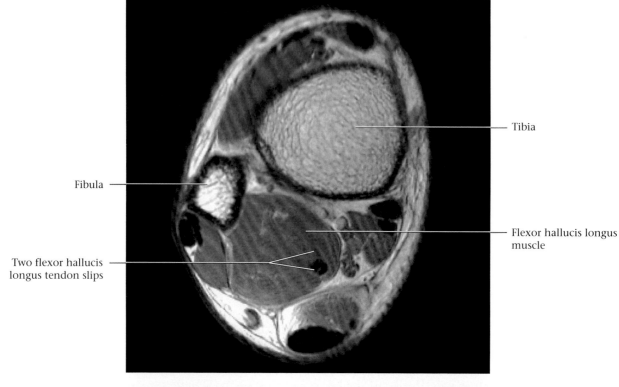

Tibia

Fibula

Flexor hallucis longus muscle

Two flexor hallucis longus tendon slips

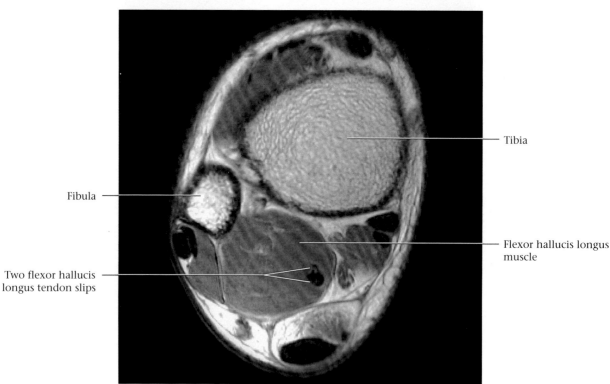

Fibula

Tibia

Flexor hallucis longus muscle

Two flexor hallucis longus tendon slips

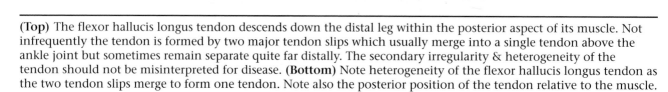

(Top) The flexor hallucis longus tendon descends down the distal leg within the posterior aspect of its muscle. Not infrequently the tendon is formed by two major tendon slips which usually merge into a single tendon above the ankle joint but sometimes remain separate quite far distally. The secondary irregularity & heterogeneity of the tendon should not be misinterpreted for disease. **(Bottom)** Note heterogeneity of the flexor hallucis longus tendon as the two tendon slips merge to form one tendon. Note also the posterior position of the tendon relative to the muscle.

TENDONS OVERVIEW

AXIAL T1 MR, RIGHT ANKLE: FLEXOR HALLUCIS LONGUS TENDON

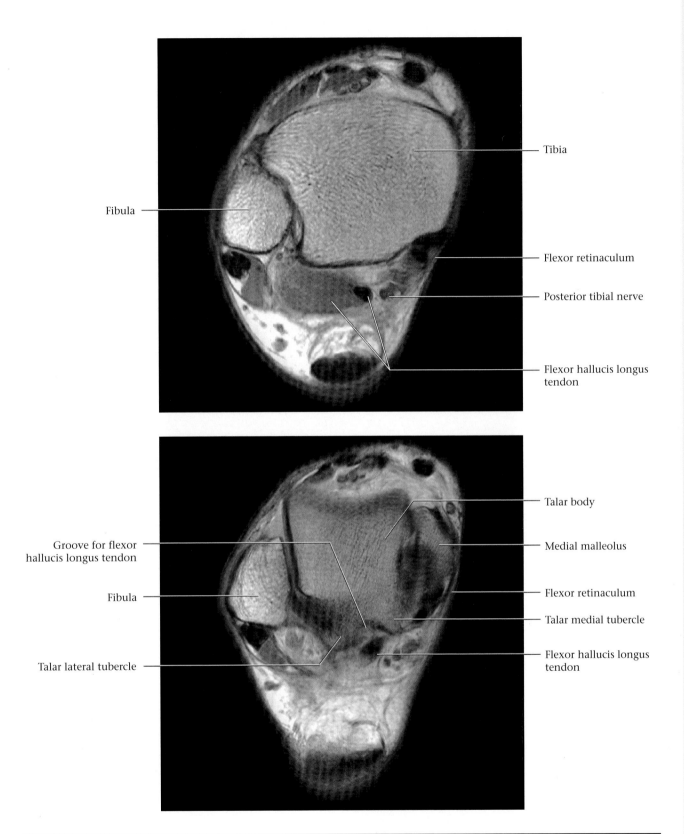

Tibia

Fibula

Flexor retinaculum

Posterior tibial nerve

Flexor hallucis longus tendon

Groove for flexor hallucis longus tendon

Talar body

Medial malleolus

Fibula

Flexor retinaculum

Talar medial tubercle

Talar lateral tubercle

Flexor hallucis longus tendon

(Top) The flexor hallucis longus tendon descends within the tarsal tunnel, deep to the flexor retinaculum. The posterior tibial nerve is typically medial to the tendon. Note that the flexor hallucis longus muscle is the only muscle of the deep flexor compartment that extends quite far distally into the ankle area. **(Bottom)** The flexor hallucis longus tendon traverses two major tunnels in the ankle and hindfoot. The tunnel is between the medial and lateral tubercles of the talus. A fibrous band converts the groove into a tunnel.

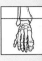

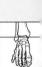

AXIAL T1 MR, RIGHT ANKLE: FLEXOR HALLUCIS LONGUS TENDON

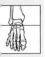

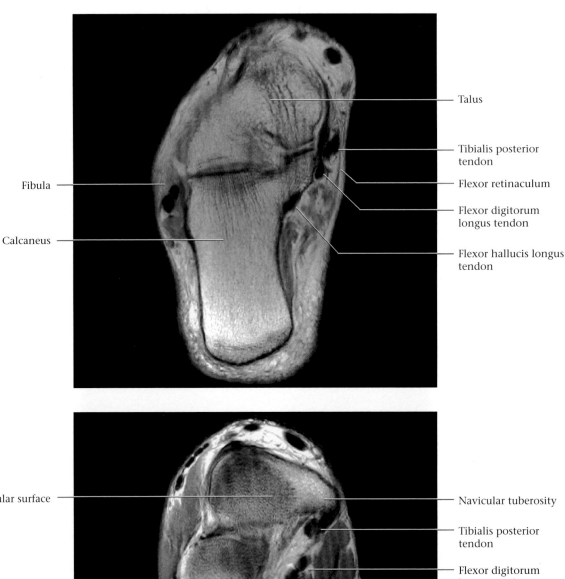

Talus

Tibialis posterior tendon

Flexor retinaculum

Fibula

Flexor digitorum longus tendon

Calcaneus

Flexor hallucis longus tendon

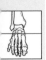

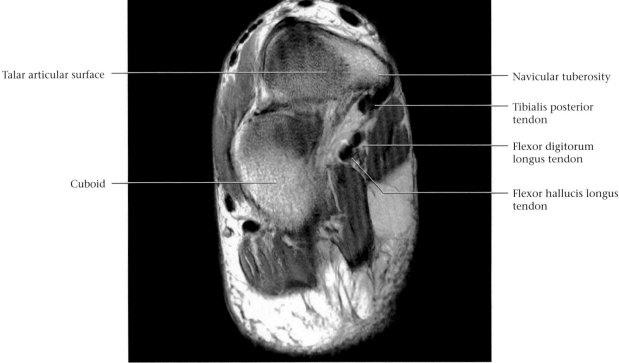

Talar articular surface

Navicular tuberosity

Tibialis posterior tendon

Flexor digitorum longus tendon

Cuboid

Flexor hallucis longus tendon

(Top) The tunnel the flexor hallucis longus traverses in the ankle and hindfoot is underneath the sustentaculum tali of the calcaneus. A fibrous band converts this groove into a tunnel. The flexor hallucis longus tendon is predisposed to tearing at the talar and sustentacular tali tunnels. **(Bottom)** As the flexor hallucis longus tendon travels into the plantar foot it takes an oblique course toward its medial insertion into the plantar base of the 1st distal toe (it traverses a third tunnel in between the sesamoid bones of the digit). Plantar to the navicular tuberosity the tendon first approaches and then crosses the flexor digitorum longus tendon as the latter takes an oblique lateral course toward its distal insertion sites.

AXIAL T1 MR, RIGHT ANKLE: FLEXOR HALLUCIS LONGUS TENDON

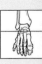

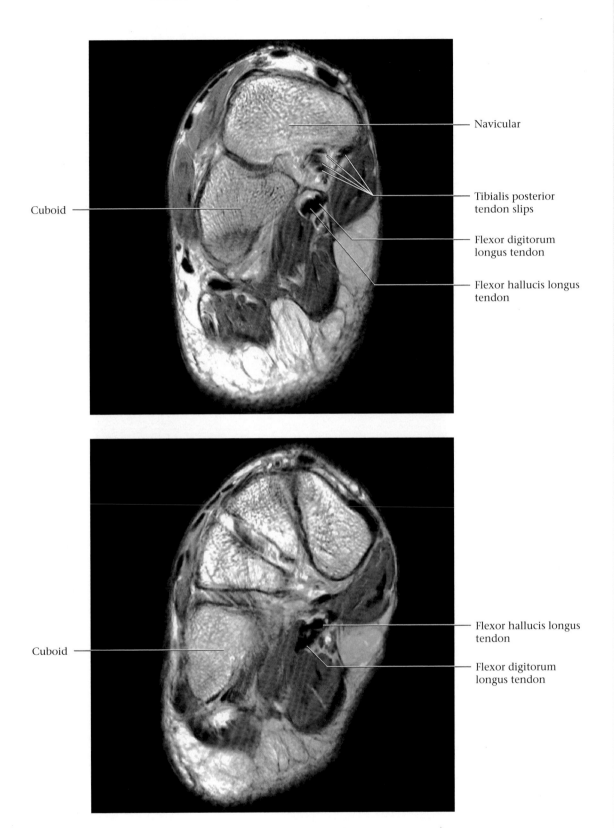

Navicular

Tibialis posterior
tendon slips

Cuboid

Flexor digitorum
longus tendon

Flexor hallucis longus
tendon

Cuboid

Flexor hallucis longus
tendon

Flexor digitorum
longus tendon

(Top) As the flexor hallucis longus tendon crosses the flexor digitorum longus tendon, (under the navicular tuberosity, at the knot of Henry), it sends a fibrous slip to the latter tendon. This slip prevents the flexor hallucis longus tendon from significant proximal retraction if it tears distal to the knot of Henry. **(Bottom)** Following the cross over, the flexor hallucis longus tendon is noted superior and medial to the flexor digitorum longus tendon.

AXIAL T1 MR, RIGHT ANKLE: FLEXOR HALLUCIS LONGUS TENDON

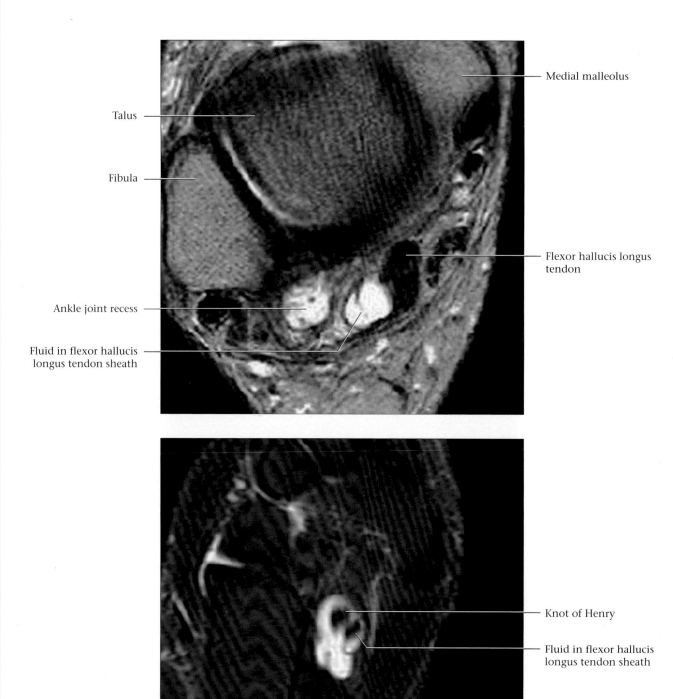

Labels (top image): Talus — Fibula — Ankle joint recess — Fluid in flexor hallucis longus tendon sheath — Medial malleolus — Flexor hallucis longus tendon

Labels (bottom image): Knot of Henry — Fluid in flexor hallucis longus tendon sheath

(Top) Communication between the flexor hallucis longus tendon & ankle joint is present in 20-30% of individuals. Thus, fluid in the flexor hallucis longus tendon sheath, in the setting of ankle joint fluid, is a frequent finding not to be misinterpreted as tenosynovitis. However, isolated fluid in the tendon sheath without ankle joint fluid is usually pathologic. Focal fluid column proximal to the flexor hallucis longus tendon's tunnels is also suspicious for disease. **(Bottom)** Fluid within the flexor hallucis longus tendon sheath may extend quite far distally into the knot of Henry. This is typically a benign finding and of no clinical significance. Isolated fluid in this area, however, without fluid proximal to it, may indicate tenosynovitis. The medial plantar nerve follows the flexor hallucis longus tendon and may be impinged upon by the fluid.

TENDONS OVERVIEW

SAGITTAL T1 MR, ANKLE: FLEXOR HALLUCIS LONGUS TENDON

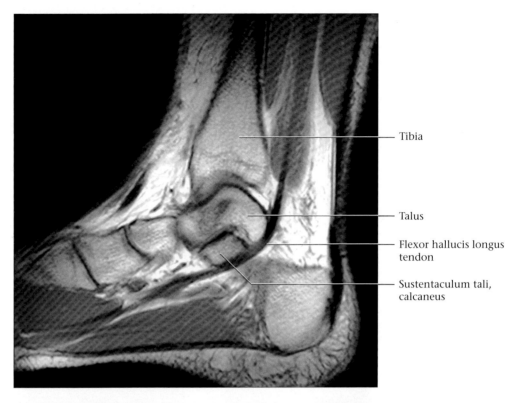

Tibia

Talus

Flexor hallucis longus tendon

Sustentaculum tali, calcaneus

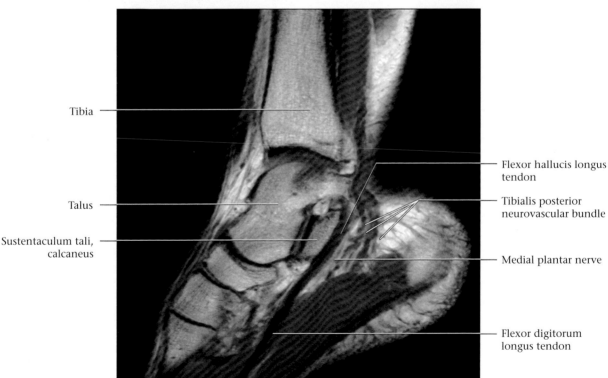

Tibia

Talus

Sustentaculum tali, calcaneus

Flexor hallucis longus tendon

Tibialis posterior neurovascular bundle

Medial plantar nerve

Flexor digitorum longus tendon

(Top) The flexor hallucis longus tendon is frequently seen on sagittal images of the ankle as it descends under the sustentaculum tali. Detecting pathology of the tendon, however, is more optimally performed on axial images. **(Bottom)** Note that the distal flexor digitorum longus tendon is typically seen on the same sagittal image in which the flexor hallucis longus tendon is noted to descend under the sustentaculum tali. This is due to the crossing over of the tendons in the knot of Henry, under the navicular tuberosity. Note also the medial plantar nerve's proximity to the flexor hallucis longus tendon.

SAGITTAL & AXIAL T1 MR, RIGHT ANKLE: FLEXOR HALLUCIS LONGUS TENDON

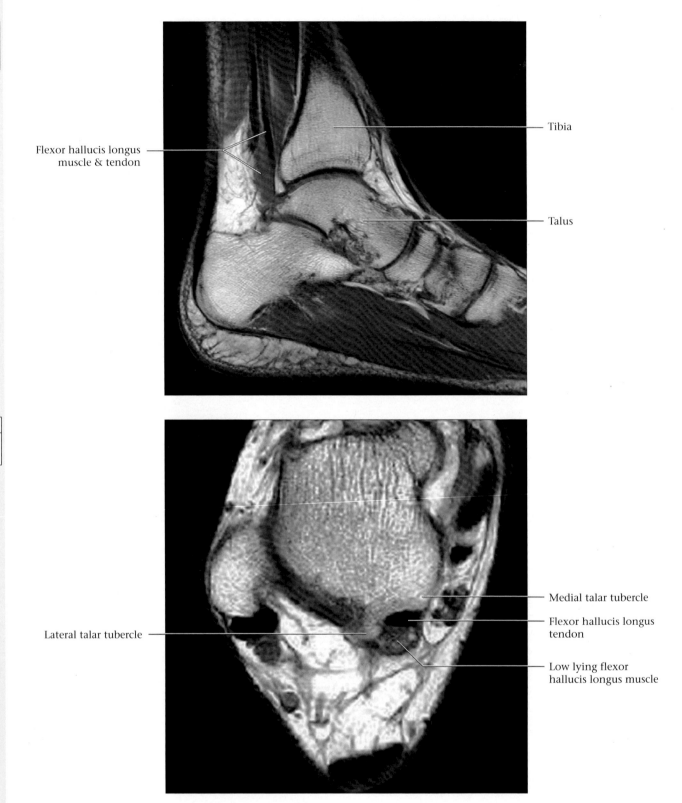

Flexor hallucis longus muscle & tendon

Tibia

Talus

Medial talar tubercle

Flexor hallucis longus tendon

Lateral talar tubercle

Low lying flexor hallucis longus muscle

(Top) Note the distal extent of the flexor hallucis muscle to below the level of ankle joint. Occasionally, further extension of the muscle into the talar tunnel may be seen and can produce symptomatic entrapment of the muscle. Care should be taken not to overcall this, however, since with ankle dorsiflexion the posterior muscles extend further distally than in plantarflexion. (Bottom) Typically the muscle of the flexor hallucis longus extends to the ankle joint and is not seen at the level of the talar groove. In a low lying flexor hallucis longus muscle, as in this patient, muscle tissue extends into the groove and may produce symptoms.

Ankle

AXIAL T1 MR, RIGHT ANKLE: PERONEAL TENDONS

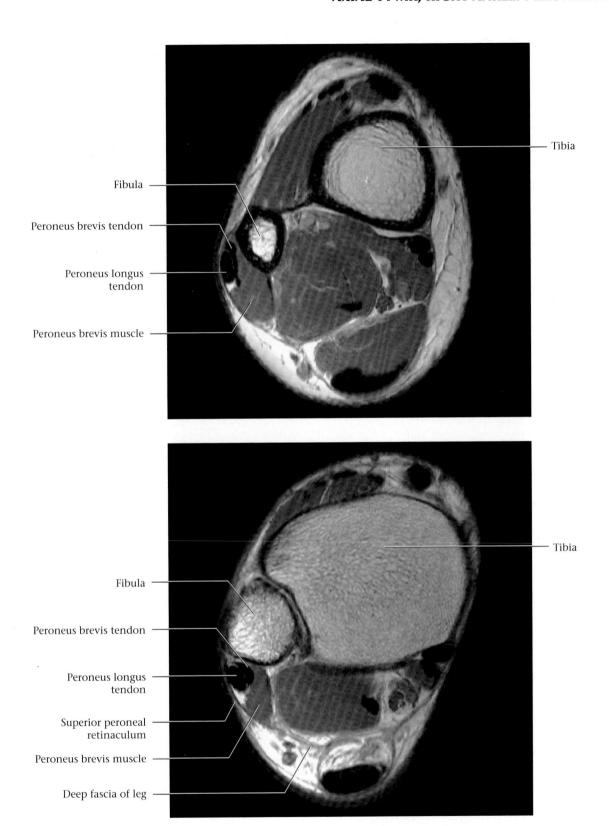

(Top) The peroneal tendons descend together in the lateral compartment of the leg. In the distal leg the peroneus longus muscle has become entirely tendinous while both muscle & tendon of the peroneus brevis are visualized. Note that in the distal leg the peroneal tendons are lateral rather than posterior to the fibula; this should not be misinterpreted as subluxation of the tendons. (Bottom) As the tendons approach the ankle they lie directly posterior to the distal fibula. The posterior surface of the fibula becomes flat or concave to form a retromalleolar groove accommodating both tendons. The peroneus brevis tendon is typically crescentic in shape & is located anteromedial to the peroneus longus tendon. The superior peroneal retinaculum extends from the distal fibula to calcaneus & deep leg fascia & maintains the peroneal tendons within the retromalleolar groove.

Ankle

VII

91

TENDONS OVERVIEW

AXIAL T1 MR, RIGHT ANKLE: PERONEAL TENDONS

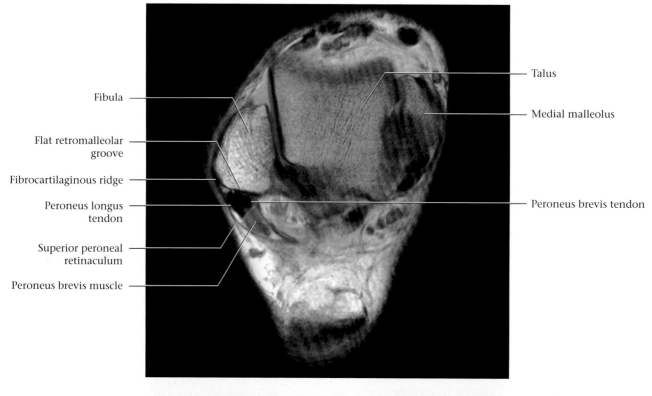

Fibula —

Flat retromalleolar groove —

Fibrocartilaginous ridge —

Peroneus longus tendon —

Superior peroneal retinaculum —

Peroneus brevis muscle —

— Talus

— Medial malleolus

— Peroneus brevis tendon

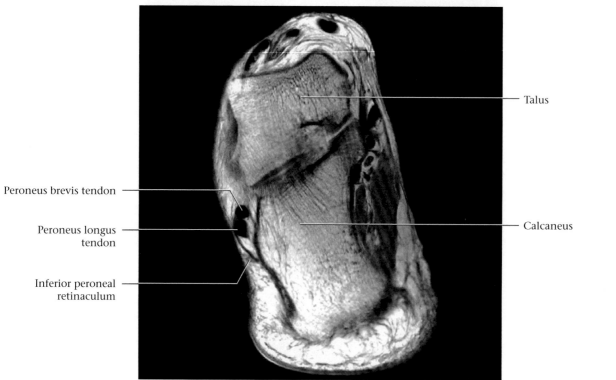

Peroneus brevis tendon —

Peroneus longus tendon —

Inferior peroneal retinaculum —

— Talus

— Calcaneus

(Top) The superior peroneal retinaculum is a reinforcement of the leg aponeurosis. It is seen as a low signal band originating from the lateral distal fibula, at the retromalleolar groove, approximately 1 cm above the fibular tip. It can be followed to its insertion to the deep fascia of the leg. Frequently, a small, low signal, triangular fibrocartilaginous or fibrous ridge is noted at or close to the fibular origin of the retinaculum. This ridge deepens the retromalleolar groove. **(Bottom)** The peroneal tendons share a common sheath at the retromalleolar groove. Along the lateral calcaneal wall the tendons & their sheath become separated by the inferior peroneal retinaculum & peroneal tubercle (when present). The inferior peroneal retinaculum is visualized as a thin, low signal structure, enveloping & in between the peroneal tendons.

TENDONS OVERVIEW

AXIAL T1 MR, RIGHT ANKLE: PERONEAL TENDONS

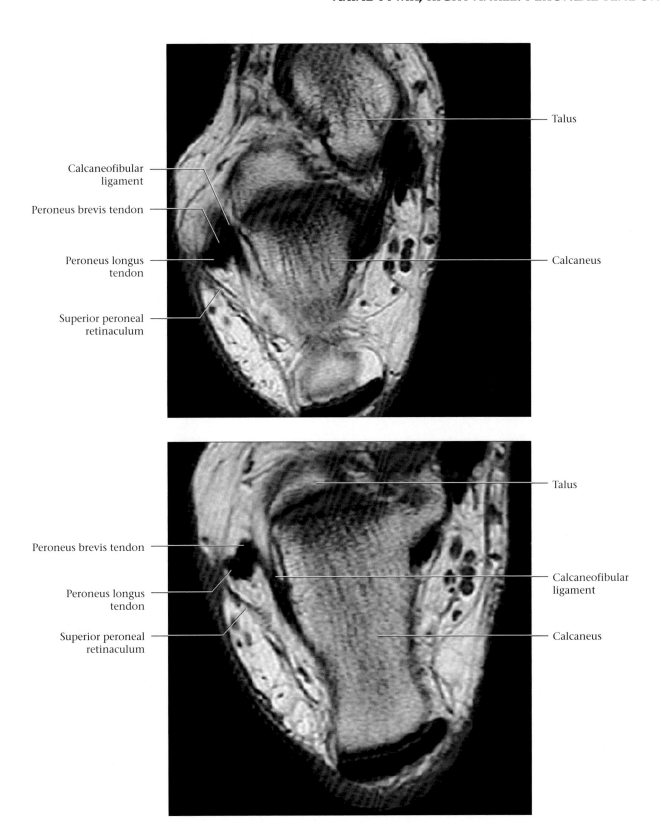

Talus

Calcaneofibular ligament

Peroneus brevis tendon

Peroneus longus tendon

Superior peroneal retinaculum

Calcaneus

Talus

Peroneus brevis tendon

Peroneus longus tendon

Superior peroneal retinaculum

Calcaneofibular ligament

Calcaneus

(Top) The calcaneofibular ligament inserts on the calcaneus deep to the peroneal tendons. The ligament may be visualized as a low signal structure in between the calcaneus & the peroneal tendons. **(Bottom)** The proximity of the peroneal tendons to the calcaneofibular ligament can result in concomitant tearing of the common peroneal tendon sheath & calcaneofibular ligament during inversion injuries. This can produce reactive fluid within the peroneal tendon sheath which should not be misinterpreted as tenosynovitis.

TENDONS OVERVIEW

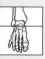

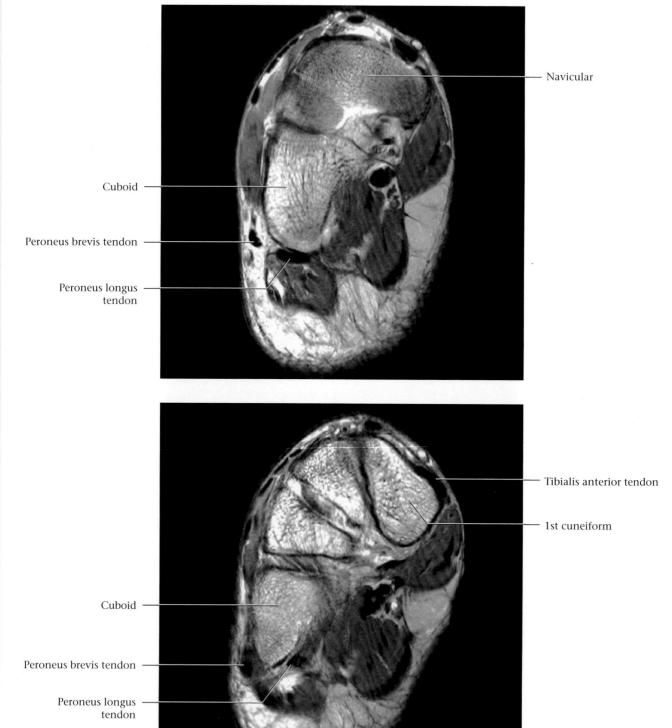

(Top) The peroneus brevis tendon continues toward its insertion on the 5th metatarsal base. The peroneus longus tendon enters the cuboid tunnel, plantar to the cuboid and continues along the sole of the foot toward its insertion on 1st cuneiform & 1st metatarsal base. **(Bottom)** The distal course of the peroneus longus tendon along the plantar surface of the foot is best seen on short axis mid foot images but may also be seen on distal axial images of the ankle. The tendon is often suboptimally seen on T1WI due to magic angle effect. Note the insertion of the tibialis anterior tendon on the 1st cuneiform.

Ankle

TENDONS OVERVIEW

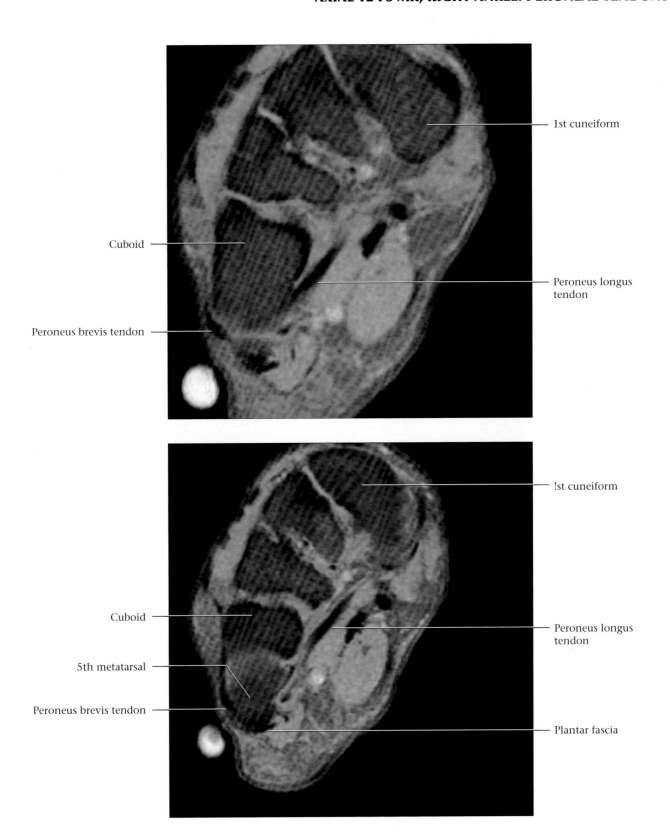

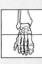

Top image labels:
- 1st cuneiform
- Cuboid
- Peroneus longus tendon
- Peroneus brevis tendon

Bottom image labels:
- !st cuneiform
- Cuboid
- 5th metatarsal
- Peroneus brevis tendon
- Peroneus longus tendon
- Plantar fascia

(Top) The course of the peroneus longus tendon along the plantar surface of the foot is frequently better seen on axial FS T2 weighted images due to the relative lack of the magic angle effect. **(Bottom)** On a more distal axial image the peroneus longus tendon continues deep to the 3rd compartment muscles. Note the insertion of the peroneus brevis tendon on the base of the 5th metatarsal. The peroneus brevis and plantar fascia insert onto the plantar base of the 5th metatarsal while the peroneus tertius tendon inserts on the dorsal base of the 5th metatarsal.

TENDONS OVERVIEW

AXIAL T2 FS MR, RIGHT ANKLE: PERONEAL TENDONS

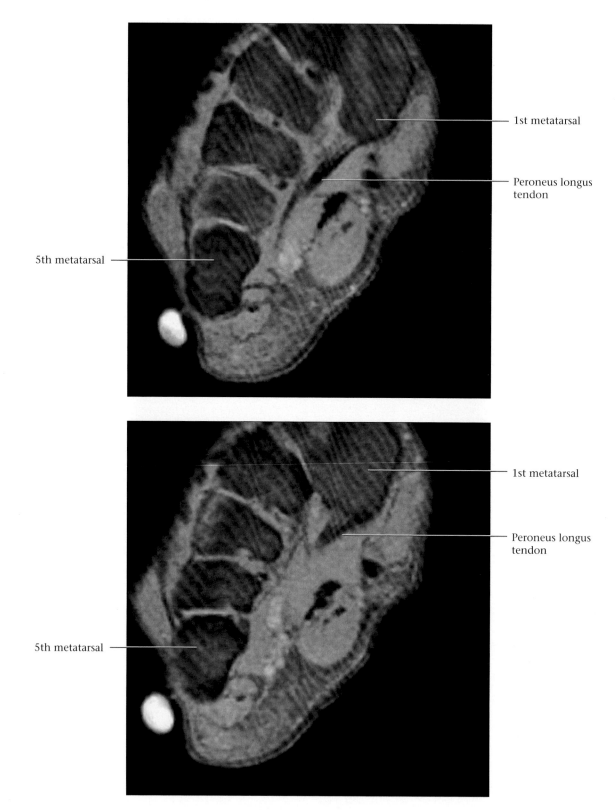

1st metatarsal

Peroneus longus
tendon

5th metatarsal

1st metatarsal

Peroneus longus
tendon

5th metatarsal

(Top) Note the striation of the very distal peroneus longus tendon. **(Bottom)** The peroneus longus tendon fans out at its insertion to the plantar base of the 1st metatarsal. It is often heterogeneous and striated at the insertion site.

TENDONS OVERVIEW

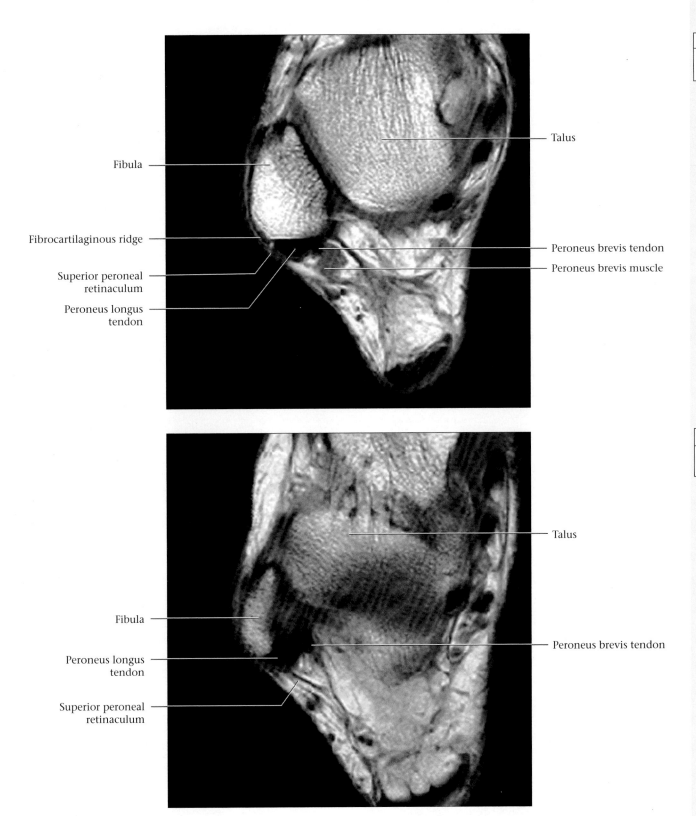

Fibula — Talus

Fibrocartilaginous ridge — — Peroneus brevis tendon
— Peroneus brevis muscle

Superior peroneal retinaculum —

Peroneus longus tendon —

Fibula — Talus

Peroneus longus tendon —

Superior peroneal retinaculum — — Peroneus brevis tendon

(Top) Usually the peroneus brevis tendon is anteromedial to the peroneus longus tendon within the retromalleolar groove. Occasionally, however, the peroneus brevis tendon is located medial to the peroneus longus tendon. In those instances, as the tendons descend distally, the peroneus brevis tendon may appear medially subluxed relative to the distal fibular tip (see next image). This is a normal finding which should not be misinterpreted for disease. **(Bottom)** Note the pseudosubluxation of the peroneus brevis tendon relative to the distal fibular tip. This is a normal finding.

TENDONS OVERVIEW

GRAPHIC & AXIAL T1, RIGHT ANKLE: PERONEUS QUARTUS MUSCLE

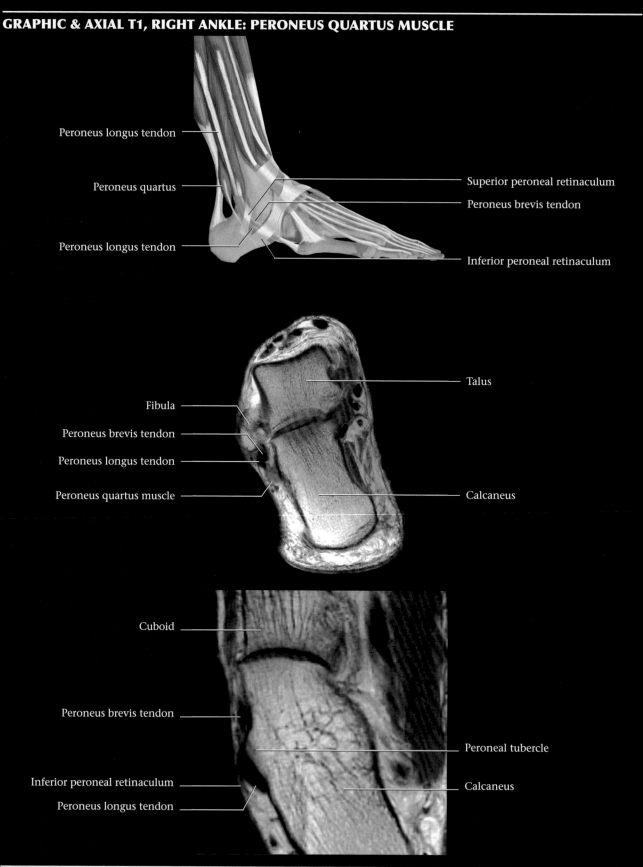

Peroneus longus tendon

Peroneus quartus

Peroneus longus tendon

Superior peroneal retinaculum

Peroneus brevis tendon

Inferior peroneal retinaculum

Fibula

Peroneus brevis tendon

Peroneus longus tendon

Peroneus quartus muscle

Talus

Calcaneus

Cuboid

Peroneus brevis tendon

Inferior peroneal retinaculum

Peroneus longus tendon

Peroneal tubercle

Calcaneus

(Top) The peroneus quartus is an accessory muscle that accompanies the peroneal tendons. It typically inserts into one of the peroneal tendons or calcaneus. It can crowd the peroneal tendons predisposing them to dislocation. **(Middle)** The peroneus quartus muscle is depicted as an accessory muscle/tendon unit adjacent to the peroneal tendons. When it inserts directly into one of the tendons it may be overlooked, as it may simulate a low lying peroneus brevis muscle with an accessory tendon slip. It should not be misinterpreted as a longitudinal split of the tendons. The presence of a peroneus quartus muscle is easiest to detect when it inserts into the calcaneus (seen here). **(Bottom)** The peroneal tubercle, a normal variant, is a calcaneal wall protuberance which separates the peroneal tendons. Hypertrophy of the tubercle predisposes to peroneus longus tendon tear.

SAGITTAL T1 MR, ANKLE: PERONEAL TENDONS

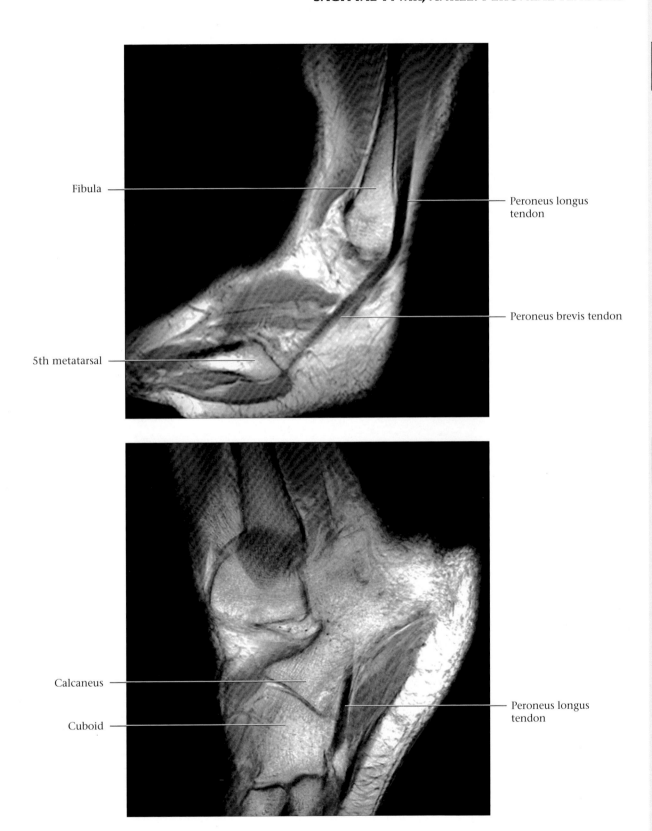

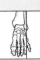

Fibula — Peroneus longus tendon

Peroneus brevis tendon

5th metatarsal —

Calcaneus —

Cuboid — Peroneus longus tendon

(Top) The peroneal tendons are optimally assessed on axial images but may be followed on sagittal images as they proceed toward their insertion sites. The peroneus brevis tendon is predisposed to friction and tearing as it descends within the fibular retromalleolar groove. **(Bottom)** The peroneus longus tendon traverses within three fibro-osseous tunnels. It first shares the retromalleolar groove with the peroneus brevis tendon. It then descends along the lateral wall of the calcaneus, where it can undergo friction posterior to the peroneal tubercle. Its final tunnel is plantar to the cuboid within the cuboid tunnel. In this image the peroneus longus tendon descends along the lateral wall of the calcaneus approaching its cuboid tunnel.

SAGITTAL T1 MR, ANKLE: PERONEAL TENDONS

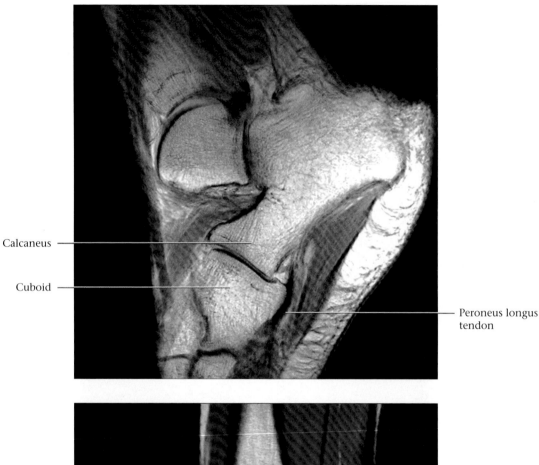

Calcaneus

Cuboid

Peroneus longus tendon

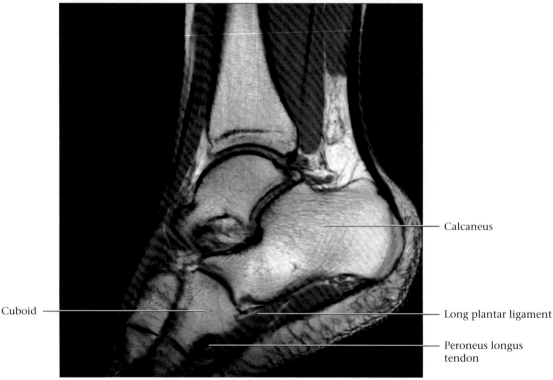

Calcaneus

Cuboid

Long plantar ligament

Peroneus longus tendon

(Top) In this image, the peroneus longus is seen starting to curve under the plantar surface of the cuboid to enter the cuboid tunnel. **(Bottom)** The peroneus longus tendon has now entered the tunnel under the cuboid. The tendon is held in place by a strong fibrous band derived from the long plantar ligament. Sequential sagittal images allow visualization of the peroneus longus tendon as it obliquely crosses the sole of the foot. The tendon is typically seen in cross section as a small linear, low signal structure deep to the plantar muscles.

Ankle

VII

TENDONS OVERVIEW

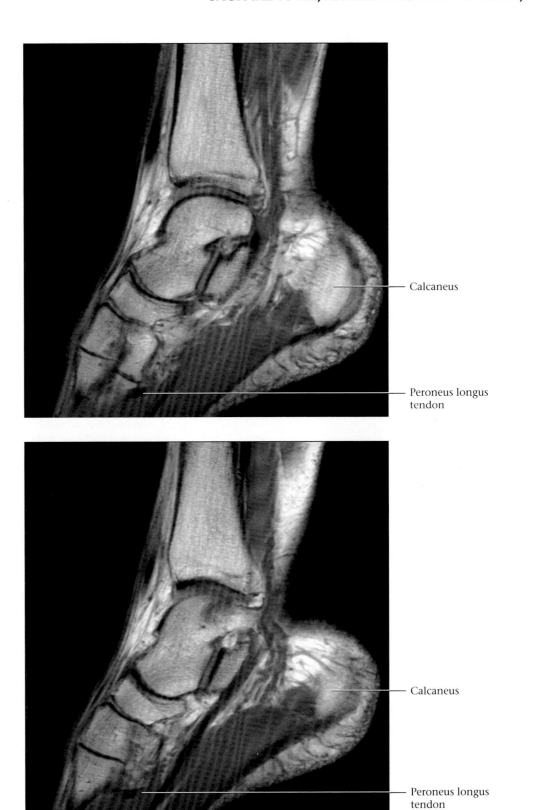

— Calcaneus

— Peroneus longus tendon

— Calcaneus

— Peroneus longus tendon

(Top) The peroneus longus tendon is seen obliquely traversing the plantar surface of the sole toward its insertion. **(Bottom)** The peroneus longus tendon is now under the 2nd metatarsal base. The insertion to the metatarsal is not always well seen on T1WI due to striation and magic angle effect.

Ankle

VII

LIGAMENTS OVERVIEW

Imaging Anatomy

Overview

- Imaging recommendations
  - Foot mildly plantar flexed: Decreases magic angle effect, visualizes calcaneofibular ligament
  - Routine T1 or PD, T2 FS axials
  - T2WI FS or GE coronals
  - T1WI & STIR sagittals
  - Axials optimal for detecting syndesmotic, lateral collateral, deltoid, spring ligaments, suboptimal for sinus tarsi ligaments
  - Sagittals optimal for sinus tarsi ligaments, inferoplantar component of spring, plantar, bifurcate; suboptimal for syndesmotic ligaments, lateral collateral ligaments, deltoid
  - Coronal images useful for all ligaments, optimal for calcaneofibular ligament & superomedial component of spring ligament
- Syndesmotic tibiofibular complex
  - Bind the fibrous distal tibiofibular joint
  - Composed of 1) anterior tibiofibular, 2) posterior tibiofibular, 3) inferior transverse, 4) interosseous tibiofibular
  - Optimally visualized on axial, coronal MR images; intermediate to low in signal
  - Anterior, posterior tibiofibular: May be heterogeneous due to fat between fascicles; oblique course, extend to level of talar dome
  - Inferior transverse: Thick, heterogeneous signal; band-like, extends distal to tibial posterior surface; tibial insertion almost at medial malleolus
  - Posterior tibiofibular ligament may simulate an intra-articular body on sagittal images
- Lateral collateral ligaments
  - Bind talus & calcaneus to fibula
  - Composed of 1) anterior talofibular ligament, 2) posterior talofibular ligament 3) calcaneofibular ligament
  - Anterior talofibular & posterior talofibular ligaments optimally visualized on axial images
  - Posterior talofibular, calcaneofibular well seen on coronal images
  - Ligaments reflect thickening of the capsule; therefore delineated by joint fluid on fluid sensitive images
  - Highlighted by fat, obliteration of fat indicative of disease
  - Insert on fibula at malleolar fossa
  - Talus is oblong shaped at level of lateral collateral ligaments
  - Posterior talofibular ligament may simulate an intra-articular body on sagittal images
  - Posterior talofibular ligament is fan shaped & striated at its insertion to fibula: Heterogeneity should not be misinterpreted for a tear
  - Anterior talofibular ligament should be straight, with a smooth undersurface
  - Calcaneofibular ligament is usually seen on axial images performed in mild plantar flexion
- Deltoid ligament
  - Subdivided into superficial & deep bands, many variations
  - Superficial subdivided into anterior tibiotalar, posterior tibiotalar, tibionavicular, tibiospring, tibiocalcaneal
  - Deep subdivided into anterior tibiotalar, posterior tibiotalar
  - Deep tibiotalar often striated
  - Superficial components originate from medial malleolus as continuous band, differentiation based on insertion sites
  - Tibiospring band continuous with superomedial component of spring ligament
  - Components highlighted by fat
- Tarsal canal & sinus tarsi ligaments
  - Limit talocalcaneal motion
  - **Cervical ligament**: Most anterior ligament, oblique course, calcaneal origin medial to extensor digitorum brevis, ascends upward, medially & anteriorly to inferolateral talar neck; whole ligament optimally visualized on coronal images; portions seen on consecutive sagittal, axial images; intermediate signal
  - **Talocalcaneal interosseous ligament**: Most medial & posterior ligament, oblique course, calcaneal origin anterior to posterior subtalar joint; ascends superiorly, medially to medial talar sulcus, intermediate to low signal
  - **Roots, inferior extensor retinaculum**: Medial: Most posterior, calcaneal insertion anterior to talocalcaneal interosseous ligament; intermediate: Calcaneal insertion posterior to cervical ligament; lateral: Calcaneal insertion lateral to extensor digitorum brevis muscle
- Spring ligament
  - Binds calcaneus to navicular, supports talar head & medial longitudinal arch
  - Superomedial, medioplantar oblique, inferoplantar longitudinal components
  - **Superomedial**: Strongest, hammock shaped; origin: Sustentaculum tali & tibiospring band of deltoid; insertion: Superomedial navicular; optimally seen on coronals, axials, lateral to tibialis posterior tendon, hugs talar head
  - **Medioplantar oblique**: Origin: Coronoid fossa; insertion: Plantar to navicular tuberosity, lateral to tibialis posterior tendon; best seen on axials; striated, oblique course
  - **Inferoplantar longitudinal**: Origin: Coronoid fossa; insertion: Navicular beak; optimally seen on axials, sagittals; short, straight course
- **Bifurcate ligament** origin: Calcaneal anterior process; insertion via two limbs to navicular & cuboid; thin, best seen on sagittal images lateral to inferoplantar longitudinal component of spring ligament
- Short & long plantar ligaments
  - Bind calcaneus & cuboid, support longitudinal arch; best seen on sagittals & axials
  - **Short plantar ligament** (plantar calcaneocuboid): Origin: Calcaneal anterior tubercle; insertion: Cuboid; very striated, medial, short
  - **Long plantar ligament**: Superficial to short plantar ligament: Origin: At & anterior to medial, lateral, anterior tubercles; insertion: Cuboid, bases 2nd-5th metatarsals; striated

GRAPHICS, TIBIOFIBULAR SYNDESMOTIC LIGAMENTS

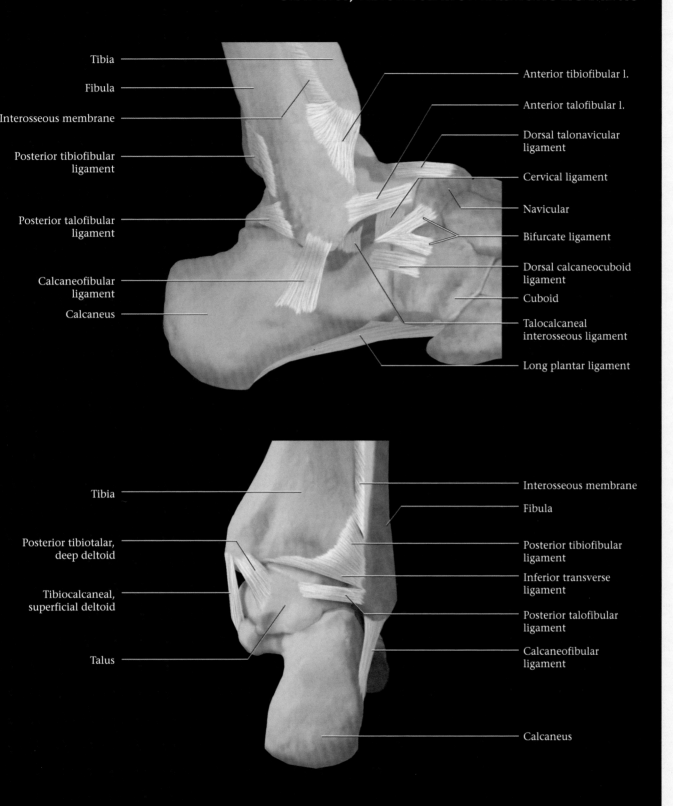

(Top) Lateral view of ankle. Two groups of ligaments support the lateral ankle: 1) the syndesmotic ligaments, including the anterior tibiofibular, posterior tibiofibular & syndesmotic ligaments & 2) the lateral collateral ligaments, including the anterior talofibular, posterior talofibular & calcaneofibular ligaments. Other ligaments that bind the hindfoot include the talocalcaneal interosseous ligament & cervical ligament in the sinus tarsi & smaller superficial talocalcaneal ligaments. Note the bifurcate ligament which extends from the calcaneus to the navicular and cuboid. **(Bottom)** Posterior view of the ankle. The tibiofibular ligaments are obliquely oriented & their fibular origin is above the fibular malleolar fossa. The inferior transverse ligament (the inferior portion of the posterior tibiofibular ligament) extends distal to the tibial posterior surface.

LIGAMENTS OVERVIEW

AXIAL T1 AND T2 FS MR, RIGHT ANKLE: TIBIOFIBULAR SYNDESMOTIC LIGAMENTS

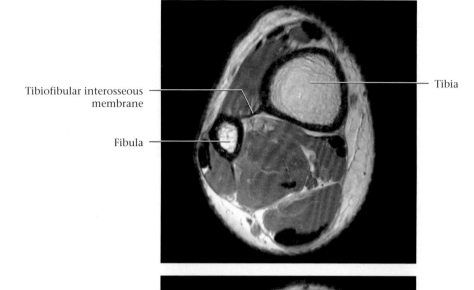

Tibiofibular interosseous membrane

Fibula

Tibia

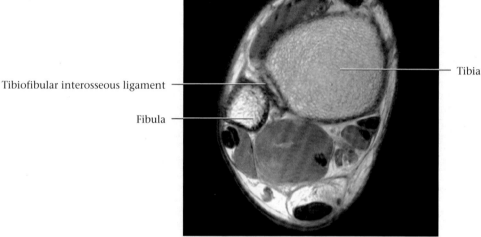

Tibiofibular interosseous ligament

Fibula

Tibia

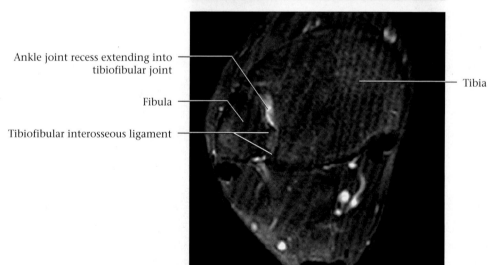

Ankle joint recess extending into tibiofibular joint

Fibula

Tibiofibular interosseous ligament

Tibia

(Top) The tibiofibular interosseous membrane. The membrane is typically visualized as a well defined, low signal structure, binding the tibia & fibula. Just above the ankle joint, the membrane becomes less defined and may even be discontinuous. (Middle) The tibiofibular interosseous ligament. The ligament is a distal thickening of the tibiofibular membrane. Occasionally, it may be visualized as a distinct structure as in this image, but often it may be poorly defined, discontinuous, and even absent. (Bottom) A fluid filled recess, measuring between 0.5-1.0 cm extends from the ankle joint into the tibiofibular fibrous joint. The tibiofibular ligament is frequently present at the superior margin of the recess. In this particular case it extends posterior to the recess.

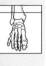

Ankle

LIGAMENTS OVERVIEW

AXIAL T1 MR, RIGHT ANKLE: TIBIOFIBULAR SYNDESMOTIC LIGAMENTS

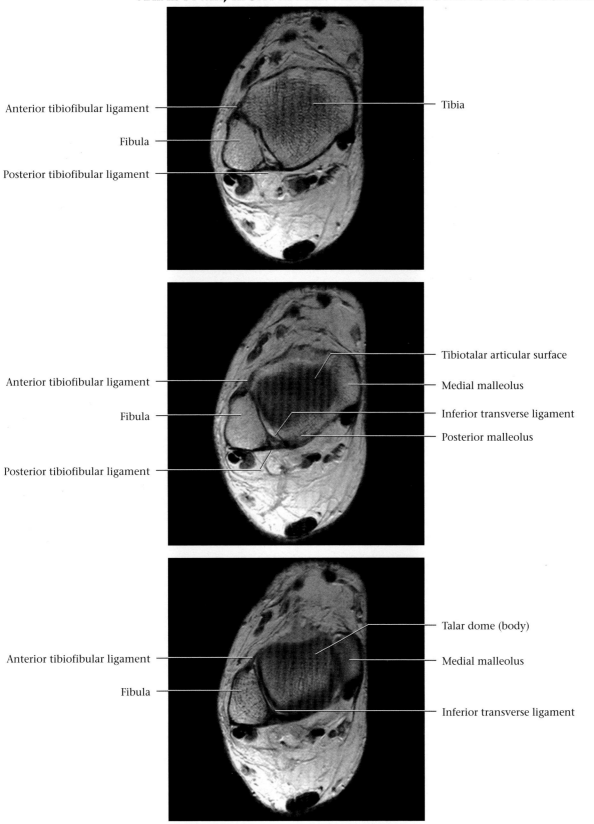

Anterior tibiofibular ligament ⎯⎯ ⎯⎯ Tibia

Fibula

Posterior tibiofibular ligament

⎯⎯ Tibiotalar articular surface

Anterior tibiofibular ligament ⎯⎯ ⎯⎯ Medial malleolus

Fibula ⎯⎯ ⎯⎯ Inferior transverse ligament

⎯⎯ Posterior malleolus

Posterior tibiofibular ligament ⎯⎯

⎯⎯ Talar dome (body)

Anterior tibiofibular ligament ⎯⎯ ⎯⎯ Medial malleolus

Fibula ⎯⎯

⎯⎯ Inferior transverse ligament

(Top) The anterior and posterior tibiofibular ligaments above the ankle joint. The ligaments are optimally seen on axial images. The anterior tibiofibular ligament is often heterogeneous and may appear discontinuous due to fat in between its fascicles. **(Middle)** Anterior and posterior tibiofibular ligaments at the ankle joint. The ligaments are visualized at, or slightly below, the ankle joint. Note that at this level, the fibula is round without the more distal medial indentation of the malleolar fossa. **(Bottom)** The anterior and posterior tibiofibular ligaments at the talar dome (talus is square at this level). The very inferior aspect of the anterior tibiofibular ligament has been coined Bassett ligament. The inferior transverse ligament is continuous with the posterior tibiofibular ligament but extends distal to the posterior tibial articular surface.

Ankle

VII

LIGAMENTS OVERVIEW

AXIAL T2 FS MR & CORONAL T1 MR: TIBIOFIBULAR SYNDESMOTIC LIGAMENTS

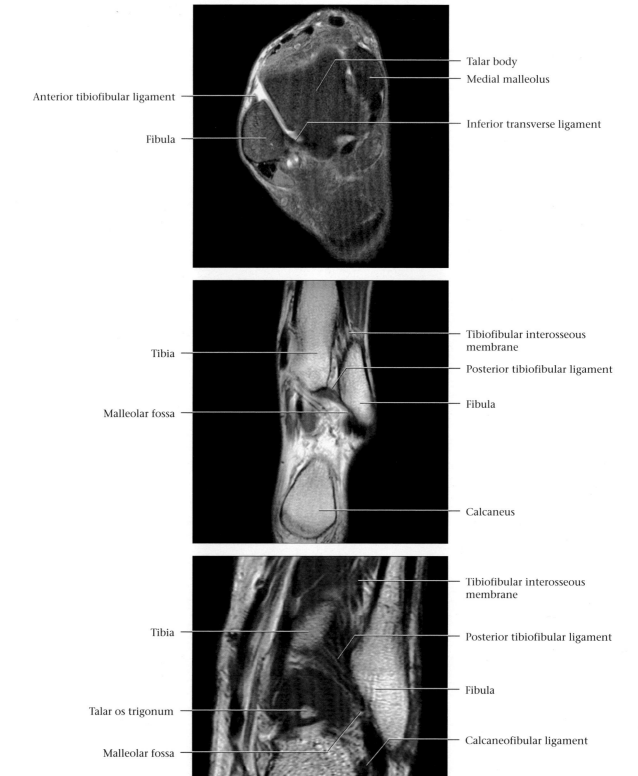

Anterior tibiofibular ligament

Fibula

Talar body

Medial malleolus

Inferior transverse ligament

Tibia

Malleolar fossa

Tibiofibular interosseous membrane

Posterior tibiofibular ligament

Fibula

Calcaneus

Tibia

Talar os trigonum

Malleolar fossa

Tibiofibular interosseous membrane

Posterior tibiofibular ligament

Fibula

Calcaneofibular ligament

Calcaneus

(Top) Axial T2 FS image of the right anterior tibiofibular ligaments at the talar dome. Note the square shape of the talus and the round shape of the fibula. Because of the oblique descent of the anterior tibiofibular ligament it may appear discontinuous at its fibular insertion as is seen in this image. This should not be misinterpreted as a tear. **(Middle)** Coronal T1 of the left ankle shows the posterior tibiofibular ligament. The downward oblique course of the ligament is best appreciated on coronal images. The ligament descends from its superior position on the tibia toward its more inferior fibular insertion. Note that the ligament inserts on the fibula above the malleolar fossa. **(Bottom)** Coronal T1 of the left ankle shows the posterior tibiofibular ligament. The striation of the ligament is due to fat interposed between its fascicles and should not be misinterpreted as a tear on axial images.

LIGAMENTS OVERVIEW

CORONAL T2 FS MR, LEFT ANKLE: TIBIOFIBULAR SYNDESMOTIC LIGAMENTS

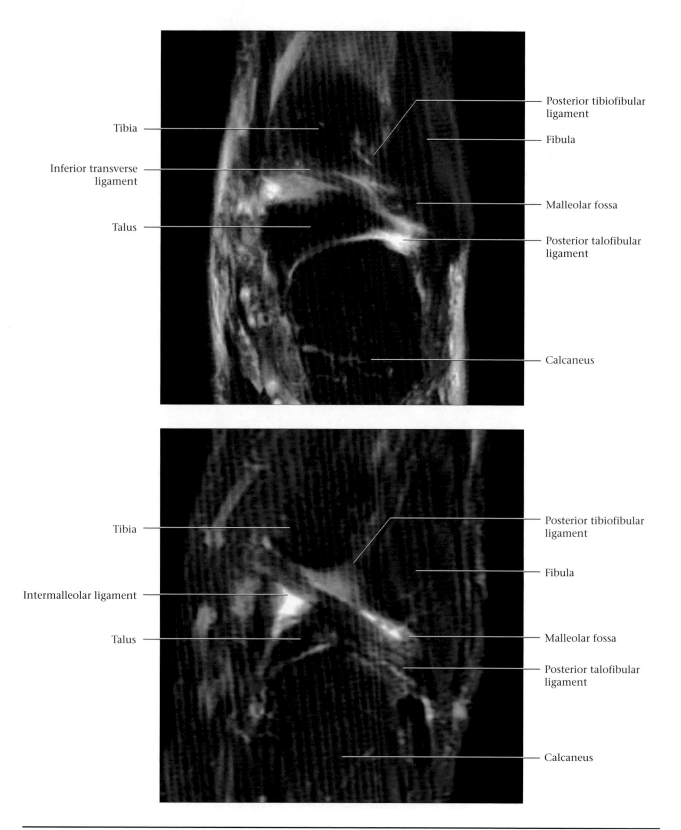

Tibia

Inferior transverse ligament

Talus

Posterior tibiofibular ligament

Fibula

Malleolar fossa

Posterior talofibular ligament

Calcaneus

Tibia

Intermalleolar ligament

Talus

Posterior tibiofibular ligament

Fibula

Malleolar fossa

Posterior talofibular ligament

Calcaneus

(Top) Posterior tibiofibular ligament on coronal fluid weighted fat suppressed image. Note that the inferior transverse ligament extends distal to the posterior tibia, forming a posterior labrum & deepening the posterior ankle joint. Its tibial insertion is quite far medial, almost to the level of the medial malleolus. The tibiofibular ligaments insert onto the fibula above the malleolar fossa while the talofibular ligaments insert below it. **(Bottom)** The intermalleolar ligament on coronal fluid weighted fat suppressed image. The intermalleolar ligament, also called the tibial slip, is a normal variant which extends from the posterior talofibular ligament almost to the tibial medial malleolus. This ligament is found between the inferior transverse and posterior talofibular ligaments. It may be difficult to distinguish it from the inferior transverse ligament.

LIGAMENTS OVERVIEW

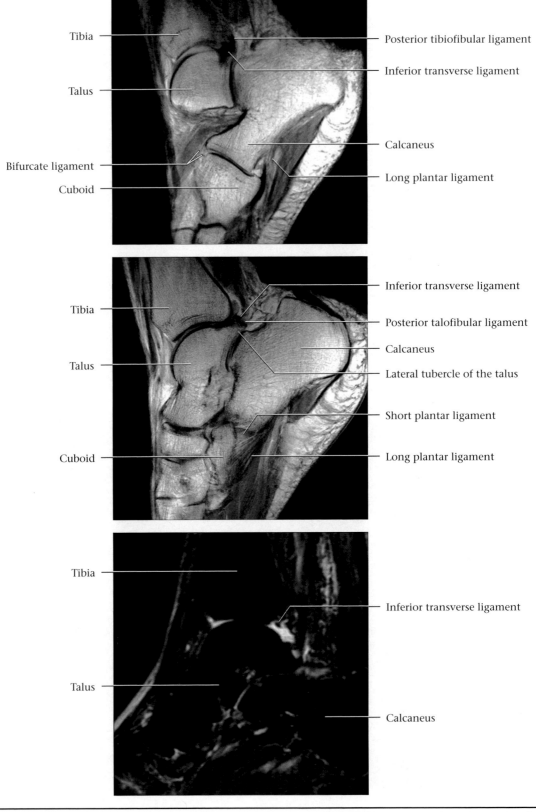

Tibia — Posterior tibiofibular ligament

Inferior transverse ligament

Talus —

Bifurcate ligament — Calcaneus

Cuboid — Long plantar ligament

Tibia — Inferior transverse ligament

Posterior talofibular ligament

Calcaneus

Talus — Lateral tubercle of the talus

Short plantar ligament

Cuboid — Long plantar ligament

Tibia —

Inferior transverse ligament

Talus —

Calcaneus

(Top) T1 weighted sagittal image demonstrates the inferior extent of the tibiofibular ligament distal to the tibial posterior surface. The sagittal images are suboptimal for visualizing the tibiofibular and talofibular ligaments. **(Middle)** On sagittal images the tibiofibular and talofibular ligaments are typically seen in cross section as small low signal intensity oval structures, posterior to the talus, and should not be misinterpreted as intra-articular bodies. Following the ligaments on sequential images will obviate this problem. Note that the posterior talofibular ligament is barely visualized as it originates from the lateral tubercle of the talus. **(Bottom)** Sagittal STIR image depicts the inferior transverse ligament surrounded by fluid, simulating an intra-articular body.

SAGITTAL & AXIAL T1 MR, RIGHT ANKLE: TIBIOFIBULAR SYNDESMOTIC LIGAMENTS

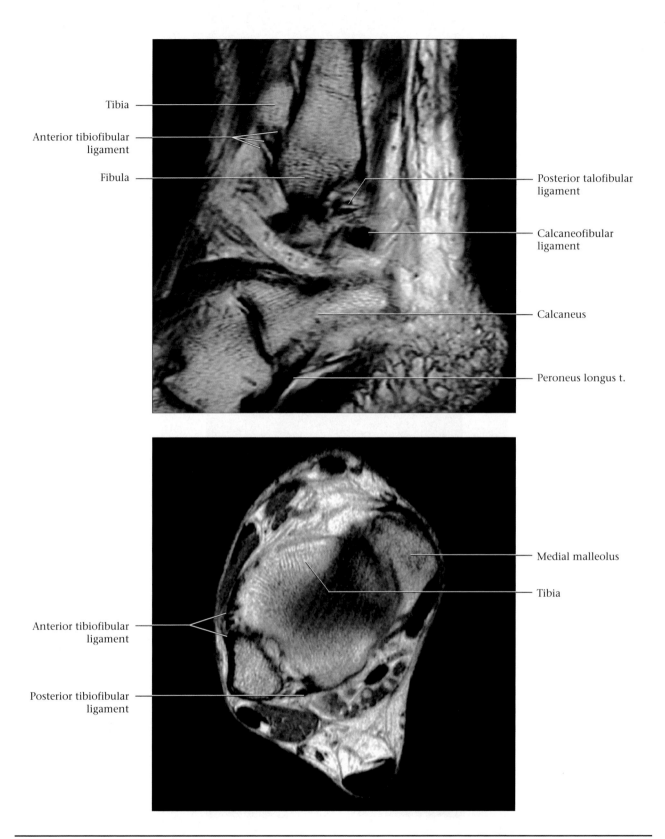

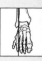

(Top) A far lateral sagittal T1WI allows a glimpse of the anterior tibiofibular ligament traversing between the tibia and fibula. Note the striation of the ligament. The calcaneofibular ligament is also visualized. **(Bottom)** Normal striation of the anterior tibiofibular ligament on axial T1WI. Because of the oblique descent of the anterior tibiofibular ligament and the fat interposed between its fascicles it may appear discontinuous. This should not be misinterpreted as a tear.

LIGAMENTS OVERVIEW

CORONAL T2 FS MR LEFT ANKLE & AXIAL T2 RIGHT ANKLE: LATERAL COLLATERAL LIGAMENTS

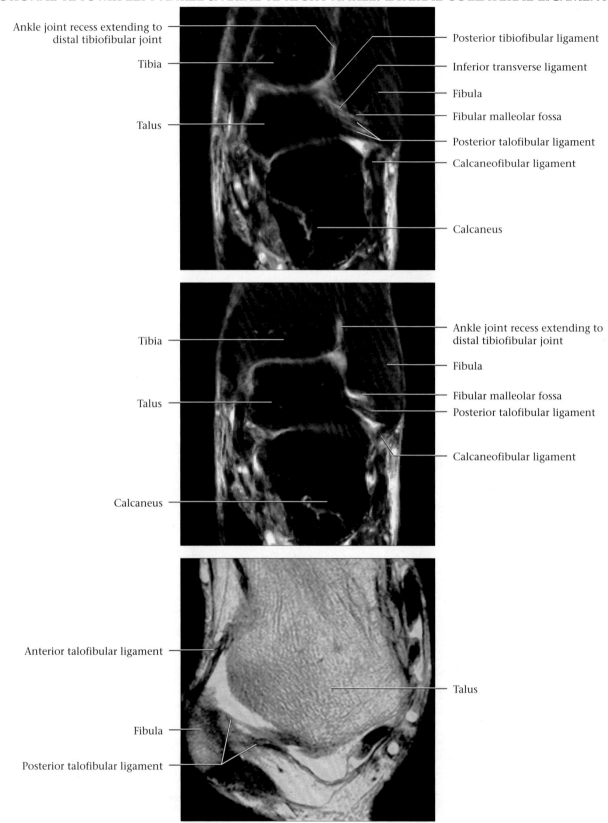

(Top) Coronal fat suppressed image of the lateral collateral ligaments. The posterior talofibular, calcaneofibular &, less frequently, anterior talofibular ligaments are well seen on coronal images. The fibular origin of the posterior talofibular ligament is at the level of the malleolar fossa. Note a normal ankle joint recess extending into the distal tibiofibular joint. (Middle) Slightly more anterior coronal fat suppressed image. The posterior talofibular ligament is visualized as a distinct structure from the posterior tibiofibular ligament. (Bottom) Lateral collateral ligaments on T2 axial image. The ligaments are optimally seen on axial images. Since these ligaments are thickening of the capsule, they are highlighted by fluid. Note the fan shaped & striated insertion of the posterior talofibular ligament which should not to be mistaken for a tear.

LIGAMENTS OVERVIEW

SEQUENTIAL CORONAL T1 MR, LEFT ANKLE: LATERAL COLLATERAL LIGAMENT

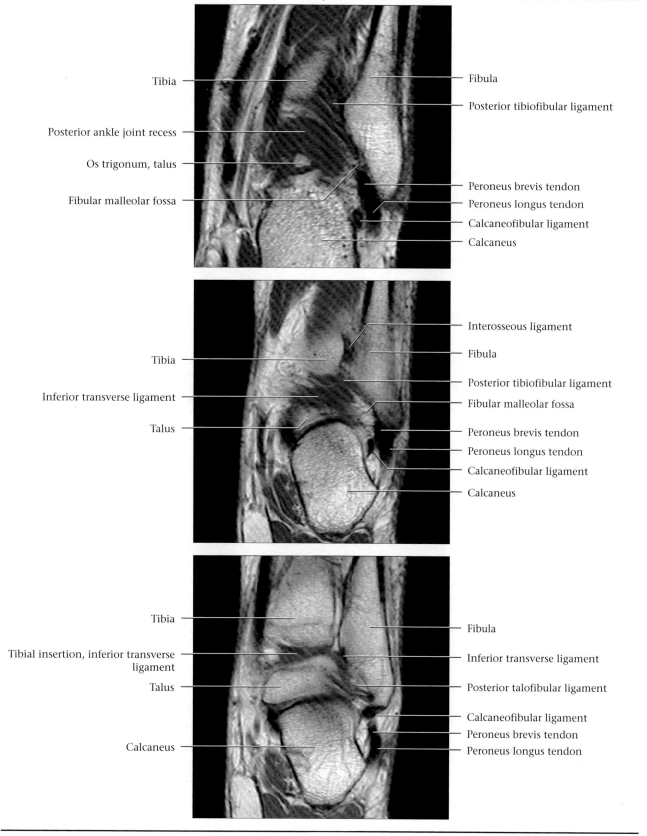

(Top) A posterior coronal T1WI of the calcaneal insertion of the calcaneofibular ligament. The ligament can be followed on sequential coronal images from its fibular origin to its calcaneal insertion. While the ligament is occasionally seen on axial images, its cross section is consistently visualized on coronal images. Note the fat surrounding the ligament; obliteration of this fat is consistent with disease of the ligament. **(Middle)** Calcaneofibular ligament on a more anterior coronal T1WI. Note proximity of the ligament to peroneal tendons, which can be used to locate the ligament. A tear of the ligament may produce reactive fluid within the common peroneal tendon sheath; this should not to be mistaken for peroneal tenosynovitis. **(Bottom)** In a more anterior image, the origin of the calcaneofibular ligament from the fibula is visualized.

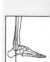

LIGAMENTS OVERVIEW

AXIAL & SAGITTAL T1 MR, RIGHT ANKLE: LATERAL COLLATERAL LIGAMENTS

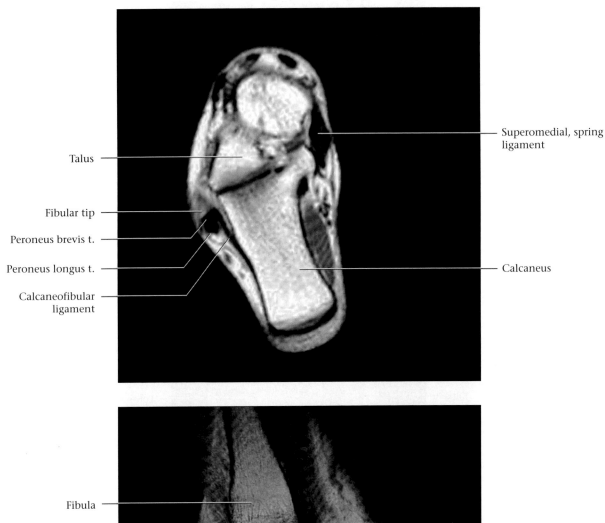

Talus

Fibular tip

Peroneus brevis t.

Peroneus longus t.

Calcaneofibular ligament

Superomedial, spring ligament

Calcaneus

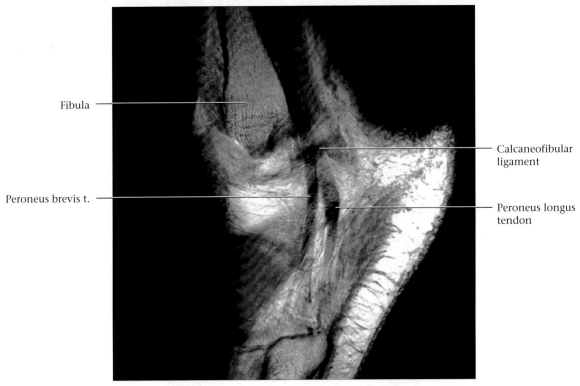

Fibula

Peroneus brevis t.

Calcaneofibular ligament

Peroneus longus tendon

(Top) Calcaneofibular ligament on axial T1WI. The calcaneofibular ligament changes orientation with ankle movements. In mild plantar flexion the ligament becomes close to horizontal in orientation and may be visualized on axial images as it hugs the calcaneus, deep to the peroneal tendons. Its location deep to the peroneal tendons is a clue in locating this ligament. (Bottom) On far sagittal image the calcaneofibular ligament may be visualized, due to partial volume averaging, as a low signal shadow superimposed on the peroneal tendons. Note that in this patient, scanned in plantarflexion, the calcaneofibular ligament is relatively horizontal. Mild plantar flexion of the ankle aids in detecting the calcaneofibular ligament on axial images because of this relatively horizontal orientation.

LIGAMENTS OVERVIEW

SAGITTAL T1 MR: LATERAL COLLATERAL LIGAMENTS

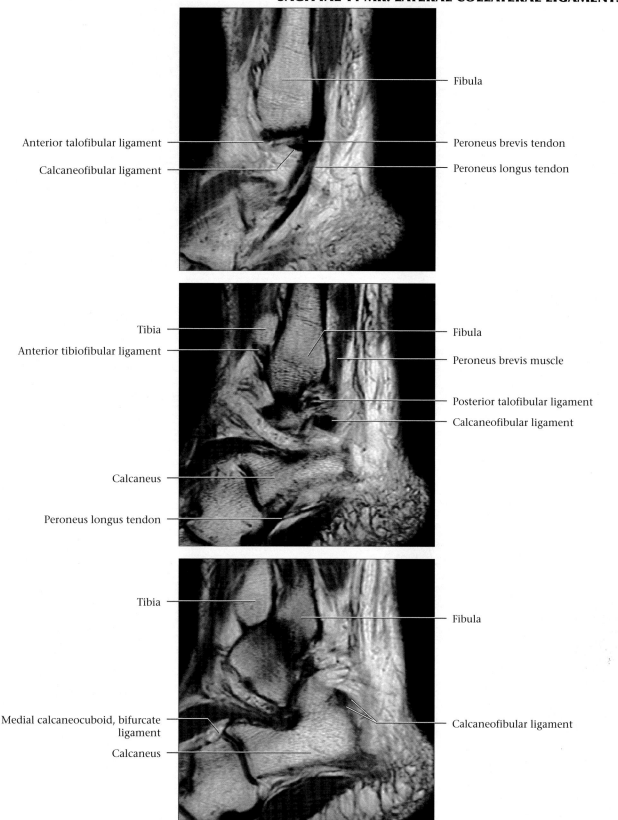

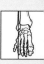
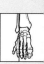

Anterior talofibular ligament — Fibula

Calcaneofibular ligament — Peroneus brevis tendon

— Peroneus longus tendon

Tibia — Fibula

Anterior tibiofibular ligament — Peroneus brevis muscle

— Posterior talofibular ligament

— Calcaneofibular ligament

Calcaneus —

Peroneus longus tendon —

Tibia — Fibula

Medial calcaneocuboid, bifurcate ligament —

— Calcaneofibular ligament

Calcaneus —

(Top) Sequential sagittal T1 weighted images of the calcaneofibular ligament, lateral to medial. Occasionally the ligament may be visualized on sequential sagittal images from its fibular origin to its posterior calcaneal insertion. **(Middle)** The calcaneofibular ligament is now visualized as it is traversing the region beneath the peroneal tendons (peroneals not well seen in this image). Note also the striated posterior talofibular ligament behind the fibula. **(Bottom)** Sagittal T1WI of the calcaneofibular ligament. The calcaneofibular ligament is now seen in cross section as it inserts onto the calcaneus.

LIGAMENTS OVERVIEW

GRAPHIC & CORONAL PD MR, RIGHT ANKLE: DELTOID LIGAMENT

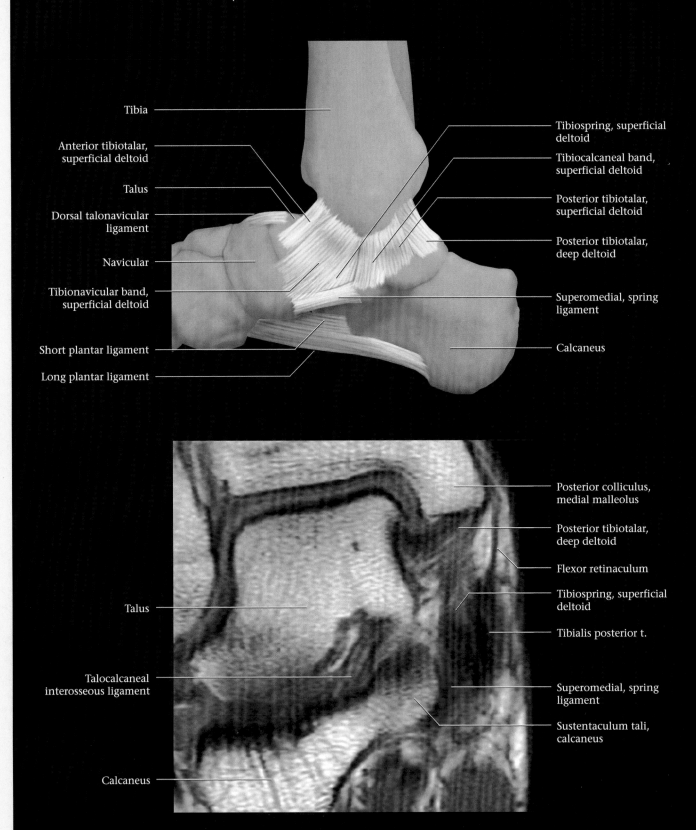

Tibia

Anterior tibiotalar, superficial deltoid

Talus

Dorsal talonavicular ligament

Navicular

Tibionavicular band, superficial deltoid

Short plantar ligament

Long plantar ligament

Tibiospring, superficial deltoid

Tibiocalcaneal band, superficial deltoid

Posterior tibiotalar, superficial deltoid

Posterior tibiotalar, deep deltoid

Superomedial, spring ligament

Calcaneus

Talus

Talocalcaneal interosseous ligament

Calcaneus

Posterior colliculus, medial malleolus

Posterior tibiotalar, deep deltoid

Flexor retinaculum

Tibiospring, superficial deltoid

Tibialis posterior t.

Superomedial, spring ligament

Sustentaculum tali, calcaneus

(Top) Medial view of ankle. The deltoid ligament has many variable bands but is commonly divided into deep & superficial components. The deep includes the anterior & posterior tibiotalar bands & the superficial includes anterior & posterior tibiotalar, tibiocalcaneal, tibiospring & tibionavicular bands. The superficial deltoid is band-like and distinction between its various components relies on their sites of insertion. (Bottom) Deep tibiotalar deltoid on coronal proton density image. Note deep location, relative horizontal orientation & striation of deep tibiotalar component. Obliteration & discontinuity of the striation is indicative of injury to ligament. The tibiospring component, partially visualized on this image, is continuous with the superomedial spring ligament. The tibialis posterior tendon is found medial to the tibiospring component of the deltoid.

AXIAL T1 MR, LEFT ANKLE: DELTOID LIGAMENT

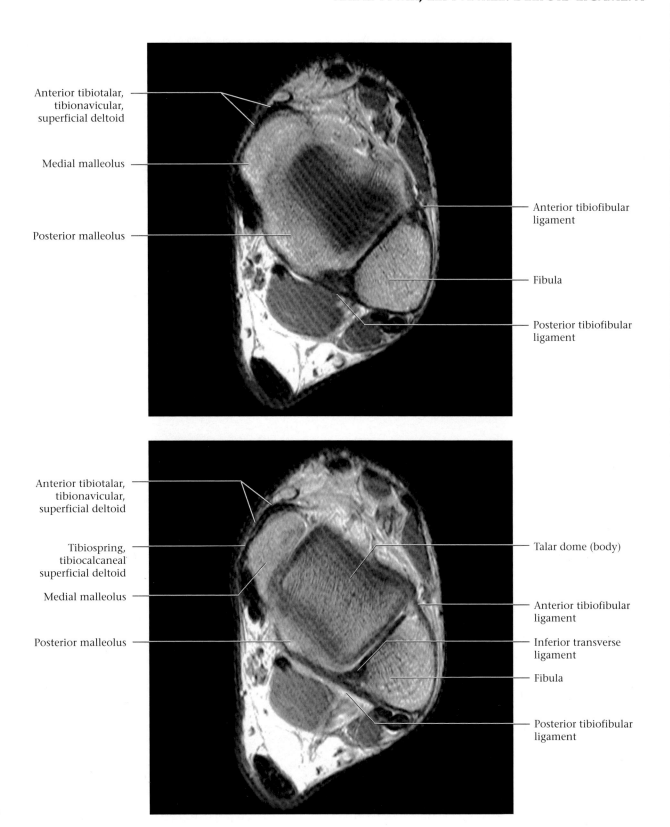

Anterior tibiotalar, tibionavicular, superficial deltoid

Medial malleolus

Posterior malleolus

Anterior tibiofibular ligament

Fibula

Posterior tibiofibular ligament

Anterior tibiotalar, tibionavicular, superficial deltoid

Tibiospring, tibiocalcaneal superficial deltoid

Medial malleolus

Posterior malleolus

Talar dome (body)

Anterior tibiofibular ligament

Inferior transverse ligament

Fibula

Posterior tibiofibular ligament

(Top) Origin of the superficial deltoid ligament on axial T1WI. The superficial deltoid ligament originates from anterior & posterior colliculi of medial malleolus as a single contiguous band. The band's various components including the tibionavicular, anterior & posterior tibiotalar, tibiospring & tibiocalcaneal have no fat planes between them & are differentiated from each other mainly based on their relative origin & insertion sites. The superficial tibionavicular and anterior tibiotalar ligaments originate together from the anterior colliculus. Their relative positions to each other is variable, therefore distinction between them on axial images is difficult. **(Bottom)** An axial T1WI located slightly more distally depicting the very origin of the tibiocalcaneal and tibiospring ligaments of the deltoid.

AXIAL T2 MR, LEFT ANKLE: DELTOID LIGAMENT

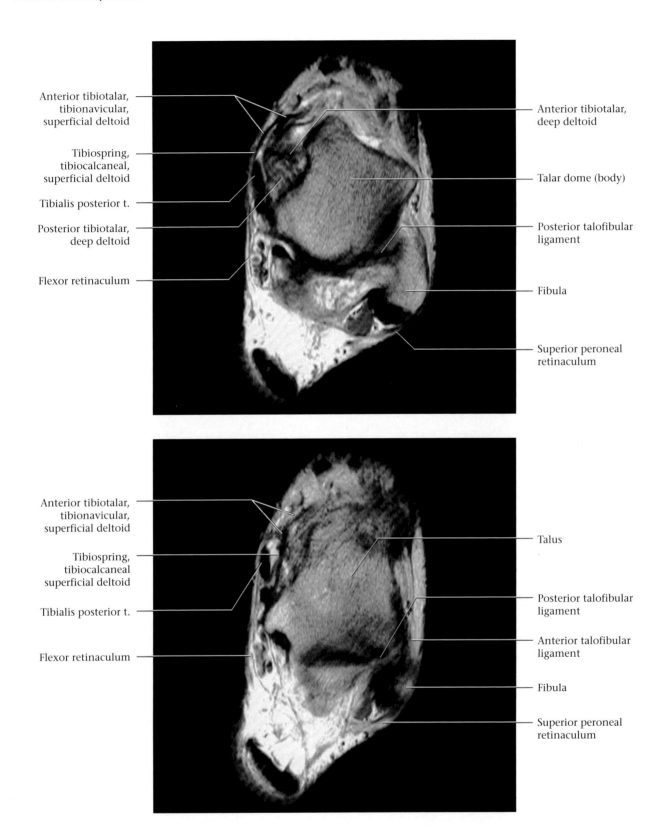

Anterior tibiotalar, tibionavicular, superficial deltoid

Tibiospring, tibiocalcaneal, superficial deltoid

Tibialis posterior t.

Posterior tibiotalar, deep deltoid

Flexor retinaculum

Anterior tibiotalar, deep deltoid

Talar dome (body)

Posterior talofibular ligament

Fibula

Superior peroneal retinaculum

Anterior tibiotalar, tibionavicular, superficial deltoid

Tibiospring, tibiocalcaneal superficial deltoid

Tibialis posterior t.

Flexor retinaculum

Talus

Posterior talofibular ligament

Anterior talofibular ligament

Fibula

Superior peroneal retinaculum

(Top) An axial T2WI at level of talar dome depicts the origin of the tibiocalcaneal and tibiospring ligaments of the deltoid. Note the striation of the deep tibiotalar deltoid. Note also the proximity of the tibialis posterior tendon to the deltoid. Fluid in the tendon sheath of the tibialis posterior ovendon may be seen following deltoid injury and should not be misinterpreted as tenosynovitis. (Bottom) An axial T2WI located slightly more distally depicts the origin of the tibiocalcaneal and tibiospring ligaments of the deltoid. Both the tibiospring & tibiocalcaneal insert on the sustentaculum tali; the tibiospring (which also inserts on the superomedial spring ligament) is anterior to the tibiocalcaneal but no fat plane is present between them & the division is almost arbitrary.

LIGAMENTS OVERVIEW

SEQUENTIAL CORONAL T1 MR, RIGHT ANKLE: DELTOID LIGAMENT

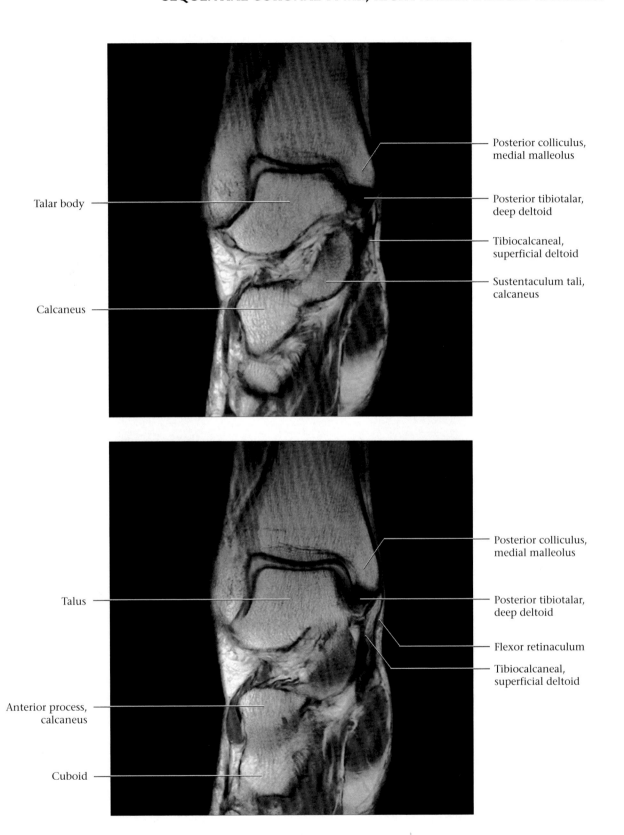

Talar body

Calcaneus

Posterior colliculus, medial malleolus

Posterior tibiotalar, deep deltoid

Tibiocalcaneal, superficial deltoid

Sustentaculum tali, calcaneus

Talus

Anterior process, calcaneus

Cuboid

Posterior colliculus, medial malleolus

Posterior tibiotalar, deep deltoid

Flexor retinaculum

Tibiocalcaneal, superficial deltoid

(Top) A posterior T1WI of the deltoid ligament depicts the deep tibiotalar band and superficial tibiocalcaneal band of the deltoid. The deep tibiotalar band of the deltoid is typically identified on coronal images as it originates from the posterior colliculus of the medial malleolus. Its fascicles tend to be more horizontal and more striated than those of the superficial band. The tibiocalcaneal band is often seen superficial to the deep tibiotalar deltoid on coronal images. **(Bottom)** A more anterior coronal T1 image still depicts the deep tibiotalar deltoid and tibiocalcaneal band of the superficial deltoid ligament. The distinction between the slightly more anterior tibiospring and the tibiocalcaneal ligaments, however, is often arbitrary.

SEQUENTIAL CORONAL T1 MR, RIGHT ANKLE: DELTOID LIGAMENT

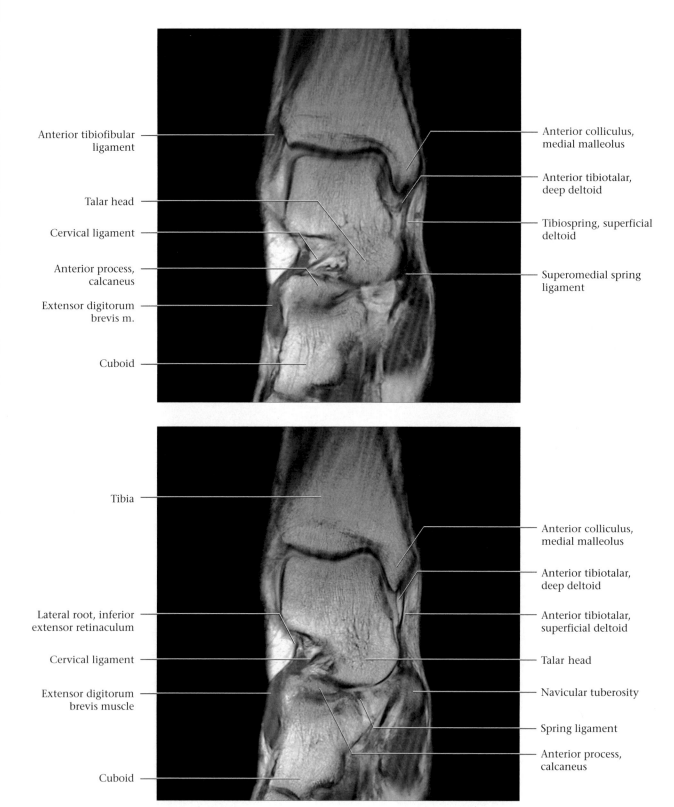

Anterior tibiofibular ligament

Talar head

Cervical ligament

Anterior process, calcaneus

Extensor digitorum brevis m.

Cuboid

Anterior colliculus, medial malleolus

Anterior tibiotalar, deep deltoid

Tibiospring, superficial deltoid

Superomedial spring ligament

Tibia

Lateral root, inferior extensor retinaculum

Cervical ligament

Extensor digitorum brevis muscle

Cuboid

Anterior colliculus, medial malleolus

Anterior tibiotalar, deep deltoid

Anterior tibiotalar, superficial deltoid

Talar head

Navicular tuberosity

Spring ligament

Anterior process, calcaneus

(Top) Slightly more anterior image of the deltoid depicting the tibiospring band. The bands of the superficial deltoid ligament are often only arbitrarily distinguished from each other on the coronal images. While this image is marked as tibiospring deltoid, it may reflect partial volume averaging with the adjacent bands of the superficial deltoid. Note a glimpse of the striated anterior tibiofibular ligament originating from the tibia. **(Bottom)** Anterior coronal image. Because of the obliquity of the superficial tibiotalar and tibionavicular bands, they are rarely seen on coronal images. The tibiotalar can occasionally be identified as a far anterior low signal band descending from the anterior colliculus of the medial malleolus.

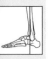

SAGITTAL T1 MR: DELTOID LIGAMENT

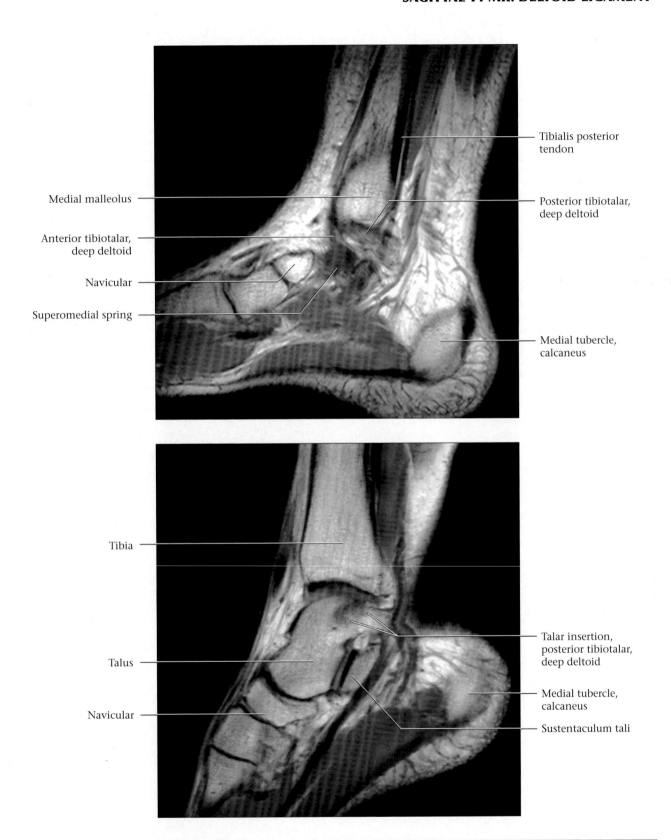

Tibialis posterior tendon

Medial malleolus

Posterior tibiotalar, deep deltoid

Anterior tibiotalar, deep deltoid

Navicular

Superomedial spring

Medial tubercle, calcaneus

Tibia

Talar insertion, posterior tibiotalar, deep deltoid

Talus

Medial tubercle, calcaneus

Navicular

Sustentaculum tali

(Top) Anterior & posterior tibiotalar bands, deep deltoid, on far medial sagittal image. The anterior & posterior tibiotalar components originate from the anterior & posterior colliculi of the medial malleolus & intercollicular area respectively. Both components are striated. The anterior tibiotalar may be small or absent. It is best seen on sagittal & axial images of the ankle. The posterior deep tibiotalar component is consistently seen on both axial & sagittal images. (Bottom) A more medial sagittal image depicts the talar insertion of the posterior tibiotalar band of deep deltoid. The low signal band should not be confused with an osteochondral talar lesion.

GRAPHICS, TARSAL CANAL & SINUS TARSI LIGAMENTS

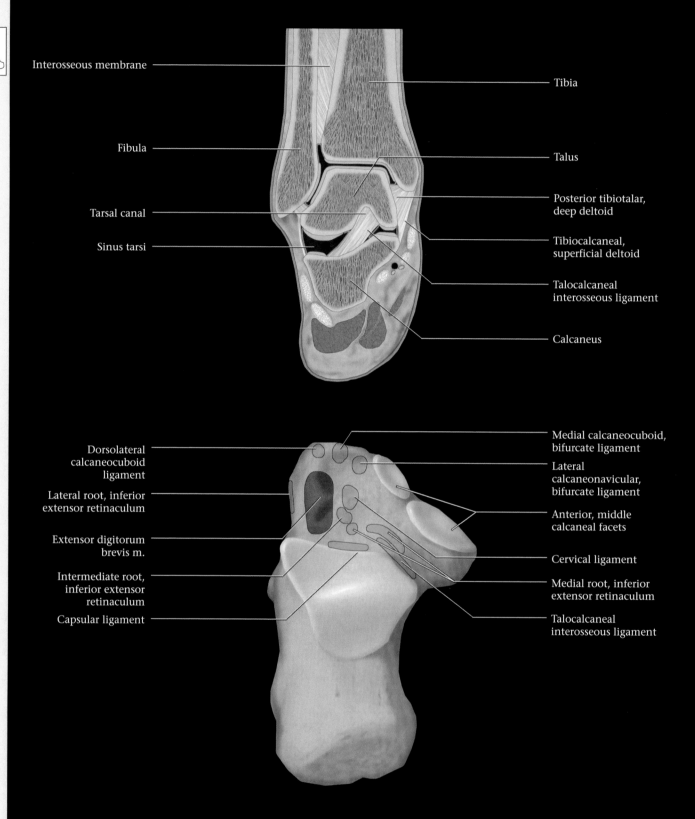

Interosseous membrane

Fibula

Tarsal canal

Sinus tarsi

Tibia

Talus

Posterior tibiotalar, deep deltoid

Tibiocalcaneal, superficial deltoid

Talocalcaneal interosseous ligament

Calcaneus

Dorsolateral calcaneocuboid ligament

Lateral root, inferior extensor retinaculum

Extensor digitorum brevis m.

Intermediate root, inferior extensor retinaculum

Capsular ligament

Medial calcaneocuboid, bifurcate ligament

Lateral calcaneonavicular, bifurcate ligament

Anterior, middle calcaneal facets

Cervical ligament

Medial root, inferior extensor retinaculum

Talocalcaneal interosseous ligament

(Top) Drawing of sinus tarsi ligaments. The tarsal canal is a space between the posterior subtalar joint & sustentaculum tali, traversed by the talocalcaneal interosseous ligament. The sinus tarsi is a more lateral space between the talus & calcaneus which is continuous with the tarsal canal. The sinus tarsi is traversed by roots of inferior extensor retinaculum & by the cervical ligament. **(Bottom)** Calcaneal insertions of sinus tarsi ligaments. The talocalcaneal interosseous ligament is most medial & posterior while cervical ligament is most anterior. The intermediate root of inferior extensor retinaculum is immediately posterior to the cervical ligament while the lateral root is lateral to the origin of the extensor digitorum brevis muscle. The medial root has 2 calcaneal & 1 talar insertions.

LIGAMENTS OVERVIEW

CORONAL T1, SAGITTAL T1 & SAGITTAL T2 FS MR: SINUS TARSI LIGAMENTS

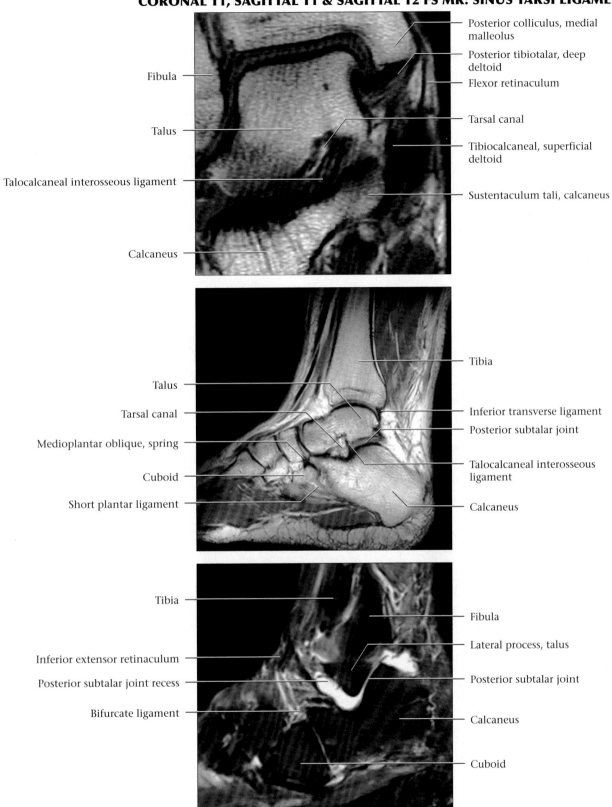

Top image labels:
- Fibula
- Talus
- Talocalcaneal interosseous ligament
- Calcaneus
- Posterior colliculus, medial malleolus
- Posterior tibiotalar, deep deltoid
- Flexor retinaculum
- Tarsal canal
- Tibiocalcaneal, superficial deltoid
- Sustentaculum tali, calcaneus

Middle image labels:
- Talus
- Tarsal canal
- Medioplantar oblique, spring
- Cuboid
- Short plantar ligament
- Tibia
- Inferior transverse ligament
- Posterior subtalar joint
- Talocalcaneal interosseous ligament
- Calcaneus

Bottom image labels:
- Tibia
- Inferior extensor retinaculum
- Posterior subtalar joint recess
- Bifurcate ligament
- Fibula
- Lateral process, talus
- Posterior subtalar joint
- Calcaneus
- Cuboid

(Top) Talocalcaneal interosseous ligament. The ligament traverses the tarsal canal and ascends obliquely & medially to insert on the talar sulcus. The ligament is best identified on coronal & sagittal images as the most posterior & medial of sinus tarsi ligaments. Its calcaneal insertion is just anterior to the posterior subtalar joint. **(Middle)** A sagittal image depicts the interosseous ligament as a band extending from the talus to the calcaneus, found anterior to the posterior subtalar joint. This ligament is typically found on the most medial sagittal images of the sinus tarsi. **(Bottom)** Sinus tarsi fluid often implies acute or chronic disease. However, a fluid filled recess may extend from the posterior subtalar joint into the sinus tarsi. This should not be misinterpreted as pathology of the sinus tarsi.

CORONAL & SAGITTAL T1 MR, LEFT ANKLE: SINUS TARSI LIGAMENTS

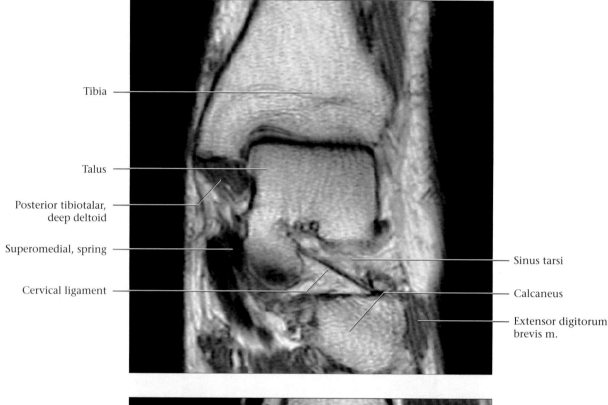

Tibia

Talus

Posterior tibiotalar, deep deltoid

Superomedial, spring

Cervical ligament

Sinus tarsi

Calcaneus

Extensor digitorum brevis m.

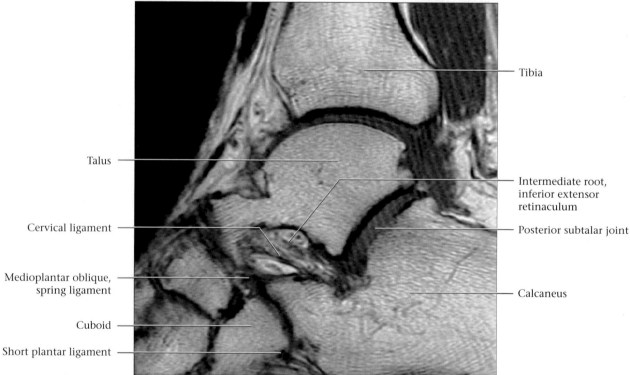

Talus

Cervical ligament

Medioplantar oblique, spring ligament

Cuboid

Short plantar ligament

Tibia

Intermediate root, inferior extensor retinaculum

Posterior subtalar joint

Calcaneus

(**Top**) Cervical ligament on coronal T1WI. The cervical ligament is the strongest ligament connecting the talus to the calcaneus. It is also the most anterior ligament of the sinus tarsi. Its calcaneal origin is medial to the origin of the extensor digitorum brevis muscle. The ligament ascends upward, anteriorly and medially to insert on the inferior aspect of the talar neck. The ligament becomes more horizontal in valgus and more vertical in varus position of the calcaneus. (**Bottom**) The cervical ligament on sagittal T1WI. The ligament's anterior course from the calcaneus to the talus is better appreciated on sagittal images. Note the intermediate root of the inferior extensor retinaculum located immediately posterior to the cervical ligament.

SAGITTAL T1 MR: SINUS TARSI LIGAMENTS

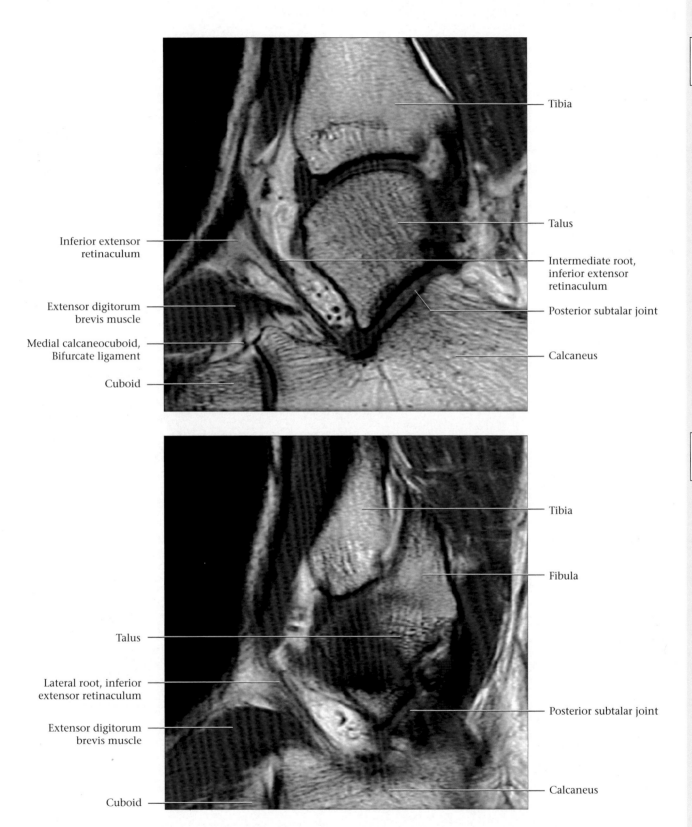

Top image labels:
- Tibia
- Talus
- Inferior extensor retinaculum
- Intermediate root, inferior extensor retinaculum
- Extensor digitorum brevis muscle
- Posterior subtalar joint
- Medial calcaneocuboid, Bifurcate ligament
- Calcaneus
- Cuboid

Bottom image labels:
- Tibia
- Fibula
- Talus
- Lateral root, inferior extensor retinaculum
- Extensor digitorum brevis muscle
- Posterior subtalar joint
- Cuboid
- Calcaneus

(Top) Roots of extensor retinaculum. The intermediate root inserts into the calcaneus slightly posterior to the cervical ligament. The medial root has medial and lateral calcaneal insertions and one talar insertion. The intermediate and lateral component of the medial root may insert very close to each other on the calcaneus but the latter is found closer to the posterior subtalar joint. **(Bottom)** The lateral root of the inferior extensor retinaculum on sagittal T1WI. The root inserts into the calcaneus lateral to the origin of the extensor digitorum brevis muscle. It is continuous with the inferior peroneal retinaculum and deep fascia. The ligament is found on very peripheral sagittal images of the sinus tarsi.

LIGAMENTS OVERVIEW

GRAPHIC & T2 FS MR, CORONAL LEFT ANKLE: SPRING LIGAMENT

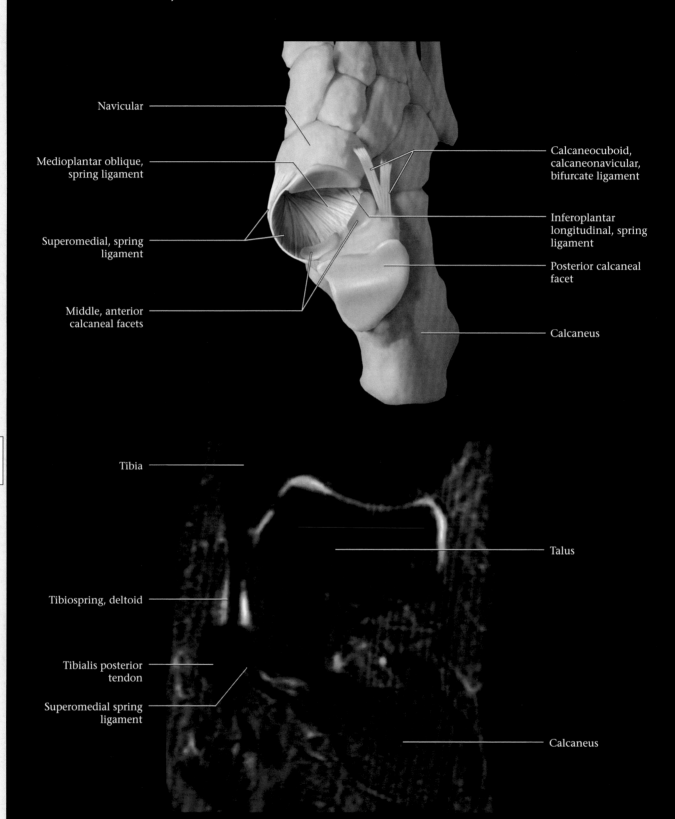

Navicular

Medioplantar oblique, spring ligament

Superomedial, spring ligament

Middle, anterior calcaneal facets

Calcaneocuboid, calcaneonavicular, bifurcate ligament

Inferoplantar longitudinal, spring ligament

Posterior calcaneal facet

Calcaneus

Tibia

Talus

Tibiospring, deltoid

Tibialis posterior tendon

Superomedial spring ligament

Calcaneus

(Top) The spring ligament is a hammock shaped structure which supports the talar head & medial longitudinal arch. Oblique coronal & sagittal images provide optimal visualization of the components of the spring ligament, however, routine ankle images are also useful. The superomedial component originates from the sustentaculum tali and inserts into superomedial navicular & the tibiospring ligament. It is best seen on coronal & axial images and occasionally on far medial sagittal image. The medioplantar oblique is best seen on axial images while the inferoplantar longitudinal is seen on both axial & sagittal images. **(Bottom)** The superomedial spring ligament on a coronal fat suppressed T2WI. The ligament hugs the talar head & is contiguous with tibiospring component of deltoid ligament. Note proximity of tibialis posterior tendon to ligament.

Ankle

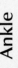

LIGAMENTS OVERVIEW

AXIAL T1 MR, RIGHT ANKLE: SPRING LIGAMENT

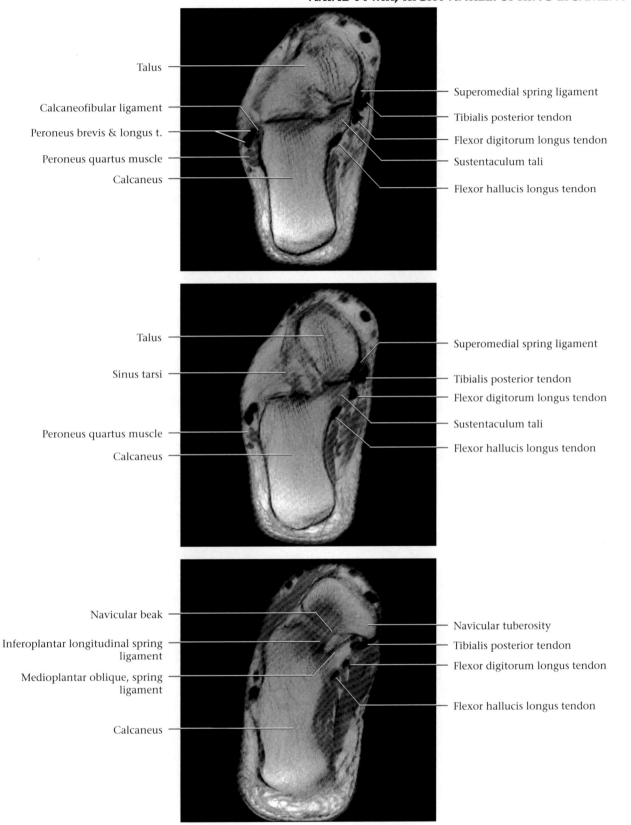

Talus — Superomedial spring ligament

Calcaneofibular ligament — Tibialis posterior tendon

Peroneus brevis & longus t. — Flexor digitorum longus tendon

Peroneus quartus muscle — Sustentaculum tali

Calcaneus — Flexor hallucis longus tendon

Talus — Superomedial spring ligament

Sinus tarsi — Tibialis posterior tendon

— Flexor digitorum longus tendon

Peroneus quartus muscle — Sustentaculum tali

Calcaneus — Flexor hallucis longus tendon

Navicular beak — Navicular tuberosity

Inferoplantar longitudinal spring ligament — Tibialis posterior tendon

Medioplantar oblique, spring ligament — Flexor digitorum longus tendon

— Flexor hallucis longus tendon

Calcaneus

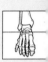
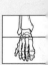

(Top) Sequential axial T1WI of the superomedial spring ligament. The superomedial spring is seen on axial images as it originates from the sustentaculum tali and curves around the talar head toward its navicular insertion (latter not seen). Notice the proximity of the tibialis posterior tendon. **(Middle)** A more distal axial T1WI of the superomedial spring ligament. **(Bottom)** A more distal axial T1WI. The medioplantar oblique and inferoplantar longitudinal components of the spring ligament originate from the calcaneus at the coronoid fossa (between the sustentaculum tali and anterior calcaneal process). The medioplantar oblique is consistently seen as it inserts into the plantar navicular, just lateral to navicular tuberosity & tibialis posterior tendon. The inferoplantar longitudinal inserts on the beak of the navicular.

Ankle

VII

125

LIGAMENTS OVERVIEW

AXIAL T1 MR, LEFT ANKLE: SPRING LIGAMENT

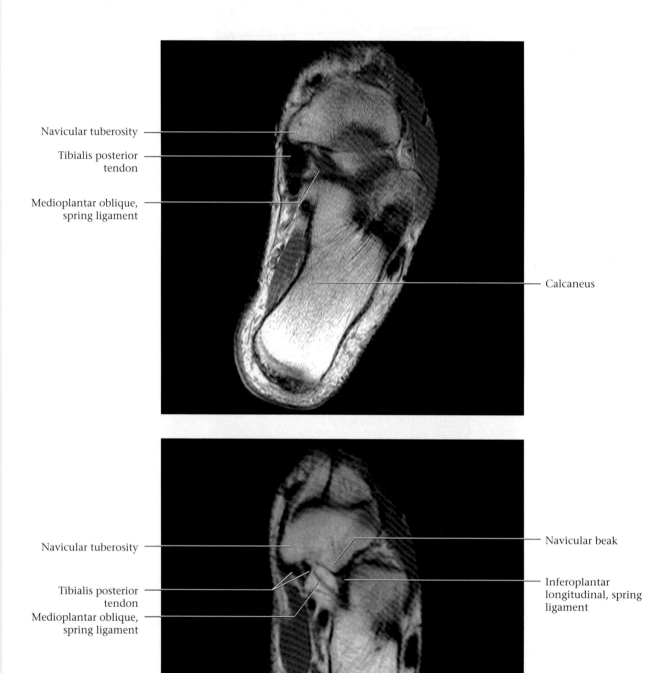

Navicular tuberosity

Tibialis posterior tendon

Medioplantar oblique, spring ligament

Calcaneus

Navicular tuberosity

Navicular beak

Tibialis posterior tendon

Medioplantar oblique, spring ligament

Inferoplantar longitudinal, spring ligament

Calcaneus

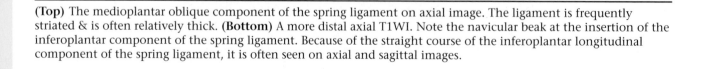

(Top) The medioplantar oblique component of the spring ligament on axial image. The ligament is frequently striated & is often relatively thick. **(Bottom)** A more distal axial T1WI. Note the navicular beak at the insertion of the inferoplantar component of the spring ligament. Because of the otraight course of the inferoplantar longitudinal component of the spring ligament, it is often seen on axial and sagittal images.

Ankle

VII

126

LIGAMENTS OVERVIEW

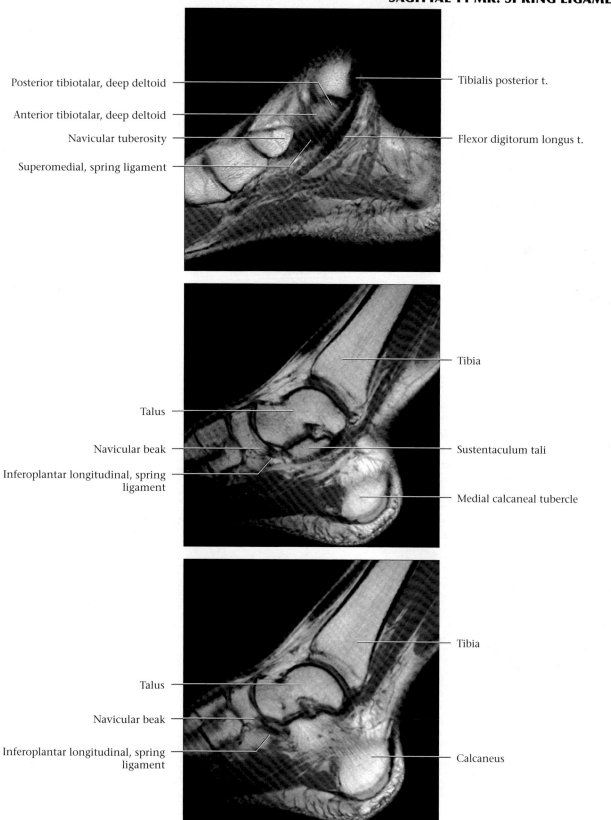

Posterior tibiotalar, deep deltoid — Tibialis posterior t.

Anterior tibiotalar, deep deltoid

Navicular tuberosity — Flexor digitorum longus t.

Superomedial, spring ligament

Talus — Tibia

Navicular beak — Sustentaculum tali

Inferoplantar longitudinal, spring ligament — Medial calcaneal tubercle

Talus — Tibia

Navicular beak

Inferoplantar longitudinal, spring ligament — Calcaneus

(Top) The superomedial component of the spring ligament is sometimes seen on a far medial image as a low signal band superomedial to the navicular tuberosity & lateral to the tibialis posterior tendon. **(Middle)** The inferoplantar longitudinal band of the spring ligament. Because of its oblique course the medioplantar oblique component of the spring ligament is difficult to identify on routine sagittal images and may been seen on cross section as an oval low signal structure. The inferoplantar longitudinal component, however, because of its straight and short course is frequently seen on sagittal images. Visualization of the beak of the navicular aids in identifying spre ligient. **(Bottom)** Inferoplantar longitudinal ligament. The ligament is a low signal band extending from the navicular beak to the coronoid fossa of the calcaneus.

LIGAMENTS OVERVIEW

GRAPHICS, BIFURCATE LIGAMENT

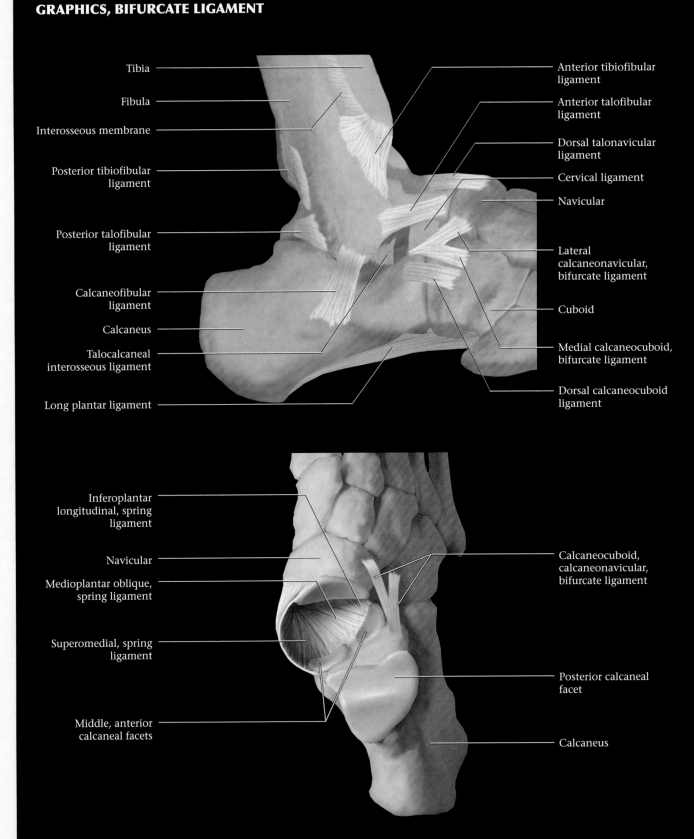

Tibia

Fibula

Interosseous membrane

Posterior tibiofibular ligament

Posterior talofibular ligament

Calcaneofibular ligament

Calcaneus

Talocalcaneal interosseous ligament

Long plantar ligament

Anterior tibiofibular ligament

Anterior talofibular ligament

Dorsal talonavicular ligament

Cervical ligament

Navicular

Lateral calcaneonavicular, bifurcate ligament

Cuboid

Medial calcaneocuboid, bifurcate ligament

Dorsal calcaneocuboid ligament

Inferoplantar longitudinal, spring ligament

Navicular

Medioplantar oblique, spring ligament

Superomedial, spring ligament

Middle, anterior calcaneal facets

Calcaneocuboid, calcaneonavicular, bifurcate ligament

Posterior calcaneal facet

Calcaneus

(Top) The bifurcate ligament is formed by the medial calcaneocuboid & lateral calcaneonavicular ligaments. These ligaments originate, close to each other, from the anterior process of calcaneus, forming a V shaped structure. The lateral calcaneonavicular ligament is stronger than the calcaneocuboid ligament. The latter may be absent. The bifurcate ligament is frequently seen on sagittal images, lateral to the spring ligament but may also be seen on axial images. **(Bottom)** Note the proximity of the bifurcate ligament to the inferoplantar longitudinal portion of the spring ligament.

LIGAMENTS OVERVIEW

SAGITTAL & AXIAL T1 MR, LEFT ANKLE: BIFURCATE LIGAMENT

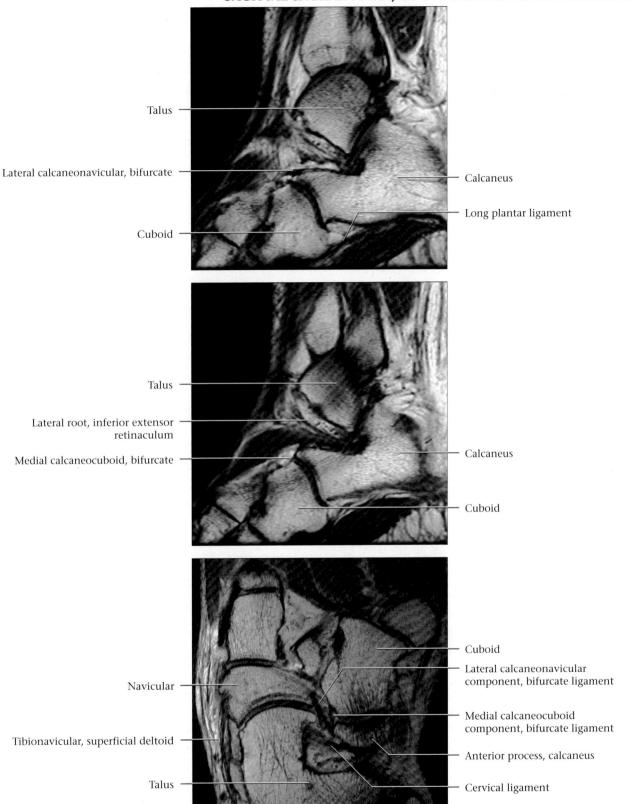

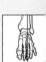

(Top) The lateral calcaneonavicular ligament of the bifurcate ligament is best seen on a sagittal image just lateral to the origin of the inferoplantar longitudinal component of the spring ligament. It is seen as a fine, curved, low signal structure originating from the anterior process of the calcaneus. **(Middle)** The medial calcaneocuboid component of the bifurcate ligament originates lateral to the lateral calcaneonavicular component. It is often quite a delicate, low signal intensity structure which may be absent in some individuals. **(Bottom)** The bifurcate ligament is occasionally seen on oblique axial images of the hindfoot.

LIGAMENTS OVERVIEW

AXIAL T1 MR, LEFT ANKLE: LONG & SHORT PLANTAR LIGAMENTS

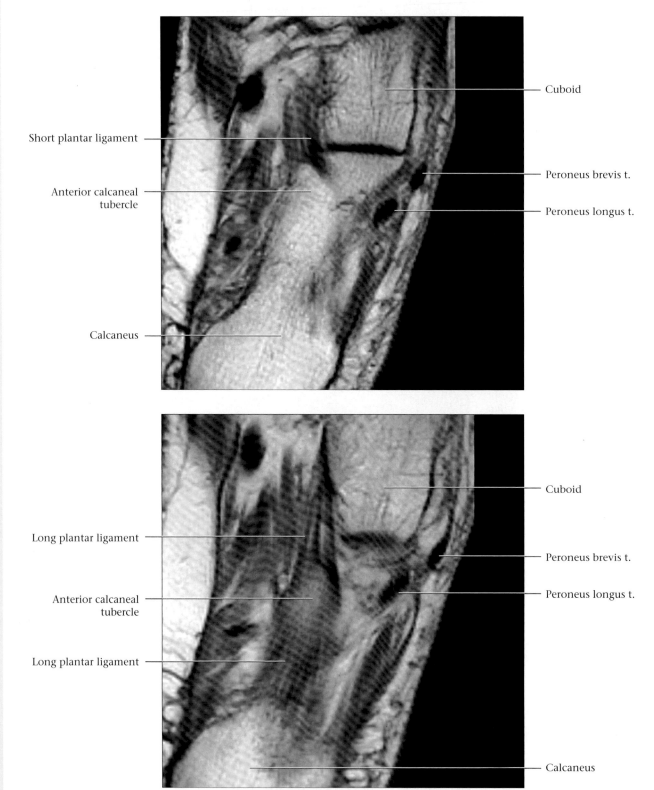

Short plantar ligament

Anterior calcaneal tubercle

Calcaneus

Cuboid

Peroneus brevis t.

Peroneus longus t.

Long plantar ligament

Anterior calcaneal tubercle

Long plantar ligament

Cuboid

Peroneus brevis t.

Peroneus longus t.

Calcaneus

(Top) The plantar calcaneocuboid ligament is subdivided into short, deep, and long superficial plantar ligaments. The short plantar ligament, also called the short plantar calcaneocuboid ligament is more medial than the long plantar ligament. It originates from the anterior tubercle of the calcaneus and inserts on the entire posterior plantar surface of and on beak of cuboid. **(Bottom)** A more distal (plantar) axial image in the same patient. The long plantar ligament originates from the anterior tubercle and more posteriorly from the anterior aspect and intertubercular segment of the posterior calcaneal tuberosities. Its deeper fibers, representing the bulk of ligament, insert to the cuboid crest and its superficial fibers form a thinner layer which forms the roof of the cuboid tunnel of the peroneus longus tendon & inserts on the 2nd-5th metatarsal bases.

LIGAMENTS OVERVIEW

SAGITTAL T1 MR: LONG & SHORT PLANTAR LIGAMENTS

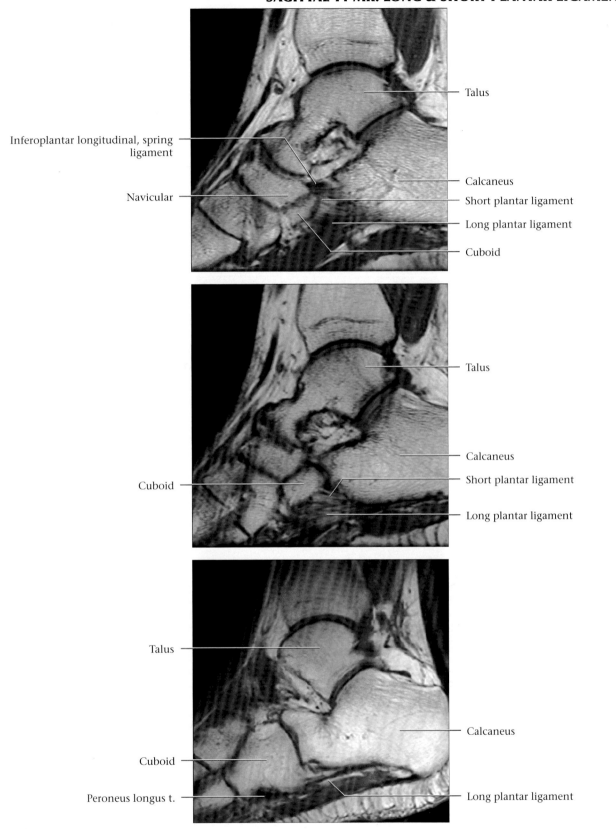

Inferoplantar longitudinal, spring ligament

Navicular

Talus

Calcaneus

Short plantar ligament

Long plantar ligament

Cuboid

Talus

Cuboid

Calcaneus

Short plantar ligament

Long plantar ligament

Talus

Calcaneus

Cuboid

Peroneus longus t.

Long plantar ligament

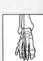

(Top) Note the proximity of the plantar component of the spring ligament to the short plantar ligament. The inferoplantar longitudinal ligament inserts into the beak of the navicular. The short plantar ligament is found more plantarly and is deeper than the long plantar ligament. It inserts on the cuboid. (Middle) A more lateral sagittal image in the same patient. Note the marked striation of both the short and long plantar ligaments. (Bottom) A more lateral sagittal image in a different patient. The superficial fibers of the long plantar ligament continue distal to the cuboid to insert onto the bases of 2nd-5th metatarsals and thus form the roof of the peroneus longus tunnel, under the cuboid.

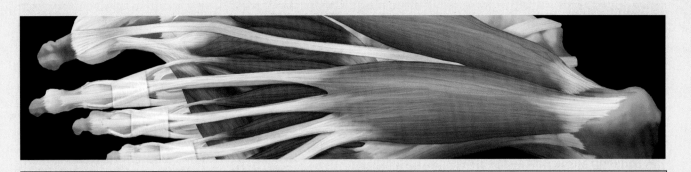

SECTION VIII: Foot

FOOT OVERVIEW

Terminology

Definitions
- **Three major divisions**
  - **Hindfoot**: Calcaneus and talus
    - Hindfoot is discussed in Ankle section
  - **Midfoot**: Navicular, cuneiforms, and cuboid
  - **Forefoot**: Metatarsals and phalanges
- **Two columns**
  - **Medial column**: Talus, navicular, cuneiforms 1-3, digits 1-3
  - **Lateral column**: Calcaneus, cuboid, digits 4 and 5
- Some authors use 2 columns in hind and midfoot as above, but divide forefoot into 3 columns
  - Medial column: 1st toe
  - Middle column: 2nd-4th toes
  - Lateral column: 5th toe

Imaging Anatomy

Overview
- Alignment of foot can only be assessed on weight-bearing radiographs

Arches of Foot
- Foot is arched from posterior to anterior, and from medial to lateral
- **Transverse arch of foot**
  - Cuneiform bones form keystone of arch due to triangular shape
  - Major supporting structures of transverse arch
    - Spring ligament
    - Lisfranc ligament and intermetatarsal ligaments
    - Intertarsal ligaments
- **Longitudinal arch of foot**
  - From posterior process calcaneus to metatarsal heads
  - Medial side is higher than lateral
  - Apex of arch is at navicular and cuneiforms
  - Metatarsals slant downward from apex of arch to metatarsophalangeal (MTP) joint from arch apex
    - This is called inclination angle
    - Inclination angle decreases from 20° at 1st to 5° at 5th metatarsal
  - Major supporting structures of longitudinal arch
    - Plantar fascia
    - Long and short plantar ligaments
    - Spring ligament
    - Posterior tibial tendon, peroneus longus tendon
- **Radiographic assessment of normal longitudinal arch**
  - Evaluate talometatarsal alignment
    - Normal: Axis of talus continues along axis of 1st metatarsal
    - Pes planus: Axis of talus falls below axis of 1st metatarsal
    - Pes cavus: Axis of talus extends above axis of 1st metatarsal

Alignment
- **Hindfoot relative to forefoot alignment**
  - Defined by axis of talus on anteroposterior radiograph
    - Axis of talus continues along axis of 1st metatarsal, or between 1st and 2nd metatarsals
- **Midfoot alignment**
  - Lateral radiograph
    - Inferior margins of calcaneus, cuboid aligned if weight-bearing
    - Pitfall: Calcaneocuboid joint usually appears subluxated on nonweight-bearing lateral radiograph
    - Cuneiforms overlap with each other
    - Lateral cuneiform overlaps with cuboid
  - Anteroposterior radiograph
    - Medial portion of navicular protrudes medially beyond margins of talar head and 1st cuneiform
    - 1st cuneiform, talar head are aligned at medial margin
    - Intercuneiform joints and cuneocuboid joints overlap
- **Forefoot alignment**
  - Lateral radiograph
    - 1st and 2nd metatarsal bases at dorsum of foot
    - Metatarsals 3-5 progressively more plantigrade
    - All MTP joints at same plantar position
    - MTP joints slightly dorsiflexed; this is most prominent at 1st MTP due to its higher inclination angle
  - Anteroposterior radiograph
    - 1st metatarsal centered on 1st cuneiform
    - 2nd metatarsal medial margin aligned to medial margin 2nd cuneiform
    - 3rd metatarsal centered on 3rd cuneiform
    - 4th metatarsal aligned to medial margin cuboid
    - 5th metatarsal styloid process extends beyond lateral border of cuboid
    - Intermetatarsal angle between 1st and 2nd metatarsals normally less than 10°
    - Slight 1st MTP abduction (hallux valgus) is normal, up to about 15°

Distribution of Weight-Bearing
- 50% of weight borne on subtalar joint and calcaneus
- Remainder transmitted via arch anteriorly to metatarsophalangeal joints, greatest weight on 1st toe

Bony Anatomy
- **Cuboid bone**
  - Roughly cuboidal shape
  - 1 ossification center: Ossifies between 9th fetal month and 6 months age
  - Articulates with calcaneus, navicular, 3rd cuneiform, 4th and 5th metatarsals, rarely head of talus
    - Dorsal ligaments (calcaneocuboid, cubonavicular, cuneocuboid, cubometatarsal) strengthen each of these articulations
    - Short and long plantar ligaments attach to plantar surface
  - Sulcus at lateral margin, under which passes peroneus longus tendon
  - 5th metatarsal base extends beyond lateral margin
- **Navicular bone**
  - Curved shape, concave proximally and convex distally
  - 1 ossification center: Ossifies in 3rd year of life
  - Articulates with talus, cuboid, cuneiforms

- Dorsal ligaments strengthen each of these articulations
- Single facet proximally for articulation with head of talus
- 3 facets distally for cuneiform articulations
- 1 facet laterally for articulation with cuboid
- Connected to anterior process of calcaneus by bifurcate ligament
- Connected to sustentaculum tali by spring ligament
  - Large median eminence for attachment of posterior tibial tendon is located more plantar than main body of navicular
- **Cuneiform bones**
  - Wedge-shaped, with base of wedge at dorsal surface of 2nd and 3rd cuneiforms, dorsomedial surface 1st cuneiform
  - In combination, form arch
  - 1st cuneiform (medial cuneiform)
    - Articulates with navicular, 2nd cuneiform, 1st metatarsal
    - 1 or 2 ossifications centers: Ossify in 2nd year of life
  - 2nd cuneiform (middle or intermediate cuneiform)
    - Articulates with navicular, 1st and 3rd cuneiforms, 2nd metatarsal
    - Smallest of cuneiforms
    - 1 ossification center: Ossifies in 3rd year of life
  - 3rd cuneiform (lateral cuneiform)
    - Articulates with navicular, 2nd cuneiform, cuboid, 3rd metatarsal
- **Metatarsal bones**
  - 2 ossifications centers: Shaft ossifies in 9th prenatal week, epiphysis in 3rd-4th years of life
    - 1st metatarsal has epiphysis at proximal end, others at distal end
  - 2nd-5th metatarsals have articulations at bases with adjacent metatarsals
  - 1st metatarsal
    - Largest of metatarsals
    - Articulates with 1st cuneiform, 1st proximal phalanx, sesamoids of metatarsal head
    - Variable articulation with 2nd metatarsal base
  - 2nd-3rd metatarsals
    - Articulate with respective cuneiforms and proximal phalanges
    - 2nd metatarsal base recessed relative to 1st and usually 3rd
  - 4th-5th metatarsals
    - Articulate with cuboid and respective proximal phalanges
    - Styloid process of 5th metatarsal extends lateral to cuboid
- **Phalanges**
  - 1st toe is biphalangeal, other toes are triphalangeal
  - 5th toe sometimes has failure of segmentation of middle and distal phalanges
  - 2 ossification centers: Shaft ossifies 9th-15th prenatal weeks, epiphysis 2nd-8th years

Musculature

- **Plantar muscles**: 4 muscle layers, numbered from superficial to deep
  - 1st layer: Abductor hallucis, flexor digitorum brevis, abductor digiti minimi, peroneus brevis
  - 2nd layer: Quadratus plantae (flexor accessorius), flexor digitorum and hallucis longus, lumbricals
  - 3rd layer: Flexor hallucis brevis, adductor hallucis, flexor digiti minimi brevis, tibialis posterior
  - 4th layer: Plantar interossei (3), dorsal interossei (4)
  - Peroneus longus courses across all layers, from superficial plantar laterally to deep plantar medially
- **Dorsal muscles**: 2 muscle layers
  - Superficial layer: Tibialis anterior, extensor hallucis longus, extensor digitorum longus, peroneus tertius
  - Deep layer: Extensor hallucis brevis, extensor digitorum brevis
  - In forefoot, long and short extensors run side by side in single layer

Compartments

- **4 plantar compartments** divided by fascial layers
  - Lateral and medial intermuscular septae determine major compartment divisions
- **Medial plantar compartment**
  - Contains abductor hallucis, flexor hallucis longus, and flexor hallucis brevis
- **Central plantar compartment**
  - Superficial subcompartment: Contains flexor digitorum brevis, distal portion of flexor digitorum longus
  - Intermediary subcompartment: Contains proximal plantar portion of flexor digitorum longus, quadratus plantae, lumbricals
  - Deep subcompartment: Limited to forefoot, contains adductor hallucis
- **Lateral plantar compartment**
  - Contains abductor and flexor digiti minimi
- **Interosseous compartment**
  - Contains plantar and dorsal interosseous muscle
- **Dorsal compartment**
  - Superficial layer: Extrinsic extensor tendon
  - Deep layer: Intrinsic extensor muscle

Major Ligaments

- Plantar fascia (aponeurosis): 3 portions extend from tuberosity of calcaneus to transverse metatarsal ligaments of toes
  - Medial band: Thin structure superficial to abductor hallucis muscle
  - Central band: Thick, strong structure superficial to flexor digitorum brevis
    - Divides into separate bands to each toe; these are linked by transverse bands
    - Distally sends septae superficially into subcutaneous fat and deep to MTP joints
  - Lateral band: Thin structure superficial to abductor digiti minimi
  - Medial and lateral bands sometimes terminate at level of mid metatarsals
- Long plantar ligament: Originates calcaneal tuberosity, inserts cuboid and bases 2nd-4th metatarsals
  - Forms retinaculum for peroneus longus tendon as it courses medially on plantar aspect of foot
- Short plantar (plantar calcaneocuboid) ligament: Deep to long ligament, inserts more proximally on cuboid

FOOT OVERVIEW

- Plantar calcaneocuboid (spring) ligament: Originates sustentaculum tali, inserts plantar aspect navicular
- Bifurcate ligament: Originates anterior process of calcaneus dorsally, inserts navicular and cuboid
- Lisfranc ligament: Originates 1st cuneiform, inserts base 2nd metatarsal
- Intermetatarsal ligaments: Dorsal and plantar ligaments between 2nd-5th metatarsal bases
- Transverse metatarsal ligaments: Superficial and deep ligaments between metatarsal heads

Nerves

- **Tibial nerve** divides into medial and lateral plantar branches at level of tarsal tunnel
  - **Medial plantar nerve**
    - Between 1st and 2nd muscle layers, accompanies medial plantar artery
    - Motor branches: Abductor hallucis, flexor digitorum and hallucis brevis, 1st lumbrical
    - Plantar digital nerves to 1st-3rd toes, medial aspect 4th toe
  - **Lateral plantar nerve**: Has deep and superficial divisions
    - Motor branches: Flexor digiti minimi brevis, lumbricals, interossei, adductor hallucis
    - Superficial lateral plantar nerve: Between 1st and 2nd muscle layers
    - Plantar digital nerves to 5th toe, lateral aspect 4th toe
    - Deep lateral plantar nerve: Between 3rd and 4th muscle layers; accompanies lateral plantar artery
- **Deep peroneal nerve**: Extends along dorsum of foot, between tibialis anterior and extensor hallucis longus
  - Motor branch: Extensor digitorum brevis
- **Superficial peroneal nerve**: Divides into medial and lateral branches at dorsum of foot
  - Sensory branches to dorsal foot
- **Sural nerve**: Lateral, superficial branch of tibial nerve
  - Extends along lateral margin of foot
  - Sensory branches to lateral foot

Arteries

- Posterior tibial artery divides into medial and lateral plantar arteries at level of tarsal tunnel
  - Plantar arteries accompany medial and deep lateral plantar nerves
- Peroneal artery accompanies superficial peroneal nerve down anterolateral aspect ankle
  - May join or replace posterior tibial artery
- Anterior tibial artery continues into foot as dorsalis pedis artery, deep to extensor retinaculum
  - Divides into multiple branches in midfoot, forming arcade

Bursae

- Extensor digitorum brevis: Between muscle and 2nd cuneiform and metatarsal bases
- Extensor hallucis longus: Between tendon and 1st cuneiform and metatarsal bases
- Abductor digiti minimi: Between muscle and tuberosity of 5th metatarsal
- Metatarsophalangeal joints: Dorsally; between metatarsal heads; and medial to 1st metatarsal head

Anatomy-Based Imaging Issues

Imaging Recommendations

- Radiographs: Weight-bearing when possible
  - Standard views: Anteroposterior (dorsoplantar), lateral, oblique
- MR: Better images obtained when field of view limited to area of concern, not entire foot
- CT: Multidetector 1 mm images with sagittal and coronal reformations

Imaging Pitfalls

- Alignment can only be reliably assessed on weight-bearing radiographs

Clinical Implications

Foot Motion

- **Supination**: Elevation of medial arch of foot
  - Combination of inversion and adduction
- **Pronation**: Depression of medial arch of foot
  - Combination of eversion and abduction
- Complex motions at multiple joints; following is a simplified description of major motions
- Chopart (calcaneocuboid and talonavicular) joint
  - These 2 joints move together on an oblique axis to produce compound motions
  - Pronation-abduction-extension to supination-adduction-flexion
- Tarsometatarsal joints
  - Dorsiflexion and plantar flexion
  - 2nd and 3rd tarsometatarsal joints relatively immobile
  - Slight abduction of 1st tarsometatarsal joint
- Metatarsophalangeal joints
  - Dorsiflexion and plantar flexion
  - Abduction and adduction at 1st metatarsophalangeal joint

Alignment

- Normal weight-bearing and gait depend on normal foot alignment
- Evaluated initially with anteroposterior and lateral weight-bearing radiographs

Malalignment

- Forefoot adductus: Medial angulation of metatarsals from axis of hindfoot
- Forefoot varus: Inversion of metatarsals resulting in shift of weight-bearing to 5th metatarsal from 1st metatarsal
- Metatarsus primus varus: Medial deviation of 1st metatarsal axis relative to 2nd
- Hallux valgus (hallux abductus): Lateral deviation of 1st proximal phalanx relative to axis of 1st metatarsal
  - Valgus refers to an angular deformity in the vertical plane, where the apex points medially
  - Abductus refers to an angular deformity in the horizontal plane, where the apex points medially
  - Therefore, hallux valgus is a misnomer, but it remains the term commonly used for hallux abductus

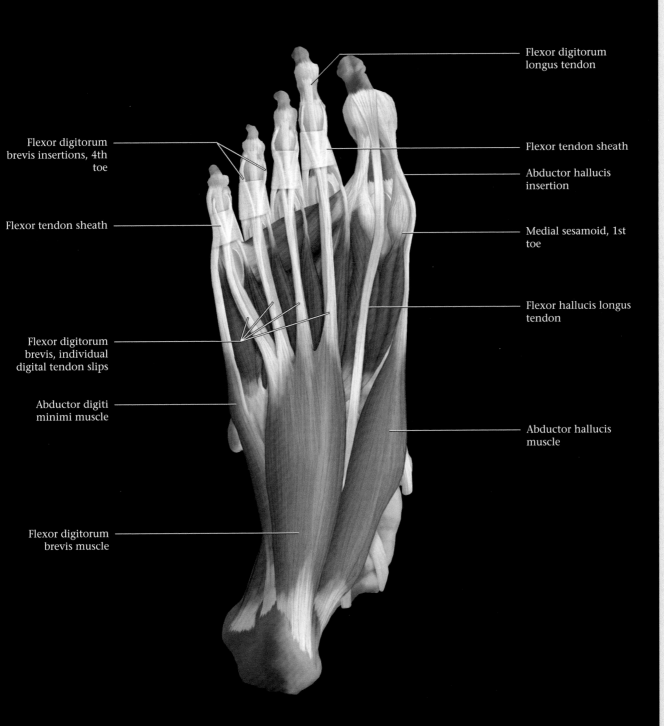

Flexor digitorum
longus tendon

Flexor digitorum
brevis insertions, 4th
toe

Flexor tendon sheath

Abductor hallucis
insertion

Flexor tendon sheath

Medial sesamoid, 1st
toe

Flexor digitorum
brevis, individual
digital tendon slips

Flexor hallucis longus
tendon

Abductor digiti
minimi muscle

Abductor hallucis
muscle

Flexor digitorum
brevis muscle

Graphic shows superficial layer of plantar foot muscles: Abductor digiti minimi, flexor digitorum brevis, and abductor hallucis. Deep muscles are partially visible deep to superficial layer. Flexor digitorum brevis tendons split in each digit (4th digit labeled), attaching at lateral aspects of middle phalangeal bases. Flexor tendon sheaths hold flexor mechanism in close proximity to phalanges.

MUSCLES OF FOOT, 2ND PLANTAR LAYER

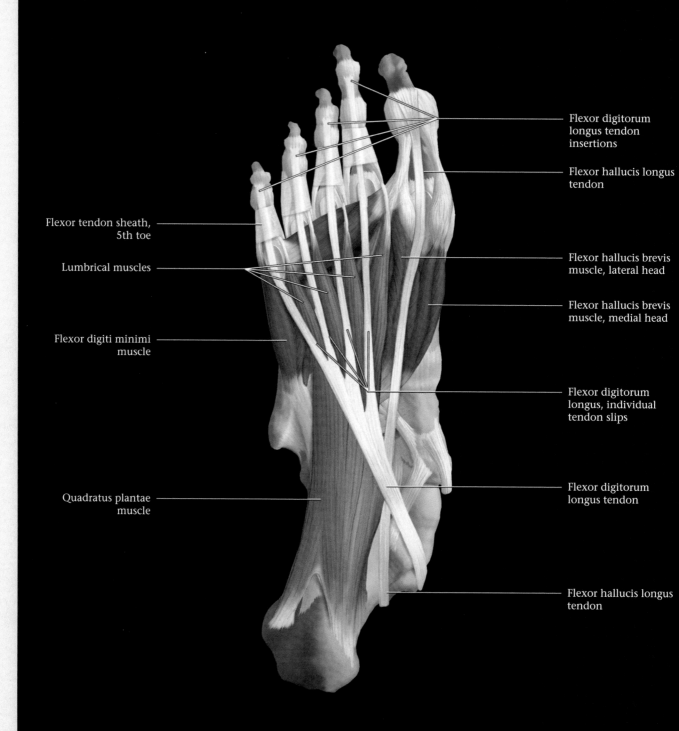

Flexor digitorum longus tendon insertions

Flexor hallucis longus tendon

Flexor tendon sheath, 5th toe

Lumbrical muscles

Flexor hallucis brevis muscle, lateral head

Flexor hallucis brevis muscle, medial head

Flexor digiti minimi muscle

Flexor digitorum longus, individual tendon slips

Quadratus plantae muscle

Flexor digitorum longus tendon

Flexor hallucis longus tendon

Graphic shows 2nd layer of plantar muscles. The interesting arrangement of interactions between flexors is well seen: Quadratus plantae inserting on flexor digitorum longus tendon, and lumbricals arising from individual flexor digitorum longus tendon slips. In toes, flexor tendons are contained with fibrous tendon sheaths.

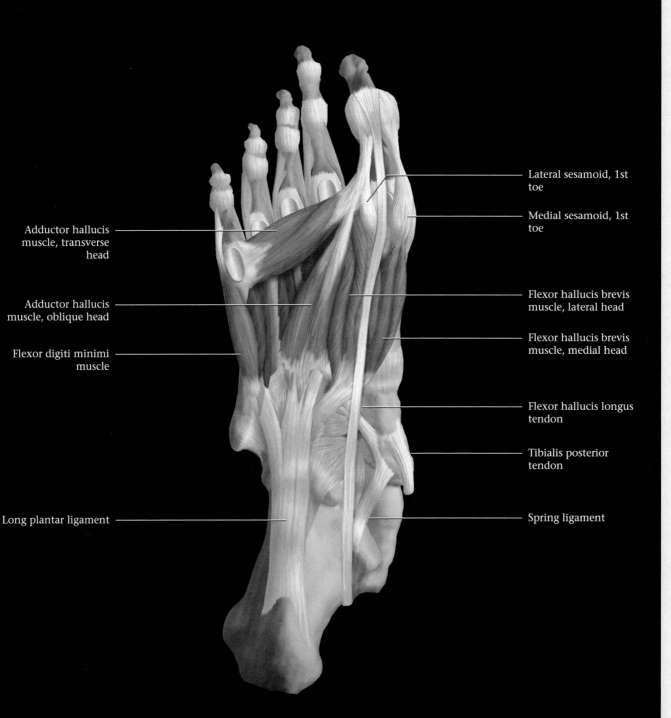

Lateral sesamoid, 1st toe

Medial sesamoid, 1st toe

Adductor hallucis muscle, transverse head

Adductor hallucis muscle, oblique head

Flexor digiti minimi muscle

Flexor hallucis brevis muscle, lateral head

Flexor hallucis brevis muscle, medial head

Flexor hallucis longus tendon

Tibialis posterior tendon

Long plantar ligament

Spring ligament

Graphic shows 3rd layer of plantar muscles. This layer contains flexor hallucis brevis and flexor digiti minimi, as well as the adductor hallucis muscle. Oblique head of adductor hallucis is thick and broad, whereas transverse head is thin, and occasionally congenitally absent.

FOOT OVERVIEW

MUSCLES OF FOOT, 4TH PLANTAR LAYER

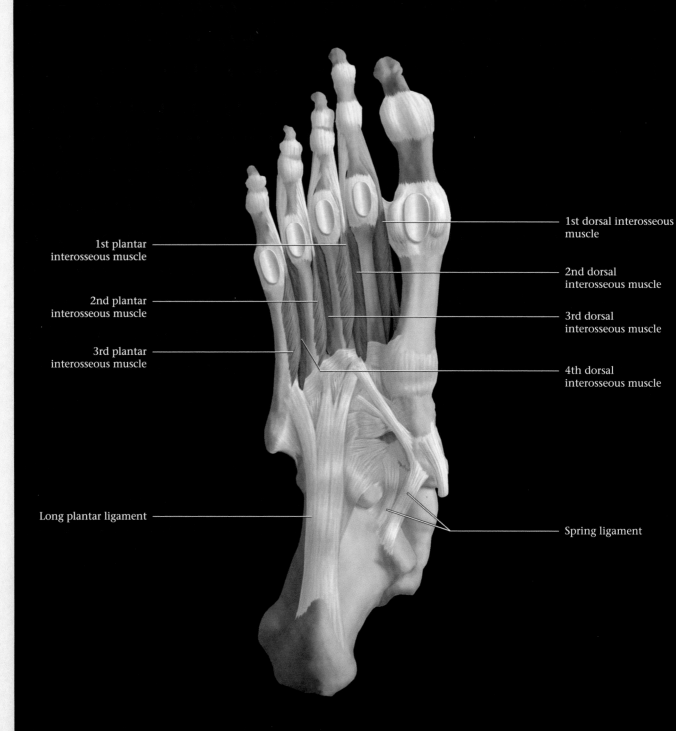

1st plantar interosseous muscle

2nd plantar interosseous muscle

3rd plantar interosseous muscle

Long plantar ligament

1st dorsal interosseous muscle

2nd dorsal interosseous muscle

3rd dorsal interosseous muscle

4th dorsal interosseous muscle

Spring ligament

Graphic shows 4th layer of plantar muscles, the interosseous muscles. There are 4 dorsal interossei. They have bipennate origins from 2 adjacent metatarsals. 1st dorsal interosseous inserts on medial side of 2nd proximal phalanx. Remaining dorsal interossei insert on lateral side of corresponding proximal phalanx. There are 3 plantar interossei. 1st plantar interosseous muscle originates from medial side of 3rd metatarsal, and inserts on medial side of 3rd proximal phalanx. 2nd and 3rd plantar interossei originate on medial sides of 4th and 5th metatarsals, respectively, and insert on medial side of corresponding proximal phalanx.

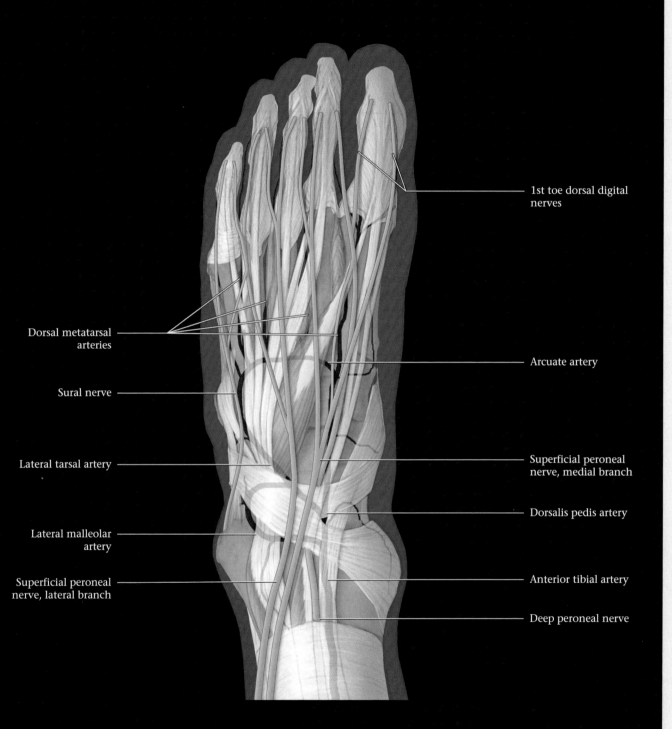

1st toe dorsal digital nerves

Dorsal metatarsal arteries

Arcuate artery

Sural nerve

Lateral tarsal artery

Superficial peroneal nerve, medial branch

Dorsalis pedis artery

Lateral malleolar artery

Superficial peroneal nerve, lateral branch

Anterior tibial artery

Deep peroneal nerve

Graphic of arteries and nerves at dorsal aspect of foot. Deep peroneal nerve accompanies anterior tibial artery. Superficial peroneal nerve divides into medial and lateral branches in distal 3rd of leg. Anterior tibial artery is called dorsalis pedis in foot. It terminates in arcuate artery, which communicates with plantar arterial arch, and in digital vessels.

FOOT OVERVIEW

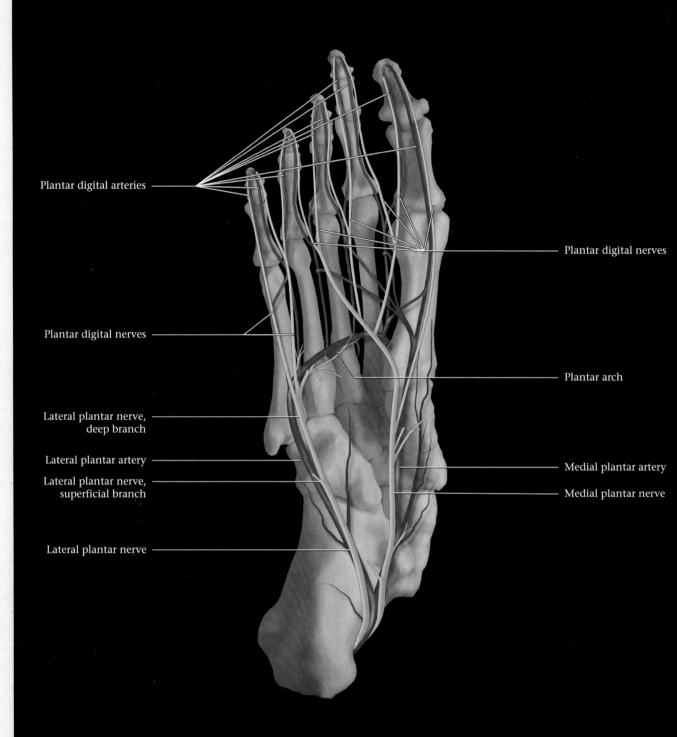

Plantar digital arteries

Plantar digital nerves

Plantar digital nerves

Plantar arch

Lateral plantar nerve, deep branch

Lateral plantar artery

Medial plantar artery

Lateral plantar nerve, superficial branch

Medial plantar nerve

Lateral plantar nerve

Graphic of arteries and nerve at plantar aspect of foot. Posterior tibial nerve and artery divide into medial and lateral plantar branches. These divide further into digital branches to medial and lateral aspects of each toe. Plantar arch sends vessels dorsally as well as to plantar aspect of toes.

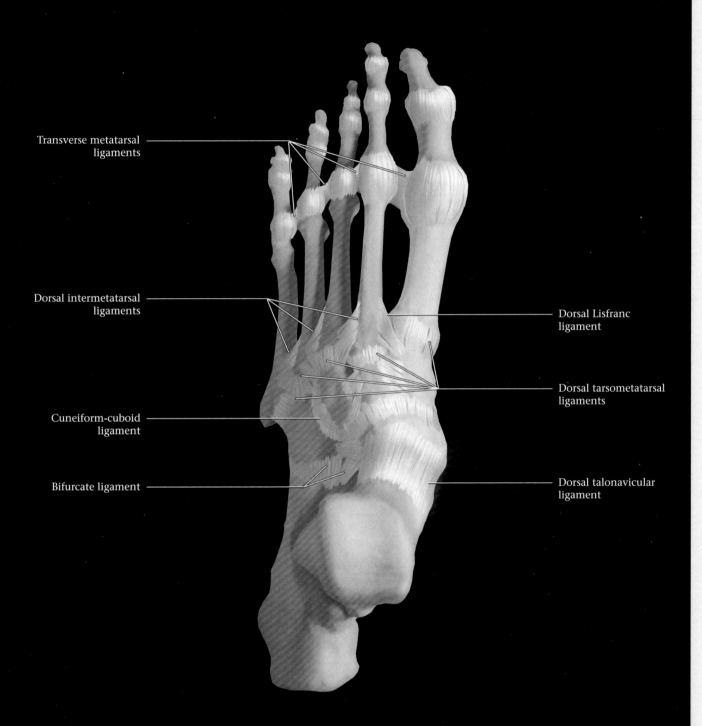

Transverse metatarsal ligaments

Dorsal intermetatarsal ligaments

Cuneiform-cuboid ligament

Bifurcate ligament

Dorsal Lisfranc ligament

Dorsal tarsometatarsal ligaments

Dorsal talonavicular ligament

Graphic of dorsal ligaments shows dense ligaments between tarsal bones, and between tarsals and metatarsals. Ligaments are generally named for the bones they bridge. Exceptions are bifurcate ligament, which extends from anterior process calcaneus to cuboid and navicular, and dorsal Lisfranc ligament, from 1st cuneiform to 2nd metatarsal.

FOOT OVERVIEW

PLANTAR LIGAMENTS OF FOOT

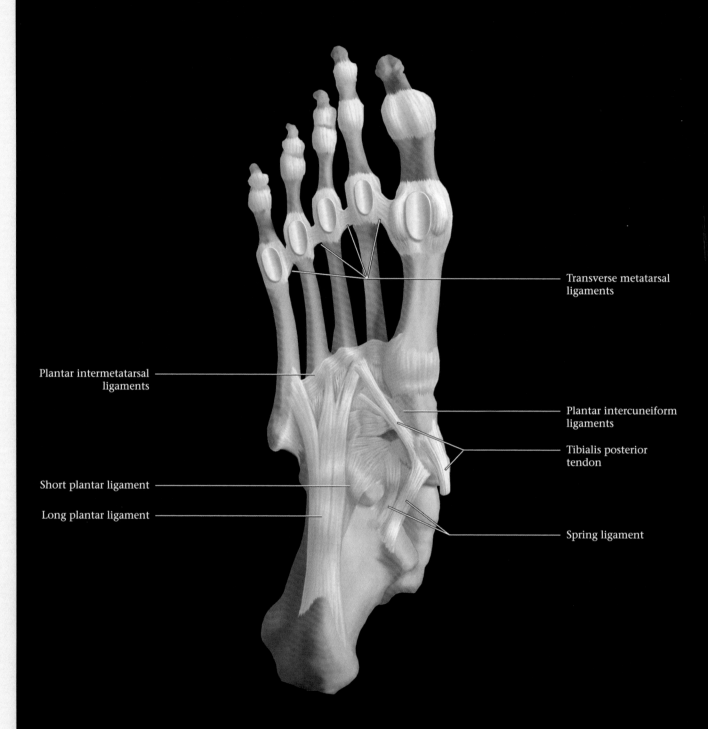

Transverse metatarsal ligaments

Plantar intermetatarsal ligaments

Plantar intercuneiform ligaments

Tibialis posterior tendon

Short plantar ligament

Long plantar ligament

Spring ligament

Graphic of plantar ligaments shows ligaments deep to plantar fascia, as well as proximal and distal attachments of tibialis posterior tendon. Spring ligament, also known as plantar calcaneonavicular ligament, originates on sustentaculum tali and anterior calcaneus, and inserts on navicular. Deep intertarsal ligaments are also shown, and are named for bones they bridge.

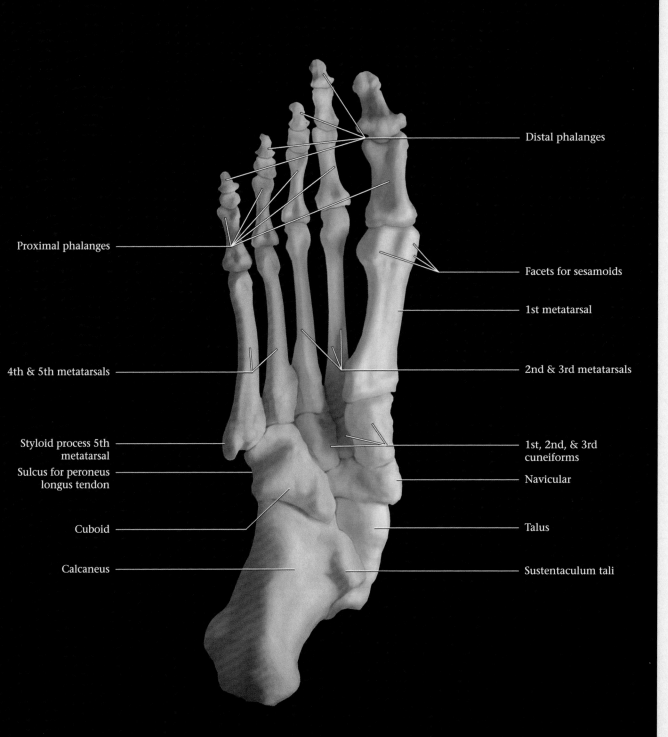

Distal phalanges

Proximal phalanges

Facets for sesamoids

1st metatarsal

4th & 5th metatarsals

2nd & 3rd metatarsals

Styloid process 5th metatarsal

1st, 2nd, & 3rd cuneiforms

Sulcus for peroneus longus tendon

Navicular

Cuboid

Talus

Calcaneus

Sustentaculum tali

Plantar view of foot shows lateral column in pink, medial column in blue. This plantar diagram is also useful for showing appearance of transverse arch created by wedge-shaped cuneiform bones. Plantar margins of cuneiforms are closely apposed, and 2nd cuneiform is recessed.

FOOT OVERVIEW

LONGITUDINAL ARCH OF FOOT

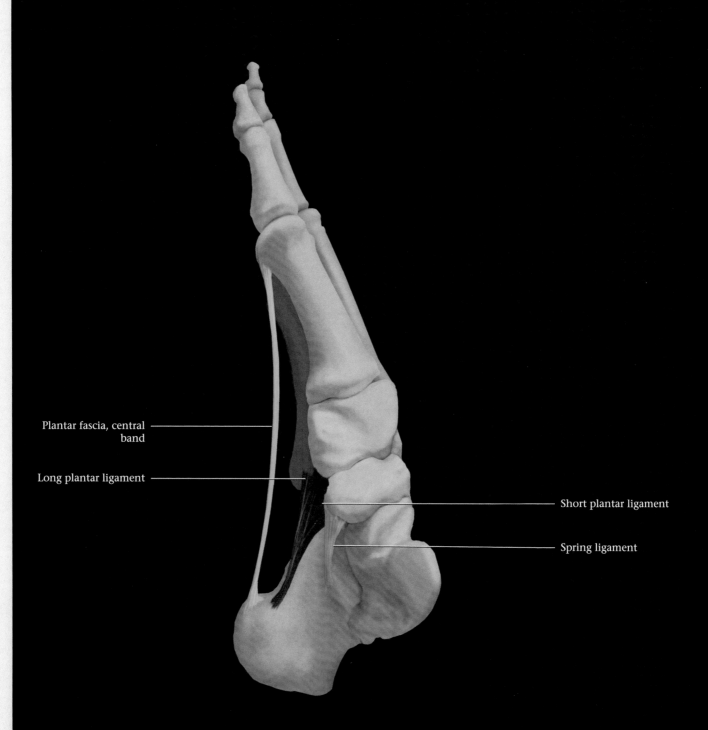

Plantar fascia, central band

Long plantar ligament

Short plantar ligament

Spring ligament

Graphic shows longitudinal arch of foot from medial side, together with schematic representation of major plantar ligaments helping maintain longitudinal arch. Plantar fascia is the most important structure for maintaining arch. It acts like a tie beam between the ends of the arch: Calcaneal tuberosity and metatarsal heads. Long and short plantar ligaments originate on calcaneus, with short plantar ligament deep to long plantar ligament. Both insert on cuboid. Long plantar ligament also sends fibers to metatarsal bases. Spring ligament extends from sustentaculum tali and adjacent anteromedial calcaneus to plantar surface of navicular.

FOOT OVERVIEW

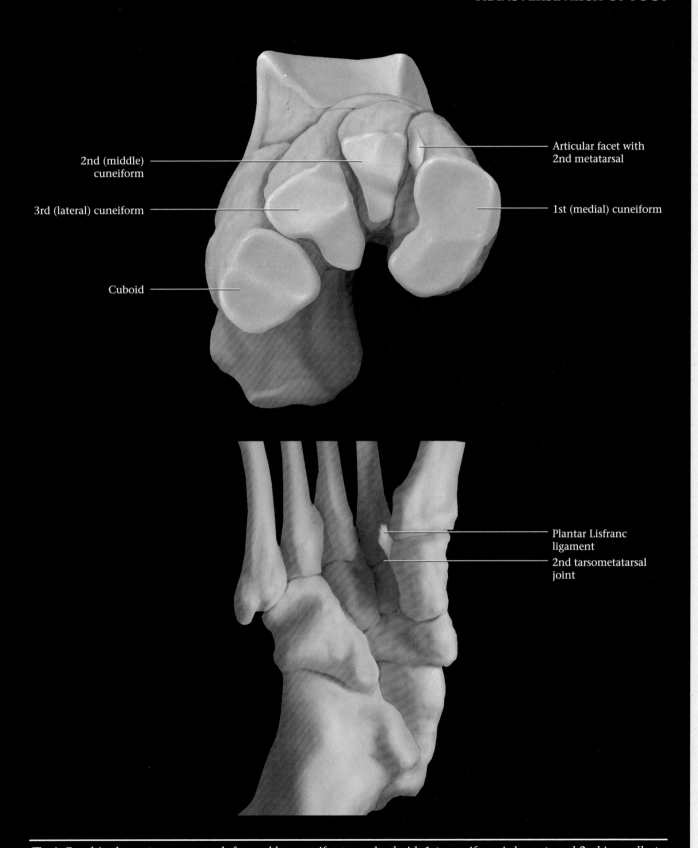

2nd (middle) cuneiform

3rd (lateral) cuneiform

Cuboid

Articular facet with 2nd metatarsal

1st (medial) cuneiform

Plantar Lisfranc ligament

2nd tarsometatarsal joint

(Top) Graphic shows transverse arch formed by cuneiforms and cuboid. 1st cuneiform is largest, and 2nd is smallest. Arch is continued anterior to this image by configuration of proximal portions of metatarsals. Interosseous and intercuneiform ligaments maintain shape of arch, together with peroneus longus tendon. Note multifaceted articular surfaces at tarsometatarsal joint. (Bottom) Graphic shows transverse arch from plantar side of foot. Arch is formed by bones, but stability is dependent on ligaments. Lisfranc ligaments are critically important in maintaining arch. There are 3 distinct Lisfranc ligaments extending from 1st cuneiform to base of 2nd metatarsal: Dorsal, interosseous, and plantar. Interosseous ligament is strongest of them and is structurally most important.

FOOT OVERVIEW

AP, OBLIQUE WEIGHT-BEARING RADIOGRAPHS

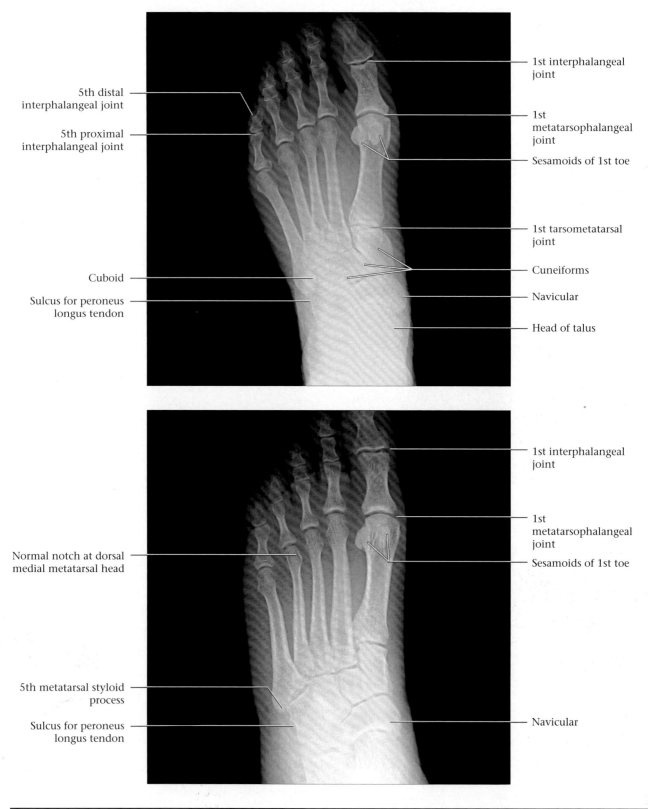

5th distal interphalangeal joint

5th proximal interphalangeal joint

Cuboid

Sulcus for peroneus longus tendon

1st interphalangeal joint

1st metatarsophalangeal joint

Sesamoids of 1st toe

1st tarsometatarsal joint

Cuneiforms

Navicular

Head of talus

Normal notch at dorsal medial metatarsal head

5th metatarsal styloid process

Sulcus for peroneus longus tendon

1st interphalangeal joint

1st metatarsophalangeal joint

Sesamoids of 1st toe

Navicular

(Top) Anteroposterior weight-bearing radiograph of foot shows normal amount of overlap of bones of midfoot. Articulations between cuboid and navicular, between cuneiforms, and between cuboid and lateral cuneiform are not seen in profile. Tarsometatarsal joints are sometimes in profile, but joints may not be visible due to obliquity of joint; this should not be mistaken for joint fusion. **(Bottom)** On oblique view, intercuneiform joints, tarsometatarsal joints and styloid process (also called tuberosity) at base of 5th metatarsal are usually better seen than on anteroposterior view. Normal notch at medial margin of metatarsal heads is often thrown into profile on this view and should not be mistaken for erosion.

FOOT OVERVIEW

LATERAL RADIOGRAPHS, WEIGHT-BEARING & NONWEIGHT-BEARING

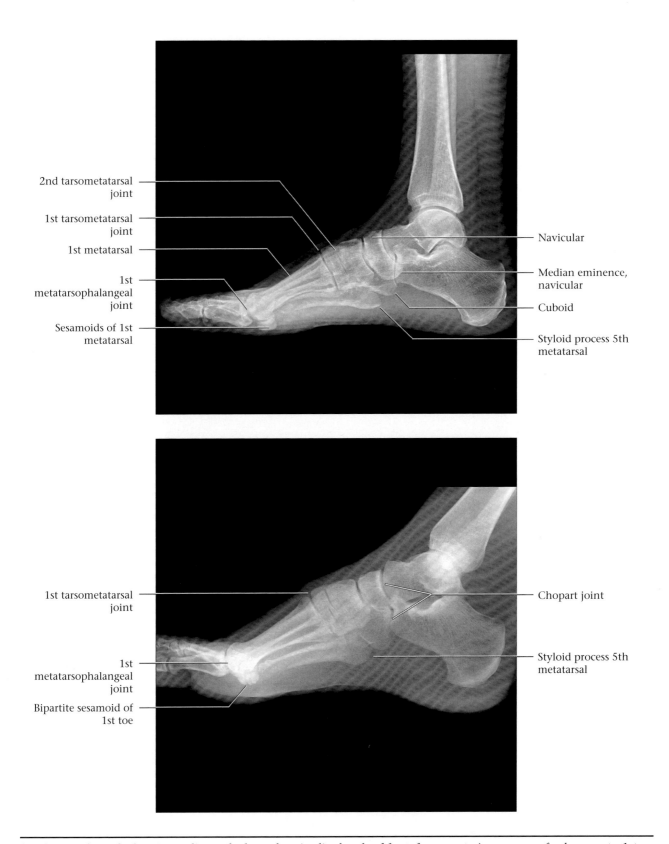

2nd tarsometatarsal joint

1st tarsometatarsal joint

1st metatarsal

1st metatarsophalangeal joint

Sesamoids of 1st metatarsal

Navicular

Median eminence, navicular

Cuboid

Styloid process 5th metatarsal

1st tarsometatarsal joint

1st metatarsophalangeal joint

Bipartite sesamoid of 1st toe

Chopart joint

Styloid process 5th metatarsal

(Top) Lateral weight-bearing radiograph shows longitudinal arch of foot, from posterior process of calcaneus to 1st MTP joint. Note relatively plantar position of median eminence of navicular. Line drawn along center of talar axis will continue along axis of 1st metatarsal in normally aligned foot. 1st and 2nd metatarsal bases are both at dorsal aspect of foot; they can be distinguished by more proximal position of 2nd metatarsal. **(Bottom)** On nonweight-bearing lateral radiograph, longitudinal arch of foot usually appears higher than on weight-bearing view. Calcaneocuboid and talonavicular joints appear subluxated inferiorly on this view but that is a normal finding which resolves on weight-bearing radiographs.

FOOT OVERVIEW

AXIAL T1 MR, PLANTAR ASPECT OF RIGHT FOOT

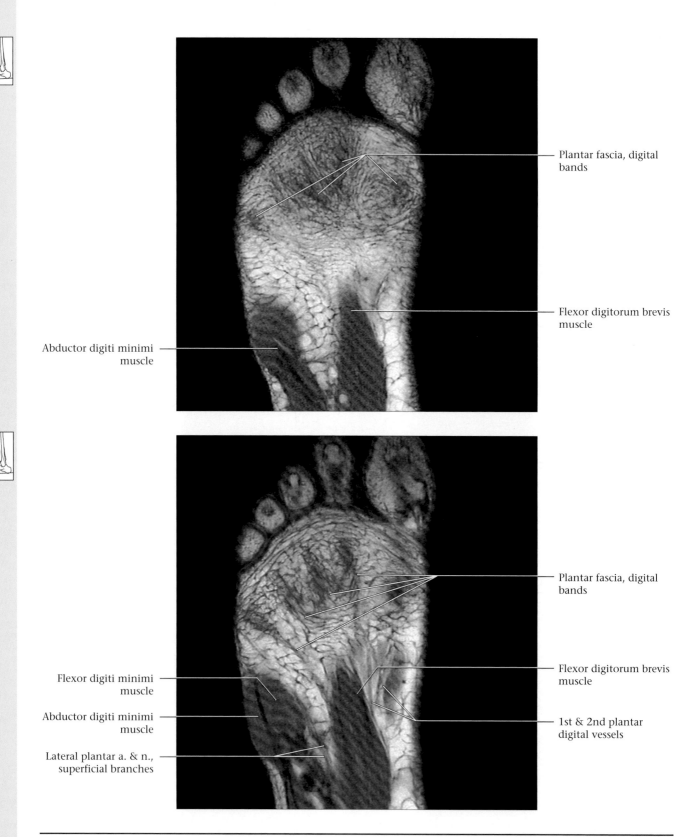

Plantar fascia, digital bands

Flexor digitorum brevis muscle

Abductor digiti minimi muscle

Plantar fascia, digital bands

Flexor digitorum brevis muscle

Flexor digiti minimi muscle

Abductor digiti minimi muscle

1st & 2nd plantar digital vessels

Lateral plantar a. & n., superficial branches

(Top) First in series of axial T1 MR images through the right foot, from plantar to dorsal. Flexor digitorum brevis and abductor digiti minimi are most plantar in position of foot muscles. **(Bottom)** Plantar fascia, superficial to flexor digitorum brevis muscle, is seen dividing into digital bands in forefoot.

FOOT OVERVIEW

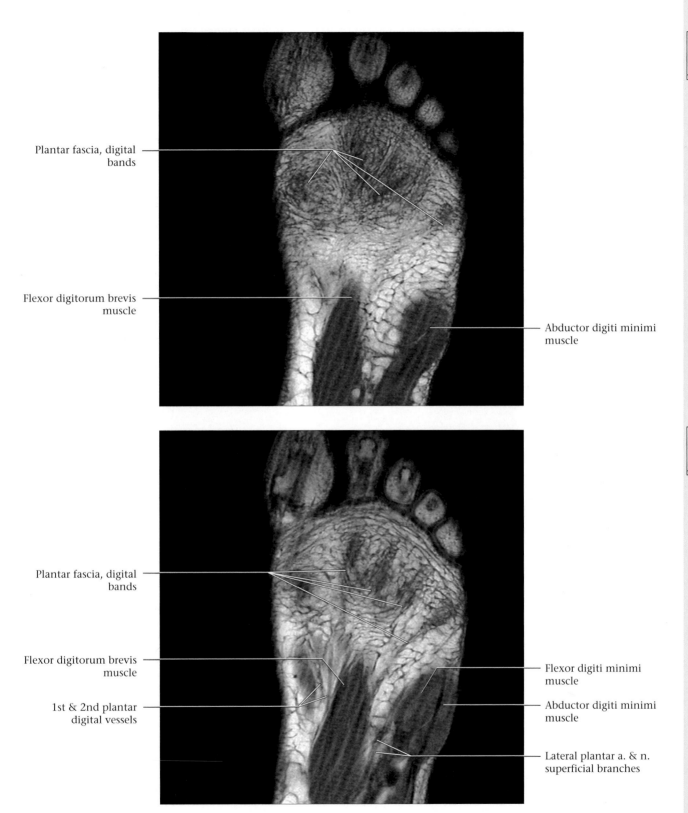

Plantar fascia, digital bands

Flexor digitorum brevis muscle

Abductor digiti minimi muscle

Plantar fascia, digital bands

Flexor digitorum brevis muscle

1st & 2nd plantar digital vessels

Flexor digiti minimi muscle

Abductor digiti minimi muscle

Lateral plantar a. & n. superficial branches

(Top) First in series of axial T1 MR images through the left foot, from plantar to dorsal. Flexor digitorum brevis and abductor digiti minimi are most plantar in position of foot muscles. **(Bottom)** Plantar fascia, superficial to flexor digitorum brevis muscle, is seen dividing into digital bands in forefoot.

FOOT OVERVIEW

AXIAL T1 MR, PLANTAR ASPECT OF RIGHT FOOT

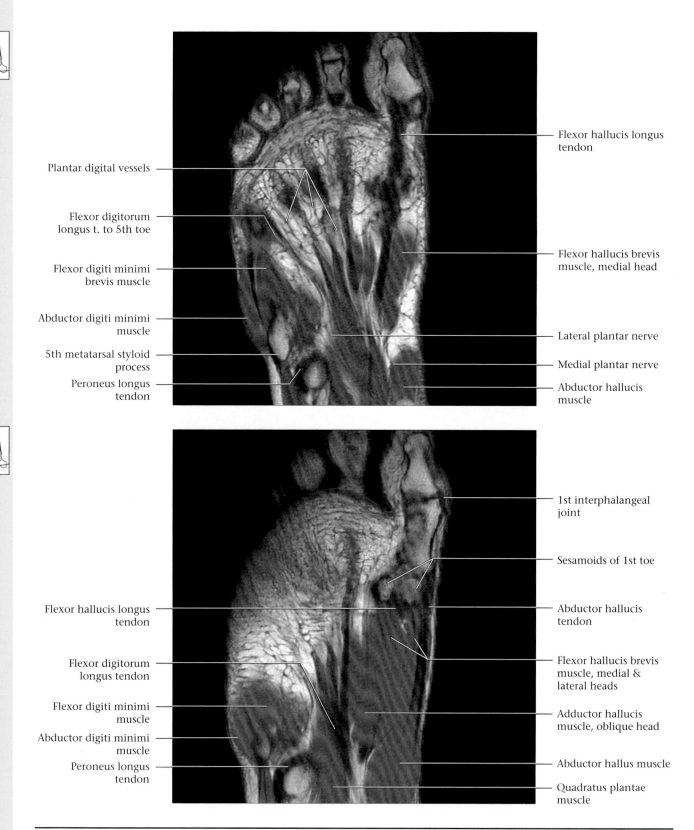

(Top) Medial plantar nerve courses lateral to medial plantar artery, between abductor hallucis and flexor digitorum brevis. Lateral plantar nerve courses between flexor digitorum brevis muscle and quadratus plantae muscle, and continues laterally, dividing into deep and superficial branches at level of 5th metatarsal base, between flexor digitorum brevis and abductor digiti minimi. **(Bottom)** Medial and lateral heads of flexor digitorum brevis muscle are seen attaching to sesamoids of 1st toe. Their distal insertion, onto base of 1st proximal phalanx, is not seen on this image.

FOOT OVERVIEW

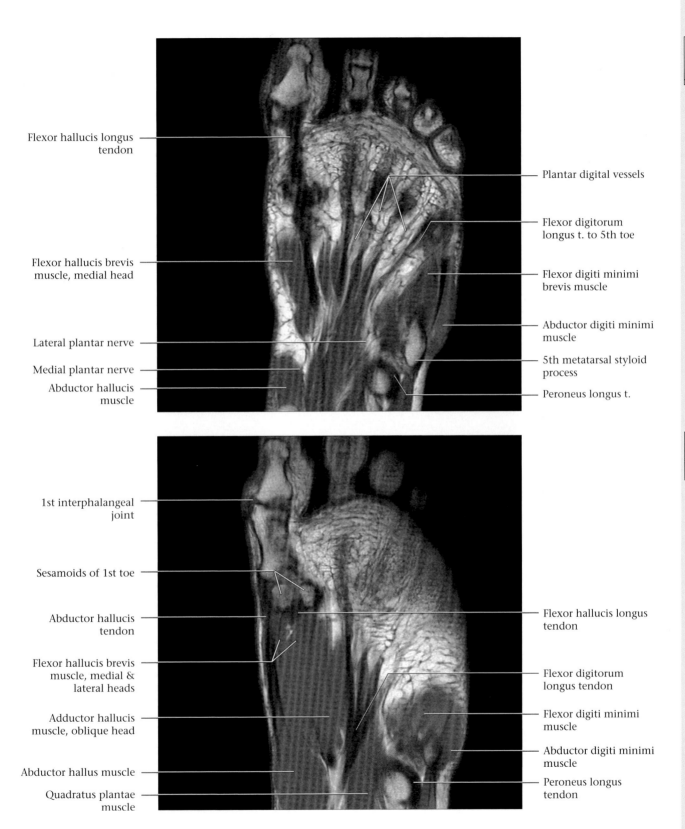

Flexor hallucis longus tendon

Flexor hallucis brevis muscle, medial head

Lateral plantar nerve

Medial plantar nerve

Abductor hallucis muscle

Plantar digital vessels

Flexor digitorum longus t. to 5th toe

Flexor digiti minimi brevis muscle

Abductor digiti minimi muscle

5th metatarsal styloid process

Peroneus longus t.

1st interphalangeal joint

Sesamoids of 1st toe

Abductor hallucis tendon

Flexor hallucis brevis muscle, medial & lateral heads

Adductor hallucis muscle, oblique head

Abductor hallus muscle

Quadratus plantae muscle

Flexor hallucis longus tendon

Flexor digitorum longus tendon

Flexor digiti minimi muscle

Abductor digiti minimi muscle

Peroneus longus tendon

(Top) Medial plantar nerve courses lateral to medial plantar artery, between abductor hallucis and flexor digitorum brevis. Lateral plantar nerve courses between flexor digitorum brevis muscle and quadratus plantae muscle, and continues laterally, dividing into deep and superficial branches at level of 5th metatarsal base, between flexor digitorum brevis muscle and abductor digiti minimi. (Bottom) Medial and lateral heads of flexor digitorum brevis muscle are seen attaching to sesamoids of 1st toe. Their distal insertion, onto base of 1st proximal phalanx, is not seen on this image.

AXIAL T1 MR, PLANTAR ASPECT OF RIGHT FOOT

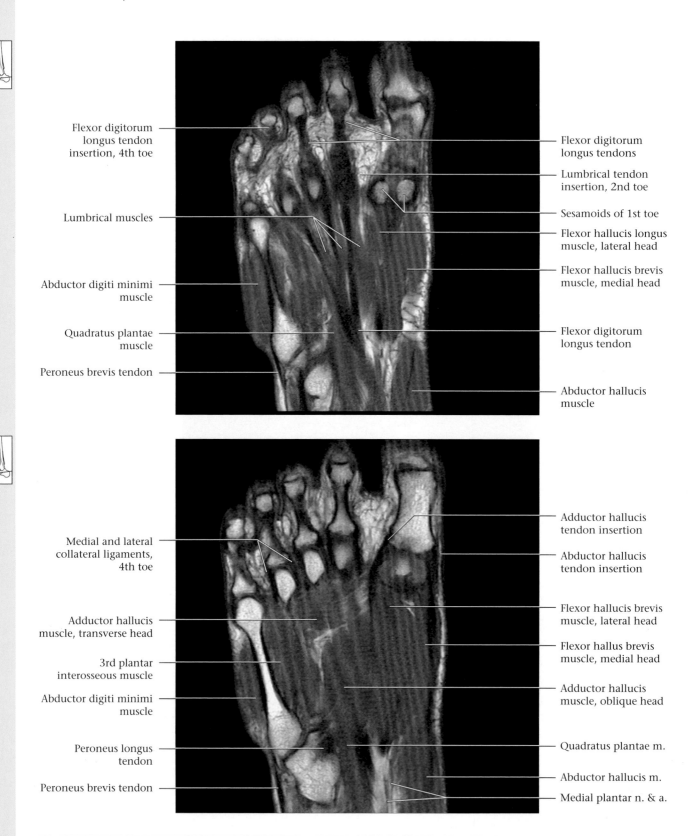

Flexor digitorum longus tendon insertion, 4th toe

Lumbrical muscles

Abductor digiti minimi muscle

Quadratus plantae muscle

Peroneus brevis tendon

Flexor digitorum longus tendons

Lumbrical tendon insertion, 2nd toe

Sesamoids of 1st toe

Flexor hallucis longus muscle, lateral head

Flexor hallucis brevis muscle, medial head

Flexor digitorum longus tendon

Abductor hallucis muscle

Medial and lateral collateral ligaments, 4th toe

Adductor hallucis muscle, transverse head

3rd plantar interosseous muscle

Abductor digiti minimi muscle

Peroneus longus tendon

Peroneus brevis tendon

Adductor hallucis tendon insertion

Abductor hallucis tendon insertion

Flexor hallucis brevis muscle, lateral head

Flexor hallus brevis muscle, medial head

Adductor hallucis muscle, oblique head

Quadratus plantae m.

Abductor hallucis m.

Medial plantar n. & a.

(Top) Note insertion of quadratus plantae muscle into flexor digitorum longus tendon just proximal to its division into slips to 4 lateral toes. Lumbrical muscles arise from individual slips of flexor digitorum longus tendon, and insert on medial aspect of proximal phalanx. A flexor digitorum longus tendon slip to 5th digit is variably present.
(Bottom) Terminology for adductor and abductor hallucis muscles becomes clear once it is remembered that abductor pulls 1st toe away from 2nd toe, and adductor pulls it toward 2nd toe. i.e., axis of reference here is foot, not entire body.

FOOT OVERVIEW

AXIAL T1 MR, PLANTAR ASPECT OF LEFT FOOT

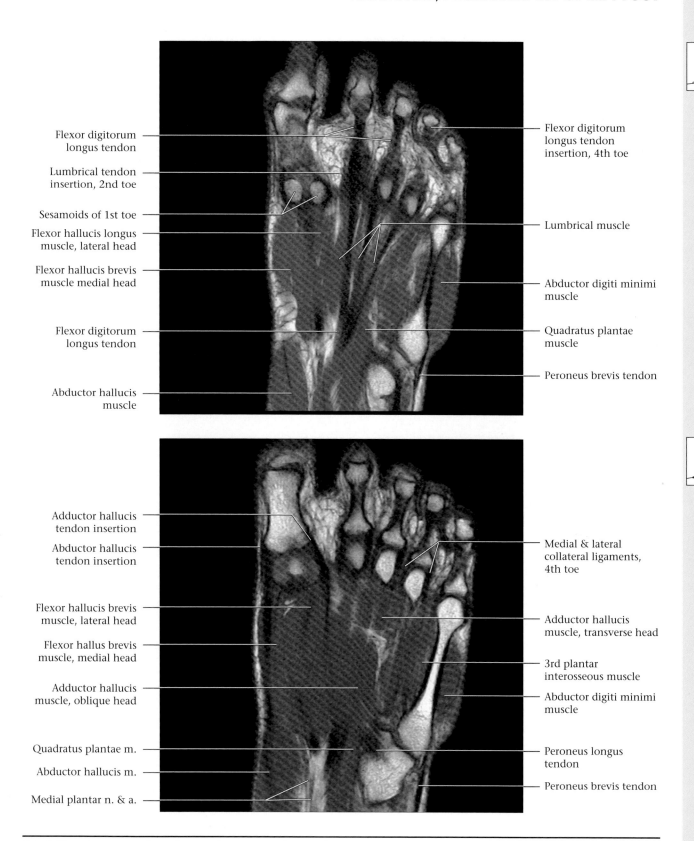

Top image labels (left):
- Flexor digitorum longus tendon
- Lumbrical tendon insertion, 2nd toe
- Sesamoids of 1st toe
- Flexor hallucis longus muscle, lateral head
- Flexor hallucis brevis muscle medial head
- Flexor digitorum longus tendon
- Abductor hallucis muscle

Top image labels (right):
- Flexor digitorum longus tendon insertion, 4th toe
- Lumbrical muscle
- Abductor digiti minimi muscle
- Quadratus plantae muscle
- Peroneus brevis tendon

Bottom image labels (left):
- Adductor hallucis tendon insertion
- Abductor hallucis tendon insertion
- Flexor hallucis brevis muscle, lateral head
- Flexor hallus brevis muscle, medial head
- Adductor hallucis muscle, oblique head
- Quadratus plantae m.
- Abductor hallucis m.
- Medial plantar n. & a.

Bottom image labels (right):
- Medial & lateral collateral ligaments, 4th toe
- Adductor hallucis muscle, transverse head
- 3rd plantar interosseous muscle
- Abductor digiti minimi muscle
- Peroneus longus tendon
- Peroneus brevis tendon

(Top) Note insertion of quadratus plantae muscle into flexor digitorum longus tendon just proximal to its division into slips to 4 lateral toes. Lumbrical muscles arise from individual slips of flexor digitorum longus tendon, and insert on medial aspect of proximal phalanx. A flexor digitorum longus tendon slip to 5th digit is variably present.
(Bottom) Terminology for adductor and abductor hallucis muscles becomes clear once it is remembered that abductor pulls 1st toe away from 2nd toe, and adductor pulls it toward 2nd toe. i.e., axis of reference here is foot, not entire body.

AXIAL T1 MR, PLANTAR ASPECT OF RIGHT FOOT

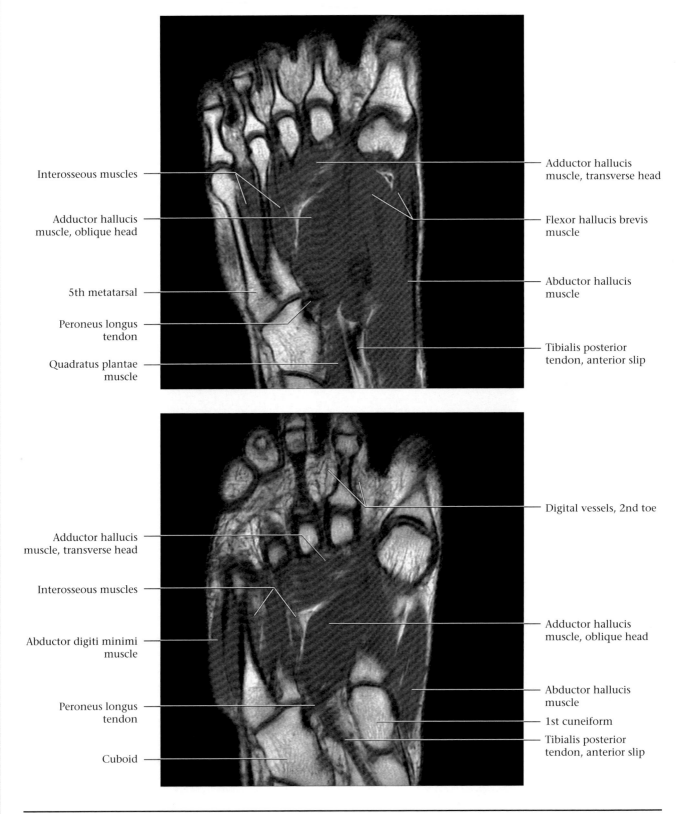

Interosseous muscles

Adductor hallucis muscle, oblique head

5th metatarsal

Peroneus longus tendon

Quadratus plantae muscle

Adductor hallucis muscle, transverse head

Flexor hallucis brevis muscle

Abductor hallucis muscle

Tibialis posterior tendon, anterior slip

Adductor hallucis muscle, transverse head

Interosseous muscles

Abductor digiti minimi muscle

Peroneus longus tendon

Cuboid

Digital vessels, 2nd toe

Adductor hallucis muscle, oblique head

Abductor hallucis muscle

1st cuneiform

Tibialis posterior tendon, anterior slip

(**Top**) Oblique head of adductor hallucis muscle is thick and broad, while transverse head is thinner, and sometimes congenitally absent. (**Bottom**) Insertion of peroneus longus tendon on 1st metatarsal is well seen. Note thread-like digital vessels at medial and lateral margins of 2nd toe.

AXIAL T1 MR, PLANTAR ASPECT OF LEFT FOOT

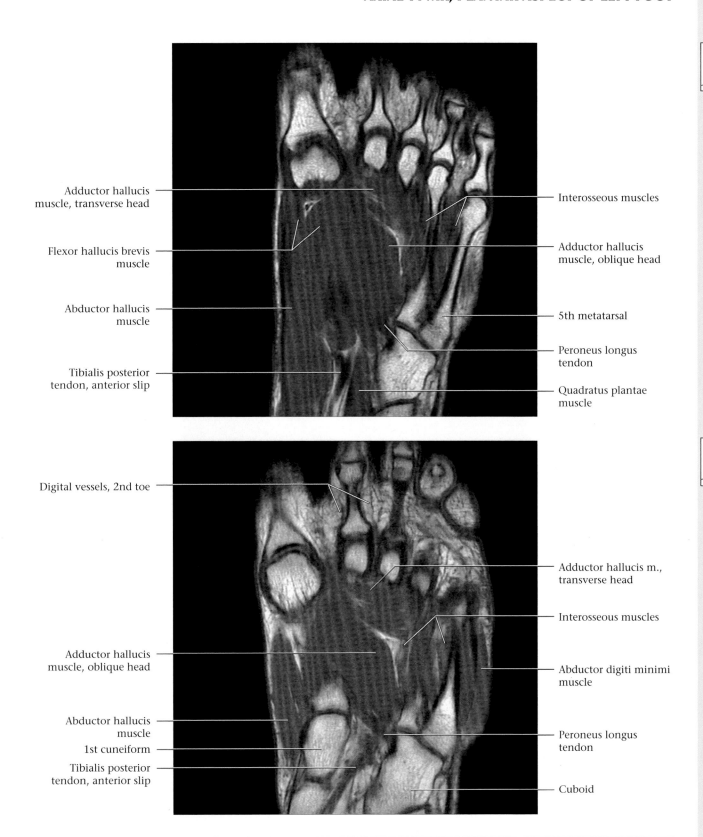

Adductor hallucis muscle, transverse head

Flexor hallucis brevis muscle

Abductor hallucis muscle

Tibialis posterior tendon, anterior slip

Interosseous muscles

Adductor hallucis muscle, oblique head

5th metatarsal

Peroneus longus tendon

Quadratus plantae muscle

Digital vessels, 2nd toe

Adductor hallucis muscle, oblique head

Abductor hallucis muscle

1st cuneiform

Tibialis posterior tendon, anterior slip

Adductor hallucis m., transverse head

Interosseous muscles

Abductor digiti minimi muscle

Peroneus longus tendon

Cuboid

(Top) Oblique head of adductor hallucis muscle is thick and broad, while transverse head is thinner, and sometimes congenitally absent. **(Bottom)** Insertion of peroneus longus tendon on 1st metatarsal is well seen. Note thread-like digital vessels at medial and lateral margins of 2nd toe.

FOOT OVERVIEW

AXIAL T1 MR, PLANTAR ASPECT OF RIGHT FOOT

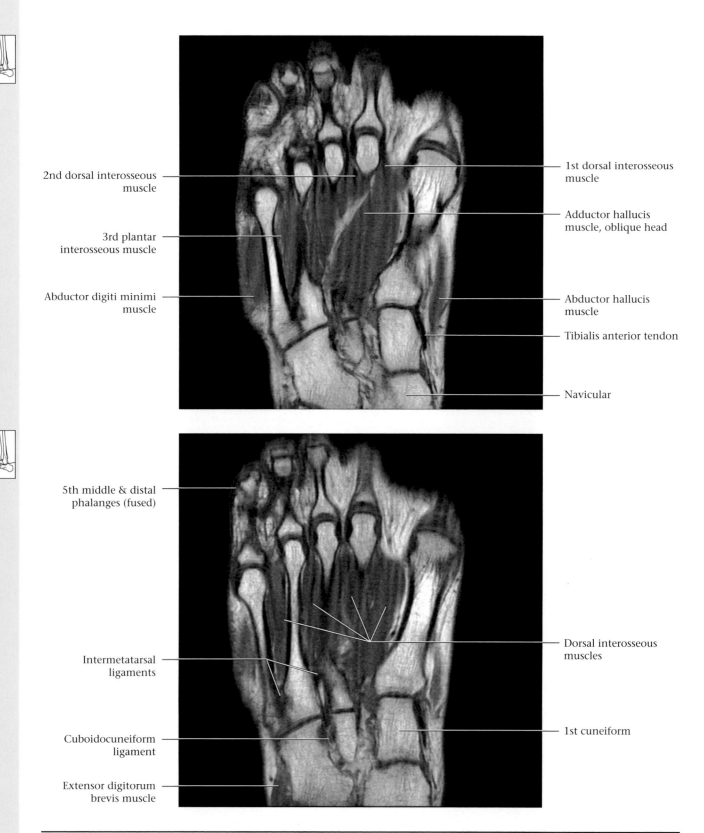

2nd dorsal interosseous muscle

3rd plantar interosseous muscle

Abductor digiti minimi muscle

1st dorsal interosseous muscle

Adductor hallucis muscle, oblique head

Abductor hallucis muscle

Tibialis anterior tendon

Navicular

5th middle & distal phalanges (fused)

Intermetatarsal ligaments

Cuboidocuneiform ligament

Extensor digitorum brevis muscle

Dorsal interosseous muscles

1st cuneiform

(Top) Plantar interossei arise from medial margin of 3 lateral toes, and insert on medial aspect of base of their respective proximal phalanges. (Bottom) There are four dorsal interosseous muscles, each with 2 heads ("bipennate") arising from bases of adjacent metatarsals. 1st dorsal interosseous inserts on medial aspect of base of 2nd proximal phalanx, and 2nd-4th to the lateral aspect of base of 2nd-4th metatarsals.

FOOT OVERVIEW

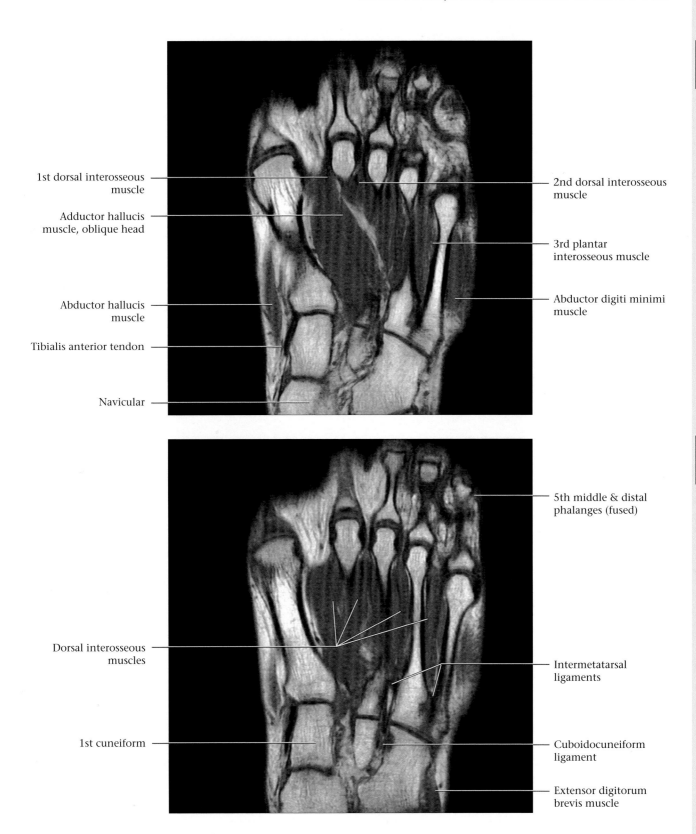

1st dorsal interosseous muscle

Adductor hallucis muscle, oblique head

Abductor hallucis muscle

Tibialis anterior tendon

Navicular

2nd dorsal interosseous muscle

3rd plantar interosseous muscle

Abductor digiti minimi muscle

5th middle & distal phalanges (fused)

Dorsal interosseous muscles

Intermetatarsal ligaments

1st cuneiform

Cuboidocuneiform ligament

Extensor digitorum brevis muscle

(Top) Plantar interossei arise from medial margin of 3 lateral toes, and insert on medial aspect of base of their respective proximal phalanges. (Bottom) There are four dorsal interosseous muscles, each with 2 heads ("bipennate") arising from bases of adjacent metatarsals. 1st dorsal interosseous inserts on medial aspect of base of 2nd proximal phalanx, and 2nd-4th to the lateral aspect of base of 2nd-4th metatarsals.

AXIAL T1 MR, DORSAL ASPECT OF RIGHT FOOT

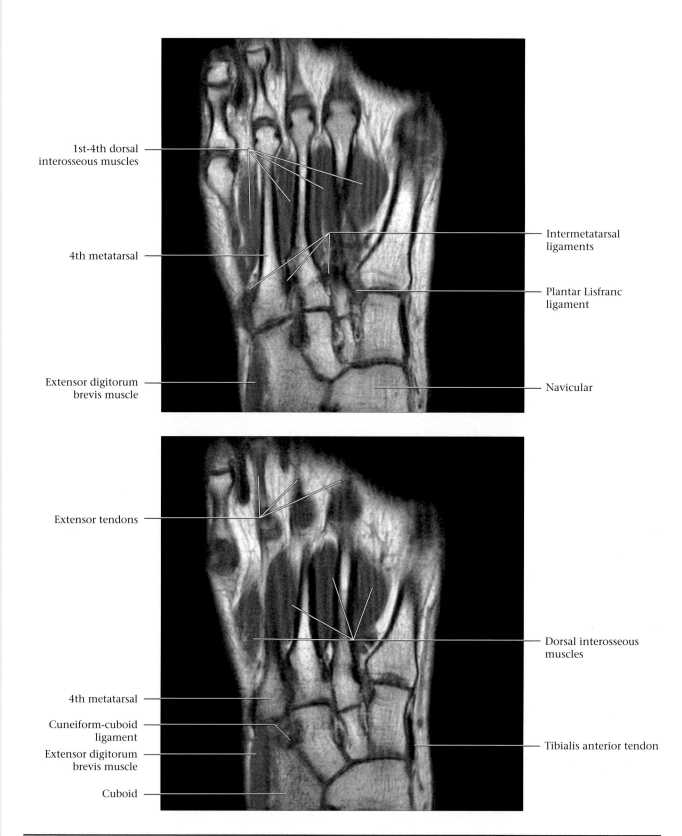

1st-4th dorsal interosseous muscles

4th metatarsal

Extensor digitorum brevis muscle

Intermetatarsal ligaments

Plantar Lisfranc ligament

Navicular

Extensor tendons

Dorsal interosseous muscles

4th metatarsal

Cuneiform-cuboid ligament

Extensor digitorum brevis muscle

Cuboid

Tibialis anterior tendon

(Top) 2nd-5th metatarsal bases are joined by dorsal, interosseous and plantar intermetatarsal ligaments. Stability between 1st and 2nd rays is achieved by 3 ligaments from 1st cuneiform to base of 2nd metatarsal: Dorsal, interosseous, and plantar. Interosseous 1st cuneiform to 2nd metatarsal ligament is broadest and strongest, and is a true Lisfranc ligament. However, "plantar" and "dorsal Lisfranc ligament" are terms which are commonly and appropriately used. **(Bottom)** Note articulations between metatarsal bases. These are constant at the lateral toes, but variability is seen in articulations between 1st and 2nd metatarsals where an articulation is variably present.

FOOT OVERVIEW

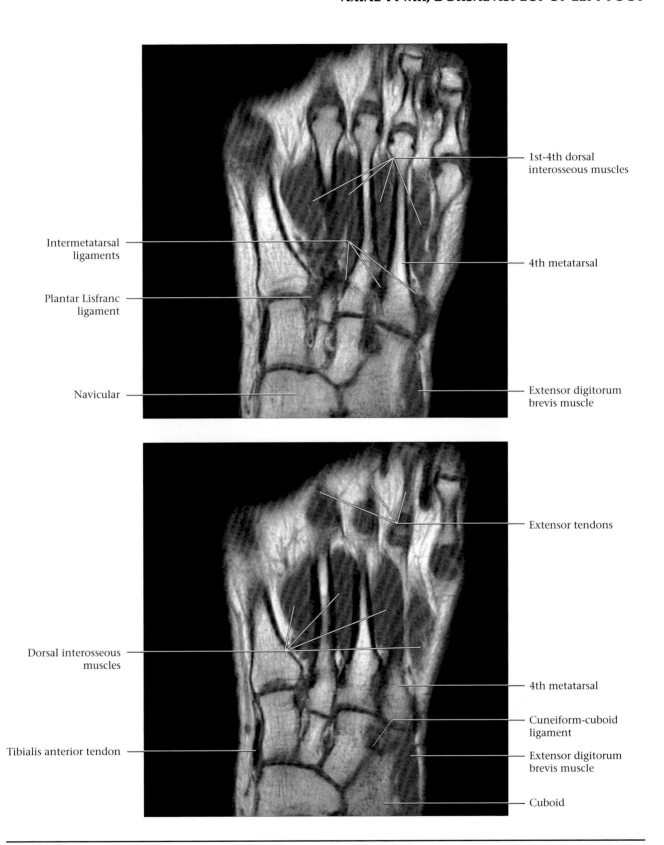

(Top labels)
- 1st-4th dorsal interosseous muscles
- 4th metatarsal
- Extensor digitorum brevis muscle
- Intermetatarsal ligaments
- Plantar Lisfranc ligament
- Navicular

(Bottom labels)
- Extensor tendons
- 4th metatarsal
- Cuneiform-cuboid ligament
- Extensor digitorum brevis muscle
- Cuboid
- Dorsal interosseous muscles
- Tibialis anterior tendon

(Top) 2nd-5th metatarsal bases are joined by dorsal, interosseous and plantar intermetatarsal ligaments. Stability between 1st and 2nd rays is achieved by 3 ligaments from 1st cuneiform to base of 2nd metatarsal: Dorsal, interosseous, and plantar. Interosseous 1st cuneiform to 2nd metatarsal ligament is broadest and strongest, and is a true Lisfranc ligament. However, "plantar" and "dorsal Lisfranc ligament" are terms which are commonly and appropriately used. **(Bottom)** Note articulations between metatarsal bases. These are constant at the lateral toes, but variability is seen in articulations between 1st and 2nd metatarsals where an articulation is variably present.

AXIAL MR, DORSAL ASPECT OF RIGHT FOOT

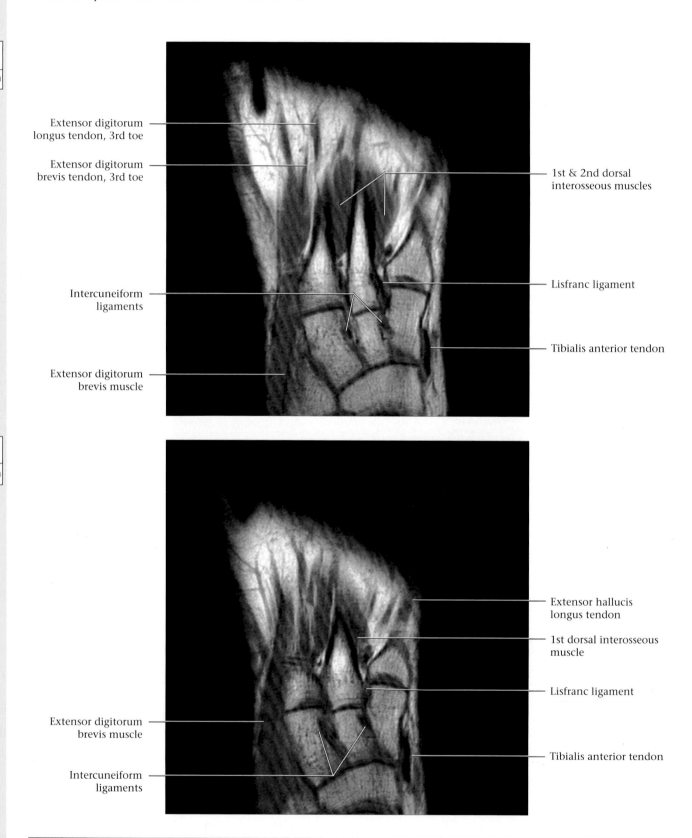

Extensor digitorum longus tendon, 3rd toe

Extensor digitorum brevis tendon, 3rd toe

Intercuneiform ligaments

Extensor digitorum brevis muscle

1st & 2nd dorsal interosseous muscles

Lisfranc ligament

Tibialis anterior tendon

Extensor hallucis longus tendon

1st dorsal interosseous muscle

Lisfranc ligament

Tibialis anterior tendon

Extensor digitorum brevis muscle

Intercuneiform ligaments

(Top) Dorsal soft tissues are much thinner than plantar, especially in forefoot. Individual extensor tendon slips are seen extending to toes, with extensor digitorum brevis tendon slips lateral to corresponding extensor digitorum longus tendon slips. Digital vessels and nerves are well outlined by subcutaneous fat. **(Bottom)** Extensor digitorum brevis muscle originates at lateral margin of calcaneus and fans out to toes. Tibialis anterior tendon wraps around 1st cuneiform to insert on its plantar surface as well as on plantar surface of 1st metatarsal.

AXIAL MR, DORSAL ASPECT OF LEFT FOOT

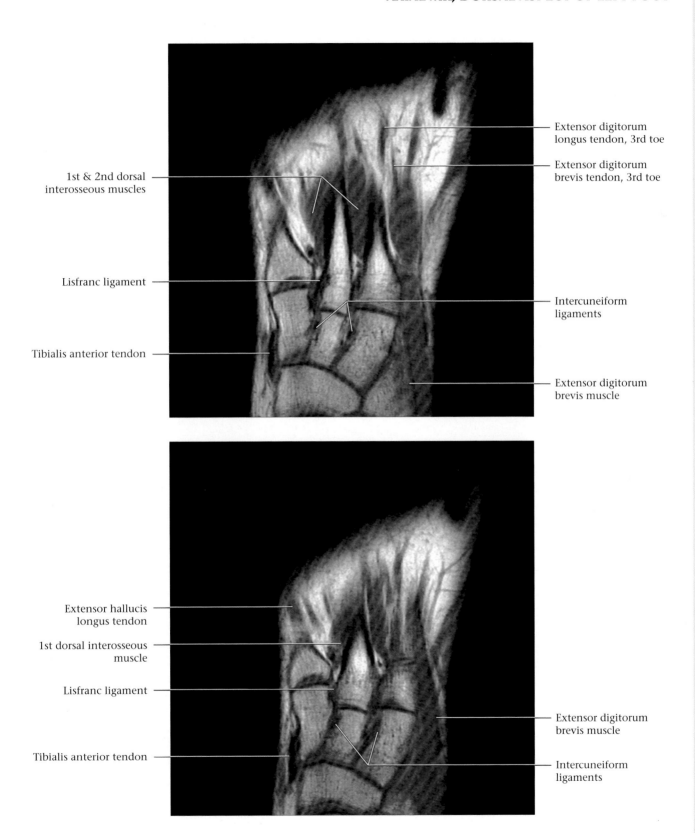

1st & 2nd dorsal interosseous muscles

Lisfranc ligament

Tibialis anterior tendon

Extensor digitorum longus tendon, 3rd toe

Extensor digitorum brevis tendon, 3rd toe

Intercuneiform ligaments

Extensor digitorum brevis muscle

Extensor hallucis longus tendon

1st dorsal interosseous muscle

Lisfranc ligament

Tibialis anterior tendon

Extensor digitorum brevis muscle

Intercuneiform ligaments

(Top) Dorsal soft tissues are much thinner than plantar, especially in forefoot. Individual extensor tendon slips are seen extending to toes, with extensor digitorum brevis tendon slips lateral to corresponding extensor digitorum longus tendon slips. Digital vessels and nerves are well outlined by subcutaneous fat. **(Bottom)** Extensor digitorum brevis muscle originates at lateral margin of calcaneus and fans out to toes. Tibialis anterior tendon wraps around 1st cuneiform to insert on its plantar surface as well as on plantar surface of 1st metatarsal.

FOOT OVERVIEW

CORONAL MR, CHOPART JOINT RIGHT FOOT

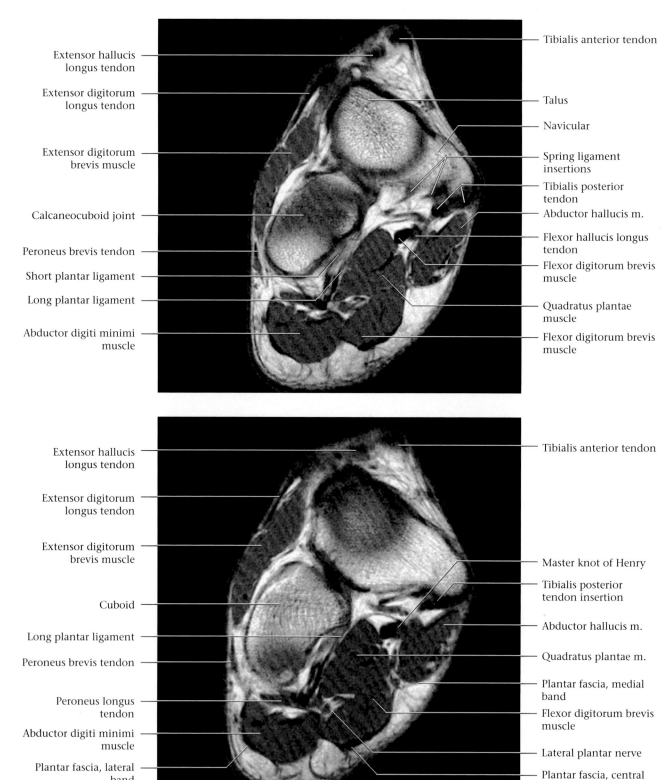

Extensor hallucis longus tendon

Extensor digitorum longus tendon

Extensor digitorum brevis muscle

Calcaneocuboid joint

Peroneus brevis tendon

Short plantar ligament

Long plantar ligament

Abductor digiti minimi muscle

Tibialis anterior tendon

Talus

Navicular

Spring ligament insertions

Tibialis posterior tendon

Abductor hallucis m.

Flexor hallucis longus tendon

Flexor digitorum brevis muscle

Quadratus plantae muscle

Flexor digitorum brevis muscle

Extensor hallucis longus tendon

Extensor digitorum longus tendon

Extensor digitorum brevis muscle

Cuboid

Long plantar ligament

Peroneus brevis tendon

Peroneus longus tendon

Abductor digiti minimi muscle

Plantar fascia, lateral band

Tibialis anterior tendon

Master knot of Henry

Tibialis posterior tendon insertion

Abductor hallucis m.

Quadratus plantae m.

Plantar fascia, medial band

Flexor digitorum brevis muscle

Lateral plantar nerve

Plantar fascia, central band

(Top) First of twenty-four sequential T1 weighted coronal MR images through the right foot from Chopart joint to phalanges. At level of talonavicular and calcaneocuboid joint (together known as Chopart joint), flexor digitorum longus and flexor hallucis longus tendons converge, exchanging fibers at master knot of Henry. **(Bottom)** Plantar fascia (aponeurosis) has 3 divisions: Medial overlies abductor hallucis, central overlies flexor digitorum brevis, and lateral overlies abductor digiti minimi. Central portion is strongest and functionally most important. Main portion of tibialis posterior tendon is seen attaching to navicular; additional slip continue anteriorly and insert on 1st cuneiform, cuboid, and 2nd-4th metatarsal bases.

FOOT OVERVIEW

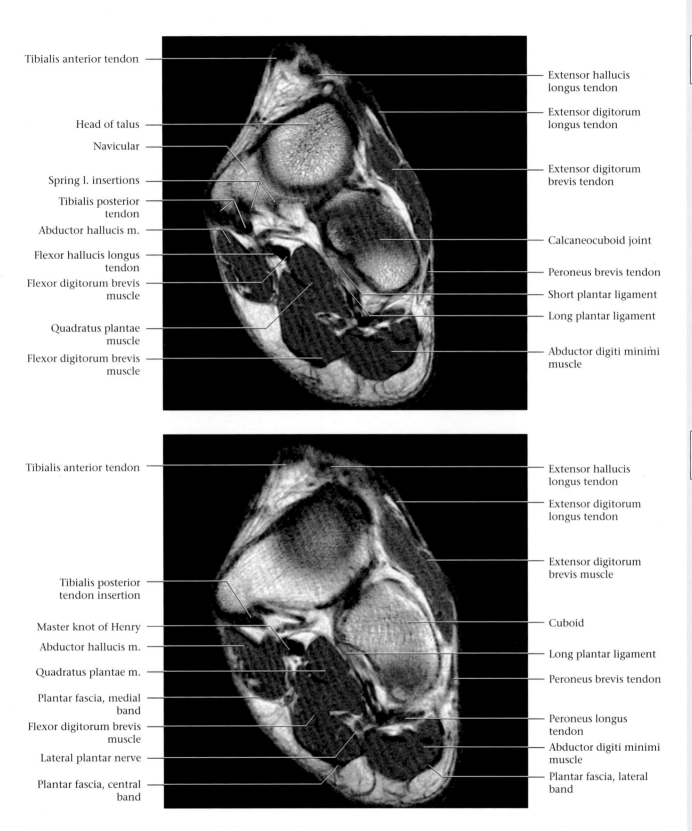

Tibialis anterior tendon

Head of talus

Navicular

Spring l. insertions

Tibialis posterior tendon

Abductor hallucis m.

Flexor hallucis longus tendon

Flexor digitorum brevis muscle

Quadratus plantae muscle

Flexor digitorum brevis muscle

Extensor hallucis longus tendon

Extensor digitorum longus tendon

Extensor digitorum brevis tendon

Calcaneocuboid joint

Peroneus brevis tendon

Short plantar ligament

Long plantar ligament

Abductor digiti minimi muscle

Tibialis anterior tendon

Tibialis posterior tendon insertion

Master knot of Henry

Abductor hallucis m.

Quadratus plantae m.

Plantar fascia, medial band

Flexor digitorum brevis muscle

Lateral plantar nerve

Plantar fascia, central band

Extensor hallucis longus tendon

Extensor digitorum longus tendon

Extensor digitorum brevis muscle

Cuboid

Long plantar ligament

Peroneus brevis tendon

Peroneus longus tendon

Abductor digiti minimi muscle

Plantar fascia, lateral band

(Top) First of twenty-four sequential coronal T1 weighted MR images through the left foot from Chopart joint to phalanges. At level of talonavicular and calcaneocuboid joint (together known as Chopart joint), flexor digitorum longus and flexor hallucis longus tendons converge, exchanging fibers at master knot of Henry. **(Bottom)** Plantar fascia (aponeurosis) has 3 divisions: Medial overlies abductor hallucis, central overlies flexor digitorum brevis, and lateral overlies abductor digiti minimi. Central portion is strongest and functionally most important. Main portion of tibialis posterior tendon is seen attaching to navicular; additional slip continue anteriorly and insert on 1st cuneiform, cuboid, and 2nd-4th metatarsal bases.

Foot

VIII

CORONAL MR, CUBOID & NAVICULAR RIGHT FOOT

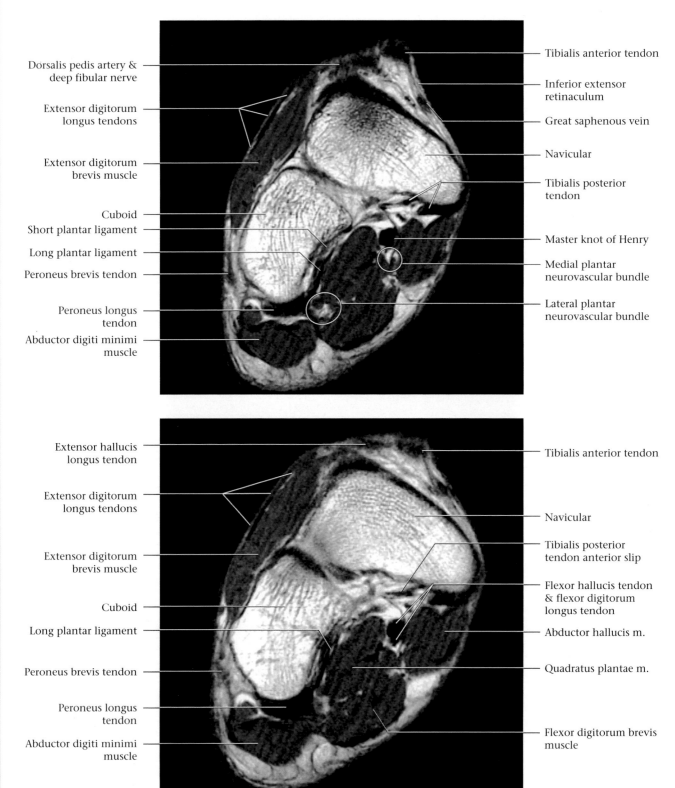

Top image labels (left):
- Dorsalis pedis artery & deep fibular nerve
- Extensor digitorum longus tendons
- Extensor digitorum brevis muscle
- Cuboid
- Short plantar ligament
- Long plantar ligament
- Peroneus brevis tendon
- Peroneus longus tendon
- Abductor digiti minimi muscle

Top image labels (right):
- Tibialis anterior tendon
- Inferior extensor retinaculum
- Great saphenous vein
- Navicular
- Tibialis posterior tendon
- Master knot of Henry
- Medial plantar neurovascular bundle
- Lateral plantar neurovascular bundle

Bottom image labels (left):
- Extensor hallucis longus tendon
- Extensor digitorum longus tendons
- Extensor digitorum brevis muscle
- Cuboid
- Long plantar ligament
- Peroneus brevis tendon
- Peroneus longus tendon
- Abductor digiti minimi muscle

Bottom image labels (right):
- Tibialis anterior tendon
- Navicular
- Tibialis posterior tendon anterior slip
- Flexor hallucis tendon & flexor digitorum longus tendon
- Abductor hallucis m.
- Quadratus plantae m.
- Flexor digitorum brevis muscle

(Top) Posterior tibial neurovascular bundle bifurcates into medial and lateral plantar divisions at origin of abductor hallucis muscle. Medial plantar neurovascular bundle courses between abductor hallucis and quadratus plantae. Lateral plantar neurovascular bundle diverges laterally between quadratus plantae and flexor digitorum brevis. **(Bottom)** Peroneus longus tendon begins to curve medially beneath plantar aspect of cuboid. Long plantar ligament superficial fibers form roof and deep fibers form floor of tunnel through which it passes.

FOOT OVERVIEW

CORONAL MR, CUBOID & NAVICULAR LEFT FOOT

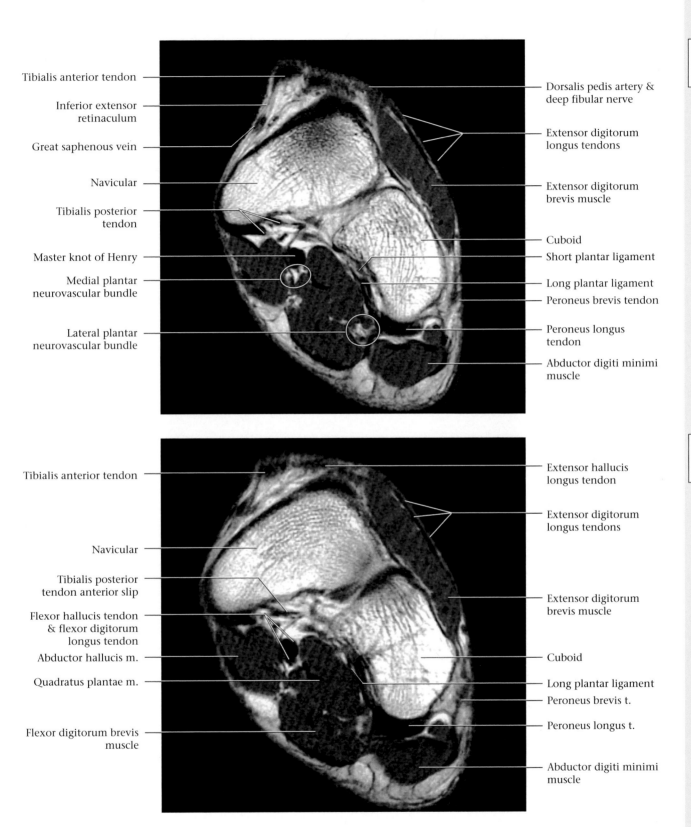

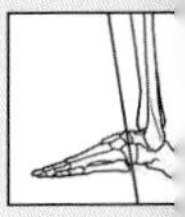

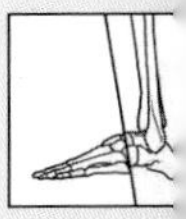

Top image labels (left):
- Tibialis anterior tendon
- Inferior extensor retinaculum
- Great saphenous vein
- Navicular
- Tibialis posterior tendon
- Master knot of Henry
- Medial plantar neurovascular bundle
- Lateral plantar neurovascular bundle

Top image labels (right):
- Dorsalis pedis artery & deep fibular nerve
- Extensor digitorum longus tendons
- Extensor digitorum brevis muscle
- Cuboid
- Short plantar ligament
- Long plantar ligament
- Peroneus brevis tendon
- Peroneus longus tendon
- Abductor digiti minimi muscle

Bottom image labels (left):
- Tibialis anterior tendon
- Navicular
- Tibialis posterior tendon anterior slip
- Flexor hallucis tendon & flexor digitorum longus tendon
- Abductor hallucis m.
- Quadratus plantae m.
- Flexor digitorum brevis muscle

Bottom image labels (right):
- Extensor hallucis longus tendon
- Extensor digitorum longus tendons
- Extensor digitorum brevis muscle
- Cuboid
- Long plantar ligament
- Peroneus brevis t.
- Peroneus longus t.
- Abductor digiti minimi muscle

(Top) Posterior tibial neurovascular bundle bifurcates into medial and lateral plantar divisions at origin of abductor hallucis muscle. Medial plantar neurovascular bundle courses between abductor hallucis and quadratus plantae. Lateral plantar neurovascular bundle diverges laterally between quadratus plantae and flexor digitorum brevis.
(Bottom) Peroneus longus tendon begins to curve medially beneath plantar aspect of cuboid. Long plantar ligament superficial fibers form roof and deep fibers form floor of tunnel through which it passes.

CORONAL MR, CUNEIFORMS RIGHT FOOT

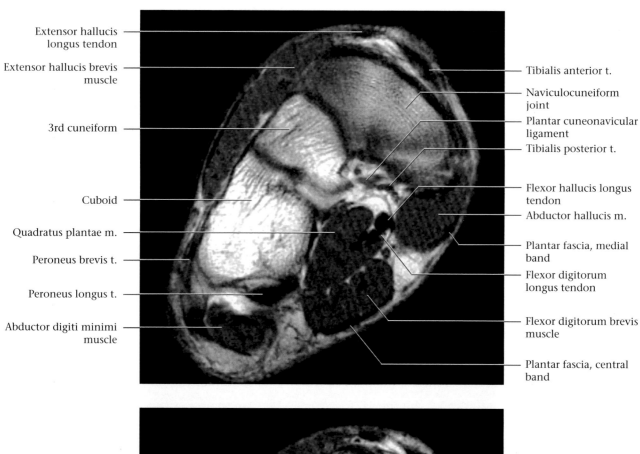

Extensor hallucis longus tendon

Extensor hallucis brevis muscle

3rd cuneiform

Cuboid

Quadratus plantae m.

Peroneus brevis t.

Peroneus longus t.

Abductor digiti minimi muscle

Tibialis anterior t.

Naviculocuneiform joint

Plantar cuneonavicular ligament

Tibialis posterior t.

Flexor hallucis longus tendon

Abductor hallucis m.

Plantar fascia, medial band

Flexor digitorum longus tendon

Flexor digitorum brevis muscle

Plantar fascia, central band

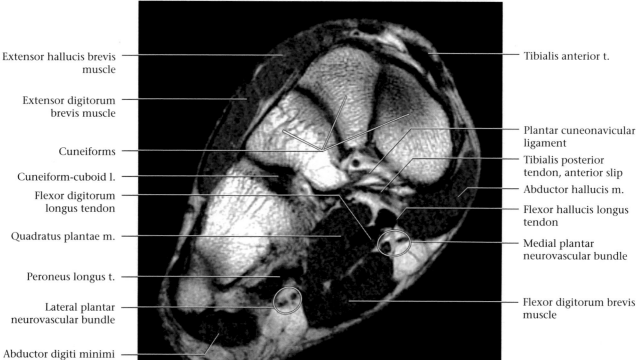

Extensor hallucis brevis muscle

Extensor digitorum brevis muscle

Cuneiforms

Cuneiform-cuboid l.

Flexor digitorum longus tendon

Quadratus plantae m.

Peroneus longus t.

Lateral plantar neurovascular bundle

Abductor digiti minimi muscle

Tibialis anterior t.

Plantar cuneonavicular ligament

Tibialis posterior tendon, anterior slip

Abductor hallucis m.

Flexor hallucis longus tendon

Medial plantar neurovascular bundle

Flexor digitorum brevis muscle

(Top) The navicular and cuneiforms are bridged by plantar cuneonavicular ligaments which lie deep to anterior slips of tibialis posterior tendon. (Bottom) Quadratus plantae muscle has a broad insertion on flexor digitorum longus tendon. Tibialis anterior tendon is turning medially towards its insertion on plantar aspect of 1st cuneiform and 1st metatarsal.

FOOT OVERVIEW

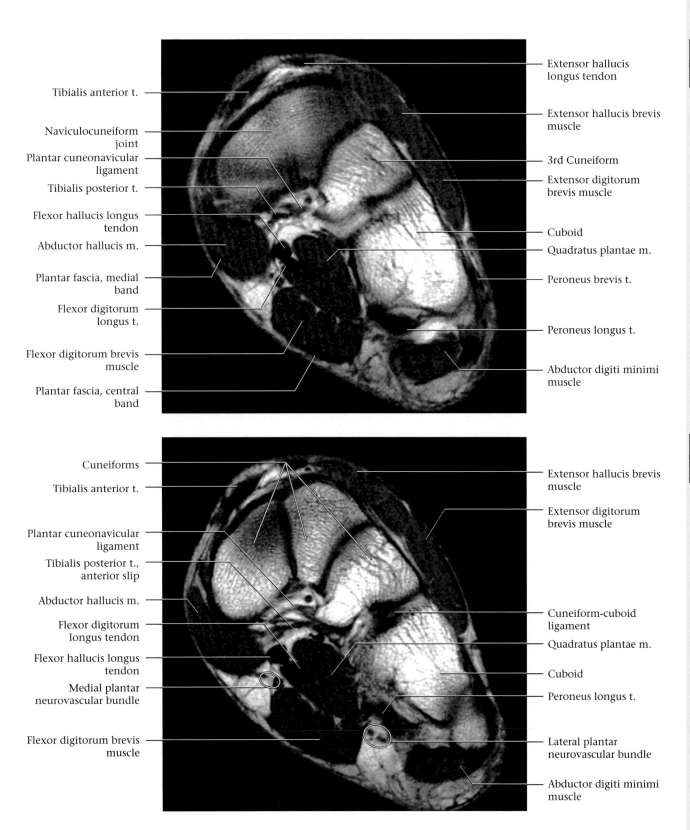

Top image labels (left):
- Tibialis anterior t.
- Naviculocuneiform joint
- Plantar cuneonavicular ligament
- Tibialis posterior t.
- Flexor hallucis longus tendon
- Abductor hallucis m.
- Plantar fascia, medial band
- Flexor digitorum longus t.
- Flexor digitorum brevis muscle
- Plantar fascia, central band

Top image labels (right):
- Extensor hallucis longus tendon
- Extensor hallucis brevis muscle
- 3rd Cuneiform
- Extensor digitorum brevis muscle
- Cuboid
- Quadratus plantae m.
- Peroneus brevis t.
- Peroneus longus t.
- Abductor digiti minimi muscle

Bottom image labels (left):
- Cuneiforms
- Tibialis anterior t.
- Plantar cuneonavicular ligament
- Tibialis posterior t., anterior slip
- Abductor hallucis m.
- Flexor digitorum longus tendon
- Flexor hallucis longus tendon
- Medial plantar neurovascular bundle
- Flexor digitorum brevis muscle

Bottom image labels (right):
- Extensor hallucis brevis muscle
- Extensor digitorum brevis muscle
- Cuneiform-cuboid ligament
- Quadratus plantae m.
- Cuboid
- Peroneus longus t.
- Lateral plantar neurovascular bundle
- Abductor digiti minimi muscle

(Top) The navicular and cuneiforms are bridged by plantar cuneonavicular ligaments which lie deep to anterior slips of tibialis posterior tendon. **(Bottom)** Quadratus plantae muscle has a broad insertion on flexor digitorum longus tendon. Tibialis anterior tendon is turning medially towards its insertion on plantar aspect of 1st cuneiform and 1st metatarsal.

CORONAL MR, CUNEIFORMS RIGHT FOOT

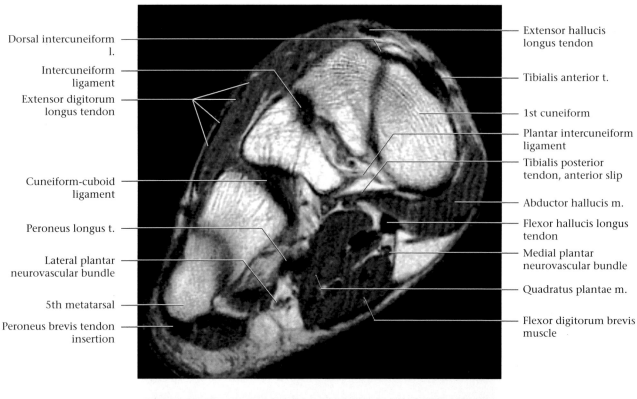

Dorsal intercuneiform l.
Intercuneiform ligament
Extensor digitorum longus tendon
Cuneiform-cuboid ligament
Peroneus longus t.
Lateral plantar neurovascular bundle
5th metatarsal
Peroneus brevis tendon insertion

Extensor hallucis longus tendon
Tibialis anterior t.
1st cuneiform
Plantar intercuneiform ligament
Tibialis posterior tendon, anterior slip
Abductor hallucis m.
Flexor hallucis longus tendon
Medial plantar neurovascular bundle
Quadratus plantae m.
Flexor digitorum brevis muscle

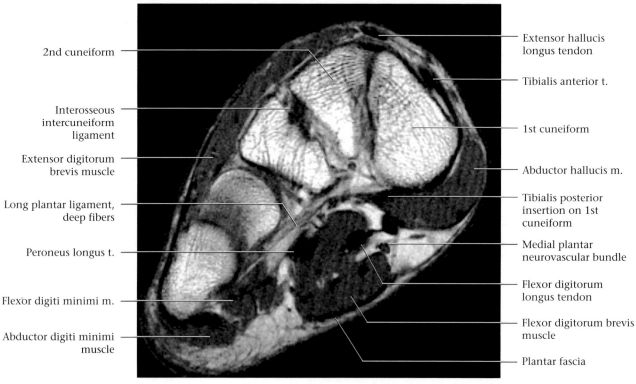

2nd cuneiform
Interosseous intercuneiform ligament
Extensor digitorum brevis muscle
Long plantar ligament, deep fibers
Peroneus longus t.
Flexor digiti minimi m.
Abductor digiti minimi muscle

Extensor hallucis longus tendon
Tibialis anterior t.
1st cuneiform
Abductor hallucis m.
Tibialis posterior insertion on 1st cuneiform
Medial plantar neurovascular bundle
Flexor digitorum longus tendon
Flexor digitorum brevis muscle
Plantar fascia

(Top) Cuneiform bones form transverse arch by virtue of their wedge shape. They are held in position by dorsal, plantar and interosseous ligaments. **(Bottom)** At this level, the 3 major compartmental divisions of plantar muscles are well seen: Medial compartment, beneath 1st ray, lateral compartment beneath 5th ray, and intermediate compartment beneath 2nd-4th rays. The compartments are separated by vertically oriented fascial layers.

CORONAL MR, CUNEIFORMS LEFT FOOT

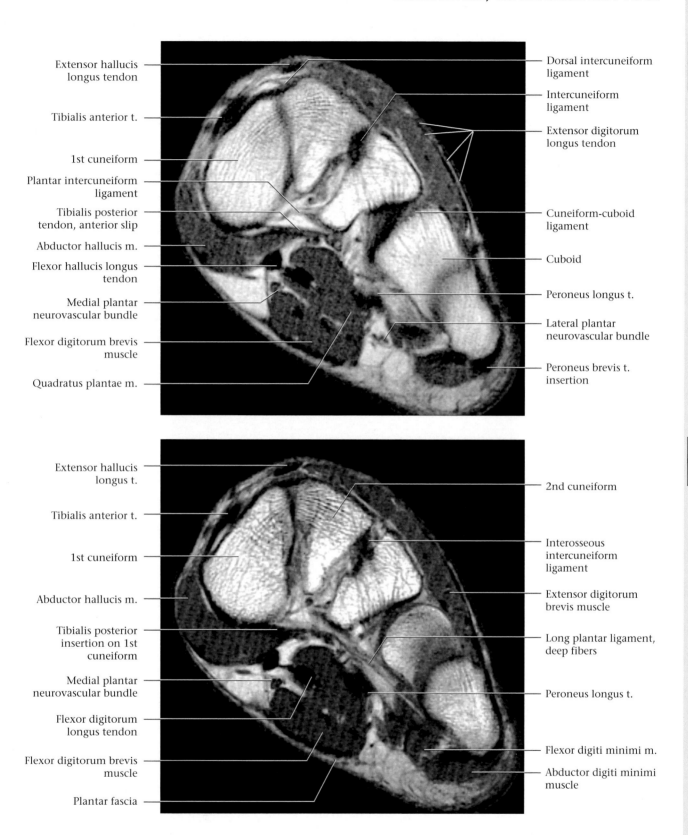

Extensor hallucis longus tendon

Tibialis anterior t.

1st cuneiform

Plantar intercuneiform ligament

Tibialis posterior tendon, anterior slip

Abductor hallucis m.

Flexor hallucis longus tendon

Medial plantar neurovascular bundle

Flexor digitorum brevis muscle

Quadratus plantae m.

Dorsal intercuneiform ligament

Intercuneiform ligament

Extensor digitorum longus tendon

Cuneiform-cuboid ligament

Cuboid

Peroneus longus t.

Lateral plantar neurovascular bundle

Peroneus brevis t. insertion

Extensor hallucis longus t.

Tibialis anterior t.

1st cuneiform

Abductor hallucis m.

Tibialis posterior insertion on 1st cuneiform

Medial plantar neurovascular bundle

Flexor digitorum longus tendon

Flexor digitorum brevis muscle

Plantar fascia

2nd cuneiform

Interosseous intercuneiform ligament

Extensor digitorum brevis muscle

Long plantar ligament, deep fibers

Peroneus longus t.

Flexor digiti minimi m.

Abductor digiti minimi muscle

(Top) Cuneiform bones form transverse arch by virtue of their wedge shape. They are held in position by dorsal, plantar and interosseous ligaments. **(Bottom)** At this level, the 3 major compartmental divisions of plantar muscles are well seen: Medial compartment, beneath 1st ray, lateral compartment beneath 5th ray, and intermediate compartment beneath 2nd-4th rays. The compartments are separated by vertically oriented fascial layers.

CORONAL MR, LISFRANC JOINT RIGHT FOOT

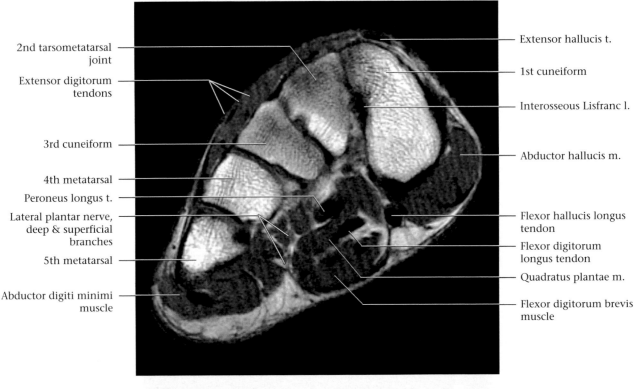

2nd tarsometatarsal joint

Extensor digitorum tendons

3rd cuneiform

4th metatarsal

Peroneus longus t.

Lateral plantar nerve, deep & superficial branches

5th metatarsal

Abductor digiti minimi muscle

Extensor hallucis t.

1st cuneiform

Interosseous Lisfranc l.

Abductor hallucis m.

Flexor hallucis longus tendon

Flexor digitorum longus tendon

Quadratus plantae m.

Flexor digitorum brevis muscle

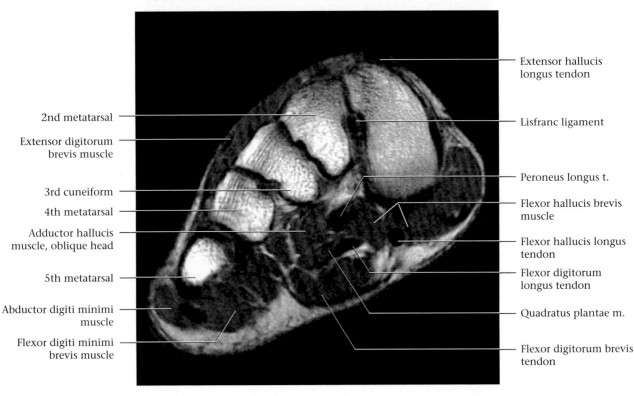

2nd metatarsal

Extensor digitorum brevis muscle

3rd cuneiform

4th metatarsal

Adductor hallucis muscle, oblique head

5th metatarsal

Abductor digiti minimi muscle

Flexor digiti minimi brevis muscle

Extensor hallucis longus tendon

Lisfranc ligament

Peroneus longus t.

Flexor hallucis brevis muscle

Flexor hallucis longus tendon

Flexor digitorum longus tendon

Quadratus plantae m.

Flexor digitorum brevis tendon

(Top) Interosseous Lisfranc ligament is seen at its origin from 1st cuneiform. **(Bottom)** Lisfranc ligament courses distally between 1st cuneiform and 2nd cuneiform, attaching to medial margin of 2nd metatarsal base.

CORONAL MR, LISFRANC JOINT LEFT FOOT

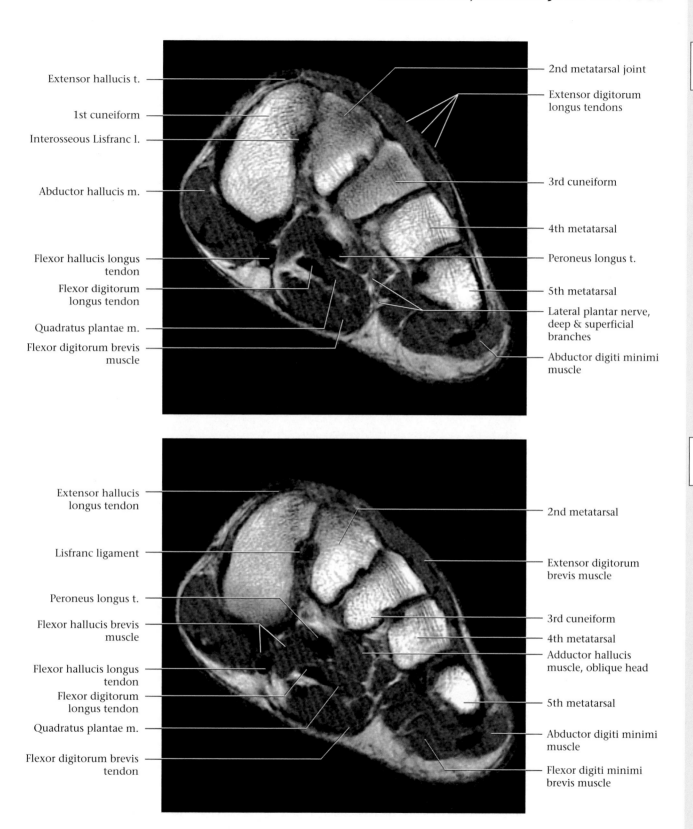

Extensor hallucis t.

1st cuneiform

Interosseous Lisfranc l.

Abductor hallucis m.

Flexor hallucis longus tendon

Flexor digitorum longus tendon

Quadratus plantae m.

Flexor digitorum brevis muscle

2nd metatarsal joint

Extensor digitorum longus tendons

3rd cuneiform

4th metatarsal

Peroneus longus t.

5th metatarsal

Lateral plantar nerve, deep & superficial branches

Abductor digiti minimi muscle

Extensor hallucis longus tendon

Lisfranc ligament

Peroneus longus t.

Flexor hallucis brevis muscle

Flexor hallucis longus tendon

Flexor digitorum longus tendon

Quadratus plantae m.

Flexor digitorum brevis tendon

2nd metatarsal

Extensor digitorum brevis muscle

3rd cuneiform

4th metatarsal

Adductor hallucis muscle, oblique head

5th metatarsal

Abductor digiti minimi muscle

Flexor digiti minimi brevis muscle

(Top) Interosseous Lisfranc ligament is seen at its origin from 1st cuneiform. **(Bottom)** Lisfranc ligament courses distally between 1st cuneiform and 2nd cuneiform, attaching to medial margin of 2nd metatarsal base.

CORONAL MR, PROXIMAL METATARSALS RIGHT FOOT

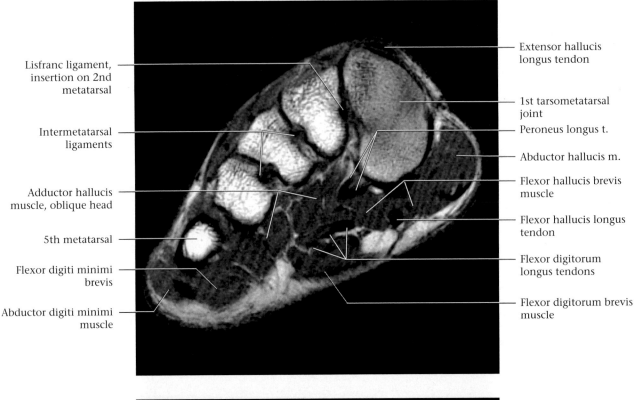

Lisfranc ligament, insertion on 2nd metatarsal

Intermetatarsal ligaments

Adductor hallucis muscle, oblique head

5th metatarsal

Flexor digiti minimi brevis

Abductor digiti minimi muscle

Extensor hallucis longus tendon

1st tarsometatarsal joint

Peroneus longus t.

Abductor hallucis m.

Flexor hallucis brevis muscle

Flexor hallucis longus tendon

Flexor digitorum longus tendons

Flexor digitorum brevis muscle

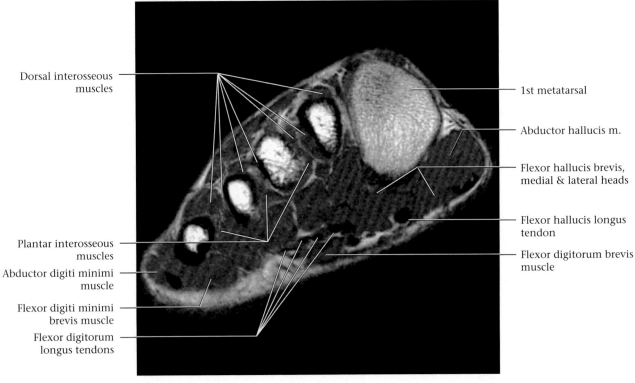

Dorsal interosseous muscles

Plantar interosseous muscles

Abductor digiti minimi muscle

Flexor digiti minimi brevis muscle

Flexor digitorum longus tendons

1st metatarsal

Abductor hallucis m.

Flexor hallucis brevis, medial & lateral heads

Flexor hallucis longus tendon

Flexor digitorum brevis muscle

(Top) Peroneus longus tendon ends in slips attaching to base of 1st metatarsal, 1st cuneiform and sometimes base of 2nd metatarsal. Oblique head of adductor hallucis muscle originates from bases of 3rd and 4th metatarsals and from tendon sheath of peroneus longus. **(Bottom)** Flexor hallucis brevis muscle has two heads, and the flexor hallucis longus tendon is centered between them. Abductor hallucis muscle is closely apposed to medial head of flexor hallucis brevis muscle.

FOOT OVERVIEW

CORONAL MR, PROXIMAL METATARSALS LEFT FOOT

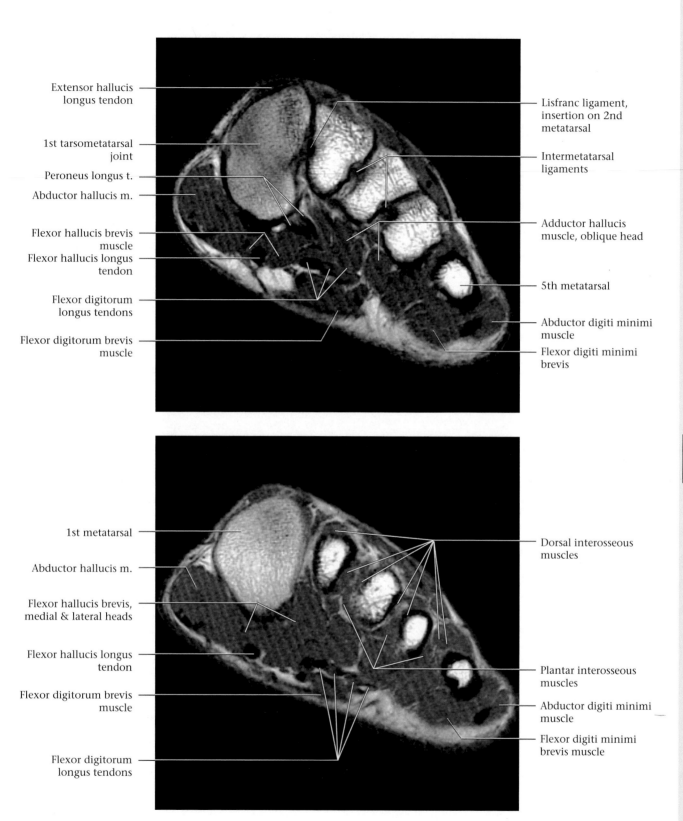

(Top) Peroneus longus tendon ends in slips attaching to base of 1st metatarsal, 1st cuneiform and sometimes base of 2nd metatarsal. Oblique head of adductor hallucis muscle originates from bases of 3rd and 4th metatarsals and from tendon sheath of peroneus longus. **(Bottom)** Flexor hallucis brevis muscle has two heads, and the flexor hallucis longus tendon is centered between them. Abductor hallucis muscle is closely apposed to medial head of flexor hallucis brevis muscle.

FOOT OVERVIEW

CORONAL MR, MID METATARSALS RIGHT FOOT

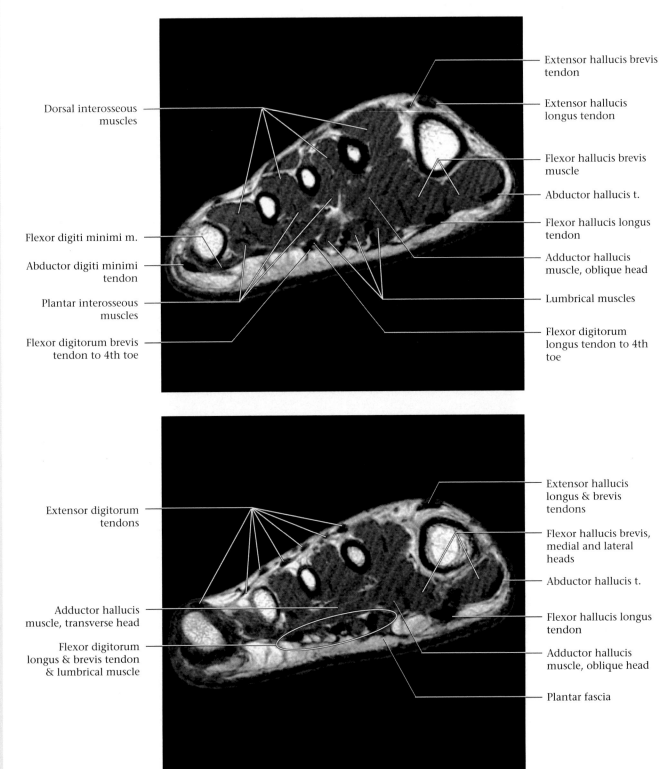

Dorsal interosseous muscles

Flexor digiti minimi m.

Abductor digiti minimi tendon

Plantar interosseous muscles

Flexor digitorum brevis tendon to 4th toe

Extensor hallucis brevis tendon

Extensor hallucis longus tendon

Flexor hallucis brevis muscle

Abductor hallucis t.

Flexor hallucis longus tendon

Adductor hallucis muscle, oblique head

Lumbrical muscles

Flexor digitorum longus tendon to 4th toe

Extensor digitorum tendons

Adductor hallucis muscle, transverse head

Flexor digitorum longus & brevis tendon & lumbrical muscle

Extensor hallucis longus & brevis tendons

Flexor hallucis brevis, medial and lateral heads

Abductor hallucis t.

Flexor hallucis longus tendon

Adductor hallucis muscle, oblique head

Plantar fascia

(Top) Flexor digitorum brevis and longus tendons have divided into individual slips to toes. Brevis tendons slips are superficial to longus. Lumbrical muscles are seen adjacent to flexor digitorum longus tendon slips. **(Bottom)** Transverse head of adductor hallucis m. supports metatarsal heads. It may be congenitally absent. Transverse and oblique heads are shown converging towards their attachment on the lateral sesamoid of the great toe.

FOOT OVERVIEW

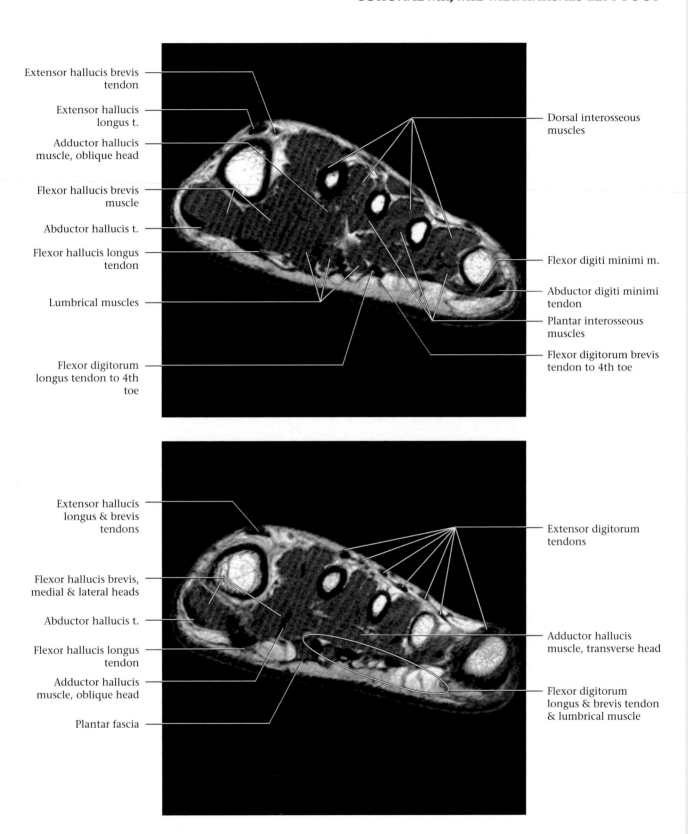

Top image labels (left side):
- Extensor hallucis brevis tendon
- Extensor hallucis longus t.
- Adductor hallucis muscle, oblique head
- Flexor hallucis brevis muscle
- Abductor hallucis t.
- Flexor hallucis longus tendon
- Lumbrical muscles
- Flexor digitorum longus tendon to 4th toe

Top image labels (right side):
- Dorsal interosseous muscles
- Flexor digiti minimi m.
- Abductor digiti minimi tendon
- Plantar interosseous muscles
- Flexor digitorum brevis tendon to 4th toe

Bottom image labels (left side):
- Extensor hallucis longus & brevis tendons
- Flexor hallucis brevis, medial & lateral heads
- Abductor hallucis t.
- Flexor hallucis longus tendon
- Adductor hallucis muscle, oblique head
- Plantar fascia

Bottom image labels (right side):
- Extensor digitorum tendons
- Adductor hallucis muscle, transverse head
- Flexor digitorum longus & brevis tendon & lumbrical muscle

(Top) Flexor digitorum brevis and longus tendons have divided into individual slips to toes. Brevis tendons slips are superficial to longus. Lumbrical muscles are seen adjacent to flexor digitorum longus tendon slips. **(Bottom)** Transverse head of adductor hallucis m. supports metatarsal heads. It may be congenitally absent. Transverse and oblique heads are shown converging towards their attachment on the lateral sesamoid of the great toe.

CORONAL MR, DISTAL METATARSALS RIGHT FOOT

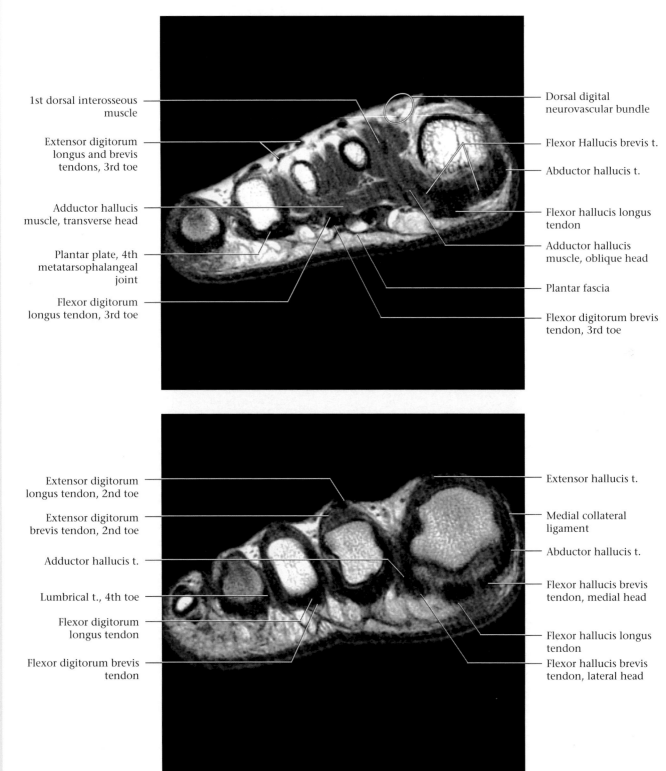

1st dorsal interosseous muscle

Extensor digitorum longus and brevis tendons, 3rd toe

Adductor hallucis muscle, transverse head

Plantar plate, 4th metatarsophalangeal joint

Flexor digitorum longus tendon, 3rd toe

Dorsal digital neurovascular bundle

Flexor Hallucis brevis t.

Abductor hallucis t.

Flexor hallucis longus tendon

Adductor hallucis muscle, oblique head

Plantar fascia

Flexor digitorum brevis tendon, 3rd toe

Extensor digitorum longus tendon, 2nd toe

Extensor digitorum brevis tendon, 2nd toe

Adductor hallucis t.

Lumbrical t., 4th toe

Flexor digitorum longus tendon

Flexor digitorum brevis tendon

Extensor hallucis t.

Medial collateral ligament

Abductor hallucis t.

Flexor hallucis brevis tendon, medial head

Flexor hallucis longus tendon

Flexor hallucis brevis tendon, lateral head

(Top) Plantar fascia sends fibers dorsally and superficially in an arborizing pattern. **(Bottom)** Flexor digitorum longus and brevis tendons are centered beneath metatarsal heads, with brevis superficial to longus, in close proximity to plantar plate of metatarsophalangeal joints. Lumbrical muscles course medial to metatarsals heads and will insert on medial margin of proximal phalanges.

CORONAL MR, DISTAL METATARSALS LEFT FOOT

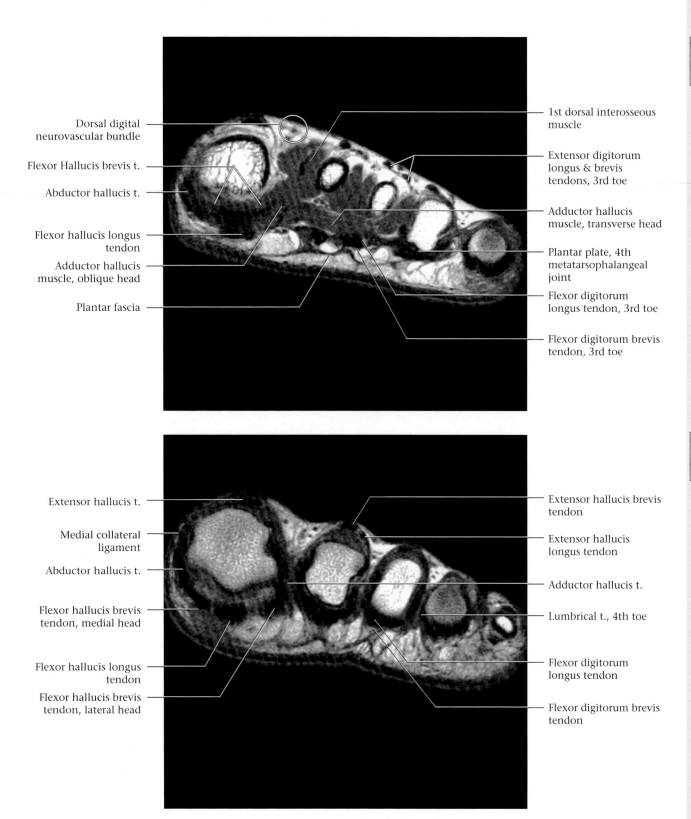

Dorsal digital neurovascular bundle

Flexor Hallucis brevis t.

Abductor hallucis t.

Flexor hallucis longus tendon

Adductor hallucis muscle, oblique head

Plantar fascia

1st dorsal interosseous muscle

Extensor digitorum longus & brevis tendons, 3rd toe

Adductor hallucis muscle, transverse head

Plantar plate, 4th metatarsophalangeal joint

Flexor digitorum longus tendon, 3rd toe

Flexor digitorum brevis tendon, 3rd toe

Extensor hallucis t.

Medial collateral ligament

Abductor hallucis t.

Flexor hallucis brevis tendon, medial head

Flexor hallucis longus tendon

Flexor hallucis brevis tendon, lateral head

Extensor hallucis brevis tendon

Extensor hallucis longus tendon

Adductor hallucis t.

Lumbrical t., 4th toe

Flexor digitorum longus tendon

Flexor digitorum brevis tendon

(Top) Plantar fascia sends fibers dorsally and superficially in an arborizing pattern. **(Bottom)** Flexor digitorum longus and brevis tendons are centered beneath metatarsal heads, with brevis superficial to longus, in close proximity to plantar plate of metatarsophalangeal joints. Lumbrical muscles course medial to metatarsals heads and will insert on medial margin of proximal phalanges.

FOOT OVERVIEW

CORONAL MR, METATARSAL HEADS RIGHT FOOT

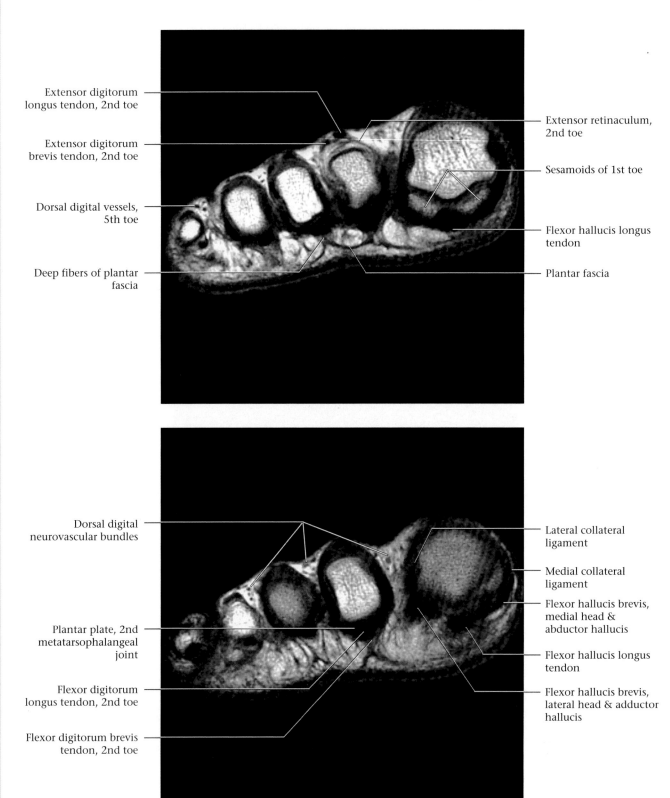

Extensor digitorum longus tendon, 2nd toe

Extensor digitorum brevis tendon, 2nd toe

Dorsal digital vessels, 5th toe

Deep fibers of plantar fascia

Extensor retinaculum, 2nd toe

Sesamoids of 1st toe

Flexor hallucis longus tendon

Plantar fascia

Dorsal digital neurovascular bundles

Plantar plate, 2nd metatarsophalangeal joint

Flexor digitorum longus tendon, 2nd toe

Flexor digitorum brevis tendon, 2nd toe

Lateral collateral ligament

Medial collateral ligament

Flexor hallucis brevis, medial head & abductor hallucis

Flexor hallucis longus tendon

Flexor hallucis brevis, lateral head & adductor hallucis

(**Top**) Medial sesamoid of 1st toe is in the tendon of medial head flexor hallucis brevis tendon, and is also attached to adductor hallucis tendon. Lateral sesamoid is in lateral head flexor hallucis brevis tendon, and also attached to abductor hallucis tendon. Flexor hallucis longus tendon courses between sesamoids. Fibrous septae extending from main portion of plantar fascia to MTP joints are well seen on this image. (**Bottom**) Plantar plate extends from metatarsal neck to base of proximal phalanx, and is an important stabilizer of the MTP joints.

CORONAL MR, METATARSAL HEADS LEFT FOOT

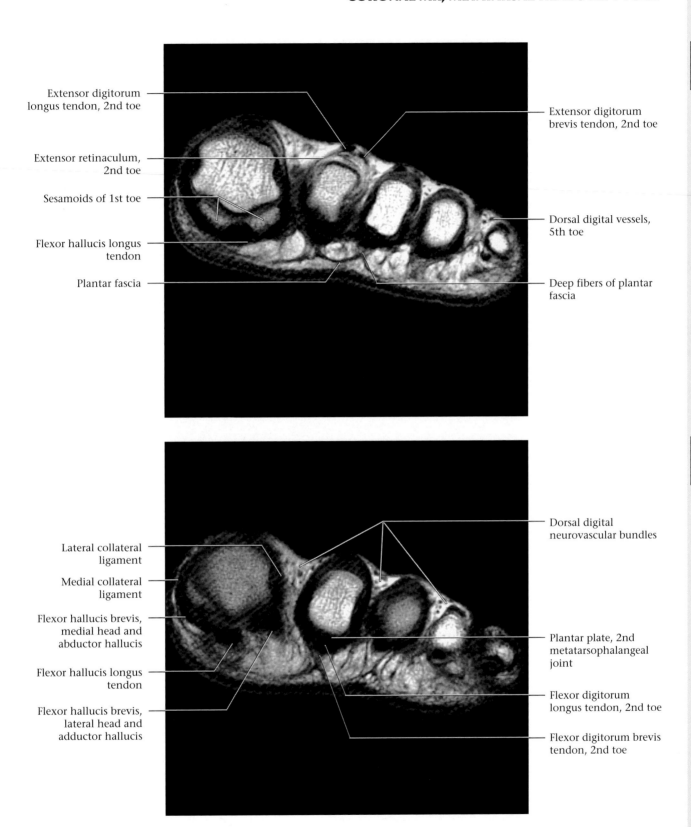

Extensor digitorum longus tendon, 2nd toe

Extensor retinaculum, 2nd toe

Sesamoids of 1st toe

Flexor hallucis longus tendon

Plantar fascia

Extensor digitorum brevis tendon, 2nd toe

Dorsal digital vessels, 5th toe

Deep fibers of plantar fascia

Lateral collateral ligament

Medial collateral ligament

Flexor hallucis brevis, medial head and abductor hallucis

Flexor hallucis longus tendon

Flexor hallucis brevis, lateral head and adductor hallucis

Dorsal digital neurovascular bundles

Plantar plate, 2nd metatarsophalangeal joint

Flexor digitorum longus tendon, 2nd toe

Flexor digitorum brevis tendon, 2nd toe

(Top) Medial sesamoid of 1st toe is in the tendon of medial head flexor hallucis brevis tendon, and is also attached to adductor hallucis tendon. Lateral sesamoid is in lateral head flexor hallucis brevis tendon, and also attached to abductor hallucis tendon. Flexor hallucis longus tendon courses between sesamoids. Fibrous septae extending from main portion of plantar fascia to MTP joints are well seen on this image. **(Bottom)** Plantar plate extends from metatarsal neck to base of proximal phalanx, and is an important stabilizer of the MTP joints.

FOOT OVERVIEW

CORONAL MR, PROXIMAL PHALANGES RIGHT FOOT

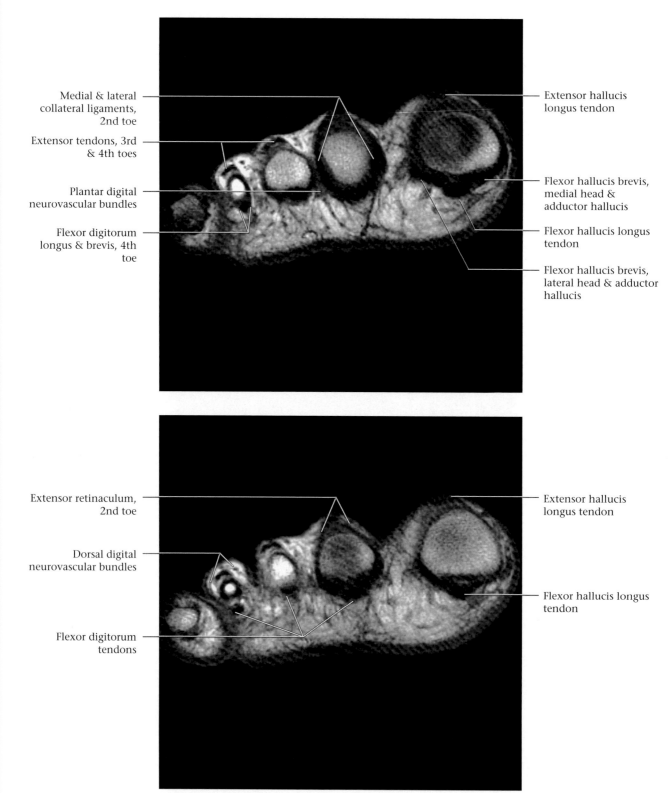

Medial & lateral collateral ligaments, 2nd toe

Extensor tendons, 3rd & 4th toes

Plantar digital neurovascular bundles

Flexor digitorum longus & brevis, 4th toe

Extensor hallucis longus tendon

Flexor hallucis brevis, medial head & adductor hallucis

Flexor hallucis longus tendon

Flexor hallucis brevis, lateral head & adductor hallucis

Extensor retinaculum, 2nd toe

Dorsal digital neurovascular bundles

Flexor digitorum tendons

Extensor hallucis longus tendon

Flexor hallucis longus tendon

(Top) Plantar vessels and nerves lie between metatarsal heads where nerves are susceptible to compression. **(Bottom)** Extensor retinacula are seen superficial to extensor tendons and attaching to dorsolateral margins of phalanges. Flexor retinacula are not well seen on this image because of their obliquity to imaging plane. At level of proximal phalanges, flexor digitorum brevis tendons split into medial and lateral slips which attach to the middle phalanges. Flexor digitorum longus tendon courses between them. The tiny slips are difficult to distinguish on MR. Dorsal digital neurovascular bundles are present at medial and lateral aspects of digits.

CORONAL MR, PROXIMAL PHALANGES LEFT FOOT

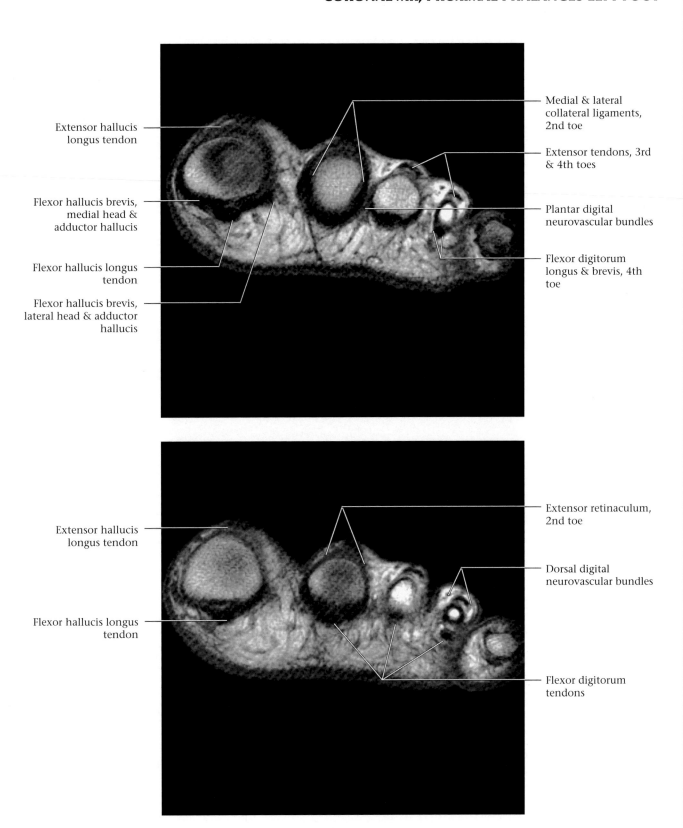

Extensor hallucis longus tendon

Flexor hallucis brevis, medial head & adductor hallucis

Flexor hallucis longus tendon

Flexor hallucis brevis, lateral head & adductor hallucis

Medial & lateral collateral ligaments, 2nd toe

Extensor tendons, 3rd & 4th toes

Plantar digital neurovascular bundles

Flexor digitorum longus & brevis, 4th toe

Extensor hallucis longus tendon

Flexor hallucis longus tendon

Extensor retinaculum, 2nd toe

Dorsal digital neurovascular bundles

Flexor digitorum tendons

(Top) Plantar vessels and nerves lie between metatarsal heads where nerves are susceptible to compression. **(Bottom)** Extensor retinacula are seen superficial to extensor tendons and attaching to dorsolateral margins of phalanges. Flexor retinacula are not well seen on this image because of their obliquity to imaging plane. At level of proximal phalanges, flexor digitorum brevis tendons split into medial and lateral slips which attach to the middle phalanges. Flexor digitorum longus tendon courses between them. The tiny slips are difficult to distinguish on MR. Dorsal digital neurovascular bundles are present at medial and lateral aspects of digits.

FOOT OVERVIEW

CORONAL MR, PHALANGES RIGHT FOOT

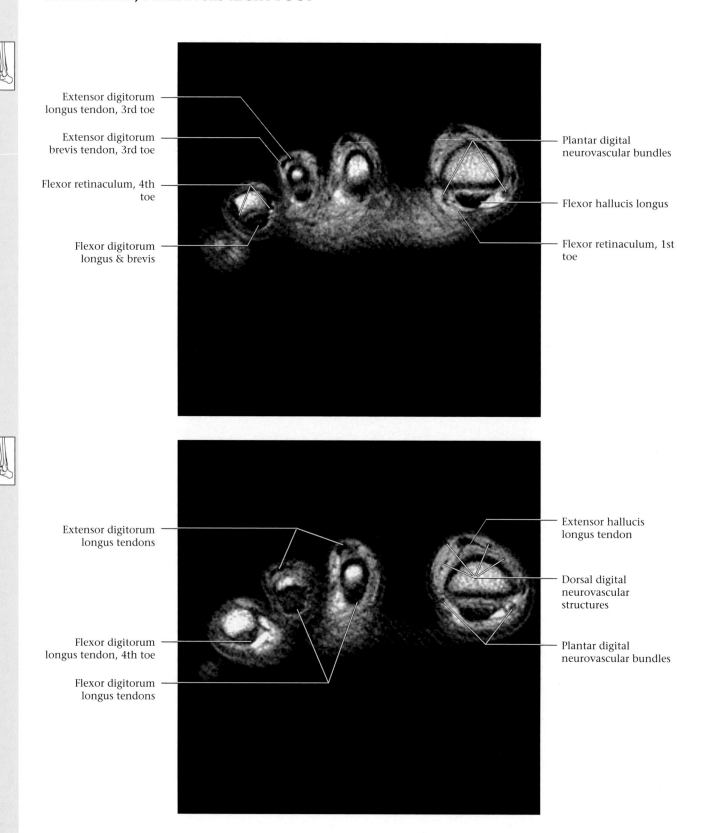

Extensor digitorum longus tendon, 3rd toe

Extensor digitorum brevis tendon, 3rd toe

Flexor retinaculum, 4th toe

Flexor digitorum longus & brevis

Plantar digital neurovascular bundles

Flexor hallucis longus

Flexor retinaculum, 1st toe

Extensor digitorum longus tendons

Flexor digitorum longus tendon, 4th toe

Flexor digitorum longus tendons

Extensor hallucis longus tendon

Dorsal digital neurovascular structures

Plantar digital neurovascular bundles

(Top) Flexor digitorum brevis divides into 2 tendon slips to each toe, inserting on middle phalanx. Flexor digitorum longus has a single slip which passes between them to insert on distal phalanx. **(Bottom)** Flexor digitorum brevis divides into 2 tendon slips to each toe, inserting on middle phalanx. Flexor digitorum longus has a single slip which passes between them to insert on distal phalanx. Extensor digitorum brevis tendon slips attach to lateral side of extensor digitorum longus tendon slips.

CORONAL MR, PHALANGES LEFT FOOT

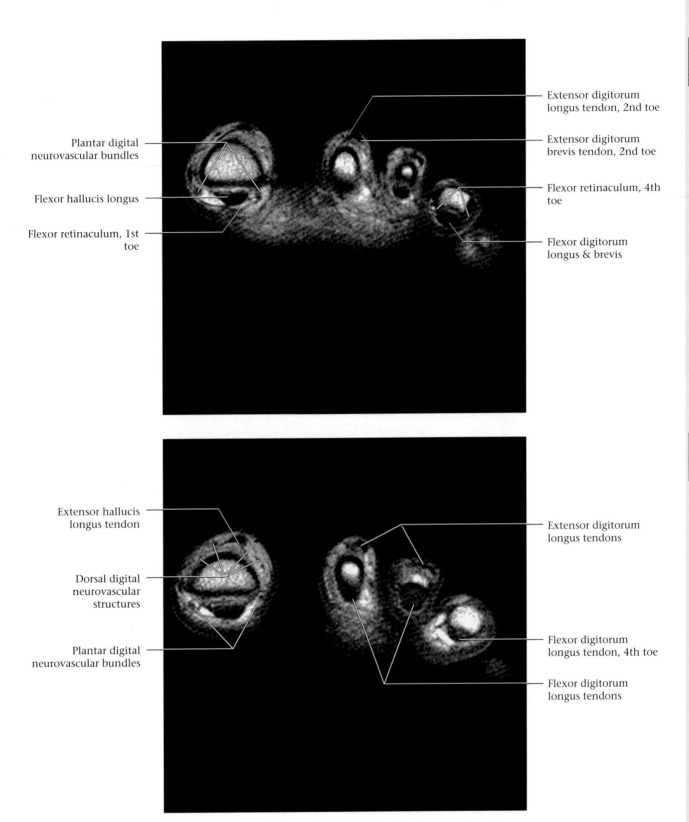

Plantar digital neurovascular bundles

Flexor hallucis longus

Flexor retinaculum, 1st toe

Extensor digitorum longus tendon, 2nd toe

Extensor digitorum brevis tendon, 2nd toe

Flexor retinaculum, 4th toe

Flexor digitorum longus & brevis

Extensor hallucis longus tendon

Dorsal digital neurovascular structures

Plantar digital neurovascular bundles

Extensor digitorum longus tendons

Flexor digitorum longus tendon, 4th toe

Flexor digitorum longus tendons

(Top) Flexor digitorum brevis divides into 2 tendon slips to each toe, inserting on middle phalanx. Flexor digitorum longus has a single slip which passes between them to insert on distal phalanx. **(Bottom)** Flexor digitorum brevis divides into 2 tendon slips to each toe, inserting on middle phalanx. Flexor digitorum longus has a single slip which passes between them to insert on distal phalanx. Extensor digitorum brevis tendon slips attach to lateral side of extensor digitorum longus tendon slips.

Foot

VIII

53

CORONAL MR, PHALANGES RIGHT FOOT

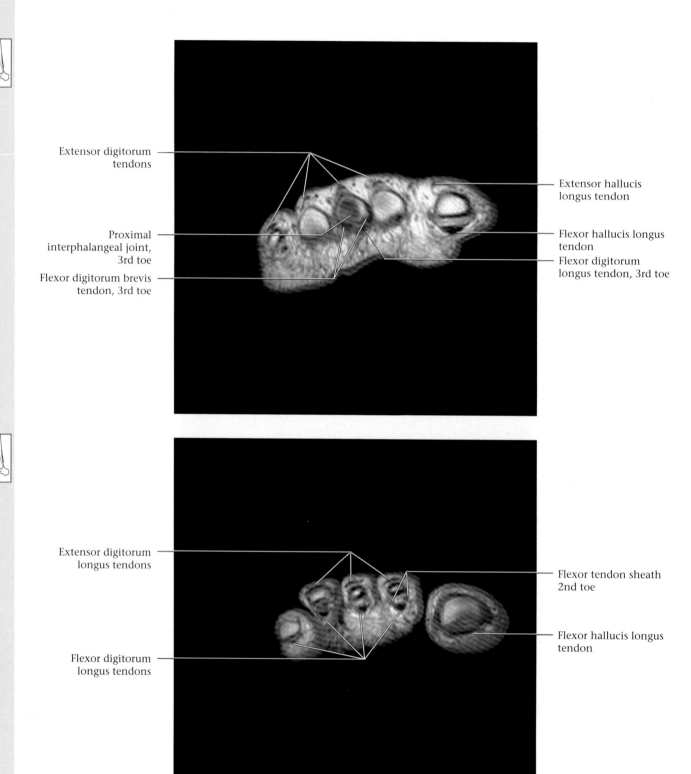

Extensor digitorum tendons

Extensor hallucis longus tendon

Proximal interphalangeal joint, 3rd toe

Flexor hallucis longus tendon

Flexor digitorum longus tendon, 3rd toe

Flexor digitorum brevis tendon, 3rd toe

Extensor digitorum longus tendons

Flexor tendon sheath 2nd toe

Flexor hallucis longus tendon

Flexor digitorum longus tendons

(Top) Flexor digitorum longus tendons run between flexor digitorum brevis and attach to distal phalanges. **(Bottom)** Distal phalanx of 4th toe and middle phalanges of 2nd-4th toes are included on this image. Flexor tendon sheaths to 2nd and 3rd toes form sling around flexor tendons.

FOOT OVERVIEW

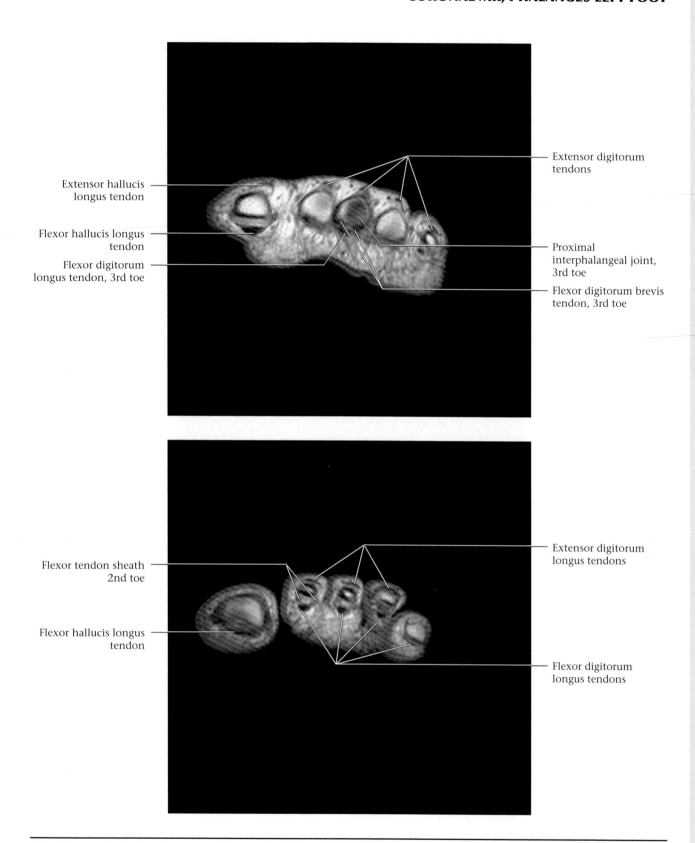

Extensor digitorum tendons

Extensor hallucis longus tendon

Flexor hallucis longus tendon

Flexor digitorum longus tendon, 3rd toe

Proximal interphalangeal joint, 3rd toe

Flexor digitorum brevis tendon, 3rd toe

Flexor tendon sheath 2nd toe

Flexor hallucis longus tendon

Extensor digitorum longus tendons

Flexor digitorum longus tendons

(Top) Flexor digitorum longus tendons run between flexor digitorum brevis and attach to distal phalanges. **(Bottom)** Distal phalanx of 4th toe and middle phalanges of 2nd-4th toes are included on this image. Flexor tendon sheaths to 2nd and 3rd toes form sling around flexor tendons.

SAGITTAL MR, 1ST RAY

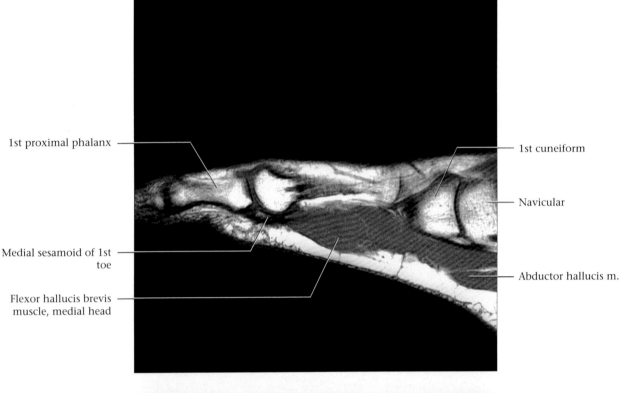

1st proximal phalanx

Medial sesamoid of 1st toe

Flexor hallucis brevis muscle, medial head

1st cuneiform

Navicular

Abductor hallucis m.

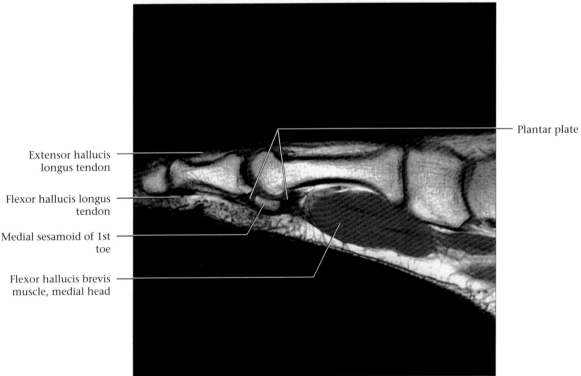

Extensor hallucis longus tendon

Flexor hallucis longus tendon

Medial sesamoid of 1st toe

Flexor hallucis brevis muscle, medial head

Plantar plate

(Top) First of sixteen sagittal MR images from medial to lateral, aligned along axis of 1st metatarsal. Abductor hallucis muscle lies medial to 1st metatarsal, while flexor hallucis brevis lies beneath it. (Bottom) Plantar plate is a strong fibrocartilaginous thickening of plantar joint capsule. It is attached to both sesamoids, to metatarsal neck, to medial and lateral collateral ligaments, and to base of proximal phalanx.

FOOT OVERVIEW

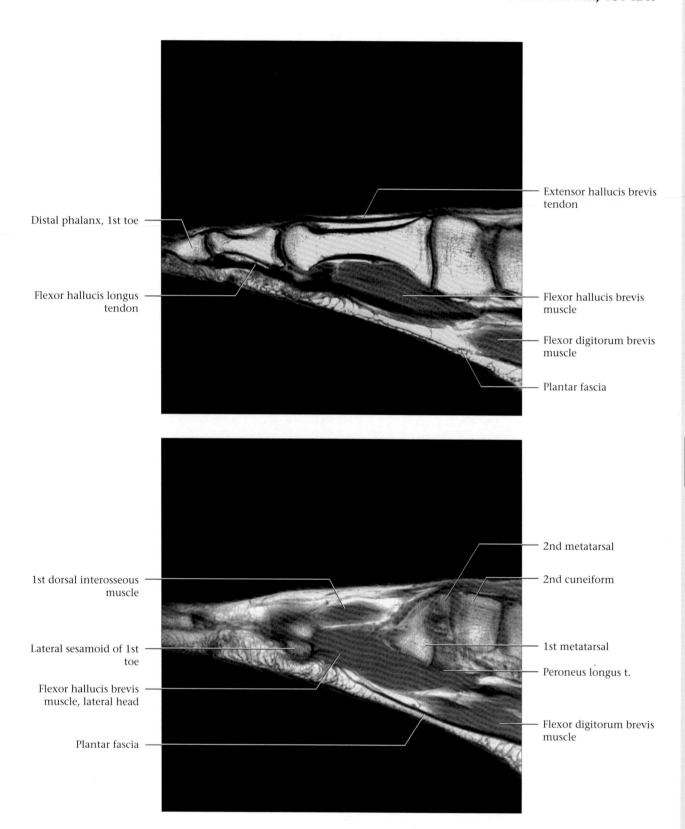

Extensor hallucis brevis tendon

Distal phalanx, 1st toe

Flexor hallucis longus tendon

Flexor hallucis brevis muscle

Flexor digitorum brevis muscle

Plantar fascia

2nd metatarsal

2nd cuneiform

1st dorsal interosseous muscle

Lateral sesamoid of 1st toe

Flexor hallucis brevis muscle, lateral head

Plantar fascia

1st metatarsal

Peroneus longus t.

Flexor digitorum brevis muscle

(Top) Flexor hallucis longus tendon courses between sesamoids of 1st toe, and inserts on distal phalanx of 1st toe. Extensor hallucis brevis tendon lies lateral to longus tendon, and inserts on proximal phalanx of 1st toe. **(Bottom)** Distal portion of peroneus longus tendon is seen attaching to 1st metatarsal base.

SAGITTAL MR, 2ND RAY

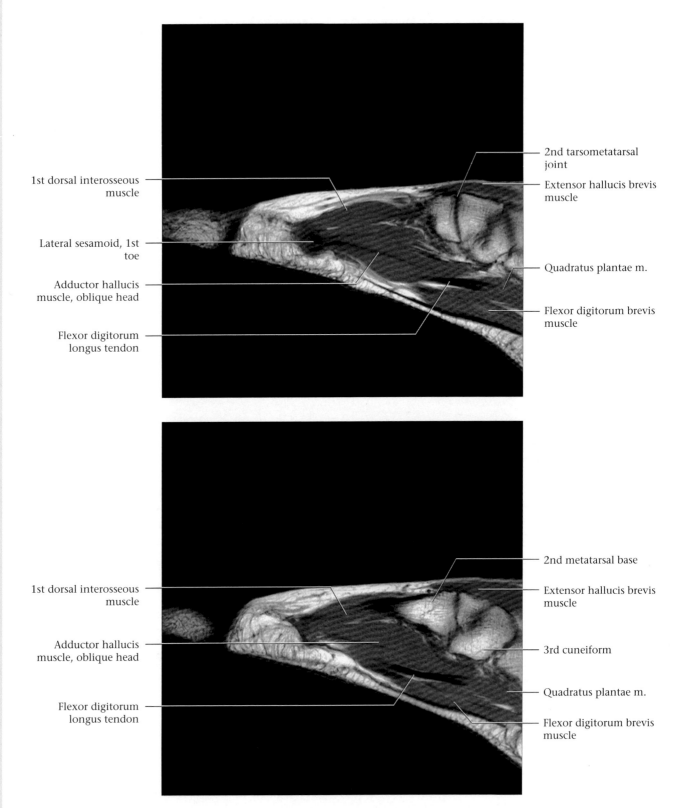

1st dorsal interosseous muscle

Lateral sesamoid, 1st toe

Adductor hallucis muscle, oblique head

Flexor digitorum longus tendon

2nd tarsometatarsal joint

Extensor hallucis brevis muscle

Quadratus plantae m.

Flexor digitorum brevis muscle

1st dorsal interosseous muscle

Adductor hallucis muscle, oblique head

Flexor digitorum longus tendon

2nd metatarsal base

Extensor hallucis brevis muscle

3rd cuneiform

Quadratus plantae m.

Flexor digitorum brevis muscle

(Top) Thick, broad adductor hallucis muscle is seen attaching to lateral sesamoid of 1st toe. Quadratus plantae muscle is seen attaching to flexor digitorum longus tendon. (Bottom) Interspace between 1st and 2nd metatarsals contains only a dorsal interosseous muscle, attaching to medial aspect of 2nd proximal phalanx. Remaining intermetatarsal interspaces contain dorsal and plantar interosseous muscles. Dorsal muscles attach to lateral aspect of proximal phalangeal bases 2-4, and plantar attach to medial aspect of proximal phalangeal bases 3-5.

FOOT OVERVIEW

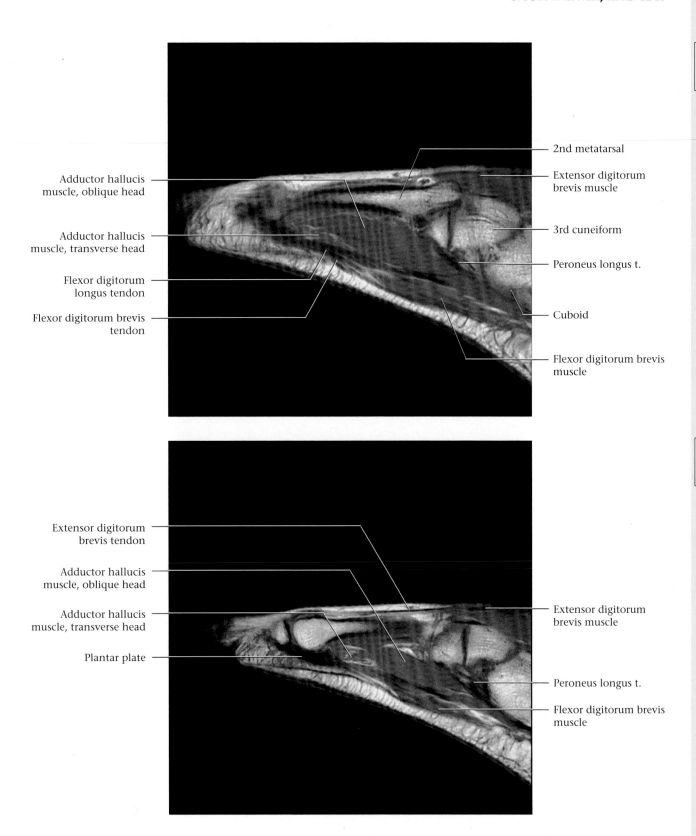

Adductor hallucis muscle, oblique head

Adductor hallucis muscle, transverse head

Flexor digitorum longus tendon

Flexor digitorum brevis tendon

2nd metatarsal

Extensor digitorum brevis muscle

3rd cuneiform

Peroneus longus t.

Cuboid

Flexor digitorum brevis muscle

Extensor digitorum brevis tendon

Adductor hallucis muscle, oblique head

Adductor hallucis muscle, transverse head

Plantar plate

Extensor digitorum brevis muscle

Peroneus longus t.

Flexor digitorum brevis muscle

(Top) Flexor digitorum brevis muscle divides into slips to toes 2-4 and sometimes 5 at level of metatarsal shafts. Tendons are superficial to flexor digitorum longus tendons. (Bottom) Extensor digitorum longus and brevis tendons run side by side in forefoot, with brevis lateral to corresponding longus tendon. Brevis tendon attaches to lateral margin of longus tendon.

SAGITTAL MR, 2ND-4TH RAYS

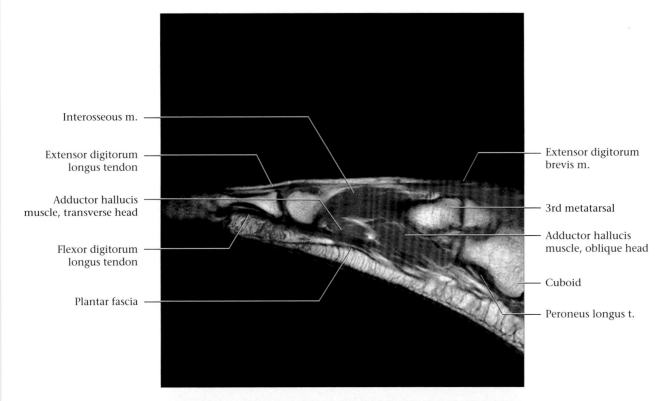

Interosseous m.

Extensor digitorum longus tendon

Adductor hallucis muscle, transverse head

Flexor digitorum longus tendon

Plantar fascia

Extensor digitorum brevis m.

3rd metatarsal

Adductor hallucis muscle, oblique head

Cuboid

Peroneus longus t.

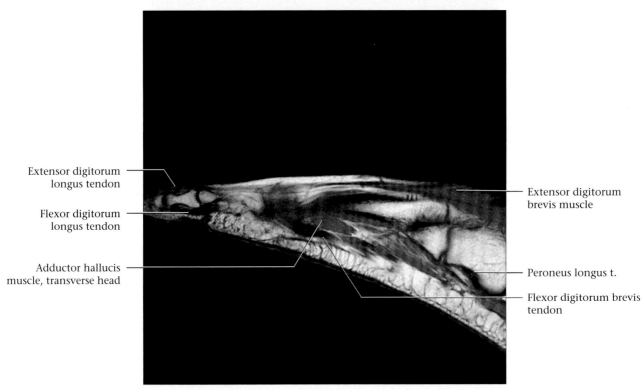

Extensor digitorum longus tendon

Flexor digitorum longus tendon

Adductor hallucis muscle, transverse head

Extensor digitorum brevis muscle

Peroneus longus t.

Flexor digitorum brevis tendon

(Top) In forefoot, plantar fascia divides into digital bands. At level of metatarsal heads, it arborizes into superficial and deep components. **(Bottom)** Peroneus longus tendon lies in groove beneath cuboid, held in place by long plantar ligament.

Foot

VIII

SAGITTAL MR, 3RD-4TH RAY

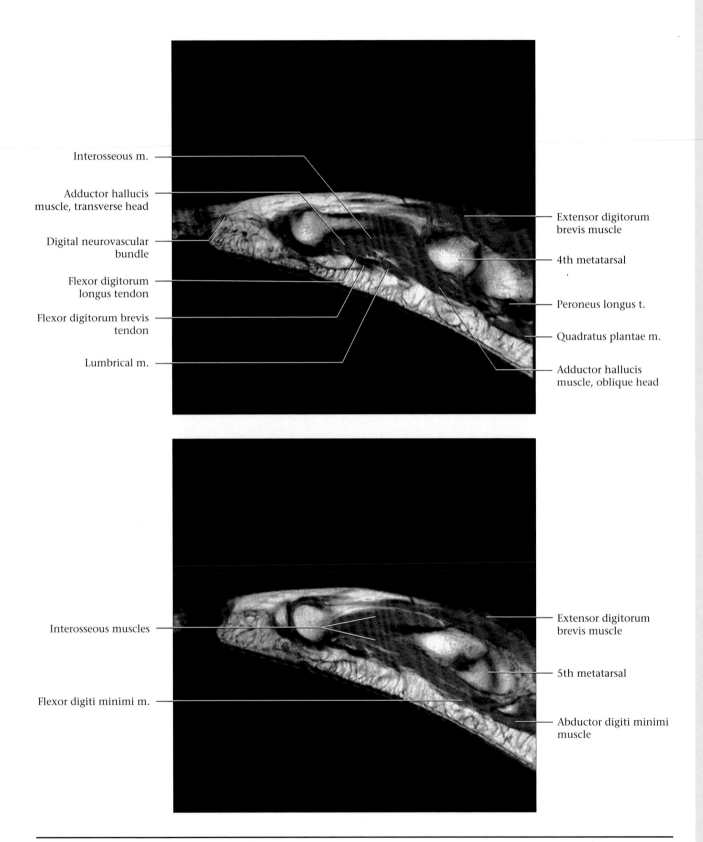

Interosseous m.

Adductor hallucis muscle, transverse head

Digital neurovascular bundle

Flexor digitorum longus tendon

Flexor digitorum brevis tendon

Lumbrical m.

Extensor digitorum brevis muscle

4th metatarsal

Peroneus longus t.

Quadratus plantae m.

Adductor hallucis muscle, oblique head

Interosseous muscles

Flexor digiti minimi m.

Extensor digitorum brevis muscle

5th metatarsal

Abductor digiti minimi muscle

(Top) Thin lumbrical muscles lie adjacent to flexor digitorum tendon slips in 2nd layer of plantar muscles. **(Bottom)** Because of normal fanning of toes, sagittal images angled to 1st metatarsal will become oblique at lateral aspect of foot, as shown on this image. 3rd metatarsophalangeal joint, 4th metatarsal and 5th metatarsal base are seen here on a single 3 mm thick slice. In clinical practice, sagittal axis for imaging forefoot will be chosen for metatarsal of concern, or as default along 1st metatarsal axis.

Foot

VIII

SAGITTAL MR, 4TH-5TH RAY

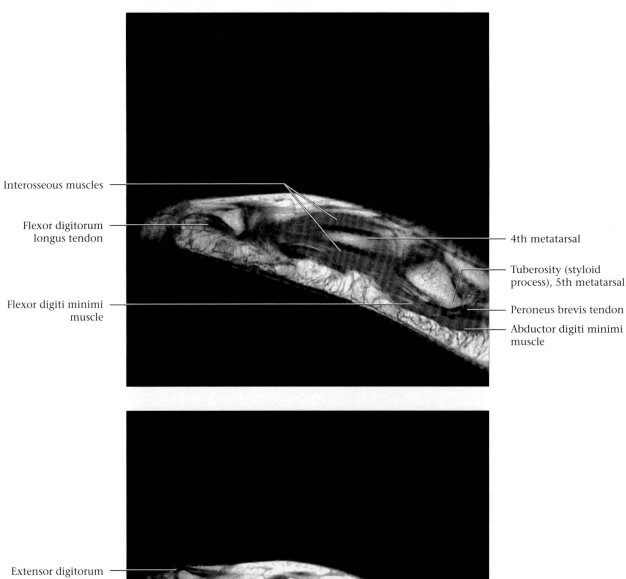

Interosseous muscles

Flexor digitorum longus tendon

Flexor digiti minimi muscle

4th metatarsal

Tuberosity (styloid process), 5th metatarsal

Peroneus brevis tendon

Abductor digiti minimi muscle

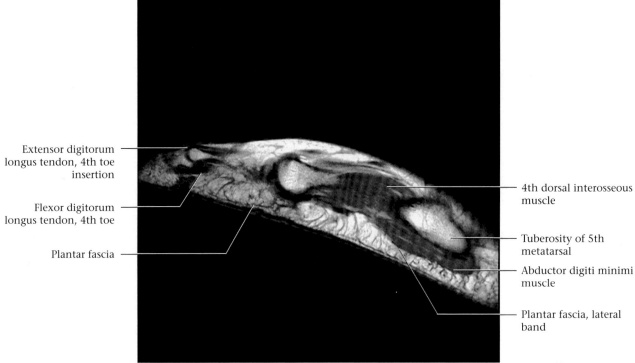

Extensor digitorum longus tendon, 4th toe insertion

Flexor digitorum longus tendon, 4th toe

Plantar fascia

4th dorsal interosseous muscle

Tuberosity of 5th metatarsal

Abductor digiti minimi muscle

Plantar fascia, lateral band

(Top) Flexor digiti minimi muscle lies at plantar aspect of 5th metatarsal, and abductor digiti minimi muscle lies at its lateral aspect. Peroneus brevis tendon attaches to tuberosity (styloid process) at lateral margin of metatarsal base. **(Bottom)** Fine digital fascial network which is distal termination of plantar fascia is well seen.

FOOT OVERVIEW

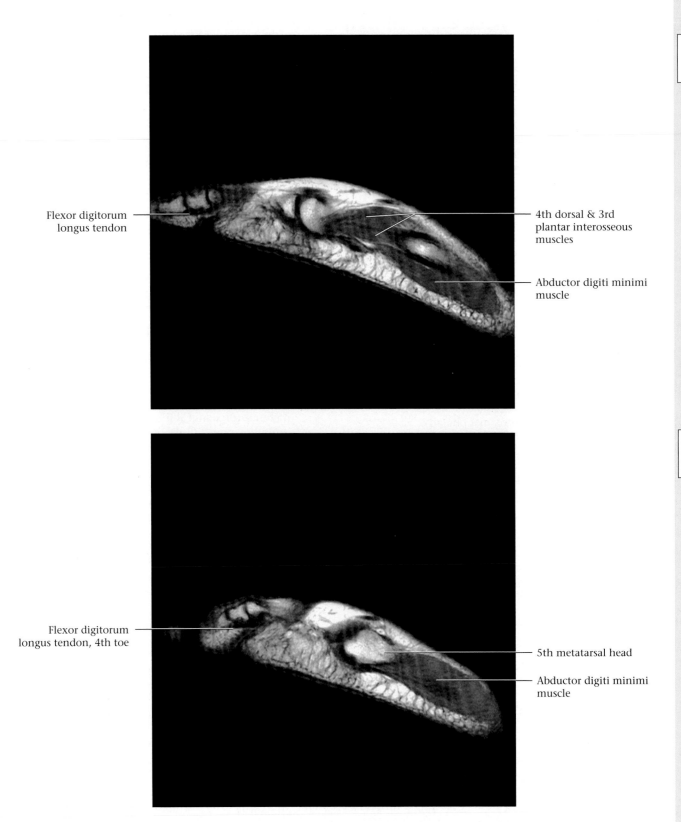

Flexor digitorum longus tendon

4th dorsal & 3rd plantar interosseous muscles

Abductor digiti minimi muscle

Flexor digitorum longus tendon, 4th toe

5th metatarsal head

Abductor digiti minimi muscle

(Top) Note that a in resting, nonweight-bearing bearing position proximal interphalangeal joint is minimally flexed, and distal interphalangeal joint is straight. **(Bottom)** Abductor digiti minimi is most lateral muscle of forefoot.

INTRINSIC MUSCLES OF THE FOOT

Gross Anatomy

Plantar Musculature

- 4 layers of muscles deep to plantar aponeurosis
- Peroneus longus tendon courses across all 4 layers from lateral to medial
- Arterial supply by network of medial and lateral plantar arteries and plantar arterial arch
- **Superficial (1st) muscle layer**
  - Abductor hallucis
    - Origin: Medial aspect posterior process calcaneus, flexor retinaculum, plantar fascia, intermuscular septum
    - Insertion: Medial sesamoid of 1st toe and medial aspect 1st proximal phalangeal base
    - Innervation: Medial plantar nerve
    - Function: Moves 1st toe medially
  - Flexor digitorum brevis
    - Origin: Posterior process calcaneus, plantar fascia, intermuscular septum
    - Divisions: 4 tendon slips split into medial and lateral tendons at metatarsophalangeals (MTPs)
    - Insertion: Medial and lateral margins of bases of middle phalanges
    - Innervation: Medial plantar nerve
    - Function: Flexes proximal interphalangeals (PIPs)
  - Abductor digiti minimi
    - Origin: Posterior process calcaneus
    - Insertion: Base 5th proximal phalanx
    - Innervation: Lateral plantar nerve
    - Function: Moves 5th toe laterally
    - Variant: Abductor ossis metatarsi quinti arises tuberosity 5th metatarsal, merges with abductor digiti minimi
- **Middle (2nd) muscle layer**
  - Tendons of 2 extrinsic muscles: Flexor digitorum longus and flexor hallucis longus
    - Fibers from these 2 tendons join at master knot of Henry, and exchange fibers
  - Quadratus plantae (also called flexor accessorius)
    - Origin: 2 heads arise from posterior process calcaneus and long plantar ligament
    - Insertion: Tendon of flexor digitorum brevis
    - Innervation: Lateral plantar nerve
    - Function: Flexes lateral 4 toes
  - 4 lumbricals
    - Origin: Tendons of flexor digitorum longus
    - Insertion: Proximal phalanges of 4 lateral toes
    - Innervation: 1st lumbrical from medial plantar nerve, others by deep branch lateral plantar nerve
    - Function: Maintain extension of interphalangeal joints
- **Deep (3rd) muscle layer**
  - Flexor hallucis brevis
    - Origin: Lateral head originates from plantar surface cuboid; medial head arises lateral division tibialis posterior and medial intermuscular septum
    - Insertion: Medial and lateral heads insert respectively on medial and lateral aspects base 1st proximal phalanx
    - Contains: Medial and lateral sesamoids of 1st toe
    - Innervation: Medial plantar nerve
    - Function: Flexes proximal phalanx of 1st toe

- Adductor hallucis
  - Origin: Oblique head originates from bases of 2nd, 3rd, and 4th metatarsals, transverse head originates from 3rd, 4th and sometimes 5th plantar MTP ligaments
  - Insertion: Lateral sesamoid of 1st toe and base of 1st proximal phalanx
  - Innervation: Deep branch lateral plantar nerve
  - Function: Stabilizes metatarsal heads, flexes proximal phalanx of 1st toe
  - Variant: Transverse head may be absent
- Flexor digiti minimi brevis
  - Origin: Base of 5th metatarsal and sheath of peroneus longus tendon
  - Insertion: Lateral margin, base of 5th proximal phalanx
  - Innervation: Superficial branch of lateral plantar nerve
  - Function: Flexes MTP joint of 5th toe
- **Interosseous (4th) layer**
  - Plantar interossei: 3 muscles, to 3rd, 4th and 5th toes
    - Origin: Medial bases of 3rd, 4th and 5th metatarsals
    - Insertion: Medial base of proximal phalanges of same toes
    - Innervation: Deep branch lateral plantar nerve
    - Function: Adduct 3rd-5th toes, flex metatarsophalangeal joints, extend proximal interphalangeal joints
  - Dorsal interossei: 4 muscles, to 2nd, 3rd, 4th, 5th toes
    - Origin: Each has 2 heads, from lateral and medial margins of 2 adjacent metatarsals
    - Insertion: 1st to medial margin 2nd proximal phalanx, 2nd-4th to lateral margin of 2nd-4th proximal phalanges
    - Innervation: Deep branch lateral plantar nerve
    - Function: Deviate toes laterally, flex MTP joints, extend PIP joints

Dorsal Muscles

- Extrinsic muscles: Tendons of tibialis anterior, extensor hallucis longus, extensor digitorum brevis, peroneus tertius
- Intrinsic muscles
  - Extensor hallucis brevis: Partially joined to extensor digitorum brevis
    - Origin: Anterior aspect calcaneus
    - Insertion: Base proximal phalanx of 1st toe
    - Innervation: Deep peroneal nerve
    - Function: Extends proximal phalanx
  - Extensor digitorum brevis
    - Origin: Anterolateral aspect calcaneus
    - Insertion: Lateral margins of extensor digitorum longus tendons to 2nd-4th digits and bases middle phalanges
    - Innervation: Deep peroneal nerve
    - Function: Extend phalanges of toes
- In hindfoot, extrinsic tendons superficial to intrinsic tendons
- In forefoot, intrinsic (brevis) tendons lateral to extrinsic (longus) tendons

INTRINSIC MUSCLES OF THE FOOT

GRAPHIC, MUSCLE ATTACHMENTS TO DORSAL ASPECT FOOT

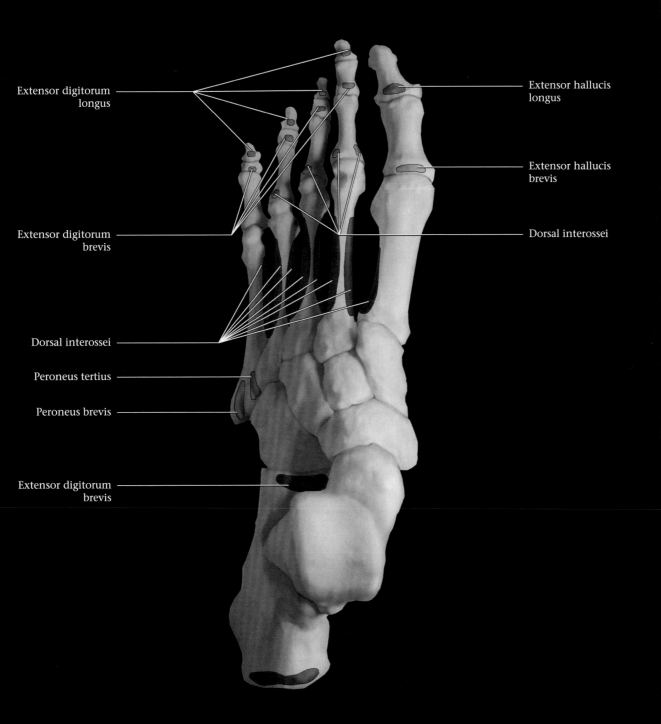

Graphic shows muscle origins (red) and insertions (blue) at dorsal surface of foot. Note that dorsal interossei insert on proximal phalangeal bases, extensor digitorum brevis on middle phalangeal bases, and extensor digitorum longus on distal interphalangeal bases.

GRAPHIC, MUSCLE ATTACHMENTS TO PLANTAR ASPECT FOOT

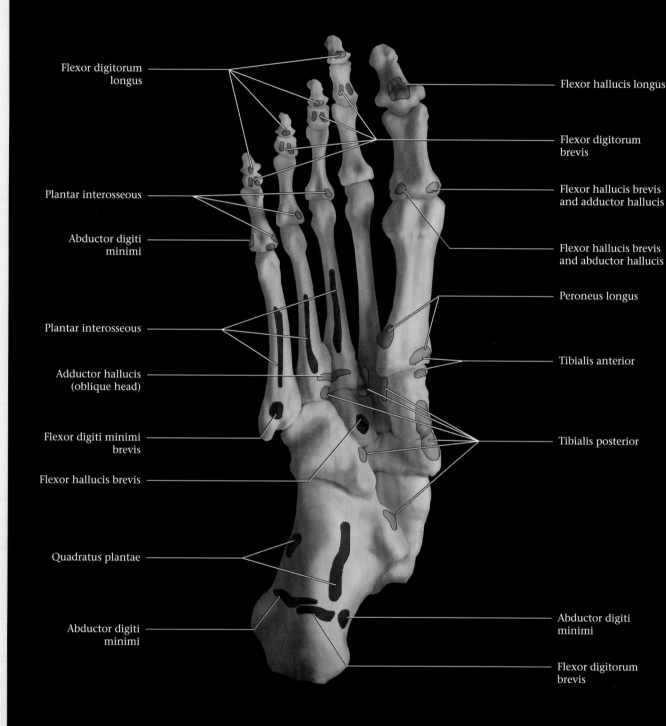

Flexor digitorum longus

Flexor hallucis longus

Flexor digitorum brevis

Plantar interosseous

Flexor hallucis brevis and adductor hallucis

Abductor digiti minimi

Flexor hallucis brevis and abductor hallucis

Peroneus longus

Plantar interosseous

Tibialis anterior

Adductor hallucis (oblique head)

Tibialis posterior

Flexor digiti minimi brevis

Flexor hallucis brevis

Quadratus plantae

Abductor digiti minimi

Abductor digiti minimi

Flexor digitorum brevis

Graphic shows muscle origins (red) and insertions (blue) at plantar surface of foot. Note multiple attachments of tibialis posterior tendon. Flexor digitorum brevis tendons to each toe split into 2 slips, attaching at plantar margins of middle phalanges, with the flexor digitorum longus tendon coursing between them to attach at base of distal phalanges.

INTRINSIC MUSCLES OF THE FOOT

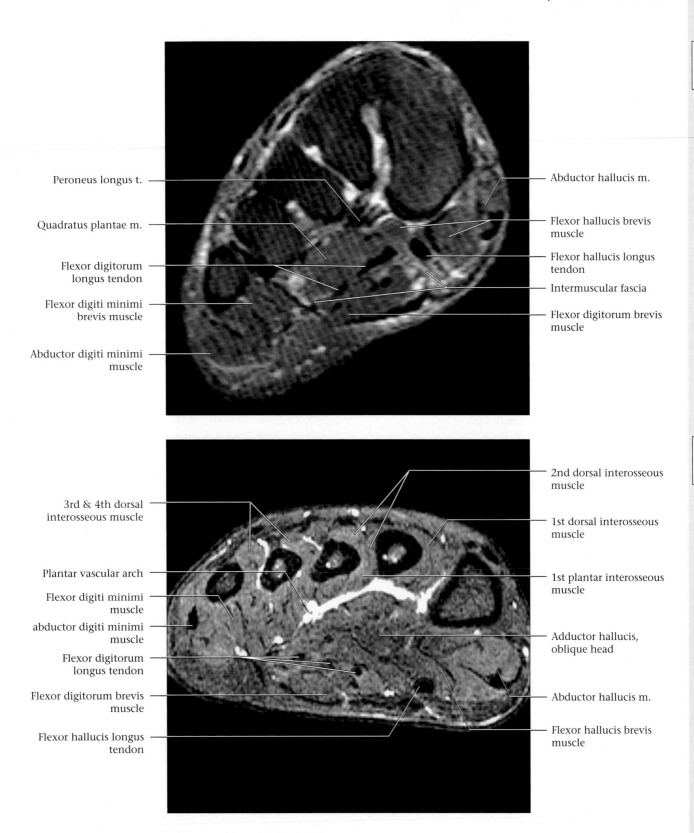

Peroneus longus t.

Quadratus plantae m.

Flexor digitorum longus tendon

Flexor digiti minimi brevis muscle

Abductor digiti minimi muscle

Abductor hallucis m.

Flexor hallucis brevis muscle

Flexor hallucis longus tendon

Intermuscular fascia

Flexor digitorum brevis muscle

3rd & 4th dorsal interosseous muscle

Plantar vascular arch

Flexor digiti minimi muscle

abductor digiti minimi muscle

Flexor digitorum longus tendon

Flexor digitorum brevis muscle

Flexor hallucis longus tendon

2nd dorsal interosseous muscle

1st dorsal interosseous muscle

1st plantar interosseous muscle

Adductor hallucis, oblique head

Abductor hallucis m.

Flexor hallucis brevis muscle

(Top) First of two non-adjacent coronal T2 MR images, at the level of cuneiforms. Division of plantar muscles into distinct medial, intermediate, and lateral compartments is well seen. Fascia dividing the compartments are often more readily apparent on T2WI than on T1WI. The four layers of plantar muscles show considerable overlap; for example abductor hallucis muscle, in 1st layer, is dorsal to flexor hallucis brevis, in 3rd layer. (Bottom) More distal image from previous image. Main plantar compartments of forefoot are readily apparent on coronal images. Abductor and flexor hallucis muscles are in medial compartment; abductor and flexor digiti minimi muscles are in lateral compartment; adductor hallucis and flexor digitorum muscles are in central compartment.

TARSOMETATARSAL JOINT

Terminology

Synonyms
- Lisfranc joint

Imaging Anatomy

Overview
- 1st-5th tarsometatarsal articulations usually considered functionally as 1 joint
- Follows transverse arch configuration established by wedge shape of cuneiforms
  - Bases of 2nd and 3rd metatarsals also have wedge shape
- In coronal plane, joint extends obliquely from anteromedial to posterolateral
  - 2nd metatarsal recessed relative to 1st and 3rd
    - This provides added bony stability ("mortise and tenon" configuration)
    - Some individuals lack recessed position of 2nd metatarsal: They have higher incidence of dislocation
  - Cuboid slightly recessed relative to 3rd cuneiform
    - Creates mortise and tenon configuration in opposite orientation to 2nd tarsometatarsal joint

Synovial Divisions
- 3 separate synovial joint cavities
  - 1st tarsometatarsal joint
  - 2nd and 3rd tarsometatarsal joint
    - Usually continuous with joint between 2nd and 3rd cuneiforms, and naviculocuneiform joint
  - 4th and 5th tarsometatarsal joint
  - Intermetatarsal joints have continuous cavity with tarsometatarsal joints

Ligaments
- **Dorsal tarsometatarsal ligaments**
  - 1st cuneiform to 1st metatarsal
  - 1st cuneiform to 2nd metatarsal (dorsal Lisfranc ligament)
  - 2nd and 3rd cuneiforms to 2nd metatarsal
  - 3rd cuneiform to 3rd metatarsal
  - Cuboid to 4th and 5th metatarsals
- **Interosseous tarsometatarsal ligaments**
  - **Lisfranc ligament**: Originates lateral surface 1st cuneiform, courses anterolaterally and slightly inferiorly, inserts lower half of medial surface of 2nd metatarsal base
    - Thick, broad ligament, and key stabilizing structure
    - Nearly 1 cm from top to bottom, 0.5 cm mediolateral
    - Ligament composed of 2 separate bands in up to 1/4 of population
  - Variable ligaments between 2nd and 3rd cuneiforms and respective metatarsals
- **Plantar tarsometatarsal ligaments**
  - 1st cuneiform to 1st metatarsal
  - **1st cuneiform to 2nd and 3rd metatarsals**
    - Act with Lisfranc ligament, also important stabilizers

- **Intermetatarsal ligaments**
  - Dorsal, interosseous and plantar ligaments between 2nd-5th metatarsal bases
  - No dorsal or plantar ligaments between 1st and 2nd metatarsal bases
    - Weak interosseous ligaments are present in this region
    - The lack of intermetatarsal ligaments between 1st and 2nd metatarsals increases importance of Lisfranc ligament

Bursae
- Bursa between 1st and 2nd metatarsal bases
- Lateral and plantar bursae at base 5th metatarsal, under abductor and flexor m. origins
- Bursa at plantar 1st tarsometatarsal joint, under origin flexor hallucis brevis
- Bursae at plantar tarsometatarsal joints, under extensor tendons

Motion
- 1st tarsometatarsal joint allows abduction, slight flexion and extension
- 2nd and 3rd tarsometatarsal joints relatively immobile
- 4th and 5th tarsometatarsal joints have about 10° of flexion and extension

Anatomy-Based Imaging Issues

Imaging Recommendations
- Radiographs must be weight-bearing to evaluate alignment
  - Abduction stress views may elicit instability
- Axial and coronal MR provide best visualization of Lisfranc ligament
  - Optimize with small surface coil placed on dorsum of foot, centered at Lisfranc joint

Imaging Pitfalls
- Interosseous Lisfranc ligament structurally most important stabilizer of Lisfranc joint
  - Since obliquely oriented, see on sequential coronal MR images
  - See on axial MR images through midportion of cuneiforms and metatarsal bases

Clinical Implications

Clinical Importance
- Injuries of Lisfranc joint commonly missed in emergency department setting
- Isolated tears of Lisfranc ligament occur with plantar flexion, axial load
- Even slight lateral displacement of 2nd metatarsal medial margin relative to medial margin of 2nd cuneiform indicates disruption of Lisfranc ligament
- Flattening of transverse and longitudinal arches of foot and osteoarthritis of Lisfranc joint develop rapidly if ligamentous disruption untreated

RADIOGRAPHS, LISFRANC JOINT

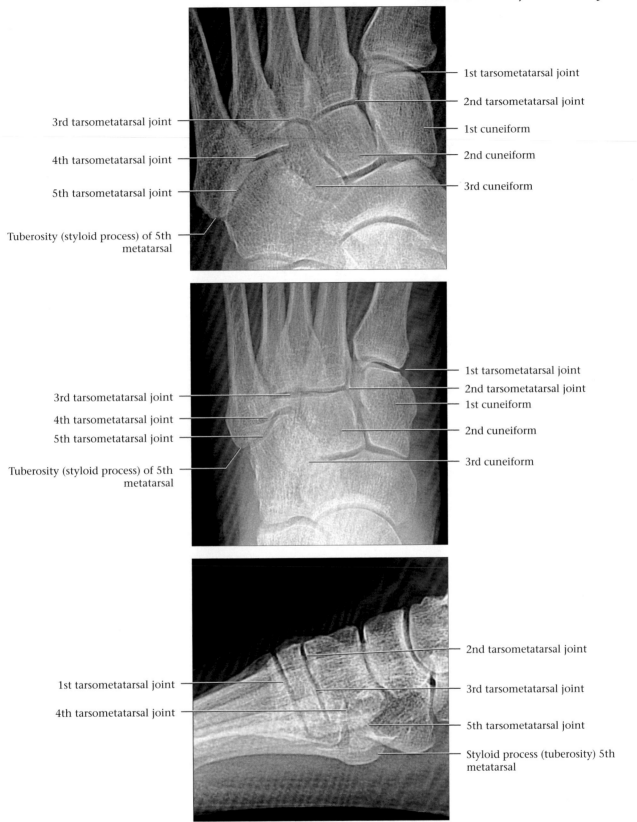

1st tarsometatarsal joint

2nd tarsometatarsal joint

1st cuneiform

2nd cuneiform

3rd cuneiform

3rd tarsometatarsal joint

4th tarsometatarsal joint

5th tarsometatarsal joint

Tuberosity (styloid process) of 5th metatarsal

1st tarsometatarsal joint

2nd tarsometatarsal joint

1st cuneiform

2nd cuneiform

3rd cuneiform

3rd tarsometatarsal joint

4th tarsometatarsal joint

5th tarsometatarsal joint

Tuberosity (styloid process) of 5th metatarsal

2nd tarsometatarsal joint

3rd tarsometatarsal joint

5th tarsometatarsal joint

Styloid process (tuberosity) 5th metatarsal

1st tarsometatarsal joint

4th tarsometatarsal joint

(Top) Anteroposterior radiograph shows zigzag configuration of tarsometatarsal joint, from anteromedial to posterolateral. 2nd metatarsal is recessed relative to 1st and 3rd, and cuboid is recessed relative to 3rd cuneiform. Tarsometatarsal joints are in profile in this subject, but in other normal subjects may not be clearly seen due to their obliquity. Metatarsal bases are overlapping, and intermetatarsal joints are not visualized. **(Middle)** Anteroposterior radiograph shows 2nd metatarsal base is not recessed relative to 3rd, a normal variant which predisposes to dislocation. **(Bottom)** On lateral radiograph, 1st and 2nd tarsometatarsal joints are at dorsum of foot, and 2nd tarsometatarsal joint is located more proximally.

SAGITTAL CT, LISFRANC JOINT

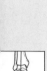

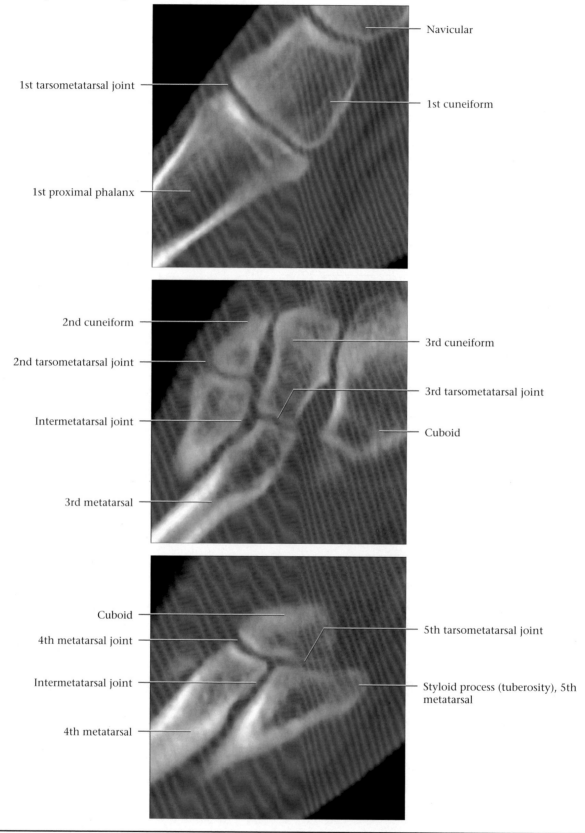

1st tarsometatarsal joint

1st proximal phalanx

Navicular

1st cuneiform

2nd cuneiform

2nd tarsometatarsal joint

Intermetatarsal joint

3rd metatarsal

3rd cuneiform

3rd tarsometatarsal joint

Cuboid

Cuboid

4th metatarsal joint

Intermetatarsal joint

4th metatarsal

5th tarsometatarsal joint

Styloid process (tuberosity), 5th metatarsal

(Top) First of three sagittal CT scans through Lisfranc joint shows bony anatomy. The 1st cuneiform, metatarsal base and tarsometatarsal joint are much larger than corresponding bones of the lateral digits. There should be no plantar or dorsal offset of the 1st proximal phalanx relative to the 1st cuneiform, even on non-weight-bearing studies. **(Middle)** Sagittal CT through 2nd and 3rd tarsometatarsal joints showing recessed position of 2nd metatarsal base relative to 3rd. Intermetatarsal joint between bases of 2nd and 3rd metatarsals is also well seen. **(Bottom)** Sagittal CT through 4th and 5th tarsometatarsal bases showing articulation of cuboid with 4th and 5th metatarsals. The tuberosity (styloid process) of 5th metatarsal extends beyond lateral margin of cuboid.

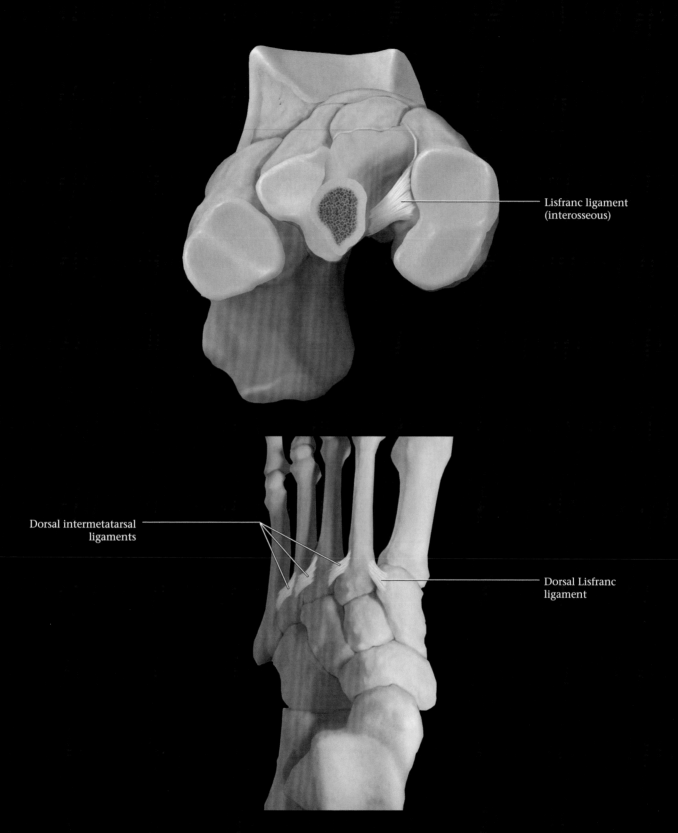

Lisfranc ligament
(interosseous)

Dorsal intermetatarsal
ligaments

Dorsal Lisfranc
ligament

(Top) Three separate ligaments extend from lateral aspect 1st cuneiform to medial aspect 2nd metatarsal: Dorsal, interosseous, and plantar. Interosseous is strongest of these. All function to prevent lateral displacement of 2nd metatarsal. **(Bottom)** Dorsally, strong intermetatarsal ligaments are seen between 2nd-5th metatarsals, but not between 1st and 2nd metatarsals. Dorsal Lisfranc ligament extends from 1st cuneiform to 2nd metatarsal.

TARSOMETATARSAL JOINT

AXIAL T1 MR, LISFRANC LIGAMENT

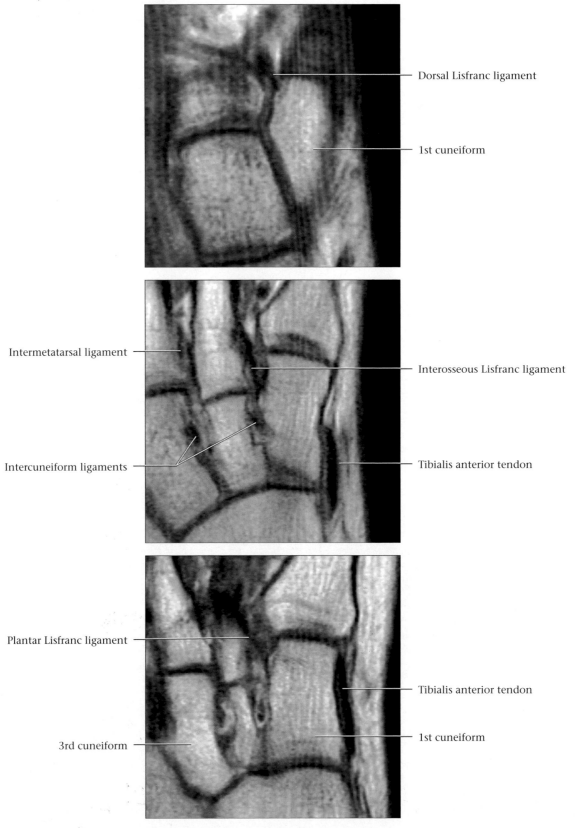

Dorsal Lisfranc ligament

1st cuneiform

Intermetatarsal ligament

Interosseous Lisfranc ligament

Intercuneiform ligaments

Tibialis anterior tendon

Plantar Lisfranc ligament

Tibialis anterior tendon

3rd cuneiform

1st cuneiform

(Top) First of three axial T1 MR images, from dorsal to more plantar positions through the Lisfranc joint. At the dorsal aspect of tarsometatarsal joint, a thin ligament extends from 1st cuneiform to 2nd metatarsal. Isolated injury to Lisfranc ligament occurs with plantarflexion of midfoot, so this ligament is 1st to be injured. **(Middle)** Interosseous Lisfranc ligament is primary stabilizer between 1st and 2nd rays. It is thick and broad when compared to other interosseous ligaments of foot. **(Bottom)** Plantar Lisfranc ligament is a thin structure paralleling dorsal and interosseous Lisfranc ligaments.

TARSOMETATARSAL JOINT

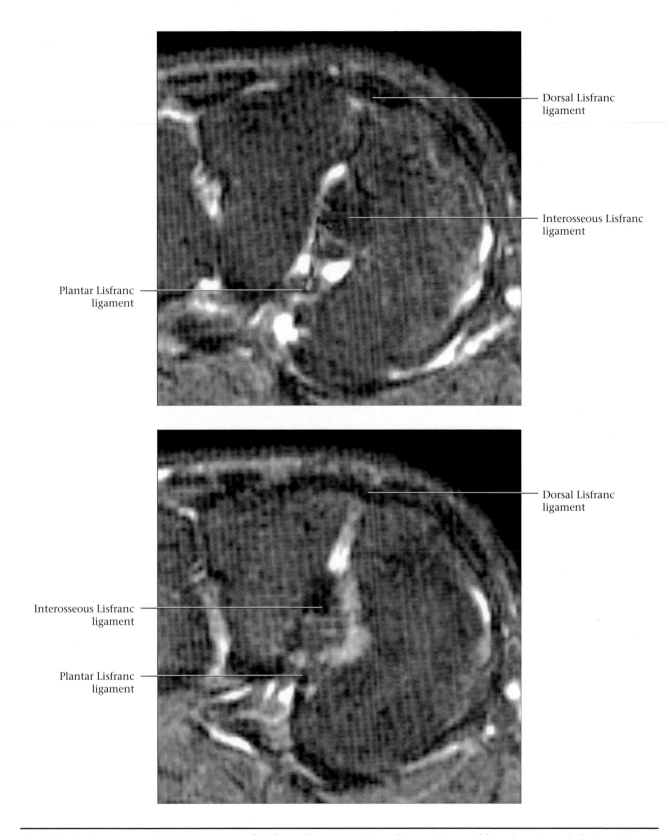

(Top) First of two coronal T2 MR images of Lisfranc ligaments. Since ligaments are obliquely oriented, their entire course will not be seen on a single coronal image. This image shows origin from 1st cuneiform. **(Bottom)** Adjacent to previous image shows insertion of interosseous Lisfranc ligament on 2nd metatarsal base.

METATARSOPHALANGEAL JOINTS

Imaging Anatomy

Overview
- In normal weight-bearing stance, all of the metatarsal heads are at same level, and all are weight-bearing
  - Metatarsophalangeal (MTP) joints are slightly extended in standing position
- Each metatarsophalangeal joint is a separate synovial cavity

1st Metatarsophalangeal Joint
- Dorsiflexion of toe important in push-off phase of gait
- Metatarsal head has 2 concave facets at plantar surface, 1 for each sesamoid, separated by ridge (crista)
- Distal articular surface of metatarsal head may be flat, rounded, or have a central prominence
- Base of proximal phalanx has concave contour
- **Sesamoids**
  - Either sesamoid may be unipartite or bipartite
  - Medial sesamoid in medial head flexor hallucis brevis and abductor hallucis
  - Lateral sesamoid in lateral head flexor hallucis brevis and adductor hallucis and deep metatarsal ligament
  - Medial and lateral sesamoids joined by intersesamoid ligament
    - Intersesamoid ligament is floor of canal in which runs flexor hallucis longus tendon
  - Both are embedded in plantar plate of joint
  - **Sesamophalangeal apparatus**
    - Sesamoids fixed in position relative to 1st proximal phalanx, move relative to 1st metatarsal
    - Therefore displaced laterally in hallux valgus
- **Plantar plate**
  - Fibrocartilaginous plantar capsular thickening extending from metatarsal neck to base proximal phalanx
  - Incorporates sesamoids

Lateral Metatarsophalangeal Joints
- Convex metatarsal head articular surface articulates with concave articular surface of proximal phalangeal base
- Plantar aspect of metatarsal head has rounded contour
- Dorsal aspect of metatarsal head is smaller than plantar aspect
  - Has concave or notched contour along medial and lateral margins
- Sesamoids variably present, most commonly at 5th toe
- **Phalangeal apparatus** is combination of plantar plate and proximal phalanx
- **Plantar plate**
  - Fibrocartilaginous plantar capsular thickening extending from metatarsal neck to base proximal phalanx
  - Attached to deep transverse metatarsal ligament, plantar fascia and flexor tendon sheath, medial and lateral collateral ligaments
  - Instability may mimic Morton neuroma

Ligaments
- Intermetatarsal ligaments: Between metatarsal heads
- Plantar fascia: Distal attachments to joint capsules

- Medial and lateral collateral ligaments: Well-defined at each digit

Bursae
- 1st metatarsophalangeal
  - Dorsal: Variably present separate from tendon sheath of extensor hallucis longus
  - Plantar: Subcutaneous, at plantar and medial aspect of metatarsal head
- Intermetatarsophalangeal
  - Located between metatarsal heads
  - Dorsal to transverse metatarsal ligament
  - Adjacent to plantar digital neurovascular bundle
    - Bursitis may irritate nerve, mimic Morton neuroma
  - Usually absent between 4th and 5th toes
- 5th metatarsophalangeal
  - Plantar: Subcutaneous, at plantar aspect of metatarsal head

Nerves
- Plantar and dorsal nerves course with arterioles along medial and lateral aspects of digits
- Plantar nerves vulnerable to impingement between metatarsal heads

Anatomy-Based Imaging Issues

Imaging Recommendations
- Sesamoid evaluation
  - Due to small size, fractures may be missed on routine examination
  - Wrist coil provides superior resolution to extremity coil
  - Toes advanced into wrist coil past metatarsal heads
  - 2 mm T1WI and T2WI through sesamoids in sagittal, axial planes

Clinical Implications

Clinical Importance
- Instability of MTP joints results in pain and deformity of forefoot

Stability of 1st MTP Joint
- Collateral ligaments
- Flexor and extensor hallucis brevis mm
- Flexor and extensor hallucis longus have a smaller contribution to stability

Stability of Lateral MTP Joints
- Collateral ligaments
- Plantar plate
  - Rupture of plantar plate results in dorsal subluxation of MTP joint and hammer toe deformity

Short 1st Metatarsal (Morton Foot)
- Normal variant but increases stress on 2nd metatarsal
- Predisposes to osteonecrosis of 2nd metatarsal head (Freiberg infraction)

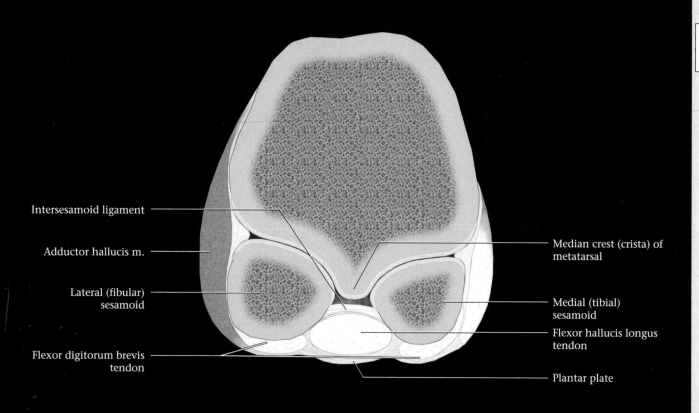

Intersesamoid ligament

Adductor hallucis m.

Lateral (fibular) sesamoid

Flexor digitorum brevis tendon

Median crest (crista) of metatarsal

Medial (tibial) sesamoid

Flexor hallucis longus tendon

Plantar plate

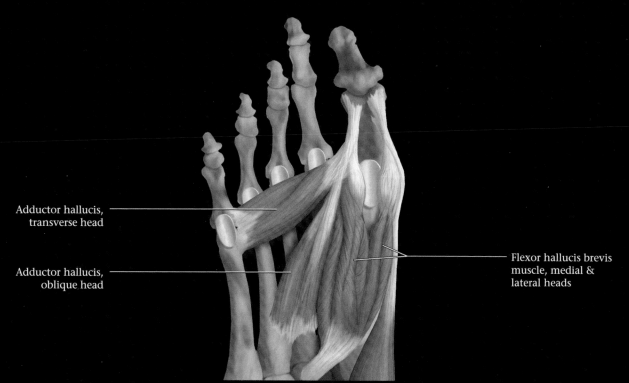

Adductor hallucis, transverse head

Adductor hallucis, oblique head

Flexor hallucis brevis muscle, medial & lateral heads

(Top) Coronal graphic shows sesamoids positioned at plantar surface of 1st metatarsal head, separated by median crest of metatarsal. Sesamoids are united by intersesamoid ligament. Intersesamoid ligament forms floor of groove between sesamoids, and flexor hallucis longus tendon runs along this groove. **(Bottom)** Axial graphic shows muscle attachments to sesamoids of 1st metatarsophalangeal joint. Abductor hallucis and medial head of flexor hallucis brevis attach to medial sesamoid. Lateral head of flexor hallucis brevis and adductor hallucis attach to lateral

RADIOGRAPH & MR, 1ST METATARSOPHALANGEAL JOINT

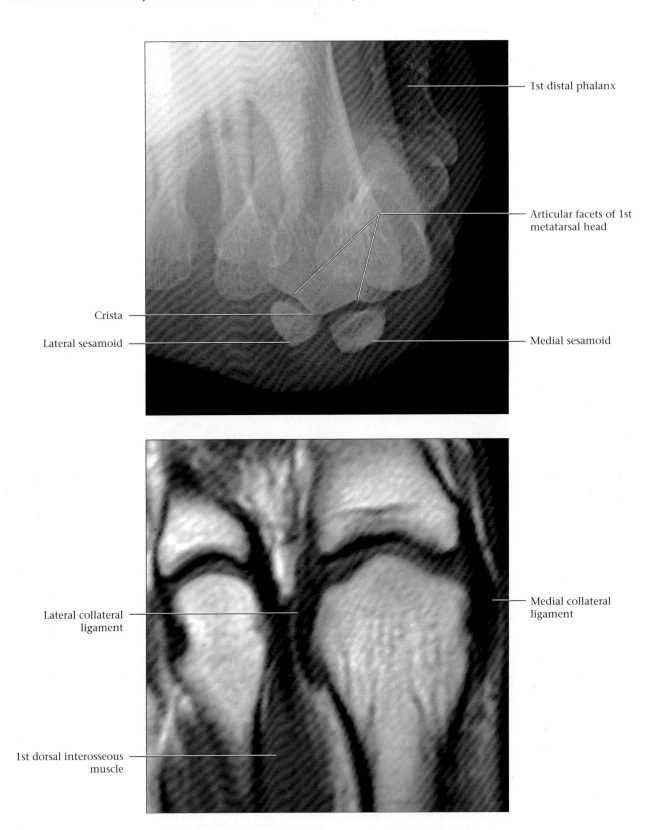

1st distal phalanx

Articular facets of 1st metatarsal head

Crista

Lateral sesamoid

Medial sesamoid

Lateral collateral ligament

Medial collateral ligament

1st dorsal interosseous muscle

(Top) Sesamoid radiograph obtained tangent to sesamoids, with toe dorsiflexed. Sesamoids are centered on articular facets of metatarsal head. **(Bottom)** Axial T1 MR in patient with conical shape of 1st metatarsal head; shape of articular surface varies from flat to round to conical in different patients.

METATARSOPHALANGEAL JOINTS

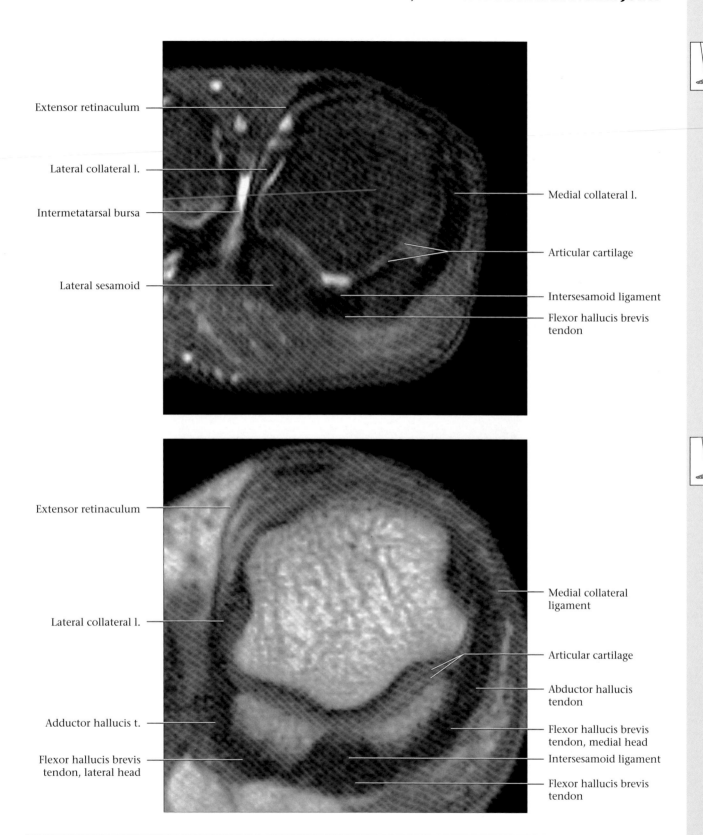

(Top) Coronal T2 MR shows normal amount of fluid outlining articular structures. Also note fluid in intermetatarsal bursa. Bursae lie between each of the metatarsal heads, and should not be mistaken for Morton neuroma. Gadolinium-enhanced MR is useful in distinguishing these two entities. **(Bottom)** Coronal T1 MR shows normal position of 1st toe sesamoids, and their stabilizing structures.

AXIAL MR, LATERAL METATARSOPHALANGEAL JOINTS

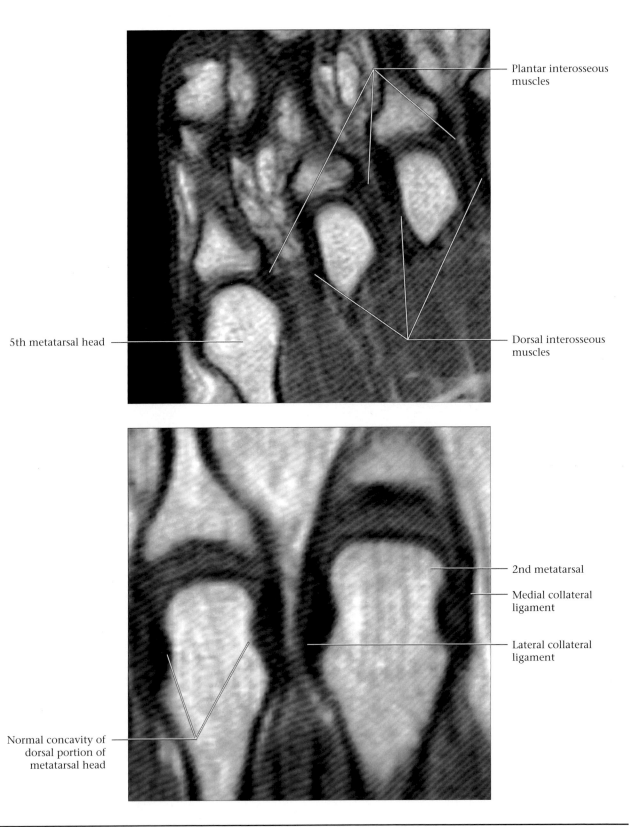

Plantar interosseous muscles

Dorsal interosseous muscles

5th metatarsal head

2nd metatarsal

Medial collateral ligament

Lateral collateral ligament

Normal concavity of dorsal portion of metatarsal head

(Top) Axial T1 MR through plantar aspects of 3rd through 5th metatarsal heads. At this level, heads have an ovoid shape. Tendons of interosseous muscles lie between metatarsal heads, with plantar interossei inserting on medial side of proximal phalangeal bases, and dorsal interossei on lateral side. **(Bottom)** Axial T1 MR through dorsal aspects of 2nd and 3rd metatarsal heads. At this level, heads have concave contour at both medial and lateral margin. These should not be mistaken for erosions. Distal articular surface is flat in contour on 2nd metatarsal compared to 3rd. This should not be mistaken for Freiberg infraction.

CORONAL & SAGITTAL MR, LATERAL METATARSOPHALANGEAL JOINTS

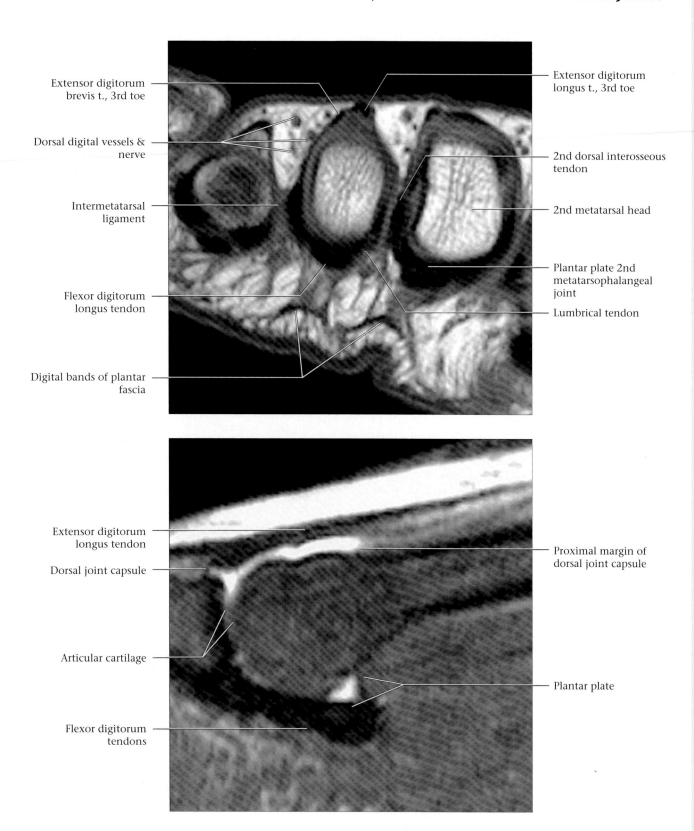

Extensor digitorum brevis t., 3rd toe

Dorsal digital vessels & nerve

Intermetatarsal ligament

Flexor digitorum longus tendon

Digital bands of plantar fascia

Extensor digitorum longus t., 3rd toe

2nd dorsal interosseous tendon

2nd metatarsal head

Plantar plate 2nd metatarsophalangeal joint

Lumbrical tendon

Extensor digitorum longus tendon

Dorsal joint capsule

Articular cartilage

Flexor digitorum tendons

Proximal margin of dorsal joint capsule

Plantar plate

(Top) Coronal T1 MR image through metatarsophalangeal joints show metatarsal heads are concave at their medial and lateral aspects, and larger at their plantar than their dorsal surface. Interosseous tendons lie between metatarsal heads, flexor and lumbrical tendons on plantar surface, and extensor tendons are dorsal. Thick plantar plate is deep to flexor tendons. Medial and lateral collateral ligaments are well seen as thickenings of joint capsule. **(Bottom)** Sagittal T2 MR through 2nd metatarsophalangeal joint shows plantar plate deep to flexor tendons. Articular cartilage ends slightly proximal to joint capsule margins, leaving an uncovered "bare area" where earliest bony erosions will be visible in cases of inflammatory arthritis.

NORMAL VARIANTS

Terminology

Definitions
- Accessory center of ossification: Variant center of ossification associated with a bone
- Sesamoid: Ossicle arising within a tendon

Imaging Anatomy

Overview
- Normal variants are commonly found in foot
- See Ankle section for description of normal variants of hindfoot

Accessory Centers of Ossification
- **Os supranaviculare** (also called os talonaviculare dorsale or Pirie bone): Dorsal, proximal margin of navicular
- **Accessory navicular** (also called os tibiale externum): Ossicle at median eminence of navicular
  - Type 1: Sesamoid in tibialis posterior tendon
  - Type 2: Accessory center of ossification joined to navicular by synchondrosis
  - Type 3 (also called cornuate or gorilloid navicular): Enlarged median eminence of navicular
- **Os intercuneiform**: Dorsal aspect foot, between 1st and 2nd cuneiforms
- **Cuboides secondarium** (secondary cuboid): Proximal medial aspect of cuboid, between cuboid and navicular
- **Pars peronea metatarsalis primi**: Plantar aspect foot, between base 1st metatarsal and 1st cuneiform
- **Os vesalianum**: Base 5th metatarsal (MT)
- **Os intermetatarseum**: Dorsal, between 1st and 2nd metatarsals
- **Os calcaneus secondarius**: Dorsal, adjacent to anterior process calcaneus

Sesamoids
- **Os peroneale** (also called os peroneum): Sesamoid within peroneus longus muscle, seen adjacent to lateral margin of cuboid
- **Sesamoids of great toe**
  - Medial (tibial) sesamoid: Beneath metatarsal head, within flexor digitorum brevis and abductor hallucis
  - Lateral (fibular) sesamoid: Beneath metatarsal head, with flexor digitorum brevis and adductor hallucis
  - 30% bipartite or multipartite (may not be symmetric on contralateral foot)
  - Medial sesamoid more frequently bipartite than lateral
  - Interphalangeal sesamoid: At interphalangeal joint, within flexor hallucis longus tendon
- **Sesamoids of 2nd-5th toes**
  - Variably present
  - May be at metatarsophalangeal or interphalangeal joints
  - May have both medial and lateral sesamoids at 5th metatarsophalangeal joint

Miscellaneous Normal Bony Variants
- Intermetatarsal joint of 1st and 2nd digits
  - Articular facet between bases of 1st and 2nd metatarsals variably present

- 35% no articular facet
- 38% small articular facet
- 27% well-developed articular facet
  - Recessed position of 2nd metatarsal relative to 3rd not universally present
- Position of 2nd tarsometatarsal joint
  - Always proximal to 1st tarsometatarsal joint
  - May be proximal to or in same plane as 3rd metatarsal joint
- Morton foot: 1st metatarsal short relative to 2nd
  - Results in increased stress on 2nd (MT)
- Failure of segmentation: Middle and distal phalanges of 5th toe commonly fail to segment

Muscle Variants
- Quadratus plantae: May be absent; may send slip to 5th toe, to 2nd-4th toes, or to 2nd-3rd toes
- Opponens digiti minimi: Variably present muscle slip of flexor digiti minimi, sharing its origin and inserting on distal 5th metatarsal shaft
- Peroneus tertius: Absent in 10% of population

Childhood Variants
- Navicular: May be sclerotic, flat, multipartite
  - Same appearance seen in symptomatic avascular necrosis of navicular
- Medial cuneiform: May have 2 ossification centers
- Metatarsals
  - May have accessory epiphysis at opposite end of bone from true epiphysis
    - 1st metatarsal: Epiphysis proximal, accessory epiphysis distal
    - 2nd-5th metatarsals: Epiphysis distal, accessory epiphysis proximal
  - Epiphyses may be bipartite

Anatomy-Based Imaging Issues

Imaging Recommendations
- Use radiographic, CT or MR criteria to distinguish normal variants from fracture
  - Fracture characteristics
    - Jagged fracture plane
    - Acute angle at fracture margin
    - Nonsclerotic margin (if acute)
    - Bone marrow edema on MR
  - Accessory ossicle/bipartite ossicle characteristics
    - Smooth, rounded margins
    - Obtuse angle at margin between ossicles
    - Surrounded by cortex
    - Bone marrow edema sometimes present on MR if injured
- Accessory centers may be symptomatic, due to injury of synchondrosis between ossicle and parent bone
  - If symptomatic, edema will be seen on MR, centered on synchondrosis

Imaging Pitfalls
- Note: Normal variants may not be bilaterally symmetric

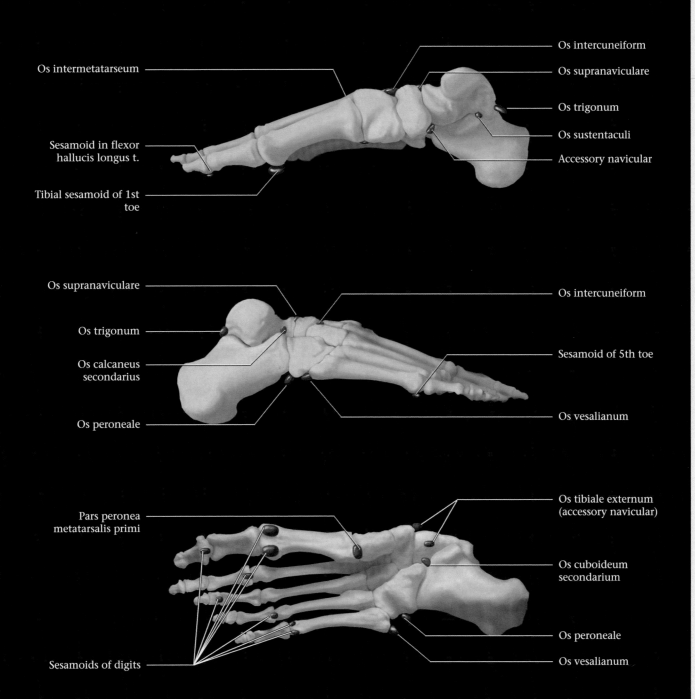

Os intermetatarseum

Os intercuneiform

Os supranaviculare

Os trigonum

Os sustentaculi

Accessory navicular

Sesamoid in flexor hallucis longus t.

Tibial sesamoid of 1st toe

Os supranaviculare

Os intercuneiform

Os trigonum

Os calcaneus secondarius

Sesamoid of 5th toe

Os peroneale

Os vesalianum

Pars peronea metatarsalis primi

Os tibiale externum (accessory navicular)

Os cuboideum secondarium

Os peroneale

Os vesalianum

Sesamoids of digits

There are multiple, variably present accessory ossicles of foot. Os sustentaculi and pars peronea metatarsalis primi are quite uncommon, while the others shown are frequently seen. Ossicles are usually called by Latin names. Os tibiale externum, however, is usually called by its simple English name, accessory navicular.

ACCESSORY NAVICULAR (OS TIBIALE EXTERNUM)

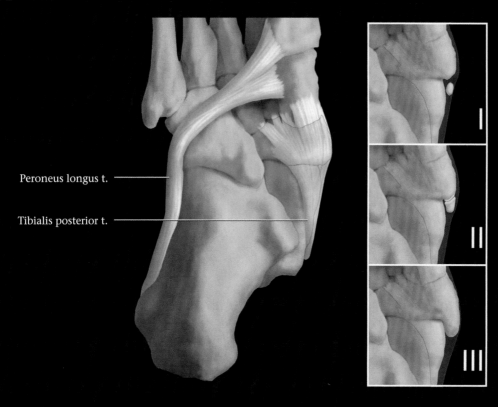

Peroneus longus t.

Tibialis posterior t.

I

II

III

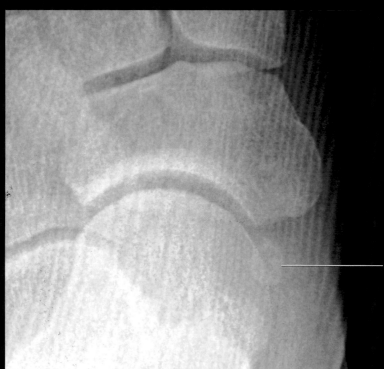

Type 1 accessory navicular

(Top) Graphic shows plantar view of accessory navicular (os tibiale externum) variants. Normally, tibialis posterior tendon attaches to plantar aspect of median eminence of navicular. A type 1 accessory navicular is a sesamoid in posterior tibial tendon. Type 2 is accessory center of ossification. Type 3 is an elongated median eminence ("cornuate navicular"). **(Bottom)** Anteroposterior radiograph shows small, rounded, type 1 accessory navicular. It is normally slightly separated from main navicular.

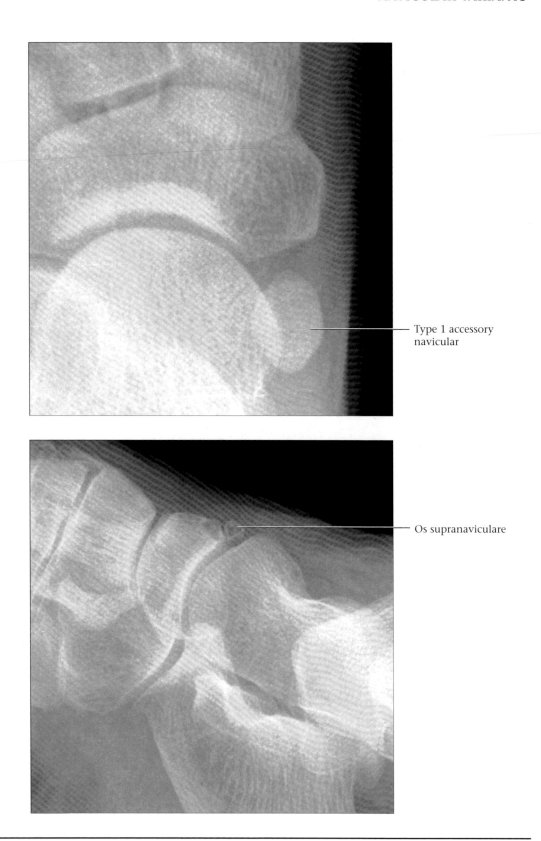

Type 1 accessory navicular

Os supranaviculare

(Top) Anteroposterior radiograph shows large type 1 accessory navicular. Despite its unusually large size it is distinguished from type 2 by the lack of an articular facet with the main navicular body. (Bottom) Lateral radiograph shows triangular ossicle at proximal, dorsal margin of navicular. Os supranaviculare is also known as os talonaviculare dorsale, or Pirie bone. Many so called cases of os supranaviculare probably represent old, nonunited fractures.

ACCESSORY NAVICULAR TYPE 2

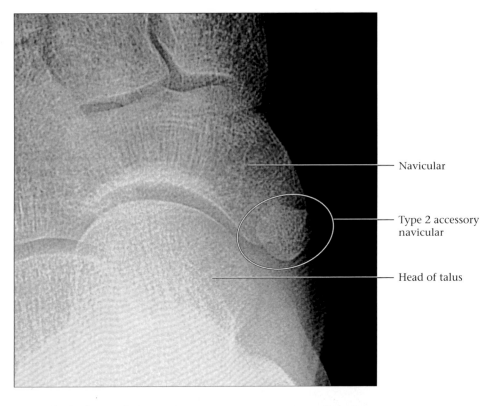

Navicular

Type 2 accessory navicular

Head of talus

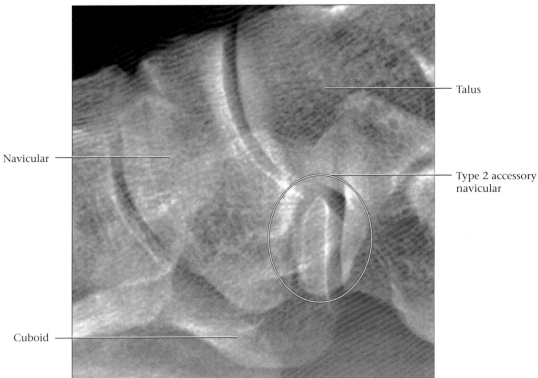

Talus

Type 2 accessory navicular

Navicular

Cuboid

(Top) Anteroposterior view shows rounded type 2 accessory navicular overlying medial eminence of navicular. Synchondrosis with navicular may or may not be seen in profile on anteroposterior view. **(Bottom)** Lateral view of same patient as previous image shows relatively plantar position of accessory navicular.

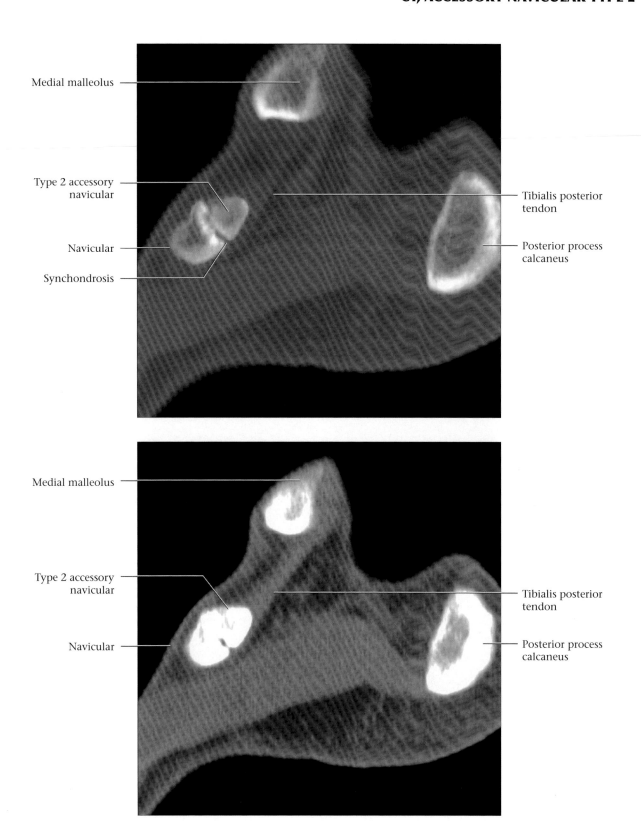

Medial malleolus

Type 2 accessory navicular

Navicular

Synchondrosis

Tibialis posterior tendon

Posterior process calcaneus

Medial malleolus

Type 2 accessory navicular

Navicular

Tibialis posterior tendon

Posterior process calcaneus

(Top) Sagittal CT shows type 2 accessory navicular and synchondrosis. Apposing bony margins of accessory navicular and main navicular are irregular and sclerotic. This appearance is common, and suggests abnormal motion at synchondrosis. **(Bottom)** Soft tissue CT window at same level better shows the normal appearing tibialis posterior tendon attaching to accessory ossicle.

MR, ACCESSORY NAVICULAR TYPE 2

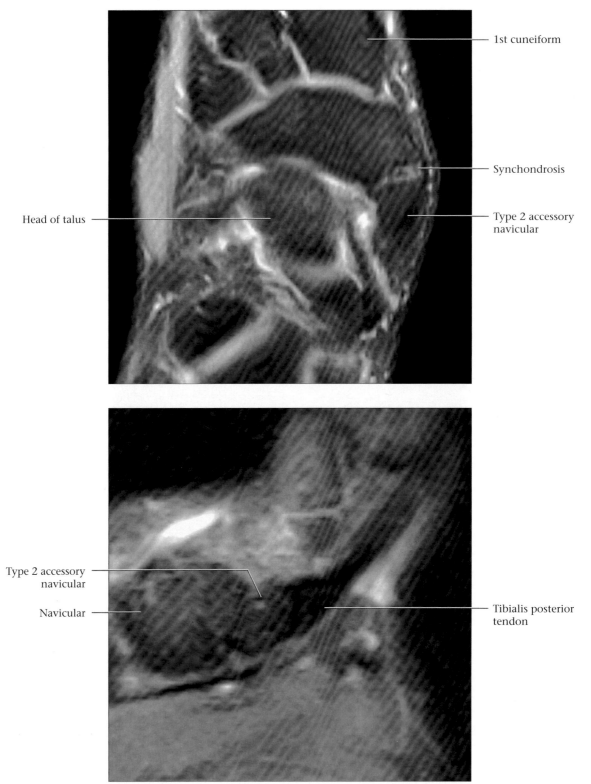

1st cuneiform

Synchondrosis

Type 2 accessory navicular

Head of talus

Type 2 accessory navicular

Navicular

Tibialis posterior tendon

(Top) Axial PD MR with FS shows type 2 accessory navicular having a flat facet joined by a synchondrosis to parent navicular. **(Bottom)** Sagittal STIR MR of same patient as previous image shows attachment of tibialis posterior tendon to accessory ossicle.

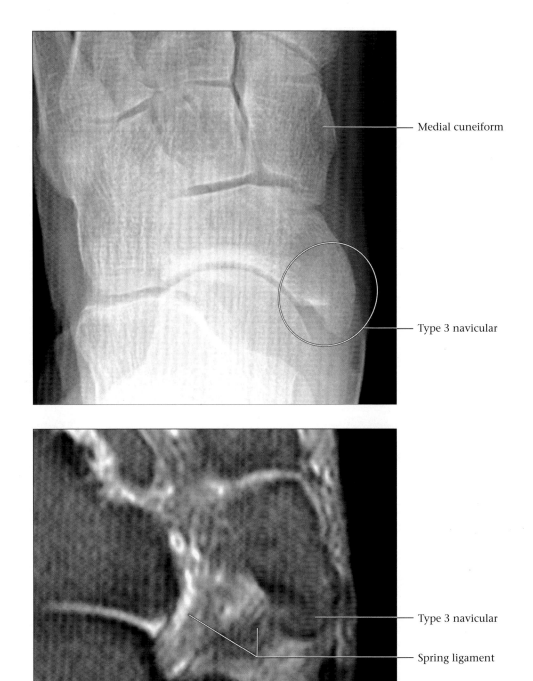

Medial cuneiform

Type 3 navicular

Type 3 navicular

Spring ligament

(Top) Anteroposterior radiograph shows type 3 navicular, also called cornuate or gorilloid. This is an assimilated accessory navicular ossicle which forms a projection at medial eminence of navicular. This configuration may cause impingement on shoes and especially on ski boots. **(Bottom)** Axial PD FS MR shows type 3 accessory navicular. Spring ligament is attaching both to the bony prominence and more medially to the main portion of the navicular.

CUBOIDES SECONDARIUM

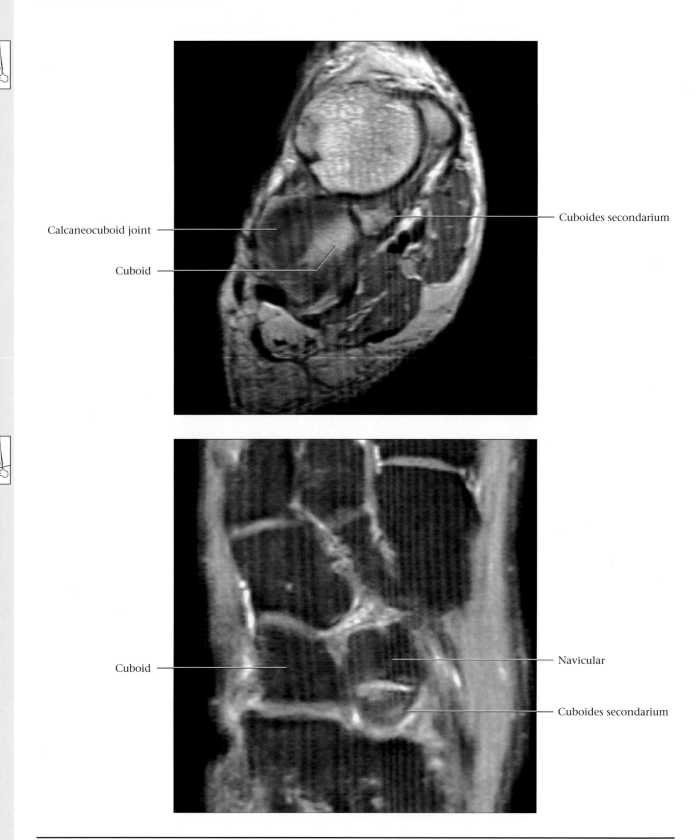

Calcaneocuboid joint

Cuboid

Cuboides secondarium

Cuboid

Navicular

Cuboides secondarium

(Top) Coronal T1 MR shows ossicle at proximal, medial, superior margin of cuboid, between cuboid and navicular. **(Bottom)** Axial PD with FS MR shows relationship of ossicle to both cuboid and navicular. This ossicle is very uncommon.

NORMAL VARIANTS

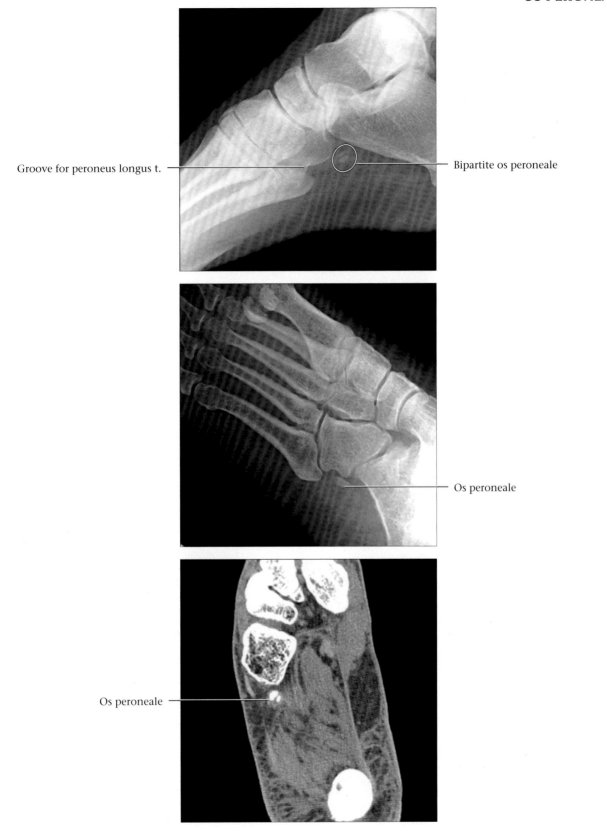

Groove for peroneus longus t. —   — Bipartite os peroneale

— Os peroneale

Os peroneale —

(Top) Lateral radiograph shows bipartite os peroneale. This ossicle may be unipartite or bipartite. It lies in peroneus longus tendon, adjacent to calcaneocuboid joint or cuboid. Proximal displacement of os peroneale can be seen as plain radiographic finding of peroneus longus tendon rupture. **(Middle)** Oblique radiograph in another patient shows unipartite os peroneale. Ossicle is just proximal to point where peroneus longus courses under cuboid groove. **(Bottom)** Axial CT, soft tissue window, shows bipartite os peroneale within peroneus longus tendon.

Foot

VIII

OS VESALIANUM

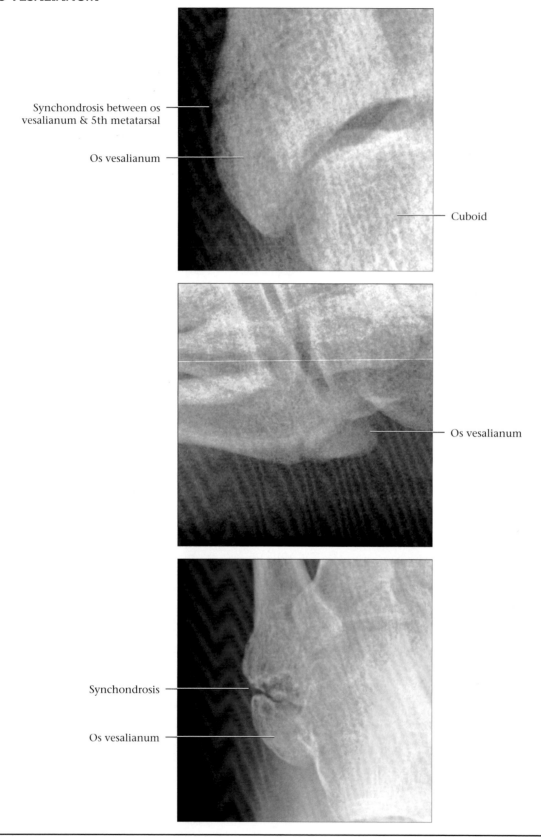

Synchondrosis between os vesalianum & 5th metatarsal

Os vesalianum

Cuboid

Os vesalianum

Synchondrosis

Os vesalianum

(Top) On anteroposterior radiograph, os vesalianum overlies styloid process of 5th metatarsal, and synchondrosis may be mistaken for fracture. **(Middle)** On lateral radiograph, rounded contour of ossicle, consistent with accessory center of ossification rather than fracture, is evident. **(Bottom)** Anteroposterior radiograph shows large os vesalianum and multiple cysts at synchondrosis.

NORMAL VARIANTS

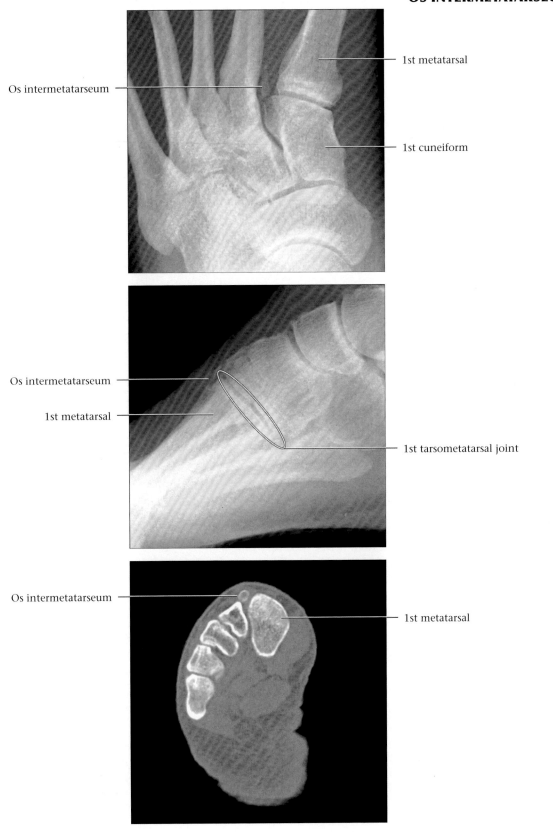

Os intermetatarseum — 1st metatarsal — 1st cuneiform

Os intermetatarseum — 1st metatarsal — 1st tarsometatarsal joint

Os intermetatarseum — 1st metatarsal

(Top) Anteroposterior radiograph shows teardrop-shaped os intermetatarseum, arising between 1st and 2nd metatarsal bases. Sometimes this ossicle will be partially assimilated to 1st metatarsal base. (Middle) On lateral radiograph, ossicle is dorsal in position, adjacent to base of 1st metatarsal. (Bottom) On coronal CT, os intermetatarseum is rounded in appearance, and no donor site from adjacent bones is visible. These signs help distinguish it from a fracture fragment.

BIPARTITE MEDIAL SESAMOID 1ST METATARSOPHALANGEAL JOINT

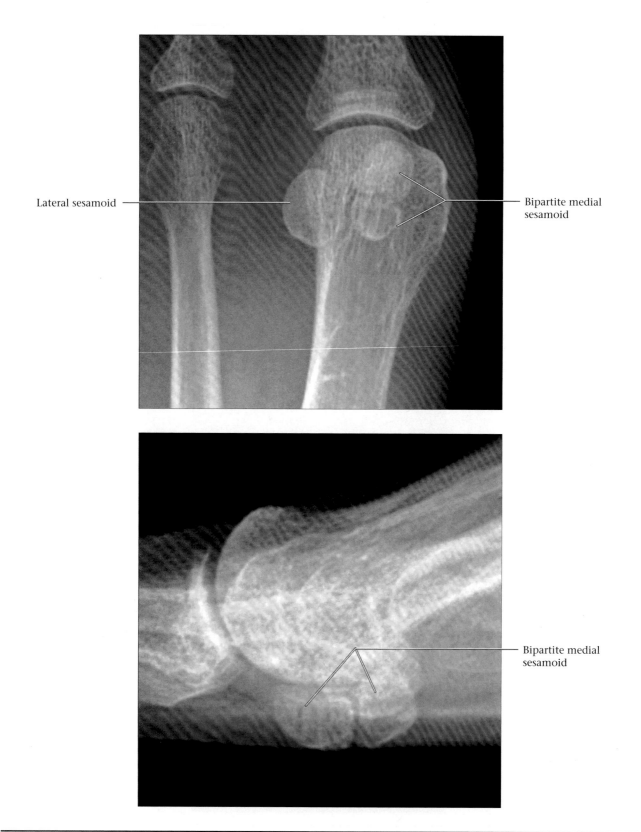

Lateral sesamoid — Bipartite medial sesamoid

Bipartite medial sesamoid

(Top) Anteroposterior radiograph shows bipartite medial sesamoid of 1st toe, and unipartite lateral sesamoid. **(Bottom)** Lateral radiograph shows rounded contour characteristic of bipartite sesamoids. Fracture fragments, in contrast, will show angular margins.

SESAMOIDS OF METATARSOPHALANGEAL JOINTS

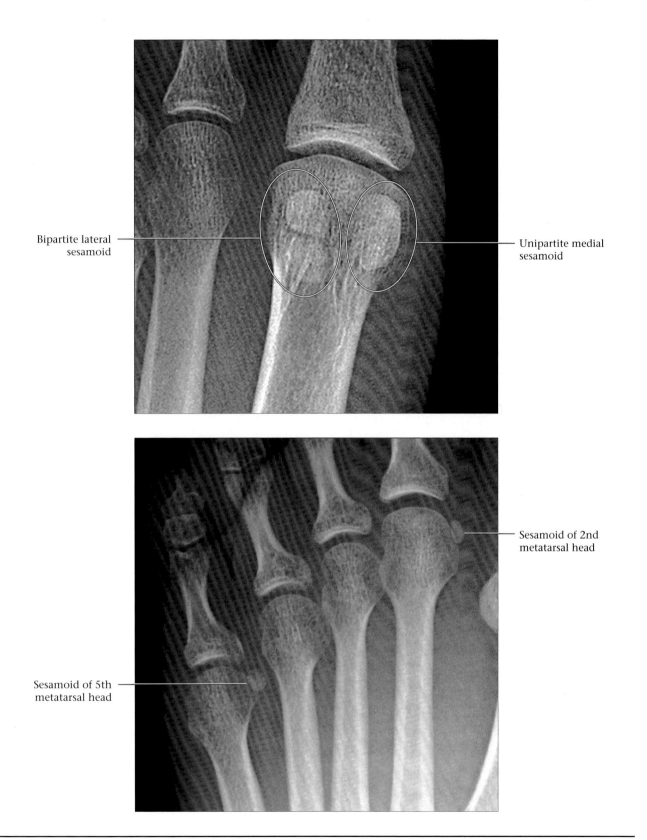

Bipartite lateral sesamoid

Unipartite medial sesamoid

Sesamoid of 2nd metatarsal head

Sesamoid of 5th metatarsal head

(Top) Anteroposterior radiograph shows bipartite lateral sesamoid of 1st toe, and unipartite medial sesamoid. Bipartite sesamoids are usually more rounded in contour than fractured sesamoids. Bipartite sesamoids are usually larger than unipartite sesamoids. Bipartite sesamoids may or may not be present on contralateral foot. (Bottom) Anteroposterior radiograph shows sesamoids of 2nd and 5th metatarsal heads. Sesamoids of lateral toes are variably present. They are always small, and may be round or oval.

MISCELLANEOUS VARIANTS

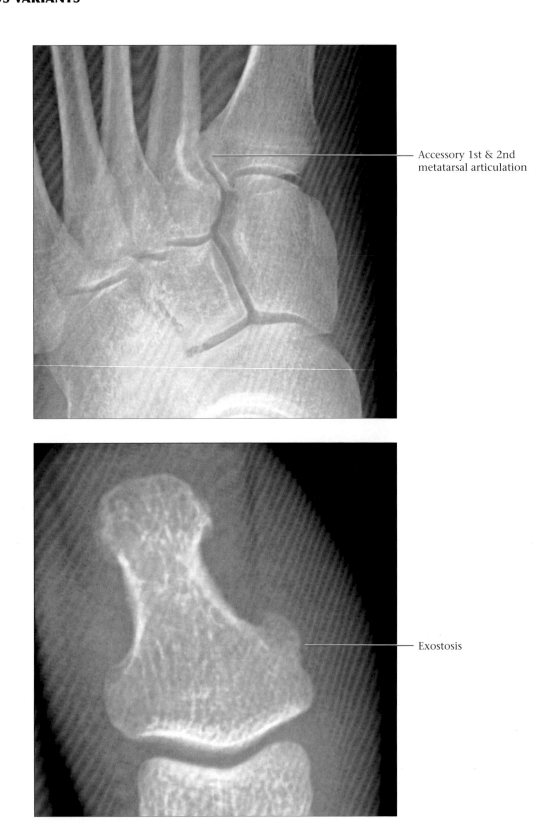

— Accessory 1st & 2nd metatarsal articulation

— Exostosis

(Top) Articulation between bases of 1st and 2nd metatarsals may be absent, small, or a fairly large joint as in this case. **(Bottom)** An exostosis is commonly seen from medial margin, base of 1st distal phalanx. Occasionally, exostosis is quite large.

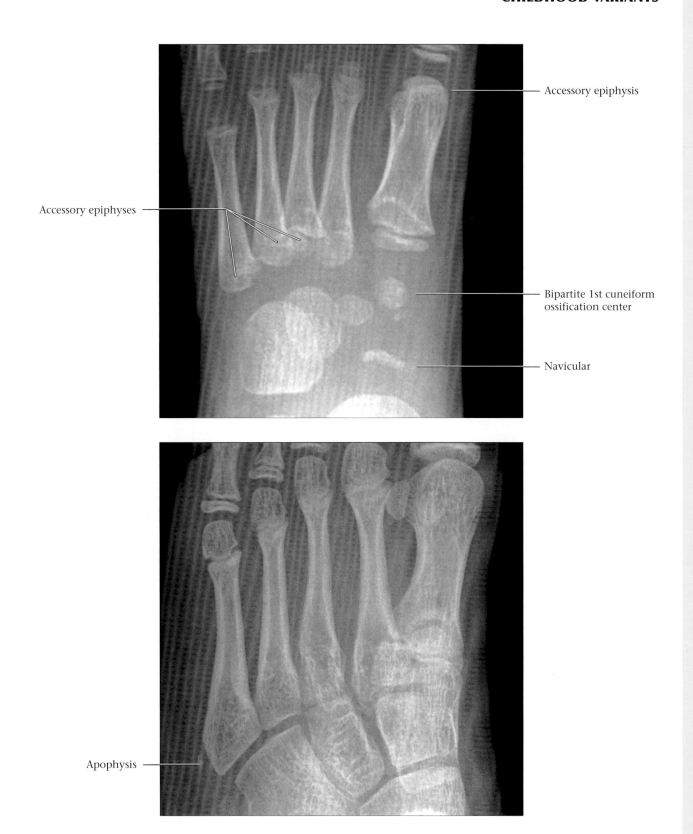

Accessory epiphysis

Accessory epiphyses

Bipartite 1st cuneiform ossification center

Navicular

Apophysis

(Top) Ossification center for 1st metatarsal is at proximal end of bone. Ossification centers of remaining metatarsals are distal. Accessory epiphyses may form at opposite end of metatarsal. This patient has further variants: Bipartite 1st cuneiform ossification center, sclerotic, fragmented appearing navicular, and bipartite metatarsal head ossification centers. **(Bottom)** Apophysis at base of 5th metatarsal. Fractures in this location tend to be horizontally oriented, while apophysis is longitudinally oriented.

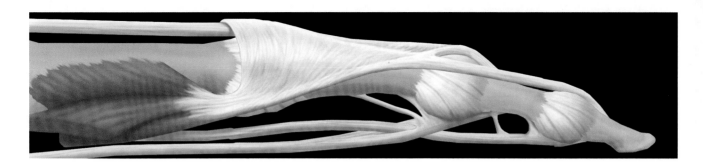

INDEX

INDEX

INDEX

INDEX

INDEX

D

INDEX

INDEX

INDEX

INDEX

INDEX

INDEX

INDEX

INDEX

INDEX

INDEX

INDEX

INDEX

INDEX

INDEX

INDEX

INDEX

INDEX

INDEX

INDEX

INDEX

INDEX